HANDBOOK OF RESEARCH IN EMOTIONAL AND BEHAVIORAL DISORDERS

HANDBOOK OF RESEARCH IN EMOTIONAL AND BEHAVIORAL DISORDERS

Edited by

Robert B. Rutherford Jr.
Mary Magee Quinn
Sarup R. Mathur

Foreword by FRANK H. WOOD

THE GUILFORD PRESS
New York   London

© 2004 The Guilford Press
A Division of Guilford Publications, Inc.
72 Spring Street, New York, NY 10012
www.guilford.com

Printed in the United States of America

This book is printed on acid-free paper.

Last digit is print number: 9 8 7 6 5 4 3 2

Library of Congress Cataloging-in-Publication Data

Handbook of research in emotional and behavioral disorders / edited by Robert B.
Rutherford Jr., Mary Magee Quinn, Sarup R. Mathur ; foreword by Frank H. Wood.
   p. cm.
  Includes bibliographical references and index.
  ISBN-10: 1-59385-056-5 ISBN-13: 978-1-59385-056-2 (hardcover : alk. paper)
  ISBN-10: 1-59385-471-4 ISBN-13: 978-1-59385-471-3 (paperback : alk. paper)
  1. Problem children—Education. 2. Emotional problems of children. 3. Behavior
disorders in children. I. Rutherford, Robert Bruce, 1943– II. Quinn, Mary M.
III. Mathur, Sarup R.
  LC4801.H35 2004
  372.94—dc22

                                         2004010864

About the Editors

Robert B. Rutherford Jr., PhD, is Professor of Special Education and Director of Graduate Programs and Research in Curriculum and Instruction at Arizona State University. Dr. Rutherford is the past president of both the Council for Children with Behavioral Disorders (CCBD) and Teacher Educators for Children with Behavior Disorders (TECBD). He is the former editor of *Behavioral Disorders* and the current coeditor (with Sarup R. Mathur) of the CCBD/TECBD Monograph Series on Severe Behavior Disorders of Children and Youth, published annually in *Education and Treatment of Children*. Dr. Rutherford is the author of numerous articles, chapters, monographs, and texts on emotional and behavioral disorders and youth with disabilities in the juvenile justice system. He is the Principal Investigator of the Office of Special Education Programs-funded Arizona State University–University of Arizona Dual University Program to Prepare Professors in Emotional and Behavioral Disorders. He was also a Fulbright Senior Scholar in Portugal in 1983 and 1992 and has been a special education consultant for the U.S. State Department and the Office of Overseas Schools in Costa Rica, Mexico, Brazil, Panama, and Colombia.

Mary Magee Quinn, PhD, is Principal Research Scientist at the American Institutes for Research. She is currently the Project Director of the Alternative Schools Project, the Systems Improvement Activities to Enhance Children's Mental Health Service Project, and the Linking Assessment Policy and Practice Project; Codirector of the Center for Effective Collaboration and Practice; and an Associate Director of the National Center on Education, Disability, and Juvenile Justice. Dr. Quinn's research interests focus on improving outcomes for children, youth, and adolescents with disabilities, especially those with emotional and behavioral disorders. She has presented at national and international conferences; authored and coauthored books, chapters, and articles; is a member of the Council for Children with Behavioral Disorders; and is the past president of Teacher Educators for Children with Behavioral Disorders.

Sarup R. Mathur, PhD, is Clinical Professor, Cluster Chair, and Initial Teacher Certification Coordinator for Special Education in Curriculum and Instruction at Arizona State University. She has extensive experience in research and developing educational programs for students with emotional and behavioral disorders. She has also published research articles and chapters on the topics of professional development, social skills training, early identification, transition, functional behavioral assessment, and behavioral intervention plans. Dr. Mathur is the coeditor (with Robert B. Rutherford) of the CCBD/TECBD Monograph Series on Severe Behavior Disorders of Children and Youth, published annually in *Education and Treatment of Children*, and coauthor of *Teacher-Mediated Behavior Management Strategies for Children with EBD* and *Effective Strategies for Teaching Appropriate Behaviors to Children with EBD*. She is also former secretary and current president of the Council for Children with Behavioral Disorders and the past president of Teacher Educators for Children with Behavior Disorders.

Contributors

Alfredo J. Artiles, PhD, Division of Curriculum and Instruction, Arizona State University, Tempe, Arizona

Renée Bradley, PhD, U.S. Department of Education, Washington, DC

Frederick J. Brigham, PhD, Department of Curriculum and Instruction, University of Virginia, Charlottesville, Virginia

Michael Bullis, PhD, Special Education Area, College of Education, University of Oregon, Eugene, Oregon

R. T. Busse, PhD, School of Education, Chapman University, Orange, California

Gwendolyn Cartledge, PhD, College of Education, The Ohio State University, Columbus, Ohio

Douglas Cheney, PhD, Department of Special Education, University of Washington, Seattle, Washington

Maureen A. Conroy, PhD, Department of Special Education, University of Florida, Gainesville, Florida

Bryan G. Cook, PhD, Department of Educational Foundations and Special Services, Kent State University, Kent, Ohio

Martha Coutinho, PhD, Department of Human Development and Learning, East Tennessee State University, Johnson City, Tennessee

Douglas Cullinan, EdD, Department of Curriculum and Instruction, North Carolina State University, Raleigh, North Carolina

R. Kenton Denny, PhD, Department of Curriculum and Instruction, Louisiana State University, Baton Rouge, Louisiana

Erik Drasgow, PhD, College of Education, University of South Carolina, Columbia, South Carolina

Lucille Eber, EdD, Illinois Emotional Behavioral Disabilities/Positive Behavior Interventions and Supports Network, La Grange, Illinois

Stephen N. Elliott, PhD, Department of Special Education, Peabody College, Vanderbilt University, Nashville, Tennessee

Steven R. Forness, EdD, Center for Health Sciences, University of California, Los Angeles, Neuropsychiatric Hospital, Los Angeles, California

James J. Fox, PhD, Center for Early Childhood Learning and Development, East Tennessee State University, Johnson City, Tennessee

Michael J. Furlong, PhD, Graduate School of Education, University of California, Santa Barbara, Santa Barbara, California

Robert A. Gable, PhD, Child Study Center, Old Dominion University, Norfolk, Virginia

Donna Gilbertson, PhD, Department of Psychology, Utah State University, Logan, Utah

Frank M. Gresham, PhD, Graduate School of Education, University of California, Riverside, Riverside, California

Eleanor Guetzloe, EdD (retired), Department of Special Education, University of South Florida, St. Petersburg, Florida

Philip L. Gunter, PhD, College of Education, Valdosta State University, Valdosta, Georgia

Jo M. Hendrickson, PhD, Division of Instruction and Curriculum, University of Iowa, Iowa City, Iowa

Peggy P. Hester, PhD, Child Study Center, Old Dominion University, Norfolk, Virginia

Charles D. Hoffman, PhD, Department of Psychology, California State University, San Bernardino, California

Kenneth W. Howell, PhD, Department of Special Education, Western Washington University, Bellingham, Washington

Keith J. Hyatt, EdD, Department of Special Education, Western Washington University, Bellingham, Washington

Shane R. Jimerson, PhD, Graduate School of Education, University of California, Santa Barbara, Santa Barbara, California

Kristine Jolivette, PhD, Department of Educational Psychology and Special Education, Georgia State University, Atlanta, Georgia

James M. Kauffman, EdD, Department of Curriculum and Instruction, University of Virginia, Charlottesville, Virginia

Kenneth A. Kavale, PhD, School of Education, Regent University, Virginia Beach, Virginia

Sandra Keenan, MEd, American Institutes for Research, Washington, DC

Kimberly T. Kendziora, PhD, American Institutes for Research, Washington, DC

Lee Kern, PhD, Department of Education and Human Services, Lehigh University, Bethlehem, Pennsylvania

Dean E. Konopasek, PhD, Anchorage School District, Anchorage, Alaska

Timothy J. Landrum, PhD, Department of Curriculum and Instruction, University of Virginia, Charlottesville, Virginia

Kathleen Lynne Lane, PhD, Department of Special Education, Peabody College, Vanderbilt University, Nashville, Tennessee

Peter E. Leone, PhD, Department of Special Education, University of Maryland, College Park, Maryland

Timothy J. Lewis, PhD, Department of Special Education, University of Missouri, Columbia, Missouri

Teri Lewis-Palmer, PhD, Educational and Community Support, University of Oregon, Eugene, Oregon

Carl J. Liaupsin, EdD, Department of Special Education, Rehabilitation Counseling, and School Psychology, University of Arizona, Tucson, Arizona

Sarup R. Mathur, PhD, Division of Curriculum and Instruction, Arizona State University, Tempe, Arizona

Richard E. Mattison, MD, Department of Psychiatry, State University of New York at Stony Brook, Stony Brook, New York

Nancy B. Meadows, EdD, School of Education, Texas Christian University, Fort Worth, Texas

Devery R. Mock, PhD, School of Education, University of Iowa, Iowa City, Iowa

Gale M. Morrison, PhD, Graduate School of Education, University of California, Santa Barbara, Santa Barbara, California

Mark P. Mostert, PhD, School of Education, Regent University, Virginia Beach, Virginia

C. Michael Nelson, EdD, Department of Special Education and Rehabilitation Counseling, University of Kentucky, Lexington, Kentucky

Lori Newcomer, PhD, Department of Special Education, University of Missouri, Columbia, Missouri

David Osher, PhD, American Institutes for Research, Washington, DC

Donald Oswald, PhD, Department of Psychiatry, Virginia Commonwealth University, Richmond, Virginia

Jeffrey M. Poirier, MA, American Institutes for Research, Washington, DC

Lewis Polsgrove, EdD, School of Education, Indiana University, Bloomington, Indiana

Mary Magee Quinn, PhD, American Institutes for Research, Washington, DC

Robert B. Rutherford Jr., PhD, Division of Curriculum and Instruction, Arizona State University, Tempe, Arizona

Edward J. Sabornie, PhD, College of Education, North Carolina State University, Raleigh, North Carolina

Terrance M. Scott, PhD, Department of Special Education, University of Florida, Gainesville, Florida

James G. Shriner, PhD, Department of Special Education, University of Illinois Urbana–Champaign, Champaign, Illinois

Stephen W. Smith, PhD, Department of Special Education, University of Florida, Gainesville, Florida

Kay B. Stevens, EdD, School of Education, Texas Christian University, Fort Worth, Texas

Janine Stichter, PhD, Department of Special Education, University of Missouri, Columbia, Missouri

Kevin S. Sutherland, PhD, Department of Special Education and Disability Policy, Virginia Commonwealth University, Richmond, Virginia

Dwight P. Sweeney, PhD, Department of Educational Psychology and Counseling, California State University, San Bernardino, California

Melody Tankersley, PhD, Department of Educational Foundations and Special Services, Kent State University, Kent, Ohio

Richard Van Acker, EdD, College of Education, University of Illinois at Chicago, Chicago, Illinois

Amanda M. VanDerHeyden, PhD, Vail School District, Vail, Arizona

Joseph H. Wehby, PhD, Department of Special Education, Peabody College, Vanderbilt University, Nashville, Tennessee

Joseph C. Witt, PhD, Department of Psychology, Louisiana State University, Baton Rouge, Louisiana

Mitchell L. Yell, PhD, College of Education, University of South Carolina, Columbia, South Carolina

Foreword

The breadth and depth of topics addressed in this handbook give those of us concerned with the education and treatment of students with emotional and behavioral disorders a sense of satisfaction at the extraordinary progress that has been made in recent years, and allow thoughtful consideration of potentially fruitful avenues for future research.

Several chapters in the volume review the history of knowledge accumulation in the past half century, during which our mental health care system moved from a hierarchically organized field dominated by psychiatrists to one where multimodal team interventions are standard best practice. Simplistic explanations of the complicated behavior problems of children and youth, which attributed primary blame to their primary caregivers, parents, and teachers, are no longer acceptable. Indeed, rather than being tolerated as "junior members" of intervention teams, teachers and parents now take leading roles in planning and carrying out treatment programs.

Psychopharmacology has a role in the treatment of children and youth only dreamed of by the pioneer researchers who observed what they called the "paradoxical effect" of stimulant medication in "damping down" the hyperactive behavior of some children. Interventions applying learning principles, originally derived from laboratory experiments using rats and pigeons as subjects, have shown extraordinary power for facilitating human learning. Identifying, measuring, and controlling key variables responsible for complex cognitive and social functioning have proved more difficult than many of us expected, but because their importance cannot be denied, the question of how to conduct needed research in this area continues to challenge practitioners and researchers.

Despite the advances in research on emotional and behavioral disorders, we still need to learn to view them in the context of the infinitely subtle differences characterizing individual human beings. We have not yet learned to describe and replicate the charisma of our master teacher–therapists or the astonishing resiliency and courage of the children and youths who grow through and beyond their problems. We remain puzzled and dismayed at the capacity of some people for inflicting serious injury on themselves or others. We also need to better understand why drugs that are therapeutic for some contribute to the criminal behavior of others. Useful though our knowledge is, much still remains to be discovered.

However, excessive self-consciousness about the limitations of our knowledge should not deter us from entering into important debates about public policy and practice. Policymakers usually weigh political considerations more heavily than advice based on knowledge of best practices when making their decisions. For example, successful field projects are chosen for replication, but budget constraints in funding make true replication impossible. Failing programs are criticized after superficial analysis of the factors that contributed to their lack of success. Parents and school officials argue about what constitutes appropriately adapted education for individual students, with parents focused on potential benefit and schools focused on program costs, while forgetting to seek shared estimates of cost and benefit. Thoughtful, balanced professional opinion is called on to inform these discussions. However, since none of us can responsibly claim to be equally well informed in all areas, we need reliable sourcebooks to supplement our knowledge. To fill this need, the chapters in this handbook provide convenient summaries of current best practices in a wide range of areas by experts in those areas.

Can we use the summary of present knowledge provided in this volume as a basis for predicting future developments? Potentially—by referring to the state of the field 50 years ago, as I recall it. At that time, the electroencephalogram was a crude tool in comparison to today's measures of brain function. Our use of medication then was based largely on trial and error. Counseling interventions were often of the "one size fits all" variety, with the method employed based solely on the therapist's personal biases or training. Recent advances in our ability to measure brain function and to influence its function by selective use of medication are remarkable. I find myself dreaming that the rapidly increasing precision of measurement in this area will enable us not only to refine and use our psychopharmacological repertoire more effectively but also to improve our nondrug interventions. It is conceivable, for example, that we may some day have a better understanding of the neurological events that determine both conduct-disordered and addictive behavior. And going a step further, how would such knowledge relate to our growing ability to map the structure of the human genome and discover ways to manipulate such basic human building blocks as the chromosome?

I predict that the interrelating of physiological measures and careful observations of behavior will have dramatic effects on every topic considered in this handbook. The possibility that such knowledge can be abused causes me some pause, but it appears that we are on this path of discovery, whether it leads to triumph or disaster. Deliberate or accidental abuse is inherent with any strong intervention, and the application of knowledge must always be subordinate to morality in a healthy society.

The editors and their collaborating authors are to be congratulated on the timeliness of this handbook. I also congratulate those who will some day in the future, when measuring their own progress, refer back to this handbook as a summary of what was known about emotional and behavioral disorders and their treatment at the beginning of the 21st century.

FRANK H. WOOD, PhD
Professor Emeritus of Educational Psychology and Special Education
University of Minnesota

Acknowledgments

The editors wish to acknowledge the contributions of each of the authors. This group of scholars has collectively contributed this corpus of chapters that define and explain research in the field of emotional and behavioral disorders. While their chapters attest to the strength of the field and confirm that much of what we know about emotional and behavioral disorders is based on sound science, all of the authors note that research and practice in their respective areas involves a continuing process in which we constantly seek to clarify and strengthen our field.

We also want to acknowledge the contributions of the five individuals who provided the section introductions for the *Handbook*. James M. Kauffman, Lewis Polsgrove, Steven R. Forness, C. Michael Nelson, and Eleanor Guetzloe have made significant contributions to the field of emotional and behavioral disorders in terms of their leadership (each is a past president of the Council for Children with Behavioral Disorders) and scholarship (collectively they have contributed over 1,000 articles, texts, chapters, and presentations relating to the education and treatment of students with emotional and behavioral disorders). These five individuals were instrumental in helping us determine the breadth and scope of the *Handbook*. Many of the contributors and chapter topics were chosen based upon their recommendations. They, along with Frank H. Wood, who wrote the Foreword, have had a profound influence on us personally and professionally over the years. We dedicate the *Handbook of Research in Emotional and Behavioral Disorders* to them.

Contents

PART V. RESEARCH METHODOLOGY

1

Overview of Foundations, Assessment, Characteristics, Interventions, and Methodology in Emotional and Behavioral Disorders Research

ROBERT B. RUTHERFORD JR., MARY MAGEE QUINN, *and* SARUP R. MATHUR

The 70 authors of the 30 chapters in this *Handbook of Research in Emotional and Behavioral Disorders* address the major foundational, assessment, characteristics, intervention, and methodological issues facing the field of emotional and behavioral disorders (EBD) of children and youth. These authors are among the top researchers, scholars, and teacher educators in the field today, and they were selected to contribute chapters related to topics to which they themselves have made major contributions in terms of research and scholarship. Because of the range and diversity of the topics covered, the *Handbook* is divided into five sections.

PART I: FOUNDATIONS OF RESEARCH

The first section of the *Handbook* focuses on the foundations and current perspectives in EBD. Following a section introduction by James M. Kauffman, five chapters address the key elements that have established the basis for research in the field. In Chapter 2, Kauffman, Brigham, and Mock make a powerful and cogent case for the continued role of the scientific method in the development of research-based practices in the field of emotional and behavioral disorders. While acknowledging that political and social ideologies have been, and continue to be, a threat to scientific discovery, the chapters in the remainder of this *Handbook* attest to the critical role that empirical validation has played and continues to play in research and practice in behavioral disorders. Kauffman and his colleagues trace historical and contemporary problems in the recognition and description of behavioral disorders in children and youth, address speculation and intervention or experimentation in behavioral disorders, and make the case that empirical evaluation of interventions is critical to the strength of our field. This chapter clearly establishes the research foundations for the remainder of the *Handbook*.

In Chapter 3, Cullinan addresses the research issues surrounding classification and definition of EBD. This chapter describes the two primary EBD classification systems—

the disease perspective exemplified by the DSM-IV and the dimensional perspective exemplified by the ASEBA system—and discusses the relative philosophical and technical merits of classification of EBD in general. Cullinan also addresses the short-comings of the Individuals with Disabilities Education Act (IDEA) definition of "emotional disturbance" and the National Mental Health and Special Education Coalition proposed definition of "emotional or behavioral disorder." He points out that the most important shortcoming of both definitions is insufficient attention to measurement. Cullinan proposes a key role for the Scale for Assessing Emotional Disturbance (SAED) in operationally defining key components of the IDEA definition of emotional disturbance. He goes on to suggest that only by measuring and researching alternative definitions of EBD will we gain a clearer understanding of the strengths, weaknesses, and implications of those definitions.

In Chapter 4, Osher, Cartledge, Oswald, Sutherland, Artiles, and Coutinho analyze issues relating to the cultural and linguistic competency and disproportionate representation of students of color in EBD programs. These authors address the issue of disproportional identification of minority children as EBD representing both the overrepresentation of African American and American Indian students and the underrepresentation of Latino and Asian American students. Osher and his colleagues state that, while thoughtful and effective responses to disproportionality have been rare in the history of special education, researchers in the field must commit to extending the knowledge base by fostering and using empirical research. They point out that the systematic collection and analysis of reliable data are absolute prerequisites to appropriate and effective responses to the problems of disproportionality.

Quinn and Poirier, in Chapter 5, focus on the costs and outcomes of the failure to prevent EBD. Research shows that youth with EBD have a higher incidence of mental health problems and substance abuse, school failure and dropout, and involvement in the justice system, and that the human and financial costs of the failure to prevent EBD are enormous. In this unique view of prevention research, the authors discuss the role of researchers and policymakers in determining how we treat children and youth with EBD; describe research on effective prevention, with a special emphasis on cost analysis; and synthesize the costs of inaction or inadequate prevention.

In the last chapter in the foundations section of the *Handbook*, Tankersley, Landrum, and Cook describe how research informs practice in the field of EBD. They assert that the field of EBD has made significant contributions in the past four decades to the research base that has led to our understanding of the nature, characteristics, and interactional patterns of children and youth with EBD. They also point out that significant empirically validated methods of intervention have been established for students with EBD. Tankersley and her colleagues lament, however, that a gap exists between what we know from the research evidence and what is put into practice in terms of implementing effective practices. They identify the extent to which evidence-based decisions are made and practices are applied in policymaking, teacher training, and classroom instruction; describe barriers to bringing research to bear upon practice; and examine ways to influence the extent to which research informs practice in the education of students with EBD.

PART II: ASSESSMENT AND EVALUATION

The second section of the *Handbook* focuses on a number of issues related to assessment of EBD. Following a section introduction by Lewis Polsgrove, six chapters describe the complex assessment factors that influence the identification of students with EBD and the factors that lead to the evaluation of the effectiveness of interventions for these students. In Chapter 7, Elliott and Busse provide a detailed review of the utility of ratings scales in the assessment and evaluation of students' behavior and intervention outcomes. They describe several frequently used behavior rating scales, discuss the validity issues commonly related to rating scales, and examine useful rating scales applications and analytical methods that may advance research and practice. The authors conclude that, while behavior rating scales are imperfect measures of human behavior, they are useful tools for screening and classification purposes and can be of great assistance in identifying target behaviors for intervention.

Fox and Gable, in Chapter 8, provide a thorough analysis of functional behavioral assessment (FBA), a relatively new process of behavioral assessment and intervention. Recognizing the controversial nature of FBA, they offer a balanced, empirically based review and describe the current state of FBA research and practice with particular regard to its application to students with EBD. They define critical terms and concepts related to FBA; present the historical development of FBA, particularly as applied to EBD students; give a succinct overview of the FBA process; review the state of the empirical knowledge regarding the various FBA methods and instruments and the effectiveness of functional hypothesis-based interventions; discuss the most effective ways in which we can prepare school personnel and others to apply this assessment—intervention technology; and, finally, discuss implications for future research and practice.

In Chapter 9, Mattison makes the case that the classification of students as *emotionally disturbed* under the IDEA definition should include both psychiatric and psychological assessment through mental health consultation. He describes how the information produced by clinical assessment can assist school multidisciplinary teams in both their evaluation of students for EBD services as well as in subsequent intervention planning. The chapter summarizes research from modern psychiatric and psychological assessment procedures, analyzes their relevance for teachers of students classified as having EBD with particular regard to classroom interventions, and discusses future research directions. Mattison makes a powerful case that special education, child psychiatry, and child psychology researchers must vigorously collaborate to incorporate scientific assessment and treatment findings from other disciplines in order to improve the future of students with EBD.

Hyatt and Howell, in Chapter 10, show how curriculum-based measurement (CBM) procedures can be used for data-based decision making for students with EBD. The authors describe CBM procedures as viable, instructionally relevant assessment alternatives to the use of commercially prepared norm-referenced tests. Hyatt and Howell define CBM, differentiate summative from formative assessment, review the research related to the validity and reliability of the measures, describe curriculum-based evaluation (CBE) that is based on CBM, and examine how CBM/CBE models might be used to address the social-behavioral concerns of students with EBD.

In Chapter 11, Conroy, Hendrickson, and Hester address early identification and the prevention of EBD. They point out that research offers solid evidence that the majority of severe and chronic problem behaviors demonstrated by school-age children and adolescents emanate from behavior patterns established during the early childhood years. They note that, unfortunately, current identification and intervention policies and practices are often *reactive*, targeting children once significant behavior problems are well established and more difficult to change. They argue that *proactive* identification of and intervention with these children earlier in life might prevent the development of EBD. Conroy, Hendrickson, and Hester provide a synthesis of key aspects of the early identification, prevention, and intervention literature pertaining to EBD in young children. They address the prevalence of EBD in young children, current identification and service delivery policies and practices, evidence-based intervention practices, and implications for future research and practice.

In the final chapter in the assessment section of the *Handbook*, Shriner and Wehby provide an analysis of accountability and assessment for students with EBD. They mention that, while there has been a significant movement toward the participation of students with disabilities in large-scale assessments, students with EBD are ill equipped to participate in these assessments. The authors provide an overview of the broad issues of assessment and accountability in the area of special education, identify the types of test accommodations that are available to students with EBD, review the literature regarding the participation and performance of students with EBD in state assessments, and identify areas of future research in the area of large-scale assessment for this population.

PART III: CHARACTERISTICS OF EMOTIONAL AND BEHAVIORAL DISORDERS

The third section of the *Handbook* focuses on research issues relating to the characteristics of EBD in children and youth. Following a section introduction by Steven R. Forness, four chapters address externalizing behaviors of aggression and violence, internalizing behavior problems, youth delinquency, and autism spectrum disorders. In Chapter 13, Furlong, Morrison, and Jimerson focus specifically on those externalizing disorders that have a primary element of aggressive or violent behavior. They present an overview of aggressive diagnostic patterns as embodied in the DSM-IV and IDEA, discuss research-derived models of how externalizing disorders involving aggressive behavior emerge from the developmental process, and focus on the context of the school as an exacerbating, buffering, or protective factor as it relates to youth aggression and violence. They then focus on future research needs for aggressive externalizing behavior. Furlong, Morrison, and Jimerson stress that research focusing on the interface of antisocial developmental patterns and the schooling process has the potential to support screening, prevention, and intervention efforts for students with EBD.

In Chapter 14, Gresham and Kern review the characteristics of internalizing disorders that, in contrast to externalizing disorders, are directed inwardly toward the individual. These authors describe and analyze various clinical and empirical classification systems for internalizing behavior problems. They critique the current Individuals with Disabilities Education Act definition of "emotional disturbance" and critique the DSM-IV on the basis of its medical model orientation, psychometric concerns, and the absence of treatment validity. They make a strong case that empirical classification systems using various multi-informant rating scales along with validated screening systems are most useful for the identification of internalizing behavior problems. Gresham and Kern conclude that, while evidence-based interven-

tion approaches are most salient for children with internalizing behavior problems, these approaches suffer from a failure to adequately address generalization of treatment effects. Few research studies describe applications of the interventions applied in natural contexts, and there is an absence of data supporting generalized effects of the interventions from clinical or analogue settings to typical everyday environments. For the most part, when present, information about generalization is limited to anecdotal accounts. Gresham and Kern further indicate that the research in internalizing disorders predominantly describes interventions implemented by researchers or clinicians in specialized settings and that an unanswered question is whether typical school personnel can implement these interventions successfully. Finally, the authors point out that information pertaining to the match between child characteristics and intervention effectiveness is notably absent. The etiology and variables that predict and play a role in occurrences of any given internalizing problem (e.g., depression) differ greatly among individuals. Thus, it is reasonable to assume that intervention effectiveness will likewise differ, depending on its match to variables that contribute to and sustain the behavior.

Chapter 15 describes prevention, intervention, and transition research for youth who are involved, or at risk of involvement, in the juvenile delinquency system. Nelson, Leone, and Rutherford point out that youth with disabilities are significantly overrepresented in the juvenile justice system and that youth with EBD make up a significant proportion of this population. These authors analyze the risk and resilience factors of youth with disabilities relative to their involvement in the juvenile delinquency system. They suggest that the schools can help these students develop resilience and avoid involvement in the justice system by providing positive and safe learning environments, setting high yet achievable academic and social expectations, and facilitating academic and social success. Nelson, Leone, and Rutherford note that youth with disabilities who are incarcerated have, with few exceptions, the same needs and rights to education and programs that are designed to promote their development as do their nonincarcerated peers. They point out that there is a dearth of research information on educational interventions for incarcerated youth and that much of the literature that does exist is descriptive and documents academic performance or social skills of youth. Finally, these authors document the relatively poor outcomes for youth returning to their communities from correctional facilities and highlight the need for immediate and sustained engagement in school, work, or both as a critical variable in avoiding recidivism and developing the resilience to succeed in school, work, and the community.

In the final chapter in the characteristics section of the *Handbook*, Sweeney and Hoffman provide a comprehensive analysis of research issues in autism spectrum disorders in children and youth. They review limitations of past autism research and, based on National Research Council best-practice recommendations for research design and methodology and American Psychological Association guidelines for the determination of treatment efficacy, they offer an ecological/family context model for program evaluation and research for autism spectrum disorders. Sweeney and Hoffman suggest that the dramatic increase in the occurrence of autism spectrum disorders in recent years indicates a compelling need for more rigorously designed and executed research in the area, particularly with regard to identifying efficacious treatment options.

PART IV: INTERVENTION AND TREATMENT RESEARCH

The fourth section of the *Handbook* focuses on intervention and treatment research with children and youth with EBD. Following a section introduction by C. Michael Nelson, 10 chapters are offered that discuss the myriad of treatment options available for students with EBD. In Chapter 17, Kendziora describes the relatively rich research base on early intervention for EBD. She states that research on early intervention is at a mature stage in which the question is not *whether* early intervention programs work but rather *how* different types of intervention affect specific outcomes for children with varied vulnerabilities and opportunities. Kendziora acknowledges the close connection between

prevention and early intervention and reviews what effective interventions for behavior disorders look like and the probable pathways through which they achieve their benefits. She identifies and discusses four major areas that have been relatively underdeveloped in this research area, including early intervention for internalizing problems, gender differences in early intervention, how to disseminate effective early interventions, and economic analysis of early interventions.

In Chapter 18, Konopasek and Forness review the research regarding the use of psychopharmacology in the treatment of EBD. They analyze the literature regarding the epidemiology and pharmacological treatment of children with EBD, address considerations surrounding the medical model as it relates to special education decision making, and address issues of collaboration and cooperation between special education providers, the family, and the medical community. Konopasek and Forness point out that advances in psychopharmacology have led to the recognition that medication plays an increasingly important role in the treatment of EBD in children and youth.

Cheney and Bullis, in Chapter 19, provide a comprehensive analysis of research findings and issues in the school-to-community transition of adolescents with EBD. They point out that research findings paint a dismal picture for many adolescents with EBD upon leaving public school, a process that is unsuccessful for most. Cheney and Bullis provide a historical and legal foundation for the transition initiative and its associated mandates and services, summarize selected follow-up studies on the transition experiences of adolescents with EBD, describe factors associated with transition success for this population, address transition-related assessment procedures and interventions, and discuss future transition research and practice.

In Chapter 20, Meadows and Stevens examine the research literature on teaching alternative behaviors to students with EBD. Teaching alternative behavior involves teaching and reinforcing prosocial behaviors to replace challenging or maladaptive behaviors. Meadows and Stevens state that research related to teaching alternative behavior has a relatively long and rich tradition in interventions for students with EBD. The authors trace the history of teaching alternative behaviors including definitions, descriptions, and research related to differential reinforcement. They then address issues of generalization and social validity related to teaching appropriate social skills and review the identification of appropriate alternative social behaviors based on outcome analysis and functional behavioral assessment.

In Chapter 21, Polsgrove and Smith identify evidence-based practices for teaching self-control to students with EBD. In reviewing the considerable research literature on behavioral self-regulation, they provide an overview of the theoretical underpinnings of self-regulation, review applied studies, and offer recommendations for training and research on self-control. Polsgrove and Smith describe both the behavioral self-control intervention and the cognitive self-control intervention literatures as they impact the teaching of self-regulation to children and youth with EBD. Although these authors remain optimistic that the teaching of self-control to students with EBD holds much promise, they believe there is a continuing need for evidence-based, reliable, and context-relevant methods to teach children to control their own behavior and thereby reduce their dependence on external methods of control.

Witt, VanDerHeyden, and Gilbertson, in Chapter 22, review the research literature on effective instruction and classroom management. These authors state that three questions must be addressed in analyzing whether effective instruction and management take place in the classroom. This pyramid model of classroom management asks: (1) "Are academic skills taught appropriately?" (2) "Are positive behavioral expectations taught appropriately?" (3) "Are teacher responses to inappropriate behavior consistent and accurate?" Witt, VanDerHeyden, and Gilbertson review foundational research and address important recent developments pertinent to classroom management and propose that comprehensive and integrated classroom management systems be implemented that evaluate both academic and behavior outcomes.

In Chapter 23, Kavale, Mathur, and Mostert analyze the social skills training research literature and describe research on teaching social behavior to students with emotional and behavioral disorders. These authors pose serious questions about the construct validity and social validity of social competence and social skills. They report the results of meta-analyses of the group and single-subject research literature on social skills training interventions with students with EBD and conclude that social skills training for these students has not produced particularly large treatment effects. They suggest that this limited efficacy, although disappointing, should not cause undue pessimism because social skills training must still be considered an *experimental* intervention that requires further specification to answer a number of theoretical, psychometric, and design questions. They recommend that social skills training should be rebuilt as part of a comprehensive treatment for students with EBD. Until that time, social skills training must be viewed as an intervention that has received limited empirical support but, nevertheless, should be viewed as one that should be refined and customized—but certainly not eliminated!

In Chapter 24, Lane reviews the literature on academic instruction and tutoring interventions for students with EBD. Building on the importance of academic instruction for students with EBD (as explicated by Witt, VanDerHeyden, and Gilbertson in Chapter 22), Lane stresses that the EBD research community must identify effective, efficient strategies and procedures for building these students' academic skills to enable maximum participation in the general education curriculum. Lane conducted an analysis of the research literature from 1990 to the present pertaining to academic interventions in the areas of reading, written expression, and mathematical skills conducted with students with or at risk of EBD and concluded that this literature provides a solid foundation from which to launch additional inquiries. She noted, however, that new research studies must address issues of unclear population focus; concerns regarding the breadth of the students involved, the scope of the content, and replication of studies; the limited presence of design features that are needed to draw accurate conclusions about intervention outcomes; and insufficient reporting procedures.

Liaupsin, Jolivette, and Scott, in Chapter

25, focus on schoolwide systems of behavior support, a relatively new area of prevention and intervention research with students with or at risk of EBD. Schoolwide systems of behavior support are processes that focus on decreasing the number of new cases of a problem behavior or situations by ensuring and maintaining the use of the most effective practices for all students. This chapter provides background information with regard to existing and emerging schoolwide systems of support and focuses on exploring the theoretical and empirical research that is typical of such programs. The authors describe the characteristics of schoolwide systems of support, identify issues surrounding the evaluation of the expected outcomes of such systems, describe the current research on positive outcomes, and identify weaknesses in the literature that should drive future research.

In the last chapter in the characteristics section of the *Handbook*, Eber and Keenan describe wraparound and systems-of-care services for children and youth with EBD. Building upon the almost universally poor transition outcomes for youth with EBD elucidated by Cheney and Bullis in Chapter 19, Eber and Keenan describe the history and development of interagency systems of care and the wraparound approach, a widely used tool for building constructive relationships and support networks among children with EBD and their families, teachers, and other caregivers. They discuss emerging interagency school and community-based models that connect effective learning and behavior change with system-of-care principles. These authors conclude by presenting evaluation data on these initiatives and make recommendations for needed research to guide system development and practices across disciplines.

PART V: RESEARCH METHODOLOGY

The final section of the *Handbook* focuses on methodological issues related to research with students with EBD. Following a section introduction by Eleanor Guetzloe, four chapters address, respectively, applied behavior analysis or single-subject research designs, experimental research designs, the role of qualitative research, and data collection in research and applications involving students with EBD. In Chapter 27, Lewis, Lewis-Palmer, Newcomer, and Stichter describe the foundations and applications of applied behavior analysis (ABA) intervention research with students with EBD. As evidenced by the fact that many of the assessment and intervention chapters in the *Handbook* report research studies that rely on this systematic, self-evaluative, performance-based method of analyzing and treating behavior, applied behavior analysis has had a significant impact on the field. The authors discuss the important contribution ABA has made in the field of EBD and the larger field of addressing problem behaviors within educational settings. They present the basic principles of behavior and provide an overview of basic ABA research designs. They then focus on the application of ABA principles and research at the individual child, classroom, and schoolwide level and explore the implications for current and future research and practice.

In Chapter 28, Van Acker, Yell, Bradley, and Drasgow describe experimental research designs in the study of children and youth with EBD. These authors point out that there have been increased efforts to ensure that teachers across the nation use instructional procedures that have been validated as effective by scientifically based research. Various reports state that education will see progress only if we build a knowledge base of educational practices that have been proven effective by rigorous experimental research. Van Acker, Yell, Bradley, and Drasgow address what constitutes sound scientific research in the field of EBD of children and youth. They provide an overview of experimental research designs and review how such designs have been applied to the scientific study of children and programs for children with EBD. They review the basic concepts of experimental research, examine factors that often affect experimental design in educational research, and offer recommendations for conducting rigorous experimental research in the field of EBD.

In Chapter 29, Sabornie addresses the role of qualitative research and its contribution to knowledge of children's emotional and behavioral disorders. Sabornie analyzes qualitative, or "naturalistic," research by contrasting it with quantitative empiricism, examining several methods typical of qualitative inquiry, reviewing the qualitative research base pertaining to EBD, and providing implications for the field of EBD drawn from the available research. He notes that, to date, the contributions of qualitative research in EBD have been relatively recent and far from abundant. While noting a number of limitations of qualitative research, Sarbornie concludes that quantitative and naturalistic research can coexist in the field of EBD and that including qualitative research in the examination of human behavior can lead to a more comprehensive picture of EBD.

The fourth chapter in the methodology section, and the last chapter in the *Handbook,* deals with data collection in research and applications involving students with EBD. Gunter and Denny make a compelling case for the continued use of formative evaluation research in EBD. They review the research literature regarding data collection procedures used in empirical investigations and classroom applications involving children and youth with EBD. They stress that applied behavior analysis procedures form the foundation for evaluation of intervention effectiveness based upon data. They review a number of simple and exhaustive data collection procedures, discuss the pragmatics of using daily data collection procedures in daily therapeutic and naturalistic settings, discuss the need to evaluate the efficiency and efficacy of data collection procedures for generalized applications, explore links relating research to the applications of data collection, and provide recommendations for future research needs regarding the development and implementation of formative evaluation data collection procedures for students with EBD.

CONCLUSIONS

In sum, through the authors of these chapters, we review the major foundational, assessment, characteristics, intervention, and methodological research issues facing the field of EBD. As Swanson, Harris, and Graham (2003) point out in their *Handbook of Learning Disabilities,* strong, theoretically based research in EBD has developed markedly over the past four decades. The breadth and depth of the content covered in these chapters attests to the vibrancy of the field and the role of empirically based research practices in the education and treatment of children and youth with emotional and behavioral disorders.

The *Handbook of Research in Emotional and Behavioral Disorders* provides a compilation of the most current information and evidence published to date. The field of EBD has made great strides and achieved noteworthy accomplishments; yet, formidable challenges lie ahead. Each chapter in the *Handbook* concludes with some of these challenges and offers directions for more scientific study and empirical research. Moreover, these chapters provide insight into the methodological issues facing researchers, the gaps in our knowledge base, and policy issues that prevent successful implementation of evidence based practices. In closing, it should be emphasized that these chapters lay out not only the quantity (how much has been done) but also the quality (relevance, soundness, and effectiveness) of research in the field of EBD.

REFERENCE

Swanson, H. L., Harris, K. R., & Graham, S. (Eds.). (2003). *Handbook of learning disabilities.* New York: Guilford Press.

PART I

FOUNDATIONS OF RESEARCH

Introduction

JAMES M. KAUFFMAN

In George Orwell's story of the world in *1984* (Orwell, 1949), an agent of the government explains that whoever controls the past controls the future. That is, history can be deconstructed and reconstructed to fit the desires and purposes of whoever has the power to construct it. The powerful people in the government of 1984 deny that there are objective historical facts and require the public to believe whatever the government says is true. Probably there is a message for all time in Orwell's story, as Pinker (2002) suggests. It is a warning that denial of objectivity carries with it a high price in moral degradation and social oppression.

> A denial of objective reality is no friend to moral progress, because it prevents one from saying, for example, that slavery or the Holocaust really took place. (Pinker, 2002, p. 416)

> It is ironic that a philosophy [postmodernism] that prides itself on deconstructing the accoutrements of power should embrace a relativism that makes challenges to power impossible, because it denies that there are objective benchmarks against which the deceptions of the powerful can be evaluated. . . . Without a notion of objective truth, intellectual life degenerates into a struggle of who can best exercise the raw force to "control the past." (Pinker, 2002, p. 426)

Although it is true that interpretations of historical facts may vary, the facts do not change; they are simply facts. But if one takes the position that factual history does not exist, then any claim can be said to be true. However, human dignity, freedom, and social justice all depend on the assumption that historical truths (facts) exist independent of anyone's interpretation of them (Wilkins, 2001).

In Chapter 2, I and my colleagues Frederick J. Brigham and Devery R. Mock have attempted to set the problem of research in emotional and behavioral disorders (EBD) in historical context. We make interpretations of the history of the field, of course, but we cannot claim to be totally objective in our interpretations (although we have tried to be as objective as we can be). However, the historical facts—who published what, when, and where, for example—cannot be changed at will without denying reality. We also try to connect historical facts and trends with contemporary issues.

We attempt to show in Chapter 2 how the field of emotional and behavioral disorders faces a stark choice between science and anti-science, between the assertion that true objectivity is unbelievable and the assertion that objectivity can be attained in meaningful degrees and that greater objectivity is usually the better choice. In short, we hope to have helped readers understand how what has become known as postmodernism is the antithesis of the assumptions on which this book is based. We agree with Spear-Swerling and Sternberg (2001), who commented:

This is not to say that science can solve every problem, or that scientific knowledge is all that matters. Many other kinds of knowledge contribute to professional growth and are important in making educational decisions, such as, for example, professional experience and judgment. However, experience alone does not necessarily lead people to correct conclusions. . . . For example, despite extensive experience with objects in the physical world, most people do not generate the laws of physics on their own. (p. 55)

Most teachers do not generate effective and efficient instructional procedures on their own, even though they may have extensive teaching experience. It is time to recognize the importance of scientific rigor in our field and to make certain that the most rigorous scientific evidence available is used in guiding interventions (Crockett, 2001).

In Chapter 3, Douglas Cullinan outlines knowledge, problems, and needed research related to issues of classification and definition. He notes the importance of classification, how it is important to recognize similarities and differences in groups and individuals. We need to classify things and people to make sense of the world, but we also need to recognize the uniqueness of the individual. As I was reading his chapter, I thought of the absolute necessity and utility of classifying music but the importance of recognizing a particular song or tune. Although there are many classifications of music into which most tunes can be put, there are always tunes that are difficult to classify or that are "sort of" but not quite the genre of interest. For example, we can easily classify some tunes as blues, but then there are tunes that are sort of bluesy.

Cullinan points out specific and important research needs, including the relevance of resilience and classification. I think these are particularly important. We need to measure the resilience of children and youth, and we need to better connect our classifications to interventions. Cullinan notes that definitions may be useful in research (deciding whom or what to study), philosophy (giving authority to statements), and administration (deciding whom to serve and how to serve them). His observation that no definition is without its limitations and problems is well taken. The definition proposed by the National Mental Health and Special Education Coalition (Forness & Knitzer, 1992) is not without its own problems, one of which is the suggestion that cultural norms for behavior are important. Cullinan discusses how, in his own research, ethnic differences showed up in some measures of EBD. Creating the cultural norms referred to in the definition proposed by the Coalition presents a particularly difficult challenge for researchers. Among those challenges are (1) the difficulty in knowing which cultures to acknowledge as needing separate norms and (2) specifying the conditions under which separate norms should be invoked. I think we should view the evidence justifying cultural norms for behavior with considerable skepticism. The issue of how culture may be related to deviant behavior leads into the topic of Chapter 4.

In Chapter 4, David Osher, Gwendolyn Cartledge, Donald Oswald, Kevin S. Sutherland, Alfredo J. Artiles, and Martha Coutinho address issues of cultural and linguistic competency and the disproportionate representation of students of various ethnicities in special education. They note that thoughtful and effective analyses of disproportionality have been rare in special education and that questions of race and language differences are always emotionally charged. There is a great temptation to say or write what is politically popular to avoid any possible charges of bias or racism. The authors of Chapter 4 intimate that it is therefore not surprising to encounter both nonscientific statements and trite observations about racial and ethnic issues. In this regard, Pinker (2002) observes that "the political messages of most postmodernist pieces are utterly banal, like 'racism is bad' " (p. 416). Historians Robert Conquest (2000) and Diane Ravitch (2003) have also noted the utter banality of postmodern views of issues relating to race, culture, and language.

Osher et al. raise interesting and difficult questions about research on issues of ethnic identity and disproportionality. Perhaps education, especially special education, is unwilling or considers it unethical to do the kind of research that Osher et al. suggest is necessary to find answers to the effects of special education (i.e., random assignment to treatment and nontreatment conditions or to treatment X and treatment Y rather than treating all identified students with whatever is presumptively effective). Osher et al. also mention, in their closing sentences, that disproportionality by ethnicity is a phenomenon in delivery of other services, namely juvenile justice and mental health. Although African American youths are disproportionately overrepresented in juvenile justice, they are clearly underrepresented in mental health. A disquieting question implicit in this observation presents itself: Is special education perceived to be more like juvenile justice than like mental health, or vice versa? To the extent that special education is a helpful service, the disproportional representation of African American students in special education for EBD is the opposite of unfairness to African Americans, unless the identification of EBD among African American students exceeds reasonable prevalence estimates. Also, Osher and colleagues recognize that the disproportionality issue must be seen in the context of the apparent underservice (by special education in the EBD category) of students of all ethnic groups. At the national level, no ethnic group is served at a percentage higher than prevalence data suggest is warranted.

Perhaps we need to ask ourselves about the cost of treatment and failure to treat individual cases of emotional and behavioral disorders regardless of the other identifying characteristics of children and youth. In Chapter 5, Mary Magee Quinn and Jeffrey M. Poirier weigh the costs of failure to serve children with emotional and behavioral disorders. They address both the human costs and the financial costs, both direct and indirect. Although cost analyses of service and nonservice are difficult, it appears that data support two conclusions: first, a substantial proportion of children and youth with EBD receive neither special education nor mental health services; second, the problems that these children and youth cause themselves and others are many and expensive. Little wonder that the idea of prevention is a topic in Kendziora's chapter (Chapter 17, this volume). We might imagine that prevention would be a relatively easy sell, given the enormous costs of letting misbehavior fester until it is intolerable. But prevention has been a topic in our field's literature for more than half a century without resulting in widespread public policies to deal with the early stages of EBD (Kauffman, 2004).

The fact is that, although prevention is a captivating idea as long as it remains an abstraction, there are many strong forces arrayed against putting prevention into practice (Kauffman, 2003, 2004, 2005a, 2005b). The inevitability of labeling, additional costs, the higher numbers of students served, more cases of uncertainty, the increased risk of false positives—all these and other typical objections to prevention must be overcome if research is to be put into practice. True, we need to know more about prevention. But in spite of our current knowledge of prevention, and perhaps in spite of what we find out, there appears to be little reason to believe that we will pay the substantial near-term human and financial costs to prevent even higher delayed costs, for reasons I have discussed previously (Kauffman, 1999).

In the final chapter in Part I, Melody Tankersley, Timothy J. Landrum, and Bryan G. Cook address the issue of what research is ultimately about—how it informs practice. They note that some special education policies are adopted in the face of contrary evidence and that other policies are not adopted in spite of evidence supporting them. Getting our field to be evidence-based is a Herculean task, particularly when anti-scientific views are popular not only among the general public but among teacher educators and advocacy organizations as well. For the foreseeable future, calls for evidence and rationality will not be unanimous among those who prepare teachers, much less among teachers themselves or the public. Science may be our best bet for finding the truth and for guiding our work, as Tankersley et al. suggest and as explained by others (e.g., Crockett, 2001; Heward, 2003; Heward & Silvestri, 2005; Spear-Swerling & Sternberg, 2001). The consequences of rejecting scientific understanding of effective teaching may be negative and severe (Mostert, Kauffman, & Kavale, 2003). Nevertheless, the insistence on evidence-based practices in special education is likely to remain a minority point of view.

Part I of this *Handbook* is intended to provide foundations for research discussed in other sections. Each chapter, including those in this section, must be read with attention to foundational knowledge in the history of our field, the nature and extent of the problem of EBD, and what scientific research can tell us about the students we serve and our attempts to help them.

REFERENCES

Conquest, R. (2000). *Reflections on a ravaged century.* New York: Norton.

Crockett, J. B. (Ed.). (2001). The meaning of science and empirical rigor in the social sciences. *Behavioral Disorders, 27*(1) [special issue].

Forness, S. R., & Knitzer, J. (1992). A new proposed definition and terminology to replace "Serious Emotional Disturbance" in the Individuals with Disabilities Education Act. *School Psychology Review, 21,* 12–20.

Heward, W. L. (2003). Ten faulty notions about teaching and learning that hinder the effectiveness of special education. *Journal of Special Education, 36,* 186–205.

Heward, W. L., & Silvestri, S. M. (2005). The neutralization of special education. In J. W. Jacobson, J. A. Mulick, & R. M. Foxx (Eds.), *Fads: Dubious and improbable treatments for developmental disabilities* (pp. 193–214). Mahwah, NJ: Erlbaum.

Kauffman, J. M. (1999). How we prevent the prevention of emotional and behavioral disorders. *Exceptional Children, 65,* 448–468.

Kauffman, J. M. (2003). Appearances, stigma, and prevention. *Remedial and Special Education, 24,* 195–198.

Kauffman, J. M. (2004). Foreword. In H. M. Walker, E. Ramsey, & F. H. Gresham, *Antisocial behavior in school: Strategies and best practices* (2nd ed.). Pacific Grove, CA: Brooks/Cole.

Kauffman, J. M. (2005a). *Characteristics of emotional and behavioral disorders of children and youth* (8th ed.). Upper Saddle River, NJ: Prentice Hall.

Kauffman, J. M. (2005b). How we prevent the prevention of emotional and behavioral difficulties in education. In P. Clough, P. Garner, J. T. Pardeck, & F. K. O. Yuen (Eds.), *Handbook of emotional and behavioral difficulties in education* (pp. 366–376). London: Sage.

Mostert, M. P., Kauffman, J. M., & Kavale, K. A. (2003). Truth and consequences. *Behavioral Disorders, 28,* 333–347.

Orwell, G. (1949). *1984.* New York: Harcourt, Brace, Jovanovich.

Pinker, S. (2002). *The blank slate: The modern denial of human nature.* New York: Viking.

Ravitch, D. (2003). *The language police: How pressure groups restrict what students learn.* New York: Knopf.

Spear-Swerling, L., & Sternberg, R. J. (2001). What science offers teachers of reading. *Learning Disabilities Research and Practice, 16,* 51–57.

Wilkins, R. (2001). *Jefferson's pillow: The founding fathers and the dilemma of black patriotism.* Boston: Beacon.

2

Historical to Contemporary Perspectives on the Field of Emotional and Behavioral Disorders

JAMES M. KAUFFMAN, FREDERICK J. BRIGHAM, *and* DEVERY R. MOCK

All scientific research follows a predictable course. First, the scientist notices a difference of some kind—a difference in appearance, behavior, or other attribute of an inanimate object or creature that can be measured. Usually, the scientist then shares this observation of difference by describing it as precisely as possible. Recognition and description prompt questions about the precise extent and nature of the difference and the particular conditions under which it can be observed. The scientist engages in speculation about the reasons for the difference and develops ways to evaluate such speculation. The evaluations are interventions to be tried out, and hypotheses about the interventions are to be tested. This is called experimentation.

Following experimentation, the scientist is confronted with a choice: (1) evaluate the outcomes on the basis of how things *did* turn out and continue the cycle of investigation running from recognition of difference to evaluation of intervention and back again or (2) evaluate the outcomes on the basis of an ideology, recognizing and interpreting differences only in ways that conform to preconceived notions of how things *should have* turned out.

Ideology may, of course, enter and corrupt the scientific process at any point. It can preclude the observation of difference (i.e., suggest so strongly that difference should not be observed that it is not) or demand the misinterpretation of differences that are observed (i.e., any differences must conform to a theory, whether it can be tested empirically or not). The most obvious cases of ideology trumping science are perhaps those of the astronomer Galileo Galilei (Sobel, 1999), the early geologist William Smith (Winchester, 2001), and the scientist Charles Darwin (e.g., Gould, 2000; Pinker, 2002; Shermer, 1997). Galileo, Smith, and Darwin all encountered religious dogma or ideology attempting to preclude their observations of differences or to insist on their interpreting the phenomena only in light of the revealed "truths" of scripture or the church. The ideologies opposing Galileo's, Smith's, and Darwin's theories proposed that reliable knowledge can be constructed without scientific inquiry. Ascientific and anti-scientific views are a hallmark of ideology (Ruscio, 2002).

Ideologies, whether political or social, have been known to corrupt knowledge in many of the sciences and humanities (see Conquest, 2000; Gould, 2000; Pinker, 2002;

Ruscio, 2002; Shattuck, 1999; Shermer, 1997, 2001). Ideologies have corrupted special education as well (see Polsgrove & Ochoa, 2004; Sasso, 2001). But ideology is not the only possible corruption of the scientific search for reliable data and its rational interpretation. Human beings are flawed creatures, prone to mistakes, sometimes honest ones. Scientific methods can be botched, and results can be misinterpreted, sometimes unwittingly, even by the best minds. However, sometimes people knowingly disavow knowledge—actually retreat from it—preferring the more comfortable "situated" or idiosyncratic "knowledge" of their personal construction (Sasso, 2001). Others may distort or misrepresent data for personal reasons of avarice, fame, ideological fidelity, or some combination of these.

Fortunately, science is a self-correcting system, although the scientific method is sometimes wrongly blamed for catastrophes because it is practiced poorly, misrepresented, set to evil purpose, or confused with pseudoscience (see Gould, 2000; Gross, 1998; Ruscio, 2002; Shermer, 1997, 2001). For example, Carlson (2003) impugned scientists in the eugenics debacle, not making clear to the unsuspecting reader either the fact that pseudosciences and ideologies created the eugenics movement or the fact that reliable science "unmasked" it as "balderdash." Scientists can be wrong or hoodwinked by pseudoscience, particularly in fields of study outside their own. But the search for truth is far better served by improved scientific understanding than by alternative ways of constructing "knowledge" (see Polsgrove & Ochoa, 2004; Sasso, 2001; Vaughn & Dammann, 2001).

Research on the behavioral disorders of children and youth has followed the usual course of scientific inquiry. It has been plagued by the same flaws as other fields of investigation. It has sometimes been misunderstood and misused. It has been confused with pseudoscience. It faces continuing challenges of its value and integrity. However, the gradual accretion of scientific understanding through research has led us from nearly total ignorance to the beginnings of understanding what behavioral disorders are, why they occur, and how we can best treat them.

The history of special education for children and youth with emotional and behavioral disorders (EBD) has been outlined in many sources (see Kauffman, 1976; Kauffman & Landrum, in press). Here we provide a brief discussion of the historical roots of research and contemporary perspectives on inquiry in the field. An important point to note is that all phases of the cycle of scientific inquiry, from recognition of difference through evaluation, are continuing and that ideological challenges to scientific thought have always been mounted.

RECOGNITION AND DESCRIPTION

Until the 19th century, recognition and description of behavioral disorders of children and youth were sketchy. However, by the middle of the 19th century, textbooks and journals contained increasingly detailed descriptions of behavior that was clearly recognized as deviant—that is, not like that of normal individuals.

> He was wholly an animal. He was without attachment; overturned everything in his way, but without courage or intent; possessed no tact, intelligence, power of dissimulation, or sense of propriety; and was awkward to excess. His *moral sentiments* are described as *null*, except the love of approbation, and a noisy instinctive gaiety, independent of the external world. . . . Devouring everything, however disgusting, brutally sensual, passionate—breaking, tearing, and burning whatever he could lay his hand upon; and if prevented from doing so, pinching, biting, scratching, and tearing himself, until he was covered with blood. He had the particularity of being so attracted by the eyes of his brothers, sisters, and playfellows, as to make the most persevering efforts to push them out with his fingers. . . . When any attempt was made to associate him with the other patients, he would start away with a sharp cry, and then come back to them hastily. (Brigham, 1845, p. 336)

Recognition and description during this era (the 19th century) were not accompanied or followed by empirical studies. We note in the next section how what now seem bizarre speculations accompanied recognition and description.

During the first half of the 20th century a classification system, or taxonomy of children's behavior disorders was devised. One of the most remarkable classifications was that of Kanner's syndrome, or early infantile autism, known today as autistic spectrum disorder (see National Research Council, 2001). Leo Kanner, the "father of child psychiatry," wrote of one of the children he saw:

> In October 1938, a 5-year-old boy was brought to my clinic from Forest, Mississippi. I was struck by the uniqueness of the peculiarities which Donald exhibited. He could, since the age of 2½ years, tell the names of all the presidents and vice-presidents, recite the letters of the alphabet forwards and backwards, and flawlessly, with good enunciation, rattle off the Twenty-Third Psalm. Yet he was unable to carry on an ordinary conversation. He was out of contact with people, while he could handle objects skillfully. His memory was phenomenal. The few times when he addressed someone—largely to satisfy his wants—he referred to himself as "You" and to the person addressed as "I." He did not respond to any intelligence tests but manipulated intricate formboards adroitly. (Kanner, 1973, p. 93)

Kanner's speculation and that of others (e.g., Bettelheim, 1950, 1967) was later found through scientific investigation to be wrong. Before 1950, however, recognition and descriptions of other differences in behavior were recorded, including schizophrenia and what is now known as *conduct disorder* (see Kauffman, 2005a; Martens & Russ, 1932). Following are descriptions of what today we might refer to as attention-deficit/hyperactivity disorder (ADHD), or traumatic brain injury:

> J.M., 7 years old: " . . . doesn't pay attention to any directions. He is unaware of anything said, yet at times he surprises me by noticing things that others don't."
> D.J., 7 years old: " . . . attention hard to hold. Asks constantly: "When can I go? Can I go now?" etc. No initiative. Little self-control. Seems high strung and nervous."
> D.H., 8 years old: " . . . has proven quite a serious problem in behavior. Has acquired the habit of throwing himself into tantrums at the slightest provocation."
> J.K., 8 years old: " . . . has made scarcely any social adjustments in relationships with other children, he loses all self-control, becoming wild and uncontrollable; he is extremely nervous and excitable; his attention span is very short and he is unable to concentrate for

more than a few minutes. During work periods he jumps from one activity to another." (Strauss & Lehtinen, 1947, p. 127)

After 1950, description included not only children's behavior but programs for them and intervention strategies as well (e.g., Grosenick, George, & George, 1987, 1988; Grosenick, George, George, & Lewis, 1991; Morse, Cutler, & Fink, 1964; Redl & Wineman, 1951, 1952; Rhodes & Head, 1974; Rhodes & Tracy, 1972a, 1972b; see Kauffman, 2005a; Kauffman & Landrum, in press, for further descriptions). The detailed description of children, conceptual models, and programs in the second half of the 20th century was invaluable in the development and evaluation of interventions.

Contemporary Problems in Recognition and Description

The recognition of children's behavioral disorders no longer consists only of observation and speculation. Researchers now use scientific study to recognize and describe these disorders with increasing reliability and validity. Such studies are exponentially more sophisticated and precise than the 19th- and early 20th-century practice of positing a causal relationship between an antecedent event (e.g., "sleeping in a barn filled with new hay") and insanity. Unfortunately, scientific knowledge does not yet reliably guide practice (see Tankersley, Landrum, & Cook, Chapter 6, this volume). Ironically, in an age of science, many practitioners are reluctant to replace conjecture with quantifiable evidence and are encouraged to abandon scientific study for ideological reasons (see Kauffman, 1999b, 2002, 2003b; Mostert, Kauffman, & Kavale, 2003).

Current research suggests that 10–20% of children experience serious mental health problems (Greenberg, Domitrovich, & Bumbarger, 1999; Kauffman, 2005a; U.S. Department of Health and Human Services, 2001; Walker, Ramsey, & Gresham, 2004); yet, less than 1% of these school-age children are identified with emotional or behavioral disabilities ("emotional disturbance," or "ED," in federal language; U.S. Department of Education, 2000). Of the more than 460,000 students in the United States who are identified with EBD, less than half are identified at the elementary school level (U.S. Department of Education, 2000). In fact, relatively stable trends indicate that referrals for EBD identification peak in the 14- to 15-year age range (Walker, Nishioka, Zeller, Severson, & Feil, 2000). Despite research demonstrating the importance of early identification and intervention, *late* identification—*the opposite of prevention*—seems to be the norm.

This norm is particularly problematic, considering that the symptoms of behavioral disorders tend to increase in intensity over time (Forness, Kavale, & Lopez, 1993). Unless students with EBD are identified early in their school careers, the risk trajectories they are on will accelerate. They are likely to become extremely aversive to others and may ultimately be pushed out of school (Walker et al., 2000). Thus, prevention, in the form of early intervention, has been found to be the most promising strategy for diverting the trajectories of these at-risk children (Walker, Stiller, Severson, Feil, & Golly, 1998; Zigler, Taussig, & Black, 1992). Such interventions are proactive in nature and therefore delivered *before*, *at*, and *just after* the point of school entry (Hester & Kaiser, 1998; Walker et al., 1998). Unfortunately, these empirically supported programs of early intervention and prevention are commonly thwarted in practice. Although there are many ways in which *prevention is prevented,* educators and professionals who are hesitant in recognizing students with EBD make prevention and remediation extremely difficult or impossible (Kauffman, 1999a, 2005b; see also Quinn & Poirier, Chapter 5, this volume).

Problems in Recognition

School personnel have difficulty recognizing and identifying students with EBD for a variety of reasons including (1) personal philosophy, (2) definitional imprecision, and (3) pragmatic concerns. Some professionals fail to identify students with EBD because of a personal distaste for labeling. Many of these individuals profess an unsubstantiated concern that the act of labeling somehow exacerbates the disability (see Kauffman, 2002, 2003a; Lambros, Ward, Bocian, MacMillan, & Gresham, 1998). In this way, disability is thought to be simply a social construction, not reflective of any inherent disorder (see Danforth & Rhodes, 1997; Elkind, 1998). Such individuals presume a causal relationship between the act of identifying disability and the patterns of aggressive behavior, noncompliance, disruptive acts, and academic deficits that seem to distinguish students with EBD. Unfortunately, pinpointing a cause, even if it is scientifically validated, often does little to improve the rather bleak long-term prognosis for students with EBD. Furthermore, unidentified behavior disorders tend to become chronic lifelong disorders that then prove refractory to intervention.

Imprecise definitions of EBD help to thwart identification of students with this disability (Forness & Kavale, 1997; Lambros et al., 1998; Tankersley & Landrum, 1997). College textbooks regularly conceptualize behavior disorders using two distinct categories: (1) externalizing behaviors and (2) internalizing behaviors (Kauffman, 2005a; Walker et al., 2004). Paradoxically, empirical studies have suggested that these categories are less clearly defined than originally thought and that students with EBD tend to demonstrate characteristics across multiple categories (Cullinan, Evans, Epstein, & Ryser, 2003; see also Cullinan, Chapter 3, this volume).

Comorbidity seems to be the rule rather than exception. The literature is rich with studies indicating the comorbid relationships between ADHD, conduct disorder, oppositional defiant disorder, learning difficulties, mood disorders, depressive symptoms, and anxiety disorders (American Psychiatric Association, 1994; Biederman, Newcorn, & Sprich, 1991; Verhulst & Van der Endè, 1993; Waldman, Rhee, Levy, & Hay, 2001). However, definitions of EBD seldom account for a disorder marked by comorbidity. As such, definitions fail to adequately describe disabling conditions in which the combined effect of multiple disorders is not additive but exponential (Tankersley & Landrum, 1997). Educators are left to recognize and respond to separate behavioral characteristics without ever addressing a disorder as a whole. Such an approach is akin to asking a mechanic to recognize and repair flat or badly worn tires without ever addressing the problems of wheel alignment and balance or nails littering the garage floor.

According to the definition stipulated in the Individuals with Disabilities Education Act (IDEA), if a student is to be identified with EBD, he or she must exhibit one or more of the characteristics listed in the definition to a marked extent and over a period of time—*and he or she must not be judged socially maladjusted but not emotionally disturbed* (Cullinan et al., 2003; see also Cullinan, Chapter 3, this volume). This exclusion is the cause of both controversy and confusion (Center, 1990; Forness & Kavale, 2000; Kauffman, 2005a). Researchers have expressed concerns that, in applying an ambiguous definition, school personnel may equate conduct disorder, externalizing behaviors, and juvenile delinquency with social maladjustment and thereby fail to identify a large number of students in need of special education services and protections—fail, in fact, to identify those students whose antisocial behavior puts them at highest risk for school failure and poor life outcomes (Lambros et al., 1998; Kauffman, 2005a; Walker et al., 2004).

Professionals are also hesitant to identify students with EBD for other reasons. Although controversial, the 1997 reauthorization of IDEA stipulated that a student with an identified disability could not be expelled from school for behaviors caused by the disability. Thus, identifying a student with EBD precludes the later expulsion of that student for the very behaviors that may later prove the most problematic for teachers. For any of these reasons, many students exhibiting symptoms of EBD are often not identified or are misidentified and served under the learning disability (LD) category (Duncan, Forness, & Hartsough, 1995). For a disability in which appropriate intervention is crucial (Lambros et al., 1998; Walker et al., 2004), ambiguous definition and delayed recognition portend dire outcomes.

Problems in Description

The contemporary science and practice of the description of behavioral disorders of children and youth (at least in the United States) cannot be considered outside of the influence of the legal regulations created in the last half of the 20th century. IDEA affects the educational services of all school-age children identified with EBD. Although IDEA does not spell out the kinds of EBD that must be assessed, it is very clear on the procedural requirements for assessment of EBD (Yell & Drasgow, 2000). Another legal influence on the identification of children and youths with EBD is the movement toward minimum competency testing that culminated in 2001 with the passage of the *No Child Left Behind Act* (NCLB; see Yell & Drasgow, 2005). A major part of NCLB is mandated assessment of student performance. Many states had such assessments in place before 2001, but NCLB increased the frequency of the tests and the importance that schools place on the information that they generate. NCLB has been described as a farcical attempt to improve schools and schooling (Kauffman, 2002, in press), but its irrationality has been noted even by mainstream media:

School administrators are also grappling with other irrationalities built into the system. States are required, for example, to bring all non-English-speaking children up to the same standards as children who are proficient in English. Yet once they are proficient in English, these children no longer count as being non-English-speaking and are tested in a different category—so there will be no demonstrable improvement. Nor does the federal law cut any slack for the children of new immigrants, who, 12 years from now, will presumably have to be proficient in English from the moment they start school, if their schools are not to be labeled "failing." The law also neglects to make distinctions between schools that fail in every category and schools that miss the targets by a small margin in a single category.

These are small points, but they matter. This is a law that will work, in practice, only as part of a larger political process. (*Washington Post*, 2003, p. A22)

Small points, perhaps, but they matter enormously in special education. Altering identification procedures and emphasizing certain aspects of the curriculum over others clearly influence the opportunities available to students in schools and the definition of tolerable behavior and acceptable performance (Brigham, Tochterman, & Brigham, 2001). Although the effects of NCLB and other changes in federal education policy have yet to be fully felt, these policies will likely affect the number of students identified with EBD as well as exacerbate the problems of schools. For example, emphasis on performance in academic skills, particularly in the formats that lend themselves to efficient administration and scoring, may eliminate or substantially reduce elements of the curriculum that enabled academically marginal students to make progress in schools. If that were to happen, those students who were previously not considered to demonstrate behavior problems would be at risk for identification as having EBD. Alternatively, the emphasis on academic testing could place new awareness of the importance of vocational education opportunities for students who are less than adept learners of abstract information contained in higher-level academics. In either case, it is clear that changes in the schools and society as a whole will affect the conditions that are recognized and described as EBD, at least at the margins separating acceptable from unacceptable behavior.

The development of functional behavioral assessment (FBA) represents a major shift in the description of students with EBD. While many of the descriptions excerpted in previous sections of this chapter focused on behavioral topography, FBA attempts to describe the purposes and conditions of maladaptive behavior and direct interventions at altering the conditions supporting maladaptive behavior and increasing conditions that support more acceptable behavior (Crone & Horner, 2003; Repp & Horner, 1999; see also Fox & Gable, Chapter 8, this volume). While the legal requirements and the calls from many advocates suggest that FBA will result in major changes in the way schools and other aspects of society view and interact with individuals with EBD, the scientific evidence has yet to fully support these assumptions (Gable, 1996; Sasso, Conroy, Stichter, & Fox, 2001).

Strength-based assessment (Epstein, 2000) represents another recent development in the description of children with EBD. Strength-based assessment can be defined as the measurement of those emotional and behavioral skills, competencies, and characteristics that (1) create a sense of personal accomplishment, (2) contribute to satisfying relationships with family members, peers, and adults, (3) enhance one's ability to deal with adversity and stress, and (4) promote one's personal, social, and academic development (Epstein & Sharma, 1998). It represents a departure from earlier models that focus on catalogs of behavioral deficiencies or excesses. The scientific evidence in support of this approach appears solid. However, the extent to which it will prove useful in schools remains to be demonstrated.

The changes in description that arise from these approaches are subtle and probably do not represent newly discovered classes of behavioral disorders. Nevertheless, the focus on the interaction of the individual and the environment is more evident in the following passages than it was in many of the preceding quotes from the 19th and early 20th centuries.

> Keith also engaged in chronic, high-rate challenging behaviors in the school setting that included aggression, tantrums, noncompliance (e.g., screaming, whining and crying, putting his head down, leaving his assigned area, refusing to walk, destroying property). When he was not engaged in challenging behaviors, Keith was able to participate in a variety of vocational and daily living tasks. However, at the time of the study, his teacher reported that Keith's problem behavior interfered with his ability to engage in these activities. (Cole & Levinson, 2002, p. 30)

or

> . . . Linda said she liked reading and math, but sometimes the work was too hard. She admitted not completing homework because it was "boring," or she didn't know what she was supposed to do. Linda liked having a teacher help her with her schoolwork, which often happened when she stayed in during recess to make up missing assignments. Linda said she didn't care whether she missed recess because the other kids didn't like her and wouldn't play with her. However, she seemed to be unaware of what she did to annoy other kids or what she could do differently to win more friends. (McConaughy, 2000, p. 189)

Both of these passages demonstrate descriptive approaches to identifying children with EBD designed to give treatment providers clear descriptions of behaviors occurring within various environments as well as clues about the relative strengths that could form the basis for intervention. However, practice in the field lags far behind these developments, with practitioners tending to rely on norm-referenced instruments that require substantially less time to complete than do more functional approaches (Landrum, 2001). Another reason for the continued reliance of many educators on more traditional measures is the distance that a norm-referenced instrument allows the evaluator to maintain from the individual being evaluated. The responsibility for statements about someone else's behavior can often be avoided by the user of normative evaluations; the evaluator is somewhat insulated by the formality of the procedure. Nevertheless, the responsibility of assessment remains. Except for extreme cases of EBD, the recognition and description of the disorder are rooted in the everyday experience, training, and tolerance of the evaluator as well as the conditions surrounding the evaluation and the behavior. As long as people continue to live and interact in groups, the recognition and description of EBD will continue to change.

SPECULATION AND INTERVENTION (EXPERIMENTATION)

By the 19th century, emotional or behavioral disorders were no longer thought to be caused by demon possession. The prevailing belief was that masturbation caused or aggravated insanity (Hare, 1962; Rie, 1971). However, although Stribling (1842) referred to masturbation as a "detestable vice" and a "degrading habit," he clearly understood that it was often mistaken as a cause of insanity. Moreover, a few writers of the day questioned the supposed cause–effect relationship between masturbation and insanity simply on logical grounds. Jarvis (1852) noted, logically, that masturbation could not be evaluated as a factor in any increase of insanity because "we have no means of knowing whether masturbation increases or diminishes" (p. 354). Even in the mid-19th century, people had the basic *idea* of correlation, although they had no statistical procedure for assessing its strength and understood that correlation did not imply causation.

Most of the time, 19th-century writers simply guessed at the causes of mental illness, and many of their guesses now seem wild and laughable indeed: "idleness and en-

nui," "pecuniary embarrassment," "sedentary and studious habits," "inhaling tobacco fumes," "gold fever," "indulgence of temper" (Stribling, 1842); "suppression of hemorrhoids," "kick on the stomach," "bathing in cold water," "study of metaphysics," "reading vile books," "license question," "preaching sixteen days and nights," "celibacy," "sudden joy," "ecstatic admiration of works of art," "mortified pride," "Mormonism," "duel," "struggle between the religious principle and power of passion" (Jarvis, 1852); "feebleness of intellect," "uterine derangement," "suppression of menses," "suppressed masturbation," "cerebral softening," "bad whiskey," "women," "worms," "politics," "Salvation Army," "novel reading," "seduction," and "laziness" (among those listed as reasons for admission to the West Virginia Hospital for the Insane at Weston, 1864–1889—noted in hospital records).

No less unsubstantiated were the 20th-century psychoanalytic assumptions about causes and interventions. Bettelheim was known to assign blame for autism to parental rejection and for deviant behavior to what seemed to empiricists to be bizarre unconscious motivations (e.g., 1950, 1961, 1967; Bettelheim & Sylvester, 1948). His hypotheses and interventions were essentially untestable, but they carried considerable influence among many professionals and lay persons who embraced the pseudoscience of psychoanalysis (see also Berkowitz & Rothman, 1960). His views and approaches to treatment are illustrated by the summary of a case described by Bettelheim.

Bertha, a four-year-old diagnosed as "psychotic" and unmanageable, was in residential treatment. She exhibited many symptoms of severe mental illness, one of which was that she frequently attempted to smash people's eyeglasses. If she was prevented from doing this, her behavior became extremely wild. The assumption of those designing a therapeutic program for Bertha was that if she were ever to be helped, they would have to understand why she engaged in this behavior; and she would have to be helped to understand her own behavior as well. To achieve this understanding, it would be necessary to simply accept her breaking glasses, not to try to suppress this symptom of her underlying mental illness. Consequently, breaking glasses was accepted for three years until Bertha was able to reveal the hidden, unconscious meaning of her behavior.

Through listening to Bertha talk about her past and observing her behavior, those responsible for her treatment arrived at the following interpretation: Bertha's mother had had chronic schizophrenia and was extremely difficult to understand. Bertha decided that because her mother wore glasses, which helped her see better and therefore understand things, she would try to understand her mother by putting on her mother's glasses. But when she put on the glasses, she saw worse instead of better. This infuriated Bertha—the injustice that her mother could see better but that she saw worse with the glasses and still could not understand her mother's behavior. She was so infuriated that she felt compelled to break all reminders or symbols of this injustice. The intervention consisted of unraveling an interpretation of the unconscious motivation of Bertha's misbehavior, not any procedures designed to control it directly. (Bettelheim, 1970, as summarized by Kauffman, 2001, pp. 114–115)

Empirically testable interventions (experimentation) followed the invention of behavioral psychology and applied behavior analysis during the middle decades of the 20th century. Pioneers in the application of behavior principles to interventions for behavior disorders included Haring and Phillips (1962, 1972), Haring and Whelan (1965), and Hewett (1964, 1965, 1967, 1968). The speculation about causes and testable interventions resulting from such speculation led researchers to investigate environmental conditions, particularly the immediate antecedents and consequences of behavior, to find the controlling factors. Although behavioral analyses were critical to the advancement of research, it also became apparent by the late 20th century that biological factors, particularly those involving brain function, must be considered in understanding the causes and treatment of many disorders (see Forness & Kavale, 2001; National Research Council, 2001; Pinker, 2002).

Contemporary Speculation and Intervention

Several influences have redirected intervention from the behavioral treatments that followed—but never completely replaced—the prescientific and psychodynamic interventions of previous decades. Among these are the increasing recognition that (1) problems are typically multiple, also known as comorbid; (2) biological factors contribute significantly to many behavioral disorders; (3) many, but not all, behavioral disorders are rooted in interactions between the individual and his or her environment; and (4) standards-based reforms and the inclusive schools movement have altered the research agenda of the field.

Comorbidity

It is increasingly clear that individuals rarely experience isolated behavioral or mental health problems. Rather, most behavioral problems occur in combination with other problems (Angold, Costello, & Erkanli, 1999; Compas, Conner, & Hinden, 1998; Cullinan & Epstein, 2001). The recognition that multiple risk factors and multiple behavior problems are important considerations in the treatment of any individual's condition has broadened the number of elements that must be considered in assessment and treatment (Loeber, Farrington, Stouthamer-Loeber, & Van Kammen, 1998).

> School psychologists or special educators may often treat disruptive behavior disorders with relatively straightforward behavioral strategies. Such approaches may not be entirely adequate, however, if such disorders are accompanied or even preceded by significant comorbidity. The gradual emergence of such comorbidity may not always be readily apparent, unless school professionals are prepared to recognize its developmental trajectory. (Forness, 2003, pp. 63–64)

Treatments for behavioral disorders need to include consideration of other conditions that coexist or preexist with the problem that brought the individual to the attention of the school or mental health officials in the first place. Often the presenting problem is actually a secondary or tertiary result of a primary, and often undiagnosed, behavioral issue. This is a substantial departure from earlier behavioral approaches that considered etiology to be of little consequence because it could not be altered. Although it is still impossible to alter the past, current approaches consider etiology to provide important clues about effective treatments as well as issues that must be addressed simultaneously with the presenting problem (Baer, MacLean, & Marlatt, 1998; Forness & Kavale, 2001; Jensen et al., 2001).

Biological Contributions to Behavioral Disorders

For much of the 20th century, psychology has ignored or denied the contributions that biology makes to our behavior and cognitive abilities (Pinker, 2002). A quick glance through the conference programs of many professional organizations shows one session after another addressing the (apparently newly discovered) idea that the brain is somehow related to learning and behavior. However, the idea that we can reliably design instruction to alter specific brain activities or even identify specific functions that can account for any given feat of learning or action are far from a reality (Pinker, 2002; Uttal, 2001). A better and more useful understanding for most behavior and learning considerations is that there are biologically based tendencies, such as temperament, that characterize each individual over the course of his or her life (Keogh, 2003).

Most people are able to adapt to a wide variety of activities and environments so that their biological tendencies, often referred to as temperaments, are not major constraints in their life. Some people have extreme tendencies toward characteristics, such as impulsiveness or hesitation in interpersonal situations, which render them unsuccessful at acquiring and executing behaviors that are relatively straightforward for their more adaptable peers. Others are able to acquire and exhibit the target behaviors but only with great effort, substantial support, and, often, with considerable discomfort. The relationship of one's temperament to behavior suggests that generalized behavior management principles cannot be applied uniformly across all students. While it is important to have effective schoolwide behavior management plans in operation, they will certainly require tailoring for many students (Brigham & Kauffman, 1998; see also Liaupsin, Jolivette, & Scott, Chapter 25, this volume). Considering biological temperaments can increase the likelihood that behavioral treatments will match individual needs (Keogh, 2003; McClowry, 1998; Teglasi, 1998).

In addition to these subtler implications, the evidence from psychiatric comorbidity studies discussed earlier and studies comparing psychopharmacological interventions with traditional treatments suggest that many organically based conditions such as hyperactivity should be treated psychiatrically as well as behaviorally for optimal treatment outcomes (Brigham & Cole, 1998; Forness & Kavale, 2001; Forness, Kavale, & Davanzo, 2002; Jensen et al., 2001; see also Konopasek and Forness, Chapter 18, this volume). Present policies for funding school-based treatments for students with EBD will clearly need to be redrawn if psychiatric interventions are to accompany traditional behavioral interventions. Currently, there is great reluctance among school personnel to request involvement of medical personnel. It is likely that some sort of public health care system will be required if such multimodal interventions are to be realized.

Interactions between the Individual and the Environment

It is clear that an individual's characteristics are valuable or detrimental in particular activities or occupations. For example, the quick reflexes and aggressive actions often associated with fighter pilots might often serve the pilot of a commercial passenger jet quite poorly. Selecting an environment in which one is very likely to be successful is a hallmark of mental health. Selecting environments to optimize one's abilities is called "niche-picking" (Scarr, 1981). Three current lines of research are related to the interactionist perspective.

First, students with EBD need to be supported in selecting optimal environments that allow them to exhibit their strengths and downplay their limitations. Some of the ways that this is currently being done are through teaching students to lead their own IEP meetings (Snyder, 2002; Snyder & Shapiro, 1997) and systematically providing students with EBD choices relevant to their school work (Jolivette, Wehby, Canale, & Massey, 2001).

Second, the behavioral repertoires of students whose maladaptive behaviors encompass many environments need expansion. This is probably the traditional view of behavioral intervention because, for a substantial number of students served in EBD programs, the hallmark of their disability is its pervasiveness. Ubiquity of maladaptive behavior suggests a strong biological component in a disorder and implies the need for the joint intervention of teachers and psychiatrists.

Third, we need to expand the behavioral repertoires for those students who have little or no choice in their environments. Whether we like it or not, successful psychological development and citizenship require individuals to do things that they just do not want to do or that they find highly tedious or odious. Children with restricted behavioral repertoires not only will encounter more challenges that they find distasteful but also, because of their maladaptive tendencies, be less likely to acquire the skills needed to manage the tasks they find distasteful (Keogh, 2003).

Standards-Based Reforms and Inclusion

The current push for standards-based reform appears to also be limiting the choices available to many students, thereby placing more and more students who were previously marginal members of the school community at risk for serious behavioral problems. These individuals require systematic instruction in social and behavioral skills that others acquire incidentally. The history of these interventions is mixed. However, the importance of the task compels continued research efforts. Several efforts appear to hold substantial promise in this area (Kamps, Tankersley, & Ellis, 2000; Overton, McKenzie, King, & Osborne, 2002; Serna, Lamros, Nielsen, & Forness, 2002; Serna, Nielsen, Mattern, & Forness, 2003; Walker et al., 2001).

It is ironic that, at the same time that researchers focusing on maladaptive behavior adopt a stronger interactionist perspective than has been evident in the past, the options that students have available to them in schools are shrinking (Hess & Brigham, 2001). Standards-based reforms are redefining what it means to be successful in schools and raising the criteria for success. Despite the rhetoric that *all* students can be success-

ful, there is little proof available for this statement. As the range of opportunities for students in general education programs is diminishing, the inclusion movement is forcing more and more students with disabilities into this environment. Often, the justifications for such actions are centered around increased opportunities for socialization and increased academic achievement. However, evidence suggests that students with EBD in self-contained special education programs are less alienated socially than are their peers in inclusive settings (Fulk, Brigham, & Lohman, 1998) and that students with strong academic learning needs fail to make satisfactory gains in many general education settings (Zigmond, 1996).

These trends will clearly affect the kind of research that is done for and with children and youths in schools. Whether we respond to what we have learned from our research or whether we act upon ideology in disregard of our knowledge is an open question. Regardless of the answer to that question, we will be judged on our decision by future generations.

EVALUATION VERSUS IDEOLOGY

Empirical evaluation of interventions—true experimentation—depended on the invention of statistical procedures applicable to group research designs (see Wert, Neidt, & Ahmann, 1954). The invention of single-case experimental designs (Sidman, 1960; see also Kazdin, 1978) greatly aided assays of interventions effects on individuals (see Alberto & Troutman, 2003; Jones, Dohrn, & Dunn, 2004; Kazdin, 2001; Kerr & Nelson, 2002).

From early in the 20th century until the late 1980s or early 1990s, scientific experimentation was clearly the dominant mode in the evaluation of interventions. Early intervention research in behavior disorders was based on a quantitative statistical model (e.g., Haring & Phillips, 1962; Hewett, 1968) or single-case experimental design (see research reported in the *Journal of Applied Behavior Analysis* dating from the late 1960s to the present or Alberto & Troutman, 2003; Krasner & Ullmann, 1965; Ullmann & Krasner, 1965). The general rules of scientific evidence, articulated in many other sources (e.g., Ruscio, 2002; Shermer, 1997, 2001), were thought to apply to research in special education and, more specifically, to behavior disorders (e.g., Crockett, 2001; Kauffman, 1999b, 2005a).

From the 1990s to the present, scientific views have been challenged by ideology, generally known by the term "postmodernism" but also called by a variety of other labels (see Heward, 2003; Kauffman, 2002, 2003b; Sasso, 2001). The ideology of postmodernism is difficult to describe clearly, as Kauffman (2002) points out, but it is generally the notions that objectivity is unbelievable and impossible, that truly scientific investigation is therefore impossible or irrelevant, that the scientific notions of universality and predictability have been discredited, and that subjective or "situated" knowledge should be considered superior to all other "ways of knowing" (for examples of postmodernism, see Danforth & Rhodes, 1997; Elkind, 1998; Gallagher, 2004; and Skrtic, Sailor, & Gee, 1996; for further examples and explanations of why postmodernism is unhelpful, see Kauffman, 2002; Koertge, 1998; Krueger, 2002; Locke, 2002; Mostert et al., 2003; Sasso, 2001; and Sokal & Bricmont, 1998).

In essence, the field of behavior disorders in the early 21st century is confronted by two competing notions of how truth or reliable information is obtained. The field is confronted by a stark choice: either (1) the notion that closer and closer approximations of reality or truth can be obtained through scientific means or (2) the idea that there are multiple realities or multiple truths (about any given phenomenon), such that no "way of knowing" is superior or privileged (except that, according to postmodern ideology, any way of knowing that *rejects* science as the most trustworthy route to truth is superior to scientific thinking). Some proponents of postmodernism may claim that a scientific view is not inferior but is simply no better than alternative ways of knowing, that all ideas must be treated as equal (see Danforth, 2001). Such an argument is clearly disingenuous and self-vitiating, as the person who makes such a suggestion is obviously arguing that his or her belief is superior to other beliefs about truth (see Kauffman, 2002, 2003a).

That is, the argument that all ideas are equal cannot be taken seriously, simply because the idea that all ideas are equal is obviously then asserted to be better than the idea that some ideas are better than others. The postmodern view of truth is an intellectual cul de sac from which the only possibility of exit is a reversal of argument. But some individuals have been led down this intellectual garden path without being informed by their leaders that their destination has no exit without turning 180 degrees. If these intellectual leaders are unaware of where they are going, then the old saying of "the blind leading the blind" applies. If these leaders are aware of where they are taking their followers, then we have a decidedly uncomplimentary view of their leadership.

We might suppose that some proponents of postmodernism will admit that the assertion that all ideas are equal is an intellectual cul de sac but argue that multiple subjectivities—multiple versions of truth—are superior and, therefore, must be adopted. That is, they might argue that multiple subjectivities are better than "objectivity," that "multiple truths" are more useful than a single truth about any given phenomenon (see Usher & Edwards, 1994). As one postmodernist writer put it, "Some disability studies and postmodern researchers, seeking a way out of what is seen as a simplifying binary of objectivity/subjectivity, look to avoid this dualism by assuming multiple subjectivities" (Smith, 2001, p. 384). Our conclusion is that such a view of truth opens the door to the most vicious human impulses and precludes by its very nature the achievement of social justice (see Koertge, 1996; Nanda, 1998; Shattuck, 1999). The most fundamental reason for this conclusion is that truth is then assumed to be made merely by the power of assertion or proclamation, a situation that Kauffman (2002), Sasso (2001), and Mostert et al. (2003) in special education and others in different disciplines (e.g., Koertge, 1996, 1998; Locke, 2002; Shattuck, 1999; Sokal & Bricmont, 1998) have argued is inimical to social justice and ethical conduct as well as to science.

Science looks for regularity, predictability, and universality in any phenomenon, including human behavior. Scientists look for the most parsimonious explanations of phenomena. Absolute regularity, predictability, or universality is seldom found, and scientists understand that objectivity is continuously distributed (meaning that, although absolute objectivity may be impossible, some observations are much more objective than are others). Postmodernism, however, eschews the scientific method in favor of whatever assertions an individual may make. Therefore, according to postmodern philosophy, "truth" or its approximation is not apprehended through scientific evaluation but through conformity to an ideology. From this ideological perspective, there is no need to try to assess the veracity of a report or the reliability of a finding through objective means or scientific methods; objectivity is not believable, so it cannot be used in the establishment of veracity or reliability.

In the early 21st century, many researchers in behavior disorders and other areas of special education continue to embrace scientific views of truth and reality (see Crockett, 2001; Heward, 2003). However, a significant minority of writers in behavioral disorders and related fields offer ideological, postmodern views that are inimical to scientific investigation (e.g., Brantlinger, 1997; Danforth, 2001; Danforth & Rhodes, 1997; Elkind, 1998; Gallagher, 1998, 2004; Skrtic, Sailor, & Gee, 1996; Smith, 2001). Some may argue (e.g., Brantlinger, 1997) that everyone is guided by ideology. However, this is just a sidestepping of the role of scientific evidence in judging claims about truth and decision making about intervention (see Sasso, 2001). Columnist William Raspberry quoted columnist Arianna Huffington in explaining how ideology can be recognized: "the utter refusal to allow anything as piddling as evidence to get in the way of an unshakable belief" (2003, p. A17).

THE FUTURE OF RESEARCH IN BEHAVIOR DISORDERS

Research in behavioral disorders may continue on the path of scientific discovery or be sidetracked or hijacked by ideologies. In this respect, the field of behavioral disorders is no different than other fields of study, such as psychology. As one writer noted of postmodernism, "All it can offer, by its own admission, is word games—word games that lead nowhere and achieve nothing. Like an-

thrax of the intellect, if allowed into mainstream psychology, postmodernism will poison the field" (Locke, 2002, p. 458). Sasso (2001) described postmodern ideology as a retreat from knowledge. Kauffman (2002) and Locke (2002) noted how postmodernism can poison the well of knowledge. Heward (2003), Heward and Silverstri (2005), and Mostert et al. (2003) detailed how the ideas associated with postmodernism harm the effectiveness of special education. Ideas have consequences, and the field of behavioral disorders must come to grips with the extremely negative consequences of postmodernism and related ideologies.

Progress may be possible, but so is regression. We hope that the future of research in emotional and behavioral disorders will be marked by a renewal of interest in and commitment to scientific investigation. That is the only hope we see of advancement or progress, which we believe means learning more about the nature of EBD and getting better at teaching students with such disorders (Jones et al., 2004).

SUMMARY

The development of scientific research in any field follows a predictable course. It begins with observation of difference, proceeds to more and more careful description and measurement of the difference, and, finally, experimentation and evaluation of the results. In the 19th and early 20th centuries, the field was characterized by raw description and ascientific speculation about causes and treatments. Since the 1960s, the field has been characterized by scientific study of EBD. Contemporary recognition and description include the study of definitional problems, comorbidity, and policy or legal issues. Contemporary speculation and intervention or experimentation include scientific studies of comorbidity, biological causal factors, interactions between individuals and their environments, standards-based reforms, and inclusion. Ideological approaches to the field, including postmodernism, are dangerous developments of the late 20th century. The field is now faced with a stark choice between ideologies and scientific study.

REFERENCES

Alberto, P., & Troutman, A. (2003). *Applied behavior analysis for teachers* (6th ed.). Upper Saddle River, NJ: Merrill/Prentice Hall.

American Psychiatric Association. (1994). *Diagnostic and statistical manual of mental disorders* (4th ed.). Washington, DC: Author.

Angold, A., Costello, E. J., & Erkanli, A. (1999). Comorbidity. *Journal of Child Psychology and Psychiatry, 40,* 57–87.

Baer, J. S., MacLean, M. G., & Marlatt, G. A. (1998). Linking etiology and treatment for adolescent substance abuse: Toward a better match. In R. Jessor (Ed.), *New perspectives on adolescent risk behavior* (pp. 182–220). New York: Cambridge University Press.

Berkowitz, P. H., & Rothman, E. P. (1960). *The disturbed child: Recognition and psychoeducational therapy in the classroom.* New York: New York University Press.

Bettelheim, B. (1950). *Love is not enough.* New York: Macmillan.

Bettelheim, B. (1961). The decision to fail. *School Review, 69,* 389–412.

Bettelheim, B. (1967). *The empty fortress.* New York: Free Press.

Bettelheim, B. (1970). Listening to children. In P. A. Gallagher & L. L. Edwards (Eds.), *Educating the emotionally disturbed: Theory to practice* (pp. 36–56). Lawrence: University of Kansas.

Bettelheim, B., & Sylvester, E. (1948). A therapeutic milieu. *American Journal of Orthopsychiatry, 18,* 191–206.

Biederman, J., Newcorn, J., & Sprich, S. (1991). Comorbidity of attention deficit hyperactivity disorder with conduct, depressive, anxiety, and other disorders. *American Journal of Psychiatry, 148,* 564–577.

Brantlinger, E. (1997). Using ideology: Cases of nonrecognition of the politics of research and practice in special education. *Review of Educational Research, 67,* 425–459.

Brigham, A. (1845). Schools in lunatic asylums. *American Journal of Insanity, 1,* 326–340.

Brigham, F. J., & Cole, J. E. (1998). Selective mutism: Developments in definition, etiology, assessment and treatment. In T. E. Scruggs & M. A. Mastropieri (Eds.), *Advances in learning and behavioral disabilities* (pp. 183–216). Greenwich, CT: JAI Press.

Brigham, F. J., & Kauffman, J. M. (1998). Creating supportive environments for students with emotional or behavioral disorders. *Effective School Practices, 17*(2), 23–33.

Brigham, F. J., Tochterman, S., & Brigham, M. S. P. (2001). Students with emotional and behavioral disorders and their teachers in test-linked systems of accountability. *Assessment for Effective Intervention, 26*(1), 19–27.

Carlson, P. (2003, February 25). A chilling triumph of "science" over sanity. *The Washington Post,* C1, C4.

Center, D. B. (1990). Social maladjustment: An interpretation. *Behavioral Disorders, 15,* 141–148.

Cole, C. L., & Levinson, T. R. (2002). Effects of within activity choices on the challenging behavior of children with severe developmental disabilities. *Journal of Positive Behavior Interventions, 4*(1), 29–37, 52.

Compas, B. E., Conner, J. K., & Hinden, B. R. (1998). New perspectives on depression during adolescence. In R. Jessor (Ed.), *New perspectives on adolescent risk behavior* (pp. 319–362). New York: Cambridge University Press.

Conquest, R. (2000). *Reflections on a ravaged century.* New York: Norton.

Crockett, J. B. (Ed.). (2001). The meaning of science and empirical rigor in the social sciences. *Behavioral Disorders, 27*(1) [special issue].

Crone, D. A., & Horner, R. H. (2003). *Building positive behavior support systems in schools: Functional behavioral assessment.* New York: Guilford Press.

Cullinan, D., & Epstein, M. H. (2001). Comorbidity among students with emotional disturbance. *Behavioral Disorders, 26,* 200–213.

Cullinan, D., Evans, C., Epstein, M. H., & Ryser, G. (2003). Characteristics of emotional disturbance of elementary school students. *Behavioral Disorders, 28,* 94–110.

Danforth, S. (2001). A pragmatic evaluation of three models of disability in special education. *Journal of Developmental and Physical Disabilities, 13,* 343–359.

Danforth, S., & Rhodes, W. C. (1997). Deconstructing disability: A philosophy for education. *Remedial and Special Education, 18,* 357–366.

Duncan, B. B., Forness, S. R., & Hartsough, C. (1995). Students identified as seriously emotionally disturbed in day treatment: Cognitive, psychiatric and special education characteristics. *Behavioral Disorders, 20,* 238–252.

Elkind, D. (1998). Behavioral disorders: A postmodern perspective. *Behavioral Disorders, 23,* 153–159.

Epstein, M. H. (2000). The Behavioral and Emotional Rating Scale: A strength-based approach to assessment. *Diagnostique, 25,* 249–256.

Epstein, M. H., & Sharma, J. (1998). *The Behavioral and Emotional Rating Scale: A strength-based approach to assessment.* Austin, TX: Pro-Ed.

Forness, S. R. (2003). Barriers to evidence-based treatment: Developmental psychopathology and the interdisciplinary disconnect in school mental health practice. *Journal of School Psychology, 41,* 61–67.

Forness, S. R., & Kavale, K. A. (1997). Defining emotional or behavioral disorders in school and related services. In J. W. Lloyd, E. J. Kameenui, & D. Chard (Eds.), *Issues in educating students with disabilities* (pp. 45–61). Mahwah, NJ: Erlbaum.

Forness, S. R., & Kavale, K. A. (2000). Emotional or behavioral disorders: Background and current status of the E/BD terminology and definition. *Behavioral Disorders, 25,* 264–269.

Forness, S. R., & Kavale, K. A. (2001). Ignoring the odds: Hazards of not adding the new medical model to special education decisions. *Behavioral Disorders, 26,* 269–281.

Forness, S. R., Kavale, K. A., & Davanzo, P. A. (2002). The new medical model: Interdisciplinary treatment and the limits of behaviorism. *Behavioral Disorders, 27,* 168–178.

Forness, S. R., Kavale, K. A., & Lopez, M. (1993). Conduct disorders in school: Special education eligibility and comorbidity. *Journal of Emotional and Behavioral Disorders, 1,* 101–108.

Fulk, B. M., Brigham, F. J., & Lohman, D. A. (1998). Motivation and self-regulation: A comparison of students with learning and behavior problems. *Remedial and Special Education, 19,* 300–309.

Gable, R. A. (1996). A critical analysis of functional assessment: Issues for researchers and practitioners. *Behavioral Disorders, 22,* 36–40.

Gallagher, D. J. (1998). The scientific knowledge base of special education: Do we know what we think we know? *Exceptional Children, 64,* 493–502.

Gallagher, D. J. (Ed.). (2004).*Challenging orthodoxy in special education: Dissenting voices.* Denver, CO: Love.

Gould, S. J. (2000). *The lying stones of Marrakech: Penultimate reflections on natural history.* New York: Three Rivers Press.

Greenberg, M. T., Domitrovich, C., & Bumbarger, B. (1999). *Preventing mental disorders in school-age children: A review of the effectiveness of prevention programs.* Prevention Research Center for the Promotion of Human Development: Pennsylvania State University.

Grosenick, J. K., George, M. P., & George, N. L. (1987). A profile of school programs for the behaviorally disordered: Twenty years after Morse, Cutler, and Fink. *Behavioral Disorders, 12,* 159–168.

Grosenick, J. K., George, N. L., & George, M. P. (1988). The availability of program descriptions among programs for seriously emotionally disturbed students. *Behavioral Disorders, 13,* 108–115.

Grosenick, J. K., George, N. L., George, M. P., & Lewis, T. J. (1991). Public school services for behaviorally disordered students: Program practices in the 1980s. *Behavioral Disorders, 16,* 87–96.

Gross, P. R. (1998). The Icarian impulse. *The Wilson Quarterly, 22,* 39–49.

Hare, E. H. (1962). Masturbatory insanity: The history of an idea. *Journal of Mental Science, 108,* 1–25.

Haring, N. G., & Phillips, E. L. (1962). *Educating emotionally disturbed children.* New York: McGraw-Hill.

Haring, N. G., & Phillips, E. L. (1972). *Analysis and modification of classroom behavior.* Upper Saddle River, NJ: Prentice Hall.

Haring, N. G., & Whelan, R. J. (1965). Experimental methods in education and management. In N. J. Long, W. C. Morse, & R. G. Newman (Eds.), *Conflict in the classroom* (pp. 389–405). Belmont, CA: Wadsworth.

Hess, F. M., & Brigham, F. J. (2001). How federal special education policy affects schooling in Virginia. In C. E. Finn Jr., A. J. Rotherham & C. R. Hokanson Jr. (Eds.), *Rethinking special education for a new century* (pp. 161–182). Washington, DC: Thomas B. Fordham Foundation and Progressive Policy Institute.

Hester, P. P., & Kaiser, A. P. (1998). Early intervention for the prevention of conduct disorder: Research issues in early identification, implementation, and interpretation of treatment outcome. *Behavioral Disorders, 24,* 57–65.

Heward, W. L. (2003). Ten faulty notions about teaching and learning that hinder the effectiveness of special education. *The Journal of Special Education, 36,* 186–205.

Heward, W. L., & Silvestri, S. M. (2005). The neutralization of special education. In J. W. Jacobson, J. A. Mulick, & R. M. Foxx (Eds.), *Fads: Dubious and improbable treatments for developmental disabilities.* Mahwah, NJ: Erlbaum.

Hewett, F. M. (1964). Teaching reading to an autistic boy through operant conditioning. *Reading Teacher, 18,* 613–618.

Hewett, F. M. (1965). Teaching speech to an autistic boy through operant conditioning. *American Journal of Orthopsychiatry, 35,* 927–936.

Hewett, F. M. (1967). Educational engineering with emotionally disturbed children. *Exceptional Children, 33,* 459–471.

Hewett, F. M. (1968). *The emotionally disturbed child in the classroom.* Boston: Allyn & Bacon.

Jarvis, E. (1852). On the supposed increase of insanity. *American Journal of Insanity, 8,* 333–364.

Jensen, P. S., Hinshaw, S. P., Kraemer, H. C., Lenora, N., Newcorn, J. H., Abikoff, H. B., et al. (2001). ADHD comorbidity findings from the MTA study: Comparing comorbid subgroups. *Journal of the American Academy of Child and Adolescent Psychiatry, 40,* 147–158.

Jolivette, K., Wehby, J. H., Canale, J., & Massey, N. (2001). Effect of choice-making opportunities on the behavior of students with emotional and behavioral disorders. *Behavioral Disorders, 26,* 131–145.

Jones, V., Dohrn, E., & Dunn, C. (2004). *Creating effective programs for students with emotional and behavioral disorders.* Boston: Allyn & Bacon.

Kamps, D. M., Tankersley, M., & Ellis, C. (2000). Social skills interventions for young at-risk students: A 2-year follow-up study. *Behavioral Disorders, 25,* 310–324.

Kanner, L. (1973). The birth of early infantile autism. *Journal of Autism and Childhood Schizophrenia, 3,* 93–95.

Kauffman, J. M. (1976). Nineteenth century views of

children's behavior disorders: Historical contributions and continuing issues. *Journal of Special Education, 10,* 335–349.

Kauffman, J. M. (1999a). How we prevent the prevention of emotional and behavioral disorders. *Exceptional Children, 65,* 448–469.

Kauffman, J. M. (1999b). The role of science in behavioral disorders. *Behavioral Disorders, 24,* 265–272.

Kauffman, J. M. (2001). *Characteristics of emotional and behavioral disorders of children and youth* (7th ed.). Upper Saddle River, NJ: Prentice Hall.

Kauffman, J. M. (2002). *Education deform: Bright people sometimes say stupid things about education.* Lahnam, MD: Scarecrow Education.

Kauffman, J. M. (2003a). Appearances, stigma, and prevention. *Remedial and Special Education, 24,* 195–198.

Kauffman, J. M. (2003b). Reflections on the field. *Behavioral Disorders, 28,* 205–208.

Kauffman, J. M. (2005a). *Characteristics of emotional and behavioral disorders of children and youth* (8th ed.). Upper Saddle River, NJ: Prentice Hall.

Kauffman, J. M. (2005b). How we prevent the prevention of emotional and behavioral difficulties in education. In P. Clough, P. Garner, J. T. Pardeck, & F. K. O. Yuen (Eds.), *Handbook of emotional and behavioral difficulties in education* (pp. 366–376). London: Sage.

Kauffman, J. M. (in press). The president's commission and the devaluation of special education. *Education and Treatment of Children.*

Kauffman, J. M., & Landrum, T. J. (in press). *Children and youth with emotional and behavioral disorders: A brief history of their education.* Austin, TX: Pro-Ed.

Kazdin, A. E. (1978). *History of behavior modification: Experimental foundations of contemporary research.* Baltimore: University Park Press.

Kazdin, A. E. (2001). *Behavior modification in applied settings* (6th ed.). Belmont, CA: Wadsworth.

Keogh, B. K. (2003). *Temperament in the classroom: Understanding individual differences.* Baltimore: Brookes.

Kerr, M. M., & Nelson, C. M. (2002). *Strategies for addressing behavior problems in the classroom* (4th ed.). Upper Saddle River, NJ: Prentice Hall.

Koertge, N. (1996). Feminist epistemology: Stalking an un-dead horse. In P. R. Gross, N. Levitt, & M. W. Lewis (Eds.), *The flight from science and reason* (pp. 413–419). Baltimore: The Johns Hopkins University Press.

Koertge, N. (Ed.). (1998). *A house built on sand: Exposing postmodernist myths about science.* New York: Oxford University Press.

Krasner, L., & Ullmann, L. P. (Eds.). (1965). *Research in behavior modification: New developments and implications.* New York: Holt.

Krueger, J. I. (2002). Postmodern parlor games. *American Psychologist, 57,* 461–462.

Lambros, K. M., Ward, S. L., Bocian, K. M., MacMillan, D. L., & Gresham, F. M. (1998). Behavioral profiles of children at-risk for emotional and behavioral disorders: Implications for assessment and classification. *Focus on Exceptional Children, 30*(5), 1–16.

Landrum, T. J. (2001). Assessment for eligibility: Issues in identifying students with emotional or behavioral disorders. *Assessment for Effective Intervention, 26*(1), 41–49.

Locke, E. A. (2002). The dead end of postmodernism. *American Psychologist, 57,* 458.

Loeber, R., Farrington, D. P., Stouthamer-Loeber, M., & Van Kammen, W. B. (1998). Multiple risk factors for multiproblem boys: Co-occurrence of delinquency, substance abuse, attention deficit, conduct problems, physical aggression, covert behavior, depressed mood, and shy/withdrawn behavior. In R. Jessor (Ed.), *New perspectives on adolescent risk behavior* (pp. 90–149). New York: Cambridge University Press.

Martens, E. H., & Russ, H. (1932). *Adjustment of behavior problems of school children: A description and evaluation of the clinical program in Berkeley, Calif.* Washington, DC: U.S. Government Printing Office.

McClowry, S. G. (1998). The science and art of using temperament as the basis for intervention. *School Psychology Review, 27,* 551–563.

McConaughy, S. (2000). Self-report: Child clinical interviews. In T. R. Kratochwill & E. S. Shapiro (Eds.), *Conducting school-based assessments of child and adolescent behavior* (pp. 170–202). New York: Guilford Press.

Morse, W. C., Cutler, R. L., & Fink, A. H. (1964). *Public school classes for the emotionally handicapped: A research analysis.* Washington, DC: Council for Exceptional Children.

Mostert, M. P., Kauffman, J. M., & Kavale, K. A. (2003). Truth and consequences. *Behavioral Disorders, 28,* 333–347.

Nanda, M. (1998). The epistemic charity of the social constructivist critics of science and why the third world should refuse the offer. In N. Koertge (Ed.), *A house built on sand: Exposing postmodernist myths about science* (pp. 286–311). New York: Oxford University Press.

National Research Council. (2001). *Educating children with autism.* Washington, DC: National Academy Press.

Overton, S., McKenzie, L., King, K., & Osborne, J. (2002). Replication of the First Step to Success model: A multiple-case study of implementation effectiveness. *Behavioral Disorders, 28,* 40–56.

Pinker, S. (2002). *The blank slate: The modern denial of human nature.* New York: Viking.

Polsgrove, L., & Ochoa, T. (2004). Trends and issues in behavioral interventions. In A. D. McCray, H. J. Rieth, & P. T. Sindelar (Eds.), *Current and emerging issues in special education* (pp. 154–179). Boston: Allyn & Bacon.

Raspberry, W. (2003, June 2). Struck dumb? *Washington Post*, A17.

Redl F., & Wineman, D. (1951). *Children who hate.* New York: Free Press.

Redl, F., & Wineman, D. (1952). *Controls from within.* New York: Free Press.

Repp, A. C., & Horner, R. H. (1999). *Functional analysis of problem behavior: From effective assessment to effective support.* Belmont, CA: Wadsworth.

Rhodes, W. C., & Head, S. (Eds.). (1974). *A study of child variance: Vol. 3. Service delivery systems.* Ann Arbor: University of Michigan.

Rhodes, W. C., & Tracy, M. L. (Eds.). (1972a). *A study of child variance: Vol. 1. Theories.* Ann Arbor: University of Michigan.

Rhodes, W. C., & Tracy, M. L. (Eds.). (1972b). *A study of child variance: Vol. 2. Interventions.* Ann Arbor: University of Michigan.

Rie, H. E. (1971). Historical perspective of concepts of child psychopathology. In H. E. Rie (Ed.), *Perspectives in child psychopathology.* Chicago: Aldine Atherton.

Ruscio, J. (2002). *Clear thinking with psychology: Separating sense from nonsense.* Pacific Grove, CA: Wadsworth.

Sasso, G. M. (2001). The retreat from inquiry and knowledge in special education. *The Journal of Special Education, 34,* 178–193.

Sasso, G. M., Conroy, M. A., Stichter, J. P., & Fox, J. J. (2001). Slowing down the bandwagon: The misapplication of functional assessment for students with emotional or behavioral disorders. *Behavioral Disorders, 26,* 282–296.

Scarr, S. (1981). Testing for children: Assessment and the many determinants of intellectual competence. *American Psychologist, 36,* 1159–1166.

Serna, L. A., Lamros, K., Nielsen, E., & Forness, S. R. (2002). Head Start children at risk for emotional or behavioral disorders: Behavior profiles and clinical implications of a primary prevention program. *Behavioral Disorders, 27,* 137–141.

Serna, L. A., Nielsen, E., Mattern, N., & Forness, S. R. (2003). Primary prevention in mental health for Head Start classrooms: Partial replication with teachers as interveners. *Behavioral Disorders, 28,* 124–129.

Shattuck, R. (1999). *Candor and perversion: Literature, education, and the arts.* New York: Norton.

Shermer, M. (1997). *Why people believe weird things: Pseudoscience, superstition, and other confusions of our time.* New York: W. H. Freeman.

Shermer, M. (2001). *The borderlands of science: Where sense meets nonsense.* New York: Oxford University Press.

Sidman, M. (1960). *Tactics of scientific research: Evaluating experimental data in psychology.* New York: Basic Books.

Skrtic, T. M., Sailor, W., & Gee, K. (1996). Voice, collaboration, and inclusion: Democratic themes in educational and social reform. *Remedial and Special Education, 17,* 142–157.

Smith, P. (2001). Inquiry cantos: Poetics of developmental disability. *Mental Retardation, 39,* 379–390.

Snyder, E. P. (2002). Teaching students with combined behavioral disorders and mental retardation to lead their own IEP meetings. *Behavioral Disorders, 27,* 340–357.

Snyder, E. P., & Shapiro, E. S. (1997). Teaching students with emotional/behavioral disorders the skills to participate in the development of their own IEPs. *Behavioral Disorders, 22,* 246–259.

Sobel, D. (1999). *Galileo's daughter: A historical memoir of science, faith, and love.* New York: Penguin.

Sokal, A., & Bricmont, J. (1998). *Fashionable nonsense: Postmodern intellectuals' abuse of science.* New York: Picador.

Strauss, A. A., & Lehtinen, L. E. (1947). *Psychopathology and education of the brain injured child.* New York: Grune & Stratton.

Stribling, F. T. (1842). Physician and superintendent's report. In *Annual Reports to the Court of Directors of the Western Lunatic Asylum to the Legislature of Virginia* (pp. 1–70). Richmond: Shepherd & Conlin.

Tankersley, M., & Landrum, T. J. (1997). Comorbidity of emotional and behavioral disorders. In J. W. Lloyd, E. J. Kameenui, & D. Chard (Eds.), *Issues in educating students with disabilities* (pp. 153–173). Mahwah, NJ: Erlbaum.

Teglasi, H. (1998). Temperament constructs and measures. *School Psychology Review, 27,* 564–585.

Ullmann, L. P., & Krasner, L. (Eds.). (1965). *Case studies in behavior modification.* New York: Holt.

U.S. Department of Education (2000). *Twenty-second annual report to Congress on the implementation of the Individuals with Disabilities Education Act.* Washington, DC: Author.

U.S. Department of Health and Human Services. (2001). *Report of the Surgeon General's conference on children's mental health: A national action agenda.* Washington, DC: Author.

Usher, R., & Edwards, R. (1994). *Postmodernism and education: Different voices, different words.* London: Routledge.

Uttal, W. R. (2001). *The new phrenology: The limits of localizing cognitive processes in the brain.* Cambridge, MA: MIT Press.

Vaughn, S., & Dammann, J. E. (2001). Science and sanity in special education. *Behavioral Disorders, 27,* 21–29.

Verhulst, F. C., & Van der Ende, J. (1993). "Comorbidity" in an epidemiological sample: A longitudinal perspective. *Journal of Child Psychology and Psychiatry, 34,* 767–783.

Waldman, I. D., Rhee, S. H., Levy, F., & Hay, D. A. (2001). Causes of the overlap among symptoms of attention deficit hyperactivity disorder, oppositional defiant disorder, and conduct disorder. In F. Levy & D. A. Hay (Eds.), *Attention, genes and ADHD* (pp. 115–138). Philadelphia, PA: Taylor & Francis.

Walker, H. M., Kavanagh, K., Stiller, B., Golly, A., Severson, H. H., & Feil, E. G. (2001). First Step to Success: An early intervention approach for preventing school antisocial behavior. In H. M. Walker & M. H. Epstein (Eds.), *Making schools safer and violence free: Critical issues, solutions, and recommended practices* (pp. 73–87). Austin, TX: Pro-Ed.

Walker, H. M., Nishioka, V. M., Zeller, R., Severson, H. H., & Feil, E. G. (2000). Causal factors and potential solutions for the persistent underidentification of students having emotional or behavioral disorders in the context of schooling. *Assessment for Effective Intervention, 26*(1), 29–39.

Walker, H. M., Ramsey, E., & Gresham, F. M. (2004). *Antisocial behavior in school: Strategies and best practices* (2nd ed.). Pacific Grove, CA: Brooks/Cole.

Walker, H. M., Stiller, B., Severson, H. H., Feil, E. G., & Golly, A. (1998). First step to success: Intervening at the point of school entry to prevent antisocial behavior patterns. *Psychology in the Schools, 35,* 259–269.

Washington Post. (2003, May 30). Editorial: Report cards due. A22

Wert, J. E., Neidt, C. O., & Ahmann, J. S. (1954). *Statistical methods in educational and psychological research.* New York: Appleton-Century-Crofts.

Winchester, S. (2001). *The map that changed the world: William Smith and the birth of modern geology.* New York: HarperCollins.

Yell, M. L., & Dragsow, E. (2000). Legal requirements for assessing students with emotional and behavioral disorders. *Assessment for Effective Intervention, 26*(1), 5–17.

Yell, M. L., & Dragsow, E. (2005). *No child left behind: A guide for professionals.* Upper Saddle River, NJ: Merrill Prentice Hall.

Zigler, E., Taussig, C., & Black, Y. (1992). Early childhood intervention: A promising preventative for juvenile delinquency. *American Psychologist, 47,* 997–1006.

Zigmond, N. (1996). Organization and management of general education classrooms. In D. L. Speece & B. K. Keogh (Eds.), *Research on classroom ecologies: Implications for inclusion of children with learning disabilities* (pp. 163–190). Mahwah, NJ: Erlbaum.

3

Classification and Definition of Emotional and Behavioral Disorders

DOUGLAS CULLINAN

Classification and definition are significant and interesting because they involve nearly all the other topics in the field of education for students with emotional and behavioral disorders (EBD). Any examination of classification or definition naturally brings up characteristics, because behaviors, emotions, and cognitions constitute the main phenomena addressed by widely used classification systems and definitions. This chapter discusses classification and definition, then suggests a way to measure important aspects of definition, including characteristics. Some significant research needs are noted in these discussions.

CLASSIFICATION

To classify is to group phenomena according to their similarities and differences. As more phenomena are observed, they may be judged similar to an existing group, or different, thus becoming the first case in a new group. Classification is a natural human activity; from early childhood we classify items and ideas. In many fields of study, advances in knowledge have depended on suitable classification of the phenomena under consideration. By analogy, in order to achieve substantial understanding in our field, we need to know how EBD of children should be classified.

Unusual and maladaptive human behaviors, emotions, and cognitions have been described and classified in various ways for thousands of years (Adams, Luscher, & Bernat, 2001). Some early classification efforts encompassed EBD such as anxiety, mania, and melancholia that resemble those seen today (Bogenshutz & Nurnberg, 2000; Segal & Coolidge, 2001). In the United States, classification systems were developed in the late 19th and early 20th centuries to survey the scope of "mental illnesses" among residents of institutions for people with EBD (American Psychiatric Association, 2000). Work on classification, including substantial attention to EBD of children, has expanded since the mid-20th century in response to observations of clinicians and other service providers, changes in theories, findings of scientific research, and other influences (Cullinan, 2002; Scotti & Morris, 2000).

Purposes of Classification

A valid classification system can serve several worthwhile purposes (Adams et al., 2001; Leckliter & Matarazzo, 1994; Mash & Wolfe, 2002; Quay, 1986; Scotti & Morris, 2000). First, it provides a consistent set of terms for communication among practitioners, researchers, policymakers, and others working in a field, increasing the chance for sharing reliable information across disciplines and points of view.

Second, good classification makes it easier to organize diverse information about EBD. The prevalence of an EBD, its demographic, biological, and psychosocial correlates, and its short- and long-term outcomes all can be clues to understanding causes and improving interventions. Categories of EBD may be distinct as to prevalence, correlates, and outcomes. Associations among these variables (e.g., whether prevalence varies according to age of child or disciplinary style of parents) can be particularly suggestive of possible causes and interventions. Classification facilitates the organization, storing, and retrieval of such key information about EBD.

Third, classification may enhance predictability of events. Outcome and intervention research may enable us to forecast various possible futures for people who evidence a particular kind of EBD, including futures modified by different interventions. Further, if we assume that no particular intervention is best for *all* instances of EBD, an important potential function of classification is to permit matching different kinds of EBD to different appropriate interventions.

To illustrate, suppose there is a simple classification system that reliably identifies three kinds of EBD of children—e.g., "Green," "Orange," and "Purple." Further, suppose research has demonstrated that children with the Green disorder return to normal functioning within a short period of time whether or not they receive intervention; that children with Orange continue to show EBD unless they receive highly structured behavior management and remedial academic intervention; and that children with the Purple kind of EBD continue to exhibit maladaptive functioning unless they receive intensive training in social skills and cognitive problem solving. To use this classification system, a practitioner would assess emotional and behavioral problems and other relevant variables about a child with maladaptive functioning. Assessment results would enable the practitioner to classify the kind of EBD involved, which in turn would indicate the preferred action to help the child return to adaptive functioning.

A fourth use of classification is to help establish a logical basis for administering services to children with EBD, including eligibility, reimbursement, and appropriate education. In the imaginary classification system above, it would be logical to direct few resources toward children classified as Green but many toward those classified as Orange and Purple. Also, we should provide certain kinds of resources to the Oranges but different kinds to the Purples.

A classification system as prognostic as the Green–Orange–Purple one is not available at present for EBD (of children or adults). Even if it were, the illustration would be an oversimplification, because each specific instance of EBD, even those within a single category, presents individualistic features (e.g., of the child, educator, education environment, and intervention feasibility); and such features might influence selection of an intervention or how it is delivered. Still, keeping this ideal classification system in mind can help clarify strengths and weaknesses of existing systems and suggest directions for research toward better ones.

Existing Classification Systems

The potential payoff of a good classification system for EBD has led to the development of a wide range of possibilities (Adams et al., 2001; Bandura, 1968; Bogenshutz & Nurnberg, 2000; Group for the Advancement of Psychiatry, 1974; Phillips, Draguns, & Bartlett, 1975; Quay, 1986; Scotti, Morris, McNeil, & Hawkins, 1996). Some classification systems have been based on a particular theory of EBD, but the most widely used ones now are fairly compatible with different theories. Their main components are nearly neutral descriptions of maladaptive and distressing behaviors, emotions, and thoughts.

The two main kinds of classification systems—disease classification and dimensional classification—stem from different perspectives about the nature of EBD. In the first perspective, an EBD is a collection of maladaptive and distressing behaviors, emotions, and thoughts that is qualitatively different from normality. Just as a person either does or does not have a particular disease, he either does or does not have a particular EBD. The disease perspective guided the creation of the most influential classification system for EBD (child and adult) in the United States and Canada, the *Diagnostic and Statistical Manual of Mental Disorders* (DSM; American Psychiatric Association, 1952, 2000).

A second perspective assumes that an EBD is a collection of problems involving behaviors, emotions, and thoughts that all people experience to some extent. Those who experience the problems to an extreme extent (unusual frequency, duration, intensity, or other aspect) are more likely to have an EBD. Among the several dimensional classification systems for EBD of children, the *Achenbach System of Empirically Based Assessment* (ASEBA; Achenbach, 1998, 2000; Achenbach & McConaughy, 1997; Achenbach & Rescorla, 2001) is in widest use and has generated the most research.

Disease Perspective

DSM was created in the mid-20th century, mainly by psychiatric authorities for fellow psychiatrists, as a modified system for classifying diseases (American Psychiatric Association, 1952). The creators of DSM saw important parallels between EBD and diseases. In general and simplified terms, a *disease* is an important health abnormality involving a syndrome, course, and etiology (Abrams, 1992; Bogenschutz & Nurnberg, 2000).

Any health abnormality is associated with subjective "symptoms" (experienced and reported by the person) and/or objective "signs" (measurable changes in body structure and function). A collection of co-occurring symptoms and signs is called a *syndrome*.

Syndromes generally change over time, in various ways. There are short- and long-term changes in overall status (e.g., decline in health to an enduring poor outcome; decline followed by return to good health; alternating periods of decline and improvement). Also, different parts of a syndrome do not necessarily change in unison (e.g., a person may report distressing symptoms before laboratory tests find any abnormal signs, or vice versa). A syndrome whose time-related changes are well known is said to have a *course*.

Evidence about heredity, abnormalities of biological structure and function, harmful aspects of the physical or social environment, and other phenomena may reveal how the health problem began and/or is maintained (its *etiology*). When a health abnormality syndrome has an established course and etiology, it qualifies as a disease.

Some EBD undoubtedly are diseases (e.g., Charney et al., 2002), but few authorities would claim that all of them are. A half-century ago, however, psychodynamic theories about EBD constituted a strong influence on psychiatric thinking. As a result, intrapsychic conflicts were readily available to serve as proposed etiologies of mental disorders for which no traditional disease-producing causes were known.

Both the disease analogy and psychodynamic theories support the idea that an EBD is a dysfunction located mainly within the person. External situational influences that might contribute to, maintain, or reduce EBD were given little consideration in early versions of DSM and remain only modestly emphasized in the current DSM (Scotti & Morris, 2000).

Mental disorder as disease, psychodynamic perspective, and intrapersonal location of EBD—these three elements have retained influence over several revisions of DSM. For example, (1) one goal in the design of DSM-IV was that its categories correspond to the International Classification of Diseases (Bogenschutz & Nurnberg, 2000). Some disease-oriented vocabulary and concepts (e.g., symptoms, course) were retained in revisions of DSM. (2) A psychodynamically oriented user may choose to code various defense mechanisms on which the client appears to be relying (American Psychiatric Association, 2000). (3) DSM continues to emphasize intrapersonal determinants of mental disorders, correspondingly putting less emphasis on context and situational factors (Scotti & Morris, 2000). This may be particularly relevant to EBD of children, in which context and situational aspects seem especially strong (e.g., often involve a family context, vary greatly across home, school, community, and other situations).

While DSM has preserved key original concepts, it also has evolved extensively, especially since about 1980. Changes in theories, feedback from clinical users, results of scientific research, and other influences have produced DSM modifications generally seen as improvements (Adams et al., 2001; Scotti

& Morris, 2000; U.S. Department of Health and Human Services, 1999). The current version reflects significant input from fields other than psychiatry, and it is used by a range of mental health professionals. There are far fewer psychodynamic suppositions about EBD but more theory-neutral descriptions of disorders, including some fairly specific criteria. This has yielded, for some DSM categories, greater consistency across diagnosticians. DSM now encourages users to clearly separate descriptions of the disorders from suspected medical and psychological etiologies and treatment considerations. Recent versions of DSM have given significant coverage to EBD of children and adolescents, generally reflecting scientific research in this area.

DSM-IV-TR. The current version, DSM-IV-TR (American Psychiatric Association, 2000), provides an update of DSM-IV (American Psychiatric Association, 1994) including information about some categories based on recent literature ("TR" stands for "text revision"). However, it did not materially change the DSM-IV approach to classification. DSM-IV calls for assessor judgments about five kinds of classification and other information, called "axes." Axis I and Axis II are used to designate one or more of about 400 categories of mental disorder and other phenomena (e.g., V["vee"]-code conditions that, although not qualifying as mental disorders, are significant problems needing intervention). Table 3.1 lists one group of DSM-IV mental disorders reserved for children and adolescents, plus a selection of other mental disorders that under some circumstances can be applied to children and adolescents. Note that the DSM concept of mental disorder includes problems that are not generally considered EBD (e.g., mental retardation).

Axis III is used for indicating the client's medical conditions that may have been a cause, complication, or consequence of the identified mental disorder or may affect its treatment. On Axis IV the assessor notes psychosocial and environmental stressors (e.g., economic, educational, social support problems) that may have caused or exacerbated the mental disorder. Finally, the assessor rates on Axis V the quality of the client's overall life functioning at the time of assess-

ment and/or in the recent past. This suggests, among other things, the client's present degree of impairment.

Proponents are confident that DSM-IV remedies many shortcomings of earlier DSMs and constitutes a useful classification system (Adams et al., 2001; Bogenschutz & Nurnberg, 2000). However, both proponents and critics recognize that important problems remain (Achenbach, 1998, 2000; Adams et al., 2001; Beutler & Malik, 2002; Doucette, 2002; Mash & Wolfe, 2002; Pine et al., 2002; Rounsaville et al., 2002; Scotti & Morris, 2000; Segal & Coolidge, 2001), specifically with DSM-IV and generally with the disease analogy as a basis for classification of EBD. Among these problems are improving the definition of mental disorder, evaluating the applicability of the disease model to various kinds of EBD, taking account of cross-cultural similarities and differences for many mental disorders, exploring the appropriateness of DSM categories for children of different ages, and studying the validity of each category in predicting improvement under different interventions. Preliminary study is under way for the next revision, DSM-V, to appear about 2010 (Kupfer & First, 2002).

Many mental health agencies, government organizations, insurance companies, medical providers, and other agents that powerfully shape our society's concepts about and services for EBD of young people consider DSM the only official classification system (Bogenschutz & Nurnberg, 2000). Often, services and reimbursements are contingent on the child or adolescent receiving a DSM diagnosis. A DSM diagnosis and related information are sometimes found in a student's school record or presented at a multidisciplinary team meeting, and various sources suggest ways to use DSM information in addressing emotional and behavioral problems of students (e.g., House, 1999). For the foregoing and other reasons, educators of students with EBD should have some knowledge of DSM-IV.

Dimensional Perspective

Dimensional (also called "empirical") classification is compatible with the viewpoint that EBD are extreme forms of ordinary behavior and emotional problems rather

TABLE 3.1. Selected DSM-IV-TR Categories and Subcategories That Can Be Applied to Children

---

Disorders Usually First Diagnosed in Infancy, Childhood, or Adolescence

Mental retardation
Learning disorders (e.g., reading, written expression)
Communication disorders
Pervasive developmental disorders (e.g., autistic disorder, Asperger's disorder)
Attention-deficit and disruptive behavior disorders (e.g., ADHD—hyperactive-impulsive
    type, ADHD—inattentive type, conduct disorder, oppositional defiant disorder)
Tic disorders (e.g., Tourette's disorder)
Elimination disorders (e.g., enuresis)
Other disorders of infancy, childhood, or adolescence (e.g., separation anxiety disorder)

Other Disorders That May Be Diagnosed among Children and Adolescents

Cognitive disorders (e.g., delirium due to head trauma)
Substance-related disorders
Psychotic disorders (e.g., schizophrenia, schizoaffective disorder)
Mood disorders (e.g., depressive disorders, bipolar disorders)
Eating disorders (e.g., anorexia nervosa)
Anxiety disorders (e.g., obsessive–compulsive disorder, posttraumatic stress disorder)
Adjustment disorders (e.g., AD with depressed mood, AD with disturbance of conduct)

V-Codes

(e.g., child or adolescent antisocial behavior, identity problem)

---

than extraordinary conditions that are different in kind from normality. Therefore, any category of EBD can be represented by some collection of problems of behavior, emotion, and thought (for brevity, "behavior problems") that tend to co-occur. In principle, no consideration is given to predictions of any theory or other preconceptions about what categories of EBD ought to be expected. Instead, identifying dimensional categories amounts to searching for groups of problems such that if a person has one of the problems he or she probably has many or even all of the other problems as well.

The first step in developing a dimensional classification system for EBD of children might be to create a large pool of items, each of which states a different measurable behavior problem that might be experienced by children. Readily measured variables other than problems could also be in the pool, although this has not ordinarily been done. Second, the investigator identifies a large group of children to be studied. To find dimensions of EBD it is generally logical to study a group of children independently identified as evidencing EBD.

Third, each child in the group is measured on every problem. Measurement can be accomplished by a variety of methods. With large samples and many behavior problems, it is often most feasible to measure via item ratings completed by someone who knows the child well (e.g., parent, teacher, peer, or the child himself).

Fourth, the resulting data on many problems of many children are examined to locate collections of items that covary, that is, tend to be scored similarly to other items within the collection but not similarly to items outside of the collection. This step is best done using computer-facilitated multivariate statistical techniques such as factor analysis. A statistically identified collection of covarying problems is called a factor or dimension. Typically, factor analysis identifies more than one dimension, each being a different collection of covarying behavior problems.

A dimension represents something in common among the individual problem items in that collection, which they do not have in common with items that are not in that collection. The "something in common" can reasonably be considered a form or category of EBD. Thus, the several dimensions in the system are each separate categories of EBD. Each dimension's name is intended to describe the essence of what is similar among many or all of its items. For instance, a dimension composed of the four problems "worries about minor things," "upset by changes," "doesn't make eye contact," and "emphasizes his or her own shortcomings" could be named "Insecure" or something similar.

Once the dimensions have been derived, this system can be used to classify behavior problems of children who did not participate in its creation. This is because each dimension is composed of scored problem items. A new child is measured on all problem items, then the scores for each item in the first dimension are combined (e.g., summed) to produce a "dimension 1" score. Next, scores for each item in the second dimension are combined to produce a "dimension 2" score, and so on until a score is computed for every dimension in the classification system.

On each dimension, some children will have a very low dimension score (i.e., low ratings on most or all problems in the dimension), some will have a moderate score, and some will have a very high score (high ratings on most or all of the problems). To help decide how high a score must be to suggest EBD, the developer can create norms for each dimension by applying the classification system to a large representative group of children. Such norms give context to the dimension scores by indicating which scores correspond to different degrees of extreme functioning (e.g., the 84th, 99th, or some other percentile of the norm group).

The fairly objective dimensional classification process becomes subjective at this point, because selecting a "cutoff point"—the percentile at which functioning should be considered "too extreme"—is largely arbitrary. In fact, different dimensional systems recommend somewhat different cutoff points. Cutoff point selection brings up a validity issue noted later.

ASEBA. The Achenbach System of Empirically Based Assessment first appeared in the early 1980s, based on prior research by Achenbach and others. It has evolved as a result of considerable research and clinical practice considerations (Achenbach, 1995, 1998, 2000; Achenbach & McConaughy, 1997; Achenbach & Rescorla, 2001). In a review of existing dimensional classification studies of EBD of children and adolescents, Achenbach & Edelbrock (1978) found about 20 different multivariate dimensions. Many of them appeared to apply mainly to a particular age or sex of child, or source of information (teacher, parent, or child perspective) (see also Achenbach, McConaughy, & Howell, 1987).

One goal of Achenbach and his colleagues was to develop a system involving a smaller number of dimensions that generally apply across ages, sexes, and informant perspectives (Achenbach, 1995; Achenbach & McConaughy, 1997). To this end they created the *Teacher's Report Form* to capture the teacher's perspective, *Child Behavior Checklist* for parent perspectives, and *Youth Self-Report* and *Semistructured Clinical Interview for Children and Adolescents* for the child's perspective (Achenbach & Rescorla, 2001; McConaughy & Achenbach, 2001). ASEBA also encompasses other forms of measurement. Data from the different informant perspectives can be combined to generate eight dimensional categories of EBD, which Achenbach calls *cross-informant syndromes* (see Table 3.2).

Using statistical and other methods it is possible to further organize the cross-informant syndromes. Two syndromes, Rule-Breaking Behavior and Aggressive Behavior, fall into a higher-order grouping Achenbach calls Externalizing. Anxious/Depressed, Withdrawn/Depressed, and Somatic Complaints syndromes fall into a grouping called Internalizing. The remaining three cross-informant syndromes—Social Problems, Thought Problems, and Attention Problems—are not grouped because they did not show statistical alignment with either Externalizing or Internalizing, or with each other (Achenbach & Rescorla, 2001).

In the ASEBA system, if a child's score on a cross-informant syndrome is above the 97th percentile of the norm group, that score is designated "clinical range," that is, of strong concern. A score below the 97th percentile but above the 93rd percentile is designated "borderline range" (of some con-

TABLE 3.2. Illustrative Emotional and Behavior Problem Items of ASEBA Cross-Informant Syndromes

Rule-Breaking Behavior	Aggressive Behavior	
Bad companions	Destroys others' property	
Lacks guilt for misbehavior	Disobedient at school	
Lying, cheating	Fights	
Steals outside home	Threatens people	

Anxious/Depressed	Withdrawn/Depressed	Somatic Complaints
Cries a lot	Enjoys very little	Dizzy
Feels worthless	Keeps things to self	Headaches
Talks about killing self	Unhappy, sad, depressed	Nausea
Too fearful or anxious	Withdrawn, not involved	Overly tired

Social Problems	Thought Problems	Attention Problems
Complains of loneliness	Can't get mind off thoughts	Can't concentrate
Feels others mistreat her/him	Hears things	Can't sit still
Jealous of peers	Strange behavior	Impulsive
Not liked by peers	Strange ideas	Poor school work

Note. Problems listed portray the essence of items concisely. For full wording of items and listings of all problem items by syndrome, see Achenbach and Rescorla (2001).

cern). Scores below the 93rd percentile are in the normal range. If corroborated by other assessment evidence, an ASEBA finding of clinical or even borderline may indicate that the child needs to be identified as EBD and receive appropriate services. Achenbach and McConaughy (2003) and McConaughy and Achenbach (2001) describe how the ASEBA may be used to address emotional and behavioral problems of students, including those who may qualify for special education according to the Individuals with Disabilities Education Act (IDEA).

Evaluating Classification

Judging the merits of classifying EBD involves important philosophical and technical issues (see, e.g., Achenbach, 1995, 1998, 2000; Adams et al., 2001; Beutler & Malik, 2002; Bogenschutz & Nurnberg, 2000; Kupfer & First, 2002; Leckliter & Matarazzo, 1994; Mash & Wolfe, 2002; Quay, 1986; Scotti & Morris, 2000; Segal & Coolidge, 2001; Wicks-Nelson & Israel, 2000). Among the philosophical issues are criticisms of the logic of classifying EBD and some undesirable results of classifying. Technical issues are too numerous and complex to cover here, but some brief comments below address reliability and validity of categories, and usability of a classification system.

Philosophical Issues

Impossible goal. To state the obvious, classification assumes that there are multiple kinds of EBD. However, some authorities have indicated that classification of EBD is an unlikely or even hopeless pursuit because categories of EBD do not actually exist (Lamiell, 1997; Rogers, 1951). Menninger (1963) embraced the position that there is really only one kind of EBD. The illusion of different kinds of EBD is created by variations in severity and diverse individual life circumstances. Szasz (1960) held that each case of what professionals call EBD is actually a "problem of living" that all people face. Just as each person is unique, each problem of living is as well, and because it makes no sense to classify unique phenomena, there can be no categories of EBD.

Even if such reservations about classification are not correct, they remind us that each child has significant individual circumstances. To achieve the benefits of classification one must overlook many aspects of individuality to focus on important similarities, but individual considerations remain crucial to appropriate assessment and intervention (Doucette, 2002).

Harmful results. Classifying EBD may lead to labels for the young person involved, and labeling can produce various unfortunate effects (DesJarlais & Paul, 1978; Phillips, Draguns, & Bartlett, 1975; Scotti & Morris, 2000; Wicks-Nelson & Israel, 2000). First, many children identified as having an EBD do not like their label. Second, a label may prompt teachers or other adults to adopt lower behavior and achievement expectations for the labeled child. If the child discovers this and performs according to the lowered expectations, there is created a "self-fulfilling prophecy" of poor behavior, achievement, and self-esteem. Similarly, identifying someone with an EBD may convey to him or her a message of reduced personal responsibility (e.g., Szasz, 1960), perhaps weakening a source of motivation to overcome problems. Third, if peers react to a label, the child may experience decreased popularity and diminished social opportunities.

Moreover, even if a label is meant to be a transient marker that qualifies a young person for services, it may endure in written or oral form, thus continuing to prejudice perceptions and efforts of peers and adults. Finally, some assert that classification serves mainly to legitimize the oppression, via isolation and therapy, of people and behaviors that threaten the powerful in society (Cockerham, 2000; Gallagher, 1995; Szasz, 1960).

Certainly it is appropriate to be concerned about detrimental effects of labeling, but exaggerating them can obstruct prevention and early intervention (Kauffman, 1999). For example, although some interventions can be applied preventively to groups, others must be focused on a particular child. Besides, even if formal labeling were to be eliminated, practitioners and peers might adopt informal identifiers of EBD and the children who exhibit them. Labeling in schools and its effects on students with EBD continue to be topics of needed research.

Technical Issues

Reliability of variables and categories. Behaviors and other variables (e.g., duration of a disorder, age when it began) are the building blocks of a classification system, so they must be measured with good reliability to be of much value. DSM's evolution toward clearer descriptions of problems, and fewer inferences about inner causes of them, has improved its reliability (e.g., consistency across users as to the presence of given symptoms). In ASEBA and other dimensional systems, the behavior problem items generally have high reliability except for those on which an adult must judge the child's thoughts and feelings (e.g., "how sad is this kid?"); these items tend to have moderate reliability. For such problems, obtaining the child's perspective is especially important (see Elliott and Busse, Chapter 7, this volume, for a discussion of self-reporting scales).

One way that a category of EBD can have low reliability is if, given the same information about a particular child, different practitioners do not make the same category assignment. That DSM calls for yes-or-no judgments about category membership works to reduce category reliability, especially when a person's problems and other information put him or her near the borderline of one mental disorder or indicate two different disorders about equally. In contrast, category reliability in dimensional systems is high because categories of EBD consist of variables with good reliability, combined according to straightforward rules that do not require yes-or-no decisions about category membership.

Validity of categories. However, a different yes-or-no issue—selection of a percentile cutoff point at which a dimension score is too extreme—brings up a category validity concern for dimensional classification. We know little about the effects of different cutoff points on false positive and false negative EBD identification decisions. The fundamental obstacle to resolving this is the lack of a gold standard for EBD; that is, we are not certain which children "really" have EBD because all known ways of determining this are imperfect. It is small consolation that a similar validity concern is common to many psychological and educational assessment decisions.

A second category-validity issue involves the likelihood that dimensional classification does not cover all forms of EBD. This issue arises from the fact that a dimension of EBD cannot be statistically derived in the first place if the problems composing it are exhibited by so few children that such problems' co-occurrence cannot be determined. That can happen with rare forms of EBD (e.g., schizophrenia among preadolescents).

Another possible validity issue for both disease perspective and dimensional classification involves comorbidity (Bogenschutz & Nurnberg, 2000). Comorbidity can be defined as one person's concurrent exhibition of multiple categories of EBD (disease perspective), or beyond-cutoff scores on multiple dimensions of EBD (dimensional perspective). Comorbidity is common among children with EBD (Nottelman & Jensen, 1995; U.S. Department of Health and Human Services, 1999). The validity issue is that, as the proportion of children comorbid for categories X and Y increases, one's confidence that X and Y are actually different forms of EBD decreases. Imagine a hypothetical ultimate manifestation of comorbidity, in which all children with EBD would be comorbid for all categories of EBD. This situation resembles the position of Menninger (1963) that there is only one kind of EBD.

We may be able to increase the validity of classification systems by broadening the range of variables from which categories and dimensions are built. For instance, it is thought that a child's competencies, social supports, and other possible sources of resilience (Epstein & Sharma, 1998; Masten & Coatsworth, 1998) may reduce the bad effects of behavior problems. That is, perhaps two children with similar behavior problems but different degrees of resilience are not equally likely to have EBD. Thus, research is needed to determine whether and which resilience variables might increase the validity of classification systems for EBD of children.

Considering the validity of categories brings us back to the purposes of classification. One important form of validity involves interactions between categories and intervention effectiveness. There is no such interaction if—to return to an earlier illustration—(1) children in Green, Orange, and Purple categories improve about equally no matter what intervention they receive, or (2) intervention Z causes the greatest improvement regardless of a child's category. In either case, all the children may as well be in one category of EBD, at least for the interventions that were evaluated. Therefore that classification system's validity would be poor in a significant way.

However, there is suggestive evidence that several interventions are more effective with some kinds of EBD than others. For example, Burns, Hoagwood, and Mrazek (1999) concluded that for children with depression, (1) several variations of cognitive behavior therapy are more effective in reducing symptoms of depression than either nondirective psychotherapy or no treatment; and (2) certain selective serotonin reuptake inhibitor (SSRI)-class medications are more effective than tricyclic-class medications. For children with ADHD, (1) intensive behavioral contingency management is more effective than cognitive behavior therapy; (2) stimulant-class medication is more effective than other medications; and (3) stimulant medication is more effective than intensive behavioral contingency management. Although the foregoing abbreviated summaries oversimplify complex results, they serve to demonstrate the feasibility of interactions between categories and intervention effectiveness and thus support the validity of classifying EBD of children and youths.

In summary, technical aspects of DSM and dimensional (including ASEBA) classification of EBD of children and adolescents have improved in recent revisions and will likely continue to do so. The relative advantages of one or the other still depend largely on the purposes of its user. Some of the DSM's advantage depends on its preference by health care payers and government sanctioning agencies. This advantage would diminish if such powerful societal forces accepted the ASEBA or other dimensional systems for official purposes. Further research in the pursuit of more reliable and valid classification will clarify the pros and cons of each form of classification, or lead to hybrid forms and other developments.

Usability. A classification system is more usable if it has enough categories to include all important forms of EBD, yet not so many categories as to be confusing or unmanageable. Usability is also related to training requirements and implementation procedures and how readily classification outcomes can be communicated. Evaluation of usability is largely subjective. DSM has hundreds of categories; is that too many? ASEBA and other dimensional systems may have too few categories because of the logistical obstacles of obtaining enough data on rare forms of EBD. Another usability consideration is training, and both DSM and ASEBA require considerable training to use properly.

Conclusions

The balance of evidence indicates that different categories of EBD of children do exist. DSM and ASEBA have various strengths and weaknesses, and each is better suited for some purposes. Classification systems as yet have limited validity for the most important purpose of classification: specifying interventions that are best suited to improve any particular form of EBD.

It is important for educators of students with EBD to have some familiarity with the purposes and processes of classification and with a few current classification systems including DSM and ASEBA, because knowledge in this field is often framed in terms of categories in one of the classification systems. Meanwhile, researchers will continue to examine the reliability, validity, usability, and other aspects of classification, in part because they expect that better classification will lead to more effective interventions, including school interventions, for young people with EBD.

At present, however, there is too little evidence to support a position that knowing a child's category of EBD is of much help in selecting an appropriate education intervention. Instead, efforts of school practitioners are better spent on identifying, measuring, and improving problems that impede the student's school and life adjustment. As new information shows how classification improves the special education endeavor, teachers can adjust their practices accordingly.

DEFINITIONS

While classification asks "Which kind(s) of EBD?," definitions of EBD address the apparently simpler question "Is this EBD?" Definitions of EBD of children can have

mainly research, authoritative, or administrative purposes. A research definition describes the participant(s) in a particular study of causes, correlates, outcomes, interventions, or some other aspect of understanding and alleviating EBD. A clear research definition helps consumers decide the extent to which study results apply to other children with EBD.

An authoritative definition expresses someone's theoretical or philosophical perspective. A clear authoritative definition can facilitate an exposition of EBD (e.g., for a text), show how an EBD is conceptualized according to a particular theory or perspective, or set the stage for a new or controversial position.

An administrative definition is created or adopted by agencies responsible for the administration of services. Assuming that the definition is implemented as written, one important purpose is to identify children who are eligible for services. If the administrative definition indicates the characteristics by which one recognizes EBD, it can play a role in determining the number and proportion of students with EBD in a school district, state, or nation. Such prevalence information influences decisions about deploying financial, personnel, and other resources for serving children with EBD. An additional purpose in some cases is to declare the nature of a program to young people participating in it, their families, personnel who will deliver services, citizens and lawmakers asked to support the program, and other interested parties.

IDEA Definition of Emotional Disturbance

IDEA directs state education administrators to ensure that students identified for special education qualify under one of the U.S. Department of Education categories of education disability. The category for which students with EBD are most likely to qualify is "emotional disturbance" (ED). The federal IDEA administrative definition of ED is as follows:

(i) The term means a condition exhibiting one or more of the following characteristics over a long period of time and to a marked degree that adversely affects a child's educational performance: (A) An inability to learn that cannot be explained by intellectual, sensory, or health factors; (B) An inability to build or maintain satisfactory interpersonal relationships with peers and teachers; (C) Inappropriate types of behavior or feelings under normal circumstances; (D) A general pervasive mood of unhappiness or depression; (E) A tendency to develop physical symptoms or fears associated with personal or school problems.

(ii) The term includes schizophrenia. The term does not apply to children who are socially maladjusted, unless it is determined that they have an emotional disturbance. (U.S. Department of Education, 1998, p. II-46)

In brief, this definition says that to qualify under the ED category, a student must exhibit at least one of the characteristics (A)–(E) in an enduring, intensive way that adversely affects her or his educational performance. Also, whether or not a student has schizophrenia or is socially maladjusted is not relevant to the ED qualification decision.

The federal definition has been thoughtfully and thoroughly criticized (e.g., Bower, 1982; Forness & Kavale, 2000; Forness & Knitzer, 1992; Grosenick & Huntze, 1980; Kauffman, 2001; Neel & Rutherford, 1981; Nelson & Rutherford, 1990; Nelson, Rutherford, Center, & Walker, 1991; Skiba & Grizzle, 1991; Wood, Cheney, Cline, Sampson, Smith, & Guetzloe, 1997). Some objections have addressed rational and philosophical deficiencies found in the definition. Others have pointed to significant practical negatives, such as that the definition could interfere with educators' efforts to identify and serve students with EBD, or even enable them to avoid serving some students with EBD. Four areas of criticism of the federal definition of ED are noted below, together with comments relevant to the objections.

1. Critics point out that important features of the federal definition are vague. This impedes clear communication among practitioners and researchers and may discourage efforts to assess important features of the definition. Of particular concern has been the ambiguity of "long period of time," "marked degree," "adversely affects educational performance," characteristics (A) and (C), and "socially maladjusted."

Comment: Many definitions of EBD contain vague concepts. It may be some consolation to those frustrated by the federal definition to consider that the DSM definition of mental disorder (see American Psychiatric Association, 2000, p. xxxi) is considerably bulkier than the ED definition, has assorted exclusions and disclaimers, but still "cannot be used as a criterion for deciding what is and is not a mental disorder" (Rounsaville et al., 2002, p. 3). This statement, along with a call for a definition that does specify what a mental disorder is, comes from a distinguished panel laying the groundwork for the next revision of DSM.

Vague concepts become less of a problem if they can be operationalized in a way that enables them to be reliably measured. How to measure the characteristics and other aspects of the federal ED definition, and possible benefits of doing so, will be considered in a later section.

2. Some features of the ED definition are viewed as illogically self-contradictory or redundant. For instance, one apparent self-contradiction is that, while children with "interpersonal relationship problems" of characteristic (B) do qualify as ED, those "who are socially maladjusted" do not necessarily qualify, even though the latter seemingly must have problems relating to other people. The phrase "adversely affects educational performance" and characteristic (A) seem to be redundant, especially if (A) is taken to mean academic achievement only.

Comment: The logic of the socially maladjusted issue is addressed in a later comment. Regarding "adversely affects," efforts to define or classify a variety of disability conditions attempt to separate the issues of (1) whether a person's functioning meets established criteria for the condition and (2) whether that person's functioning is thereby substantially disabled. For instance, DSM calls for separate consideration of whether an individual meets criteria for a mental disorder (Axes I and II) and whether that individual's life functioning is impaired (Axis V). In determinations of mental retardation, the American Association on Mental Retardation calls for separate consideration of whether a person evidences impairments in intellectual functioning and in everyday life adaptive functioning.

Two related purposes of separating these two issues may be to encourage independent consideration of information that should not be confounded during the decision-making process, and to reduce false identifications. The federal ED definition's phrase "adversely affects educational performance" appears to be conceptually similar. Conceivably, a student could show one of the characteristics of ED to an extreme extent and yet not be adversely affected in educational functioning. The extent to which IEP (individualized education program) teams consider a student's characteristics of ED separate from adverse effects on education performance is an interesting issue for research. It may also be important to study what "adversely affects" denotes to educators of students with ED, perhaps with an eye to improving consistency in the phrase's meaning.

3. A further criticism is that the five ED qualifying characteristics (A)–(E) seem to have been arbitrarily chosen and to lack support from scientific research. At the same time there are said to be other behavior problems not found in the ED definition but for which research support exists.

Comment: The true nature of EBD is open to diverse perspectives, of course, but the characteristics in the federal definition of ED appear to correspond to widely accepted aspects of EBD of children. Table 3.3 presents some varieties of EBD found in the DSM-IV-TR and ASEBA classification systems that seem to correspond to the five characteristics and two other stated conditions of interest in the federal definition (many additional DSM categories and subcategories could also fit in Table 3.3). Table 3.3 assumes that ED characteristic (C) involves aggressive, defiant, and destructive behavior at school. Justification for this assumption is presented later.

In addition, there is research evidence that the five characteristics of ED in the federal definition actually do discriminate between students with and without ED. Table 3.4 lists research that addresses characteristics (A)–(E) in which children and adolescents identified as having ED by schools (not clinics or other agencies) had greater problems than peers who were not identified as having ED.

4. Critics have been especially troubled by the term and concept "socially maladjusted." Its ambiguity is underscored by the fact that different authorities have given it diverse interpretations (Center, 1990). Critics doubt that a logical or scientific basis exists for differentiating social maladjustment from ED.

Aside from philosophical controversies, the definition's possible implication that socially maladjusted students are disqualified from services has significant practical ramifications. Slenkovich (1983) combined legal arguments, interpretations of the DSM, and the socially maladjusted clause in the federal definition to assert that students with various conduct and antisocial behavior problems must not be identified with ED. Based on this and similar reasoning, some education agencies have declined to identify students as having ED if they were determined to be socially maladjusted (Cheney & Sampson, 1990). Yet, young people with chronic aggression and conflict with authorities tend to have poor adjustment in school and adult life (Loeber, Farrington, Stouthamer-Loeber, & Van Kammen, 1998; McMahon & Wells, 1998), so it may be that they are among those who most need intervention.

Comment: The federal definition does not say that socially maladjusted students—whatever that means—cannot be identified with the ED education disability. It says that students do not qualify as ED just because they are socially maladjusted.

As Table 3.3 suggested, classification information provides scientific and logical support for discriminating social maladjustment from other emotional and behavioral problems. ASEBA separates aggressive and defiant behavior problems from rule breaking and delinquent behavior problems. The same is true in other dimensional classification systems (e.g., Quay & Peterson, 1996; Reynolds & Kamphaus, 1992, 2002; see also Achenbach & Edelbrock, 1978; Quay, 1986). That is, the multivariate analyses of data on which such systems are based support separate categories of antisocial child behavior more strongly than a single category. In DSM, some patterns of delinquent and antisocial behavior can qualify as a mental disorder (e.g., conduct disorder)

TABLE 3.3. Potential Correspondence among Emotional and Behavior Problems of Children in the Federal Definition of ED and Two Classification Systems

ED definition terms	DSM-IV mental disorders	ASEBA syndromes
• (A) An inability to learn that cannot be explained by intellectual, sensory, or health factors	• Learning disorders • Communication disorders • ADHD—inattentive type	• Attention problems
• (B) An inability to build or maintain satisfactory interpersonal relationships with peers and teachers	• No specific DSM disorder but an important part of many	• Withdrawn/depressed • Social problems
• (C) Inappropriate types of behavior or feelings under normal circumstances	• ADHD—hyperactive-impulsive type • Conduct disorder • Oppositional-defiant disorder • Bipolar I disorder • Adjustment disorder with disturbance of conduct	• Aggressive behavior
• (D) A general pervasive mood of unhappiness or depression	• Depressive disorders • Adjustment disorder with depressed mood • Other mental disorders with depressive features	• Anxious/depressed • Withdrawn/depressed
• (E) A tendency to develop physical symptoms or fears associated with personal or school problems	• Separation anxiety disorder • Anxiety disorders • Somatoform disorders	• Anxious/depressed • Somatic complaints
• Schizophrenia (specifically included)	• Schizophrenia and most psychotic disorders • Mood disorders accompanied by psychotic features	• Thought problems
• Socially maladjusted (if sole problem, does not qualify as ED)	• Conduct disorder • Child or adolescent antisocial behavior (V-code)	• Rule-breaking behavior

while others are considered a focus of concern (V-code) but not a mental disorder.

The existence of scientific and logical support for differentiating ED from social maladjustment does not necessarily mean that it is wise and desirable to do so. Socially maladjusted students are entitled to a proper education, and it is difficult to refute arguments that they are more likely to receive one if provided the services and protections afforded under IDEA (Kauffman, 2001; Nelson & Rutherford, 1990; Wood et al., 1997). But what constitutes a proper education for students with social maladjustment? And is it the same as an appropriate education for students with ED? Research is needed to clarify the relative merits of various interventions for students with social maladjustment and those with ED. Such re-

search presumes, of course, a sound way to measure both social maladjustment and ED.

Definition Proposed by the National Mental Health and Special Education Coalition

Dissatisfied with the federal ED definition, the Council for Children with Behavioral Disorders and other professional and advocacy groups have cooperated to try to change it. Operating as the National Mental Health and Special Education Coalition, they proposed an alternative definition (Forness & Knitzer, 1992; also see *Federal Register*, 1993, February 10, p. 7938) and petitioned Congress—so far unsuccessfully—to substitute it for the existing one

TABLE 3.4. Selected Research Supporting the Five Federal Definition Characteristics as Discriminators of Students with and without ED

IDEA definition characteristic	Research support
(A) An inability to learn that cannot be explained by intellectual, sensory, or health factors	Bower (1969); Cullinan, Evans, Epstein, & Ryser (2003); Cullinan & Sabornie (in press); Cullinan, Schloss, & Epstein (1987); Ellen (1989); Epstein, Kinder, & Bursuck (1989); Gresham, Elliott, & Black (1987); Merrell, Johnson, Merz, & Ring (1992); Trout, Nordness, Pierce, & Epstein (2003); Wagner (1995)
(B) An inability to build or maintain satisfactory interpersonal relationships with peers and teachers	Bower (1969); Bullis, Nishioka-Evans, Fredericks, & Davis (1993); Cullinan et al. (2003); Cullinan & Epstein (1985); Cullinan, Epstein, & Kauffman (1984); Cullinan & Sabornie (in press); Gresham et al. (1987); Lopez, Forness, MacMillan, Bocian, & Gresham (1996); Merrell et al. (1992); Sabornie (1987); Sabornie, Kauffman, & Cullinan (1990); Sabornie, Thomas, & Coffman (1989); Schonert-Reichl (1993)
(C) Inappropriate types of behavior or feelings under normal circumstances	Bower (1969); Cullinan et al. (2003); Cullinan & Epstein (1985); Cullinan et al. (1984); Cullinan & Sabornie (in press); Cullinan et al. (1984); Ellen (1989); Epstein, Cullinan, & Rosemier (1983); Farmer & Hollowell (1994); Tobin & Sugai (1999)
(D) A general pervasive mood of unhappiness or depression	Bower (1969); Cullinan et al. (2003); Cullinan et al. (1984); Cullinan et al. (1987); Cullinan & Sabornie (in press); Maag & Behrens (1989); Miller (1994); Newcomer, Barenbaum, & Pearson (1995)
(E) A tendency to develop physical symptoms or fears associated with personal or school problems	Bower (1969); Cullinan et al. (2003); Cullinan et al. (1984); Cullinan & Sabornie (in press); Ellen (1989); Newcomer et al. (1995)

(Forness & Kavale, 2000). The Coalition-proposed definition is as follows:

(i) The term emotional or behavioral disorder means a disability characterized by behavioral or emotional responses in school so different from appropriate age, cultural, or ethnic norms that they adversely affect educational performance. Educational performance includes academic, social, vocational, and personal skills. Such a disability (A) is more than a temporary, expected response to stressful events in the environment; (B) is consistently exhibited in two different settings, at least one of which is school-related; and (C) is unresponsive to direct intervention in general education or the child's condition is such that general education interventions would be insufficient.

(ii) Emotional and behavioral disorders can co-exist with other disabilities.

(iii) This category may include children or youth with schizophrenic disorders, affective disorders, anxiety disorders, or other sustained disorders of conduct or adjustment when they adversely affect educational performance in ac-cordance with section (i). (Forness & Knitzer, 1992, p. 13)

The Coalition-proposed definition is admirable for various reasons. One is that it is far easier to find fault with a definition of EBD than to create a worthy alternative. Still, potential problems of this definition require consideration.

For one thing, the Coalition proposal contains material similar to some of the criticized parts of the federal definition of ED. Table 3.5 summarizes some of the similarities in coverage of the IDEA and Coalition definitions. A vaguely-stated or illogical concept that is objectionable in the IDEA definition should be similarly objectionable in the Coalition definition.

A second possible problem is inherent in the Coalition definition phrase "different from appropriate age, cultural, or ethnic norms." As presently stated, this may be no more than a nonspecific caution to assessors and decision teams (a similar statement is found in DSM-IV-TR). But particularly as

TABLE 3.5. Similarities in Coverage of the Federal Definition and Coalition-Proposed Definition

Coalition definition wording	IDEA definition wording
"so different from appropriate . . . norms"	"inappropriate . . . behavior or feelings under normal circumstances"
"adversely affect educational performance"	"adversely affects . . . educational performance"
"more than a temporary, expected response to stressful events" and "sustained disorders"	"over a long period of time and to a marked degree"
"may include . . . schizophrenic disorders"	"includes schizophrenia"
"may include . . . affective disorders"	"pervasive mood of unhappiness or depression"
"may include . . . anxiety disorders"	"physical symptoms or fears"

evidence accumulates on age, cultural, and ethnic variations in behavior problems and use of services (Alarcon et al., 2002; U.S. Department of Health and Human Services, 2001), a nonspecific caution may not be sufficient. Instead, serious consideration of this part of the Coalition proposal would seem to necessitate development of normative data on behavior problems for various ages, cultures, and ethnicities.

Creating these norms would present some practical challenges. Regarding age norms, perhaps as few as two levels would be required—say, elementary and secondary. Regarding cultural or ethnic subgroups, many government agencies and other organizations recognize five: African American, Asian/Pacific Islander, European American, Hispanic, and Native American (or equivalent terms). Some may object that European Americans residing in Old Greenwich and Muskogee do not really belong to the same ethno-cultural group, or point out that the most recent census allowed respondents to designate membership in any of more than two dozen ethnic or cultural subgroups. Assuming just five ethno-cultural groups, would the Coalition proposal require at minimum ten sets of nationally representative norms, one for each of two age levels within five ethno-cultural groups?

This phrase of the Coalition definition brings up a philosophical issue as well—specifically, is it proper for a U.S. government agency to establish behavior and emotional expectations that systematically vary according to an individual's culture and ethnicity?

A third reservation involves phrase (B), which specifies that, to qualify, the problems must be "consistently exhibited in two different settings." This feature might help to avoid identifying students caught up in conflicts with a particular teacher or experiencing other school problems not of a pervasive nature. At the same time, it suggests interesting complications. For example, what constitutes a "setting"? Many elementary teachers supervise their students on the playground; in this case, do classroom and playground constitute two different settings? Further, might there be circumstances in which a student should qualify for emotional or behavioral disorder even though her or his problem is exhibited in only one setting (e.g., extreme disruption or anxiety, but only in the cafeteria)?

Also needing further examination is phrase (C) of the Coalition definition, "is unresponsive to direct intervention in general education." The intent evidently is to require prereferral interventions, widely accepted as a sound practice to reduce needless identifications. The question is, should this concept be part of a definition of EBD? Its implementation would mean that whether or not a particular student qualifies as ED is determined in part by the abilities of other people—prereferral team members and other educators—to cope with his or her behavior problems.

But the most important shortcoming of the Coalition proposal is the same one that bedevils the IDEA definition—insufficient attention to its measurement. As with the IDEA definition, significant parts of the Coalition proposal should be carefully operationalized and measured in order to judge its psychometric and other merits. This may show that it is the improved alternative its creators anticipate and/or may point to needed modifications to increase its value and strengthen the case for its adoption.

MEASUREMENT AND RESEARCH ON ED

Most of the needed research on the IDEA and Coalition administrative definitions presumes sound ways to measure significant aspects of them. Nominations and ratings by teachers and peers, structured and semistructured interviews, objective personality assessment, and target-behavior recording (e.g., Breen & Fiedler, 2003; Cullinan, 2002; Merrell, 2003) are among the potentially useful measurement methods for this task. This section illustrates how some important features of the IDEA definition can be measured in order to pursue research issues that may be of interest.

The Scale for Assessing Emotional Disturbance (SAED) operationally defines key components of the federal ED definition of emotional disturbance, including characteristics (A)–(E) and "socially maladjusted" (Epstein & Cullinan, 1998; Epstein, Cullinan, Ryser, & Pearson, 2002). One of its purposes is to facilitate research on this definition.

Six of the SAED subscales are based on teacher ratings of their student's behavior problems. *Inability to Learn* measures problems with achievement and behaviors that can facilitate it (e.g., "Does not independently complete assigned schoolwork"). *Relationship Problems* addresses a student's difficulties in establishing and maintaining relationships with peers and teachers; for example, "Lacks skills needed to be friendly and sociable." *Inappropriate Behavior* focuses on defiant and aggressive behaviors toward others, such as "Makes threats to others." *Unhappiness or Depression* measures the student's negative affect and thinking, for instance, "Experiences little pleasure or joy." *Physical Symptoms or Fears* is concerned with problems of anxiety and physical distress (e.g., "Anxious, worried, tense"). *Socially Maladjusted* subscale pertains to antisocial behaviors taking place outside of school (e.g., "Steals in the community or at home").

The scale development process and other research have indicated good reliability and validity for the SAED (Cullinan, Harniss, Epstein, & Ryser, 2002; Epstein & Cullinan,

1998; Epstein, Cullinan, Harniss, & Ryser, 1999; Epstein, Cullinan, et al., 2002; Epstein, Nordness, Cullinan, & Hertzog, 2002). Table 3.6 briefly explains why the SAED authors operationalized the definition's characteristic (C) and the "socially maladjusted" phrase as they did.

Research on Definitions: An Example

The following abbreviated analysis is intended to illustrate how interesting and potentially important questions relating to the federal ED definition can be pursued empirically. It is based on data obtained during SAED norming. The present results have not been published, and specific findings should not be used to address any issue about the topics involved.

Participants. Participants were students who had been identified by their school systems as ED according to federal and applicable state criteria. There were 1,089 students with ED, female and male, ages 6–18, attending schools in 32 states across the United States. An educator who knew the student provided race, placement, and other information, and completed the SAED.

Grouping variables. Participants were of two races, African American and European American. They were being educated in one of four "placements" (i.e., settings): "General Class" (in a regular school, no more than 20% of the time outside of general education classes); "Resource Room" (regular school, 21–60% of the time outside of general classes); "Separate Class" (regular school, 61–100% outside of general classes); and "Alternative School" (in a special or alternative public school).

Dependent variables. The five characteristics of ED plus the socially maladjusted condition were measured via subscales of the SAED. This instrument's 45 behavior and emotional problem items are rated on a four-point scale (higher ratings mean greater problems). Different groups of items constitute subscales corresponding to the dependent variables (previously described).

Analysis. To explore how the federal definition variables may vary by student race

TABLE 3.6. Federal Definition Characteristic (C) and Socially Maladjusted as Measured by SAED

Why should the global and ambiguous wording of the federal ED definition's characteristic (C) be taken to represent aggression, defiance, and disruption? Analysis of data collected during SAED development (Epstein & Cullinan, 1998; Epstein, Cullinan, Ryser, & Pearson, 2002) identified six multivariate dimensions. The items in four dimensions corresponded to definition characteristics (A), (B), (D), and (E), while items in a fifth corresponded to "socially maladjusted." But the strongest (highest eigenvalue) dimension was composed of items describing aggression, oppositional behavior, and disruption. Although this dimension has no particular logical relationship to the wording of characteristic (C), there was no other federal definition characteristic for this dimension to represent, and no other dimension remained to represent characteristic (C). Thus, by a process of elimination the SAED dimension featuring aggression, oppositional behavior, and disruption was left to represent federal definition characteristic (C).

This match makes sense: nearly every multivariate analysis of young people's emotional and behavior problems has identified a dimension—often, the strongest dimension identified—that includes defiance and aggression (Achenbach & McConaughy, 1997; Quay, 1986). Logically, the federal ED definition must include such a characteristic. Examination of item content shows that SAED Inappropriate Behavior subscale closely resembles subscales pertaining to defiance and aggression found on other rating scales. Moreover, in a study of students with ED (Cullinan, Harniss, Epstein, & Ryser, 2002), (C) Inappropriate Behavior—but not the other SAED characteristics subscales—was found to be highly correlated with the Conduct Disorder subscale of the Behavior Problem Checklist—Revised (RBPC; Quay & Peterson, 1996) and the Aggressive Behavior subscale of the ASEBA Teacher's Report Form (Achenbach, 1991).

Table 3.3 presented evidence on classification of children's EBD that supports differentiating socially maladjusted from other behavior problems, including student defiance and aggression. SAED Socially Maladjusted subscale operationalizes social maladjustment in terms of antisocial acts *outside of school*. This decision was made for two reasons: to underscore the definition's point that whether or not a student is socially maladjusted has no bearing on identification as ED and to block the possibility that a student whose school problems should qualify him as ED could be disqualified because he was also deemed to be socially maladjusted.

and placement, a 2×4 (race $\times$ placement) analysis of variance was performed separately on each of the six dependent variables, with follow-up comparisons using the Tukey HSD. Alpha was set at .05. Some SAED items were left blank for a few students, so N varied across analyses.

Inability to Learn results. The analysis of variance of Inability to Learn revealed no main effect for Race or Placement, but there was a Race $\times$ Placement interaction effect, $F (3, 1033) = 2.86$, $p = .0359$. Follow-up comparisons showed that this interaction arose because the races showed Inability to Learn to similar extents in all placements except Alternative School, where African Americans showed greater problems than European Americans, $Q = 3.04$, $p < .05$.

Relationship Problems results. The analysis of variance of Relationship Problems revealed a main effect for Race, $F (1, 1058) = 5.00$, $p < .0001$ (European Americans had greater Relationship Problems than African

Americans, regardless of placement). The Placement main and Race $\times$ Placement interaction effects were not significant.

Inappropriate Behavior results. The analysis of variance of Inappropriate Behavior revealed no main effect for Race, but there was a Placement main effect, $F (3, 1044) = 2.87$, $p = .0357$. Follow-up analysis showed ED students in Alternative School placements showed greater Inappropriate Behavior than those in General Class placements, $Q = 2.57$, $p < .05$, but other pairs of placements did not differ. The Race $\times$ Placement interaction effect was not significant.

Unhappiness or Depression results. On Unhappiness or Depression there was a main effect for Race, $F (1, 1042) = 6.97$, $p < .0001$; European Americans exhibited greater Unhappiness or Depression than African Americans, regardless of placement. The Placement and Race $\times$ Placement effects were not significant.

Physical Symptoms or Fears results. On Physical Symptoms or Fears there was a main effect for Race, F (1, 1053) = 10.92, $p < .0001$. Regardless of placement, European Americans with ED manifested greater Physical Symptoms or Fears than African Americans. The Placement and Race × Placement effects were not significant.

Socially Maladjusted results. On Socially Maladjusted there was no effect for race but there was a Placement effect, F (3, 1046) = 4.08, $p = .0068$. Students with ED in Alternative School placements evidenced Socially Maladjusted to a greater extent than those in General Class placements, $Q = 2.57$, $p < .05$, but contrasts of the other pairs of placements revealed no differences. The Race × Placement interaction was not significant.

In summary, on the characteristics of ED there were race differences in one of the four placements on Inability to Learn, and in all placements on Relationship Problems, Unhappiness or Depression, and Physical Symptoms or Fears. On Inappropriate Behavior, there were no race differences but there were placement differences. On Socially Maladjusted there were also placement differences.

These results suggest some follow-up questions: (1) Would measuring characteristics of ED via direct observation or student self-report yield similar race and placement findings? (2) Why did the various characteristics of ED and socially maladjusted show race and/or placement differences? Do the characteristics play a role in placement decisions? Instead, do placements shape the behavior, emotion, and learning problems exhibited by students with ED? Or is it both? (3) Are there implications for assessment or intervention if characteristics of ED are differentially exhibited across settings and/or student races? Whether or not these particular questions merit investigation, it should be evident that research on the federal definition has potential to clarify issues about students with ED, including significant aspects of their education.

Debates and decisions about the value of any definition of ED must rely heavily on logic and argument, but these should be supplemented by research based on operationally defining and measuring key parts of the definition. Such research exists for the IDEA definition (see Table 3.4) but not in sufficient scope and quantity to substantially inform judgments about it.

Potentially important research questions about the IDEA definition include the following: (1) What can we learn from measuring the five characteristics using different methods, including information from both teacher and student perspectives? (2) How can "long period of time" and "marked degree" be quantified for more accurate assessment? Do these modifiers vary across characteristics (e.g., should duration criteria for characteristics (B) and (D) be different?)? (3) What does "adversely affects . . . educational performance" mean to teachers, students, and assessors? How is "adversely affects" related to the characteristics of ED and selection of school interventions? (4) Is it feasible and advantageous to use repeated measurements of the characteristics as progress and outcome indicators? (5) Does knowledge of a student's measured functioning on any ED characteristic or "socially maladjusted" provide information that helps educators select interventions that are most likely to be successful? (6) Some students exhibit multiple characteristics of ED (Cullinan & Epstein, 2001). Should they receive a combination of interventions that have been shown to be successful for each of the characteristics singly, or do comorbid characteristics of ED require entirely different interventions? (7) To what extent are DSM and ASEBA categories of EBD congruent with the federal definition characteristics of ED? Is a clinical and/or community intervention that is effective for a particular category of EBD also likely to be effective in school for students with the congruent characteristic of ED? Does congruence between categories of EBD and characteristics of ED have implications for coordinating multisystem or wraparound interventions? (8) How might a student's resilience or other personal and social resources be measured and used in identification and intervention decisions?

A body of research may also exist that addresses key features of the Coalition definition, although to date research findings have not played much of a role in efforts to substitute it for the IDEA definition. Nevertheless, the Coalition definition, like the federal definition, merits empirical study via measurement of its significant aspects.

Potentially important research questions about the Coalition definition include the following: (1) What, specifically, are the age, cultural, and ethnic variations in students' behavioral or emotional responses? For accommodating age, cultural, and ethnic variations in responses, are there scientifically verifiable, practically usable alternatives to data-based norms? If needed, how would multiple sets of data-based norms for different age, cultural, and ethnic groups be obtained and used? Should consideration also be given to other potential influences on behavior and emotions in developing norms (e.g., gender)? (2) What are reliable definitions of "different settings"? Does the use of alternative definitions of different settings affect the prevalence of ED? (3) What interventions are likely to be used in prereferral situations for students with emotional and behavioral problems? What interventions are most likely to be successful (e.g., divert students from referral) and for what kinds of problems? For some students the prereferral process will be successful, for others it will not (i.e., they will be referred and identified as ED); how are educational outcomes different for these two groups of students?

Defining EBD is frustrating but, as the research questions imply, important. Nearly any administrative definition of EBD of students is likely to—perhaps even ought to—raise objections and prompt controversies. Measuring and researching alternative definitions can lead to a clearer understanding of the strengths, weaknesses, and implications of each. From this process may come a definition that is more useful to the practitioners who implement it and more beneficial to the students whom it describes.

REFERENCES

Abrams, G. D. (1992). General concepts of disease: Health versus disease. In S. A. Price & L. M. Wilson (Eds.), *Pathophysiology: Clinical concepts of disease processes* (4th ed., pp. 3–5). St. Louis: Mosby-Year Book.

Achenbach, T. M. (1991). *Manual for the Teacher's Report Form and 1991 profile*. Burlington, VT: University of Vermont, Department of Psychiatry.

Achenbach, T. M. (1995). Developmental issues in assessment, taxonomy, and diagnosis of child and adolescent psychopathology. In D. Cicchetti & D. J. Cohen (Eds.), *Developmental psychopathology: Vol. 1. Theory and methods* (pp. 57–80). New York: Wiley.

Achenbach, T. M. (1998). Diagnosis, assessment, taxonomy, and case formulations. In T. H. Ollendick & M. Hersen (Eds.), *Handbook of child psychopathology* (3rd ed., pp. 63–87). New York: Plenum.

Achenbach, T. M. (2000). Assessment of psychopathology. In A. J. Sameroff, M. Lewis, & S. M. Miller (Eds.), *Handbook of developmental psychopathology* (2nd ed., pp. 41–56). New York: Kluwer Academic/Plenum.

Achenbach, T. M., & Edelbrock, C. S. (1978). The classification of child psychopathology: A review and analysis of empirical efforts. *Psychological Bulletin, 85,* 1275–1301.

Achenbach, T. M., & McConaughy, S. H. (1997). *Empirically based assessment of child and adolescent psychopathology: Practical applications* (2nd ed.). Thousand Oaks, CA: Sage.

Achenbach, T. M., & McConaughy, S. H. (2003). *School based practitioners' guide for the ASEBA.* Burlington, VT: University of Vermont, Research Center for Children, Youth, & Families.

Achenbach, T. M., McConaughy, S. H., & Howell, C. T. (1987). Child/adolescent behavioral and emotional problems: Implications of cross-informant correlations for situational specificity. *Psychological Bulletin, 101,* 213–232.

Achenbach, T. M., & Rescorla, L. A. (2001). *Manual for ASEBA school-age forms and profiles.* Burlington, VT: University of Vermont, Research Center for Children, Youth, and Families.

Adams, H. E., Luscher, K. A., & Bernat, J. A. (2001). The classification of abnormal behavior: An overview. In P. B. Sutker & H. E. Adams (Eds.), *Comprehensive handbook of psychopathology* (3rd ed., pp. 3–28). New York: Kluwer Academic/Plenum.

Alarcon, R. D., Bell, C. C., Kirmayer, L. J., Lin, K-M., Ustun, B., & Wisner, K. L. (2002). Beyond the funhouse mirrors: Research agenda on culture and psychiatric diagnosis. In D. J. Kupfer, M. B. First, & D. A. Regier (Eds.), *A research agenda for DSM-V* (pp. 219–281). Washington, DC: American Psychiatric Association.

American Psychiatric Association. (1952). *Diagnostic and statistical manual of mental disorders.* Washington, DC: Author.

American Psychiatric Association. (2000). *Diagnostic and statistical manual of mental disorders* (4th ed., text rev.). Washington, DC: Author.

Bandura, A. (1968). A social learning interpretation of psychological dysfunctions. In P. London & P. Rosenhan (Eds.), *Foundations of abnormal psychology* (pp. 293–344). New York: Holt, Rinehart & Winston.

Beutler, L. E., & Malik, M. L. (Eds.). (2002). *Rethinking*

the DSM: A psychological perspective . Washington, DC: American Psychological Association.

Bogenschutz, M. P., & Nurnberg, H. G. (2000). 9.1 Classification of mental disorders. In B. J. Sadock & V. A. Sadock (Eds.), *Kaplan and Sadock's comprehensive textbook of psychiatry* (7th ed., vol. 1, pp. 824–839). Philadelphia: Lippincott, Williams & Wilkins.

Bower, E. M. (1969). *Early identification of emotionally handicapped children in school* (2nd ed.). Springfield, IL: Thomas.

Bower, E. M. (1982). Defining emotional disturbances: Public policy and research. *Psychology in the Schools, 19,* 55–60.

Breen, M. J., & Fiedler, C. R. (Eds.). (1996). *Behavioral approach to assessment of youth with emotional/behavioral disorders* (2nd ed.). Austin: Pro-Ed.

Bullis, M., Nishioka-Evans, V., Fredericks, H. D., & Davis, C. (1993). Identifying and assessing the job-related social skills of adolescents and young adults with emotional and behavioral disorders. *Journal of Emotional and Behavioral Disorders, 1,* 236–250.

Burns, B. J., Hoagwood, K., & Mrazek, P. J. (1999). Effective treatment for mental disorders in children and adolescents. *Clinical Child and Family Psychology Review, 2,* 199–254.

Center, D. B. (1990). Social maladjustment: An interpretation. *Behavioral Disorders, 15,* 141–148.

Charney, D. S., Barlow, D. H., Botteron, K., Cohen, J. D., Goldman, D., Gur, R. E., et al. (2002). Neuroscience research agenda to guide development of a pathophysiologically based classification system. In D. J. Kupfer, M. B. First, & D. A. Regier (Eds.), *A research agenda for DSM-V* (pp. 31–83). Washington, DC: American Psychiatric Association.

Cheney, C. O., & Sampson, K. (1990). Issues in identification and service delivery for students with conduct disorders: The "Nevada Solution." *Behavioral Disorders, 15,* 174–179.

Cockerham, W. C. (2000). *Sociology of mental disorder* (5th ed.). Upper Saddle River, NJ: Prentice Hall.

Cullinan, D. (2002). *Students with emotional and behavior disorders: An introduction for teachers and other helping professionals.* Upper Saddle River, NJ: Merrill/Prentice Hall.

Cullinan, D., & Epstein, M. H. (1985). Adjustment problems of mildly handicapped and nonhandicapped students. *Remedial and Special Education, 6(2)* 5–11.

Cullinan, D., & Epstein, M. H. (2001). Comorbidity among students with emotional disturbance. *Behavioral Disorders, 26,* 200–213.

Cullinan, D., Epstein, M. H., & Kauffman, J. M. (1984). Teachers' ratings of students' behaviors: What constitutes behavior disorder in school? *Behavioral Disorders, 10,* 9–19.

Cullinan, D., Evans, C., Epstein, M. H., & Ryser, G. (2003). Characteristics of emotional disturbance of elementary school students. *Behavioral Disorders, 28,* 94–110.

Cullinan, D., Harniss, M. K., Epstein, M. H., & Ryser, G. (2002). The Scale for Assessing Emotional Disturbance: Concurrent validity. *Journal of Child and Family Studies, 10,* 449–466.

Cullinan, D., & Sabornie, E. J. (in press). Characteristics of emotional disturbance of middle and high school students. *Journal of Emotional and Behavioral Disorders.*

Cullinan, D., Schloss, P. J., & Epstein, M. H. (1987). Relative prevalence and correlates of depressive characteristics among seriously emotionally disturbed and nonhandicapped students. *Behavioral Disorders, 12,* 90–98.

DesJarlais, D. C., & Paul, J. L. (1978). Labeling theory: Sociological views and approaches. In W. C. Rhodes & J. L. Paul (Eds.), *Emotionally disturbed and deviant children: New views and approaches* (pp. 171–189). Englewood Cliffs, NJ: Prentice-Hall.

Doucette, A. (2002). Child and adolescent diagnosis: The need for a model-based approach. In L. E. Beutler & M. L. Malik (Eds.), *Rethinking the DSM: A psychological perspective* (pp. 201–220). Washington, DC: American Psychological Association.

Ellen, A. S. (1989). Discriminant validity of teacher ratings for normal, learning-disabled, and emotionally handicapped boys. *Journal of School Psychology, 27,* 15–25.

Epstein, M. H., & Cullinan, D. (1998). *Scale for Assessing Emotional Disturbance.* Austin, TX: Pro-Ed.

Epstein, M. H., Cullinan, D., Harniss, M. K., & Ryser, G. (1999). The Scale for Assessing Emotional Disturbance: Test–retest and interrater reliability. *Behavioral Disorders, 24,* 222–230.

Epstein, M. H., Cullinan, D., & Rosemier, R. A. (1983). Behavior problems of behaviorally disordered and normal adolescents. *Behavioral Disorders, 8,* 171–175.

Epstein, M. H., Cullinan, D., Ryser, G., & Pearson, N. (2002). Development of a scale to assess emotional disturbance. *Behavioral Disorders, 28,* 5–22.

Epstein, M. H., Kinder, D., & Bursuck, B. (1989). The academic status of adolescents with behavioral disorders. *Behavioral Disorders, 14,* 157–165.

Epstein, M. H., Nordness, P. D., Cullinan, D., & Hertzog, M. (2002). Scale for Assessing Emotional Disturbance: Long term test–retest reliability and convergent validity with kindergarten and first grade students. *Remedial and Special Education, 23,* 141–148.

Epstein, M. H., & Sharma, J. M. (1998). *Behavioral and Emotional Rating Scale: A strength based approach to assessment.* Austin, TX: Pro-Ed.

Farmer, T. W., & Hollowell, J. H. (1994). Social networks in mainstream classrooms: Social affiliations and behavioral characteristics of students with EBD. *Journal of Emotional and Behavioral Disorders, 2,* 143–155.

Federal Register. (1993). February 10, p. 7938.

Forness, S. R., & Kavale, K. A. (2000). Emotional or behavioral disorders: Background and current status of the E/BD terminology and definition. *Behavioral Disorders, 25,* 264–269.

Forness, S. R., & Knitzer, J. (1992). A new proposed definition and terminology to replace "Serious Emotional Disturbance" in Individuals with Disabilities Education Act. *School Psychology Review, 21,* 12–20.

Gallagher, B. J. (1995). *The sociology of mental illness* (3rd ed.). Englewood Cliffs, NJ: Prentice Hall.

Gresham, F. M., Elliott, S. N., & Black, F. L. (1987). Teacher-rated social skills of mainstreamed mildly handicapped and nonhandicapped children. *School Psychology Review, 16,* 78–88.

Grosenick, J. K., & Huntze, S. L. (1980). *National needs analysis in behavior disorders: Severe behavior disorders.* Columbia: University of Missouri.

Group for the Advancement of Psychiatry, Committee on Child Psychiatry. (1974). *Psychopathological disorders in childhood: Theoretical considerations and a proposed classification.* New York: Aronson.

House, A. E. (1999). *DSM-IV diagnosis in the schools.* New York: Guilford Press.

Kauffman, J. M. (1999). How we prevent the prevention of emotional and behavioral disorders. *Exceptional Children, 65,* 448–468.

Kauffman, J. M. (2001). *Characteristics of emotional and behavioral disorders of children and youth* (7th ed.). Columbus, OH: Merrill.

Kupfer, D. F., & First, M. B. (2002). Introduction. In D. J. Kupfer, M. B. First, & D. A. Regier (Eds.), *A research agenda for DSM-V* (pp. xv–xxiii). Washington, DC: American Psychiatric Association.

Lamiell, J. T. (1997). Individuals and the differences between them. In R. Hogan, J. A. Johnson, & S. Briggs (Eds.), *Handbook of personality psychology* (pp. 117–141). New York: Academic Press.

Leckliter, I. N., & Matarazzo, J. D. (1994). Diagnosis and classification. In V. B. Van Hasselt & M. Hersen (Eds.), *Advanced abnormal psychology* (pp. 3–18). New York: Plenum.

Loeber, R., Farrington, D. P., Stouthamer-Loeber, M., & Van Kammen, W. B. (1998). *Antisocial behavior and mental health problems.* Mahwah, NJ: Erlbaum.

Lopez, M. F., Forness, S. R., MacMillan, D. L., Bocian, K. M., & Gresham, F. M. (1996). Children with attention deficit hyperactivity disorder and emotional or behavioral disorders in primary grades: Inappropriate placement in the learning disability category. *Education and Treatment of Children, 19,* 286–299.

Maag, J. W., & Behrens, J. T. (1989). Depression and cognitive self-statements of learning disabled and seriously emotionally disturbed adolescents. *Journal of Special Education, 23,* 17–27.

Mash, E. J., & Wolfe, D. A. (2002). *Abnormal child psychology* (2nd ed.). Belmont, CA: Wadsworth.

Masten, A. S., & Coatsworth, J. D. (1998). The development of competence in favorable and unfavorable environments: Lessons from research on successful children. *American Psychologist, 53,* 205–220.

McConaughy, S. H., & Achenbach, T. M. (2001). Manual for the *Semistructured Clinical Interview for Children and Adolescents* (2nd ed.). Burlington, VT: University of Vermont, Research Center for Children, Youth, and Families. (Available at: *http://www.ASEBA.org*).

McMahon, R. J., & Wells, K. C. (1998). Conduct problems. In E. J. Mash & R. A. Barkley (Eds.) *Treatment of childhood disorders* (pp. 111–207). New York: Guilford Press.

Menninger, K. (1963). *The vital balance.* New York: Viking.

Merrell, K. W. (2003). *Behavioral, social, and emotional assessment of children and adolescents* (2nd ed.). Mahwah, NJ: Erlbaum.

Merrell, K. W., Johnson, E. R., Merz, J. M., & Ring, E. N. (1992). Social competence of students with mild handicaps and low achievement: A comparative study. *School Psychology Review, 21,* 125–137.

Miller, D. (1994). Suicidal behavior of adolescents with behavior disorders and their peers without disabilities. *Behavioral Disorders, 20,* 61–68.

Neel, R. S., & Rutherford, R. B. (1981). Exclusion of the socially maladjusted from services under PL 94-142. In F. H. Wood (Ed.), *Perspectives for a new decade: Education's responsibility for seriously emotionally disturbed and behaviorally disordered youth* (pp. 79–84). Reston, VA: Council for Exceptional Children.

Nelson, C. M., & Rutherford, R. B. (1990). Troubled youth in the public schools: Emotionally disturbed or socially maladjusted? In P. E. Leone (Ed.), *Understanding troubled and troubling youth* (pp. 38–60). Newbury Park, CA: Sage.

Nelson, C. M., Rutherford, R. B., Center, D. B., & Walker, H. M. (1991). Do public schools have an obligation to serve troubled children and youth? *Exceptional Children, 57,* 406–415.

Newcomer, P. L., Barenbaum, E., & Pearson, N. (1995). Depression and anxiety in children and adolescents with learning disabilities, conduct disorders, and no disabilities. *Journal of Emotional and Behavioral Disorders, 3,* 27–39.

Nottelmann, D. D., & Jensen, P. S. (1995). Comorbidity of disorders in children and adolescents: Developmental perspectives. In T. H. Ollendick & R. J. Prinz (Eds.), *Advances in clinical child psychology* (Vol. 17, pp. 109–155). New York: Plenum.

Phillips, L., Draguns, J. G., & Bartlett, D. P. (1975). Classification of behavior disorders. In N. Hobbs (Ed.), *Issues in the classification of children* (Vol. 1, pp. 26–55). San Francisco: Jossey-Bass.

Pine, D. S., Alegria, M., Cook Jr., E. H., Costello, E. J., Dahl, R. E., Koretz, D., et al. (2002). Advances in developmental science and DSM-V. In D. J. Kupfer, M. B. First, & D. A. Regier (Eds.), *A research agenda for DSM-V* (pp. 85–122). Washington, DC: American Psychiatric Association.

Quay, H. C. (1986). Classification. In H. C. Quay & J. S. Werry (Eds.), *Psychopathological disorders of childhood* (3rd ed., pp. 1–34). New York: Wiley.

Quay, H. C., & Peterson, D. R. (1996). *Revised Behavior Problem Checklist, PAR Edition: Professional manual.* Odessa, FL: Psychological Assessment Resources.

Reynolds, C. R., & Kamphaus, R. W. (1992). *Behavior Assessment System for Children.* Circle Pines, MN: American Guidance Service.

Reynolds, C. R., & Kamphaus, R. W. (2002). The clinician's guide to *The Behavior Assessment System for Children.* New York: Guilford Press.

Rogers, C. R. (1951). *Client-centered therapy.* Boston: Houghton-Mifflin.

Rounsaville, B. F., Alarcon, R. D., Andrews, G., Jackson, J. S., Kendell, R. E., & Kendler, K. (2002). Basic nomenclature issues for DSM-V. In D. J. Kupfer, M. B. First, & D. A. Regier (Eds.), *A research agenda for DSM-V* (pp. 1–29). Washington, DC: American Psychiatric Association.

Sabornie, E. J. (1987). Bi-directional social status of behaviorally disordered and nonhandicapped elementary school pupils. *Behavioral Disorders, 13,* 45–57.

Sabornie, E. J., Kauffman, J. M., & Cullinan, D. A. (1990). Extended sociometric status of adolescents with mild handicaps: A cross-categorical perspective. *Exceptionality, 1,* 197–209.

Sabornie, E. J., Thomas, V., & Coffman, R. M. (1989). Assessment of social/affective measures to discriminate between BD and nonhandicapped early adolescents. *Monograph in behavior disorders: Severe behavior disorders in children and youth, 12,* 21–32.

Schonert-Reichl, K. A. (1993). Empathy and social relationships in adolescents with behavioral disorders. *Behavioral Disorders, 18,* 189–204.

Scotti, J. R., & Morris, T. L. (2000). Diagnosis and classification. In M. Hersen & R. T. Ammerman (Eds.), *Advanced abnormal child psychology* (2nd ed., pp. 15–32). Mahwah, NJ: Erlbaum.

Scotti, J. R., Morris, T. L., McNeil, C. B., & Hawkins, R. P. (1996). DSM-IV and disorders of childhood and adolescence: Can structural criteria be functional? *Journal of Consulting and Clinical Psychology, 64,* 1177–1191.

Segal, D. L., & Coolidge, F. L. (2001). Diagnosis and classification. In M. Hersen & V. B. Van Hasselt (Eds.), *Advanced abnormal psychology* (2nd ed., pp. 5–22). New York: Kluwer Academic/Plenum.

Skiba, R., & Grizzle, K. (1991). The social maladjustment exclusion: Issues of definition and assessment. *School Psychology Review, 20,* 577–595.

Slenkovich, J. (1983). *PL 94-142 as applied to DSM III diagnoses: An analysis of DSM III diagnoses in special education law.* Cupertino, CA: Kinghorn.

Szasz, T. S. (1960). The myth of mental illness. *American Psychologist, 15,* 113–118.

Tobin, T. J., & Sugai, G. M. (1999). Discipline problems, placements, and outcomes for students with serious emotional disturbance. *Behavioral Disorders, 24,* 109–121.

Trout, A. L., Nordness, P. D., Pierce, C. D., & Epstein, M. H. (2003). Research on the academic status of children with emotional and behavioral disorders: A review of the literature from 1961 to 2000. *Journal of Emotional and Behavioral Disorders, 11,* 198–210.

U.S. Department of Education. (1998). *Twentieth annual report to Congress on the implementation of the Individuals with Disabilities Education Act.* Washington, DC: Author.

U.S. Department of Health and Human Services. (1999). *Mental health: A report of the Surgeon General.* Rockville, MD: Substance Abuse and Mental Health Services Administration, Center for Mental Health Services, National Institutes of Health.

U.S. Department of Health and Human Services. (2001). Mental health: Culture, race, and ethnicity— A supplement to *Mental health: A report of the Surgeon General.* Rockville, MD: Public Health Service, Office of the Surgeon General.

Wagner, M. M. (1995). Outcomes for youths with serious emotional disturbance in secondary school and early adulthood. *The Future of Children, 5*(2), 90– 112. Retrieved August 2000 from *http://www. futureofchildren.org/cri/07cri.pdf.*

Wicks-Nelson, R., & Israel, A. C. (2000). *Behavior disorders of childhood* (4th ed.). Upper Saddle River, NJ: Prentice Hall.

Wood, F. H., Cheney, C. O., Cline, D. H., Sampson, K., Smith, C. R., & Guetzloe, E. C. (1997). *Conduct disorders and social maladjustment: Policies, politics, and programming.* Reston, VA: Council for Children with Behavioral Disorders.

4

Cultural and Linguistic Competency and Disproportionate Representation

DAVID OSHER, GWENDOLYN CARTLEDGE,
DONALD OSWALD, KEVIN S. SUTHERLAND,
ALFREDO J. ARTILES, *and* MARTHA COUTINHO

The disproportionate representation of children of color in programs for emotional and behavioral disorders (EBD) is part of a broader long-term concern regarding racial disproportionality (Artiles & Trent, 1994; Dunn, 1968). Although earlier critiques focused primarily on disproportionate representation in mental retardation and learning disabilities, concerns now include the disproportionate representation of children of color in EBD categories (Sims, 1996). The issue was seen as so important that the *National Agenda for Improving Results for Children and Youth with Serious Emotional Disturbance* made it both a target and a crosscutting theme (Osher & Hanley, 1997; Singh, Williams, & Spears, 2002; U.S. Department of Education [DOE], 1994).

Although often treated as a problem of assessment, disproportionality is better conceptualized multidimensionally (Artiles, Osher, & Ortiz, 2003; Skiba, Knesting, & Bush, 2002). It involves myriad transactions between and among adults in schools, the students, and families. These transactions, in turn, are structured, mediated, or both by cultural factors (e.g., bias) as well as the capacity and social capital of families and schools.

Disproportionality should also be understood historically. It occurs in a society shaped by a long history of institutionalized racism (Delpit, 1995), segregation (Artiles et al., 2003), ethnocentrism (Takaki, 1993), and race-related labor market segmentation (Wilson, 1997). Other important factors include tracking in schools (Campbell-Whatley & Comer, 2000; Oaks, 1995); deficit-oriented, victim-blaming approaches to service delivery (McKnight, 1995; Ryan, 1972); and the stigmatization of individuals who are poor, have mental illness, or are parents of children with EBD (Osher & Osher, 1996; U.S. Public Health Service, 1999). Disproportionality is more than a technical matter; it involves segregating students in restrictive settings, labeling them with a stigmatizing marker, and limiting their access to services. The first section of this chapter discusses factors critical to reducing disproportionate representation in special education: identification rates, service disparities, school effects, cultural competence, and collaboration with families. Four sections follow it on school practice, policy and law, teacher training, and research.

IDENTIFICATION RATES

Minority disproportionality has been defined globally as pertaining to "minority students" or "students of color." The results, however, are different for various disability categories and for children from various ethnic groups and genders (Caseau, Luckasson, & Kroth, 1994; Zahn-Waxler, 1993) and may include under- as well as overrepresentation. For example, Fierros and Conroy's (2002) analyses of Office for Civil Rights (OCR) data found that, while black students were overrepresented in EBD (as well as mental retardation) categories, Latino students were underrepresented. Similarly, Parish (2002) (analyzing U.S. Department of Education data) determined that, while Asians and Latinos were less likely than Caucasians to be identified as having EBD (having risk ratios of 0.74 and 0.29 compared with those of Caucasians), the risk ratio for African Americans was 1.92 and the risk ratio for American Indians was 1.24 (Parrish, 2002). General education data and anecdotal reports from mental health and special education suggest that more finely grained analyses might also identify disproportionality among various Latino, Asian, and Pacific Islander groups, as well as among various immigrant "generations" (Lee, 2001; Rong & Brown, 2001; Valenzuela, 1999). For example, Fierros and Conroy (2002) found that in Connecticut (where a large proportion of Latino students are Puerto Rican, and many are second, third, and fourth generation) Latino students are disproportionately identified as having EBD.

Identification rates vary by state and district. For example, state risk ratios for black students identified as having EBD ranged from a high of 6.06 in Nebraska to a low of 0.65 in Idaho, with a black student being at least twice as likely to be identified as a Caucasian student in 29 states (Parrish, 2002). Similarly, American Indian EBD risk ratios ranged from a high of 4.83 in Nebraska to a low of 0 in Arkansas, and Latino risk ratios ranged from a high of 2.33 in New York to a low of 0.25 in Arkansas. The risk ratio for Asian-Pacific Islanders exceeded 1 (i.e., 1.16) in only one state, Hawaii (Parrish, 2002). Rates also vary by school district. For example, in an analysis of OCR data, Cohen and Osher (1994) found that black students were likely to be overidentified in districts in which they constituted a minority of the student body and underidentified in districts in which they were a majority.

The identification rate for EBD has remained stable at approximately 0.9% since OSEP began collecting data in 1976 (Oswald & Coutinho, 1995). This rate is significantly less than the predicted prevalence of EBD within schools (DOE, 1980). Many experts believe that an identification rate of 3–6% would be more accurate (Friedman, Kutash, & Duchnowski, 1996; Kauffman, 2001). In fact, mental health epidemiological studies suggest even higher rates of diagnosable psychological and psychiatric impairments in youth (Costello et al., 1988; Friedman et al., 1996). Therefore, it is possible that although African American and American Indian students are overidentified in comparison with other students, they may still be underidentified in terms of need and access to preventive and early behavioral supports in the general education setting (Osher, Woodruff, & Sims, 2002).

Placement data for Latinos(as) and English language learners (ELLs) have traditionally reflected an underrepresentation pattern in high incidence disabilities (including EBD) at the national level (Artiles, Trent, & Palmer, 2004). There is, however, a scarcity of placement research on subgroups of students within Latino communities (e.g., by nationality or generation in the United States), and empirical evidence on ELL special education placement is almost nonexistent. Recent district-level data from California suggest the number of Latino ELLs placed in special education has tripled in a 6-year period (1993–1999) (Rueda, Artiles, Salazar, & Higareda, 2002); this research also reflected overrepresentation patterns, particularly at the middle and high school levels. It should be noted, however, that placement data at the state level in LD and EBD reflected underrepresentation patterns. Artiles, Rueda, Salazar, and Higareda (2002, in press) examined data from the same districts in California for the year when bilingual education programs were abolished. They found different configurations of overrepresentation patterns in various high incidence categories, depending on the indicators used to gauge this problem. Grade level and type of language support mediated overrepresentation patterns for certain subgroups of ELLs. More specifically, students in middle and high school grades, students receiving less primary language support, and ELLs who lacked proficiency in both their first language and English had a greater chance to be placed in special education. Interestingly, overrepresentation was not observed in the EBD category.

SERVICE DISPARITIES

Although policy debate has frequently focused on disproportionate representation, disparate services and disparate outcomes should be of equal concern (Losen & Orfield, 2002). For example, a reanalysis of NLTS data for students with EBD (Valdes, Williamson, & Wagner, 1990) found that fewer black students received counseling than their Caucasian student counterparts and that, among those who did, the average dosage was less (Osher et al., 2002). Similarly, analyses revealed that children of color were disproportionately placed in restrictive settings. Finally, analyses of mobility, dropout, and graduation data for identified African American children and youths found that they were more likely to experience nonnormative mobility and to drop out and less likely to graduate than their Caucasian counterparts (Osher, Morrison, & Bailey, 2003a, 2003b; Osher & Osher, 1996).

These disparities are nested within general education. School structure and culture, as well as teacher capacity, affect student behavior and outcomes (Teddlie & Reynolds, 2000). Cultural discontinuity, both between teachers and students and between schools and students, can place children at risk of developing EBD or being inappropriately identified as having EBD (Boykin, 1983; Gay, 2000). This discontinuity can include a lack of understanding of behavioral and learning styles and may contribute to disproportionate rates of disciplinary referrals, suspensions, and expulsions (Skiba,

Michael, Nardo, & Peterson, 2000; Webb-Johnson, 2003).

Although disparities have usually been examined within special education (e.g., Donovan & Cross, 2002; Losen & Orfield, 2002), the data are consistent with disparities in other service domains (Osher, 2002). For example, black, Latino, and American Indian youths are more likely to receive punitive and segregating interventions and to interact with overworked, underpaid, demoralized professionals and paraprofessionals in child welfare, juvenile justice, and mental health, as well as in education than Caucasian students (Barton, 2003; Osher et al., 2002; Sheppard & Benjamin-Coleman, 2001; Snyder & Sickmund, 1999). African American, Latino, and American Indian children also have less access to appropriate health and mental health services than their Caucasian peers (Institute of Medicine, 2002; U.S. Public Health Service, 2001). Similarly, black children are disproportionately removed from their birth families by the child welfare system, and this disproportionality exists even when one controls for reported abuse (Fluke, Ying-Ying, Hedderson, & Curtis, 2003; Needell, Brookhart, & Lee, 2003). Finally, black youths are disproportionately incarcerated in the juvenile justice and adult correctional system, and this disproportionality is not sufficiently explained by rates of offending (Snyder & Sickmund, 1999). Unfortunately, evidence on service disparities for ELLs is not available.

SCHOOL EFFECTS

Teacher perceptions, judgment, and capacity play a powerful role in referring students for identification (Foster, 1990; Lomotey, 1990; Sims, 1996). They also play a key role in setting the stage for, and maintaining or exacerbating, academic and behavior problems—factors that place students at risk for subsequent referral and identification (Flores-Gonzalez, 1999; Kellam, Ling, Merisca, Brown, & Ialongo, 1998; Kellam, Mayer, Rebok, & Hawkins, 1998). Teacher attitudes, perceptions, and understanding of student behavior, and teachers' ability to interact with students, are mediated by gender, ethnicity, and socioeconomic status

(SES) (Casteel, 1998, 2000). Although it is possible for teachers from different racial, ethnic, and socioeconomic groups to teach students of color successfully (Ladson-Billings, 1994), cultural incapacity and separation from student communities present challenges (Bacon, Jackson, & Young, 2003; Delpit, 1998; Noguera, 1995; Valenzuela, 1999).

Once referred, students may be evaluated with instruments and procedures that have psychometric limitations (Figueroa, 1983; Hilliard, 1991; Reynolds, Lowe, & Saenz, 1999). In addition, the assessment may take place in a context that introduces its own biases, and data may be interpreted by individuals lacking appropriate cultural knowledge (Skiba, Knesting, & Bush, 2002; Taylor, 1988).

Although individual teacher and examiner bias is a problem (Artiles et al., 2003), the greater problem may be structural and systemic. Although schools can provide nurturing contexts that buffer the impact of risk factors (Mehan, Villanueva, Hubbard, & Lintz, 1996), schools can also function as risk factors and subject students to what Valenzuela (referring to Mexican American youths) conceptualizes as *subtractive schooling*. Schools that (1) enable students and adults to connect among and with one another, (2) help students develop appropriate self-regulatory skills, (3) employ positive behavioral supports, and (4) provide appropriate curricula and instruction are likely to reduce the likelihood that students will be referred to, or be identified as having, EBD (Dwyer & Osher, 2000; Greenberg, Domitrovich, & Bumbarger, 1999). Similarly, reducing class size in early grades (Donovan & Cross, 2002; Finn & Achilles, 1999) and providing students with access to efficacious early interventions (see Osher, Dwyer, & Jackson, 2003, for examples of such interventions) can also reduce the likelihood that students will have discipline problems or be identified as needing special education services.

CULTURAL COMPETENCE

Culture mediates school and mental health processes and outcomes (Anderson et al., 2003; Demmert & Towner, 2003; U.S. Public Health Service, 2001). Cultural competence is frequently recommended as a mechanism for bridging the cultural disconnect between teachers, other professionals, schools, students, and families and for reducing service disparities (Cross, Bazron, Dennis, & Isaacs, 1989; U.S. Public Health Service, 1999). Cultural competence has been defined as a set of congruent behaviors, attitudes, and policies that come together in a system, in a school, in an agency, or among professionals and enables that system, school, or agency or those professionals to work effectively in cross-cultural situations (Cross et al., 1989; Isaacs & Benjamin, 1991). Cultural competence is having the capacity to "step outside of our own framework" (Harry, 1992a, p. 334) and to treat individuals individually while respecting and acknowledging their cultural beliefs and values. An OSEP work group operationalized cultural competency as the integration and transformation of knowledge about individuals and groups of people into specific standards, policies, practices, and attitudes used in appropriate cultural settings to increase the quality of services, thereby producing better outcomes (Sims, King, & Osher, 1999).

COLLABORATING WITH FAMILIES

Families can play a key role in improving education and mental health outcomes (Henderson & Mapp, 2002; Lewis, 2001; Osher & Osher, 2002). The cultural disconnect between schools and families is a key challenge (Harry, 1992a; Osher, 2000; Project Forum at NASDSE, 1993), particularly in the EBD area where parents are often blamed for their children's behavior (Friesen & Osher, 1996). The *National Agenda* called for culturally competent, family-driven approaches (Cheney & Osher, 1997; DOE, 1994), and a synthesis of OSEP-funded research projects identified a link between family collaboration, cultural competence, and disproportionate identification (Sims et al., 1999). Promising and efficacious culturally competent interventions have been developed to engage culturally and linguistically diverse families of children with and at risk of EBD (Kratochwill, McDonald, & Levin, 2003; Rumberger & Larson, 1994), and prevention researchers have demonstrated the ability to tailor outreach and interventions to engage families and improve results (Strader, Davenport, & Kumpfer, 2003).

SCHOOL PRACTICE

Students with EBD have the poorest outcomes of all the students in our schools, and disaggregated outcomes for African American, Latino American, and Native American students are even more depressed (Losen & Orfield, 2002). The prognosis is especially poor for black males, who are disproportionately identified for EBD placements (DOE, 1998, 2000; Kehrberg, 1994). The factors contributing to school and later life failure (e.g., criminality, unemployment, underemployment, mental health disorders, institutionalization, and homelessness) are multifaceted, but a determining factor pertains to the quality of their schooling (Osher et al., 2002).

Academic Preparation

With few exceptions, the majority of students with EBD perform below grade level in most academic areas (Kauffman, 2001). These conclusions hold for students with EBD, whether at elementary (Mastropieri, Jenkins, & Scruggs, 1985) or secondary levels (Epstein, Kinder, & Bursuck, 1989) or in residential facilities (Farrel, Critchley, & Mills, 1999). Although, in some cases, this academic failure may be attributed to underlying learning disabilities, a more critical focus needs to be on the educational programming for students with EBD. Public school placements for students with EBD tend to be dominated by the curriculum of control, where teachers are much more focused on maintaining order, moving students along a level system through points and other reinforcers, than capitalizing on the smaller class sizes to provide individualized, meaningful, and stimulating lessons (Knitzer, Steinberg, & Fleisch, 1990). The instructional day is too often characterized by worksheets and workbooks, and it is not uncommon to find students spending long periods idly waiting on the teacher or even sleeping (Steinberg & Knitzer, 1992; Vaughn, Levy, Coleman, & Bos, 2002). This lack of emphasis on effective instruction may reflect a deficit in research as well as training. Indeed, Gunter, Denny, and Venn (2000) bemoan the paucity of studies for students with EBD that address instructional modifications compared with the preponderance of studies that analyze the effects of consequences, such as reinforcers or punishments.

The link between academic performance and EBD is powerful, and the absence of effective academic instruction within classrooms for students with EBD is particularly disconcerting. Authorities have begun to place greater emphasis on academic instruction for students with EBD, theorizing that students who fail to receive sufficient instruction to be successful will find academic tasks aversive and that disruptive behavior will function as a means to escape (see Lane, Chapter 24, this volume). Furthermore, academic interventions can be a highly effective means for bringing about more adaptive academic and social behavior (Gunter et al., 2000; Scott, Nelson, & Liaupsin, 2001).

No studies were found comparing school programs for children of color with EBD with those for majority-group youths, but it would be appropriate to assume that such studies would produce findings comparable to those for mainstream students. Poor minority children present the greatest educational need and are the least likely to receive effective instruction. The existing data indicate that they come to school with more educational deficits than their majority peers, they receive a lower quality and quantity of instruction than that in higher-income schools, and the achievement gaps between them and their more privileged peers systematically widens as they progress through the grades (Greenwood, Delquadri, & Hall, 1989; Hart & Risley, 1995, 1999).

Reading and Behavior Disorders

The role of reading disorders in EBD is not clearly delineated, but the fact that they coexist is undisputed. Levy and Chard (2001) assert that reading and behavior problems are the two most common childhood disorders and report research findings where students with EBD scored significantly below nondisabled peers in reading, with the gap systematically increasing with grade levels.

One speculation is that many students labeled EBD are principally acting out frustrations that are due to the inability to read. The reverse can be argued as well; that is, behavior disorders interfere with the opportunities to learn to read. Kellam and his colleagues found considerable overlap between problems in reading and mathematics achievement, aggression, shy/withdrawn behavior, peer relations, and depressive symptoms among first graders; further, raising reading scores lowered the level of aggressive behavior in boys and lowered the levels of depression in girls over the course of first grade (Kellam, Mayer, et al., 1998). This chicken-and-egg dispute may never be fully resolved, but we do know that reading and behavior disorders can be exacerbated by their comorbidity. This may be especially true for students from culturally diverse backgrounds. Intervention research can be designed to determine the mechanisms that link behavioral and academic performance as well as the mediators and moderators of intervention effects.

The reading report card for many culturally diverse students in our schools depicts a failing grade and a discouraging prognosis for the near future if we continue with our current schooling practices. The 2000 federal survey of student achievement, the National Assessment of Educational Progress (NAEP), shows that reading levels for 63% of African American, 58% of Latino, and 57% of Native American fourth graders were below basic, compared with 27% for Caucasian children and 22% for Asian/Pacific Islander children (National Center for Education Statistics, 2001). These figures underscore the poor reading performance of children of color in our society. Although African American children have made some gains since 1992 (dropping from 67% below basic to 63% below basic), the only group with significant increases on the fourth-grade reading measure was Asian/Pacific Islander children, who dropped from 41% below basic in 1992 to 22% below basic in 2000. The NAEP report also documents that females performed better (33% below basic) than males (42% below basic), suggesting that the most failure-prone reader in our schools is the African American male.

Reading success depends on systematic instruction in phonics, phonemes, word analysis, fluency, and comprehension (Vaughn et al., 2002). Unfortunately, those students with the greatest need in reading often receive relatively little instruction, sometimes only a few minutes a day (Levy & Chard, 2001). The existing evidence on reading lessons in classrooms for students with EBD verifies an overall poor quality of reading instruction with little time devoted to the reading of text or direct instruction on reading skills or comprehension (Vaughn et al., 2002). Studies are needed on the effects of effective reading practices on children's behavior disorders. Would scientifically validated reading instruction implemented in grades K–3 (e.g., Kame'enui, Carnine, Dixon, Simmons, & Coyne, 2002) not only produce better readers but also correspondingly moderate children's behavior problems? Little is known of the beneficial impact that scientifically effective practices within a general education classroom would have on children's emotional and behavioral disturbances. Other related questions could focus on the ways effective instruction, especially in reading, is used as a primary mode of intervention in early and intensive interventions. That is, once problem behaviors have emerged, would individualized or intensive reading interventions in general or special education settings aid in producing more adaptive behaviors that would warrant placements in more normalized environments? Such investigations are especially important for children from culturally and linguistically diverse (CLD) backgrounds, who show disproportionality in both of these areas (i.e., reading difficulties and EBD).

Although limited, some preliminary research in this area suggests that instruction in reading fluency (Scott & Shearer-Lingo, 2002) or in early literacy (Lane et al., 2002) can bring about both increases in reading performance and reductions in disruptive behavior for students with or at risk for EBD. Students of color were included in at least one of these studies, but much more research is needed along these lines, documenting the immediate and long-term effects on reading and behavioral progress.

Early Intervention

An obvious implication of the preceding discussion is the importance of early interventions both in terms of programming for young children and intervening at the earliest signs of problem behavior among school-age children. Scott and colleagues (2001) argue that the stage for poor school performance is set at birth for impoverished children of color. There is good evidence that we can reduce disruptive classroom behavior through early identification and academic intervention for learning problems (Osher, Dwyer, & Jackson, 2003).

Quality early childhood programs have long held much attraction for special educators and other professionals in our quest to improve children's options for school success. Such interventions are indicated for culturally diverse children born into families with specific markers associated with severe school failure (e.g., extreme poverty, premature parenting, parent criminality, family disorganization) and include wraparound services such as family support and education, health services, sustained high-quality care, and cognitive stimulation. Recent scientific reports show that high-quality preschool intervention, including child care, has a lasting effect on cognitive and academic development even into adulthood (Campbell, Pungello, Miller-Johnson, Burchinal, & Ramey, 2001; Strain & Timm, 2001). While some research has included particular ethnic groups (e.g., Weikart, Bond, & McNeil, 1978), replications should examine the effectiveness of different interventions with other ethnic groups.

Hettleman (2003) argues that public schools are discriminating against the nation's poor and minority students by not providing interventions sufficiently early to avoid failure and special education. The problem, according to Hettleman, centers on low expectations and the use of IQ scores and discrepancies. Most urban and minority learners do not achieve IQ scores that are sufficiently high to produce a discrepancy score that warrants early intervention. This practice underscores "the conventional educational wisdom that early reading difficulties including dyslexia are rare and mysterious disorders found predominantly in the IQ elite" (p. 4).

The issue of early intervention in the primary (K–3) grades is particularly contentious, where general educators insist that early childhood classrooms need only employ "developmentally appropriate" practices and the reading skills of these children will eventually emerge (Hettleman, 2003; Kame'enui et al., 2002). As noted previously, specialized services often are not made available until the intermediate grades (or later) when the student is several grade levels behind and reading disabilities are accompanied by behavior problems. Specialized interventions tend to be less beneficial for students in higher grades.

Some modest studies at the preschool and primary levels are promising, indicating that early identification and intervention for academic learning problems reduce the likelihood that students will engage in disruptive classroom behavior (Lane et al., 2002; Scott et al., 2001). Evidence-based instructional practices are potentially useful in preventing and modifying children's behavior problems. Large-scale investigations that inform the pedagogy of both general and special educators are imperative.

Constructive and Proactive Approaches to Discipline

A major goal in establishing *disciplined schools* with positive, nurturing environments is to empower school personnel to be *proactive* rather than reactive. Proactive, child-centered approaches are based on the theoretical model that most behavior is learned, and plans are designed to promote children's social development. The emphasis is on motivating children to want to be adaptive in their behavior, and there is evidence of beneficial schoolwide returns (Carr et al., 1999; Metzler, Biglan, Rusby, & Sprague, 2001).

Without proactive supports, schools employ a purely punitive disciplinary system (Lewis & Sugai, 1999), which is ominous for students of color, especially African American students who are disproportionately represented in EBD programs (DOE, 1998, 2000), suspended from school more frequently and for longer durations (Cartledge, Tillman, & Talbert-Johnson, 2001; Skiba et al., 2000), and punished more severely in school (Office for Civil Rights, 1992). Currently, we have no evidence that our students, with or without disabilities, are well served by harsh disciplinary systems (Skiba & Peterson, 2000), but we do have evidence that current disciplinary practices contribute to disproportionately high rates of dropouts and incarceration for black, Latino, and Native American children (Osher et al., 2002).

Collaborative and Respectful Relationships with Families

Many families of culturally diverse backgrounds are distrustful of schools, often complaining that schools are quick to place their children in special education and are unlikely to recommend their children for gifted or advanced schooling. They also complain that schools contact them only to report some infraction on the part of their child. Poor minority parents, unduly stressed by the everyday problems of living, tend to assign the full responsibility for their children's achievement to the schools (Paratore, 2001). Furthermore, a history of discrimination, rejection, criticism, and poor services cause many low-income minority families to be reluctant to trust public agencies and schools (Unger, Jones, Park, & Tressell, 2001). Teachers, in turn, are challenged by the difficulties of teaching children with learning and behavior problems and are likely to view the parents as uncaring and their instructional efforts as futile. Thus, a pervasive and unhealthy tension seems to exist between teachers and families of children from diverse backgrounds.

Without specialized and concentrated intervention, the gulf between school and home is likely to grow to the detriment of the learner. Kutash, Duchnowski, Sumi, Rudo, and Harris (2002) present a school, family, and community collaborative program where participants were trained to develop and implement a strengths-based plan to guide a productive educational program for middle school students with EBD. The authors report positive effects of this training on the school performance of the students with EBD and family involvement. Unger and colleagues (2001) found support from their child's teacher to be a facilitating factor in the involvement of urban, predominantly African American caregivers. Qualities valued by the parents were honesty, a no-blaming attitude, supportiveness, and inclusion in decision making. Research on family involvement suggests that other keys

to working with families of color include recognizing and proceeding on the assumption that all parents, regardless of income, education level, or cultural background, want their children to do well, adopting a no-fault policy that includes high expectations for all families, demonstrating respect and compassion for family members and respect for families' cultures and experiences, and sharing power with families (Henderson & Mapp, 2002; Osher & Osher, 2002).

Addressing the needs of students of color requires "working reciprocal relationships" with families and the community (Trickett, 1997, p. 141). Policies can support systemic reform to change the relationship between culturally and diverse low-income families and schools (Comer & Haynes, 1991; Epstein & Dauber, 1991). These systemic changes can include support for family involvement as well as parent–teacher collaborations in planning. Policies can also support the effective involvement of families, including families of color, in developing, evaluating, implementing, and disseminating research (Osher, Van Kammen, & Zaro, 2001).

POLICY AND LAW

Special education is a civil right, which, when implemented well, can ensure that all children receive a free appropriate public education. Unfortunately, inappropriate education perpetuates the segregation of children of color with and at risk for EBD (Losen & Orfield, 2002). This paradox can be eliminated by developing and implementing appropriate public and school policies that ensure that students of color have access to appropriate curriculum and instruction and that schools have the capacity to support their learning and behavior. Schools need to employ culturally competent approaches, use assessment efficiently, and collaborate with families.

Appropriate Curriculum and Instruction

Students of color with or at risk for EBD are more likely than their peers to be subjected to a general education curriculum of control (Fine, 1991; Valenzuela, 1999). They often lack access to appropriate instruction and engaging curricula in reading and mathematics (Delpit, 1995; Donovan & Cross, 2002). In addition, the pedagogy, curricula, and materials provided do not align with the linguistic backgrounds and cultural resources of many students of color (Hoover, 1998; Valenzuela, 1999). Further, they frequently attend schools that fail to provide learning opportunities that help them develop social and emotional skills that will enable them to succeed in school and the community. Also, compared with their peers, these students have less access to assistive technology, and when they do have access, it is less likely to be used to support higher-order thinking skills (Coley, Cradler, & Engel, 1997). These gaps contribute to poor academic performance, which, in turn, exacerbates behavioral problems, nonnormative mobility, grade retention, and school dropout. These academic problems are heightened in an era of standards-based reform in which schools are starting to discipline students for academic-related issues (Morrison, 2002) and in which students are losing hope about their ability to pass graduation tests.

Public and school policy should ensure that students of color have access to linguistically and culturally appropriate pedagogy, curricula, and opportunities to learn that enable them to develop the social, emotional, and intellectual competencies necessary for school and postsecondary success. These opportunities include access to evidence-based approaches in reading and mathematics; tutorial support; individual adaptation, when required; and intensive academic support (including extra, rather than diminished, opportunities to learn) when necessary. They also should include access to the social and self-regulatory skills that mediate school success.

Evidence-based interventions exist regarding what works, what may work, and what is unlikely to work in preventing and treating behavioral problems and mental disorders (Greenberg, Domitrovich, & Bumbarger, 1999). Lists of evidence-based practices should address ecological validity (Hoagwood, 1997; Schoenwald & Hoagwood, 2001) and treatment effects with different populations of children (Osher, Dwyer, & Jackson, 2003). Policy should (1) support effectiveness and transportability research to determine how evidence-based interventions can be effectively used or refined so that they can produce good outcomes with culturally diverse populations and (2) ensure that schools employ appropriate interventions and provide staff with the training and support to implement these interventions effectively.

Prevention, Screening, Assessment, and Intervention

Student support is linked to academic performance (Learning First Alliance, 2001), particularly for students challenged by multiple risk factors. Even when appropriate interventions are employed, they are often fragmented or insufficiently powerful to overcome the impact of aversive school environments characterized by chaos, low staff morale, and inexperienced teachers (e.g., Balfanz, Spiridakis, Neild, & Legters, 2003). Policy should enable schools to develop a comprehensive three-level approach to prevention and intervention, which provides a strong relational foundation for success, intervenes early when students are at risk of academic or social failure, and provides intensive interventions for those students who are at high level of need (Osher, Sandler, & Nelson, 2001; Osher, Dwyer, & Jackson, 2003). Policy change is necessary to eliminate racial and cultural biases in school discipline, which disproportionately affect students of color (Skiba et al., 2000).

Policy also should support universal screening for learning and behavioral problems (Donovan & Cross, 2002), awarness of early warning signs (Dwyer & Osher, 2002), and culturally and linguistically competent assessments. Assessments should be strengths- as well as needs-based and be implemented in a manner that guides early and intensive interventions.

Some interventions can be done in groups. For example, the Positive Adolescent Choices Training (PACT) is a culturally sensitive violence prevention training program developed specifically for African American adolescents. It is designed to be implemented in an intensive small-group setting with African American students who are at risk for becoming victims or perpetrators of violence

(Yung & Hammond, 1996). STEP (School Transitional Environment Program) is a selective early intervention that focuses on providing supports to students who are at risk for potential problems at predictable school transition times (Felner & Adan, 1989). Other interventions are individual-based (e.g., functional assessment). Finally, intensive, individualized, ecological family- and community-based interventions that address the multiple determinants of serious antisocial behavior include Multisystemic Therapy (MST) and wraparound (Henggeler, Schoenwald, Borduin, Rowland, & Cunningham,1998; Kendziora, Bruns, Osher, Pacchiano, & Mejia, 2001; Woodruff et al., 1999).

Cultural Competency

Both bias and limited understanding of cultural differences and dynamics can lead to the misidentification and inappropriate treatment of children of color, which reduces the likelihood that interventions will work or that students will connect to the school and its staff. Bias and ignorance can also create environments hostile to staff and families of color. Policy should ensure the operationalization of cultural competency at all levels of education—research, staff recruitment and training, pedagogy and curriculum, screening and assessment, interaction with families, and the school environment.

INITIAL TEACHER PREPARATION

There is a significant underrepresentation of individuals from minority groups pursuing careers in special education (Tyler & Smith, 2000). Townsend (2000) notes that social class, generational differences, and differing life experiences can affect teacher–student relationships, even when the teacher and the student share similar ethnic backgrounds. This "representational mismatch" may lead to teachers unfamiliar with school behaviors of students from minority groups and different social classes misinterpreting cultural difference for behavioral deviance (Townsend, 2000; Utley, Kozleski, Smith, & Draper, 2002). School failure may occur when

educators fail to recognize or effectively address students' cultural, social, or linguistic characteristics, and these characteristics may exacerbate problem behaviors in school (Kea & Utley, 1998). While recruiting and retaining highly qualified teachers from culturally and linguistically diverse (CLD) backgrounds has been a priority for many years (Smith, McLeskey, Tyler, & Saunders, 2002), there is a large disproportion between the number of students and teachers of color (Townsend, 2000; Tyler & Smith, 2000). Further, all teachers, regardless of cultural background, must be prepared to provide high-quality, evidence-based, culturally competent academic and social skills instruction to all students.

Understanding and Confirming Cultural Competence

The ability to understand and confirm cultural competence allows educators to appreciate the relationships among the cognitive, motivational, and value-belief systems of children of color in order to enhance their ongoing learning and development (Cartledge & Milburn, 1996). At the same time, an inability to be culturally competent may result in attributing poor school performance to deficient ability levels within the child or to problematic home environments (Cartledge, Kea, & Ida, 2000).

Training programs should provide opportunities for teachers to explore cultural differences in educational contexts. For example, black students might exhibit behaviors, such as "stage-setting" behaviors prior to beginning a task, and exhibit verbal and nonverbal language that might conflict with the expectations of their nonblack teachers (Townsend, 2000). Townsend suggests that teachers identify some general behavioral styles that may create dissonance between their experiences, values, and belief systems and those of their students. Training should thus help teachers become both knowledgeable about the subject matter and respectful and responsive to the experiences of the students that they will teach (Webb-Johnson, 2003). Culturally competent teachers are knowledgeable about both their own and their students' cultures. They use characteristics of their students' experiences as beginning points to better contextualize instruction (Gay, 1993). Research should examine the impact of training on improving outcomes for children of color in order to develop approaches that produce the most positive impact. This research can determine what level of awareness and knowledge changes behavior.

Cartledge and colleagues (2000) identified several additional components of cultural competence, including learning about family structures, strengths, traditions, and the unique relationship between families and the "contentious relationship between special education and minority parents" (p. 33). Research has shown that African American and Puerto Rican American parents have broader parameters of normalcy than were allowed by educational evaluations (Harry, 1992b) and that this disconnect can further contribute to a contentious relationship between schools and families. Cartledge and colleagues suggest that teachers of culturally diverse students with EBD need to facilitate more communication with parents to promote positive home–school connections. The transactional nature of social interchanges, in which an individual is influenced by another individual's behavior to do something that he or she might not otherwise have done (Sameroff, 1983), provides a framework for teachers to better understand the perspectives of parents of students from CLD backgrounds with EBD. Teachers' ability to recognize their own cultural biases, manifested in part by their expectations of and interactions with the families of their students, is critical. For example, Harry (1995) found that school personnel contributed to decreased African American parental involvement in the special education process through power dynamics, such as teachers' use of technical jargon, ignoring parents' questions and concerns, and scheduling conferences without parental input, which may be experienced in a racialized manner. Training programs can help teachers become more culturally competent by providing multiple opportunities for trainees to meet with both practicing teachers and families of students from CLD backgrounds, with both pre- and follow-up self-assessments to provide relevant opportunities for personal growth.

Due to the interrelated systems that im-

pact the development of students with EBD, and particularly those from CLD backgrounds, training programs should address multiple factors that affect students to maximize the impact of service delivery. Training teachers to recognize the impact of various systems on the academic and social growth of their students will help teachers avoid placing the blame for a student's poor school performance on a particular system, such as the family, which hinders opportunities for positive home–school connections. This is important because teacher practices and attempts to involve parents are as (or more) important than race or ethnicity, social class, and marital status in determining how parents become involved in their children's education (Epstein, 1996). Moreover, through increased parental involvement, teachers may enhance their knowledge base of the sociocultural context of the community served by the school (Haynes & Ben-Avie, 1996), and this knowledge base may be further enhanced through home visits (McCarthey, 2000). For example, increased exposure to families may help a teacher develop an understanding of the family strengths of African American students, such as the importance of the extended family, spirituality, and resilience in the face of racism, poverty, inadequate education, and violence (Day-Vines, 2000). An ability to use family strengths, while recognizing and supporting growth in areas of need, will help teachers improve transactions between families and the school, resulting in improved outcomes for their students.

Evidence-Based and Culturally Competent Methods

Teachers require training in helping CLD students make relevant connections among themselves, the academic material, and the tasks they are asked to perform (Salend, Duhaney, & Montgomery, 2002). There also is a pressing need for personnel preparation in evidence-based academic instruction for students with EBD (Gunter & Denny, 1998). Methods that have been suggested that meet these criteria include positive interventions, functional assessment, social skills instruction, individual management systems, and peer-mediated strategies such as peer tutoring and cooperative learning (Cartledge,

2002; Greenwood, Horton, & Utley, 2002). Further, providing high-quality, evidence-based instruction (particularly in reading, writing, and mathematics) that is based on appropriate curriculum-based measurement (CBM), is crucial for all children with learning problems, particularly those from CLD backgrounds (Cartledge, 2002). Training programs must infuse these competencies in coursework, with subsequent demonstrations by trainees in sustained fieldwork experiences.

It is critical that teachers use appropriate assessments, both formal and CBM, to determine what and how to best teach students (Deno, 1998). The systematic use of CBM allows teachers to make instructional decisions on the basis of actual student progress rather than poorly supported personal judgments that may be affected by personal bias (Walker et al., 1998). Similarly, functional behavioral assessment (FBA) allows the teacher, in collaboration with other professionals, to make data-based decisions when confronted with a student's problem behavior (Quinn, Gable, Rutherford, Nelson, & Howell, 1998; Utley et al., 2002). We believe that, to be most effective, the FBA process must take the student's culture into account (Townsend & Osher, 2002) "because the social context of learning and the attitudes, values, and behaviors of the family, peer group, and community profoundly influence students' emotional, behavioral, moral and cognitive development" (Utley et al., 2002, p. 199). Trainees must learn how to conduct and interpret academic and behavioral assessments in their coursework, understanding the role that cultural differences may play in both the behaviors emitted by students and the interpretational bias of observers and raters.

Sustained Field Experience

Training programs should expose trainees to evidence-based, culturally competent instructional practices in coursework and expect trainees to demonstrate competence in selecting and implementing appropriate practices in their field experiences. Therefore it is critical that sustained field experiences occur in multicultural school settings (Kozleski, Sands, & French, 1993). Moreover, trainees should demonstrate their cul-

tural and instructional competence at both conducting behavioral and academic assessments and making instructional decisions that are based on assessment results, writing lesson plans, delivering instruction, and working with families (Anderson et al., 2003). To facilitate trainees' acquisition of competencies, family members should be given opportunities during the course of a training program to guest lecture in classes, participate in panel discussions and on staff development teams, and make decisions regarding increasing the family-centeredness of the program (Harry, 2002).

To support the development of culturally competent, evidence-based practices, university supervisors and cooperating teachers should systematically evaluate trainees in their application of competencies and skills in classroom settings throughout their field experience, focusing on skills such as academic and behavioral assessments, implementation of peer-mediated interventions, social skills instruction, and communications with families. Sileo (2000) also suggests additional learning activities, such as learning journals and videotaped reflections that may be used during field experiences to further facilitate the development of competencies of trainees in diverse settings. The provision of sustained, multiple field-based experiences in schools in multicultural settings affords trainees opportunities to experience culturally responsive interactions with students, teachers, family members, and other school personnel. The integration of culturally competent training, opportunities to experience relevant professional experiences, and systematic feedback from university and public school personnel will increase the likelihood of producing culturally responsive teachers (Artiles, Trent, Hoffman-Kipp, & López-Torres, 2000).

RESEARCH

Thoughtful and effective responses to disproportionality have been relatively rare in the history of special education. Questions of race and language difference are always politically and emotionally charged, and a strong temptation exists to choose a politically popular response, regardless of its demonstrated efficacy. In such a context, a commitment to extending the knowledge base by fostering and using empirical research becomes even more important. The systematic collection and analysis of reliable data, and the thoughtful interpretation of the resultant findings, may be viewed as absolute prerequisites to appropriate and effective responses to the problem of disproportionality.

Understanding the Causes of Disproportionality

First among the goals of disproportionality research continues to be the clarification of the basis of the phenomenon. While it is unlikely that a single cause will ever fully and convincingly account for any single instance of disproportionality (much less for the wide range of situations in which it occurs), there is reason to hope that important contributing factors can be isolated and that indicators can be identified that will pinpoint likely causal factors in a given situation. Such a hope, however, rests on a more complete knowledge base than that which currently exists (Artiles et al., 2004).

Useful research in pursuit of a comprehensive understanding of disproportionate representation requires a commitment to several fundamental principles. First, the importance of a coherent and well-articulated conceptual framework within which to view the problem cannot be overstated if the field is to overcome the divisiveness that marks the current state of the dialogue. Second, the responsible use of data is essential to the accurate representation of the extent of the problem and the outcome of efforts to address it. Finally, the research dialogue must be informed by an appreciation of the complex sociopolitical history and current context of race and education in the United States.

Building on these principles, a number of specific lines of inquiry emerge that must be followed to move the field forward. The fundamental issue of causality can be reduced to a single global question: To what extent, and under what circumstances, does racial/ethnic disproportionality reflect (1) differential susceptibility to educational disability based on observed, individual child differences, as opposed to (2) the operation of bias in the educational practices (Osher et al., 2002) as well as special education referral, assessment, and eligibility process (Coutinho, Oswald, Best, & Forness, 2002)?

The notion of differential susceptibility suggests a need to understand the role that demographic, social, economic, and educational experience factors play in the etiology of educational disability, the extent to which those risk factors are evenly distributed across racial/ethnic groups, and the extent that efficacious interventions exist to buffer or eliminate the impact of the risk factors (Osher, Dwyer, & Jackson, 2003). For example, children of color are disproportionately exposed to potentially toxic environmental influences; this fact represents a critical feature of our society that cannot be ignored. Yet, the relationship between this differential exposure to harmful influences and the disproportional identification of educational disability, as well as the mechanisms that contribute to that relationship, is largely unknown.

Improved understanding of the bias hypothesis requires investigation of how *specific* system characteristics (e.g., the prereferral, referral, assessment, evaluation, and eligibility process; teacher characteristics and belief; community values and expectations) interact with child characteristics (ethnicity, gender, SES, achievement, ability, and adaptive behavior) to produce a special education eligibility decision. One promising approach to clarifying this interaction involves community-level, follow-along studies that seek to investigate both the operation of bias and the differential susceptibility to disability. Such an approach might select sites that are "at risk" for significant overrepresentation of minority children with regard to predictors such as poverty and percentage of minority enrollment, but which vary with respect to disproportional representation (i.e., some demonstrating high disproportionality, others with none or very low rates). Individual child samples should include students with EBD who remain in, or return to, general education; those who receive Title I services; and those students served through inclusive or pull-out special education arrangements. Student and system information should be collected so that (1) the special education referral and eligibility process is examined for bias and (2) student characteristics, educational placements, and outcomes are documented to test the hypothesis of differential susceptibility.

Research should examine the short- and long-term implications of school effects. For example, Kellam's work suggests that poor teacher behavioral management in first grade contributes to later academic and behavioral problems that drive special education identification (Kellam, Ling, et al., 1998). Similarly, research should examine the short- and long-term implications of placement decisions, including tracking and detracking, on diverse students of color. Although some segregating interventions may be effective in one domain, they may have iatrogenic effects in others (Dishion, McCord, & Poulin, 1999; Osher et al., 2002).

Disproportionality research can be conceptualized to examine the implications of the transactions contributing to disproportionality (Artiles et al., 2003; Osher et al., 2002). This research should align quantitative study with ethnography to explore the implications of cross-sectional analyses (Cohen & Osher, 1994; Harry, Klingner, Sturges, & Moore, 2002). Research designs should be more finely grained to deal with the interaction of race, language, social class, type of community, and years within the United States.

Examining the Role of Poverty

Particular attention is warranted with respect to understanding the relationship between individual child poverty and identified educational disability. Fujiura and Yamaki (2000) noted that the "locus of increased risk for disability was among constituencies defined by poverty and single-parent headed families" (p. 194). Parker, Greer, and Zuckerman (1988) described the association between poverty and both prenatal and perinatal effects on the child that make normal development less likely: "An increase in poverty will result in not only more children with environmental risk factors but also more children with biological or established risk who come from families with multiple critical needs" (p. 187).

Poverty may produce multigenerational impact through persistent lack of economic resources, lack of appropriate prevention interventions, lack of access to quality education or social services, and physiologic deprivation. African American and other minority children are at an increased risk for disability owing to the cumulative effects of deleterious postnatal factors, including lead exposure or anemia. Further, some maternal medical conditions that may increase the risk of disability are more common in African American women, including anemia, elevated lead levels, hypertension, diabetes, chronic renal disease, and sickle cell anemia (Yeargin-Allsopp, Drews, Decoufle, & Murphy, 1995). Differences in access to health care may lead to differences in early treatment of maternal or pediatric conditions that affect the risk of developing disabling conditions (Blendon, Aiken, Freeman, & Corey, 1989).

The National Research Council placed considerable emphasis on the role of poverty, and the risk factors associated with economic disadvantage, as a principal cause of disproportionality (Donovan & Cross, 2002). To the extent that they are important in the etiology of disability, poverty and associated risk factors unquestionably have the potential to exacerbate disproportionate representation of minority students in special education. Appropriate responses to disproportionality, that is, responses that improve the educational outcomes of minority children, will depend on additional research to obtain a better understanding of factors that influence differential susceptibility to disability and public advocacy to implement appropriate responses. Because poverty-related risk factors may play a key role, developmental epidemiological approaches (Kellam, Koretz, & Moscicki, 1999) may be useful.

Nonetheless, concern persists that systemic and cultural biases that continue to plague society generally play a role in the overrepresentation of minority children in special education (e.g., Artiles, 1998). While the role of poverty in the etiology of disability cannot be denied, it is premature to abandon investigation of such bias, to reduce our vigilance in monitoring potentially discriminatory practices, or to deemphasize the development of evidence-based means to increase cultural competence.

Emphasizing Outcomes

Equally important as a goal for disproportionality research is the thorough investigation of the outcomes of special education. Little is known about the effectiveness of educational programs for minority students who are identified and served as disabled compared with those who display similar educational and behavioral profiles but are not so identified. Differences among ethnic groups with respect to the academic and social progress of students both within and outside of special education must be better understood in order to improve educational success and identify essential changes in general and special education programs. There is a need to better understand the factors that limit the effectiveness of both education services, particularly for children of color, including (in some school districts) the overwhelming number of children in need, and insufficient resources and alternatives available through general education (Gottlieb & Alter, 1994).

Responding appropriately to disproportionate representation entails a commitment to improving outcomes for minority students and is inextricably linked to the extent to which regular and special education programs yield consistent, measurable, and socially meaningful educational progress. Because outcomes are so important, families, educators, and researchers of color, as well as representatives of community-based organizations, should be involved in the identification and operationalization of outcomes. The goal of improved outcomes demands research that is guided by the outcomes criterion to ensure that efforts to reduce disproportionality are associated with student benefits (Reschly, 1988). Reforms to address overrepresentation of children of color in special education must include an emphasis on evidence-based practices that improve student competencies and expand educational opportunities. If changes in assessment practices are introduced, they must be linked to effective interventions in special and regular education settings that lead to improved outcomes. And such reforms and changes demand careful research to document the impact on educational outcomes for minority students served in special and regular education programs and to describe the progress of identified and nonidentified minority students.

An emphasis on outcomes will lead to the careful investigation of a number of specific scenarios: if the outcomes of minority students identified as students with EBD are positive (i.e., equal to or better than outcomes for other EBD students) and are better than outcomes for comparable minority students who are not identified, then even substantial disproportionality may be less important because such outcomes demonstrate the effectiveness of special education interventions and the positive impact those interventions produce in the lives of students of color. If the outcomes for comparable identified and nonidentified minority students are similarly unsatisfactory, then the emphasis belongs not on disproportionality but on improving the educational experiences of all minority students, perhaps involving larger-scale social changes (Garcia & Malkin, 1993).

If the outcomes for identified minority children are measurably inferior to the outcomes of similar children who do not receive special education, then the quality of the special education service is indicted, and disproportionality in such a system may indeed be discriminatory. Finally, if minority and majority special education student outcomes are unequal, even if there is no disproportionality, attention should shift to the quality of special education services. The special education experience may be differentially ineffective for minority students; even if these students are appropriately identified, if their outcomes are measurably inferior to those of majority students, then it cannot be said that they are receiving a free appropriate education under the Individuals with Disabilities Education Act (IDEA).

English Language Learner Placement

There is an urgent need to conduct research on the special educational needs of ELLs (Artiles & Ortiz, 2002). We do not know, for instance, the potential impact that the emerging movement to abolish bilingual education will have on disproportionality. The available evidence suggests these students are overrepresented as disabled in districts that serve large numbers of ELLs (Artiles et al., 2002, in press; Rueda et al., 2002). It will be important to track whether ELL placement in the EBD category changes over time as language support is withdrawn. Research with adolescent ELLs is sorely needed, as research suggests that dropout rates increase in secondary schools and that these students grapple with issues related to identity, ethnic affiliation, and peer pressure. It is not clear whether the traditional underrepresentation of ELLs (and of Latinos, who constitute the largest ethnic group in the ELL population) in EBD will change for adolescent ELLs as policy changes limit the educational resources available for this population.

Other Research-Related Issues

In addition to the larger questions of causality, language differences, and outcomes, other fundamental issues are relevant to disproportionality research. One such issue is the basic question of how disproportionality shall be characterized. Recent efforts to catalog and review the methods for calculating disproportionality have highlighted this issue (Willis, Garrison-Mogren, & Schroll, 2002). Progress in this area would be furthered if educational administrators, researchers, and advocates were to establish a common metric for characterizing the extent of disproportionality; in the absence of such agreement, it is essential for all who work and write on the issue to carefully describe their calculation method to ensure clear communication.

Researchers in the EBD field also need to articulate and use more complex views of culture in their work. Future research must be based on a systematic understanding of the link between culture, behavior, and power, particularly because we are referring to groups of students who have been historically oppressed (Artiles, 2003). A sizable proportion of the literature in the EBD field tends to emphasize a view of culture that is bounded by racial, ethnic, or linguistic differences. From this perspective, culture is treated as a categorical variable. An important consequence is that most research has not accounted for the dynamic dimension of culture that is encoded in individuals' and

institutional practices. The emerging evidence on school disciplinary sanctions, for example, compels us to understand the cultural contexts in which decisions about disciplinary practices are enacted. That is, we must conduct research that accounts for a view of culture that honors both the unique toolkits of various groups and the material practices that individuals produce and reproduce in institutional contexts (Artiles, 2002, 2003).

The key issue is what intervention works for what type of child in what type of context (Osher, Dwyer, & Jackson, 2003). Children with EBD are not a singular group; they have a variety of behavioral, emotional, and co-occurring disorders. Culture, ethnicity, and language and the historical impact of race further complicate the challenge. Research with some students of color has demonstrated the effectiveness of universal interventions that build a strong classroom and school community and connect students to the school (e.g., Solomon, Battistich, Watson, Schaps, & Lewis, 2000) as well as those that develop students' social and emotional skills (e.g., McMahon, Washburn, Felix, Yakin, & Childrey, 2000). Meta-analyses suggest that many other interventions work successfully across racial and cultural groups (e.g., Dubois, Holloway, Valentine, & Harris, 2002; Wilson, Lipsey, & Soydan, 2003). However, the issue remains an empirical question with regard to particular interventions (U.S. Public Health Service, 2001), and we need to know more about how risk factors and treatment results vary within and across different cultural subgroups, social classes, and genders (Kellam & Langevin, 2003). For example, research suggests youths of color are more likely to drop out of treatment and had worse treatment outcomes in community treatment-as-usual settings (Weersing & Weisz, 2002) and that premature treatment dropout, which affects outcomes, is linked to a cultural divide between families and therapists (Kazdin & Wassall, 1998; Malgady, Rogler, & Costantino, 1990).

Several highly individualized interventions have demonstrated equivalent effectiveness across cultural groups (Chamberlain & Reid, 1998; Henggeler, Melton, & Smith, 1992; Kendziora et al., 2001), and other interventions have demonstrated efficacy with black and white children (Kazdin, Siegel, & Bass, 1992; Kendall, 1994). Some specifically designed interventions have demonstrated efficacy with Latino and black youths (Santisteban et al., 2003; Yung & Hammond, 1996). However, not all evidence-based interventions have been examined for differential effects across cultural groups or their impact in diverse settings (Hoagwood, Burns, Kiser, Ringeisen, & Schoenwald, 2001). Research should include sufficient numbers of children from particular groups so that studies have the statistical power to examine the differential impact of interventions across children of different cultures. Research should also examine how the cultural competence of school and agency staff and their ability to collaborate with families affect outcomes. Finally, since adaptation is likely, particularly when working with different culture groups, research should also identify the effects of modifying interventions as well as the impacts of adding new elements to the interventions.

Minority overrepresentation must still be viewed in the context of pervasive under-identification of students with emotional and behavioral disorders. EBD identification rates fall far short of prevalence estimates (Institute of Medicine, 1989) and approach zero for some groups (e.g., Asian/Pacific Islander children and Latinas). Further investigation must consider whether appropriate responses to disproportionate representation should be designed to raise identification rates for underserved subpopulations.

Finally, the investigation of disproportionality in special education may contribute to understanding similar phenomena in other services. There is evidence that race plays an important role in the delivery of mental health services and in the operation of the juvenile justice system (Cohen, Parmelee, Irwin, & Weisz, 1990). Indeed, a comprehensive analysis of the issue undoubtedly requires a multidisciplinary approach examining the entire system of care.

ACKNOWLEDGMENTS

David Osher acknowledges the support of Dr. Kimberly Kendziora, American Institutes for Research. Alfredo J. Artiles acknowledges the support of the National Center for Culturally Responsive Educational Systems (NCCRES) under Grant No. H326E020003 awarded by the U.S. Department of Education, Office of Special Education Programs.

REFERENCES

Anderson, M., Beard, K., Delgado, B., Kea, C. D., Raymond, E. B., Singh, N. N., Sugai, G., Townsend, B. L., Voltz, D., & Webb-Johnson, G. (2003). Excerpts from working with culturally and linguistically diverse children, youth, and their families: Promising practices in assessment, instruction, and personnel. *Beyond Behavior, 12*(2), 12–16.

Artiles, A. J. (1998). The dilemma of difference: Enriching the disproportionality discourse with theory and context. *Journal of Special Education, 32,* 32–36.

Artiles, A. J. (2002). Culture in learning: The next frontier in reading difficulties research. In R. Bradley, L. Danielson, & D. P. Hallahan (Eds.), *Identification of learning disabilities: Research to policy* (pp. 693–701). Hillsdale, NJ: Erlbaum.

Artiles, A. J. (2003). Special education's changing identity: Paradoxes and dilemmas in views of culture and space. *Harvard Educational Review, 73,* 164–202.

Artiles, A. J., & Ortiz, A. (Eds.). (2002). *English language learners with special needs: Identification, placement, and instruction.* Washington, DC: Center for Applied Linguistics.

Artiles, A. J., Osher, D., & Ortiz, A. (2003, April). *"Context" and "culture" in the 2002 NRC report: Challenges and risks for future special education research and practice.* Paper presented at the annual meeting of the American Educational Research Association, Chicago.

Artiles, A. J., Rueda, R., Salazar, J., & Higareda, I. (2002). English-language learner representation in special education in California urban school districts. In D. Losen & G. Orfield (Eds.), *Racial inequity in special education* (pp. 117–136). Cambridge, MA: Harvard Education Press.

Artiles, A. J., Rueda, R., Salazar, J., & Higareda, I. (in press). Within-group diversity in minority disproportionate representation: English language learners in urban school districts. *Exceptional Children.*

Artiles, A. J., & Trent, S. C. (1994). Overrepresentation of minority students in special education: A continuing debate. *Journal of Special Education, 27,* 410–437.

Artiles, A. J., Trent, S. C., Hoffman-Kipp, P., & López-Torres, L. (2000). From individual acquisition to cultural-historical practices in multicultural teacher education. *Remedial and Special Education, 21,* 79–89.

Artiles, A. J., Trent, S. C., & Palmer, J. (2004). Culturally diverse students in special education: Legacies and prospects. In J. A. Banks & C. M. Banks (Eds.), *Handbook of research on multicultural education* (2nd ed., pp. 716–735). San Francisco: Jossey-Bass.

Bacon, E., Jackson, F., & Young, K. (2003, April). *African American and European American teachers' perceptions of schooling African American males with behavior problems.* Paper presented at the annual meeting of the American Educational Research Association, Chicago.

Balfanz, R., Spiridakis, K., Neild, R., & Legters, N. (2003, May). *High poverty secondary schools and the juvenile justice system: How neither is helping the other and how that could change.* Paper presented at Reconstructing the School-to-Prison Pipeline: Charting Intervention Strategies of Prevention and Support for Minority Children, The Civil Rights Project, Harvard University, Cambridge, MA.

Barton, P. E. (2003, November). *Parsing the achievement gap: Baselines for tracking progress.* Princeton, NJ: Educational Testing Service.

Blendon, R. J., Aiken, L. H., Freeman, H. E., & Corey, C. R. (1989). Access to medical care for black and white Americans: A matter of continuing concern. *Journal of the American Medical Association, 261,* 278–281.

Boykin, A. W. (1983). The academic achievement performance of Afro-American children. In J. Spence (Ed.), *Achievement and achievement motives* (pp. 324–371). San Francisco: Freeman.

Campbell, F. A., Pungello, E. P., Miller-Johnson, S., Burchinal, M., & Ramey, C. T. (2001). The development of cognitive and academic abilities: Growth curves from an early childhood educational experiment. *Developmental Psychology, 37,* 231–242.

Campbell-Whatley, G. D., & Comer, J. (2000). Self-concept and African-American student achievement: Related issues of ethics, power and privilege. *Teacher Education and Special Education, 23,* 19–31.

Carr, E., Horner, R. H., Turnbull, A. P., Marquis, J. G., McLaughlin, D. M., McAtee, M. L., Smith, C. E., Ryan, K. A., Ruef, M. B., Doolabh, A., & Braddock, D. E. (1999). *Positive behavior support for people with developmental disabilities: A research synthesis.* Washington, DC: U.S. Department of Education, Office of Special Education Programs.

Cartledge, G. (2002). Issues of disproportionality for African American learners. In G. Cartledge, K. Y. Tam, S. A. Loe, A. H. Miranda, M. C. Lambert, C. D. Kea, & E. Simmons-Reed (Eds.), *Culturally and linguistically diverse students with behavioral disorders* (pp. 15–24). Arlington, VA: Council for Children with Behavioral Disorders.

Cartledge, G., Kea, C. D., & Ida, D. J. (2000). Anticipating differences—celebrating strengths: Providing culturally competent services for students with serious emotional disturbance. *Teaching Exceptional Children, 32*(3), 30–37.

Cartledge, G., & Milburn, J. F. (1996). *Cultural diversity and social skills instruction: Understanding eth-nic and gender differences.* Champaign, IL: Research Press.

Cartledge, G., Tillman, L. C., & Talbert-Johnson, C. (2001). Professional ethics within the context of student discipline and diversity. *Teacher Education Special Education, 24,* 25–37.

Caseau, D. L., Luckasson, R., & Kroth, R. L. (1994). Special education services for girls with serious emotional disturbance: A case of gender bias? *Behavioral Disorders, 20,* 51–60.

Casteel, C. A. (1998). Teacher–student interactions and race in integrated classrooms. *Journal of Educational Research, 92,* 115–121.

Casteel, C. A. (2000). African American students' perceptions of their treatment by Caucasian teachers. *Journal of Instructional Psychology, 27,* 143–149.

Chamberlain, P., & Reid, J. B. (1998). Comparison of two community alternatives to incarceration for chronic juvenile offenders. *Journal of Consulting and Clinical Psychology, 66,* 624–633.

Cheney, D., & Osher, T. (1997). Collaborate with families. *Journal of Emotional and Behavioral Disorders, 5,* 36–44.

Cohen, J., & Osher, D. (1994). *Race and SED Identification: An analysis of OCR data.* Technical paper prepared for Division of Innovation and Development, Office of Special Education Programs, U.S. Department of Education.

Cohen, R., Parmelee, D. X., Irwin, L., & Weisz, J. R. (1990). Characteristics of children and adolescents in a psychiatric hospital and a corrections facility. *Journal of the American Academy of Child and Adolescent Psychiatry, 29,* 909–913.

Coley, R., Cradler, J., & Engel, P. K. (1997). *Computers and classrooms: The status of technology in U.S. schools, policy, and information report.* Princeton, NJ: Educational Testing Service.

Comer, J., & Haynes, M. (1991). Parent involvement in schools: An ecological approach. *Elementary School Journal, 91,* 271–278.

Costello, E. J., Edelbrock, C., Costello, A. J., Dulcan, M. K., Burns, B. J., & Brent, D. (1988). Psychopathology in pediatric primary care: The new hidden morbidity. *Pediatrics, 82,* 415–424.

Coutinho, M. J., Oswald, D. P., Best, A. M., & Forness, S. R. (2002). Gender and sociodemographic factors and the disproportionate identification of minority students as emotionally disturbed. *Behavioral Disorders, 27,* 109–125.

Cross, T., Bazron, B., Dennis, K., & Isaacs, M. (1989). *Towards a culturally competent system of care: A monograph on effective services for minority children who are seriously emotionally disturbed.* Washington, DC: Georgetown University Child Development Center, National Technical Assistance Center for Children's Mental Health.

Day-Vines, N. L. (2000). Ethics, power, and privilege: Salient issues in the development of multicultural competencies for teachers serving African-American children with disabilities. *Teacher Education and Special Education, 23*, 3–18.

Delpit, L. (1995). *Other people's children*. New York: The New Press.

Delpit, L. (1998). What should teachers do? Ebonics and culturally responsive instruction. In T. Perry & L. Delpit (Eds.), *The real Ebonics debate* (pp. 17–26). Boston: Beacon.

Demmert, W. G., & Towner, J. C. (2003). *A review of the research literature on the influences of culturally based education on the academic performance of Native American students*. Portland, OR: Northwest Regional Educational Laboratory.

Deno, S. L. (1998). Academic progress as incompatible behavior: Curriculum-based measurement (CBM) as intervention. *Beyond Behavior, 9*(3), 12–17.

Dishion, T. J., McCord, J., & Poulin, F. (1999). When interventions harm: Peer groups and problem behavior. *American Psychologist, 54*, 755–764.

Donovan, M., & Cross, C. (2002). *Minority students in special and gifted education*. Washington, DC: National Academy Press.

Dubois, D. L., Holloway, B. E., Valentine, J. C., & Harris, C. (2002). Effectiveness of mentoring programs for youths: A meta-analytic review. *American Journal of Community Psychology, 30*, 157–197.

Dunn, L. M. (1968). Special education for the mildly retarded: Is much of it justifiable? *Exceptional Children, 35*, 5–22.

Dwyer, K., & Osher, D. (2000). *Safeguarding our children: An action guide*. Washington, DC: U.S. Department of Education.

Epstein, J. L. (1996). Perspectives and previews on research and policy for school, family, and community partnerships. In A. Booth & J. F. Dunn (Eds.), *Family-school links: How do they affect educational outcomes* (pp. 209–246). Mahwah, NJ: Erlbaum.

Epstein, J. L., & Dauber, S. (1991). School programs and teacher practices of parent involvement in inner-city elementary and middle schools. *Elementary School Journal, 91*, 289–306.

Epstein, M. H., Kinder, D., & Bursuck, D. (1989). The academic status of adolescents with behavioral disorders. *Behavioral Disorders, 14*, 157–165.

Farrel, P., Critchley, C., & Mills, C. (1999). The educational attainments of pupils with emotional and behavioural difficulties. *British Journal of Special Education, 26*, 50–53.

Felner, R. D., & Adan, A. M. (1989). The school transitional environment project: An ecological intervention and evaluation. In R. H. Price, E. L. Cowen, R. P. Lorion, & J. Ramos-McKay (Eds.), *14 ounces of preventions: A casebook for practitioners*. Washington, DC: American Psychological Association.

Fierros, E. G., & Conroy, J. E. (2002). Double jeopardy: An exploration of restrictiveness of race in special education. In D. Losen (Ed.), *Minority issues in special education* (pp. 39–70). Cambridge, MA: The Civil Rights Project, Harvard University and the Harvard Education Publishing Group.

Figueroa, R. A. (1983). Test bias and Hispanic children. *Journal of Special Education, 17*, 431–440.

Fine, M. (1991). *Framing dropouts*. New York: Teachers College Press.

Finn, J. D., & Achilles, C. M. (1999). Tennessee's class size study: Findings, implications, misconceptions. *Educational Evaluation and Policy Analysis, 21*, 97–109.

Flores-Gonzalez, N. (1999). Puerto Rican high achievers: An example of ethnic and academic identity compatibility. *Anthropology and Educational Quarterly, 30*, 343–362.

Fluke, J. D., Ying-Ying, T. Y., Hedderson, J., & Curtis, P. A. (2003). Disproportionate representation of race and ethnicity in child maltreatment: Investigation and victimization. *Children and Youth Services Review, 25*, 365–379.

Foster, H. (1990). Ethnocentrism and racism: The disproportionate representation of minorities and poor in special education programs for the emotionally disturbed. *Perceptions, 25*(2), 16–19.

Friedman, R. M., Kutash, K., & Duchnowski, A. J. (1996). The population of concern: Defining the issues. In B. Stroul (Ed.), *Children's mental health: Creating systems of care in a changing society*. Baltimore: Brookes.

Friesen, B. J., & Osher, T. W. (1996). Involving families in change: Challenges and opportunities. Co-published simultaneously in *Special Services in the Schools, 11*, 187–207, and R. J. Illback & C. M. Nelson (Eds.), *Emerging school-based approaches for children with emotional and behavioral problems: Research and practice in service integration*. New York: Haworth.

Fujiura, G. T., & Yamaki, K. (2000). Trends in demography of childhood poverty and disability. *Exceptional Children, 66*, 187–199.

Garcia, S. B., & Malkin, D. H. (1993). Towards defining programs and services for culturally and linguistically diverse learners in special education. *Teaching Exceptional Children*, Fall, 52–58.

Gay, G. (1993). Building cultural bridges: A bold proposal for teacher education. *Education and Urban Society, 25*(3), 45–51.

Gay, G. (2000). *Culturally responsive teaching: Theory, research and practice*. New York: Teachers College Press.

Gottlieb, J., & Alter, M. (1994). *An analysis of referrals, placement, and progress of children with disabilities who attend New York City public schools*. New York: New York University, School of Education (ERIC Document Reproduction Service No. ED 414 372).

Greenberg, M. T., Domitrovich, C., & Bumbarger, B. (1999). *Preventing mental disorder in school-aged children: A review of the effectiveness of prevention programs* (Report submitted to the Center for Mental Health Services [SAMHSA]). State College, PA: Pennsylvania State University, Prevention Research Center.

Greenwood, C. R., Delquadri, J. C., & Hall, R. V. (1989). Longitudinal effects of classwide peer tutoring. *Journal of Educational Psychology, 81*, 371–383.

Greenwood, C. R., Horton, B. T., & Utley, C. A. (2002). Academic engagement: Current perspectives on research and practice. *School Psychology Review, 31*, 328–349.

Gunter, P. L., & Denny, R. K. (1998). Trends and issues in research regarding academic instruction of students with emotional and behavioral disorders. *Behavioral Disorders, 24*, 44–50.

Gunter, P. L., Denny, R. K., & Venn, M. L. (2000). The modification of instructional materials and procedures for curricular success of students with emotional and behavioral disorders. *Preventing School Failure, 44*, 116–121.

Harry, B. (1992a). *Cultural diversity, families and the special education system: Communication and empowerment.* New York: Teachers College Press.

Harry, B. (1992b). Restructuring the participation of African American parents in special education. *Exceptional Children, 59*, 123–131.

Harry, B. (1995). Communication versus compliance: African-American parents' involvement in special education. *Exceptional Children, 61*, 364–377.

Harry, B. (2002). Trends and issues in serving culturally diverse families of children with disabilities. *Journal of Special Education, 36*, 131–138, 147.

Harry, B., Klingner, J., Sturges, K., & Moore, R. (2002). Of rocks and soft places: Using qualitative methods to investigate disproportionality. In D. Losen & G. Orfield (Eds.), *Racial inequity in special education* (pp. 71–92). Cambridge, MA: The Civil Rights Project at Harvard University, Harvard Education Press.

Hart, B., & Risley, T. R. (1995). *Meaningful differences in the everyday experience of young American children.* Baltimore: Brookes.

Hart, B., & Risley, T. R. (1999). *The social world of children learning to talk.* Baltimore: Brookes.

Haynes, N. M., & Ben-Avie, M. (1996). Parents as full partners in education. In A. Booth & J. F. Dunn (Eds.), *Family-school links: How do they affect educational outcomes* (pp. 45–55). Mahwah, NJ: Erlbaum.

Henderson, A. T., & Mapp, K. L. (2002). *A new wave of evidence: The impact of school, family, and community connections on student achievement.* Austin, TX: National Center for Family and Community Connections with Schools.

Henggeler, S. W., Melton, G. B., & Smith, L. (1992). Family preservation using multisystemic therapy: An effective alternative to incarcerating serious juvenile offenders. *Journal of Consulting and Clinical Psychology, 60*, 953–961.

Henggeler, S. W., Schoenwald, S. K., Borduin, C. M., Rowland, M. D., & Cunningham, P. B. (1998). *Multisystemic treatment of antisocial behavior in children and adolescents.* New York: Guilford Press.

Hettleman, K. R. (2003). *The invisible dyslexics: How public school systems in Baltimore and elsewhere discriminate against poor children in the diagnosis and treatment of early reading difficulties.* Baltimore: Abell Foundation.

Hilliard, A. G. (Ed.). (1991). *Testing African American students: Special re-issue of The Negro Educational Review.* Morristown, NJ: Aaron.

Hoagwood, K. (1997). Ecological validity and the assessment of children's psychopathology and functioning workshop. Rockville, MD: National Institute of Mental Health.

Hoagwood, K., Burns, B. J., Kiser, L, Ringeisen, H., & Schoenwald, S. K. (2001). Evidence-based practice in child and adolescent mental health services. *Psychiatric Services, 52*, 1179–1189.

Hoover, M. R. (1998). Ebonics: Myths and realities. In T. Perry & L. Delpit (Eds.), *The real Ebonics debate* (pp. 196–208). Boston: Beacon.

Institute of Medicine. (1989). *Research on children and adolescents with mental, behavioral, and developmental disorders: Mobilizing a national initiative.* Washington, DC: National Academy Press.

Institute of Medicine. (2002). *Unequal treatment: Confronting racial and ethnic disparities in health care.* Washington, DC: Author.

Isaacs, M., & Benjamin, M. (1991). *Towards a culturally competent system of care: Vol. 2. Programs which utilize culturally competent principles.* Washington, DC: Georgetown University Child Development Center, CASSP Technical Assistance Center.

Kame'enui, E. J., Carnine, D. W., Dixon, R., Simmons, D. C., & Coyne, M. D. (2002). *Effective teaching strategies that accommodate diverse learners* (2nd ed.). Upper Saddle River, NJ: Prentice Hall.

Kauffman, J. M. (2001). *Characteristics of emotional and behavioral disorders of children and youth* (7th ed.). Columbus, OH: Merrill.

Kazdin, A. E., Siegel, T. C., & Bass, D. (1992). Cognitive problem-solving skills training and parent management training in the treatment of antisocial behavior in children. *Journal of Consulting and Clinical Psychology, 60*(5), 733–747.

Kazdin, A. E., & Wassell, G. (1998). Treatment completion and therapeutic change among children referred for outpatient therapy. *Professional Psychology: Research and Practice, 29*(4), 332–340.

Kea, C. D., & Utley, C. A. (1998). To teach me is to know me. *Journal of Special Education, 32*, 44–47.

Kehrberg, R. S. (1994). Behavioral disorders and gender/sexual issues. In R. L. Peterson & S. Ishii-Jordan (Eds.), *Multicultural issues in the education of students with behavioral disorders* (pp. 184–195). Cambridge, MA: Brookline Books.

Kellam, S. G., Koretz, D., & Moscicki, E. K. (1999). Core elements of developmental epidemiologically based prevention research. *American Journal of Community Psychology, 27*, 463–482.

Kellam, S. G., & Langevin, D. G. (2003). A framework for understanding "evidence" in prevention research and programs. *Prevention Science, 4*(3), 137–153.

Kellam, S. G., Ling, X., Merisca, R., Brown, C. H., &

Ialongo, N. (1998). The effect of the level of aggression in the first grade classroom on the course and malleability of aggressive behavior into middle school. *Development and Psychopathology, 10*, 165–185.

Kellam, S. G., Mayer, L. S., Rebok, G. W., & Hawkins, W. E. (1998). The effects of improving achievement on aggressive behavior and of improving aggressive behavior on achievement through two prevention interventions: An investigation of causal paths. In B. Dohrenwend (Ed.), *Adversity, stress and psychopathology* (pp. 486–505). Arlington, VA: American Psychiatric Press.

Kendall, P. C. (1994). Treating anxiety disorders in children: Results of a randomized clinical trial. *Journal of Consulting and Clinical Psychology, 62*(1), 100–110.

Kendziora, K. T., Bruns, E., Osher, D., Pacchiano, D., & Mejia, B. (2001). *Wraparound: Stories from the field.* Washington, DC: American Institutes for Research, Center for Effective Collaboration and Practice.

Knitzer, J., Steinberg, Z., & Fleisch, B. (1990). *At the schoolhouse door: An examination of programs and policies for children with behavioral and emotional problems.* New York: Bank Street College of Education.

Kozleski, E. B., Sands, D. J., & French, N. K. (1993). Preparing special educators for urban environments. *Teacher Education and Special Education, 16*, 14–22.

Kratochwill, T. R., McDonald, L., & Levin, J. R. (2003). *Families and Schools Together (FAST): An experimental analysis of a parent-mediated early intervention program for elementary school children.* Madison: Wisconsin Center for Education Research.

Kutash, K., Duchnowski, A. J., Sumi, W. C., Rudo, Z., & Harris, K. (2002). A school, family, and community collaborative program for children who have emotional disturbances. *Journal of Emotional and Behavioral Disorders, 10*, 99–107.

Ladson-Billings, G. (1994). What we can learn from multicultural education research. *Educational Leadership, 51*(8), 22–26.

Lane, K. L., Wehby, J. H., Menzies, H. M., Gregg, R. M., Doukas, G. L., & Munton, S. M. (2002). Early literacy instruction for first-grade students at-risk for antisocial behavior. *Education and Treatment of Children, 25*, 438–458.

Learning First Alliance. (2001). *Every child learning: Safe and supportive schools.* Washington, DC: Author.

Lee, S. J. (2001). More than "model minorities" or "delinquents": A look at Hmong American high school students. *Harvard Education Review, 71*, 505–528.

Levy, S., & Chard, D. J. (2001). Research on reading instruction for students with emotional and behavioural disorders. *International Journal of Disability, Development and Education, 48*, 429–444.

Lewis, A. (2001). *Add it up: Using research to improve education for low-income and minority students.*

Washington, DC: Poverty and Race Research Action Council.

Lewis, T. J., & Sugai, G. (1999). Effective behavior support: A systems approach to proactive school wide management. *Focus on Exceptional Children, 31*(6), 1–24.

Lomotey, K. (1990). An interview with Booker Peek. In K. Lomotey (Ed.), *Going to school: The African American experience* (pp. 13–29). New York: SUNY Press.

Losen, D. J., & Orfield, G. (Eds.). (2002). *Racial inequity in special education.* Cambridge, MA: Harvard Education Press.

Malgady, R. G., Rogler, L. H., & Costantino, G. (1990). Culturally sensitive psychotherapy for Puerto Rican children and adolescents: A program of treatment outcome research. *Journal of Consulting and Clinical Psychology, 58*, 704–712.

Mastropieri, M. A., Jenkins, V., & Scruggs, T. E. (1985). Academic and intellectual characteristics of behaviorally disordered children and youth. In R. B. Rutherford, Jr., C. M. Nelson, & S. R. Forness (Eds.), *Severe behavior disorders of children and youth* (Vol. 8, pp. 86–104). San Diego, CA: College-Hill.

McCarthey, S. J. (2000). Home-school connections: A review of the literature. *Journal of Educational Research, 93*, 145–152.

McKnight, J. (1995). *The careless society: Community and its counterfeits.* New York: Basic Books.

McMahon, S. D., Washburn, J., Felix, E. D., Yakin, J., & Childrey, G. (2000). Violence prevention: Program effects on urban preschool and kindergarten children. *Applied and Preventive Psychology, 9*, 271–281.

Mehan, H., Villanueva, I., Hubbard, L., & Lintz, A. (1996). *Constructing school success: The consequences of untracking low-achieving students.* Cambridge, UK: Cambridge University Press.

Metzler, C. W., Biglan, A., Rusby, J. C., & Sprague, J. R. (2001). Evaluation of a comprehensive behavior management program to improve school-wide positive behavior support. *Education and Treatment of Children, 24*, 448–479.

Morrison, G. M. (2002). *Turning points for students experiencing discipline problems in schools: Individual profiles and contextual processes.* Paper presented at the annual conference for Teacher Educators for Children with Behavior Disorders, Tempe, AZ.

National Center for Education Statistics. (2001, April). *The National Assessment of Educational Progress (NAEP).* Washington, DC: U.S. Department of Education, Institute of Education Sciences. Available at *http://nces.ed.gov/nationsreportcard/.*

Needell, B., Brookhart, A., & Lee, S. (2003). Black children and foster care placement in California. *Children and Youth Services Review, 25*, 399–414.

Noguera, P. (1995). Preventing and producing violence: A critical analysis of responses to school violence. *Harvard Educational Review, 65*, 189–212.

Oaks, J. (1995). Two cities' tracking and within-school segregation. *Teachers College Record, 96,* 681–691.

Office for Civil Rights. (1992). *Elementary and secondary civil rights survey, 1990: National summaries.* Arlington, VA: DBS.

Osher, D. (2000). Breaking the cultural disconnect: Working with families to improve outcomes for students placed at risk of school failure. In I. Goldenberg (Ed.), *Urban education: Possibilities and challenges confronting colleges of education* (pp. 4–11). Miami: Florida International University.

Osher, D. (2002, September). *Disparities across other disciplines and services systems.* Paper presented at the Children's Bureau Research Roundtable on Children of Color in the Child Welfare System, Washington, DC.

Osher, D., Dwyer, K., & Jackson, S. (2003). *Safe, supportive, and successful schools step by step.* Longmont, CO: Sopris West.

Osher, D., & Hanley, T. V. (1997). Building on emergent social service delivery paradigm. In L. M. Bullock & R. A. Gable (Eds.), *Making collaboration work for children, youth, families, schools, and communities* (pp. 10–15). Reston, VA: Council for Exceptional Children.

Osher, D., Morrison, G. M., & Bailey, W. (2003a). *Mobility and students with emotional and behavioral disorders.* Presentation at the 2nd National Summit on the IDEA, Crystal City, VA.

Osher, D., Morrison, G. M., & Bailey, W. (2003b). Exploring the relationship between students: Mobility and dropout among students with emotional and behavioral disorders. *Journal of Negro Education, 72*(1), 79–96.

Osher, D., & Osher, T. W. (1996). The national agenda for children and youth with serious emotional disturbance (SED). In C. M. Nelson, R. B. Rutherford, Jr., & B. I. Wolford (Eds.), *Comprehensive and collaborative systems that work for troubled youth: A national agenda* (pp. 149–164). Richmond, KY: Eastern Kentucky University, National Juvenile Detention Association.

Osher, T. W., & Osher, D. (2002). The paradigm shift to true collaboration with families. *Journal of Child and Family Studies, 11*(1), 47–60.

Osher, D., Sandler, S., & Nelson, C. M. (2001). The best approach to safety is to fix schools and support children and staff. *New Directions in Youth Development, 92,* 127–154.

Osher, T. W., Van Kammen, W., & Zaro, S. M. (2001). Family participation in evaluating systems of care: Family, research, and service system perspectives. *Journal of Emotional and Behavioral Disorders, 9*(1), 63–70.

Osher, D., Woodruff, D., & Sims, A. (2002). Schools make a difference: The relationship between education services for African American children and youth and their overrepresentation in the juvenile justice system. In D. Losen (Ed.), *Minority issues in special education* (pp. 93–116). Cambridge, MA:

The Civil Rights Project, Harvard University and the Harvard Education Publishing Group.

Oswald, D., & Coutinho, M. (1995). Identification and placement of students with serious emotional disturbance. Part I: Correlates of state child-count data. *Journal of Emotional and Behavioral Disorders, 3,* 224–229.

Paratore, J. R. (2001). *Opening doors, opening opportunities: Family literacy in an urban community.* Boston: Allyn & Bacon.

Parker, S., Greer, S., & Zuckerman, B. (1988). Double jeopardy: The impact of poverty on early childhood development. *Pediatric Clinics of North America, 35,* 1227–1240.

Parrish, T. (2002). Racial disparities in the identification, funding, and provision of special education. In D. Losen (Ed.), *Minority issues in special education* (pp. 15–38). Cambridge, MA: The Civil Rights Project, Harvard University and the Harvard Education Publishing Group.

Project FORUM at NASDSE. (1993). *Disproportionate participation of students from ethnic and cultural minorities in special education classes and programs: Forum to examine current policy.* Alexandria, VA: The National Association of State Directors of Special Education.

Quinn, M. M., Gable, R. A., Rutherford, Jr., R. B., Nelson, C. M., & Howell, K. W. (1998). *Addressing student problem behavior: An IEP team's introduction to functional behavioral assessment and behavior intervention plans.* Washington, DC: Center for Effective Collaboration and Practice, American Institutes for Research.

Reschly, D. J. (1988). Assessment issues, placement litigation, and the future of mild mental retardation classification and programming. *Education and Training in Mental Retardation, 23,* 285–301.

Reynolds, C. R., Lowe, P. A., & Saenz, A. L. (1999). The problem of bias in psychological assessment. In C. R. Reynolds & T. B. Gutkin (Eds.), *The handbook of school psychology* (3rd ed., pp. 549–596). New York: Wiley.

Rong, X. L., & Brown, F. (2001). The effects of immigrant generation and ethnicity on educational attainment among young African and Caribbean Blacks in the United States. *Harvard Education Review, 71,* 536–565.

Rueda, R., Artiles, A. J., Salazar, J., & Higareda, I. (2002). An analysis of special education as a response to the diminished academic achievement of Chicano/Latino students: An update. In R. R. Valencia (Ed.), *Chicano school failure and success: Past, present, and future* (2nd ed., pp. 310–332). London: Routledge/Falmer.

Rumberger, R. W., & Larson, K. W. (1994). Keeping high-risk Chicano students in school: Lessons from a Los Angeles middle school dropout prevention program. In R. J. Rossi (Ed.), *Schools and students at risk: Context and framework for positive change* (pp. 141–162). New York: Teachers College Press.

Ryan, W. (1972). *Blaming the victim.* New York: Vintage Books.

Salend, S. J., Duhaney, L. M. G., & Montgomery, W. (2002). A comprehensive approach to identifying and addressing issues of disproportionate representation. *Remedial and Special Education, 23,* 289–299.

Sameroff, A. J. (1983). Developmental systems: Contexts and evolution. In P. H. Mussen (Gen. Ed.) & W. Kessen (Vol. Ed.), *Handbook of child psychology: Vol. 1. History, theory, and methods* (4th ed., pp. 237–294). New York: Wiley.

Santisteban, D. A., Coatsworth, J. D., Perez, V., Vidal, A., Kurtines, W. M., Schwartz, S. J., LaPerriere, A., & Szapocznik, J. (2003). Efficacy of brief strategic family therapy in modifying Hispanic adolescent behavior problems and substance use. *Journal of Family Psychology, 17,* 121–133.

Schoenwald, S. K., & Hoagwood, K. (2001). Effectiveness, transportability, and dissemination of interventions: What matters when? *Psychiatric Services, 52,* 1190–1197.

Scott, T. M., Nelson, C. M., & Liaupsin, C. J. (2001). Effective instruction: The forgotten component in preventing school violence. *Education and Treatment of Children, 24,* 309–322.

Scott, T. M., & Shearer-Lingo, A. (2002). The effects of reading fluency instruction on the academic and behavioral success of middle school students in a self-contained EBD classroom. *Preventing School Failure, 46,* 167–175.

Sheppard, V. B., & Benjamin-Coleman, R. (2001). Determinants of service placement patterns for youth with serious emotional and behavioral disturbances. *Community Mental Health Journal, 37*(1), 53–65.

Sileo, T. W. (2000, May). Reform and restructuring in special education teacher preparation: Multicultural considerations. In J. Smith-Davis & K. Murray (Eds.), *Eighth Annual CSPD Conference on Leadership and Change: Monograph of proceedings* (pp. 59–69). Alexandria, VA: National Association of State Directors of Special Education.

Sims, A. (1996). *Individual and group characteristics associated with the disproportionate representation of African-American students classified as seriously emotionally disturbed.* Unpublished doctoral dissertation, Howard University.

Sims, A., King, M., & Osher, D. (1999). *What is cultural competency?* Washington, DC: Center for Effective Collaboration and Practice.

Singh, N. N., Williams, E., & Spears, N. (2002). To value and address diversity: From policy to practice. *Journal of Child and Family Studies, 11*(1), 35–45.

Skiba, R. J., Knesting, K., & Bush, L. D. (2002). Culturally competent assessment: More than nonbiased tests. *Journal of Child and Family Studies, 11*(1), 61–78.

Skiba, R. J., Michael R., Nardo, A., & Peterson, R. (2000). *The color of discipline: Gender and racial disparities in school punishment.* Bloomington, IN: Indiana Education Policy Center.

Skiba, R. J., & Peterson, R. L. (2000). School discipline at a crossroads: From zero tolerance to early response. *Exceptional Children, 66,* 335–346.

Smith, D. D., McLeskey, J., Tyler, N. C., & Saunders, S. (2002). *The supply and demand of special education teachers: The nature of the chronic shortage of special education teachers. COPSEE Report.* Gainesville, FL: University of Florida.

Snyder, H. N., & Sickmund, M. (1999). *Juvenile offenders and victims: 1999 national report.* Washington, DC: Office of Juvenile Justice and Delinquency Prevention.

Solomon, D., Battistich, V., Watson, M., Schaps, E., & Lewis, C. (2000). A six-district study of educational change: Direct and mediated effects of the Child Development Project. *Social Psychology of Education, 4,* 3–51.

Steinberg, Z., & Knitzer, J. (1992). Classrooms for emotionally and behaviorally disturbed students: Facing the challenge. *Behavioral Disorders, 17,* 145–156.

Strader, T., Davenport, P., & Kumpfer, K. (2003, June). *Implementing SAMHSA model programs with multiethnic families.* Presentation at the annual meeting of the Society for Prevention Research, Washington, DC.

Strain, P. S., & Timm, M. A. (2001). Remediation and prevention of aggression: An evaluation of the Regional Intervention Program over a quarter of a century. *Behavioral Disorders, 26*(4), 297–313.

Takaki, R. (1993). *A different mirror: A history of multicultural America.* Boston: Little Brown.

Taylor, S. M. (1988). Community reactions to deinstitutionalization. In C. Smith & J. Giggs (Eds.), *Location and stigma: Contemporary perspectives on mental health and mental health care* (pp. 224–245). Boston: Unwin Hyman.

Teddlie, C., & Reynolds, D. (2000). *The international handbook of school effectiveness research.* London: Falmer Press.

Townsend, B. L. (2000). The disproportionate discipline of African-American learners: Reducing school suspensions and expulsions. *Exceptional Children, 66,* 381–391.

Townsend, B. L., & Osher, D. (2002, April). *Cultural competence in functional behavioral assessment.* Presentation at the annual meeting of the Council for Exceptional Children, New York.

Trickett, E. J. (1997). Developing an ecological mindset on school–community collaboration. In J. L. Swartz & W. E. Martin, Jr. (Eds.), *Applied ecological psychology for schools within communities: Assessment and intervention* (pp. 139–166). Mahwah, NJ: Erlbaum.

Tyler, N., & Smith, D. D. (2000). Welcome to the TESE special issue: Preparation of culturally and linguistically diverse special educators. *Teacher Education and Special Education, 23,* 261–263.

Unger, D. G., Jones, C. W., Park, E., & Tressell, P. A. (2001). Promoting involvement between low-income single caregivers and urban early intervention programs. *Topics in Early Childhood Special Education*, *21*, 197–212.

U.S. Department of Education. (1980). *Second annual report to Congress on the implementation of Public Law 94-142: The Education for All Handicapped Children Act*. Washington, DC: Author.

U.S. Department of Education. (1994). *National agenda for achieving better results for children and youth with serious emotional disturbance*. Washington, DC: U.S. Department of Education, Office of Special Education Programs.

U.S. Department of Education, Office of Special Education Programs. (1998). *Twentieth annual report to Congress on the implementation of the Individuals with Disabilities Education Act*. Washington, DC: Author.

U.S. Department of Education, Office of Special Education Programs. (2000). *Twenty-second annual report to Congress on the implementation of the Individuals with Disabilities Education Act*. Washington, DC: Author.

U.S. Public Health Service. (1999). *Mental health: A report of the Surgeon General*. Washington, DC: Author.

U.S. Public Health Service. (2001). *Mental health: Culture, race, ethnicity: A supplement to the Surgeon General's Report on Mental Health*. Washington, DC: Author.

Utley, C. A., Kozleski, E., Smith, A., & Draper, I. L. (2002). Positive behavior support: A proactive strategy for minimizing behavior problems in urban multicultural youth. *Journal of Positive Behavior Interventions*, *4*, 196–208.

Valdes, K., Williamson, C., & Wagner, M. (1990). *The National Longitudinal Transition Study of Special Education Students: Statistical almanac, Vol. 1, Overview*. Palo Alto, CA: SRI International.

Valenzuela, A. (1999). *Subtractive schooling: U.S.–Mexican youth and the politics of caring*. Albany: State University of New York Press.

Vaughn, S., Levy, S., Coleman, M., & Bos, C. S. (2002). Reading instruction for students with LD and EBD: A synthesis of observation studies. *Journal of Special Education*, *36*, 2–13.

Walker, H. M., Forness, S. R., Kauffman, J. M., Epstein, M. H., Gresham, F. M., Nelson, C. M., & Strain, P. S. (1998). Macro-social validation: Referencing outcomes in behavioral disorders to societal issues and problems. *Behavioral Disorders*, *24*, 7–18.

Webb-Johnson, G. (2003). Behaving while black: A hazardous reality for African-American learners? *Beyond Behavior*, *12*(2), 3–7.

Weersing, V. R., & Weisz, J. R. (2002). Community clinic treatment of depressed youth: Benchmarking usual care against CBT clinical trials. *Journal of Consulting and Clinical Psychology*, *70*, 299–310.

Weikart, D. P., Bond, J. T., & McNeil, J. T. (1978). *The Ypsilanti Perry Preschool Project: Preschool years and longitudinal results through fourth grade*. Ypsilanti, MI: High/Scope Press.

Willis, S. P., Garrison-Mogren, R., & Schroll, K. M. (2002). *Final report on special populations: Disproportionality in special education*. (Prepared under contract to the U.S. Department of Education). Rockville, MD: Westat.

Wilson, S. J., Lipsey, M. W., & Soydan, H. (2003). Are mainstream programs for juvenile delinquency less effective with minority youth than majority youth?: A meta-analysis of outcomes research. *Research on Social Work Practice*, *13*, 3–26.

Wilson, W. J. (1997). *When work disappears: The world of the new urban poor*. New York: Knopf.

Woodruff, D., Osher, D., Hoffman, C., Gruner, A., King, M., Snow, S., & McIntire, J. (1999). *The role of education in a system of care: Effectively serving children with emotional or behavioral disorders. Systems of care: Promising practices in children's mental health*, 1998 Series, Volume III. Washington, DC: American Institutes for Research, Center for Effective Collaboration and Practice.

Yeargin-Allsopp, M., Drews, C. D., Decoufle, S. D., & Murphy, C. C. (1995). Mild mental retardation in black and white children in metropolitan Atlanta: A case-control study. *American Journal of Public Health*, *85*, 324–328.

Yung, B. R., & Hammond, W. R. (1996). Breaking the cycle: A culturally sensitive violence prevention program for African American children and adolescents. In J. R. Lutzker (Ed.), *Handbook of child abuse research and treatment* (pp. 289–321). New York: Plenum.

Zahn-Waxler, C. (1993). Warriors and worriers: Gender and psychopathology. *Development and Psychopathology*, *5*, 79–89.

5

Linking Prevention Research with Policy

Examining the Costs and Outcomes of the Failure to Prevent Emotional and Behavioral Disorders

MARY MAGEE QUINN *and* JEFFREY M. POIRIER

PREVENTION RESEARCH: WHAT ARE WE PREVENTING?

Left to progress without appropriate treatment, young children with emotional and behavioral disorders (EBD) are at increased risk for serious mental health problems, substance abuse, truancy, delinquency, and adult crime (Robins & Ratcliff, 1978–1979); furthermore, within the realm of education, adolescents with EBD are at risk for school failure (Wagner et al., 1991). From an economic perspective, school failure and delinquency are particularly significant consequences of EBD. In fact, the Office of Justice and Delinquency Prevention estimates that "allowing one youth to leave school for a life of crime and of drug abuse costs society $1,700,000 to $2,300,000 annually" (Juvenile Justice and Delinquency Prevention Act of 2002). Economics is only one aspect of this issue.

Longitudinal research suggests that, if left untreated, these children and adolescents will have unhappy adulthoods plagued with marital problems (Caspi, Elder, & Bem, 1987), erratic employment (Robins & Ratcliff, 1978–1979), and heightened risk for multiple arrests, drug and alcohol abuse, and institutionalization for crimes or mental

health disorders (Caspi et al., 1987). Further, the effects of ongoing patterns of EBD and the resulting antisocial behaviors are likely to continue for generations. Robins, West, and Herjanic (1975) found that "antisocial" grandparents had significantly more children who were arrested and significantly more grandchildren who were delinquent than did grandparents not exhibiting antisocial behavior. Left without some form of intervention, those with EBD are likely to lead frustrating lives in which they are "loved by and love few" (Klein, Lewinsohn, & Seeley, 1997).

One of the primary concerns about identifying and treating children and adolescents with EBD stems from the multiple agencies involved in their care and the lack of coordination among and between those agencies. To further complicate matters, these agencies often have different missions, eligibility criteria, intake procedures, and staff members who are generally trained to view a problem through a particular professional lens (Bruner, 1991; Dunkle & Nash, 1989; Leone, Quinn, & Osher, 2002). In fact, service fragmentation has been blamed as the root cause of many of the problems associated with treating and preventing EBD. This fragmentation of services inevitably leads to ineffective and costly interventions by agencies (due to overlap) such as schools, social welfare, and juvenile justice because the lack of collaboration leads to less comprehensive services (Bickman et al., 1996).

This chapter (1) examines the consequences of the failure to prevent emotional and behavioral disorders, including mental health/substance abuse, school failure and dropout, and involvement in the justice system; (2) discusses the role of researchers and policymakers in determining how the United States treats children and adolescents with EBD, and the need to inform policy with research; (3) describes research on effective prevention, with a special emphasis on cost analysis; and (4) synthesizes the salient costs of inaction or inadequate prevention.

The Potential Consequences of Inaction or Inadequate Intervention

Mental Health/Substance Abuse

Research supports the notion that children and adolescents with mental health problems that are left un- or underaddressed will face lifelong difficulties. Research has found that a significant number of children with conduct disorder have other psychiatric and medical problems when they are adults. These problems contribute to unemployment, broken marriages, criminality, and imprisonment. Other studies have linked childhood mental problems with schizophrenia (Hollis, 1995), hyperactivity (Klein & Slomkowski, 1993), obsessional disorders (Rapoport, Swedo, & Leonard, 1994), depression, and higher use of health services as adults (Harrington, Fudge, Rutter, Pickles, & Hill, 1990).

Self-reports of adults who were identified as having antisocial behavior that went untreated show that they tend to punish their children physically (Patterson, Reid, & Dishion, 1992). "They inflict pain, misery, and sorrow on the people who are close to them. They tend to have low self-esteem and rely increasingly on drugs and alcohol to fill the gaps in their lives" (Patterson et al., 1992, p. 25). Others have also found that many adolescents with EBD will have problems with drug abuse (Wagner, Blackorby, Cameto, & Newman, 1993).

Education

In educational settings in the United States, a diagnosis of emotional or behavioral disorders is based on the functional impairment of the disability on the student's academic performance. "Emotional disturbance" is defined in the Individuals with Disabilities Education Act (IDEA) as a condition exhibiting one or more of various characteristics over a long period of time and to a marked degree that adversely affects a child's educational performance. These characteristics may include, among others, an inability to learn that cannot be explained by intellectual, sensory, or health factors; an inability to build or maintain satisfactory interpersonal relationships with peers and teachers; or a general pervasive mood of unhappiness or depression (C.F.R. 300.7 [a] 9). According to the 23rd Annual Report to Congress on the Implementation of IDEA (U.S. Department of Education, 2001), approximately 0.74% of children and adolescents between the ages of 3 and 21 are served under the emotional disturbance category. However, the Methodology for Epidemiology of Mental Disorders in Children and Adolescents (MECA) Study puts the prevalence of diagnosable mental or addictive disorders that cause extreme functional impairment among 9- to 17-year-olds in the United States at about 5%. In addition, about 11% of these children have significant functional impairments, and almost 21% are at least minimally impaired by diagnosable mental or addictive disorders (Shaffer et al., 1996).

Although less than 1% of adolescents in the United States are receiving services for emotional disturbance from education agencies, research has shown, surprisingly, that education agencies are the mental health provider for these children and adolescents more often than are specialists in mental health agencies (Burns et al., 1995). Again, the MECA study found that education agencies provided mental health services for 11% of children and adolescents, while the health sector (including general medicine as well as mental health services) serviced only 9% (Shaffer et al., 1996).

Alarming statistics describe the educational future of students categorized as having emotional disturbance. Research has shown that about 50% of these students will drop out of school (Wagner et al., 1991). The lack of a high school diploma may also be the reason that most students with EBD are likely to have multiple short-term jobs during their lives (Wagner, D'Amico, Marder, Newman, & Balckorby, 1992). This erratic employment profile means that these students will earn less than students categorized in any other disability category (Frank & Sitlington, 1997).

Juvenile Justice

Research also has shown that children and adolescents with EBD are at a greater risk for involvement in the juvenile justice system; within 3 years of dropping out of school, approximately 70% of students with EBD are arrested (Jay & Padilla, 1987). This contributes to the overrepresentation of children and adolescents with disabilities, especially those with EBD, involved in the juvenile justice system. To study this issue, the Center for Effective Collaboration and Practice (CECP) at the American Institutes for Research (AIR) and the National Center on Education, Disability, and Juvenile Justice (EDJJ) recently completed a national survey of juvenile detention facilities and state departments of juvenile corrections to investigate the prevalence of children and adolescents with disabilities in these settings. The CECP/EDJJ survey found that those with specific learning disabilities (SLD) and emotional disturbance (ED) were overrepresented in both detention facilities and correctional systems (Quinn, Rutherford, Leone, Osher, & Poirier, in press). Sixty-four percent of detention facilities responded and indicated that approximately 8% of all children and adolescents in these facilities, which account for 42% of those eligible for special education and related services as mandated by IDEA, had SLD as a primary disability. Another 8% of the total number of detained children and adolescents, accounting for 40% of those eligible for services under IDEA, had ED. Similarly, 71% of state departments of juvenile corrections responded to the survey and indicated that about 12% of all incarcerated adolecents, which accounted for 49% of adolescents, eligible for services under IDEA, had ED. Nine percent of the total number of incarcerated adolescents in juvenile corrections,

accounting for 36% of adolescents eligible for services under IDEA, had SLD as a primary disability. This raises two critical issues: first, the prevalence of students identified as eligible for special education and related services in detention and correctional facilities is approximately four times that of the general population, and second, the proportion of students with disabilities that have a primary disability of ED is eight times higher in detention and correctional facilities than in the general school-age population.

Researchers have identified four primary theories to explain how disability affects the tendency toward delinquent behavior. *School failure theory* (Murray, 1977; Post, 1981) states that delinquent behavior is a secondary result of disability: disability leads to school failure, subsequently causing a negative self-image. This poor sense of self, in turn, contributes to behavior that precipitates school suspension and dropout (or push-out, as some believe). This tends to provide the adolescent with unstructured and unsupervised time because he or she is not in school and lacks the skills (and high school diploma) to secure meaningful employment. This, it is believed, is a prime breeding ground for delinquent behavior because these adolescents are likely to spend their free time with peers who also have dropped out of school and are unemployed. Research has shown a correlation between school failure, early onset of delinquent behavior, substance abuse, and serious and chronic juvenile offending (Schumacher & Kurz, 2000).

Disability → School →
                failure

          → Negative → Suspension
             self-image   Dropout
                           Delinquency

According to *susceptibility theory* (Keilitz & Dunivant, 1987; Murray, 1977), delinquency stems from behaviors that are a direct result of the defining characteristics of the disability. These characteristics (e.g., personality traits, cognitive deficits) lead to a lack of impulse control, suggestibility, and poor perceptions of social cues, which in turn put these children and adolescents at greater risk for delinquent behavior.

Disability → Personality → traits/ cognitive deficits

→ Poor impulse → Delinquency control

Suggestibility

Poor perception of social cues

Metacognitive deficits theory (Larson, 1988; Larson & Turner, 2002) states that, as a result of the disability, the student lacks the interpersonal skills necessary to build relationships with his or her peers. To gain social status, these students engage in behaviors to impress their peers. Unfortunately, many of these behaviors are delinquent.

Disability → Poor interpersonal → skills

Attempts to gain social status

→ Delinquent acts

Differential treatment theory (Keilitz & Dunivant, 1987; Leone & Meisel, 1997) holds that adolescents with disabilities commit as many delinquent acts as adolescents without disabilities. However, because of certain personality traits that result from the disability, these adolescents frustrate justice personnel (including arresting officers, judges and other court personnel, and corrections staff) and behave in ways that may potentially result in miscommunication with these personnel. This may result in the adolescents with disabilities receiving harsher treatment such as higher incarceration rates, longer sentences, or higher rates of transfer from juvenile to criminal court than their peers without disabilities.

Average → Personality → levels of traits delinquent impact behavior justice personnel

→ Differential → Overrepresentation treatment

Summary

The theories discussed here elucidate how disability is a factor in delinquent behavior or in differential treatment within the juvenile justice system. This raises serious concerns about the need for prevention and treatment, and raises questions about the implications of the failure to prevent EBD and the costs of such failure. Based on research, we know that adolescents with EBD are likely to have higher incidence of mental health and substance abuse, school failure and dropout, and involvement in the justice system. Because of different terminologies and measurements across the mental health, education, and juvenile justice fields, comparisons of data at the level of adolescents with EBD is difficult. In addition, because agencies do not disaggregate their data to the level of age and disability category, generalizations of data to adolescents with EBD are not feasible. Given such constraints, we present in this chapter available data to illustrate the potential costs across these areas where negative outcomes emerge. We first begin with mental health/substance abuse, followed by school failure and dropout and finally delinquency.

IMPLICATIONS OF EBD: WHY PREVENT?

Mental Health/Substance Abuse

Estimates of the number of children in the United States who are in need of mental health services vary widely. Padgett, Patrick, Burns, Schlesinger, and Cohen (1993) estimate a prevalence rate of between 5 and 22%; Brandenburg, Friedman, and Silver (1990) report an estimate ranging from 14 to 20%; and Costello (1989) estimates a rate of between 17 and 22% needing mental health services. Although many of the estimates are dated, a more important implication of the validity of these estimates is that, because of improvements in epidemiological techniques (Knapp, 1997), the number of children and adolescents identified as needing mental health service is rising (Friedman & Kutash, 1992).

In tandem with issues of underidentification are issues of underservice. Costello and colleagues (Costello, Burns, Argold, & Leaf, 1993) argue that community studies reveal that this population of children and adolescents are underserved. They state that approximately 20% of children have a DSM disorder while 10% have a mental health disorder that significantly impairs functioning. However, only 5% of children receive care for mental health problems.

Perhaps the main reason that children and adolescents in need of mental health services often "slip through the cracks" is the reality that there is no strategic plan for identifying and providing services to them. One attempt to address this problem was presented by the Health Advisory Service (1995) of the United Kingdom, which recommended a four-tiered approach to the identification and service of children and adolescents in need of mental health services. The first tier involves professionals whose primary role is not mental health (e.g., social workers, teachers, police officers, primary-care doctors) but, because of their interactions with children and adolescents, are in a prime position to make referrals to the second tier. The second tier involves professionals who work with children and adolescents and their families on a peripatetically or specialty basis (e.g., school psychologists, specialty social workers, mental health professionals). The third tier offers a multidisciplinary team treatment approach (e.g., wraparound, systems of care) for those children and adolescents who are in need of more specialized and intensive services. Finally, the fourth tier is available to those children and adolescents who need very specialized care (e.g., inpatient care).

Although this is an excellent strategic plan, it is rarely the reality in the United States, where Matthews (1991) observed that the levels of service provision are more likely to be categorized as follows:

- Negligence—a lack of services or the provision of inadequate services because of a failure to recognize need.
- Skimping—the provision of inadequate services as an intentional attempt to save money.
- Supplier-induced demand—the provision of unnecessary services because of the service-providers' attempt to make money.
- Indulgence—the provision of too many or inappropriate services that are not supported by professionals but are provided because of the demands of the child or family member.

Unfortunately, as discussed above, mental health services for children and adolescents often fall into the negligence categories. This may be a direct result of a lack of a strategic plan for identifying children and adolescents in need. Further, skimping may occur because the services received, and often the prices paid for those services, are driven by the insurance reimbursement system (McGuire, 1989). Therefore, the real need for mental health services and the extent of the population that could benefit from those services is difficult to determine. Given the problems with negligence and skimping, and the determination by insurance companies of what constitutes allowable services, any attempt to determine the real cost of mental health problems would be a conservative estimate.

One symptom of mental health problems that is particularly relevant in this discussion of adolescents with EBD is substance abuse. Longitudinal research suggests that, if mental health issues are untreated, these adolescents are at heightened risk for drug and alcohol abuse (Caspi et al., 1987). While we are uncertain about the exact prevalence of adolescents with EBD who abuse substances, we do have such estimates for adolescents ages 12–17 overall from the 2002 National Survey on Drug Use and Health conducted by the U.S. Department of Health and Human Services, which found that 11.6% of adolescents ages 12–17 were current illicit drug users[1] in 2001 (DHHS, 2003). This survey also found that 17.6% of adolescents in this age group used alcohol during the month prior to the survey interview, and that almost 11% were binge drinkers and 2.5% were heavy drinkers. Arguably the percentage of adolescents with

EBD who abuse substances is likely to be greater than the percentage of adolescents without EBD, but further research is needed. Regardless, both mental health and substance abuse yield significant costs, which are now discussed.

Costs

Mental health services are funded through a variety of means. A few patients are seen in what economists call the "nonmarket" sector. These include psychiatric services provided by the Veterans Administration (adults only) or public mental health hospitals. The patients themselves pay for most services through private insurance, Medicare, or Medicaid (McGuire, 1989). Federal, state, and local governments provide mental health services as well. Of all contributions made by the government, the federal level shoulders the major burden at 59.5% (e.g., Medicare, Medicaid, Title XX, public housing), while states fund 37.8% through direct allocations and Medicaid, and the local level funds about 2.7% of mental health services (Goldman, 1987).

Economists break down the costs of having mental health disorders into direct and indirect costs. For those identified and treated, direct costs include expenditures such as hospitalization, outpatient treatment, and psychopharmaceuticals. Indirect costs include lost productivity, disability payments, housing and food subsidies, social services, and police services. These are important costs to consider when examining the implications of EBD. It is estimated that the United States paid more than $99 billion (in 1990 dollars) on direct costs for treatment of those with mental disorders, with approximately half of that spent on 15–20% of patients (Mark, McKusick, King, Harwood, & Genuardi, 1998). Less than 5% of patients with chronic mental illness consume some 37% of all resources. Of those having chronic mental illness, approximately 57% ($4.2 billion) is spent on specialty services, 34% ($2.5 billion) on general medical providers, and 9% ($670 million) on human service agencies. Goldman (1987) estimates that another $3.7 billion is used in indirect costs to support people with chronic mental illness. These figures are dated, and the costs of mental health care have risen since Goldman calcu-

lated his estimates. In fact, from 1982 to 1995, costs for mental health care rose from 6 to 15% of the nation's spending on all health care (Staton, 1989), and by 1998 more than 3% ($19.3 billion) of state revenues alone were spent on mental health programs and programs for the developmentally disabled (National Center on Addiction and Substance Abuse at Columbia University, [CASA], 2001) (see Table 5.1). Mental health-related costs consume from less than 1% of state budgets in 6 states to between 4 and 12% of 11 state budgets (CASA, 2001).[2]

Service providers may indicate that the best way to reduce the indirect costs of mental illness would be to increase spending on direct costs. Goldman (1987) argues that the phenomenon of diminishing returns disputes the efficiency of this approach. He states that at some point investing in direct services will not have as great an impact on the costs as it initially does. For this reason, he postulates that, to be truly efficient (i.e., provide the best services possible within a given budget), society will have to tolerate some symptomology in some children and adolescents. The real question, then, is: What are the most beneficial investments? (That is, where should we invest to make the greatest amount of change, over the greatest population, for the least amount of money? This question can be answered through cost–benefit analysis. Unfortunately, much work needs to be done before there can be a comprehensive evaluation of interventions. As Bickman and colleagues (1996) indicate in their evaluation of mental health care at Fort Bragg, research and data are needed to determine the cost-effectiveness of interventions, but these are currently lacking. The importance of these evaluative data cannot be overstated. Without this information, policymakers and insurance companies are left to make decisions on mental health services based on initial costs only.

Although evaluative data are important, such data are not always easy to acquire. Whatever the problems associated with the collection and analysis of these data, we must not let ourselves become "pennywise and pound foolish." We must keep in mind the findings of Light and Bailey (1993): "Nine-tenths of these disturbed and abused children will run up large costs as they stum-

TABLE 5.1. Total State Expenditures and Type of Expenditure as a Percent of Total Expenditures

	Total state expenditures (in millions)	Juvenile justice	Adult corrections/ judiciary	Mental health/ developmentally disabled	Spending related to substance abuse[a]
Alabama	$9,178	0.7%	3.2%	2.0%	13.0%
Alaska	$3,291	0.0%	4.7%	2.2%	9.8%
Arizona	$9,683	0.7%	5.7%	2.1%	9.6%
Arkansas	$6,658	0.5%	3.1%	1.4%	7.8%
California	$68,483	0.6%	6.7%	2.1%	16.0%
Colorado	$6,821	N/A[b]	6.8%	1.8%	12.4%
Connecticut	$11,428	0.2%	3.4%	0.1%	7.6%
Delaware	$3,604	0.1%	4.4%	3.1%	10.2%
Florida	$32,568	1.5%	4.8%	0.9%	9.7%
Georgia	$16,205	N/A	4.3%	3.1%	9.7%
Hawaii	$5,100	0.1%	3.4%	2.6%	8.6%
Idaho	$2,188	1.5%	4.1%	2.3%	10.8%
Illinois	$22,727	0.4%	3.5%	3.5%	12.6%
Indiana	N/A[b]	N/A	N/A	N/A	N/A
Iowa	$7,810	0.5%	4.1%	2.1%	9.4%
Kansas	$6,208	0.9%	3.1%	4.1%	9.4%
Kentucky	$10,216	0.5%	2.6%	2.4%	9.4%
Louisiana	$10,533	0.8%	4.1%	1.7%	10.1%
Maine	N/A	N/A	N/A	N/A	N/A
Maryland	$12,260	0.9%	4.7%	5.2%	10.5%
Massachusetts	$15,517	0.1%	6.1%	9.9%	17.4%
Michigan	$22,460	0.1%	6.0%	0.5%	12.3%
Minnesota	$12,848	0.2%	1.6%	2.0%	8.1%
Mississippi	$5,196	N/A[b]	4.0%	4.0%	9.4%
Missouri	$10,599	0.5%	7.7%	4.9%	12.9%
Montana	$1,665	1.1%	4.3%	12.1%	15.4%
Nebraska	$3,560	0.4%	2.1%	3.2%	8.2%
Nevada	$5,195	0.3%	4.2%	1.9%	9.1%
New Hampshire	N/A	N/A	N/A	N/A	N/A
New Jersey	$19,577	0.3%	4.8%	4.9%	10.4%
New Mexico	$4,683	1.0%	3.4%	2.3%	10.0%
New York	$48,243	0.6%	7.7%	3.3%	18.0%
North Carolina	N/A	N/A	N/A	N/A	N/A
North Dakota	$1,218	0.4%	1.3%	4.6%	8.1%
Ohio	$28,518	0.8%	5.2%	5.5%	10.3%
Oklahoma	$6,709	1.1%	5.5%	3.5%	10.5%
Oregon	$10,010	0.6%	4.6%	3.4%	9.0%
Pennsylvania	$24,237	0.4%	5.5%	5.5%	14.5%
Rhode Island	$2,643	0.9%	5.1%	3.9%	11.3%
South Carolina	$9,046	1.0%	1.1%	0.5%	6.6%
South Dakota	$1,183	1.0%	3.9%	4.3%	10.9%
Tennessee	$9,310	0.6%	4.3%	0.8%	10.0%
Texas	N/A	N/A	N/A	N/A	N/A
Utah	$4,293	1.1%	5.0%	1.9%	11.6%
Vermont	$1,098	0.2%	4.8%	3.9%	12.3%
Virginia	$15,315	1.4%	6.3%	4.9%	11.7%
Washington	$13,874	0.7%	2.8%	3.4%	10.9%
West Virginia	$3,229	0.2%	1.8%	0.4%	10.5%
Wisconsin	$15,028	0.7%	3.8%	1.4%	9.5%
Wyoming	$1,486	1.1%	2.7%	1.1%	7.8%

Note. Data from National Center on Addiction and Substance Abuse at Columbia University (CASA, 2001).

[a] Costs related to substance abuse are part of the state expenditures on juvenile justice, adult corrections/judiciary, and mental health/developmentally disabled programs.

[b] N/A indicates data not provided by states.

ble through school and work" and face difficulty creating their own families (p. 18). Clearly, we must address the social costs to the families of mentally ill parents, who experience more problems with obstetric complications; divorce and separation; productivity, absenteeism, and unemployment; poor educational attainment; truancy and delinquency of their children; an increased need for special health, social care, and educational services; and an increased need for informal care, including care by their own children (Cox, 1994; Gopfert, Webster, & Seemen, 1995).

Unfortunately, there is a dearth of research on substance abuse prevention since it is a relatively new field. As Woodward (1998) argues, research on the cost-effectiveness of substance abuse prevention is needed to persuade policymakers that effective substance abuse prevention is a sensible investment. Regardless, we do know that substance abuse is costly.

In fact, "every sector of society spends hefty sums of money shoveling up the wreckage of substance abuse and addiction" (CASA, 2001, p. i). In a comprehensive study of state spending on substance abuse, CASA found that, of the $620 billion spent in 1998 by 45 states, the District of Columbia, and Puerto Rico, more than 13% ($81.3 billion) was spent, in total, on substance abuse and addiction. Of the latter amount, only 3.7% was invested in prevention, treatment, and research intended to reduce the incidence of substance abuse and its consequences, while the remainder was spent on the burden of substance abuse on public programs such as education, the mental health system, and the criminal/juvenile justice system. Further, states spent approximately $24.9 billion in 1998 on the costs of substance abuse to children, with less than 9% of this amount invested in prevention or treatment. These costs do not include federal or local spending on substance abuse, or the human costs of substance abuse—such as the impact on the individuals and their families.

Various state agencies incur the costs of substance abuse. CASA (2001) found that in 1998 states spent $39.7 billion on justice programs, of which 77% was related to substance abuse. States also spent $4.4 billion on juvenile justice-related costs (i.e., deten-

tion and corrections), of which about two-thirds was spent on adolescent substance abusers. Substance abuse also impacts state education budgets, of which about 10% of the $165 billion states spent on elementary and secondary education in 1998 was used to deal with adolescents who abused substances, as well as state mental health budgets, of which more than one-fourth of the $60.4 billion spent by states for health care in 1998 was used for substance abuse-related costs (CASA, 2001).

The costs of substance abuse to states is significant—not to mention federal and local governments as well as individuals themselves. Adolescents with EBD are vulnerable to substance use, but effective treatment and prevention has a role in diminishing the number of adolescents who experience EBD and substance abuse. While we have no direct data on the costs for the treatment of adolescents with EBD and co-occurring substance abuse issues, we can only infer that because substance abuse itself is a costly problem as a whole that it is also costly in the case of adolescents with EBD.

Education

In addition to mental health and substance abuse-related problems, adolescents with EBD are five times more likely to drop out of school than are students in the general population. According to the National Center for Educational Statistics, 10.7% of students between the ages of 16 and 24 in 2001 dropped out of school in the United States (U.S. Department of Education, National Center for Educational Statistics, 2003, Table 108). In contrast, during the 1999–2000 school year, more than half (51.4%) of students with emotional and behavioral disorders dropped out (U.S. Department of Education, 2001). Further, of all the disability categories, students with EBD have the highest dropout rate. This is particularly salient from an economic perspective since dropping out of high school is costly for individuals who do not earn a diploma, as well as their families, communities, and society.

More costly than a good education is a poor one. Nobody epitomizes this reality more than adolescents who have untreated or "undertreated" EBD. Indeed, research has shown that dropping out of high school is costly not only to the individuals who do not earn a diploma but also in terms of adverse consequences, to their families, communities, and society as well. Research also has shown that most dropouts have difficulty finding and keeping meaningful employment that can enable them to rise above dependence on public assistance (Rumberger & Lamb, 2003). Unemployment rates for high school dropouts in 2001 were 60% higher than for graduates (U.S. Department of Education, 2003, Table 380). Further, when dropouts *are* employed, they earn less than graduates, with one-third earning less than the official poverty rate (U.S. Bureau of the Census, 1992). High school dropouts also engage in more criminal activities and are more dependent on welfare than graduates (Rumberger, 1987). One study found that in one U.S. city alone dropouts cost over $3.2 billion in lost earnings and more than $400 million in social services in 1 year (Catterall, 1987).

Paradoxically, attempts to make schools more accountable for students who fail or drop out are likely to worsen this costly problem rather than improve it (National Research Council, 1999). This movement, which has brought about policies that reduce "social" promotion and require exit exams for graduation, are likely to increase the number of students who give up trying to earn a diploma or who decide to earn an alternative exit credential instead. In fact, the number of students earning such credentials (e.g., GED) has already increased (U.S. Department of Education, 2000, Table 6); unfortunately, these high school equivalency credentials do not greatly improve an individual's economic prospects (Cameron & Heckman, 1993; Murnane, Willett, & Boudett, 1995, 1997; Murnane, Willett, & Tyler, 2000; Rumberger & Lamb, 2003; Tyler, Murnane, & Willett, 2000). The lack of a high school diploma—or even substituting an alternative credential for a diploma—consequently makes the future for adolescents and young adults with EBD bleak and costly for themselves and society.

Juvenile Justice

Educational problems (such as EBD), for reasons that are not entirely clear, greatly impact an adolescent's propensity for involvement in the juvenile justice system. In fact, research has shown that adolescents with EBD are disproportionately involved in the justice system (Jay & Padilla, 1987; Quinn et al., in press; Rutherford, Bullis, Anderson, & Griller-Clark, 2002), and therefore juvenile delinquency is a potential outcome when EBD is not prevented. School failure, susceptibility to dropping out, and metacognitive deficits all increase the likelihood of delinquency. Therefore, it is important to treat the human and monetary costs of delinquency as a significant consequence of not preventing EBD.

Although total violent crime has remained relatively static over the past 20 years, violent juvenile crime has increased significantly (Sprague & Walker, 2000). Juveniles are defined as adolescents at or below the oldest age[3] at which a juvenile court has original jurisdiction over the individual for law violating behavior. In 2001, juveniles were involved in about 1 in 10 arrests for murder, 1 in 8 arrests for a drug abuse violation, and 1 in 3 arrests for larceny-theft, burglary, or motor vehicle theft (Snyder, 2003). The Bureau of Justice Statistics reports that the juvenile contribution to overall crime has declined; however, "The relative responsibility of juveniles and adults for crime is hard to determine [because] research has shown that crimes committed by juveniles are more likely to be cleared by law enforcement than are crimes by adults . . . [which] is likely to give a high estimate of the juvenile responsibility for crime" (Snyder, 2002, p. 10). In other words, because many juvenile crimes are cleared before they actually go to trial, some are not counted in the overall breakdown between the juvenile and adult proportion of crime. This makes estimates of the actual rate of juvenile crime difficult to determine.

Juvenile crime, however, is a reality, and it is important to examine the extent of this problem. According to the U.S. Department of Justice, there were 1.757 million delinquency cases[4] in juvenile courts in 1998, which represents a 44% increase since 1989 (Stahl, 2001). Of the more than 1 million cases brought before judges in 1998, juveniles were adjudicated (i.e., found guilty for a delinquent act) in 63% of these cases. Of those adjudicated, 26%, or 163,800 juveniles, were placed in residential facilities (Stahl, 2001).

Between 1992 and 2001, the number of juvenile arrests decreased by 3%, but in 2001, there were still 2.3 million juvenile arrests (those under the age of 18), and juveniles accounted for anywhere from 1 (driving under the influence of substances) to 49% (arson) of all arrests for various types of crime[5] (see Table 5.2) (Snyder, 2003). In a study designed to examine the extent of juvenile violent crime in Pennsylvania, researchers found juveniles were responsible for 25% of the 377,000 estimated violent crimes in that state (Miller, Fisher, & Cohen, 2001). This finding is supported by government statistics that indicate juveniles were involved in, on average, 25% of serious violent victimizations each year between 1973 and 1997 (U. S. Department of Justice, 1999b).

The Costs of Juvenile Delinquency and a Lifetime of Crime

Data disaggregating the costs of crime by adult and juvenile offenders are not available. However, one can cautiously infer these costs. If total government expenditures for criminal and civil justice were $147 billion in 1999 (Gifford, 2002) and juveniles accounted for 17% of all arrests (see Table 5.2), an estimate of the portion of costs attributable to juvenile crime would be about $25 billion.

However, it is possible to estimate the direct costs to victims due to juvenile crime using two sources of extant data: the total estimated direct costs of certain types of crime and the proportion of total crime attributed to juveniles. Using this approach, an estimated $396.5 million (in 1992 dollars) was lost in 2000 because of juvenile crime (see Table 5.3). In addition, researchers and policymakers must also consider the nonmonetary loss attributable to juvenile crime (e.g., pain and suffering). Although these estimates are not available, the extent of economic loss resulting from juvenile crime is clearly significant. For example, the Pennsylvania study also looked at the costs of juvenile violent crime and estimated the victim costs of juvenile violence in that state to be $2.6 billion (Miller, Fisher, & Cohen, 2001). It is important to recognize when examining these costs that we do not know whether delinquent acts committed by adolescents with EBD are more or less serious, or more or less costly, than those committed by adolescents without EBD. This is a question that deserves further study.

Juveniles who continue into a lifetime of crime as an adult, that is, chronic juvenile offenders, represent a significant cost. To

TABLE 5.2. Number of Juvenile Arrests, 2001; Percent Change in Number of Arrests, 1992–2001, and Juvenile Arrests as a Percentage of Total Arrests, 2001

Type of arrest	Number of juvenile arrests in 2001	Percent change in number of arrests, 1992–2001	Juvenile arrests as a percentage of total arrests, 2001
Total	2,273,500	–3%	17%[a]
Murder and nonnegligent manslaughter	1,400	–62%	10%
Forcible rape	4,600	–24%	17%[a]
Robbery	25,600	–32%	24%
Aggravated assault and other assaults	64,900, aggravated 239,000, other	–14% aggravated 30%, other	14%, aggravated 18%, other
Larceny-theft	343,600	–27%	30%
Burglary	90,300	–40%	31%
Motor vehicle theft	48,200	–51%	33%
Stolen property	26,800	–45%	22%

Note. Data from Snyder (2003) and U.S. Department of Justice (1994).

[a] These indicate the percentage of crimes cleared by juvenile arrests, rather than juvenile arrests as a percentage of total arrests.

TABLE 5.3. Estimated Direct Costs to Crime Victims Due to
Juvenile Crime, in 1992 Dollars

Selected crimes	Estimated direct costs[a]
Forcible rape	$1.1 million
Robbery	$14.2 million
Aggravated and other assaults	$37.7 million
Larceny-theft	$75.9 million
Burglary	$75.3 million
Motor vehicle theft	$192.3 million

Note. Data from U.S. Department of Justice (1994) and Snyder (2003).

[a] The monetary loss is calculated using the 1992 mean loss per crime
and the number of juvenile arrests in 2001; this is only an estimate of the
monetary loss due to juvenile crime. These costs include loss from property theft or damage, cash losses, medical expenses, and amount of pay
lost because of injury or activities related to the crime. Many types of juvenile arrests are not included (e.g., fraud, arson, vandalism) due to limited data on victim costs of these crimes.

calculate the average cost of a criminal career, Cohen (1998) uses a formula that includes the mean number of offenses, victim
costs, criminal justice and incarceration
costs, average number of days served, and
opportunity costs of the offender's time in a
given year. A juvenile career of crime assumes one to four offenses[6] per year and a
criminal career of 4 years. Using this methodology, Cohen estimates the average costs
of juvenile delinquency of adolescents ages
14–17 to be between $83,000 and $335,000,
about a quarter of which is criminal justice
costs (see Table 5.4). For those juvenile offenders who become adult offenders, the total estimated cost to society of a lifetime of
crime is estimated at $1.5–$1.8 million (Cohen, 1998).

Summary

The key objectives in this section are to support the claim that the costs of mental health
and substance abuse problems, school failure and dropout, and delinquency and criminality should be examined when building
support for policies intended to prevent EBD
and their co-occurring symptomologies. It
should be carefully noted, though, that we
have not provided evidence that adolescents
with EBD would be less symptomatic even if
their disability were prevented. This is another area that requires further study.

LINKING PREVENTION RESEARCH AND POLICY CHANGE

Research on the costs of EBD and its co-
occurring symptomologies can be used to
buttress support for EBD prevention policy.
Traditionally, the funding of prevention programs has been a battle between social scientists, who champion efforts to fund programs that are more effective for children
and adolescents, and policymakers, who
have an obligation to those they are elected
to represent to be circumspect and efficient
with public funds. As with many investments, though, funding for the research and
implementation of prevention interventions
might save money from different "pots"
(e.g., education funding may save future dollars spent on juvenile justice) and then may
not yield returns for several decades—long
after the policymaker has left office.

The nature of politics often makes the
funding of many prevention programs impossible. Policymakers must be *socially* responsive to the desires of voters and interest
groups even if that means funding what the
public "thinks" it wants rather than what
the public really needs. Currently, the public
agenda in the United States has been to "get
tough on crime." Unfortunately, with the
growing popularity of reporting violence in
the media, news agencies have convinced the
American public that crime and violence are
a major problem in the United States (Quinn,

TABLE 5.4. Lifetime Cost of a Career Criminal, in 1997 Dollars

Cost category	Total costs[a]
Juvenile career	
Victim costs	$62,000–$250,000
Criminal justice costs	$21,000–$84,000
Total juvenile career costs	$83,000–$335,000
Adult career	
Victim costs	$1,000,000
Criminal justice costs	$335,000
Lost offender productivity	$64,000
Total adult career costs	$1,400,000
Adult and juvenile career combined	
Total juvenile and adult career costs	$1.5–$1.8 million

Note. Data from Cohen (1998).

[a]According to Cohen (1998), the low end of this range is based on actual convictions while the other is based on self-reports.

2000). In response, the American public has demanded that policymakers address this issue with a legislative agenda that includes punitive policies such as "three strikes, you're out," boot camps, and "zero tolerance." This myopic response to the media's and the public's dogmatic overemphasis on violence inhibits the provision of coordinated and effective services for children and adolescents with or at risk of developing EBD.

In addition to being responsive to public demands, policymakers must be *fiscally* responsive to the taxpayers (i.e., tax-paying "voters"). When fiscal resources are tightest, however, it is the programs with the most distant payoffs, such as prevention treatments, that are the most vulnerable to not being funded during the appropriations process. This leads to policies that often appear inexpensive, at least in the immediate future, because the term limits of most state policymakers in the United States are relatively short (2–6 years). This encourages a policy cycle in which programs are funded because they are both inexpensive and perceived as tough on crime rather than because of their long-term benefits (e.g., reduced recidivism, fewer victims) and savings to society (i.e., reduced costs owing to fewer crimes). This is problematic.

Because of these social and fiscal pressures on policymakers, the public often funds programs that they think will work rather than

what is really best. One clear example is the current public interest in boot camps for delinquent adolescents. At first glance, boot camps meet both the requirements of getting tough on crime and of being less expensive than alternatives. However, research on boot camps using random-assignment evaluations has shown that they are ineffective at reducing juvenile (and adult) recidivism at best and may even increase the likelihood that participants will recidivate (Parent, 2003). When the taxpayer and victim costs of higher recidivism rates are considered, boot camps are costly in comparison to less punitive alternatives (Aos, Phipps, Barnoski, & Lieb, 2001).

Aligning Policy with Research

CASA (2001) argues that the government must adopt strategies to prevent and reduce rather than just manage substance abuse. On a similar note, the government should also implement policy that prevents rather than manages EBD and its co-occurring symptomologies. Two issues must be addressed before social scientists are able to improve policymakers' and the public's confidence in the argument that prevention works. First, scientific-based evidence must be used to show that these programs are effective. Policymakers must be convinced that treatment programs that are not perceived as tough on criminals will indeed be tough on crime. Further, taxpayers must be confident that prevention dollars invested today are invested *wisely* and will ultimately yield a greater benefit than if those same dollars were merely "managing symptomologies."

This is where "pure" science must meet reality. If social scientists really want research to make a difference, they must move from a mindset of "research for the sake of research," through "research to practice," and to "research to change policy." Because policymakers are often left to examine all alternatives for scarce resources, we must employ a methodology that allows them to make more informed decisions—one such framework is *cost analysis*. As Levin and McEwan (2001, p. 3) point out, "Policy decisions in the public sector must be based increasingly upon a demonstrated consideration of both the cost and effects of such decisions."

Paradoxically, the argument to increase the rigor of research so that it more effectively informs policy change may be aided by a change in federal policy that encourages more rigorous research. The No Child Left Behind Act of 2001 legislated the federal policymakers' preference for educational programs and practices based on rigorous scientific evidence. In fact, one of the four major pillars of the legislation, focusing on what works, requires federally supported programs to use effective methods and instructional strategies grounded in scientifically based research. Fortunately, several federal offices have supported the evaluation of prevention programs to identify those with evidence of their effectiveness.

PREVENTION RESEARCH: IDENTIFYING EFFECTIVE PROGRAMS

Although there currently have been no attempts to create a database of scientifically based programs that specifically address EBD, programs that address behaviors pertinent to the educational, mental health/substance abuse, and delinquency needs of students with EBD have been identified. In particular, the U.S. Departments of Health and Human Services, Education, and Justice have each invested in the identification and recognition of effective scientifically based programs.

Mental Health/Substance Abuse

The U.S. Surgeon General released a 1999 report on mental health and mental illness. A collaborative effort by the Substance Abuse and Mental Health Services Administration and the National Institute of Mental Health, two federal agencies, this report examined more than 3,000 research articles and firsthand experiences of mental health providers and consumers. The report suggests several broad courses of action that should be addressed by researchers. These include:

- Continue to build a science base.
- Overcome stigma.
- Improve public awareness of effective treatment.
- Ensure the supply of mental health services and providers.
- Ensure delivery of state-of-the-art treatments.
- Tailor treatment to age, gender, race, and culture.
- Facilitate entry into treatment.
- Reduce financial barriers to treatment.

In addition to these considerations, the report establishes criteria for categorizing interventions and treatments as well established: "For a psychotherapy to be well established, at least two experiments with group designs or similar types of studies must have been published to demonstrate efficacy" (U.S. Department of Health and Human Services, 1999, p. 11). Further, the authors recognize the use of meta-analysis as a way of combining and evaluating the results of several studies to statistically determine the significant effects of treatments. The U.S. Department of Education also examined the need for evidence-based treatment.

Education

In response to the Education, Research, Development, Dissemination, and Improvement Act of 1994, the Office of Safe and Drug-Free Schools at the U.S. Department of Education set up a 15-member expert panel to review 124 recommended programs designed to reduce adolescent violence and substance abuse. The U.S. Department of

Education directed the panels to review the programs and determine if there were "empirical data to demonstrate that the program was effective and should be designated as exemplary or . . . whether there was sufficient evidence to demonstrate that the program showed promise for improving student achievement and should be designated as promising" (U.S. Department of Education, 2001, p. 1). The expert panel excluded pre- and postdesigns that did not include comparison groups as well as posttest only comparison studies that did not include randomization or some other effort to control for threats to internal validity and case studies that did not include comparison groups (U.S. Department of Education, 2002). The panel identified 9 programs as exemplary and 33 as promising. Although there are no ongoing efforts to update the list, the programs and any potential updates can be located through the U.S. Department of Education's website at *http://www.ed.gov.*

Juvenile Justice

The Office of Juvenile Justice and Delinquency Prevention of the U.S. Department of Justice supports the Center for the Study and Prevention of Violence at the University of Colorado at Boulder in identifying research-based violence and drug prevention programs. Designated as Model or Promising, these Blueprint Programs are subjected to rigorous scientific evaluation. Through a strong research design, each nominated program must show evidence that it has a deterrent effect. The seven-member advisory board prefers evaluation studies that include random assignment but will consider studies that use control groups that are matched on relevant characteristics or studies that use control groups and statistical techniques to control for initial differences on key variables. Nominated programs also must show sustainability of effects, multiple site replication, analysis of mediating factors that may change the violent behavior, and proof that the program's expected benefits are greater than its costs. To date over 600 programs have been reviewed, and only 11 have been designated as Model Blueprint Programs and another 21 as Promising Programs. The list of Model and Promising Practices is up-

dated as new research is completed and is available at *www. colorado.edu/cspv/.*

Summary

As a nation, we are embracing more and more the use of practices and programs based on rigorous research. As a research community, we need to increase the likelihood that our research efforts will be recognized and implemented by increasing the quality of our research designs. In addition, the inclusion of components to evaluate the costs and benefits of various interventions will enable us to make wiser decisions about the effectiveness of interventions. The use of cost analysis will help further this end, in addition to leading to a more efficient use of our mental health, education, and juvenile justice resources.

PREVENTION RESEARCH: COST ANALYSIS

Two approaches to cost analysis are cost-effectiveness analysis, which evaluates the costs and outcomes of programs designed to produce the *same* outcome, and cost–benefit analysis, which evaluates the costs and benefits of *different* programs in monetary terms (Barnett, 1998; Levin & McEwan, 2001). In cost-effectiveness analysis, programs with identical goals are compared using a common assessment measure. For instance, cost-effectiveness could be used to compare several dropout prevention programs and determine, given the costs of each program, how effective each is in preventing school dropout. On the other hand, cost–benefit analysis can be used to determine the monetary benefits of graduating from high school (e.g., better jobs, higher wages, less dependence on social services) and to compare these benefits with the costs of the dropout prevention program. This would show whether the costs of the dropout prevention programs are economically worth the benefits to their recipients and to society.

These techniques, especially cost–benefit analysis, are useful because they can show the long-term savings for intervention programs. Because all costs and benefits (both direct and indirect, tangible and intangible) are ideally assigned a monetary value in cost–benefit analysis, policymakers are able to better understand which programs are likely to produce benefits that exceed program costs and are better able to choose between alternatives. The potential outcome of policy decisions informed by cost analyses is noteworthy: the passage of policy that will use taxpayer dollars more efficiently even if it appears costly in the short term. Although cost analyses result in additional costs for program evaluations, these costs may be small when compared with the costs of poorly informed policy decisions (Barnett, 1998).

The Washington State Institute for Public Policy (WSIPP) conducted a noteworthy analysis of the costs and benefits of prevention programs. Directed by the legislature of the state of Washington to evaluate the costs and benefits of prevention programs, among others, WSIPP conducted a meta-analysis of more than 400 evaluations of prevention programs published during the preceding 25 years (Aos et al., 2001). WSIPP identified studies that used methodologies of a high standard to evaluate prevention and measured whether the programs reduced delinquency relative to control or comparison groups. WSIPP then examined programs meeting these criteria by looking at the costs and the benefits of reduced criminal activity of program participants.

Although WSIPP uses cost estimates (adjusted to 2000 dollars) for the state of Washington to predict the costs and savings of programs *for* Washington State residents, the findings offer strong indicators of the potential savings for programs implemented in other states. WSIPP found that a significant number of the prevention programs it examined yielded total benefits greater than program costs (see Table 5.5). Although some programs may seem costly in terms of up-front costs, the payoffs more than compensate for these costs. Two popular "get tough on crime" programs, juvenile boot camps and "scared straight" programs, were estimated to yield costs that *exceed* program benefits, thereby costing the taxpayer more money in the long run.

In its analysis, WSIPP examined two programs that traditionally address the needs of children and adolescents with EBD: Functional Family Therapy (FFT) and Multisystemic Therapy (MST). The estimated net cost of FFT is $2,161 per participant (Aos et al., 2001). Using outcome data from seven studies meeting the criteria for inclusion in its cost–benefit analysis, WSIPP found that the estimated value of reduced criminal justice costs exceeded the program cost by $14,149 per participant. When the estimated value of reduced victim costs were also considered, benefits increased to $59,067. With a benefit–cost ratio of $27.33, every

TABLE 5.5. Comparison of Prevention Program Costs, Benefits, and Benefit–Cost Ratios

Program	Net program cost, per participant	Net taxpayer and crime victim benefits, per participant	Benefit–cost ratio[a]
Aggression replacement training	$738	$33,143	$44.91
Functional Family Therapy	$2,161	$59,067	$27.33
Juvenile boot camps	−$15,424	−$3,587	N/A
Multidimensional Treatment Foster Care	$2,052	$87,622	$42.70
Multisystemic Therapy	$4,743	$131,918	$27.81
Nurse home visitation	$7,733	$15,918	$2.06
Perry Preschool Program[b]	$14,716	$105,000	$7.16
"Scared straight" programs	$51	−$24,531	N/A
Seattle Social Development Project	$4,355	$14,169	$3.25

[a] The report by Aos et al. appears to compute benefit–cost ratios by dividing the sum of estimated program benefit *and* program costs by total program cost. We have adjusted the reported ratios by directly dividing estimated benefits by costs and not including costs in the numerator. We believe that this approach makes benefit–cost ratios more comparable to those reported in other studies.

[b] These data are taken from Schweinhart (2003).

dollar invested in FFT is estimated to yield approximately $27 in total benefits.

Three studies passed WSIPP's criteria for inclusion in the cost–benefit analysis of MST, which was estimated to have a net cost of $4,743 per participant (Aos et al., 2001). WSIPP estimated that the value of reduced crime outcomes of participants yields benefits to taxpayers of $31,661 in reduced criminal justice costs. When the value of reduced victim costs was considered along with that of reduced criminal justice costs, benefits increased to $131,918. With a benefit–cost ratio of $27.81, every dollar invested in MST is estimated to yield almost $28 in total benefits.

Concomitant with research on effectiveness, cost analyses such as the work of WSIPP are integral to linking and, thus, bridging the gap between research and policy change. This research and these analyses will likely help to develop political will in support of funding prevention and facilitate the redeployment of resources wasted on ineffective or even harmful programs (Osher, Quinn, Poirier, & Rutherford, 2003). Cost analyses specifically might help to reframe issues so that policymakers are more attentive to the need for long-term benefits of effective prevention and are, therefore, more likely to view it as a wise investment.

FUTURE DIRECTIONS

Future research is needed to further expand what is known about the efficacy of prevention and early intervention programs for children and adolescents with or at risk of developing EBD. In particular, long-term longitudinal studies with randomized experimental designs or at least strong statistical control of variables designs should be conducted to examine the impact of prevention and early intervention programs on mental health problems, substance abuse, academic achievement, delinquency, and crime. Cost–benefit analyses should also be conducted to further build support for prevention programs.

The use of this methodology in studying early intervention and prevention programs is still emerging. However, this evaluative approach appears to have a potentially strong role in helping researchers to incorporate their findings into efforts not only to change practice but also to gain the support of public opinion and influence policy decisions. The combination of program evaluation with the collection of cost data will require strong collaboration between prevention and intervention researchers and economists (and perhaps those responsible for making and funding policy). This collaboration cannot come after program research has begun, but rather must be in place during the early stages of the design of the research to ensure that appropriate data are collected.

In addition to including cost analyses with new research efforts, researchers and policymakers would be wise to replicate and scale up the work of the Washington State Institute for Public Policy to develop cost and savings estimates for prevention at the national or regional (e.g., the Northeast or the Midwest) levels or even for other states, metropolitan areas, or individual localities. According to the Juvenile Justice Evaluation Center (2002), cost–benefit analyses can provide invaluable input as decisions are made regarding which prevention programs should be funded, expanded, or terminated and can help "decision makers choose courses of action that have the best chance of producing favorable returns on taxpayer dollars" (p. 14). In conducting cost–benefit analyses, researchers should examine four aspects of prevention programs, as described by the Center: the monetary benefits of at least two programs, their costs, the difference between their benefits and costs to produce and compare their cost–benefit ratios, and the risk of the conclusions relative to assumptions made in the estimates of costs and benefits.

Researchers at RAND reported that "no attempt has been made to compare the costs and effectiveness of various early-intervention approaches with each other and with incarceration" (Greenwood, Model, Rydell, & Chiesa, 1998, p. 3). RAND contributed to this body of research with its study *Diverting Children from a Life of Crime: Measuring Costs and Benefits*, which concluded that some crime prevention strategies designed for at-risk adolescents are potentially more cost-effective in reducing serious crime when compared with long mandatory sentences for repeat offenders. More such analyses are needed.

CONCLUSION

The aforementioned theories suggest how disability is a factor in delinquent behavior or in differential treatment within the juvenile justice system. Further, research shows that adolescents with EBD are likely to have higher incidence of mental health and substance abuse, school failure and dropout, and involvement in the justice system. This raises serious concerns about the need for prevention and treatment of EBD, and raises questions about the implications of the failure to prevent and the costs of such failure. For example, research shows that money spent on child psychiatry services provides a wide range of indirect savings to health, education, the justice system, and social welfare and that long-term benefits include improvement in the quality of life of the child and his or her family, poverty prevention, reductions in adult criminality, and fewer self-induced injuries and illnesses (Knapp, 2001).

Policymakers encounter various social and fiscal pressures as they formulate and adopt policy, making the public policy process complex and difficult to navigate when pursuing an issue not already on the agenda of policymakers. This chapter lays out the key issues that can be used to move prevention of EBD onto the institutional agenda of policymakers: EBD has been defined as a public problem worth addressing but this must be brought to the attention of policymakers and moved onto their agenda before meaningful policy emerges (Anderson, 2003). Researchers and empirical research designs related to adolescents with EBD are integral to this effort.

NOTES

1. This includes nine forms of illicit drug use: cocaine, hallucinogens, heroin, inhalants, marijuana, nonmedical use of prescription-type pain relievers, sedatives, stimulants, and tranquilizers.
2. Data were not available for five states: Indiana, Maine, New Hampshire, North Carolina, and Texas.
3. This age is 15 in three states, 16 in ten states, and 17 in the remaining 37 states and the District of Columbia (Snyder & Sickmund, 1999).
4. These cases are based on data from approximately 2,100 courts that have jurisdiction over almost 70% of the U.S. juvenile population. One adolescent can account for more than one case.
5. It is important to emphasize that these data are estimates since the reporting of juvenile arrests varies by state. For example, 16 states had reporting coverage of 90% or greater, while Kansas and the District of Columbia had no coverage and nine states (Georgia, Illinois, Kentucky, Mississippi, New Mexico, New York, South Carolina, South Dakota, and Wisconsin) had coverage of less than 50%. Therefore, the number of juvenile arrests would be higher with full reporting.
6. According to Cohen (1998), the low end of this range is based on actual convictions while the other is based on self-reports.

REFERENCES

Anderson, J. E. (2003). *Public Policymaking* (5th ed.). Boston: Houghton Mifflin.

Aos, S., Phipps, P., Barnoski, R., & Lieb, R. (2001). *The comparative costs and benefits of programs to reduce crime.* Olympia, WA: Washington State Institute for Public Policy.

Barnett, W. S. (1998). Benefit–cost analysis and related techniques. In A. J. Reynolds & H. J. Walberg (Eds.), *Advances in educational productivity* (Vol. 7, pp. 241–261). New York: JAI Press.

Bickman, L., Guthrie, P. R., Foster, E. M., Lambert, E. W., Summerfelt, W. T., Breda, C. S., & Heflinger, C. A. (1996). *Evaluating managed mental health services: The Fort Bragg experiment.* New York: Plenum.

Brandenburg, N. A., Friedman, R., & Silver, S. E. (1990). The epidemiology of childhood psychiatric disorders: Prevalence findings from recent studies. *Journal of the American Academy of Child and Adolescent Psychiatry, 29,* 76–83.

Bruner, C. (1991). *Thinking collaboratively: Ten questions and answers to help policy makers improve children's services.* Washington, DC: Education and Human Services Consortium.

Burns, B. J., Costello, E. J., Angold, A., Tweed, D., Stangl, D., Farmer, E. M. Z., & Erkanli, A. (1995). Children's mental health service use across service sectors. *Health Affairs, 14*(3), 147–159.

Cameron, S. V., & Heckman, J. J. (1993). The nonequivalence of high school equivalents. *Journal of Labor Economics, 11,* 1–47.

Caspi, A., Elder, G. H., & Bem, D. J., (1987). Moving against the world: Life course patterns of explosive children. *Developmental Psychology, 23*, 308–313.

Catterall, J. S. (November 1987). On the social costs of dropping out of school. *The High School Journal, 71*, 19–30.

Cohen, M. A. (1998). The monetary value of saving a high-risk youth. *Journal of Quantitative Criminology, 14*(1), 5–33.

Costello, E. J. (1989). Developments in child psychiatric epidemiology. *Journal of the American Academy of Child and Adolescent Psychiatry, 28*, 836-841.

Costello, E. J., Burns, B. J., Angold, A., & Leaf, P. J. (1993). How can epidemiology improve mental health services for children and adolescents? *Journal of American Academy of Child and Adolescent Psychiatry, 32*, 1106–1114.

Cox, A. (1994). Social factors in child psychiatric disorder. In M. Rutter, E. Taylor, & L. Hersov (Eds.), *Child and adolescent psychiatry: Modern approaches*. Oxford, UK: Blackwell.

Dunkle, M., & Nash, M. (1989, March 15). Creating effective interagency collaboratives. *Education Week, 35*, 44.

Frank, A. R., & Sitlington, P. L. (1997). Young adults with behavioral disorders: Before and after IDEA. *Behavioral Disorders, 23*, 40–56.

Friedman, R. M., & Kutash, L. (1992). Challenges for child and adolescent mental health. *Health Affairs, 11*, 125–136.

Gifford, S. L. (2002). *Justice expenditure and employment in the United States, 1999*. (NCJ Publication No. 191746). Washington, DC: U.S. Department of Justice, Office of Justice Programs, Bureau of Justice Statistics.

Goldman, H. H. (1987). Financing the mental health system. *Psychiatric Annals, 17*(9), 580–585.

Gopfert, M., Webster, J., & Seeman, M. V. (Eds.). (1995). *Disturbed mentally ill parents and their children*. Cambridge, UK: Cambridge University Press.

Greenwood, P. W., Model, K. E., Rydell, C. P., & Chiesa, J. (1998). *Diverting children from a life of crime: Measuring costs and benefits*. Santa Monica, CA: RAND.

Harrington, R. C., Fudge, H., Rutter, M. L. Pickles, A., & Hill, J. (1990). Adult outcomes of childhood and adolescent depression. *Archives of General Psychiatry, 47*, 465–473.

Health Advisory Service. (1995). *Child and adolescent mental health services: Together we stand*. London: HMSQ.

Hollis, C. (1995). Child and adolescent (juvenile onset) schizophrenia: A case control study of premorbid developmental impairments. *British Journal of Psychiatry, 166*, 489–495.

Jay, D. E., & Padilla, C. L. (1987). *Special education dropouts*. Menlo Park, CA: SRI International.

Juvenile Justice and Delinquency Prevention Act of 2002, 42 U.S.C. 5601, 2002.

Juvenile Justice Evaluation Center, Justice Research and Statistics Association, Office of Juvenile Justice and Delinquency Prevention. (2002). *Cost–benefit analysis for juvenile justice programs*. Washington, DC: Author.

Keilitz, I., & Dunivant, N. (1987). The learning disabled offender. In C. M. Nelson, R., B., Rutherford, & B. I. Wolford (Eds.), *Special education in the criminal justice system* (pp. 120–137). Columbus, OH: Merrill.

Klein, D. N., Lewinsohn, P. M., & Seeley, J. R. (1997). Psychosocial characteristics of adolescents with a past history of dysthymic disorder: Comparison with adolescents with past histories of major depressive and non-affective disorders, and never mentally ill controls. *Journal of Affective Disorders, 42*, 127–135.

Klein, R. G., & Slomkowski, C. (1993). Treatment of psychiatric disorders in children and adolescents. *Psychopharmacology Bulletin, 29*(4), 525–535.

Knapp, M. (1997). Economic evaluations and interventions for children and adolescents with mental health problems. *Journal of Child Psychology and Psychiatry, 38*, 3–25.

Knapp, M. (2001). Economic evaluation and conduct disorders. In J. Hill & B. Maughan (Eds.), *Conduct disorders in childhood and adolescence* (pp. 478–506). Cambridge, UK: Cambridge University Press.

Larson, K. A. (1988). A research review and alternative hypothesis explaining the link between learning disabilities and delinquency. *Journal of Learning Disabilities, 21*, 257–263, 369.

Larson, K. A., & Turner, D. (2002). *Best practices for serving court involved youth with learning, attention, and behavioral disorders*. Washington, DC: Center for Effective Collaboration and Practice, National Center for Education, Disability, and Juvenile Justice.

Leone, P. E., & Meisel, S. (1997). Improving education services for students in detention and confinement facilities. *Children's Legal Rights Journal, 17*, 1–12.

Leone, P. E., Quinn, M. M., & Osher, D. (2002). *Collaboration in the juvenile justice system and youth serving agencies: Improving prevention, providing more efficient services, and reducing recidivisim for youth with disabilities*. Washington, DC: Center for Effective Collaboration and Practice.

Levin, H. M., & McEwan, P. J. (2001). *Cost-effectiveness analysis* (2nd ed.). Thousand Oaks, CA: Sage.

Light, D., & Bailey, V. (1993). Pound foolish. *Health Science Journal, 11*, 16–18.

Mark, T., McKusick, D., King, E., Harwood, H., & Genuardi, J. (1998). *National expenditures for mental health, alcohol, and other drug abuse treatment, 1996*. Rockville, MD: Substance Abuse and Mental Health Service Administration.

Matthews, R. C. O. (1991). The economics of professional ethics: Should the professions be more like business? *Economic Journal, 101*, 737–750.

McGuire, T. G. (1989). Financing and reimbursement for mental health services. In C. Taube, D. Mechanic, & A. Hohmann (Eds.). The future of mental health services research (pp. 87–111). (DHHS Publication No. (ADM) 89-1600). Washington, DC: U.S. Government Printing Office.

Miller, T. R., Fisher, D. A., & Cohen, M. A. (2001). Costs of juvenile violence: Policy implications. Retrieved April 28, 2003, from *http://www.pediatrics.org/cgi/content/full/107/*.

Murnane, R. J., Willett, J. B., & Boudett, K. P. (1995). Do high school dropouts benefit from obtaining a GED? *Educational Evaluation and Policy Analysis, 17*, 133–147.

Murnane, R. J., Willett, J. B., & Boudette, K. P. (1997). Does acquisition of a GED lead to more training, post-secondary education, and military service for school dropouts? *Industrial and Labor Relations Review, 51*, 100–116.

Murnane, R. J., Willett, J. B., & Tyler, J. H. (2000). Who benefits from obtaining a GED?: Evidence from high school and beyond. *The Review of Economics and Statistics, 82*, 23–37.

Murray, C. A. (1977). *The link between learning disabilities and juvenile delinquency: Current theory and knowledge.* Washington, DC: U.S. Government Printing Office.

National Center on Addiction and Substance Abuse at Columbia University (CASA). (2001). *Shoveling up: The impact of substance abuse on state budgets.* New York: Author.

National Research Council. (1999). *Making money matter.* Washington, DC: National Academy Press.

Osher, D. M., Quinn, M. M., Poirier, J. M., & Rutherford, R. B. (2003). Deconstructing the pipeline: Using efficacy and effectiveness data and cost-benefit analyses to reduce minority youth incarceration. In J. Wald & D. J. Losen (Issue Eds.), *New direction for youth development: Deconstructing the school-to-prison pipeline* (pp. 91–120). San Francisco: Jossey-Bass.

Padgett, D. K., Patrick, C., Burns, B. J., Schlesinger, H. J., & Cohen, J. (1993). The effect of insurance benefit changes on use of child and adolescent outpatient mental health services. *Medical Care, 31*, 96–110.

Parent, D. G. (2003). *Correctional boot camps: Lessons from a decade of research.* Washington, DC: U.S. Department of Justice, Office of Justice Programs.

Patterson, G. R., Reid, J. B., & Dishion, T. J. (1992). *Antisocial boys.* Eugene, OR: Castalia.

Post, C. H. (1981). The link between learning disabilities and juvenile delinquency: Cause, effect and "present solutions." *Juvenile and Family Court Journal, 32*, 58–68.

Quinn, M. M. (2000). Creating safe, effective, and nurturing schools: New opportunities and new challenges for serving all students. In L. M. Bullock & R. A. Gable (Eds.). *Positive academic and behavioral supports: Creating safe, effective, and nurturing schools for all students.* Reston, VA: Council for Children with Behavioral Disorders.

Quinn, M. M., Rutherford, R. B., Leone, P. E., Osher, D., & Poirier, J. M. (in press). Students with disabilities in detention and correctional settings. *Exceptional Children.*

Rapoport, J. L., Swedo, S., & Leonard, H. (1994). Obsessive-compulsive disorder. In M. Rutter, E. Taylor & L. Hersov (Eds.), *Child and adolescent psychiatry: Modern approaches* (pp. 441–454). Oxford: Blackwell.

Robins, L. N., & Ratcliff, K. S. (1978–1979). Risk factors in the continuation of childhood antisocial behaviors into adulthood. *International Journal of Mental Health, 7(3–4)*, 96–116.

Robins, L. N., West, P. A., & Herjanic, B. L. (1975). Arrests and delinquency in two generations: A study of black urban families and their children. *Journal of Child Psychology and Psychiatry, 16* , 125–140.

Rumberger, R. W. (1987). High school dropouts: A review of issues and evidence. *Review of Educational Research, 57*, 101–121.

Rumberger, R. W., & Lamb, S. P. (2003). The early employment and further education experiences of high school dropouts: A comparative study of the United States and Australia. *Economics of Education Review, 22*, 353–356.

Rutherford, R. B., Bullis, M., Anderson, C. W., & Griller-Clark, H. M. (2002). *Youth with Disabilities in the correctional system: Prevalence rates and identification issues.* Washington, DC: Center for Effective Collaboration and Practice/Center for Education, Disability, and Juvenile Justice.

Schumacher, M., & Kurz, G. A. (2000). *The 8% solution: Preventing serious, repeat juvenile crime.* Thousand Oaks, CA: Sage.

Schweinhart, L. (2003, April). Benefits, costs, and explanation of the High/Scope Perry Preschool Program. Paper presented at the meeting of the Society for Research in Child Development, Tampa, FL.

Shaffer, D., Fisher, P., Dulcan, M. K., Davies, M., Piacentini, J., Schwab-Stone, M. E., et al. (1996). The NIMH Diagnostic Interview Schedule for Children Version 2.3 (DISC-2.3): Description, acceptability, prevalence rates, and performance in the MECA study. Methods for the epidemiology of child and adolescent mental disorders study. *Journal of the American Academy of Child and Adolescent Psychiatry, 35*, 865–877.

Snyder, H. N. (2002). *Juvenile arrests 2000.* (NCJ Publication No. 191729). Washington, DC: U.S. Department of Justice, Office of Justice Programs, Bureau of Justice Statistics.

Snyder, H. N. (2003). *Juvenile arrests 2001.* (NCJ Publication No. 201370). Washington, DC: U.S. Department of Justice, Office of Justice Programs, Bureau of Justice Statistics.

Snyder, H. N., & Sickmund, M. (1999). *Juvenile offenders and victims: 1999 national report.* Washington, DC: Office of Juvenile Justice and Delinquency Prevention.

Sprague, J., & Walker, H. M. (2000). Early identification and intervention for youth with antisocial and violent behavior. *Exceptional Children, 66,* 367–379.

Stahl, A. L. (2001). *Delinquency cases in juvenile courts, 1998* (OJJDP Fact Sheet #31). Washington, DC: U.S. Department of Justice, Office of Justice Programs, Office of Juvenile Justice and Delinquency Prevention.

Staton, D. (1989). Mental health care economics and the future of psychiatric practice. *Psychiatric Annals, 19,* 421–427.

Tyler, J. H., Murnane, R., & Willett, J. B. (2000). Estimating the labor market signaling value of the GED. *The Quarterly Journal of Economics, 115,* 431–468.

U.S. Bureau of the Census. (1992). *Workers with low earnings.* Washington, DC: U.S. Government Printing Office.

U.S. Department of Education. (2000). *Digest of education statistics, 1999.* Washington, DC: U.S. Government Printing Office.

U.S. Department of Education. (2001). *Twenty-third annual report to Congress on the implementation of the Individuals with Disabilities Education Act.* Washington, DC: Author.

U.S. Department of Education. (2002). *Exemplary and promising safe, disciplined, and drug-free school programs.* Washington, DC: Office of Special Educational Research and Improvement, Office of Reform Assistance and Dissemination.

U.S. Department of Education, National Center for Educational Statistics. (2003). *Digest of education statistics, 2001.* Washington, DC: U.S. Government Printing Office.

U.S. Department of Health and Human Services. (1999). *Mental health: A report of the Surgeon General.* Rockville, MD: Author.

U.S. Department of Health and Human Services (DHHS), Substance Abuse and Mental Health Services Administration, Office of Applied Studies. (2003). *Results from the 2002 National Survey on Drug Use and Health: National findings.* Washington, DC: Author.

U.S. Department of Justice, Office of Justice Programs, Bureau of Justice Statistics. (1994). *The costs of crime to victims: Crime Data Brief.* NCJ Publication No. 145865. Washington, DC: Author.

U.S. Department of Justice, Office of Justice Programs, Office of Juvenile Justice and Delinquency Prevention. (1999a). *OJJDP statistical briefing book.* Retrieved March 2, 2003, from *http://ojjdp.ncjrs.org/ojstatbb/html/qa085.html.*

U.S. Department of Justice, Office of Justice Programs, Office of Juvenile Justice and Delinquency Prevention. (1999b). *OJJDP statistical briefing book.* Retrieved March 2, 2003, from *http://ojjdp.ncjrs.org/ojstatbb/html/qa136.html.*

Wagner, M., Blackorby, J., Cameto, R., & Newman, L. (1993). *What makes a difference? Influences in school outcomes of youth with disabilities.* Menlo Park, CA: SRI International.

Wagner, M., D'Amico, R., Marder, C., Newman, L., & Blackorby, J. (1992). *What happens next?: Trends in postschool outcomes of youth with disabilities. The second comprehensive report from the National Longitudinal Transition Study of Special Education Students.* Menlo Park, CA: SRI International.

Wagner, M., Newman, L., D'Amico, R., Jay, E. D., Butler-Nalin, P., & Marder, C., (Eds.). (1991). Youth with disabilities: How are they doing? In *The first comprehensive report from the National Longitudinal Transition Study of Special Education Students.* Menlo Park, CA: SRI International.

Woodward, A. (1998). Overview of methods: Cost-effectiveness, cost-benefits, and cost-offsets of prevention. In W. J. Bukoski & R. I. Evans (Eds.), *Cost-benefit/cost-effectiveness research of drug abuse prevention: Implications for programming and policy* (NIDA Research Monograph 176). Rockville, MD: U.S. Department of Health and Human Services, National Institutes of Health.

6

How Research Informs Practice in the Field of Emotional and Behavioral Disorders

MELODY TANKERSLEY, TIMOTHY J. LANDRUM, *and* BRYAN G. COOK

The recent focus on the legitimacy of special education has engendered critics and professionals alike to challenge the efficacy and efficiency of the field (see Kauffman, 1999a). Finn and Rotherham (2001), for example, reported that "special education has become not a road to life but a cul-de-sac where they [students] are stopped before they get the help they need to do as well as they can" (p. B13). Yet, despite such attacks, there is much that is right about special education (see Hockenbury, Kauffman, & Hallahan, 1999–2000). Through empirical research, the field of special education has accumulated vast knowledge and achieved significant outcomes in relation to shaping public policy and providing educational services for students with exceptional learning needs. Mostert and Crockett (1999–2000) consider examples of achievement such as professional and parental advocacy, legal safeguards and policies, effective educational interventions, and social and societal acceptance of persons with disabilities as evidence of the positive influence special education has had to date. The base of rigorous, scientifically determined research that provides the foundation for special education is a significant achievement and signifies one of the things that is most right about the field.

Although a relatively new subspecialty within the special education field (dating from the early 1960s; see Wood, 1999), researchers in the area of emotional and behavioral disorders (EBD) have accomplished much in little time. As Walker, Sprague, Close, and Starlin (1999–2000) outline, the field of EBD has made significant contributions to the research base that provide a growing understanding of the nature, characteristics, and interactional patterns of children and youths with EBD. Through empirical investigation, the complex and systemic nature of the problems faced by students with EBD, their families, schools, and communities can be described reliably and validly.

Research has shown, for example, that students with EBD are more likely than students without behavioral problems to underachieve academically, engage in aggressive acts, receive less positive attention from teachers, and be rejected by their peers (e.g., Hinshaw, 1992; Kauffman, 2001; Shores et al., 1993; Walker, Colvin, & Ramsey, 1995). Scholarly pursuits for understanding characteristics of children and youths with EBD have also led to the identification of comorbid conditions between and within facets of behavioral and learning problems (e.g., Gresham, Lane, et al., 2001; Kaiser &

98

Hester, 1997; Tankersley & Landrum, 1997). Moreover, students with EBD are among those most likely to drop out of school and grow up to become adults who are unemployed, involved in criminal behavior, and abuse substances (e.g., Carson, Sitlington, & Frank, 1995; Frank, Sitlington, & Carson, 1991; Kazdin, 1987; Marder, 1992; Wagner, D'Amico, Marder, Newman, & Blackorby, 1992).

Along with identifying descriptive features and outcomes associated with EBD, researchers have also developed theoretical and conceptual models for describing and explaining interactional patterns of behavior of children and youths with EBD. For example, Patterson (1982) and colleagues (e.g., Patterson, Reid, & Dishion, 1992) generated and substantiated a theory of children's antisocial behavior based on a coercive interactive pattern of noncompliance, and Colvin (1993) developed a conceptual model of behavioral escalation that describes characteristic behavior at each phase.

Because of sustained research efforts, educators and other school-related professionals have empirically validated approaches to guide their decision making for identifying and assessing students with EBD (see Lane, Gresham, & O'Shaughnessy, 2002). Instruments for detecting risk for EBD, such as the Systematic Screening for Behavior Disorders (Walker & Severson, 1992) as well for identifying the behavioral and social profiles of children and youth, such as the Child Behavior Checklist (Achenbach, 1991) and the Walker–McConnell Scale of Social Competence and School Adjustment (Walker & McConnell, 1995), provide researchers and practitioners the means to describe, quantify, and compare critical areas of child development.

In addition to identifying descriptive characteristics, building theoretical explanations, and developing assessment tools, researchers in the field of EBD have produced and evaluated methods for intervening with students' academic and behavioral concerns (see Dunlap & Childs, 1996). In a recent review, Landrum, Tankersley, and Kauffman (2003) cited interventions associated with improving the outcomes of students with EBD in three defining areas—inappropriate behavior, academic learning problems, and ineffectual interpersonal relationships. When con-

sidering the extent to which a set of effective practices to address these areas of concern, Landrum et al. concluded that substantial empirically validated methods of intervention have been established.

Due to the relentless efforts of professionals in the field of EBD, an assemblage of reliable and valid empirically tested practices that improve the social and academic behaviors of children and youths with behavioral and learning problems is available. We (Cook, Landrum, Tankersley, & Kauffman, 2003; Landrum et al., 2003) and others (e.g., Dunlap & Childs, 1996; Shinn, Walker, & Stoner, 2002) have recognized and discussed examples of effective practices elsewhere— for example, token economies have been shown to increase positive social behaviors (Smith & Farrell, 1993; Walker, Hops, & Fiegenbaum, 1976); response cost (Proctor & Morgan, 1991) and time out from positive reinforcement (Salend & Gordon, 1987) have been shown to decrease aggressive behavior; precision requests have been shown to increase compliance (Neville & Jenson, 1984); curriculum-based measurement has been shown to be effective for monitoring academic progress (Deno, 2003); the Good Behavior Game has been shown to decrease disruptive behaviors (Darveaux, 1984); self-monitoring has been shown to increase on-task behavior and academic productivity (Lloyd, Bateman, Landrum, & Hallahan, 1989); and Classwide Peer Tutoring has been shown to increase rates of academic engagement (Delquadri, Greenwod, Whorton, Carta, & Hall, 1986). It seems clear that effective practices for alleviating many of the behavioral and learning challenges associated with EBD have been developed.

Although the field of EBD has created a significant empirical foundation of knowledge, the use of that knowledge to inform practice has not been fully realized. Indeed, "researchers can justly claim that even 'quality' findings are routinely ignored" (Carnine, 1997, pp. 513–514). And if our hope is to ameliorate those social, behavioral, and academic conditions that affect students with EBD described previously, we must turn to research as "the best trick we know" (Crockett, 2004) for identifying and implementing effective practices. This gap between what is known and what is applied is frequently bemoaned throughout special education (Carnine, 1997; Espin & Deno, 2000; Greenwood & Abbott, 2001; Kauffman, 1996), and at no other time in its history has the field paid more attention to the issues related to the gap than now. As Cook et al. (2003) highlighted, special series of journals have been devoted to issues of bridging the research to practice gap (e.g., *Teacher Education and Special Education*; Greenwood, 2001), granting agencies have directed funds toward developing and sustaining models for using research knowledge to improve practice (e.g., National Science Foundation, Office of Special Education Programs), and public policy has included directives to use research in practice (e.g., the No Child Left Behind Act)—all within the past few years. Thus, substantial effort and energy have clearly been committed to this topic. The results of these efforts have been to (1) identify the extent to which evidence-based decisions are made and practices are applied in policy and in classrooms, (2) describe barriers to bringing research to bear upon practice, and (3) examine ways to influence the extent to which research informs practice.

The purpose of this chapter is to discuss these themes in relation to the education of students with EBD. We delineate three interrelated types of practice involved in providing optimal services to students with EBD—policy, teacher training, and classroom instruction—and discuss the gap between our knowledge base and its application to these areas of practice. Discussions of barriers to and directions for addressing the research-to-practice gap in each area then follow.

THE EXTENT TO WHICH EVIDENCE-BASED DECISIONS AND PRACTICES ARE APPLIED

As presented at the beginning of this chapter, the field of EBD has developed an impressive library of empirical work that describes characteristics and outcomes of students, builds theory and conceptual models, validates assessment instruments, and determines effective interventions. But the ultimate utility of this body of work lies in its application to the education and treatment of students. As Cook and Schirmer (2003) state, "Iden-

tifying effective practices is only meaningful to the extent that they are applied (and applied with fidelity) with children and youth with disabilities" (p. 203). Fuchs and Fuchs (1995), Hallahan and Kauffman (2003), and Hockenbury et al. (1999–2000) agree that it is the *use* of empirically identified practices that makes special education *special*.

Clearly, the concern with not using evidence-based practices in the classroom is that children and youths will not reach their potential—a risk that students receiving special education services already bear given the nature of disability. Whereas nondisabled students may progress despite the lack of effective instruction, students with disabilities may actually regress in skill (Chall, 2000). Such an effect would be particularly detrimental for students with EBD who, it can be argued, remain at a great disadvantage even with the most powerful intervention practices in place.

The process of bringing research knowledge to bear upon practice, however, is not confined to the classroom setting—although most of the discussions that frame the research-to-practice issue tend to focus on the application of instructional practices in classroom settings. Using empirically based information should be the norm in developing and instituting policy and training teachers, as well as in delivering instruction to students. The interactional, reinforcing nature of these three areas suggests that optimal use of research in one will influence and reinforce use of research in another. Unfortunately, there exist gaps between what is known and what occurs in policy, teacher training, and in the classroom.

The Research-to-Policy Gap

Educational policies provide the structure and support for the day-to-day practice of teaching students with EBD and are established through such means as legislation, educational reform initiatives, local (e.g., school board) mandates, and administrative decisions. Through policy, the conditions for practice are set. In examining some of the policies related to students with EBD, there seem to be gaps between what we know and what legislation, case law, and local procedures decree. Some policies have been established in direct opposition to what is known through empirical support, other policies have been established even though a critical base of empirical support has not been acquired, and some policies have yet to be established despite strong evidence of their need (see also Quinn & Poirier, Chapter 5, this volume).

Policies Established That Oppose Research Results

Perhaps one of the foremost examples of policies established in opposition to what research supports is the federal definition of emotional disturbance (Individuals with Disabilities Education Act [IDEA], 1997). The definition identifies five criteria for classifying a student as having emotional disturbance (see Forness & Kavale, 1997, 2000; see also Cullinan, Chapter 3, this volume). These criteria were adopted from a definition developed by Bower (1981) through his empirical work with thousands of students during the 1950s. In addition to Bower's five adapted criteria, the federal definition of emotional disturbance continues and states that "The term does not include children who are socially maladjusted unless it is determined that they have an emotional disturbance" (34 C.F.R. 300.7[9]§602[3][b][8] [ii] of IDEA). This exclusionary clause in the definition has been the source of much discussion because it effectively negates the criteria that delineate the term "emotionally disturbed"; that is, if a student is found to meet the characteristic criteria listed in the definition, that student is—by any credible interpretation of the definition (Kauffman, 2001)—socially maladjusted (Bower, 1982; Cline, 1990). The definitional criteria that identify students for services employ an exclusionary statement that may then exclude these very same students.

Although the definitional criteria included were based on Bower's (1981) research, adding the exclusionary clause opposes what is known about the characteristics of children and youths who have EBD (e.g., Duncan, Forness, & Hartsough, 1995; Kauffman, 2001). Research has failed to show that there is a reliable and valid distinction between social maladjustment and emotional disturbance, but has shown that the behavioral and academic characteristics typically associated with social maladjustment and emotional disturbance often coexist (e.g., Costenbader & Buntaine, 1999; Forness, Kavale, King, & Kasari, 1994). In short, there appears to be no separate, distinguishable diagnostic criteria between social maladjustment and emotional disturbance. Yet, in direct opposition to what research has determined, the definition requires such a distinction.

Policies Established without Full Empirical Support

Whereas some policies may be established in opposition to what is known, other policies may be established without a complete research base or with a misapplied research base. For example, one of the requirements added to the 1997 Amendments of IDEA was the provision for implementing functional behavioral assessments (FBAs) when a student with a disability becomes the subject of school disciplinary proceedings (Tilly, Knoster, & Ikeda, 2000). In a Forum series in the journal *Behavioral Disorders* (Armstrong & Kauffman, 1999), several scholars in the field discussed the application of this legislative requirement to use FBA in designing behavioral interventions for students with EBD. In general, the contributors to the Forum agreed on two points: (1) there is much to recommend the use of FBA to understand the motivating factors and antecedent/consequent events that set the occasion for and maintain problem behavior; and (2) there is insufficient research regarding effectiveness of FBA with students with EBD. Although FBAs provide a means for developing potentially effective interventions (see Gresham, Watson, & Skinner, 2001), the research to date has been primarily conducted with students with low-incidence disabilities, instituted in clinical settings, and conducted by researchers (see Nelson, Roberts, Mathur, & Rutherford, 1999). At this time, research has not credibly demonstrated either the treatment validity (the extent to which FBA can be used to address the problem behavior of students with EBD) or the external validity (the extent to which FBA can be generalized to public school settings and their practitioners with fidelity) of this procedure (Braden & Kratochwill, 1997; Gresham, Watson, et al., 2001; Lane et al., 2002; Nelson et al., 1999; Sasso, Conroy, Stichter, & Fox, 2001).

Another example of policy without a substantive research base is the movement toward inclusion of students with disabilities in general education classrooms. The available empirically derived outcomes of inclusive educational placements for students with disabilities in general are not convincing, and for students with behavioral disorders are almost nonexistent. For example, Klingner, Vaughn, Hughes, Schumm, and Elbaum (1998) and Zigmond et al. (1995) found that, even in inclusion programs with atypically high levels of support, included students with learning disabilities made less-than-appropriate gains in academic achievement. These students also have been found to be poorly accepted by their nondisabled peers when included (Ochoa & Olivarez, 1995; Swanson & Malone, 1992). In fact, Baker and Zigmond (1995) concluded that decreased outcomes in inclusive environments are to be expected for many students with learning disabilities, because the intense and individualized nature of special education was not present in the inclusive environments they observed.

We know much less about the effectiveness of inclusion on the academic and behavioral success of students with EBD (McMillan, Gresham, & Forness, 1996). We do know that meta-analytic results have shown that effect sizes for special classes for students with learning or behavior problems are higher than for all special classroom placement (Lloyd, Forness, & Kavale, 1998) and that effect sizes are greater for academic achievement of students with EBD in more restrictive settings (Schneider & Leroux, 1994). Such results may be related to the contextual variables that can characterize a separate class for students with EBD. For example, Kauffman, Bantz, and McCullough (2002) describe the structure, intensity, precision, and relentlessness with which teachers in successful special classes for students with EBD deliver, monitor, and adapt instruction—characteristics which seem beyond that which would be possible in a regular classroom (Baker & Zigmond, 1995).

Policies Not Established

Whereas some policies are established in contradiction to what is known and others are instituted prior to substantiation of their validity and reliability, the presence of compelling evidence may also be ignored by policymakers and fail to find its way into policy. For example, the need for earlier and better services for young children before they develop emotional or behavioral disorders is well established in the empirical literature. Longitudinal studies show that students identified as having EBD have recognizable problem behavior even before entering first grade (Achenbach, Howell, McConaughy, & Stranger, 1995; McConaughy, Stranger, & Achenbach, 1992). Moreover, these behaviors were found to be stable through 3- and 6-year follow-ups—a pattern of stability that led Moffitt (1994) to term the early onset of problem behavior as *life-course-persistent*. Given the early beginning of problem behaviors, their stability, and the life-altering impact of their occurrence, it is heartening to know that early intervention efforts can be effective in ameliorating and/or reducing the effects of EBD (e.g., Forness et al., 2000; Kellam & Rebok, 1992; Mastropieri, Scruggs, & Casto, 1985; Reid, 1993; Tankersley, Kamps, Mancina, & Weidinger, 1996; Walker, Kavanagh, et al., 1998).

Although research has identified appropriate means for detecting and intervening early to prevent and/or lessen the occurrence and/or magnitude of problem behavior, it is unfortunate that policies that mandate, encourage, or take account of practices related to the early identification of and intervention with children at risk of or who have developed EBD are not readily available. Special education does little by means of early detection or primary prevention when efforts could be most influential (Forness & Kavale, 2000; Forness, Kavale, MacMillan, Asarnow, & Duncan, 1996), focusing instead on reactive interventions after the behavioral patterns are well established and often intractable. As Kauffman (1999b) has lamented, we do much to prevent the prevention of EBD.

Discussion

Because policy sets the conditions for practice, the use, misuse, or disregard of research in determining policy can have direct consequences for practice—as evidenced by the preceding examples. When policies ignore or misapply research findings, the potential for implementing practices that are not optimally effective—or that impede progress or even harm students—increases. The most advantageous association between research and policy is one in which research is brought to bear upon legislative, reform, or administrative decisions and successful practices are designed, mandated, and applied in educational practice. In turn, research-based policies then foster the implementation of evidence-based practices and improve student outcomes.

Yet, to be candid, there is not always a direct relationship between policy and classroom practice (Elmore, 1997), and there may, in fact, be little application of policy in practice. Of course, this may constitute good news when the policy is not based on empirical evidence. Policy mandates typically circumscribe the activities of teachers. There are often things that teachers cannot do and resources they cannot access due to policy. By making certain resources available, policies also encourage certain activities. However, there exists little control or direct supervision of teachers in schools. Even if an administrator mandates a particular procedure, or if a practice becomes codified as law, these policies are largely unenforceable. Within reason, teachers can do largely what they want in their own classrooms. Indeed, educators—or street-level bureaucrats—can be quite adept at avoiding or transforming policies that require great change or are difficult to implement (e.g., Weatherley & Lipsky, 1977). The heightened emphasis on accountability in education may enhance the ability of policies to dictate practice. However, given the "decoupled" or "loosely coupled" nature of our public schools (see Gamoran & Dreeben, 1986; Meyer & Rowan, 1977), it is likely that teachers will always have a large degree of autonomy in their instructional decision making and activities. As such, in addition to improving the connection between research and policy, it is imperative that we bridge the gap between research and practice in the classroom and in teacher preparation in order to improve the outcomes of children and youths with EBD.

The Research-to-Teacher Training Gap

One of the most straightforward means for ensuring that effective practices are used in the day-to-day education of students with EBD is to train teachers in such a way that they can access, understand, and implement empirically validated practices. Although repeated calls for improved, empirically driven teacher preparation programs have been expressed (e.g., Whelan & Simpson, 1996), teacher training programs are also susceptible to misapplying research, using faulty research bases, or ignoring the empirical research base.

Teacher educators are, perhaps, the most direct source of translating research to practice for future teachers. Indeed, Greenwood and Maheady (2001) argue that the role of all teacher educators is to construct and foster in their university students an attitude that teaching is based on scientific principles. Unfortunately, teacher educators may actually succeed in doing quite the opposite. Gersten (2001) presents the example of teacher training programs with faculty who support conflicting approaches to teaching reading and math, all of which claim empirical support. "As a result, many students of education leave universities feeling bewildered, betrayed, or both" in regard to the utility and validity of educational research (p. 45).

In addition to being presented with confusing interpretations of the research base, some preservice educators may leave their training programs without vital information in key areas of teaching. For example, the literature suggests that regular education teachers are not trained to teach social skills and manage behavior of their students (see Kauffman & Wong, 1991). This lack of training is even more disconcerting considering that demonstrated competency in classroom management is probably the most critical skill necessary to teach students with EBD. Research shows that not only do regular educators lack preparation in this area but also teachers of students with EBD routinely report insufficient training in empirically sound practices of managing and intervening with problem behavior (e.g., Bullock, Ellis, & Wilson, 1994; George, George, Gersten, & Grosenick, 1995). In fact, Jack et al. (1996) found that only 5% of the teachers of students with EBD in their study credited their college coursework as the source of the management strategies they use.

Not only are gaps between research and preservice teacher education evident, but the same gulf is apparent between research and inservice teacher training. The traditional top-down, one-shot approach to professional development trainings may offer exposure to evidence based practices, but their effects are not long-lasting (e.g., Fuchs & Fuchs, 2001; Sindelar & Brownell, 2001).

Regardless of their level of experience, the *practice* of effective practices often seems missing in the learning equation. Teachers (preservice or experienced) have infrequent opportunities for learning how to implement practices by watching them modeled or by receiving instructive feedback on their use of the practices (Gersten, Morvant, & Brengelman, 1995). Even though preservice teachers have field-based and student teaching experiences incorporated into their training program, the extent to which and the fidelity with which supervising teachers use effective practices is often unknown—yet, these supervising teachers are very influential in new teachers' determinations of which practices to employ in their own classrooms (Cook, 2003).

The Research-to-Classroom Practice Gap

Perhaps the ultimate test of the efficacy and effectiveness of the research base in the education of students with EBD is the extent to which research is brought to bear on improving their outcomes (Cook & Schirmer, 2003). As discussed earlier, the field of EBD can take pride in an established research base that has accumulated reliable and valid interventions that positively influence the academic, behavioral, and social outcomes of children and youths with EBD (e.g., Landrum et al., 2003). Unfortunately, there is similar evidence that those same empirically supported procedures are not routinely implemented in practice (e.g., Meadows, Neel, Scott, & Parker, 1994; Shores et al., 1993). In fact, Kauffman (1996) has suggested that there may even be an inverse relationship be-

tween the effectiveness of a practice and its level of implementation.

Possibly the most explicit examples of the gap between research and classroom practice is the use of contingent teacher attention, or praise. Praise has been shown repeatedly to influence the social and academic behavior of students positively. Twenty years ago, the strength of the research base on the positive student outcomes of use of praise was summarized by Strain, Lambert, Kerr, Stagg, and Lenkner (1983): "Literally hundreds of classroom based studies have shown that teachers' delivery of social reinforcement can result in improved academic performance . . . rule-following and good school deportment . . . cognitive and linguistic performance . . . and increased social responsiveness" (p. 243). Regardless, then as now, the use of praise is not a routine practice in classrooms. For example, Strain et al. (1983) found that for merely 10% of the time did teacher attention follow student compliance, and for the 82% of the children in their study who were rated low in social adjustment, no positive consequences for compliance ever occurred. In classrooms for students with EBD, Shores et al. (1993) found teacher praise rates as low as one per hour. Given these and similar results from other studies, Wehby, Symons, Canale, and Go (1998) have concluded that "teacher praise . . . is almost nonexistent in classrooms for children with E/BD" (p. 51).

That teachers do not use effective practices at a high rate is troublesome; however, a further concern is that teachers often do not implement practices with integrity. As Malouf and Schiller (1995) noted, "When research does find its way into practice, it is often misapplied" (p. 419). For example, time out from positive reinforcement has a corpus of literature demonstrating its effective use for decreasing problem behavior (e.g., Martin & Pear, 2003); yet, time out is very likely to be implemented incorrectly in classroom settings (see Nelson & Rutherford, 1983). Intervention integrity, also known as treatment fidelity or intervention adherence (Moncher & Prinz, 1991), is an important aspect in effecting research-based practices given that the extent to which interventions are implemented as designed is directly associated with the extent of behavior change noted (e.g., Allinder & Oats, 1997; Gansle & McMahon, 1997; Greenwood, Terry, Arreaga-Mayer, & Finney, 1992; Gresham, Gansle, Noell, Cohen, & Rosenblum, 1993). In other words, if an effective practice is implemented incorrectly, its positive impact is likely to be diminished or completely destroyed. Precision in implementation is one of the defining characteristics of effective classroom procedures for teaching students with EBD (Kauffman et al., 2002).

Discussion

The research-to-practice gap that plagues education is often presented as a classroom-level implementation phenomenon. We contend, however, that it is the misuse or disregard of research at multiple levels of decision making and action that accounts for many students with EBD not benefiting from the interventions known to be effective. If teachers are not taught to use effective practices and policy does not mandate or promote them, teachers are not likely to incorporate effective practices in their classrooms. The interrelated nature of policy, teacher education, and classroom instruction requires that efforts be aimed at bridging the research-to-practice gaps in each of these areas concurrently; in fact, for improved outcomes for children and youths with EBD, it is almost certainly a necessity.

BARRIERS TO AND DIRECTIONS FOR BRINGING RESEARCH TO BEAR UPON PRACTICE

Unquestionably, an important goal in educational research is to develop, evaluate, and disseminate work that directly influences the instructional activities of children and youths in classrooms so that positive outcomes in academic and social learning occur. However, problems in bringing research to bear upon practice are many, and obstacles are often present throughout the strata of policy, teacher training, and classroom instruction (Malouf & Schiller, 1995). When taking into account the ways in which research can be used, misused, or ignored and the complexities of educational practice, it seems that issues related to how knowledge is identified, disseminated, used, and maintained are important considerations for bridging the research-to-practice gap. In the following sections, we discuss these considerations as well as suggest directions for addressing the gap.

Identifying Knowledge: Using Science to Establish Desired Practice

Regardless of whether developing policy, championing reform movements, teaching preservice educators, or instructing students with EBD in the classroom, science (public testing of verifiable data) and its resulting conclusions should be the guiding basis for action (Kauffman, 1999a). Yet, how do policymakers, preservice educators, teacher trainers, and classroom teachers identify the conclusions of existing bodies of scientific knowledge so that they can set priorities, enact legislation, train teachers, and deliver instruction? Greenwood and Maheady (2001) suggest developing and using standards of practice to identify the scientific knowledge base.

Standards of practice are common in other professions to delineate specific practices that have been shown to produce the best outcomes (Carnine, 1995). The importance of standards is that they set the norms for best practices and products. Many professions within the basic sciences (e.g., medicine, engineering) and social sciences (e.g., psychology) have determined which practices are linked empirically to the best results. Such standards of practice provide a unified approach to guiding the profession, training professionals, and affecting consumers in scientifically determined ways; as well as a means for the public to evaluate and support the actions of the profession and its members (Walker, Forness, et al., 1998).

In contrast to other professional groups, Greenwood and Maheady (2001) point out that "education has no public, agreed-upon process for identifying practices that should be included in and excluded from" standards of practice (p. 336). To date, no agreed-upon teaching behaviors, instructional procedures, intervention techniques, or organizational structure has been acknowledged as standard practice, nor have any agreed-upon methods for determining how standard practice should be identified been advocated. As Vaughn and Dammann (2001) point out, "A base of rigorous scientifically determined research does exist, but the implications of the research have not been recognized, agreed upon, or implemented" (p. 21).

Given our considerable and strong research literature, standards of practice in special education (and in the field of EBD) could be assembled and applied, thereby providing a scientific knowledge base to guide educational decisions, training, and classroom instruction. In fact, this process seems to be under way, as a relatively large number of literature syntheses have been conducted recently in attempts to summarize the effectiveness of specific interventions and practices using meta-analytic techniques (e.g., Forness & Kavale, 1996; Forness, Kavale, Blum, & Lloyd, 1997; Quinn, Kavale, Mathur, Rutherford, & Forness, 1999; Talbott, Lloyd, & Tankersley, 1994). The results of meta-analyses include an effect size for each study in the synthesis that examines a particular intervention. An average effect size is then calculated based on the number of studies in the synthesis, providing an indication of the strength of that intervention (Forness et al., 1997).

Another way to summarize the literature is by determining whether specific practices have sufficient empirical support regarding their efficacy and/or utility by applying a set of criteria to the body of literature. For example, Division 12 Task Force of the American Psychological Association developed a model of criteria for establishing which treatments and practices warrant implementation, promotion, and dissemination. Two sets of criteria were established for defining a treatment as empirically supported: that it be well established or probably efficacious (Chambless et al., 1998). Treatments receiving either of these designations represent those for which there is demonstrated efficacy in outcome. Other professional organizations also employ or are considering similar techniques for summarizing their knowledge base (e.g., Council for Exceptional Children, The Task Force on Evidence-Based Interventions in School Psychology, U.S. Department of Education's Institute of Education Sciences).

The importance of determining standards of practice is that they set the norms for action in the field: the empirical knowledge base becomes the guide for policy, teacher preparation, and classroom instruction. Standards of practice make it apparent which practices have solid empirical support and which do not (Greenwood & Maheady, 2001; Mostert & Crockett, 1999–2000); using standards of practice, stakeholders (e.g., parents, teachers, politicians, administrators, teacher trainers, researchers) have a guide for discerning between research-supported practices and those without a scientific foundation. Without actively determining, advocating, and using empirically based standards of practice, the most substantial evidence we have for affecting child learning and behavioral outcomes may be ignored or misused.

Disseminating Knowledge: Connecting Positive Student Outcomes to the Use of Effective Practices

The empirical literature base in special education does not, and probably cannot ever (Cook & Cook, 2004), permit us to conclusively determine the efficacy of every known instructional technique with every child who may be taught in a school. The social sciences simply do not result in such perfect predictions. However, it is almost certainly true that, as Mostert and Crockett (1999–2000) suggest, we now know more about effective practices in special education than ever before—and researchers are continually expanding and improving upon that research base. Although much work is left to be accomplished in determining and applying standards of practice, we believe that this goal can and will be accomplished in the near future. However, determining what works does not necessarily entail that practitioners—who bear the responsibility for implementing effective practice—know and value that information.

Currently, teachers receive a barrage of information about what and how to teach—much of it with no empirical basis (see Landrum & Tankersley, 2004). This happens at both the preservice and inservice levels. And because most teachers have not been extensively trained in research, they are unable to evaluate the scientific merits of claims that a given procedure works. Indeed, teaching has been described as a profession that is particularly cynical about research (Gersten, 2001). One avenue for ameliorating teachers' neglect of and even hostility toward research is changing how research is disseminated or reported.

Teachers do not tend to value reports of research. Most are not experts in research methodology or in interpreting statistics. Moreover, even for those who understand the methods, reports of research are extremely difficult to translate into practice (Carnine, 1997). Knowing that a procedure had a statistically significant effect on an outcome does not go very far toward being able to use it with a classroom full of students tomorrow. We have begun to investigate the types of information that teachers most value. Not surprisingly, teachers appear to place more worth on information that comes from other teachers than research reports (Cook, 2003; Landrum, Cook, Tankersley, & Fitzgerald, 2002). Thus, it appears that inundating teachers with more and more reports of research is unlikely to be productive. Researchers and teacher educators might consider (1) embedding research findings in stories and anecdotes from teachers illustrating how to effectively use a given procedure and the effectiveness of the technique with their students and (2) providing repeated practice in effective techniques so that evidence-based practices become the experiential basis from which teachers make the many instantaneous decisions that are needed in a typical school day (Cook & Cook, 2004).

Implementing Knowledge: Bringing Research to Bear upon Practice

Establishing and disseminating standards of practice that are connected to student outcomes provides policymakers, teacher educators, and classroom teachers the means for using the knowledge base. A further consideration is bringing research to bear upon practice in the classroom. Research shows that teachers are not likely to use research as a means for determining what instructional and management techniques they use. For example, Jack et al. (1996) found that most teachers sought their colleagues' advice on classroom management concerns instead of

referring to university coursework. Similarly, Landrum et al. (2002) found that preservice and experienced teachers rated university classes and research literature as less trustworthy and helpful resources than other teachers for identifying effective teaching techniques. Given that research is often presented in confusing ways (Gersten, 2001) and may be difficult or impossible to translate meaningfully into practice (Abbott, Walton, Tapia, & Greenwood, 1999; Carnine, 1997), it is little wonder that teachers seek other avenues to inform their practice.

Unfortunately, getting research through the classroom door is not a simple matter of informing teachers of effective practices (Gersten, Chard, & Baker, 2000). The results of sponsored projects focusing on increasing the implementation of empirically validated practices with students with disabilities provide a number of specific recommendations for assisting teachers and school personnel in increasing their use of these practices. Among the recommendations, Gersten, Vaughn, Deshler, and Schiller (1997) specified that the context of supportive and professional peer interactions is a critical element for enacting change of teacher practice and implementing effective practices in classrooms (see also Abbott et al., 1999; Boudah, Logan, & Greenwood, 2001; Gersten & Dimino, 2001). Additionally, teachers were found to be more likely to embrace change with the support of colleagues.

As the realities of classrooms, teachers, and students inevitably differ, no one prescription for effective teaching will meet the needs of all teachers and students. One theme that resonates throughout the literature on implementation is that teachers need to adapt effective practices to best match the needs of their students, their teaching strengths, and the available resources (Abbott et al., 1999; Boudah et al., 2001; Gersten & Dimino, 2001; Gersten et al., 1997; Speece, MacDonald, Kilsheimer, & Krist, 1997). Abbott et al. (1999) noted that successful support and implementation of effective practices, based on a model of consultative problem solving, provides a means to take individual needs into consideration. Consultative problem solving is a conceptual framework for dyadic and team problem solving and planning based on a model that serves as the foundation for most contemporary collaborative consultation endeavors in schools (e.g., student-study teams) (see Bergan, 1995; Kratochwill, Elliott, & Rotto, 1995). This empirically validated model calls for teams to describe the problem, specify measurable goals, analyze the problem, select an effective practice for intervention, formulate a plan for action, and develop a monitoring and evaluation system (see Kampwirth, 1999; Telzrow, 1995). The problem-solving model, then, seeks empirically based interventions specified because of known student outcomes, and devises a plan for supporting the implementation of the identified interventions in the classroom. Such a model addresses many of the identified barriers to bringing research to bear upon practice.

Maintaining and Sustaining Knowledge in Practice

Engendering supportive environments that use the collaborative problem-solving model will increase the likelihood of evidence-based practices making their way into schools and classrooms (Kratochwill, Elliott, & Callan-Stoiber, 2002; Sheridan, Welch, & Orme, 1996). However, it is important to realize that school-based support is "steady work" (Boudah et al., 2001; Gersten & Dimino, 2001; Gersten et al., 1997). Teachers will confront a number of unanticipated challenges in implementing effective practices with their students (Gersten et al., 1995). Without easily accessible, frequent, and regular support, many teachers will revert to their traditional practices that are not based on evidence of effectiveness.

Monitoring and evaluative efforts that link the implementation of effective practices to improvements in student behavior and performance are also necessary for sustained implementation of effective practices (Abbott et al., 1999; Gersten et al., 1997). Systematically collecting and analyzing information regarding student progress in relation to intervention implementation will validate the use of the practice. In this way, teachers directly link the two phenomena. Once they are convinced that their efforts are resulting in improved outcomes for their students, most teachers are likely to continue to implement and refine the effective

practices employed. Use of formative performance-monitoring techniques, such as curriculum-based measurement (CBM; see Deno, 2003) and direct observation and analysis techniques, such as single-subject research methods (see Kazdin, 1982), provides educators a means for making the direct connection between their use of effective practices and changes in student behavior and learning.

In addition to providing supports to individual teachers, there must be a commitment to a more widespread adoption of empirically based instructional methods. The supports just noted have been associated with teachers adopting effective practices. But the projects that utilized these supports were successful with individual teachers, not entire school systems. It is unlikely that this method—supporting individual teachers one by one—will ever result in whole school systems (let alone whole states or countries) pervasively bridging the gap between research and practice. Fuchs and Fuchs (1998, 2001) provide suggestions for "scaling up" efforts for implementing effective teaching practices. One strategy involves working with a small, select group of teachers in a large number of schools. By selecting only a small group of motivated and talented teachers, the probability of successfully adopting effective practices among initial participants is heightened. After witnessing the success of these teachers, others are more likely to embrace the idea. Furthermore, the initial participants can serve as mentors to others in their schools to facilitate the diffusion of research-based procedures.

CONCLUSION

Increasing the extent, consistency, and ease with which research informs practice is a formidable challenge in the field of EBD. As we seek to improve practice, areas of policy, teacher education, and classroom instruction must be concurrent considerations. The interactional nature of the three can result in dissonance and impede the use of effective practices or can act in concert and facilitate the use of effective practices on a widespread basis. It is only in the synchronization of policy, teacher education, and classroom practices can far-reaching effects be actualized—

and for the effects to be optimal, decisions and actions must be based on the empirical evidence available. Further, eliminating the barriers that seem to be related to how knowledge is identified, disseminated, used, and maintained will go a long way toward bringing research to bear upon the education of children and youths with EBD.

With even this cursory examination of the status of research in the field of EBD, we can garner two truths: (1) we have accumulated and continue to generate knowledge sufficient for improving the academic and behavioral outcomes of students with EBD, and (2) we have much work ahead of us in ensuring that this knowledge is used in policy making, teacher education, and classroom instruction. The fact that EBD is a relatively young profession is an important consideration in relation to our knowledge base: the research focus has been primarily on—and probably rightly so—the identification of student characteristics, validating assessments, building theoretical explanations, and developing and evaluating interventions. Now attention must turn to getting the established empirical knowledge base used as the guide for determining policy, training teachers, and intervening with children and youths with EBD.

We must build a foundation of science so that our practices are clearly tied to what is known through our knowledge base. Developing standards of practice and connecting practice to positive outcomes for children and youths with EBD will provide the field and its stakeholders guidelines to direct practice and demonstrate accountability. Using science to determine practice for policy, personnel preparation, and student instruction also elevates the field to that of a profession (Walker, Forness, et al., 1998).

REFERENCES

Abbott, M., Walton, C., Tapia, Y., & Greenwood, C. R. (1999). Research to practice: A "blueprint" for closing the gap in local schools. *Exceptional Children, 65,* 339–352.

Achenbach, T. M. (1991). *The Child Behavior Checklist: Manual for the teacher's report form.* Burlington. University of Vermont, Department of Psychiatry.

Achenbach, T., Howell, C., McConaughy, S. H., &

Stranger, C. (1995). Six-year predictors of problems in a national sample: 1. Cross-informant syndromes. *Journal of the American Academy of Child and Adolescent Psychiatry, 34,* 336–347.

Allinder, R. M., & Oats, R. G. (1997). Effects of acceptability on teachers' implementation of curriculum-based measurement and student achievement in mathematics computation. *Remedial and Special Education, 18,* 113–120.

Armstrong, S. W., & Kauffman, J. M. (1999). Functional behavioral assessment: Introduction to the series. *Behavioral Disorders, 24,* 167–168.

Baker, J. M., & Zigmond, N. (1995). The meaning and practice of inclusion for students with learning disabilities: Themes and implications from the five cases. *The Journal of Special Education, 29,* 163–180.

Bergan, J. R. (1995). Evolution of a problem-solving model of consultation. *Journal of Educational and Psychological Consultation, 6,* 111–124.

Boudah, D. J., Logan, K. R., & Greenwood, C. R. (2001). The research to practice projects: Lessons learned about changing teacher practice. *Teacher Education and Special Education, 24,* 290–303.

Bower, E. M. (1981). *Early identification of emotionally handicapped children in school* (3rd ed.). Springfield, IL: Thomas.

Bower, E. M. (1982). Defining emotional disturbance: Public policy and research. *Psychology in the Schools, 19,* 55–60.

Braden, J., & Kratochwill, T. (1997). Treatment utility of assessment: Myths and realities. *School Psychology Review, 26,* 475–485.

Bullock, L. M, Ellis, L. L., & Wilson, M. J. (1994). Knowledge/skills needed by teachers who work with students with severe emotional/behavior disorders: A revisitation. *Behavioral Disorders, 19,* 108–125.

Carnine, D. (1995). Trustworthiness, useability, and accessibility of educational research. *Journal of Behavioral Education, 5,* 251–258.

Carnine, D. (1997). Bridging the research-to-practice gap. *Exceptional Children, 63,* 513–521.

Carson, R. R., Sitlington, P. L., & Frank, A. R. (1995). Young adulthood for individuals with behavioral disorders: What does it hold? *Behavioral Disorders, 20,* 127–135.

Chall, J. S. (2000). *The academic achievement challenge.* New York: Guilford Press.

Chambless, D. L., Baker, M. J., Baucom, D. H., Beutler, L., Calhoun, K. S., Crits-Christoph, P., Daiuto, A., DeRubeis, R., Detweiler, J., Haaga, D. A. F., Bennett-Johnson, S., McCurry, S., Mueser, K. T., Pope, K. S., Sanderson, W. C., Shoham, V., Stickle, T., Williams, D. A., & Woody, S. A. (1998). Update on empirically validated therapies II. *Clinical Psychologist, 51,* 3–16.

Cline, D. H. (1990). A legal analysis of policy initiatives to exclude handicapped/disruptive students from special education. *Behavioral Disorders, 15,* 159–173.

Colvin, G. (1993). *Managing acting out behavior.* Eugene, OR: Behavior Associates.

Cook, B. G., & Cook, L. (2004). Bringing science into the classroom by basing craft on research. *Learning Disabilities Research and Practice, 37,* 240–247.

Cook, B. G., Landrum, T. J., Tankersley, M., & Kauffman, J. K. (2003). Bringing research to bear on practice: Effecting evidence-based instruction for students with emotional or behavioral disorders. *Education and Treatment of Children, 26,* 345–361.

Cook, B. G., & Schirmer, B. R. (2003). What is special about special education? Overview and analysis of the topical issue [special issue]. *Journal of Special Education, 37,* 200–205.

Cook, L. (2003, April). *Influences on special education student teachers' instructional choices.* Paper presented at the annual meeting of the Council for Exceptional Children. Seattle, WA.

Costenbader, V., & Buntaine, R. (1999). Diagnostic discrimination between social maladjustment and emotional disturbance: An empirical study. *Journal of Emotional and Behavioral Disorders, 7,* 2–10.

Crockett, J. B. (2004). Taking stock of science in the schoolhouse: Four ideas to foster effective instruction. *Journal of Learning Disabilities, 37,* 189–199.

Darveaux, D. X. (1984). The Good Behavior Game plus merit: Controlling disruptive behavior and improving student motivation. *School Psychology Review, 13,* 510–514.

Delquadri, J. C, Greenwood, C. R., Whorton, D., Carta, J. J., & Hall, R. V. (1986). Classwide peer tutoring. *Exceptional Children, 52,* 535–542.

Deno, S. L. (2003). Developments in curriculum-based measurement. *Journal of Special Education, 37,* 184–192.

Duncan, B. B., Forness, S. R., & Hartsough, C. (1995). Students identified as seriously emotionally disturbed in school-based day treatment: Cognitive, psychiatric, and special education characteristics. *Behavioral Disorders, 20,* 238–252.

Dunlap, G., & Childs, K. E. (1996). Intervention research in EBD: An analysis of studies from 1980-1993. *Behavioral Disorders, 21,* 125–136.

Elmore, R. F. (1997). The politics of education reform. *Issues in Science and Technology, 14,* 41–49.

Espin, C. A., & Deno, S. L. (2000). Introduction to the special issue of *Learning Disabilities Research & Practice*: Research to Practice: Views from researchers and practitioners. *Learning Disabilities: Research and Practice, 15,* 67–68.

Finn, C. E., Jr., & Rotherham, A. J. (2001, December 26). Give special ed a road map to success. *Los Angeles Times,* p. B13.

Forness, S. R., & Kavale, K. A. (1996). Treating social skill deficits in children with learning disabilities: A meta-analysis of the research. *Learning Disabilities Quarterly, 19,* 1–13.

Forness, S. R., & Kavale, K. A. (1997). Defining emotional or behavioral disorders in school and related services. In J. W. Lloyd, E. J., Kameenui, & D. Chard (Eds.), *Issues in educating students with disabilities* (pp. 45–61). Mahwah, NJ: Erlbaum.

Forness, S. R., & Kavale, K. A. (2000). Emotional or behavioral disorders: Background and current status of the E/BD terminology and definition. *Behavioral Disorders, 25,* 264–269.

Forness, S. R., & Kavale, K. A. (2001). Reflections on the future of prevention. *Preventing School Failure, 45,* 75–81.

Forness, S. R., Kavale, K. A., Blum, I. M., & Lloyd, J. W. (1997). What works in special education and related services: Using meta-analysis to guide practice. *Teaching Exceptional Children, 29*(6), 4–9.

Forness, S. R., Kavale, K. A., King, B. H., & Kasari, C. (1994). Simple versus complex conduct disorders: Identification and phenomenology. *Behavioral Disorders, 19,* 306–312.

Forness, S. R., Kavale, K. A., MacMillan, D. L., Asarnow, J. R., & Duncan, B. B. (1996). Early detection and prevention of emotional or behavioral disorders: Developmental aspects of systems of care. *Behavioral Disorders, 21,* 226–240.

Forness, S. R., Serna, L. A., Nielson, E., Lambros, K., Hale, M. J., & Kavale, K. A. (2000). A model for early detection and primary prevention of emotional or behavioral disorders. *Education and Treatment of Children, 23,* 325–345.

Frank, A. R., Sitlington, P. L., & Carson, R. (1991). Transition of adolescents with behavioral disorders: Is it successful? *Behavioral Disorders, 16,* 180–191.

Fuchs, D., & Fuchs, L. S. (1995). What's "special" about special education? *Phi Delta Kappan, 76,* 522–530.

Fuchs, D., & Fuchs, L. S. (1998). Researchers and teachers working together to adapt instruction for diverse learners. *Learning Disabilities Research and Practice, 13,* 126–137.

Fuchs, L. S., & Fuchs, D. (2001). Principles for sustaining research-based practice in the schools: A case study. *Focus on Exceptional Children, 33*(6), 1–14.

Gamoran, A., & Dreeben, R. (1986). Coupling and control in educational organizations. *Administrative Science Quarterly, 31,* 612–632.

Gansle, K. A., & McMahon, C. M. (1997). Component integrity of teacher intervention management behavior using a student self-monitoring treatment: An experimental analysis. *Journal of Behavioral Education, 7,* 405–419.

George, N. L., George, M. P., Gersten, R., & Grosenick, J. K. (1995). To leave or stay? An exploratory study of teachers of students with emotional and behavioral disorders. *Remedial and Special Education, 16,* 227–236.

Gersten, R. (2001). Sorting out the roles of research in the improvement of practice. *Learning Disabilities Research and Practice, 16,* 45–50.

Gersten, R., Chard, D., & Baker, S. (2000). Factors enhancing sustained use of research-based instructional practices. *Journal of Learning Disabilities, 33,* 445–457.

Gersten, R., & Dimino, J. (2001). Realities of translating research into classroom practice. *Learning Disabilities: Research and Practice, 16,* 120–130.

Gersten, R., Morvant, M., & Brengelman, S. (1995). Close to the classroom means close to the bone: Coaching as a means to translate research into classroom practice. *Exceptional Children, 62,* 52–67.

Gersten, R., Vaughn, S., Deshler, D., & Schiller, E. (1997). What we know about using research findings: Implications for improving special education practice. *Journal of Learning Disabilities, 30,* 466–476.

Greenwood, C. R. (Ed.). (2001). Bridging the gap between research and practice in special education: Issues and implications for teacher preparation [Special issue]. *Teacher Education and Special Education, 24*(4).

Greenwood, C. R., & Abbott, M. (2001). The research to practice gap in special education. *Teacher Education and Special Education, 24,* 276–289.

Greenwood, C. R., & Maheady, L. (2001). Are future teachers aware of the gap between research and practice and what should they know? *Teacher Education and Special Education, 24,* 333–347.

Greenwood, C. R., Terry, B., Arreaga-Mayer, C., & Finney, R. (1992). The classwide peer tutoring program: Implementation factors moderating students' achievement. *Journal of Applied Behavior Analysis, 25,* 101–116.

Gresham, F. M., Gansle, K. A., Noell, G. H., Cohen, S., & Rosenblum, S. (1993). Treatment integrity of school-based intervention studies: 1980–1990. *School Psychology Review, 22,* 254–272.

Gresham, F. M., Lane, K. L., McIntyre, L. L., MacMillan, D. M., Lambros, K. M., & Bocain, K. (2001). Risk factors associated with the co-occurrence of hyperactivity–impulsivity–inattention and conduct problems. *Behavioral Disorders, 26,* 189–199.

Gresham, F. M., Watson, T. S., & Skinner, C. H. (2001). Functional behavioral assessment: Principles, procedures, and future directions. *School Psychology Review, 30,* 156–172.

Hallahan, D. P., & Kauffman, J. M. (2003). *Exceptional learners: Introduction to special education* (9th ed.). Boston: Allyn & Bacon.

Hinshaw, S. P. (1992). Externalizing behavior problems and academic underachievement in childhood and adolescence: Causal relationships and underlying mechanisms. *Psychological Bulletin, 111,* 127–155.

Hockenbury, J. C., Kauffman, J. M., & Hallahan, D. P. (1999–2000). What is right about special education. *Exceptionality, 8,* 3–11.

Jack, S. L., Shores, R. E., Denny, R. K., Gunter, P. L., DeBriere, T., & DePaepe, P. (1996). An analysis of the relationship of teachers' reported use of classroom management strategies on types of interactions. *Journal of Behavioral Education, 6,* 67–87.

Kaiser, A., & Hester, P. P. (1997). Prevention of conduct disorders through early intervention: A social-communicative perspective. *Behavioral Disorders, 22,* 117–130.

Kampwirth, T. J. (1999). *Collaborative consultation in the schools: Effective practices for students with learning and behavior problems.* Upper Saddle River, NJ: Prentice Hall.

Kauffman, J. M. (1996). Research to practice issues. *Behavioral Disorders, 22,* 55–60.

Kauffman, J. M. (1999a). Commentary: Today's special education and its messages for tomorrow. *Journal of Special Education, 32,* 244–254.

Kauffman, J. M. (1999b). How we prevent prevention of emotional and behavioral disorders. *Exceptional Children, 65,* 448–468.

Kauffman, J. M. (2001). *Characteristics of emotional and behavioral disorders of children and youth* (7th ed.). Upper Saddle River, NJ: Merrill/Prentice Hall.

Kauffman, J. M., Bantz, J., & McCullough, J. (2002). Separate and better: A special public school class for students with emotional and behavioral disorders. *Exceptionality, 10,* 149–170.

Kauffman, J. M., & Wong, K. L. H. (1991). Effective teachers of students with behavioral disorders: Are generic teaching skills enough? *Behavioral Disorders, 16,* 225–237.

Kazdin, A. E. (1982). *Single-case research designs: Methods for clinical and applied settings.* New York: Oxford University Press.

Kazdin, A. E. (1987). *Conduct disorders in childhood and adolescence: Vol. 9.* Beverly Hills, CA: Sage.

Kellam, S. G., & Rebok, G. W. (1992). Building developmental and etiological theory through epidemiologically based preventive intervention trials. In J. McCord & R. E. Tremblay (Eds.), *Preventing antisocial behavior: Interventions from birth through adolescence* (pp. 162–195). New York: Guilford Press.

Klingner, J. K., Vaughn, S., Hughes, M. T., Schumm, J. S., & Elbaum, B. (1998). Outcomes for students with and without learning disabilities in inclusive classrooms. *Learning Disabilities Research and Practice, 13,* 153–161.

Kratochwill, T. R., Elliott, S. N., & Callan-Stoiber, K. (2002). Best practices in school-based problem-solving consultation. In A. Thomas & J. Grimes (Eds.), *Best practices in school psychology* (4th ed., pp. 583–608). Bethesda, MD: National Association of School Psychologists.

Kratochwill, T. R., Elliott, S. N., & Rotto, P. C. (1995). Best practices in school-based behavioral consultation. In A. Thomas & J. Grimes (Eds.), *Best practices in school psychology* (3rd ed., pp. 519–538). Washington, DC: National Association of School Psychologists.

Landrum, T. J., Cook, B. G., Tankersley, M., & Fitzgerald, S. (2002). Teacher perceptions of the trustworthiness, useability, and accessibility of information from different sources. *Remedial and Special Education, 23,* 42–48.

Landrum, T. J., & Tankersley, M. (2004). Science in the

schoolhouse: An uninvited guest. *Learning Disabilities Research and Practice, 37,* 207–212.

Landrum, T. J., Tankersley, M., & Kauffman, J. M. (2003). What's special about special education for students with emotional or behavioral disorders? *Journal of Special Education, 37,* 148–156.

Lane, K. L., Gresham, F. M., & O'Shaughnessy, T. E. (2002). Serving students with or at-risk for emotional and behavior disorders: Future challenges. *Education and Treatment of Children, 25,* 507–521.

Lloyd, J. W., Bateman, D. F., Landrum, T. J., & Hallahan, D. P. (1989). Self-recording of attention versus productivity. *Journal of Applied Behavior Analysis, 22,* 315–323.

Lloyd, J. W., Forness, S. R., & Kavale, K. A. (1998). Some methods are more effective than others. *Intervention in School and Clinic, 33,* 195–200.

Malouf, D. B., & Schiller, E. P. (1995). Practice and research in special education. *Exceptional Children, 61,* 414–424.

Marder, C. (1992). Education after secondary school. In M. Wagner, R. D'Amico, C. Marder, L. Newman, & J. Blackorby (Eds.), *What happens next?: Trends in postschool outcomes of youth with disabilities. The second comprehensive report from the National Longitudinal Transition Study of Special Education Students* (pp. 3-1–3-39). Menlo Park, CA: SRI International.

Martin, G., & Pear, J. (2003). *Behavior modification: What it is and how to do it* (7th ed.). Upper Saddle River, NJ: Prentice Hall.

Mastropieri, M. A., Scruggs, T. E., & Casto, G. (1985). Early intervention for behaviorally disordered children: An integrative review. In R. B. Rutherford (Ed.), *Monograph in Behavior Disorders* (Vol. 9, pp. 27–35). Reston, VA: Council for Children with Behavioral Disorders.

McConaughy, S. H., Stranger, C., & Achenbach, T. M. (1992). Three-year course of behavioral/emotional problems in a national sample of 4- to 16-year-olds: I. Agreement among informants. *Journal of the American Academy of Child and Adolescent Psychiatry, 31,* 932–940.

McMillan, D. L., Gresham, F. M., & Forness, S. R. (1996). Full inclusion: An empirical perspective. *Behavioral Disorders, 21,* 145–159.

Meadows, N. B., Neel, R. S., Scott, C. M., & Parker, G. (1994). Academic performance, social competence, and mainstream accommodations: A look at mainstreamed and nonmainstreamed students with serious behavioral disorders. *Behavioral Disorders, 19,* 170–180.

Meyer, J. W., & Rowan, B. (1977). Institutionalized organizations: Formal structure as myth and ceremony. *American Journal of Sociology, 83,* 340–363.

Moffitt, T. (1994). Adolescence-limited and life-course persistent antisocial behavior: A developmental taxonomy. *Psychological Review, 100,* 674–701.

Moncher, F. J., & Prinz, R. J. (1991). Treatment fidelity in outcome studies. *Clinical Psychology Review, 11,* 247–266.

Mostert, M. P., & Crockett, J. B. (1999–2000). Reclaiming the history of special education for more effective practice. *Exceptionality, 8,* 133–143.

Nelson, C. M., & Rutherford, R. B. (1983). Timeout revisited: Guidelines for its use in special education. *Exceptional Education Quarterly, 3*(4), 56–67.

Nelson, J. R., Roberts, M. L., Mathur, S. R., & Rutherford, R. B. (1999). Has public policy exceeded our knowledge base?: A review of the functional behavioral assessment literature. *Behavioral Disorders, 24,* 169–179.

Neville, M. H., & Jenson, W. R. (1984). Precision command and the "sure I will" program: A quick and efficient compliance training sequence. *Child and Family Behavior Therapy, 6,* 61–65.

Ochoa, S. H., & Olivarez, A. (1995). A meta-analysis of peer rating sociometric studies of pupils with learning disabilities. *Journal of Special Education, 29,* 1–19.

Patterson, G. R. (1982). *Coercive family process: Vol. 3. A social learning approach.* Eugene, OR: Castalia.

Patterson, G. R., Reid, J. B., & Dishion, T. J. (1992). *Antisocial boys.* Eugene, OR: Castalia.

Proctor, M. A., & Morgan, D. (1991). Effectiveness of a response cost raffle procedure on the disruptive behavior of adolescents with behavior problems. *School Psychology Review, 20,* 97–109.

Quinn, M. M., Kavale, K. A., Mathur, S. R., Rutherford, R. B., & Forness, S. R. (1999). A meta-analysis of social skills interventions for students with emotional or behavioral disorders. *Journal of Emotional and Behavioral Disorders, 7,* 54–64.

Reid, J. (1993). Prevention of conduct disorder before and after school entry: Relating interventions to developmental findings. *Development and Psychopathology, 5,* 243–262.

Salend, S. J., & Gordon, B. D. (1987). A group-oriented timeout ribbon procedure. *Behavioral Disorders, 12,* 131–137.

Sasso, G., Conroy, M. A., Stichter, J., & Fox, J. J. (2001). Slowing down the bandwagon: The misapplication of functional assessment for students with emotional or behavioral disorders. *Behavioral Disorders, 26,* 282–296.

Schneider, B. H., & Leroux, J. (1994). Educational environments for the pupil with behavioral disorders: A 'best evidence' synthesis. *Behavioral Disorders, 19,* 494–501.

Sheridan, S. M., Welch, M., & Orme, S. F. (1996). Is consultation effective? A review of outcome research. *Remedial and Special Education, 17,* 341–354.

Shinn, M. R., Walker, H. M., & Stoner, G. (Eds.). (2002). *Interventions for academic and behavior problems: II. Preventive and remedial approaches.* Bethesda, MD: National Association of School Psychologists.

Shores, R. E., Jack, S., Gunter, P. L., Ellis, D., DeBriere, T., & Wehby, J. H. (1993). Classroom interactions of children with behavioral disorders. *Journal of Emotional and Behavioral Disorders, 1,* 27–39.

Sindelar, P. T., & Brownell, M. T. (2001). Research to practice dissemination, scale, and context: We can do it, but we can we afford it? *Teacher Education and Special Education, 24,* 348–355.

Smith, S., & Farrell, D. (1993). Level system use in special education: Classroom intercvention with prima facie appeal. *Behavioral Disorders, 18,* 251–264.

Speece, D. L., MacDonald, V., Kilsheimer, L., & Krist, J. (1997). Research to practice: Preservice teachers reflect on reciprocal teaching. *Learning Disabilities Research and Practice, 12,* 177–187.

Strain, P. S., Lambert, D. L., Kerr, M. M., Stagg, V., & Lenkner, D. A. (1983). Naturalistic assessment of children's compliance to teachers' requests and consequences for compliance. *Journal of Applied Behavior Analysis, 16,* 243–249.

Swanson, H. L., & Malone, S. (1992). Social skills and learning disabilities: A meta-analysis of the literature. *School Psychology Review, 21,* 427–443.

Talbott, E., Lloyd, J. W., & Tankersley, M. (1994). Reading comprehension interventions for students with learning disabilities. *Journal of Learning Disabilities, 17,* 223–232.

Tankersley, M., Kamps, D., Mancina, K., & Wiedinger, D. (1996). Social interventions for Head Start children with behavioral risks: Implementation and outcomes. *Journal of Emotional and Behavioral Disorders, 4,* 171–181.

Tankersley, M., & Landrum, T. J. (1997). Comorbidity of emotional and behavioral disorders. In J. W. Lloyd, E. J. Kameenui, & D. Chard (Eds.), *Issues in educating students with disabilities* (pp. 153–173). Mahwah, NJ: Erlbaum.

Telzrow, C. F. (1995). Best practices in facilitating intervention adherence. In A. Thomas & J. Frimes (Eds.), *Best practices in school psychology* (3rd ed., pp. 501–510). Washington, DC: National Association of School Psychologists.

Tilly, W. D., Knoster, T. P., & Ikeda, M. J. (2000). Functional behavioral assessment: Strategies for positive behavior support. In C. F. Telzrow & M. Tankersley (Eds.), *IDEA Amendments of 1997: Practice guidelines for school-based teams* (pp. 151–197). Washington, DC: National Association of School Psychologists.

Vaughn, S., & Dammann, J. E. (2001). Science and sanity in special education. *Behavioral Disorders, 27,* 21–29.

Wagner, M., D'Amico, R., Marder, C., Newman, L., & Blackorby, J. (1992). *What happens next?: Trends in postschool outcomes of youths with disabilities. The second comprehensive report from the National Longitudinal Transition Study of Special Education Students.* Menlo Park, CA: SRI International.

Walker, H. M., Colvin, G., & Ramsey, E. (1995). *Antisocial behavior in school: Strategies and best practices.* Pacific Grove, CA: Brooks/Cole.

Walker, H. M., Forness, S. R., Kauffman, J. M., Epstein, M. H., Gresham, F. M., Nelson, C. M., & Strain, P. S. (1998). Macro-social validation: Referencing outcomes in behavioral disorders to societal issues and problems. *Behavioral Disorders, 24,* 7–18.

Walker, H. M., Hops, H. & Fiegenbaum, E. (1976). Deviant classroom behavior as a function of combinations of social and token reinforcement and cost contingency. *Behavior Therapy, 7,* 76–88.

Walker, H. M., Kavanagh, K., Stiller, B., Golly, A., Severson, H. H., & Feil, E.G. (1998). First Step to Success: An early intervention approach for preventing school antisocial behavior. *Journal of Emotional and Behavioral Disorders, 6,* 66–80.

Walker, H. M., & McConnell, S. (1995). *The Walker–McConnell Scale of Social Competence and School Adjustment—Elementary Version.* San Diego, CA: Singular.

Walker, H. M., & Severson, H. H. (1992). *Systematic Screening for Behavior Disorders: User's guide and technical manual.* Longmont, CO: Sopris West.

Walker, H. M., Sprague, J. R., Close, D. W., & Starlin, C. M. (1999–2000). What is right with behavior disorders: Seminal achievements and contributions of the behavior disorders field. *Exceptionality, 8,* 13–28.

Weatherley, R., & Lipsky, M. (1977). Street level bureaucrats and institutional innovation: Implementing special-education reform. *Harvard Educational Review, 47,* 171–197.

Wehby, J. H., Symons, F. J., Canale, J. A., & Go, F. J. (1998). Teaching practices in classrooms for students with emotional and behavioral disorders: Discrepancies between recommendations and observations. *Behavioral Disorders, 24,* 51–56.

Whelan, R. J., & Simpson, R. L. (1996). Preparation of personnel for students with emotional and behavioral disorders: Perspectives on a research foundation for future practice. *Behavioral Disorders, 22,* 49–54.

Wood, F. M. (1999). CCBD: A record of accomplishment. *Behavioral Disorders, 24,* 273–283.

Zigmond, N., Jenkins, J. R., Fuchs, L. S., Deno, S., Fuchs, D., Baker, J. N., Jenkins, L., & Coutinho, M. (1995). Special education in restructured schools: Findings from three multi-year studies. *Phi Delta Kappan, 76,* 531–540.

PART II

ASSESSMENT AND EVALUATION

Introduction

LEWIS POLSGROVE

This section of the *Handbook* concerns issues on assessment of children and youth who may be "at risk" for or have been identified as having emotional and/or behavioral disorders (EBD). I use the qualifier "and/or" here to call attention to the notion that some children—hose with anxiety and mood disorders, for example—have difficulty controlling their emotions, while others may have good emotional control but display considerable antisocial behaviors and instrumental aggression. Others, perhaps most, may exhibit difficulty controlling *both* their emotions and behavior. Both the type and degree of EBD varies along a continuum. Thus, lines drawn between EBD and children whose emotional and behavioral development falls within normal developmental parameters, and between different categories and subtypes of EBD, are frequently subjective and context-specific (Kauffman, 2001).

These points may seem belabored, even superfluous. I make them to remind readers weighing material in these chapters of the political and arbitrary nature of various assessment activities. The authors in this section of the *Handbook* deal with such recurrent issues as identification and early intervention with students "at risk" for EBD; whether a youngster "has" EBD; what type of EBD a child or youth displays; the development of instruments that provide the most effective and useful information; use of systematic academic assessment and individualization of instruction on students' performances; application of multimodal assessment approaches for developing and evaluating interventions; and the effects of testing on students with EBD.

Thus, readers will be exposed to a considerable amount of material on assessment. The body of evidence presented by the authors in this section may seem somewhat incoherent and, for the uninitiated reader, even disparate. However, as an organizational schema, the content can be parsed into essentially two main issues: the goals and procedures of various assessment approaches and the viability of these approaches.

GOALS AND PROCEDURES OF ASSESSMENT

As documented by the authors of the six chapters in this section, assessment of students with EBD assumes a number of forms and is undertaken for various reasons. These can be categorized in terms of various functions. *First,* educators may conduct a "screening" of a student body using various methods to identify students who are struggling in their academic and/or behavioral development. This information may be used to determine the need for prereferral intervention and to monitor their progress. In Chapter 11, Maureen A. Conroy, Jo M. Hendrickson, and Peggy P. Hester point out the irony of the current federal policy of requiring children to have "serious" emotional disorders as a condition for accessing services and present the case for screening and early intervention as measures for preventing or reducing the onslaught of these disorders.

A *second* function of assessment involves determining whether a student identified through screening or referral exhibits academic, emotional, or behavioral disorders significant enough to qualify him or her for special services. Typically, this process is initiated when prereferral efforts such as curriculum modification, contingency management, and behavior modification in general educational settings have not addressed the student's needs successfully. In most states identification of a child as having a disability or disorder significant enough to qualify him or her for ongoing special services requires an extensive psychological and educational assessment and a "differential diagnosis" to determine the type of disability the child demonstrates. Richard E. Mattison, in Chapter 9, describes procedures for identification and differential diagnosis. He makes a case for determining the "comorbidity" of symptoms a student displays as critical to the intervention planning process and the importance of educational personnel being able to recognize symptoms of various diagnostic entities for assessing disorders and developing intervention services.

Behavior ratings by parents, teachers, and, in some cases, the students themselves are perhaps the most widely used instruments for aiding diagnosis of children's EBD and monitoring the effectiveness of interventions. Stephen N. Elliot and R. T. Busse, in Chapter 7, contribute a comprehensive review pertaining to the construction, appropriate uses, and provisos related to these devices, including synopses of five of those most commonly used in educational settings.

While behavioral rating scales offer, indirectly, more molar information on students' behavior, observational approaches provide direct and fine-grained records of a student's behavior in various settings. These instruments allow service providers to identify certain target behaviors, formulate hypotheses concerning environmental variables that occasion and maintain them, establish a preintervention baseline on problem and prosocial behaviors, and offer accurate, low-inference data on the effectiveness of interventions.

The advantages, procedures, and issues related to using observational assessment methods are provided in the chapters by James J. Fox and Robert A. Gable (Chapter 8); Conroy, Hendrickson, and Hester (Chapter 11); and Elliot and Busse (Chapter 7).

The *third* and arguably the most important form of assessment undertaken with students who are at risk or who have been identified as having EBD concerns development and monitoring of academic and behavioral intervention plans by a prereferral or multidisciplinary team of professionals. This process is epitomized by functional behavioral analysis or ecological-behavioral assessment. This approach uses information from a variety of sources and is a complex and ongoing process. The goals are to both identify variables contributing to a student's problem behaviors and use these data to develop and monitor effective intervention programs.

Figure II.1 offers a conceptual framework depicting variables that research has linked to academic and/or behavioral disorders. The model could be used as a guide for collecting pertinent information in a particular case, formulating explanatory hypotheses, and developing interventions. It assumes four major "causative" and interactive sources for observed disorders. *Physiological variables* include temperament, biological state, and arousal level. *Environmental variables* include such stimuli as setting location, type and "schedule" of consequences, influence of significant others, and explicit or implicit demand characteristics of the setting. *Behavioral variables* include previous reinforcement history, response repertoire, and response history. *Cognitive variables* include "private events" such as situational interpretation, self-instructions, level of commitment, personal standards, self-evaluative statements, and cognitive and metacognitive strategies.

For example, the response that a student with EBD may make to, say, a teacher's academic assignment—whether he or she begins work immediately, creates a disruption, or ignores the demand—depends on certain "trait-state" physiological or biological conditions (P) as to whether he or she is inherently oppositional or compliant, physically healthy or ill, fatigued, medicated, anxious, or angry. Too, characteristics of the immediate environment (E) such as setting location

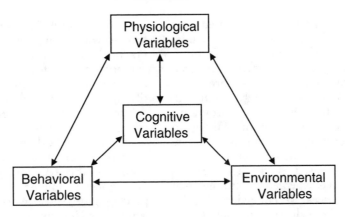

FIGURE II.1. Conceptual model for assessing emotional and behavioral disorders.

(e.g., self-contained vs. inclusive classroom), availability of reinforcers (e.g., points, preferred activities), and history of teacher–pupil interactions determine the student's motivation to perform. The behavioral "component" (B) also affects the probability of the occurrence of a particular response or response pattern. Present behavior is strongly correlated with prior behavior. Thus, whether the child has a particular skill in his or her academic or behavioral "repertoire," can identify appropriate responses required in a situation, has met with prior success or failure at a similar task, and has recently emitted appropriate responses (i.e., behavioral momentum) all influence reactions to current circumstances. Finally, although they are frequently covert, the presence or absence of certain cognitive stimuli (C) also interact with the foregoing variables. The student who interprets a task as too difficult, declares himself or herself uninterested in it, or who lacks the metacognitive skills for task analysis, self-direction, performance evaluation, and motivational support has diminished capacity for responding appropriately.

The applications of such a multifactor approach to assessment are extensive. While it is impossible to completely understand, explain, and predict behavior of a child in all settings, it is important to collect as much information as time and expense will allow in order to grasp general behavioral tendencies and to narrow down the probable motivation factors. Ideally, a comprehensive assessment of a child's behavior for case problem solving should be conducted across

the entire ecology in which he or she operates. To accomplish this, information is collected not just in the classroom or school, but from multiple sources such as medical records, agency service histories, and significant others in other ecological settings (i.e., home, community, and organizations). Such an approach to assessment is critical to developing effective long-term interventions and for planning "wraparound" services.

The chapters contributed by Conroy, Hendrickson, and Hester (Chapter 11) and Fox and Gable (Chapter 8), between them, provide extensive reviews of instruments and descriptions of procedures for conducting a complete functional behavioral assessment for case problem solving. Mattison (in Chapter 9) also supports greater attention to treatment of EBD involving family therapy and the use of a multimodal approach to determining outcomes. Although academic interventions are often overshadowed by emotional and behavioral considerations, they are critical components of school-based change programs for children with EBD. Considerable evidence supports the effectiveness of curriculum-based measurement (CBM) for designing low-failure individualized instructional programs for students with various types of educational disabilities. In Chapter 10, Keith J. Hyatt and Kenneth W. Howell provide a comprehensive overview of the process, issues, and research related to the use of CBM for academic interventions with students identified as EBD.

A *fourth* reason for assessment of students with EBD is wrapped up in the school accountability movement that has gradually emerged over the past decade. Related state and federal policies have resulted in mandatory monitoring of pupils' academic progress in school systems across the country. School districts whose students score above average on measures of progress stand to gain additional funding for their programs. Districts or individual schools failing to show adequate progress stand to lose state and federal funding and/or even incur program closure. Thus, the term High Stakes Testing (HST) has emerged describing such assessment practices. Recent federal legislation requires school districts to include test data on the progress of students with disabilities. Little is known, however, about the effects of such HST practices on students with EBD. In Chapter 12, James G. Shriner and Joseph H. Wehby provide an overview of issues related to HST, its impact on children with EBD, and offer recommendations for making HST accommodations for this population.

VIABILITY OF ASSESSMENT APPROACHES

The field of children's mental health has advanced considerably, especially over the past couple of decades, toward understanding the nature of emotional and behavioral disorders of children and youths and their treatment. Assessment has played an important role in this progress. We have psychological measures that can reliably identify developmentally deviant patterns of behavior and characterize their nature. We have an arsenal of formal and informal identification and diagnostic procedures. We can reliably identify academic and behavioral difficulties. Most importantly, we have an array of effective empirically based interventions that can be used to ameliorate various psychological disorders of children and youths (Kazdin & Weisz, 2003; Polsgrove & Ochoa, 2003).

Professionals entering the field in the 21st century will receive the legacy of an extensive body of evidence-based information related to assessment and intervention of EBD. They also will inherit an array of procedures that have been shaped considerably by political, historical, and, in some cases, arbitrary influences. In addition to building on previous work, future researchers will devote efforts to winnowing nonviable from effective practices and selecting out "nonreactive" components of effective practices. The ultimate goal of these activities will be to identify the most informative, socially valid, culturally sensitive, efficient, and fiscally accountable assessment system possible.

Like the medical profession that heavily influences our efforts, the ultimate "end-users" of this technology are educational practitioners: administrators, teachers, school psychologists, social workers, and guidance counselors. Ideally, we anticipate that the practices that produce positive outcomes will become, through scientific selection, more widely used by practitioners than "unwieldy," ineffectual, or detrimental practices.

Each of the chapters in this section of the *Handbook* can be viewed as contributing in one way or the other to this continuing evolution. The authors present arguments concerning the importance of using a particular assessment instrument or approach. In some cases the downside aspects of these are explored; in others they are accepted uncritically. Thus, it remains for readers to determine the worth or viability of these practices for benefiting children and youths with EBD. Exposure to such a wealth of information presented by such talented and informed scholars may absorb readers so thoroughly that they lose sight of certain "meta" considerations regarding assessment. To encourage critical analysis of the material to follow, therefore, I thought it appropriate to assume the role of a provocateur, posing questions about assessment practices of students who are "at risk" or identified as EBD. I urge them to think critically as they pore over this material and ponder in the process such questions as:

- Is this procedure supported by convincing empirical data, or is it an artifact of convention or tradition?
- Is the procedure essential to planning effective interventions?
- Does this approach or instrument encompass culturally sensitive issues?
- Would educators adopt this approach in the face of competing or traditional alternatives?
- How cost-effective are these practices?
- Could identical or better results be achieved

with a more cost-effective, empirically validated approach?

- What are the long-range benefits of using this approach for assessment of children with EBD?
- Do the benefits outweigh the risks of identifying students at risk for EBD?

PERSPECTIVE

I feel confident that readers will find, as did I, that the wealth of information provided in this section of the *Handbook* is not just "informative" but also definitive in scope. Although material in individual chapters overlaps somewhat in some cases, each chapter provides a unique perspective on various topics and issues related to school-based assessment of children and youths both at risk for and identified as EBD. These contributions will serve as a prime reference on the topic for years to come.

REFERENCES

Kazdin, A. E., & Weisz, J. R. (Eds.). (2003). *Evidence-based psychotherapies for children and adolescents.* New York: Guilford Press.

Kauffman, J. M. (2001). *Characteristics of emotional and behavioral disorders of children and youth* (7th ed.). Columbus, OH: Merrill/Prentice Hall.

Polsgrove, L., & Ochoa, T. (2003). Trends and issues in behavioral interventions. In A. M. Sorrells, H. J. Rieth, & P. T. Sindelar (Eds.), *Critical issues in special education* (pp. 154–179). Boston: Allyn & Bacon.

7

Assessment and Evaluation of Students' Behavior and Intervention Outcomes

The Utility of Rating Scale Methods

STEPHEN N. ELLIOTT *and* R. T. BUSSE

Rating scales are efficient tools for representing summary characterizations of individuals' observations of other people or their own behavior. They are imperfect "mirrors" for reflecting images of individuals' social, emotional, and personal functioning; yet, in many cases, the information reflected by a well-constructed rating scale can be very useful to researchers and practitioners alike. Rating scale technology has advanced considerably over the past two decades and today represents one of the primary and most efficient methods used by researchers to (1) describe and categorize children's behaviors and attitudes and (2) evaluate the integrity and effects of interventions designed to improve children's functioning.

Behavior rating scales and inventories are versatile assessment tools and are the most common methods for quantifying teacher and parent judgments (Edelbrock, 1983; Elliott, Busse, & Gresham, 1993; Merrell, 2003). Consequently, rating scales are useful tools for researchers interested in studying child behavior at school or in the community. For several powerful constructs concerning the self-system (e.g., self-efficacy,

anxiety), rating scales are valuable tools for communicating with individual child clients or research participants. Well-designed behavior rating scales essentially are raters' summary characterizations of recent observations and experiences with children or youth. Rating scales can be used repeatedly, across settings, and by numerous sources (i.e., teachers, parents, therapists, children themselves) to provide multiple indicators of a wide range of behavior. As with any assessment tool, rating scales have limitations and must be used as part of a more comprehensive database to increase the likelihood that their resulting scores are reliable and valid.

In this chapter, we discuss validity issues commonly related to rating scales, describe several frequently used behavior rating scales, and examine some useful rating scales applications and analytical methods that may advance research and practice. Before discussing the rationale and technical aspects of behavior rating scale assessment, we present six fundamental assumptions that should be kept in mind when using and interpreting behavior rating scales.

FUNDAMENTAL ASSUMPTIONS REGARDING BEHAVIOR RATING SCALES

Well-designed behavior rating scales are surprisingly complex assessment tools that comply with the tenets of good assessment (i.e., *Standards for Educational and Psychological Testing*; American Educational Research Association [AERA], 1999). Rating scales are more than a *checklist* or *inventory* of children and youth's observable behaviors or self-reported emotions or attitudes. They are also more than a *survey* or *questionnaire* about individuals' functioning. Yet, rating scales often have much in common with checklists and surveys or questionnaires. The following six assumptions help to differentiate rating scales from less rigorous assessment tools and serve as part of the defining attributes for the rating scales we discuss later in this chapter.

• *Assumption 1: Ratings are efficient summaries of observations of specific behaviors or response classes of behavior. These observations typically feature the frequency dimension of human behavior.* On most rating scales, the summary ratings emphasize the relative frequency of a child's behavior. For example, one student may exhibit cooperative behavior three times a day, whereas a second student performs the same behavior once a day. Although these students exhibit different rates of behavior, when their teacher is asked to rate how often the behavior occurs, the teacher may characterize both students on a rating scale as exhibiting the behavior with equal frequency. In short, the precision of measurement with rating scales is relative, not absolute, and often needs to be supplemented by more direct methods of assessment such as direct observation and interview procedures. Ratings of behavior, however, are an efficient way to determine which specific behaviors need to be observed directly and provide a sense of the relative frequency of key behaviors.

• *Assumption 2: Ratings of behavior are evaluative judgments affected by the environment and a rater's standards for behavior.* An individual's behavior may change depending on the situation. Such variability has led researchers to characterize many behaviors as situationally specific rather than as traits or permanent characteristics of the individual (Achenbach, McConaughy, & Howell, 1987; Kazdin, 1979). In addition to environmental influences, behaviors deemed important in one setting may be largely determined by the standards of behavior established by the adult(s) who regulate the setting. Because both the rater's standards for behavior and the situation will influence the actual rating, one should use multiple raters in the assessment process.

• *Assumption 3: Multiple raters of the child's behavior may agree only moderately.* This statement is based on three facts. First, many behaviors are situationally specific. Second, all measures of behavior are made with some degree of error. Third, rating scales use rather simple frequency response categories for quantifying behaviors that may vary widely in their frequency, intensity, and duration. The work of Achenbach et al. (1987), and more recently Elliott and associates (Kettler, Elliott, Bolt, & DiPerna, 2003; Ruffalo & Elliott, 1997), provides empirical support for this assumption. Moderate agreement should not be taken as an indictment of the use of multiple raters. Rather, it suggests that different raters perceive behaviors in various settings differently. Collectively, such ratings may tell us more about a child than only one rater from one setting.

• *Assumption 4: Rating scales can be used to make both norm-referenced and criterion-referenced decisions.* Most published behavior rating scales have been developed using classic test theory and yield scores that are interpreted against a normative sample of individuals similar in age and gender to those assessed with the instrument. Such assessment results are characterized as norm-referenced. A norm group is a useful framework for interpreting rating results, particularly when the purpose of the assessment is to identify deviance and/or to provide a relative classification of performance. With recent advances in intervention evaluation and events within standards-based educational accountability, however, it is likely that more users also will value a criterion-referenced interpretation framework. Rating scales have the flexibility to be adapted, so both criterion-referenced and norm-referenced interpretive approaches can be used.

• *Assumption 5: The social validity of behaviors assessed and possibly treated should be understood. Socially valid behaviors are those behaviors that society considers important, encourages, and reinforces.* The social validity of a behavior is reflected in the *importance* attributed to it by society or adults who regulate specific settings in which the child functions (Wolf, 1978). Social validity can also refer to the *tolerance* for a given behavior in a given setting. Problem behaviors such as fighting, inattention, disruptive behavior, shyness, and so forth are tolerated to different degrees by different persons in different settings and cultures. For example, being quiet and shy may be tolerated in a library but not in situations requiring verbal communication and social interaction. Similarly, being assertive may be tolerated by parents at home but not by teachers at school. Thus, in interpreting and using behavior ratings, it is important to consider the social validity of the behaviors being assessed and identified for potential intervention.

• *Assumption 6: The user's purpose and theoretical framework are compatible with those of the rating scale he or she selects to use.* Assessment instruments are designed for a variety of purposes. Some instruments are primarily used to screen large groups of students; others are intended to facilitate classification of students or to help identify target behaviors for intervention. Still other assessment instruments primarily are used to evaluate outcomes of interventions. Users must be cognizant of the stated and validated purpose(s) for which an assessment has been designed and use the instrument accordingly. In addition, many assessment instruments have been strongly influenced by a particular theoretical orientation—behavioral, social-cognitive, cognitive-behavioral—which, in turn, influences the particular constructs assessed, item content, and, in some cases, the treatment utility of the results. Thus, users are also expected to understand the theoretical orientation that has guided the development and potential use of a rating scale.

TECHNICAL CONSIDERATIONS FOR THE VALIDITY OF BEHAVIOR RATING SCALES RESULTS

There are two basic approaches to constructing behavior rating scales. The first approach is called the *empirical* approach because the final items appearing on the scale are selected on empirical or quantitative grounds. Most behavior rating scales are constructed on the basis of a statistical procedure known as factor analysis. In factor analysis, items belonging to a factor (or scale) are retained if they correlate highly with that factor or scale. Items showing little or no correlation with a particular factor or scale are either deleted from the final version or are moved to another factor with which they highly correlate.

The second approach to building a behavior rating scale is termed the *rational* approach. In a rational approach, behaviors on rating scales are selected on the basis of theoretical notions of what behaviors tend to co-occur. There is no basis, other than rational considerations, for including or excluding specific behaviors from behavior rating scales constructed in this manner. Edelbrock (1983) indicated that behavior rating scales constructed using a rational approach may have less predictive power than empirically derived behavior rating scales.

The construction of behavior rating scales varies according to a number of factors, including what is to be assessed, response scaling, standardization procedures, item type, and scores. These development factors impact the validity of the rating scale results. We briefly examine key aspects of rating scales and some related research that should influence thinking about the use of behavior rating scales.

Content Assessed

Behavior rating scales assess a variety of content areas or constructs, including childhood psychopathology, social skills, depression, hyperactivity, anxiety, and behavior disorders. Some behavior rating scales assess a number of these areas whereas other scales focus on only one or two content areas. Items for behavior rating scales may be derived from a variety of sources. These sources might include clinical case records, experts (e.g., psychologists, psychiatrists, mental health professionals), school records, and the research literature. These items may be revised, rewritten, or discarded based on readability and clarity. Edelbrock (1983) indicated that good items for behavior rating scales are written in terms of overt, easily observable events, behaviors, or characteristics.

The relative "grain size" and specificity of items also are important considerations when selecting a rating scale. Some items can be considered molar, that is, they describe a combination of behaviors or require several discrete and observable behaviors within a rating. An example of a molar item is "Makes friends easily." This item is actually an outcome of a series of behaviors—perhaps involving sharing, listening, helping, and talking nicely—and is one of the top loading items from the *Social Skills Rating System—Teacher Version* (Gresham & Elliott, 1990). By comparison, some items on a rating scale are much more molecular in nature. That is, the item is narrow or focuses on only one discrete skill such as "Takes turns" or "Shares his or her possessions with others." Both molar and molecular items have advantages and disadvantages, but in general we have found that molar items are useful for purposes of classification, whereas molecular items are more prescriptive and have better treatment utility (Gresham, Noell, & Elliott, 1996; Ruffalo & Elliott, 1997).

Response Scaling

Behaviors on behavior rating scales typically are quantified in some way to convey meaning. Response scales may include two-point (e.g., Yes/No; Agree/Disagree; Present/Absent), three-point (e.g., Never/Sometimes/Frequently), four-point, five-point scales, and even more points. The majority of the most popular behavior rating scales employ a 3-point scale. Although a 3-point scale can result in some restriction of range issues when conducting correlational research, it seems that humans are more efficient at making decisions using a 3-point versus a 5- or 7-point scale. Moreover, a smaller response range is likely to enhance the reliability, as determined by agreement methods, for a given measure. As noted in our assumptions, behavior rating scales measure behavior in *relative* rather than in *absolute* terms. Raters are typically not asked to report on the specific number of times a given

behavior occurs or an estimate of its duration or intensity.

Dimensions of behavior other than frequency that can be used to build scales with descriptive anchor points have been identified for use with goal attainment scales (to be discussed later in this chapter; also see Figure 7.2 on p. 135). These dimensions may include a variety of behavioral descriptors such as duration, intensity, quality, accuracy, and effort. Possibilities for scaling various dimensions of behavior are almost limitless. The challenge is to create a scale that communicates consistently and in a meaningful way with users. The majority of published rating scales, however, focus on the *frequency* dimension of behavior, given that it is the cornerstone dimension of direct observations and often the dimension of greatest concern to educators and parents.

Standardization and Normative Characteristics

The standardization and normative characteristics of behavior rating scales exhibit a great deal of variability. Some behavior rating scales have no normative data and, as such, are limited in the types of comparisons that can be made. Basically, such scales provide results about the relative frequency of behaviors within one individual. In many ways, then, ratings without norms are simply a summary of observations about an individual. One of the important contributions of rating scales to observation-based assessments is the development and use of norms to facilitate interpretation of results. This is particularly important for purposes of screening and classification. Behavior rating scales that have normative data vary in terms of how the norms are stratified. For example, scales may be stratified according to sex, age, disability group membership, or a combination of demographic characteristics. The decision to stratify a behavior rating scale according to certain demographic variables depends on whether the variable influences the scores obtained from the scale, and on the desired level of generalizability of the scores to a given population. Thus, if sex, age, or disability status influence scores derived from behavior rating scales, then the scale is typically stratified according to these variables.

Informant Considerations

A key issue in using behavior rating scales is who the informant should be that completes the rating scale. Typically, informants are teachers, parents, and children themselves. Some behavior rating scales are for teachers only, other rating scales are for parents only or children only, and still others utilize all three informants. Some informants are in a better position to rate certain behaviors. For instance, teachers are in a better position to rate attention span, classroom behaviors, social interactions in school settings, and the like. Parents are likely to be more knowledgeable about behaviors such as sleep disturbances, sibling interactions, mealtime behaviors, and so forth.

The best practice in using behavior rating scales is to employ multiple informants to rate the same child's behavior to provide a more complete view of a child's behavior across situations and settings (Edelbrock, 1983; Gresham & Elliott, 1990). By using multiple informants, one can discern which behaviors tend to occur across a variety of situations and which behaviors appear to be situationally specific. This information can be of use in classification decisions as well as for intervention planning. Of course, researchers have repeatedly found that multiple informants often agree only moderately at best (Achenbach et al., 1987; Ruffalo & Elliott, 1997; Schneider & Byrne, 1989).

Validity Issues with Direct and Indirect Observational Data

As with any assessment instrument, the scores from a rating scale need to be validated. Given that behavior rating scales are intended to be indirect observational measures, it is logical that an important part of the validation effort for a rating scale is to compare its results with those from direct observations of the same target child. This logic is especially true within a behavioral model of assessment wherein direct observation is considered the "gold standard" for which all other assessments should be compared (Witt, Elliott, Daly, Gresham, & Kramer, 1998). Few authors of behavior rating scales, however, report information about the relationships between ratings and observations. This fact may surprise many read-

ers, but most direct observation systems and behavior rating scales differ in several significant ways that result in only a modest comparability of results. For example, a key difference is that behaviors targeted for direct observation are often far more molecular or discrete than those operationalized by items on a rating scale. Another difference is that the results from a direct observation of behavior are rarely aggregated across response classes or factors as they are on most behavior rating scales. In addition, behavior assessed via a direct observation is often limited to one or two discrete skills, whereas on a rating scale it is common to gather information on 50 or 60 behaviors or skills. These differences in coverage and scoring reduce the comparability of the results of direct and indirect observational assessments and decrease concurrent validity estimates.

The research data are limited regarding how much observational data one should collect to gain a representative sample of behavior, whereas many behavior rating scales suggest the rater summarize his or her observations over the past month or two. Barton and Ascione (1984) reported that, in general, the more data that can be gathered, the more likely the results will be representative of the target child's behavior. Too few data could threaten the validity and reliability of the observations. To ensure representativeness, an observational procedure should acquire a sufficiently large sample of behavior, but it can only be estimated how often the periods of observation should occur and how long they should last (Johnston & Pennypacker, 1980). How, then, should one go about arriving at that estimation, confident that the decision yields a sample of behavior representative of a child's typical behavior?

Doll and Elliott (1994) addressed the issue of how much observational data are enough in a study with preschoolers. They used a correlational research design to examine the number of classroom observations it takes to gain an accurate and representative sample of a preschool child's social behavior. Twenty-four children were observed using a partial-interval sampling procedure. Observations were conducted over 6 weeks, and each child was observed for nine 20-minute periods in his or her classroom through one-way mirrors during free-play periods. Doll and Elliott compared early observation sessions to later sessions using correlations and kappa coefficients, and they compared the results of the complete set of nine observation sessions to those of the first session, the first two sessions, the first three sessions, and so on. Results from these comparisons indicated that neither two nor three observation sessions were sufficient to describe a consistent pattern of social behavior. After five observations, six out of eight behaviors correlated highly ($r = .80$) with the total observation record. From these data, the authors concluded that at least five 20-minute observation sessions across several weeks would adequately represent students' social behavior. Doll and Elliott also found that the type of behavior accounted for the variation in predictability of behaviors. Some behaviors, such as directed play or physical aggression, were much more consistent in their occurrence than others. A less consistent social behavior, like sharing, often depended more on context or setting events than did other behaviors and was therefore difficult to predict even with seven or eight observations. The authors concluded that "depending upon the behaviors of interest for a particular child, observational records might need to be quite lengthy before a sufficiently consistent description of child behavior can be recorded" (Doll & Elliott, 1994, p. 234).

As noted in one of our fundamental assumptions about rating scales, it is considered a best practice to use a multisource, multimethod approach in the assessment of children's social-emotional behavior (McConaughy & Ritter, 1995; Preator & McAllister, 1995). One must recognize, however, that variance exists in all assessments. Common sources of variance stem from different methods, informants, settings, and times. Given this variance, it is important to consider two fundamental measurement principles: there is error in all measures, and tests are samples of behavior.

The reaction to these principles has been to use multiple sources and multiple methods to reduce error and gain more representative samples, despite the chance that there may not be high agreement among the methods or sources. For example, Achenbach et al. (1987) performed a meta-analysis to study agreement among informants' ratings of children's behavior. In a review of 119 studies, they found that the mean correlations between all types of informants were statistically significant, yet moderate in magnitude. Similar informants (i.e., pairs of teachers, pairs of mental health workers) had the highest correlations (mean $r = .64$ and mean $r = .54$, respectively). Informants with different roles (i.e., teacher/parent pairs) had lower correlations, but still significant, with the highest occurring between teacher and observer pairs (mean $r = .42$). Mean agreement between pairs of observers was $r = .57$.

Though different informants using the same assessment method can have significant levels of agreement, it is another issue to conclude that different assessment methods share consistency. Merrell (1993a) found correlations between the *Child Behavior Checklist—Direct Observation Form* (CBC-DOF; Achenbach, 1986) and the *School Social Behavior Scale* (SSBS; Merrell, 1993b) were weak to moderate between teachers and observers for problem behavior scores ($r = -.06$ to $-.39$) and moderate for on-task ratings ($r = .26–.52$). Likewise, Elliott, Gresham, Freeman, and McCloskey (1988) found that teachers' and observers' ratings on the *Social Skills Rating System—Teacher Version* (SSRS-T; Gresham & Elliott, 1990) and observers' observations correlated moderately with observed behaviors.

Research conducted with observation systems designed to be used with a specific rating scale also has shown only moderate correlations between the two methods. Robertson (1993) and Racine (1994) both researched the relationship between observations and ratings using an observation system designed by Robertson to be used with the SSRS-T. Robertson found moderate correlations between teachers' and observers' ratings (mean $r = .58$), yet low to moderate correlations (mean $r = .38$) between teachers' ratings and observers' observations.

In summary, behavior rating scales appear to be more than an aggregation of a series of structured direct observations. The rater often is a "participant" in the environment where the target child behaves, and the behavior to be rated is often a more comprehensive collection of skills than typically operationalized via a direct observation system. Rating scales offer an efficient means for collecting data to create a relatively comprehensive picture of functioning. These differences in observational methods does not make one method better than the other; rather, they highlight that the "gold standard" for the validation of behavior rating scales is not likely to be a typical direct observation system.

FREQUENTLY USED BEHAVIOR RATING SCALES

In this section, we briefly review selected published behavior rating scales that are frequently used to assess the social-emotional behavior of children and youth and represent an array of psychological constructs of interest to many researchers studying students with behavior disorders. Some of these rating scales are part of a system of rating instruments designed to be used by multiple respondents, whereas others are completed by a single rater. The instruments we review provide normative information and have well-established psychometric characteristics.

Teacher or Parent Rating Scales

Systematic Screening for Behavior Disorders

The Systematic Screening for Behavior Disorders (SSBD; Walker & Severson, 1992) is a device for the identification of children with behavior disorders. The SSBD is known as a "multiple-gating" device because it contains a series of progressively more involved and precise assessments, or "gates." The first gate of the SSBD uses teacher nominations, in which teachers identify three students in their class who match profiles of externalizing or internalizing behavior patterns. The second gate of the SSBD involves teacher ratings of the three children ranked the highest on externalizing problems and three children ranked the highest on internalizing problems (for a total of six students). Teachers rate these children on a Critical Events Checklist that assesses whether a student has exhibited any of 33 externalizing and internalizing behavior problems within the past 6 months. The second rating involves the Combined Frequency Index, which measures how often the student exhibits specific adaptive and maladaptive behaviors. Those students exceeding the normative criteria in the second

gate of the SSBD are then independently assessed in gate three.

In the third gate of the SSBD, a school professional (e.g., school psychologist, guidance counselor, social worker) assesses students on two measures of school adjustment, using direct observation procedures. The first measure is known as academic engaged time (AET), which is recorded during independent seatwork periods. The second measure is the peer social behavior observation, which measures the quality and nature of students' social behavior during recess periods. Students exceeding normative criteria on these two measures are considered to "pass" gate three and are referred for a formal assessment of behavior disorders.

The SSBD was nationally standardized on 4,500 cases on the Gate 2 measures and approximately 1,300 cases on the Gate 3 measures. The SSBD appears to have an adequate standardization sample for the purposes for which it is to be used. The SSBD technical manual presents a large amount of data supporting the reliability and validity of the measure. For example, the SSBD correlates with measures of behavior problems, social skills, and sociometric status. It reliably differentiates students with and without behavioral disorders and distinguishes among externalizers, internalizers, and nonreferred students.

The SSBD is a well-conceptualized and well-researched instrument designed for the identification of students with behavior disorders. Its multiple-gating procedure represents an efficient method of identifying students with behavior problems and is designed to save time and money in the assessment process. We believe that the SSBD serves as one of the best examples of how assessment methods (teacher nominations, teacher ratings, and direct observations of behavior in naturalistic settings) can be combined to identify students in potential need of special services and to identify target behaviors for intervention. To date, there is no better instrument for the screening and identification of students with behavior disorders.

Social Skills Rating System

The Social Skills Rating System (SSRS; Gresham & Elliott, 1990) provides a broad, multirater assessment of student social behaviors that can affect teacher–student relations, peer acceptance, and academic performance. The SSRS documents behaviors that influence a student's development of social competence and adaptive functioning at school and at home. The SSRS components include three behavior rating forms (teacher, parent, and student versions) and an integrative assessment and intervention planning record. Teacher and parent forms are available for three developmental levels: preschool, grades K–6, and grades 7–12. The SSRS assesses the domains of social skills, problem behavior, and academic competence.

The Social Skills Scale has five subscales: Cooperation, Assertion, Responsibility, Empathy, and Self-Control. All social skills items are rated on two dimensions: *frequency* and *importance*. The inclusion of an importance dimension allows raters to specify how important each social skill is for classroom success (teacher ratings), for their child's development (parent ratings), and for the student's relationships with others (student ratings).

The Problem Behavior Scale has three subscales that measure Externalizing Problems, Internalizing Problems, and Hyperactivity. The Academic Competence domain concerns student academic functioning and consists of a small, yet critical, sample of relevant behaviors. Items are rated on a 5-point scale that corresponds to percentage clusters (1 = lowest 10%, 5 = highest 10%). This domain includes items measuring reading and mathematics performance, motivation, parental support, and general cognitive functioning. This scale appears on the teacher form at the elementary and secondary levels.

The SSRS is a well-constructed and well-researched multirater approach for measuring social skills, problem behaviors, and academic competence for children between the ages of 3–18 years. The SSRS has a representative national standardization and extensive evidence for reliability and validity. One of the most attractive features of the SSRS is its utility in selecting target behaviors for intervention purposes, a feature not common to most behavior rating scales. An intervention guide (Elliott & Gresham, 1991) that provides a manualized approach to teaching and improving over 40 social skills coordinates with the SSRS results.

Child Behavior Checklist

The Child Behavior Checklist (CBCL; Achenbach & Rescorla, 2001) is one of the most widely known and used parent rating scales for children's behavior problems. The CBCL assesses two broad-band domains of behavior, externalizing behavior and internalizing behavior, and a variety of narrow-band domains (e.g., Anxious/Depressed, Aggressive Behavior). The CBCL consists of two forms: a 118-item checklist for children ages 6–18 and a separate 100-item checklist for children ages 1.5–5 (Achenbach & Rescorla, 2000). The CBCL is part of an empirically derived system of assessment that includes the Teacher's Report Form (TRF) and Youth Self-Report Form (YSR) for adolescents. All three of the scales contain similar problem behaviors and provide a method for ascertaining cross-informant data. These rating scales have been extensively studied and have been shown to be well-constructed measures that possess adequate reliability and validity.

These checklists, which are part of the Achenbach System of Empirically Based Assessment (ASEBA), share common features with other well-known, current behavior rating scale systems. For example, the system focuses on problem behaviors within a variety of behavioral domains and provides for cross-informant data through the use of student and teacher ratings. One unique characteristic is the inclusion of a competence scale within each measure. These scales are designed to provide data regarding a child's social and academic functioning. Another unique characteristic is the preschool version of the CBCL for young children.

The ASEBA forms have been used in over 5,000 published studies and have been translated into 69 languages (Retrieved from ASEBA website: *http://www.ASEBA.org*. The strengths of the Achenbach system are that the rating scales are empirically derived, possess good psychometrics, provide for cross-informant and cross-method data, the checklists are relatively simple to complete, and the system includes a useful website. The system's major limitations include a lack of strong evidence in support of the competence scales and limited data on the use of the young children's scales.

Behavior Assessment System for Children

The Behavior Assessment System for Children (BASC; Reynolds & Kamphaus, 1992) consists of the Parent Rating Scales (PRS), the Teacher Rating Scales (TRS), and the Self-Report of Personality (SRP). The PRS and TRS have three forms for children ages 4–5, 6–11, and 12–18 that measure Externalizing Problems, Internalizing Problems, School Problems, Adaptive Skills, and "Other" Problems. The SRP has two forms for children ages 8–11 and 12–18 designed to assess Clinical Maladjustment, School Maladjustment, Personal Adjustment, and "Other" Problems. The BASC scales are well constructed and possess adequate reliability and validity.

The BASC shares several commonalities with other omnibus, broad-based measures such as the CBCL. It focuses on behavior problems and provides for cross-informant information. The system also includes a Structured Developmental History measure that can be used in interview or questionnaire format, and the system includes an observation form. There are unique characteristics of the BASC that set it apart from similar measures. One positive, unique aspect is the inclusion of a veracity scale. Another unique component is a mixture of items phrased in a socially positive and socially negative manner.

The strengths of the BASC are that it possesses solid psychometrics, provides separate forms and norms for a variety of age groups, includes a veracity measure, includes positively worded items and scales, provides for cross-informant and cross-method data, and it includes a computer-based portable observation system. The limitations of the BASC are that the level of cross-informant information is limited between children and adults, and there are limited research data on the usefulness of the observation and interview components.

Behavioral and Emotional Rating Scale

The Behavioral and Emotional Rating Scale (BERS; Epstein & Sharma, 1998) is a 52-item scale designed to be a "strength-based" assessment of children's behaviors. The BERS consists of an adult rater form. As on the SSRS, the items focus on positive, prosocial behaviors that provide five factors: Interpersonal Strength, Family Involvement, Intrapersonal Strength, School Functioning, and Affective Strength. The scale appears to possess adequate psychometric properties. A newer edition of the BERS will soon be available that includes parent, teacher, and youth self-report forms, although this revised edition requires further reliability and validity studies. The BERS-2 and its predecessor were developed relatively recently and are less known and used; thus, it is an emerging tool that may prove useful in research and practice. We have included the BERS, albeit briefly, because of its focus on prosocial behaviors, and, for adolescents, the newer version contains a vocational strength index that provides a unique and potentially useful screening measure.

Self-Report Rating Scales

Self-report measures require individuals to provide standardized information about themselves, such as thoughts, feelings, and physical experiences (Eckert, Dunn, Guiney, & Codding, 2000). They allow researchers and practitioners to gain information about an individual's own perceptions, which can "provide 'red flags' that may be indicative of general social or emotional distress," and in some cases they can isolate specific areas of concern in which additional assessment is needed (Merrell, 2003, p. 180). Self-report information can be used in screening and can aid in making diagnoses and formulating interventions.

Self-report rating scales are an important means of gathering information about children's internal states of which no one else may be cognizant. Kazdin (1986) recommended the use of self-reports in the assessment of children's internalizing symptoms, and several researchers have documented the utility of children assessing their own anxiety levels (Edelbrock, Costello, Dulcan, Kalas, & Conover, 1985).

A number of concerns about the use of self-report measures have been noted. First, self-report measures require individuals to provide information about their own perceptions, which are relatively subjective (McConaughy & Ritter, 1995), are often retrospective in nature (Kratochwill & Shapiro, 2000), and are often setting-specific

(Kazdin, 1979). Self-report measures of behavior also need to be developmentally appropriate for their intended population (Eckert et al., 2000). Thus, it is important for researchers to consider respondents' cognitive, language, and reading abilities. These factors may play a significant role in determining whether responses are valid. Another set of factors that influence the validity of respondents' completion of a self-report scale are commonly referred to as response bias factors, including faking, acquiescence, or social desirability (Merrell, 2003).

Despite criticism or concerns about self-report measures, they play a role in research and the comprehensive assessment and treatment of students with social emotional difficulties. The multidimensional scales presented above (i.e., SSRS, CBCL, BASC) include self-report measures that can be used in a multi-axial assessment. We now briefly review two specific examples of self-rating scales.

Revised Children's Manifest Anxiety Scale

The Revised Children's Manifest Anxiety Scale (RCMAS; Reynolds & Richmond, 1985) is one of the most widely used self-report measures of anxiety and related emotional concerns. The RCMAS can be used with a population between the ages of 6–19, and can be administered in groups for children 9½ or older who have appropriate reading levels. There are 37 items on the RCMAS, each requiring "yes" or "no" responses. The RCMAS has four subscales: Physiological Anxiety, Worry/Oversensitivity, Social Concerns/Concentration, and a Lie subscale.

The RCMAS has been used in over 250 published studies and is a frequently used screening tool. Laurent, Hadler, and Stark (1994) administered the RCMAS to 758 students in grades 4–7 and featured it in a three-stage screening procedure to identify 83 students who qualified as having severe anxiety disorders. The RCMAS ratings were the primary indicator in Stage 1 and Stage 2, and a clinical interview using the Schedule for Affective Disorders and Schizophrenia for School-Age Children (K-SADS; Puig-Antich & Chambers, 1986) was used in Stage 3 of the screening. The RCMAS has been used in similar ways to screen for anxiety and emotional difficulties by a number of other investigators (Stavrakaki, Williams, Walker, & Roberts, 1991). It is consistently found to yield scores with high reliability (test–retest) and good predictive validity.

Student Self-Concept Scale

The Student Self-Concept Scale (SSCS; Gresham, Elliott, & Evans-Fernandez, 1992) is a 72-item group or individually administered multidimensional measure of self-concept. The SSCS provides a norm-referenced measure of self-concept for children and adolescents in grades 3–12 and documents the perceived *confidence* and *importance* of specific behaviors influencing the development of students' self-concepts.

The SSCS conceptualizes self-concept as being multidimensional in nature in that individuals categorize their self-perceptions into facets or domains (e.g., academic, social). The SSCS defines self-concept as an individual's perception that he or she can perform certain behaviors that will result in certain outcomes. Self-concept is multidimensional and is determined by an individual's perceptions of efficacy in performing certain behaviors and the importance of these behaviors for that individual.

The SSCS provides users several unique features to facilitate more comprehensive assessment and intervention services for children experiencing difficulties in self-concept. First, the SSCS provides norms based on a large, representative sample for boys and girls in grades 3–12. Second, the SSCS is theoretically based, which provides more specific behavioral information regarding a child's self-concept. Finally, the SSCS represents the first self-concept scale to utilize joint ratings of confidence and importance for each behavior on the scale. The inclusion of importance ratings facilitates intervention planning for children and adolescents who have problems with their self-concept.

EMERGING RATING SCALE METHODS FOR MONITORING AND EVALUATING TREATMENTS

In this section, we present emerging technologies predicated on the logic of criterion-referenced rating scale methods that can be used to facilitate assessment and intervention. We first examine the application of rating scale methods in the assessment of intervention implementation.

Ratings of Intervention Integrity

Standardization, or procedural specification of an intervention, refers to the development of formal guidelines, procedural protocols, and/or manuals when the intervention is implemented. Use of a standardized format for intervention has several advantages for research (Kratochwill & Stoiber, 2000). First, standardization of an intervention will allow replication of intervention procedures developed and empirically supported in research for dissemination in practice. Second, standardization of interventions facilitates training in specific intervention skills. A major shortcoming of some intervention techniques is the lack of specific procedures for training individuals in their use. Some empirical work has indicated that a standardized approach focused on competency-based criteria can be used to train school psychologists in consultation (e.g., Kratochwill, Elliott, & Busse, 1995; LePage, Kratochwill, & Elliott, 2004) and for preservice and in-service preparation of classroom and special education

teachers (West, Idol, & Cannon, 1987). The use of standardized formats in training and practice would appear to be essential in the empirical development of effective techniques.

Once intervention procedures have been specified or procedurally standardized, a major issue that must be addressed is implementation integrity—the degree to which an intervention is implemented as intended. Researchers have stressed that when an intervention is implemented, it must be carried out as originally intended to ensure the internal validity of the treatment (Yeaton & Sechrest, 1981). Integrity, or fidelity, can be evaluated at several levels. First, it must be demonstrated that the intervention agent is implementing the intervention program as prescribed. This is the level at which intervention integrity usually has been evaluated through assessment of the intervention agent and through data on the client's responsiveness to the intervention. In practice, direct and indirect observational assessment data can be gathered to determine intervention integrity. For example, Gresham (1989) presented a rating scale format that can be completed by the intervention agent, consultant, and/or by an independent observer (see Figure 7.1). The example refers to a response

Consultee: _____ Date: _____ Consultant: _____

Response Cost Lottery

	Strongly disagree				Strongly agree
1. Described system to students.	1	2	3	4	5
2. Displayed and described reinforcers.	1	2	3	4	5
3. Placed 3 × 5 card on students' desks.	1	2	3	4	5
4. Card taped on three sides.	1	2	3	4	5
5. Four slips of colored paper inserted (different colors for each student).	1	2	3	4	5
6. Lottery in effect for ½ hour.	1	2	3	4	5
7. Slips removed contingent on rule violations.	1	2	3	4	5
8. Teacher restated rule contingent on violation.	1	2	3	4	5
9. Remaining tickets placed in box.	1	2	3	4	5
10. Drawing occurred on Friday.	1	2	3	4	5
11. Winner selected reinforcer on Friday.	1	2	3	4	5

FIGURE 7.1. Example of a behavior rating scale for treatment integrity. Adapted from Gresham (1989). Copyright 1989 by the National Association of School Psychologists. Adapted by permission of the publisher.

cost lottery program implemented in a classroom for a student with behavior difficulties. Finally, if a child is involved in implementing an intervention (e.g., a self-control strategy), program implementation and its integrity can be self-monitored at the client level.

Ratings of Intervention Outcomes

Questions about intervention effectiveness are relevant before, during, and after the implementation of a given intervention. Prior to selecting a specific intervention, one must identify an intervention procedure that is theoretically consistent or empirically linked with the intended approach to change, then focus on what challenges, social competencies, and the populations with which the intervention has been used, and finally examine the relative effectiveness of the intervention in comparison with several other interventions. Psychologists, special educators, and other intervention agents ethically are bound to monitor the effects (both intended and unintended) of their intervention procedures during intervention and after termination of the intervention. Decisions about intervention outcomes should involve information from many sources (e.g., parents, teachers, peers, self-report) about changes in the client's problematic behavior and social competencies. Information about the trend and the magnitude of change is difficult to interpret without some comparative standard or criterion. In academic domains, outcome criteria are usually available in the form of curriculum mastery tests, lists of essential grade skills, or assigned learning objectives. In contrast, outcome criteria in social/emotional domains are less standardized and more variable across settings. Therefore, comparisons with typical peers, with intervention goals established a priori, and with behavior standards established by significant adults are the primary criteria by which behavioral changes are interpreted. Additional criteria for a successful intervention are maintenance of the change over time and generalization of the behavior across settings.

One useful strategy for assessing treatment outcomes that is receiving increasing attention is performance or progress monitoring (Gettinger, Stoiber, & Lange, 1999;

Stoiber & Kratochwill, 2001). Intervention progress monitoring fits within the framework of determining the child's responsiveness to the intervention. Ongoing data regarding how the child is progressing toward a desired intervention goal or outcome are collected in conjunction with the implementation of the intervention. Ongoing performance or progress monitoring should contribute to a better understanding of whether and which components of an intervention, including instructional or environmental modifications, are effective. Another intent of performance/progress monitoring is that it provides a purposeful structure for guiding the development of alternative interventions if the present intervention is not successful. Finally, progress monitoring data are essential when a child's response to an intervention is used for making decisions about the child's psychological or educational needs, or for determining a child's disability status (Reschly, Tilly, & Grimes, 1999).

Much of what is known about the usefulness of rating scales is based on data within a group design format. Whether researchers have explored diagnostic or intervention issues, the predominant method for examining outcomes relies on single rating scale differences that are analyzed via group variance statistical methods (e.g., ANOVA, correlations). Whereas traditional group difference statistical procedures provide valuable information, group data obfuscate individual differences, which are considered part of error variance within group design methods. Moreover, using a single rating scale does not take into account variances that may be evident across raters, settings, and methods of assessment. To address these issues, we examine goal attainment scales, and two data analytic methods that can be used with single-case or group designs.

Goal Attainment Scales

Goal attainment scales (GAS) provide an individualized, criterion-referenced rating scale approach to documenting changes in behaviors (Kiresuk, Smith, & Cardillo, 1994). When this technique is used in educational contexts, teachers, parents, consultants, or students can complete GAS ratings to provide an indirect measure of academic or social behavior performance. Kiresuk and

Sherman (1968) developed the original GAS method for use in evaluating the effectiveness of mental health services. The original conceptualization of GAS resulted in a technique that promoted individualized idiographic measurement of clients' actual progress toward treatment goals and that allowed for comparisons between different therapists and treatment programs.

The basic methodology of GAS involves the following steps: (1) selecting a target behavior, (2) describing the desired behavior or academic outcome in objective terms, and (3) developing three to five descriptions of the probable outcomes from "least favorable" to "most favorable" (Elliott, Sladeczek, & Kratochwill, 1995). By using numerical ratings for each of the descriptive

levels of functioning, a rater can provide a daily or weekly report of student progress. These criterion-referenced reports can accompany direct indicators of progress (e.g., direct observations or permanent products) and other indicators such as work samples, student self-reports, or rating scales from parents or other individuals. An example of a GAS for a student who needs to improve his ability to work cooperatively with others is provided as Figure 7.2. In Figure 7.3, we have summarized the steps for designing an individualized GAS.

Although there has been substantial investigation and implementation of GAS in a variety of mental health and medical fields over the past 35 years, there has been less extensive research and application of GAS

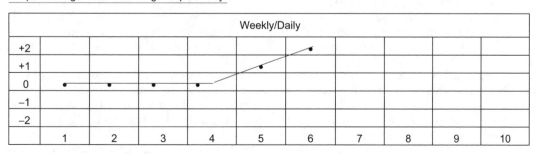

Student: _Eddie Jensen_ Date of birth: _April 6, 1990_

Today's date: _March 2, 2002_ Grade: _6th_ Gender: ☒ Male ☐ Female

Teacher: _Mrs. Williams_ School: _Bailey Elementary_

Target Behavior(s):
Eddie will demonstrate his ability to work cooperatively with a small group of classmates on a project without prompts or cues from an adult.

Goal Attainment Scale with Descriptive Criteria for Monitoring Behavior Change

+2   *When it is time to work with his project team, Eddie works cooperatively more than 80% of the time during the entire period, without an adult prompting or cueing him to do so.*

+1   *When it is time to work with his project team, Eddie works cooperatively 60–80% of the time during the entire period, with only minimal prompting or cueing from an adult.*

 0   *When it is time to work with his project team, Eddie works cooperatively 40–60% of the time during the entire period, with periodic prompting or cueing from an adult.*

−1   *When it is time to work with his project team, Eddie works cooperatively 20–40% of the time during the entire period, with frequently and strong prompting or cueing from an adult.*

−2   *When it is time to work with his project team, Eddie works cooperatively less than 20% of the time during the entire period, regardless of the amount of prompting and cueing from an adult.*

Graph of Progress on "Working Cooperatively"

	Weekly/Daily									
+2										
+1										
0										
−1										
−2										
	1	2	3	4	5	6	7	8	9	10

FIGURE 7.2. Example of a goal attainment scale worksheet.

Step 1. Identify concerns. Teacher(s) identify academic or social behavior strengths, performance problems, and acquisition problems by considering data on performance gathered via standardized assessments, observations, and/or work samples.
Step 2. Analyze concerns. Teacher(s) identify a target behavior and define it in objective terms so it can be read and accurately paraphrased.
Step 3. Plan instruction or intervention. First, teacher(s) establish the instructional or intervention goal, defining the desired outcome in concrete terms. In many cases, the target behavior and desired outcome will be the same. After identifying the desired outcome, teacher(s) describe the general instruction or intervention strategy that will be used to achieve this goal.
Step 4. Constructing the Goal Attainment Scale. The basic elements of GAS are a five-point scale ranging from +2 to –2 and descriptions of the target behavior and instructional support that correspond with the following conditions: Best Possible Outcome (+2), No Change in Behavior/Performance (0), and Worst Possible Outcome (-2). The following characteristics or dimensions may be helpful in developing descriptions for the different GAS rating points: • Frequency (Never—Sometimes—Very Often—Almost Always—Always) • Quality (Poor—Fair—Good—Excellent) • Development (Not present—Emerging—Developing—Accomplished—Exceeding) • Usage (Unused—Inappropriate Use—Appropriate Use—Exceptional Use) • Timeliness (Late—On Time—Early) • Percent complete (0%—25%—50%—75%—100%) • Accuracy (Totally Incorrect—Partially Correct—Totally Correct) • Effort (Not Attempted—Minimal Effort—Acceptable Effort—Outstanding Effort) • Engagement (None—Limited—Acceptable—Exceptional) A template to facilitate the development of GAS ratings is provided as Figure 7.1.
Step 4. Implement instruction or intervention.
Step 5. Evaluate instruction or intervention. Graph the GAS ratings (collected daily or weekly) of student progress.

FIGURE 7.3. A framework for developing and utilizing GAS ratings.

by school-based psychologists and special educators. For example, GAS was not included in a review of assessment methods commonly used by school psychologists or special educators (Wilson & Reschly, 1996). This lack of familiarity with GAS as an assessment technique is unfortunate because of its utility as an element of multidimensional behavioral assessment (Shapiro & Kratochwill, 2000). Within the continuum of behavioral assessment developed by Shapiro and Browder (1990), student GAS self-ratings can function as either self-monitoring (a form of direct assessment, completed as behavior occurs) or self-report (a less direct measure of an individual's perception of their behavior). GAS ratings completed by teachers and other adults function as informant reports, which are also indirect measures of behavior. Moreover, because of its emphasis on operationalizing target behaviors and ongoing (i.e., time-series) evaluation of academic progress, GAS is a particu-

larly useful tool for monitoring students' progress and for verifying the need for additional support or intervention (Elliott, DiPerna, & Shapiro, 2001).

Kratochwill and Elliott (discussed in Kratochwill, Elliott, & Rotto, 1995) used a modified version of GAS as part of a U.S. Department of Education research project entitled "An Experimental Analysis of Teacher/Parent Mediated Interventions for Preschoolers with Behavioral Problems." Beyond its utility as a follow-up measure of clinician or program effectiveness, Kratochwill and Elliott conceptualized GAS as a formative assessment that could be repeated periodically to monitor students' academic or behavior progress. Using GAS as a repeated measure of students' progress required changes in the original scaled descriptions developed by Kiresuk and Sherman. Although Kratochwill and Elliott maintained the five-point scale, the modified GAS included initial assessments to establish a baseline, which was subsequently assigned a score of "0." Thus, the new scale levels ranged from the best possible outcome (+2) to the worst possible outcome (–2). In addition, the modified GAS allowed for ratings of both over- and underattainment of behavioral or academic objectives (Kratochwill, Elliott, & Rotto, 1995).

GAS is a versatile assessment method that can be used to evaluate both classwide or schoolwide interventions or interventions for individual students. Maher's (1982) evaluation of the *Goal-Oriented Approach to Learning* (GOAL) program indicated that students who completed GAS self-ratings achieved higher goal attainment scores than peers who did not self-evaluate, and were more likely to achieve the "Expected Outcome" level for their goals. A follow-up investigation (Maher, 1982) demonstrated that student and adult (i.e., guidance counselor) GAS ratings of school adjustment and achievement "did not differ significantly in terms of estimating goal attainment" (p. 533). Single-case studies utilizing GAS ratings have been conducted with students with autism (Oren & Ogletree, 2000), traumatic brain injuries (Mitchell & Cusick, 1998), and conduct problems (Sladeczek, Elliott, Kratochwill, Robertson-Mjaanes, & Stoiber, 2001). In each case, consultants and consultees reported GAS ratings helped to clarify intervention goals and document student progress toward those goals.

Acceptability research with school and mental health professionals indicates that GAS is perceived as highly acceptable and useful in a variety of settings. Robertson-Mjaanes (1999) asked professionals (including teachers, N = 36) to rate the ease of use and acceptability of GAS. The results indicate that most teachers (94%) endorsed GAS as "very feasible" or "feasible" to use with their students. Moreover, Robertson-Mjaanes found that 70% of the teachers believed that most professionals would find GAS "easy" or "very easy" to use for monitoring intervention progress and outcomes. Carr (1979) found that special education teachers who participated in an evaluation project described the time necessary to construct an individual GAS as "worthwhile" and valuable for specifying goals and facilitating the inclusion process. Cardillo (1994) reported that the existing research on the

implementation of GAS in mental health settings suggests study participants experienced the GAS process as "an unexpected, but beneficial learning experience, with respect to both goal setting and treatment planning" and as leading "to an enhanced awareness of and respect for documentation requirements" (p. 59).

An example of a rating scale assessment tool that uses the GAS method to structure the outcome evaluation process of a school-based intervention program is *Outcomes: Planning, Monitoring, Evaluating* (Outcomes: PME; Stoiber & Kratochwill, 2001). Outcomes: PME is built on an evidence-based framework and is a general assessment instrument designed to facilitate the design, implementation, and monitoring of academic and social-behavioral interventions in virtually any domain of performance across traditional educational and mental health settings. Outcomes: PME uses a goal-attainment framework but allows the assessor to integrate multiple sources of progress monitoring data for purposes of making decisions about the efficacy of interventions. The structure of Outcomes: PME lends itself to (1) prereferral or early intervention activities typically performed by school-based collaborative teams, (2) intervention planning and monitoring activities, and (3) special education decision making that occurs through the individualized education program (IEP) team process. An important characteristic of Outcomes: PME is that it can be applied both for documenting and determining the effectiveness of interventions and for determining eligibility for special programs based on a consensus-building framework called convergent evidence scaling (CES). Another unique feature of Outcomes: PME is that it incorporates diverse progress-monitoring components and the recording of intervention results based on multiple data sources (e.g., direct observation, goal attainment ratings, anecdotal records, work samples) that are graphically presented in hard copy or handheld computer formats. In addition, it can be used in conjunction with traditional assessment and alternative assessment procedures, such as functional assessment of social performance, and with the assessment of academic and social competencies.

In summary, we strongly urge that more

attention be paid to the integrity of interventions and to systematic progress monitoring. Methods such as component checklists or rating scales may provide the necessary information to decide whether an intervention has been implemented with integrity. Without such information, modification to interventions may be misguided. Rating scale technology also can be easily applied to progress monitoring with methods such as goal attainment scaling. To further our discussion on the use of rating scale technology in progress monitoring we conclude with a presentation of two data analytic methods, Reliable Change Index and Convergent Evidence Scaling.

Reliable Change Index

Reliable Change Index (RCI) is a method that can be readily applied to rating scale research for providing an effect size or indicator of change from pretest–posttest data that can be used to represent statistical as well as clinical or social significance (Jacobson, Follette, & Revenstorf, 1984; Jacobson & Truax, 1991; Nunnally & Kotsche, 1983). The basic procedure proposed by Nunnally and Kotsche (1983) involves subtracting one standard score from another and dividing by the standard error of measurement (SEM), which is the standard deviation of measurement error. Therefore the method uses the *logic* of other statistics and procedures such as z scores and t tests by examining the difference between scores in relation to variance. Thus, the RCI may be interpreted as significant and reliable at ± 1.96 ($p \leq .05$) and, as with GAS ratings, changes can be evaluated in either direction (positive or negative). The method also allows for the construction of confidence intervals by adding the obtained standard score to the confidence term (i.e., $\underline{X}$ ± 1.96 [SEM]).

Because the RCI method relies on the standard error of measurement, it is useful for standardized measures, most of which provide internal reliability estimates on which SEM is based, along with SEMs that are typically reported in a technical manual. For measures that are empirically derived and may not report internal reliability estimates but are well constructed and are deemed to demonstrate strong internal consistency due to de facto internal reliability,

we suggest a conservative estimate index of 5 may be used to approximate the SEM. Alternative methods are to use the standard error of estimate, or the standard error of difference.

The strengths of the RCI are that the method allows for quantifiable changes for individuals, reliable changes are indexed by an error term, confidence intervals can be constructed that take into consideration the reliability of a measure and may help to avoid overinterpretation, and data can be aggregated to evaluate group changes. The limitations of the RCI method are that low reliability estimates of a given measure may result in nonsignificance even though large changes may be evident or, conversely, significant results based on a measure with poor reliability may not be valid, and the method typically is limited to pre–post designs.

Although the RCI method is used to provide an index of statistical and clinical change, it seldom is used as an index of magnitude of change. Drawing on the logic of GAS ratings, RCI magnitude potentially can be used to evaluate moderate or no change from pretest to posttest. For example, an RCI of +1 may be indicative of change in the direction of a goal. From a social significance vantage, magnitude data can provide valuable information toward determining whether a given treatment has an effect, albeit not a strong one.

Other applications are to use the RCI method to evaluate sustained change (or lack of change) or to evaluate magnitude of change within a group. For example, a low RCI from treatment to follow-up would be indicative of sustained change across time. Individual RCIs can be used to provide mean or median RCIs and deviations in change indices to evaluate group outcomes. These applications should be used with caution, however, and must be interpreted within a context that takes into consideration limitations with using repeated measures without controlling for error, and the current lack of research on the use of magnitude of effects.

Convergent Evidence Scaling

Convergent Evidence Scaling (CES) is an emerging method we have specifically constructed for converging outcomes derived from multiple indices (see Busse, Elliott, & Kratochwill, 1995). A similar method is used by Stoiber and Kratochwill (2001) in *Outcomes: PME*. The method for CES follows the logic of goal attainment scaling and provides a common metric for aggregating data. The basic elements are a 5-point scale from +2 to −2 and descriptions of outcomes that correspond to the following conditions: treatment goal fully met (+2); treatment goal partially met (+1); no progress toward goal (0); treatment goal unmet, behavior somewhat worse (−1); treatment goal unmet, behavior significantly worse (−2). As with GAS ratings, each outcome index is operationalized and converted into the 5-point scale. CES is designed to combine data from multiple sources and methods into a single quantitative index of effect size that reflects magnitude of change.

For example, consider a study wherein data are gathered from a child, parents, teachers, and an observer. These data may include pretest–posttest rating scale outcomes, GAS ratings, and single-case time-series observational data. Each outcome provides a different type of data that can account for source, setting, and method variance that traditionally are "converged" through visual inspection and decisions about the magnitude of effects. CES provides a systematic method for converging data such as these. Each outcome index is converted into the +2 to −2 scale. First, each index is operationalized with regard to magnitude of effect. For example, pre–post RCIs ≥ 1.6 may be deemed a strong effect (CES rating +2; treatment goal significantly met), RCIs ≥ .6 to 1.5 are indicative of a moderate effect (CES rating of +1; goal partially met), RCIs ≥ −.5 to .5 indicate no effect (CES = 0; goal unmet), RCIs ≥ −1.5 to −.6 indicate a moderate negative effect (CES = −1; goal unmet, somewhat worse), and RCIs <− 1.6 indicate a strong negative effect (CES = −2; goal unmet, significantly worse). For a 5-point GAS rating, the average rating may follow a similar magnitude conversion. For the observational data, a single-case effect size can be calculated (see Busk & Serlin, 1992; Busse et al., 1995) and converted, i.e., an effect size ≥ +1 may be deemed a strong effect with a CES rating of +2; an effect size of .4 to .9, a moderate effect with a CES rating of +1; and

so on. To aggregate these data, each outcome index is converted into an individual CES rating. Next, the mean rating is computed to provide an overall CES outcome. To clarify the method, let us consider the following composite single-case example of treatment outcomes for aggressive behavior.

For this simple example, data are based on teacher and parent ratings, and observations of aggressive behavior at baseline and treatment. Teacher ratings on the BASC Aggression subscale at pretest and posttest yield an RCI of +3, parent GAS ratings average +.44, and observations of aggressive behavior yield a single-case effect size of 1.8. Based on the operationalized magnitude conversions for CES, the BASC CES = +2, GAS CES = 0, and the effect size CES = +2. The mean of these individual CES ratings is 1.33, which is operationalized as an overall CES outcome rating of 1 (overall moderate effect).

This method of converting multiple outcome indices into a common metric and then converting into an overall converged outcome has several advantages. First, the method allows for converging data from indices that have different magnitudes— somewhat akin to converting raw scores to standard scores—thereby providing an overall quantity from which to base decisions on treatment effect. This overall CES also can be used within a meta-analytic study to compare treatment outcomes from studies that use different methods of data collection (e.g., rating scales vs. observations) and can be used within a given study to combine treatment outcomes.

The major limitations of CES include difficulty with decision making when individual indices indicate mixed outcomes, which are averaged in the overall CES rating (although this could be indicative of an overall moderate effect or situation-specific factors), and the magnitude of effects and subsequent CES operationalizations are in need of validation. At this point in its evolution, CES should be considered an experimental method that requires further study and discussion on its use.

SUMMARY AND CONCLUSIONS

Behavior rating scales can be versatile, economical, reliable, and valid tools for assessing human behavior. They can be used for screening purposes, for classification purposes, and can be of great assistance in identifying target behaviors for intervention. Behavior rating scales, however, are imperfect mirrors of human behavior. Like all observation-based assessments, behavior rating scales only sample behavior and are affected by measurement error and rater bias or reactivity. Their validity occasionally has been questioned because of only modest correspondence with direct observation data and varying degrees of interrater agreement for same-subject assessments. These concerns withstanding, behavior rating scales have become established tools in the research and practice of educators and psychologists interested in the social-emotional functioning of children and adolescents who experience behavior difficulties.

Rating scale technology has also been shown to be useful in the assessment of intervention procedures and outcomes. As documented in this chapter, some of the most interesting advances in the use of rating scale methodology concern the assessment of intervention integrity and progress monitoring. Specifically, the basic integrity or fidelity checklist has been expanded to include performance scales for evaluating degree of compliance with the recommended intervention steps. In addition, goal attainment scaling was discussed and recommended as a method for assessing intervention progress and outcomes. Goal attainment scales have a substantial and positive history in mental health research, but have rarely been used in school-based intervention work. Finally, two data synthesis techniques, RCI and CES, were described and recommended as methods for analyzing rating scale results for intervention outcomes. These are relatively simply data analysis techniques that are useful for both single-participant and group interventions.

Behavior rating scales have been part of emotional and behavioral disorders research and practice for more than two decades. With increasing interest in school-based intervention programs and emphasis on progress monitoring, rating scale technology is destined to further improve and to continue as a cornerstone of good research and practice.

REFERENCES

Achenbach, T. M. (1986). *Child Behavior Checklist—Direct Observation Form*. Burlington, VT: University of Vermont, Department of Psychiatry.

Achenbach, T. M., McConaughy, S. H., & Howell, C. T. (1987). Child/adolescent behavioral and emotional problems: Implications of cross-informant correlations for situational specificity. *Psychological Bulletin, 101*, 213–232.

Achenbach, T. M., & Rescorla, L. A. (2000). *Manual for the ASEBA preschool forms and profiles*. Burlington: University of Vermont, Research Center for Children, Youth, and Families (Available from *http://www.ASEBA.org*.)

Achenbach, T. M., & Rescorla, L. A. (2001). *Manual for the ASEBA school age forms and profiles*. Burlington: University of Vermont, Research Center for Children, Youth, and Families (Available from *http://www.ASEBA.org*.)

American Educational Research Association. (1999). *Standards for educational and psychological testing*. Washington, DC: American Psychological Association.

Barton, E. J., & Ascione, F. R. (1984). Direct observation. In T. Ollendick & M. Hersen (Eds.), *Child behavioral assessment: Principles and procedures* (pp. 166–194). New York: Pergamon.

Busk, P. L., & Serlin, R. C. (1992). Meta-analysis for single-case research. In T. R. Kratochwill & J. R. Levin (Eds.), *Single-case research design and analysis* (pp. 187–212). Hillsdale, NJ: Erlbaum.

Busse, R.T., Elliott, S.N., & Kratochwill, T.R. (1999). Influences of verbal interactions during behavioral consultations on treatment outcomes. *Journal of School Psychology, 37*, 117–143.

Busse, R. T., Kratochwill, T. R., & Elliott, S. N. (1995). Meta-analysis for single-case consultation outcomes: Applications to research and practice. *Journal of School Psychology, 33*, 269–285.

Cardillo, J. E. (1994). Goal setting, follow-up, and goal monitoring. In T. J. Kiresuk, A. Smith, & J. E. Cardillo (Eds.), *Goal Attainment Scaling: Application, theory, and measurement* (pp. 39–60). Hillsdale, NJ: Erlbaum.

Carr, R. A. (1979). Goal attainment scaling as a useful tool for evaluating progress in special education. *Exceptional Children, 46*, 88–95.

Doll, B., & Elliott, S. N. (1994). Representativeness of observed preschool social behaviors: How manny data are enough? *Journal of Early Intervention, 18*, 227–238.

Eckert, T. L., Dunn E. K., Guiney, K. M., & Codding, R. S. (2000). Self-reports: Theory and research in using rating scale measures. In E. S. Shapiro & T. R. Kratochwill (Eds.), *Behavioral assessment in schools: Theory, research, and clinical foundations* (2nd ed., pp. 288–352). New York: Guilford Press.

Edelbrock, C. (1983). Problems and issues in using rating scales to assess child personality and psychopathology. *School Psychology Review, 12*, 293–299.

Edelbrock, D., Costello, A. J., Dulcan, M. K., Kalas, R., & Conover, N. C. (1985). Age differences in the reliability of the psychiatric interview of the child. *Child Development, 56*, 265–275.

Elliott, S. N., Busse, R. T., & Gresham, F. M. (1993). Behavior rating scales: Issues of use and development. *School Psychology Review, 22*, 313–321.

Elliott, S. N., DiPerna, J. C., & Shapiro, E. S. (2001). *Academic Intervention Monitoring System*. San Antonio, TX: Psychological Corporation.

Elliott, S. N., & Gresham, F. M. (1991). *Social skills intervention guide: Practical strategies for social skills training*. Circle Pines, MN: American Guidance Service.

Elliott, S. N., Gresham, F. M., Freeman, T., & McCloskey, G. (1988). Teacher and observer ratings of children's social skills: Validation of the social skills rating scales. *Journal of Psychoeducational Assessment, 6*, 152–161.

Elliott, S. N., Sladeczek, I., & Kratochwill, T.R. (1995). *Goal attainment scaling: Its use as a progress monitoring and outcome effectiveness measure in behavioral consultation*. Paper presented at the Annual Convention of the American Psychological Association, New York, New York.

Epstein, M. H., & Sharma, H. M. (1998). *Behavioral and Emotional Rating Scale*. Austin, TX: Pro-Ed.

Gettinger, M., Stoiber, K. C., & Lange, J. (1999). Collaborative investigation of inclusive early education practices: A blueprint for teacher–researcher partnership. *Journal of Early Intervention, 22*, 257–265.

Gresham, F. M. (1989). Assessment of intervention integrity in school consultation and prereferral interventions. *School Psychology Review, 18*, 37–50.

Gresham, F. M., & Elliott, S. N. (1990). *Social Skills Rating System*. Circle Pines, MN: American Guidance Service.

Gresham, F. M., Elliott, S. N., & Evans-Fernandez, S. (1992). *Student Self-Concept Scales*. Circle Pines, MN: American Guidance Service.

Gresham, F. M., Noell, G. H., & Elliott, S. N. (1996). Teachers as judges of social competence: A conditional probability analysis. *School Psychology Review, 25*, 108–117.

Jacobson, N. S., Follette, W. C., & Revenstorf, D. (1984). Psychotherapy outcome research: Methods for reporting variability and evaluating clinical significance. *Behavior Therapy, 15*, 336–352.

Jacobson, N. S., & Truax, P. (1991). Clinical significance: A statistical approach to defining meaningful change in psychotherapy research. *Journal of Consulting and Clinical Psychology, 59*, 12–19.

Johnston, J. M., & Pennypacker, H. S. (1980). *Strategies and tactics of human behavioral research*. Hillsdale, NJ: Erlbaum.

Kazdin, A. E. (1979). Situational specificity: The two-edged sword of behavioral assessment. *Behavioral Assessment, 1*, 57–75.

Kazdin, A. E. (1986). Comparative outcome studies of psychotherapy: Methodological issues and strategies. *Journal of Consulting and Clinical Psychology, 54*, 95–105.

Kettler, R. J., Elliott, S. N., Bolt, D..M., & DiPerna, J. C. (2003). *Teacher and student ratings of academic competence: An examination of cross-informant agreement and classification accuracy*. Unpublished manuscript, University of Wisconsin–Madison.

Kiresuk, T. J., & Sherman, R. E. (1968). Goal attainment scaling: A general method for evaluating community mental health programs. *Community Mental Health Journal, 4*, 443–453.

Kiresuk, T. J., Smith, A., & Cardillo, J. E. (Eds.). (1994). *Goal attainment scaling: Application, theory, and measurement* (pp. 135–160). Hillsdale, NJ: Erlbaum.

Kratochwill, T. R., Elliott, S. N., & Busse, R. T. (1995). Behavioral consultation training: A five-year evaluation of consultant and client outcomes. *School Psychology Quarterly, 10*, 87–117.

Kratochwill, T. R., Elliott, S. N., & Rotto, P. (1995). Best practices in school-based behavioral consultation. In A. Thomas & J. Grimes (Eds.), *Best practices in school psychology* (3rd ed., pp. 519–538). Washington, DC: National Association of School Psychologists.

Kratochwill, T. R., & Shapiro, E. S. (2000). Conceptual foundations of behavioral assessment in schools. In E. S. Shapiro & T. R. Kratochwill (Eds.), *Behavioral assessment in the schools: Theory, research, and clinical foundations* (2nd ed., pp. 3–15). New York: Guilford Press.

Kratochwill, T. R., & Stoiber, K. C. (2000). Empirically supported interventions and school psychology: Conceptual and practice issues: Part II. *School Psychology Quarterly, 15*, 233–253.

Laurent, J., Hadler, J. R., & Stark, K. D. (1994). A multiple stage screening procedure for the identification of childhood anxiety disorders. *School Psychology Quarterly, 9*, 239–255.

LePage, K., Kratochwill, T. R., & Elliott, S. N. (2004). Competency-based consultation training: An evaluation of consultation outcomes, treatment effects and consumer satisfaction. *School Psychology Quarterly, 19*(1), 1–28.

Maher, C. A. (1982). Learning disabled adolescents in the regular classroom: Evaluation of a mainstreaming procedure. *Learning Disability Quarterly, 5*, 82–84.

McConaughy, S. H., & Ritter, D. R. (1995). Multidimensional assessment of emotional or behavioral disorders. In A. Thomas & J. Grimes (Eds.), *Best practices in school psychology III* (pp. 865–877). Washington, DC: National Association of School Psychologists.

Merrell, K. W. (1993a). Using behavior rating scales to assess social skills and antisocial behavior in school settings: Development of the school social behavior scales. *School Psychology Review, 22,* 115–133.

Merrell, K. W. (1993b). *School Social Behavior Scales.* Austin, TX: Pro-Ed.

Merrell, K. W. (2003). *Behavioral, social, and emotional assessment of children and adolescents.* Mahwah, NJ: Erlbaum.

Mitchell, T., & Cusick, A. (1998). Evaluation of a client-centered pediatric rehabilitation programme using goal attainment scaling. *Australian Occupational Therapy Journal, 45,* 7–17.

Nunnally, J., & Kotsche, W. (1983). Studies of individual subjects: Logic and methods of analysis. *British Journal of Clinical Psychology, 22,* 83–93.

Oren, T., & Ogletree, B. T. (2000). Program evaluation in classrooms for students with autism: Student outcomes and program processes. *Focus on Autism and Other Developmental Disabilities, 15,* 170–175.

Preator, K. K., & McAllister, J. R., (1995). Assessing infants and toddlers. In A. Thomas & J. Grimes (Eds.), *Best practices in school psychology III* (pp. 775–788). Washington, DC: National Association of School Psychologists.

Puig-Antich, J., & Chambers, W. (1986). *The Schedule for Affective Disorders and Schizophrenia for School-Age Children (Kiddie-SADS).* New York: New York State Psychiatric Institute.

Racine, C. N. (1994). *The relationship between observations and ratings of children's social behavior: An extension of the accuracy–reliability paradigm.* Unpublished master's thesis, University of Wisconsin–Madison.

Reschly, D. J., Tilly, W. D., & Grimes, J. P. (Eds.). (1999). *Special education in transition: Functional assessment and noncategorical programming.* Longmont, CO: Sopris West.

Reynolds, C. R., & Kamphaus, R. W. (1992). *Behavior Assessment System for Children.* Circle Pines, MN: American Guidance Service.

Reynolds, C. R., & Richmond, B. O. (1985). *Revised Children's Manifest Anxiety Scale.* Los Angeles: Western Psychological Services.

Robertson, S. L. (1993). *The relationship between observations and ratings of children's social behavior.* Unpublished master's thesis, University of Wisconsin–Madison.

Robertson-Mjaanes, S. L. (1999). *An evaluation of goal attainment scaling as an intervention monitoring and outcome evaluation technique.* Unpublished doctoral dissertation: University of Wisconsin–Madison.

Ruffalo, S. L., & Elliott, S. N. (1997). Teachers' and parents' ratings of children's social skills: A closer look at the cross-informant agreements through an item analysis protocol. *School Psychology Review, 26,* 489–501.

Schneider, B. H., & Byrne, B. M. (1989). Parents rating children's social behavior: How focused the lens? *Journal of Clinical Child Psychology, 18,* 237–241.

Shapiro, E. S., & Browder, J. L. (1990). Behavioral assessment: Applications for persons with mental retardation. In J. L. Matson (Ed.), *Handbook of behavior modification with the mentally retarded* (pp. 93–120). New York: Plenum.

Shapiro, E. S., & Kratochwill, T. R. (Eds.). (2000). *Conducting school-based assessments of child and adolescent behavior.* New York: Guilford Press.

Sladeczek, I. E., Elliott, S. N., Kratochwill, T. R., Robertson-Mjaanes, S., & Stoiber, K. C. (2001). Application of goal attainment scaling to a conjoint behavioral consultation case. *Journal of Educational and Psychological Consultation, 12,* 45–58.

Stavrakaki, C., Williams, E., Walker, S., & Roberts, N. (1991). Pilot study of anxiety and depression in prepubertal children. *Canadian Journal of Psychiatry, 36,* 332–338.

Stoiber, K. C., & Kratochwill, T. R. (2001). *Outcomes PME: Planning, monitoring, and evaluating.* San Antonio: Psychological Corporation.

Walker, H. M., & Severson, H. H. (1992). *Systematic Screening for Behavior Disorders (SSDB) technical manual* (2nd ed.). Longmont, CO: Sopris West.

West, J. G., Idol, L., & Cannon, G. (1987). *A curriculum for preservice and inservice preparation of classroom and special education teachers in collaborative consultation.* Austin: The University of Texas at Austin, Research and Training Project on School Consultation.

Wilson, M. S., & Reschly, D. J. (1996). Assessment in school psychology training and practice. *School Psychology Review, 25,* 9–23.

Witt, J. C., Elliott, S. N., Daly, E. J., Gresham, F. M., & Kramer, J. J. (1998). *Assessment of at-risk and special needs children* (2nd ed.). Boston: McGraw-Hill.

Wolf, M. M. (1978). Social validity: The case for subjective measurement or how applied behavior analysis is finding its heart. *Journal of Applied Behavior Analysis, 11,* 203–214.

Yeaton, W. H., & Sechrest, L. (1981). Critical dimensions in the choice and maintenance of successful interventions: Strength, integrity, and effectiveness. *Journal of Consulting and Clinical Psychology, 49,* 156–167.

8

Functional Behavioral Assessment

JAMES J. FOX *and* ROBERT A. GABLE

Two subjects guaranteed to start an argument are religion and politics. We suspect that one could also add "functional behavioral assessment" (FBA) to that list. Debate among professionals over issues ranging from the definition, essential procedures, brief versus extended assessment, clinical utility, and broader legal implications of FBA, can be and has been spirited, to say the least. Indeed, the specific terminology (e.g., functional assessment, functional behavioral assessment, functional analysis, etc.) that various professionals use to refer to this assessment process itself has been the subject of disagreement (see, for example, Dunlap & Kincaid, 2001) as well as the specific procedures that define the necessary and sufficient conditions of FBA (e.g., Scott, Meers, & Nelson, 2000).

Recognizing the controversial nature of FBA, we will attempt to offer a sufficiently balanced, empirically based review and to shed further light on the current state of FBA research and practice, with particular regard to its application to students with emotional and behavioral disorders (EBD). In this chapter, we (1) define critical terms and concepts related to FBA; (2) review the historical development of FBA, particularly as applied to EBD students; (3) give a succinct overview of the FBA process; (4) review the state of our empirical knowledge regarding the various FBA methods and instruments and the effectiveness of functional hypothesis-based interventions; (5) discuss ways in which we can most effectively prepare school personnel and others to apply this assessment–intervention technology; and finally, (6) discuss implications for future research and practice.

DEFINITION OF TERMS AND CONCEPTS IN FUNCTIONAL BEHAVIORAL ASSESSMENT

One can take a pragmatic view in defining functional assessment. O'Neill et al. (1997) defined FBA as "a process for gathering information that can be used to maximize the effectiveness and efficiency of behavioral support" (p. 3). O'Neill and his colleagues further elaborated this definition by referring to "five primary outcomes" of this process: (1) a clear description of the problem behavior; (2) identification of the events, times, and situations that predict when the problem behavior will and will not occur; (3) identification of the consequences that maintain the problem behavior; (4) development of summary statements or hypotheses describing the problem behavior, the specific situations in which it occurs, and the outcomes that maintain the behavior in those situations; and (5) collection of direct observation data that support the summary statements. Others have taken an equally pragmatic view of FBA, defining it as a process designed to develop more effective interventions by identifying the situations and events that influence the occurrence of challenging behavior (e.g., Bambara & Knoster, 1998; Demchak & Bossert, 1996; Nelson, Roberts, & Smith, 1998).

Generally, there seems to be agreement that FBA is a process rather than a single specific set of procedures or instruments (Dunlap & Kincaid, 2001). There also seems to be recognition that "functional assessment" includes a relatively broad range of processes (including indirect and direct descriptive assessment strategies and experimental analytic strategies), whereas the term "functional analysis" is reserved for that component of FBA that specifically involves planned, systematic manipulation of classroom factors (especially the consequences of behavior) and that more exactly identifies how the manipulation of these variables may negatively or positively affect the challenging behavior (e.g., Sasso, Conroy, Stichter, & Fox, 2001).

While the immediate purpose of FBA is to identify the specific conditions that trigger and maintain challenging behavior, most authorities advocate some form of positive programming, if not as a necessity, then as highly desirable. Response equivalence and response efficiency (e.g., Carr & Kemp, 1989; Horner & Day, 1991; Horner, Sprague, O'Brien, & Heathfield, 1990; Skinner, Belfiore, Mace, Williams-Wilson, & Johns, 1997) are integral to both the assessment and the behavior intervention processes. The first concept, response equivalency, refers to selecting replacement behaviors that can serve the same function as the challenging behavior. The second concept, response efficiency, is concerned with ensuring that the replacement behaviors achieve the functional outcome at least as quickly, consistently, and with the same quality of maintaining consequence as the challenging behavior. Viewed together, these concepts provide an underpinning for the more pragmatic, time-honored ABA injunction known as the "fair pair rule" (White & Haring, 1980), which dictates that for every behavior that you decrease you should increase a behavior in its place. These concepts provide the conceptual integration of functional assessment with positive behavior support.

There are several areas of significant disagreement or differences in emphasis between researchers and practitioners of FBA.

These include the relative role of descriptive/structural methods versus functional analysis methods in assessing challenging behavior (e.g., Lerman & Iwata, 1993), and the degree to which the existing FBA technology effectively addresses the myriad behavior challenges presented by children and youths with EBD (e.g., Nelson, Mathur, & Rutherford, 1999; Peck, Sasso, & Stambaugh, 1998; Sasso et al., 2001). Definitive answers to these issues, especially the necessary and sufficient components of FBA, would yield a more explicit definition, and we will attempt to address them in subsequent sections of this chapter.

HISTORICAL OVERVIEW OF FUNCTIONAL BEHAVIORAL ASSESSMENT AND STUDENTS WITH EBD

The essentials of FBA are not new but have been a part of analyzing and intervening on challenging behaviors since the inception of applied behavior analysis (ABA). The history of FBA can be traced to the early days of ABA. The conceptual statements regarding the seven dimensions of applied behavior analysis by Baer, Wolf, and Risley (1968) and methodological statements such as Bijou, Peterson, and Ault's (1968) description of the procedures for and the analysis of A–B–C (antecedent–behavior–consequence) recording of naturalistic observations of child behavior have clearly shaped the FBA process.

Attempting to identify beginning points in the application of FBA to students with EBD is more problematic. The child in the Allen, Hart, Buell, Harris, and Wolf (1964) investigation was, other than her isolation from peers, a typically developing preschooler. Most FBA studies have been conducted with children and youths having low-incidence, moderate to severe developmental disabilities such as mental retardation or autism while relatively few have included children or youths clearly identified as EBD (Fox, Conroy, & Heckaman, 1998; Heckaman, Conroy, Fox, & Chait, 2000; Lane, Umbreit, & Beebe-Frankenberger, 1999; Reid & Nelson, 2002; Sasso et al., 2001). In part, this is the result of the changing and imprecise definition of what constitutes EBD.

There are several early reports that applied the basic principles of FBA to children without developmental delays but who exhibit serious challenging behaviors.

Zimmerman and Zimmerman (1962) described two case studies of boys in self-contained classrooms of a residential treatment program. Both boys were 11 years old and diagnosed as emotionally disturbed but presented different behavior challenges (i.e., intentionally and repeatedly misspelling words on a spelling assignment, crumpling and throwing away task materials, and severe aggressive tantrums). Although the investigators reported no formal data on the potential antecedents or consequences of the behaviors, informal observations led them to hypothesize that social attention (by the teacher in the first case and by residential staff in the second case) functioned to maintain their behaviors. Based upon these hypotheses, Zimmerman and Zimmerman implemented planned ignoring along with social attention to appropriate task behaviors. Subsequently, the students' challenging behaviors reportedly decreased and task performance improved; however, no formal data were provided to verify these outcomes.

The first study of a child exhibiting serious challenging behaviors that also included empirical documentation may be that of Zeilberger, Sampen, and Sloane (1968), who analyzed a young boy's aggressive and disobedient behavior at home with peers and his mother. Although there was no formal diagnosis of EBD, the boy's challenging behaviors were long-standing, had resulted in his dismissal from two preschool programs, and were frequent and of high intensity. Informal and formal data collection suggested the boy's challenging behaviors were maintained at least in part by the mother's reprimands and extended explanations of the inappropriateness of his behavior. The mother applied a package of behavioral procedures including differential attention to appropriate play and compliance, as well as time out for the unacceptable behaviors. A reversal design provided validation of the parent social attention hypothesis and of the effectiveness of the intervention package. While the overall amount of parent attention did not change, reductions in attention following the challenging behaviors correlated well with reductions in the challenging behaviors.

Looking at these studies as empirical benchmarks for FBA, it is important to note that none of the investigators referred to their procedures as "functional assessment" or "functional behavioral assessment." This is not surprising since the term did not have significance until more than 20 years later. Also, most early reports reflect rich textual descriptions of the case analysis (e.g., Risley, 1968; Zimmerman & Zimmerman, 1963). Few of the more formal elements we have come to associate with FBA (e.g., structured interviews, scatterplots, functional assessment rating scales, sequential recording of antecedents, consequences, and behavior, or structured analog analyses) were described. These formal processes and instruments are more recent developments. What is evident, however, across these early reports and what links them directly to current FBA practices is: (1) their focus on attempting to identify the environmental triggers and maintaining consequences for challenging behavior; (2) basing a motivational hypothesis on this informal analysis; and (3) developing an intervention based on that hypothesis that eliminated the environmental supports for the challenging behavior or altering the arrangement of those environmental events to support alternative appropriate behavior. Put another way, in these early studies researchers "behaviorally diagnosed" the maladaptive behavior–environment relationship and then "prescribed" an intervention and behavioral target for intervention based upon that empirically derived diagnosis (Bailey & Pyles, 1989). This general process is the essence of what constitutes FBA. In this sense, these early case studies and experimental analyses can be legitimately viewed as the progenitors of contemporary FBA.

Perhaps one of the clearest applications of the emerging FBA technology to students with EBD in school settings was that reported by Dunlap et al. Those investigators described the application of several different FBA assessment procedures. The FBA procedures included: (1) the *Functional Analysis Interview Form* (FAIF) developed by O'Neill et al. (1997), (2) A–B–C recording of the antecedents and consequences of the subjects' challenging behaviors in the classroom, (3) development of hypothesis statements of potential classroom factors (e.g., staff attention and praise, proximity of staff, choice-making opportunities), and (4) functional analysis hypothesis testing of those suspected antecedent triggers and maintaining consequences.

OVERVIEW OF THE FUNCTIONAL BEHAVIORAL ASSESSMENT PROCESS

Before reviewing the empirical status of FBA as applied to children and youths with EBD, it will be helpful to describe briefly the overall FBA process to ensure a common reference point. There are several ways in which this process can be categorized. One very simple categorization is to view FBA as composed of three major assessment stages: (1) indirect assessment, (2) direct descriptive assessment, and (3) hypothesis development and validation, or functional behavioral analysis (Watson & Steege, 2003). Generally, these stages proceed in that order.

Indirect assessment involves the gathering of information from existing data bases (school records, other assessment reports, disciplinary referrals, etc), and soliciting informant reports about the student via interviews and rating scales completed by teachers, other school personnel, parents, peers, and the student him- or herself. In this stage, the assessor(s) casts a wide net and attempts to gather all potentially relevant information from a number of diverse sources. Although indirect methods contain a number of inherent limitations (e.g., selective or biased recall and imprecise summary reports of behavioral and environmental events), this stage of the process is important for several reasons. First, indirect FBA is the point at which critical definitions of target behaviors, potential antecedent triggers, maintaining consequences, and enabling setting events are first developed. Clear definition of challenging behaviors in "action-object" terms and the description of potential environmental events in concrete, objective terms are absolutely essential to successful FBA.

Second, indirect FBA affords an initial opportunity to compare and contrast information from different sources and situations. The consistency (interinformant reliability) of the indirect data in terms of the nature and severity of the student's behavior as well as the consistency of the events reported to trigger and maintain those behaviors is eval-uated. This is also the first opportunity to identify the people present, situations, and times in which the student's challenging behavior is reported most likely and least likely to occur. Indirect analysis facilitates the ongoing process of functional hypothesis development and narrows the contexts, events, and behaviors that will be the focus of the next stage of direct assessment. A third purpose of indirect FBA is to assess those challenging behaviors that are significant but may be of low or irregular frequency or that may occur in circumstances that make direct assessment more difficult to implement (e.g., smoking, stealing, sexual behavior).

The second stage of FBA, *direct assessment procedures*, like indirect assessment, is largely descriptive. The goals are to: (1) document the current level of the challenging behaviors and (2) identify specific setting events, antecedents, and consequences as they currently occur in the student's natural environment and that may be functionally related to the behavior. This stage includes measures such as the scatterplot (Touchette, MacDonald, & Langer, 1985) to detect times and activities associated with the challenging behavior, structured multicategory observation systems (e.g., Bijou et al., 1968; Gable, Hendrickson, & Sealander, 1998; O'Neill et al., 1997; Slate & Saudargas, 1986; Scott & Sugai, 1994) to assess specific antecedents and consequences, and setting event checklists (Conroy & Fox, 1994; Fox & Conroy, 1995; Gardner, Cole, Davidson, & Karan, 1986; Kennedy & Itkonen, 1993) that track contextual variables associated with challenging behavior(s).

The third stage of FBA is *hypothesis development and validation*. This stage involves the summary and analysis of data compiled during indirect and direct assessment into a more coherent statement of the apparent function(s) of the challenging behavior(s). Various methods have been introduced to accomplish that task. Data triangulation (Gable et al., 2002) is an analytic strategy borrowed from quantitative research that involves evaluating the consistency among different sources and levels of FBA data and the degree to which these different sources point to a common behavior function(s). Once a team identifies one or more function(s), a "problem pathway analysis" or "competing pathway analysis" chart (Gable et al., 2002; Sugai, Lewis-Palmer, & Hagan, 1998) is used to construct behavior–environment time lines. These pathway statements consist of the possible sequences of setting events, antecedents, challenging behaviors, and consequences that provide an opportunity for, trigger, and maintain the challenging behavior.

Because more than one function of the behavior and pathway may be suggested by the assessment data, the events depicted on the pathway chart represent the conditions that are systematically manipulated in the next step, *hypothesis validation*. Ordinarily, single-subject experimental designs (or some modification) are used to isolate the differential effects of those manipulations on the challenging behavior. Variously known as experimental analysis, functional analysis, or environmental manipulation, this analytic (as opposed to the previous two descriptive stages of indirect and direct assessment) component of the FBA process serves several related purposes. First, it evaluates the degree to which each of the previously hypothesized functions is valid. Second, it previews the effectiveness of an intervention based on the specific variables manipulated in that functional analysis. Third, used in conjunction with problem pathway analysis, functional analysis enables the interventionist to determine replacement behaviors that may serve the same function as the challenging behavior but that are more socially/educationally acceptable.

There are two basic approaches to accomplishing hypothesis validation. Analogue probes are specially constructed and highly controlled presentations of the suspected triggering and maintaining events. These probes are most often conducted in clinic or specially created conditions, and usually involve a single student and one or more specially trained assessment personnel. Probe sessions are comparatively brief (5–15 minutes long) and consist of a relatively standard set of conditions such as those originally reported by Iwata, Dorsey, Slifer, Bauman, and Richman (1982): (1) a social attention condition, in which the adult interacts briefly with the student whenever the challenging behavior occurs; (2) an escape condition, in which the adult permits the student to briefly stop the task

or removes the task contingent upon the challenging behavior; (3) a sensory condition, in which few or no materials are available and the adult is present but does not interact in any way with the student and ignores the behavior; and (4) an alone condition, in which the student is placed in the assessment room alone to serve as a control condition.

Environmental manipulations are conducted within a classroom (or other naturalistic environment) and may be implemented by specially trained assessment personnel or by natural environment agents such as the teacher or parent. Also, the manipulated conditions may replicate the social attention–escape–sensory reinforcement–tangible reinforcement model originally reported by Iwata et al. (1982), or the process may consist of systematic changes in antecedents, consequences, or setting events (or some combination of all three) that typify that student's classroom.

Gable et al. (2002) further elaborated the FBA process, describing it as a 10-step process. The first 6 steps consist of the literal functional assessment activities: (1) describe and verify the problem's seriousness; (2) refine the problem behavior definition; (3) collect information on possible functions of the problem behavior; (4) analyze information using data triangulation and problem pathway analysis; (5) generate a hypothesis statement of the probable function of the problem behavior; and (6) test the hypothesis statement regarding the problem behavior function. The final four steps describe developing, applying, and evaluating the function-based intervention that results from the first six steps: (7) develop and implement a behavioral intervention plan; (8) monitor the faithfulness of plan implementation; (9) evaluate effectiveness of the intervention; and (10) modify the intervention as needed. This 10-step sequence serves as a task analysis FBA and emphasizes that FBA is not a single event or instrument. Rather, FBA is a process that should lead to an intervention or intervention package that takes advantage of the challenging behavior's function and that evaluates the validity of that intervention (and the underlying hypothesis) through ongoing direct assessment of the student's and alternative behaviors. We now turn to a review and analysis of the existing research on some of the key instruments or components of this process.

INDIRECT ASSESSMENT IN FUNCTIONAL BEHAVIORAL ASSESSMENT

As we noted earlier, indirect assessment is accomplished in various ways, including methods that rely on examination of existing data records of a student's behavior (e.g., incident reports, discipline referrals, psychological or educational assessments, treatment or management plans or an anecdotal narrative compiled notes kept by a teacher). Another common strategy is to solicit reports from significant others (e.g., teachers, instructional assistants, parents, other students) about some aspect of the student's behavior. Usually these reports are obtained through some form of face-to-face interview or by having the informant(s) complete a structured behavior-situation rating scale. Indirect assessment may also include the student reporting about his or her own behavior by means of a student-focused interview and/or completion of a rating scale. This assumes the student has the necessary cognitive and verbal communication skills and is willing cooperate with the assessor.

FBA Interviews

A modest body of empirical research suggests that functional interviews are a useful tool for identifying the source(s) of student behavior problems. There are a number of specific interview protocols including (but not limited to) the *Behavioral Diagnosis and Treatment Form* (Bailey & Pyles, 1989), the *Functional Assessment Interview Form* (FAIF; O'Neill et al., 1997), the *Student-Assisted Interview Form* (SAIF; O'Neill et al., 1997), the *Student-Assisted Interview* (SAI; Kern, Dunlap, Clarke, & Childs, 1994), the *Functional Behavioral Assessment Interview/Self-Report Form* (Nelson et al., 1998), and a series of interview forms developed by Watson and Steege (2003). Researchers have often developed these and other interviews for use with different student populations, types of informants (teachers, parents, the student), and settings

(residential institutions vs. classrooms). Consequently, the interview protocols vary in length, structure, and the specific types and scope of questions, depending, for example, on whether the student being assessed has milder or more severe disabilities.

Most FBA interviews were developed for use with people with developmental disabilities. While many of the questions or areas of information sought on these interviews are applicable across disability groups, some questions, either because of the specific information sought or the way in which they are asked, may have limited applicability to students with EBD. For example, the interview developed by Bailey and Pyles (1989) includes questions such as "Could the client be signaling some deprivation condition?" and "Does the behavior cause serious tissue damage?" Similarly, the FAIF (O'Neill et al., 1997) contains questions that relate to communicative competence (e.g., use of signing, communication boards, electronic devices) and imitative skills that, while appropriate for chronologically young or developmentally delayed students, may have less relevance for older students with mild or no developmental delays. To their credit, O'Neill et al. (1997) encouraged users to adapt the FAIF to the particular needs of the specific child or adolescent.

When attempting to evaluate the reliability of most FBA interview protocols, difficulties arise in applying typical methods of reliability analyses. Existing interviews usually combine open-ended, free-response, and forced-choice response formats. Thus, an informant's response to some interview items (e.g., "What are the behaviors of concern?") is likely to result in a description that may literally differ from that of another informant with regard to the specific language used to characterize the behavior ("he's disruptive in class"). This difference may be true even when the interviewer asks for more concrete "action-object" descriptors of the behavior ("he talks to peers, plays with objects on his desk, makes loud verbal complaints about the assignment"). Were the second informant to label the general category of behavior differently ("he's off-task") and/or use somewhat different action-object descriptors (e.g., the informant refers to "talking to peers" but does not mention playing with objects or refers to verbally refusing to do the assignment rather than making verbal complaints), it is unclear whether or not the informants' responses will be considered to be in agreement. In these instances, it may be necessary for someone to independently judge the extent to which the informants' responses are in agreement and how much confidence to attach to those data.

Few published studies have analyzed the reliability of FBA interviews. Reed, Thomas, Sprague, and Horner (1997) had 10 students in grades 5–8 and their teachers (some special education, some general education) independently complete the O'Neill et al., (1997) Student-Guided Functional Assessment Interview. All students had a history of office referrals for challenging behaviors, three currently had individualized education programs (IEPs), and two had been diagnosed as having attention-deficit/hyperactivity disorder (ADHD). The experimenters coded teachers' and students' statements during the interview and developed hypothesis statements based on that interview information. Students reported slightly more challenging behaviors for themselves than did teachers. Overall agreement on behaviors was 85%. Analyzing only those behaviors reported by both students and teachers, Reed et al. (1997) found 77% agreement on both antecedents and consequences, while agreement on setting events was much lower (26%). Overall, Reed and colleagues indicated that students and teachers were in agreement on 66% of the interview items.

Kinch, Lewis-Palmer, Hagan-Burke, and Sugai (2001) analyzed data from eight students in grades 6–8 identified by their teachers as exhibiting high rates of problem behavior in certain classes and low rates of that behavior in other classes. Direct classroom observations and explicit quantitative criteria were used to confirm the high and low rates of behavior in each class. The challenging behaviors encompassed disruptive, noncompliant, task-related, and aggressive behaviors. Teachers completed a shortened version of the FAIF (O'Neill et al., 1997), while students completed the SAIF (O'Neill et al., 1997). Independent raters categorized teachers' and students' specific responses as being in agreement or disagreement on be-

haviors and environmental events. Raters exhibited 80% or better agreement on their judgments of teachers' and students' concurrence. In the high-risk (rate) classrooms, teachers and students were in agreement on 79% of the challenging behaviors, and when the environmental events associated with those behaviors were examined, teachers and students agreed on 100% of the antecedents, 91% of the consequences, but only 21% of the setting events. In contrast, in the low-risk (rate) classrooms, student and teacher agreement was lower: 46% agreement on behaviors, 31% agreement on antecedents, 46% agreement on the consequences, and 40% on setting events. Across the classroom teachers (the high- and low-risk classrooms), there was 83% agreement on antecedents, 100% agreement on consequences, yet only 43% agreement on the setting events for the behaviors identified for the students.

The preceding studies evaluated interinformant (teacher–student and teacher–teacher) reliability of the instrument assessed. We were unable to find any other published studies of the reliability of those particular interview forms (the FAIF and the SAIF) or of any other interview protocols used for conducting functional assessment. A few investigators have looked at what might be considered the concurrent validity of FBA interviews and other FBA instruments. These studies have been conducted, however, with populations of students or adults with developmental disabilities rather than those with EBD. For example, Cunningham and O'Neill (2000) examined the congruence between several FBA methods (the FAIF, the FAOF, the Motivation Assessment Scale (MAS), and analogue functional analyses) in identifying the function of challenging behaviors of three young boys with autism and challenging behaviors (self-injury, screaming, tantrums, and aggression to others). Each boy's teacher and an instructional assistant were interviewed using the FAIF. These staff also completed MASs on each student and teachers collected direct observational data on the challenging behaviors, antecedents, and consequences, using the FAOF (O'Neill et al., 1997). At the same time the experimenters conducted analog functional analyses using the procedures developed by Iwata et al. (1982). The results showed agreement on the function of challenging behaviors between the interview protocol, direct observations, and analogues. Girolami and Scotti (2001) relied on parents as informants to functionally assess food refusal (throwing food, slapping hand of server, spitting food out, turning head away, aggression to server) in three young children (28–32 months old) with mental retardation. The assessment procedures included the FAIF, the MAS, A–B–C observations, and analogue functional analyses. For two of the children, all four methods indicated an escape function. For the third child, analogue and MAS data indicated that the behavior was motivated by access to tangible objects, whereas the interview and A–B–C observations indicated the behaviors occurred to access attention.

To summarize the current the technical adequacy of FBA interviews with students who have EBD has been evaluated in surprisingly few studies. The existing studies of interinformant agreement suggest moderate to high reliability of the FAIF and the SAIF with regard to the behaviors, antecedents, and maintaining consequences, but very low agreement on important contextual or setting events. There are many qualifications for these data. Despite the number of different specific interview protocols that have been developed, only the FAIF and SAIF (O'Neill et al., 1997) have been analyzed for their reliability, and this has been limited to interinformant agreement (Kinch et al., 2001; Reed et al., 1997). It is unclear to what extent agreement on these specific instruments might predict agreement that might be obtained on conceptually similar but structurally different instruments. Furthermore, it is possible that agreement is affected by the frequency of the challenging behaviors (Kinch et al., 2001). The implication of this latter finding is that the technical adequacy of existing interviews might be compromised for low incidence but significant challenging behaviors (e.g., fighting, smoking, weapons possession), the very behaviors for which many students with disabilities are subjected to more restrictive and intrusive interventions (e.g., suspension, homebound instruction, alternative schools).

The empirical situation for validity of FBA interviews seems even worse. We were unable to find any published studies on the concurrent or predictive validity of FBA interviews for EBD students. Indeed, there have been very few such analyses even for students with other cognitive/developmental disabilities (Cunningham & O'Neill, 2000; Girolami & Scotti, 2001; Yarbrough & Carr, 2000). Generally, these studies have shown acceptable levels of concurrence between behavior functions identified through interview information and other concurrently or sequentially applied instruments (behavior–situation rating scales, direct observations, functional analyses). Unfortunately, most instruments against which FBA interviews have been compared have themselves received little or no formal evaluation of reliability or validity. Suffice it to say there is as yet no standard FBA assessment instrument or technique that has sufficiently documented technical adequacy so as to serve as a validity standard.

Behavior–Situation Rating Scales

Several instruments have been developed that allow informants to rate the likelihood of a specific challenging behavior in particular types of situations. These instruments include the *Motivational Assessment Scale* (MAS; Durand & Crimmins, 1988, 1992), the *Problem Behavior Questionnaire* (PBQ; Lewis, Scott, & Sugai, 1994), and the *Questions about Behavior Function* (QABF; Matson, Bamburg, Cherry, & Paclawskyj, 1999).

As one of the best-known and frequently researched behavior–situation rating scales, the MAS is a 16-item scale that was originally developed to identify motivational conditions for chronic severe behavior problems, such as self-injury, stereotypy, and aggression. In an early study of the technical adequacy of the MAS, Durand and Crimmins (1988) found significant and high interrater agreement (.89–.98) between the teachers and aides as well as high test–retest reliability (.82–.99).

There have been a number of subsequent studies of the psychometric characteristics of the MAS. Although conducted across a wide range of ages, settings, and challenging behaviors, these studies have been restricted to subject populations with developmental disabilities (mental retardation, autism), with levels of functioning in the moderate to profound range. Generally, these studies have only partially replicated the reliability results originally reported by Durand and Crimmins (1988). However, various investigators have reported moderate to high internal consistency for the MAS (Akande, 1994; Bihm, Kienlen, Ness, & Poindexter, 1991; Conroy, Fox, Bucklin, & Good, 1996; Newton & Sturmey, 1991). Unfortunately, the accumulated literature shows that the interrater reliability and agreement have not held up as well as the internal consistency of the MAS (Akande, 1994; Conroy, Fox, Bucklin, & Good, 1996; Duker & Sigafoos, 1998; Kearney, 1994; Newton & Sturmey, 1991; Sigafoos, Kerr, & Roberts, 1994; Thompson & Emerson, 1995; Zarcone, Rodgers, Iwata, Rourke, & Dorsey, 1991).

Other investigations, using similar or different methods of evaluating validity of the MAS, have produced mixed results (Duker & Sigafoos, 1998; Durand & Crimmins, 1988; Crawford, Brockel, Schauss, & Miltenberger, 1992; Girolami & Scotti, 2001; Cunningham & O'Neill, 2000) and suggest that, as with reliability analyses, the validity of the MAS has received only partial and inconsistent replication with persons with developmental disabilities.

There have been scattered reports of other behavior–situation rating scales. Matson and his colleagues (Matson et al., 1999; Paclawskyj, Matson, Rush, Salls, & Vollmer, 2000) reported initial reliability and validity data for the Questions about Behavioral Function Scale. The reliability data (test–retest, interrater, internal consistency) were quite high, and treatment validity data were impressive. Interventions derived from functions identified by the QABF were reported to be more effective than standard treatment control subjects. These positive findings are tempered somewhat by the fact that the QABF development and evaluation research, like the MAS, was conducted with subjects with developmental disabilities, not students with EBD. Also, these initial positive reports about the QABF's technical adequacy are not unlike those initial, very positive reports for the MAS. The QABF may be a promising instrument, but it will require systematic replication by other investigators, and its utility for students with EBD remains to be tested.

The Problem Behavior Questionnaire is one of the few instruments that was designed for use with students with higher-incidence disabilities. The PBQ was developed by Lewis et al. (1994) through a series of activities to develop potential situational factors that involved accessing and escaping peer and adult attention as well as possible setting events for challenging behaviors. Lewis et al. described application of the PBQ in a case study of a 7-year-old first-grade student but did not present any formal analysis of the PBQ's reliability or validity.

Barton-Arwood, Wehby, Gunter, and Lane (2003) reported an analysis of intrarater reliability (consistency within raters over time) of the MAS and the PBQ for 27 students with EBD between 5 and 12 years old in self-contained public school classrooms. Barton-Arwood and colleagues reported that: (1) item-by-item correlations for the MAS were statistically significant but of moderate magnitude across the administrations; (2) the size of the MAS correlations declined over time similar to that reported by Conroy, Fox, Bucklin, and Good (1996); (3) item-by-item correlations for the PBQ were more variable and yielded fewer significant correlations; (4) item-by-item exact percentages of agreement were lower and more variable than adjacent agreement; (5) fewer than half of the exact percentages of agreement reached acceptable levels (i.e., 80%), while exact agreement was somewhat higher for adjacent agreement; (6) the primary function remained constant across the three administrations for less than half of the students on either scale; and, (7) the correlation between the MAS and PBQ results depended upon the particular type of function identified for a student (e.g., MAS escape and PBQ adult escape being positively and significantly correlated and the MAS escape and the PBQ peer escape being negatively correlated). Barton-Arwood et al. (2003) called for further research to evaluate factors related to the stability of MAS and PBQ scores over time, strongly urging practitioners to understand the technical limits of both instruments and to use them only as part of a more comprehensive set of FBA procedures.

The current psychometric status of behavior–situation rating scales such as the MAS and PBQ appears to be highly limited and qualified. With the exception of the Barton-Arwood et al. (2003) study, research evaluating the technical adequacy of behavior–situation rating scales has been conducted with populations having developmental disabilities and functioning within the moderate to severe range of mental retardation. Data from the Barton-Arwood et al. study confirm the questionable status of these scales for students with EBD since fewer than half of the students exhibited consistent functions over time on either scale. The Barton-Arwood et al. study did not address the issue of interrater reliability/agreement, but the data from studies with developmentally disabled populations have not been positive in this regard. Among the studies we reviewed, researchers were unable to find technically adequate interobserver reliability or agreement, while the factor structure and predictive or concurrent validity of the instrument received inconsistent support. Although indirect assessment options are of growing popularity, especially in applied settings, we found little reason to believe they yield data that can stand alone and be consistently useful to the FBA process.

DIRECT ASSESSMENT IN FUNCTIONAL BEHAVIORAL ASSESSMENT

Direct observation is one of the most common and perhaps most critical elements in FBA. Previous literature reviews underscore that in applied research studies with students with developmental disabilities (O'Neill & Johnson, 2000) and students with EBD (e.g., Fox et al., 1998; Sasso et al., 2001), direct observation is the most frequently reported assessment procedure. The two most universally applied, the scatterplot and direct multicategory observation systems, differ in their purpose and application. For this reason, we will present separately the research on these two procedures.

Scatterplot

Introduced by Touchette et al. (1985), the scatterplot divides a student's day into successive time blocks (e.g., every 30 minutes) and/or activity sequences. Observers record the occurrence of a challenging behavior by making either frequency tallies within each of these time/activity periods or by using some summary procedure (e.g., using a series of symbols to indicate whether the behavior did not occur at all, occurred 1 to 2 times, or 3 to 4 times during that interval). Recording is continued each day of the week for at least 1 week, preferably for 2 or 3 weeks, to identify patterns of challenging behavior within times and/or days of the week. Scatterplots are often recorded by classroom personnel, though they may also be implemented by researchers or consultants. Once the times/conditions during which the challenging behavior is most likely to occur are identified, other direct observation systems can be deployed and the particular antecedents and consequences of challenging behavior can be more precisely identified.

We found few other authoritative reports on scatterplot agreement/reliability. O'Reilly (1995) reported reliability data of 100% on the scatterplot. In one of the few large-scale studies on the usefulness of the scatterplot in identifying temporal patterns of challenging behavior in persons with mental retardation, Kahng et al. (1998) reported that mean interobserver agreement, calculated by the occurrence-plus-nonoccurrence method, was 80.6%, ranging from 29.6 to 97.1%. The only analysis of the scatterplot with EBD students was reported by Symons, McDonald, and Wehby (1998). Percentage agreement (occurrence-plus-nonoccurrence formula) averaged 93% for one subject (range 75–100%) and 90.5% for the other subject (range 89–100%).

Because it is frequently used as a component or adjunctive instrument in FBA, it is difficult to evaluate the validity of the scatterplot. Few studies have examined separately the specific contribution of the scatterplot to the functional assessment process. One sign of the "validity" of the scatterplot is the degree to which it can identify a clear activity or time-related pattern in a student's challenging behavior. Generally, the preceding case studies (O'Reilly, 1995; Symons et al., 1998; Touchette et al., 1985) successfully identified time/activity patterns in subjects' challenging behaviors, although one of the three subjects in the Touchette et al. report did not show a clear pattern. The larger scale study by Kahng et al. (1998) indicated that 12 of 15 subjects for whom there was adequate interobserver agreement also demonstrated clear patterns in their challenging behaviors. Validity of the scatterplot may also be shown if interventions based on these data lead to positive behavioral outcomes. The case study reports of O'Reilly (1995), Symons et al. (1998), and Touchette et al. (1985) indicate that function-based interventions based in part on the data from the scatterplot analysis were moderately to highly successful in reducing challenging behaviors of subjects. There is, however, one caveat. Since data from other formal or informal assessment sources were analyzed to develop the interventions, it is unclear to what extent treatment success specifically validated the scatterplot analyses. We were unable to find any other formal, published systematic comparisons of the scatterplot with other FBA instruments or procedures. In addition, with the exception of the subjects with EBD in the Symons et al. (1998) study, the existing research on the scatterplot has been conducted with populations with developmental disabilities.

Direct, Systematic Observational Recording

Because the purpose of FBA is to identify particular antecedent triggers and maintaining consequences as well as contextual variables that influence challenging behavior, the broad time interval and activity setting descriptors of the scatterplot usually are insufficient for such a precise analysis. Instead, multicategory direct observation systems that assess specific environmental stimuli and events, as well as the student's behavior(s), are an essential part of the FBA process. Typically, the forms of challenging behavior and the environmental events associated with them are defined for specific individual student cases. For that reason, unlike interviews and behavior–situation rating scales, there are few standard direct observation systems in FBA. Instead, there are observation schemata or procedures that may be used, while the specific environmental events and behaviors are likely to vary from one study to the next. The reliability and validity of these observation procedures usually are assessed on an individual case or research report basis.

Few standard observation protocols have been developed specifically for use in con-

ducting FBA. The *Functional Analysis Observation Form* (FAOF; O'Neill et al., 1997) is more a suggested observation form rather than a standard set of behavior and event categories. Although the published example does have some behavior, antecedent, setting event, and consequence categories labeled, the FAOF, like most direct observation systems used in FBA, is meant to provide a recording procedure in which the various behaviors and environmental events identified through indirect assessment and informal observation can be entered into the form. The recording procedure is continuous and sequential, preserving the frequency of the behaviors and events as well as their temporal sequence. Such recording permits a conditional probability analysis of the student's challenging behavior(s) in which the setting events and antecedents most likely to precede a challenging behavior and the consequences most likely to follow that behavior can be readily identified. O'Neill et al. (1997) did not report statistical information for the FAOF; however, Cunningham and O'Neill (2000) did evaluate the interobserver agreement for the FAOF as part of a study of comparative outcomes of different FBA methods/instruments in young children with autism. Percentage agreement reportedly ranged from 80–100% across the subjects.

Gable, Hendrickson, and Sealander (1998) described an "Eco-behavioral Observation" system that consisted of a matrix recording procedure. The columns of the matrix are divided among various challenging (e.g., aggression, disruption, off task, out of seat) and appropriate behaviors (e.g., asking questions, answering questions, attention, task participation). The rows are various environmental setting variables or factors (e.g., paper and pencil, listen–lecture, discussion, or manipulative activities). Behavior frequencies are recorded in the appropriate behavior–setting cell. Although Gable et al. caution that users should establish the reliability of such observations, they reported no such data for their matrix.

Scott and Sugai (1994) reported a somewhat simpler direct observation matrix recording procedure, the *Classroom Ecobehavioral Assessment Instrument* (CEAI). This instrument consists of two parts, a set of standard ("permanent") teacher and student behaviors, and an optional section in which the user can specify additional ("teacher-defined") events or behaviors. The permanent behaviors were developed from a research literature review pertaining to variables associated with effective learning environments and student achievement. They include "active" (questioning, discussing, modeling, giving feedback) and "passive" (grading papers, making transitions, supervising independent study) teaching and "on-task" (reading, writing, answering questions, discussing) and "off-task" (not following teacher directions or rules, interrupting a task or presentation by the teacher, interrupting other students) behaviors. As with the Gable et al. (1998) ecological matrix, Scott and Sugai's (1994) matrix is completed by frequency tallies within the appropriate student behavior–teaching behavior cell. Various development activities were completed for this observation system, including review by several experts in the field of behavioral assessment and interobserver agreement analysis. Interobserver agreement for videotaped sessions reportedly had a mean of 91% (range 82–100%), while comparable data for live classroom observation had a mean of 88% (range of 79–95%).

Although not developed specifically for FBA, there are standard observation systems that include both student behaviors and teacher or peer behavior categories that may be useful in functional assessment and that have been evaluated for certain of their psychometric characteristics. For example, Slate and Saudargas (1986) reported on the development and evaluation of the *State–Event Classroom Observation System* (SECOS), consisting of 14 child and 6 teacher behavior categories. SECOS allows observers to capture both behavioral "states" (durational behaviors such as engagement in school work, looking around, out of seat) using momentary time sampling and "event" behaviors (discrete behaviors such as hand raising, calling out, aggression toward other children) using frequency recording within short time intervals. Teacher behaviors included approaching the target student when he or she is engaged or not engaged in a task as well as giving directions, approvals, and disapprovals. What may make SECOS useful to FBA is that Slate and Saudargas conducted a discriminant analysis of the observation categories and found that several

student and teacher behaviors toward those students clearly and significantly discriminated EBD from the behavior of typical students.

Validity of Direct Observational Assessment

Few articles have been published in which direct observation systems are the primary focus of a validity analysis. Researchers apparently have relied on the "face" validity of the observational behavior, antecedent, consequence, and setting event categories. When it has been assessed, the validity analysis of direct assessment has been accomplished in different ways. Some have examined the agreement between an FBA observation instrument and one or more other instruments. Scott and Sugai (1994) assessed the concurrent validity between A–B–C recording and their CEBAI matrix system and found that four of the six observers identified the same function across the two observation systems. Girolami and Scotti (2001) reported that observers using an A–B–C recording system identified the same target behavior function as that identified by other FBA methods (MAS, FAIF, functional analysis) for two subjects but only matched that of the FAIF for the third subject. Similarly, Cunningham and O'Neill (2000) reported that, in analyzing the behavior of three young children with autism, the primary behavior function identified using FAOF observations matched that indicated by the MAS, the FAIF and analogue functional analyses for two subjects but not for a third subject.

Scott, Desimone, Fowler, and Webb (2000) did not attempt to validate A–B–C recording but did use data collected from those observations to develop function-based interventions for the challenging behaviors of students with learning disabilities. These function-based interventions increased appropriate task-related behavior and assignment completions, suggesting that not only the behaviors but also the triggering and maintaining events identified through A–B–C recording were valid. Notwithstanding its clinical appeal, judging the validity of an observation system by the effects of an intervention package based on data from that observation protocol, of course, is not an unequivocal demonstration of validity. Such validation would require at least a side-by-side comparison (within or between subjects) of the effects of A–B–C derived function interventions with behavior change brought about by other behavioral interventions that were not based on function or that were contraindicated.

When we look at studies specifically directed at assessing the reliability of standard observation systems that have been or could be used in FBA, the research is generally positive, albeit sparse. When such observation systems have been evaluated, they have shown acceptable or high reliability/agreement as well as some amount of documented concurrent or treatment validity. Unfortunately, there is a paucity of studies of standardized observation systems with students with high-incidence disabilities, and even fewer with EBD students, the results of Slate and Saudargas (1986) and Symons et al. (1998) being the exceptions. Scott and Sugai (1994) used an unidentified population of students to evaluate the reliability and validity of their CEBAI, while Scott, Desimone, et al. (2000) focused on students with learning disorders. As with the other FBA instruments, we continue to lack sufficient information about the reliability and validity of direct observational assessment instruments for students with EBD.

FUNCTIONAL ANALYSIS

Over the past 5 years there have been several reviews of research on FBA for students with EBD (Fox et al., 1998; Heckaman et al., 2000; Lane et al., 1999; Reid & Nelson, 2002; Sasso et al., 2001). Despite variations in the criteria for inclusion of studies and in the particular questions addressed, these reviews expressed strikingly similar conclusions: (1) comparatively little FBA research has been conducted with students with mild disabilities or EBD; (2) studies with EBD populations have generally involved male students in elementary through middle school ages with multiple challenging behaviors; (3) in most studies the functional analysis and intervention development were primarily conducted by researchers rather than classroom teachers or other natural environment agents; and (4) for those studies with function-based interventions, reductions were obtained in challenging behaviors and/or

increases were obtained in more appropriate target behaviors. This last finding would seem to support the "treatment validity" of functional analysis procedures, since some type of analogue or environmental manipulation within the natural environment was one of the most frequently used FBA procedures in these studies (Heckaman et al., 2000; Lane et al., 1999).

The exact status of functional analysis as an FBA procedure is not, however, entirely clear. Most FBA studies in general and with EBD students in particular have used multiple procedures and instruments (i.e., some combination of two or more interviews, ratings, observation and functional analysis). Thus, it is unclear the extent to which the interventions that were developed and that produced the behavior change were based upon the results of the functional analysis alone or upon the data from the combined procedures. The assumption would be that a functional analysis (analogue or naturalistic), given its controlled nature, would provide the clearest, most reliable, and valid data, but this is an empirical question. Also, there are several levels of reliability and validity against which functional analysis procedures can and should be evaluated, including: (1) the reliability or interobserver agreement of direct observational measures behaviors, (2) the consistency with which functional analyses demonstrate reliable differences between variables or functions within that study over time (i.e., experimental control); (3) the degree to which functional analysis results concur with functions identified by other FBA instruments/procedures; (4) the extent to which function-based interventions result in both immediate and long-term changes in behaviors; and (5) the degree to which investigators show that the components of the intervention were in fact implemented (i.e., treatment integrity) (Fox et al., 1998; Heckaman et al., 2000; Lane et al., 1999; Reid & Nelson, 2002; Sasso et al., 2001).

Reliability of Functional Analysis Results

The reliability of functional analysis results is addressed in two basic ways. First, direct measures of change in the dependent variable(s) must be shown to have sufficient interobserver agreement. The second major way in which reliability of functional analysis is an issue concerns the consistency of results, the extent to which the different variables or conditions of the analysis produce clearly different results (i.e., clearly indicate one or more functions of a behavior).

Concurrence of Functional Analysis Results with Other FBA Methods

Another way to evaluate the validity is the extent to which functional analysis results concur with the results of other functional assessment techniques or procedures (interviews, rating scales, descriptive observations). Overall, it appears that across a wide range of challenging behaviors, situations, apparent functions, and types of functional analysis (analogue and naturalistic), there has been considerable agreement between the hypothesized functions of behavior identified through interviews, rating scales, and/or descriptive observations and the results of functional analyses in populations of EBD or at-risk students (e.g., Blair, Umbreit, & Eck, 2000; Broussard & Northup, 1995, 1997; Burke, Hagan-Burke, & Sugai, 2003; Dunlap, Kern-Dunlap, Clarke, & Robbins, 1991; Dunlap et al., 1993; Ervin, Dupaul, Kern, & Friman, 1998; Kern, Childs, Dunlap, Clarke, & Falk, 1994; Lewis & Sugai, 1996; Umbreit, 1995, 1996; Umbreit & Blair, 1997).

High agreement between functional analysis and other FBA techniques may, however, be somewhat misleading. These studies were ones in which the interview, rating scale, and descriptive observations were implemented first to identify the specific variables for manipulation in the functional analysis. Furthermore, the functional analyses were developed and/or implemented by researchers or their staff who were aware of some or all of the results of the prior assessment. To clearly and objectively evaluate the concurrence between descriptive and functional FBA analysis procedures would require that those implementing the functional analysis procedures, for example, be independent of those who implemented the prior descriptive observational assessment component.

There is evidence that functional analyses and other FBA techniques/instruments do not always identify the same function in students with other types of disabilities. For example, Girolami and Scotti (2001) and Cunningham and O'Neill (2000) reported agreement between functional analysis and other FBA assessment procedures for some but not all subjects. Analyzing the data for subjects who exhibited clear behavioral differences during analogue functional analyses, Conroy, Fox, Crain, Jenkins, and Belcher (1996) reported that analogue analyses and direct classroom observations concurred on the function of one subject but not for a second subject.

Immediate and Long-Term Behavior Change

A second way to evaluate the validity of functional analysis results is to determine the degree to which interventions based upon the identified function do in fact result in behavior change. Treatment validity is a criterion against which any intervention research, particularly that in ABA, must ultimately be judged. Not only should function-based interventions reduce challenging behaviors and/or increase functionally equivalent alternative behaviors when initially applied, but, if they address some or all of the significant maintaining variables for challenging behavior, one would expect these interventions to lead to durable behavior change (i.e., "maintenance"). Reviews of the literature on FBA with EBD students have reached very similar conclusions (Heckaman et al., 2000; Lane et al., 1999; Reid & Nelson, 2002; Sasso et al., 2001). First, in most cases, FBA-based interventions have substantially reduced challenging behaviors and/or increased appropriate alternative behaviors. Second, while the durability of these behavior changes has been evaluated in only a few studies, generally these results have also been positive with maintenance being assessed anywhere from 7 to 30 weeks (Broussard & Northup, 1997; Kern, Dunlap, et al., 1994; Skinner et al., 2002; Umbreit, 1995; Umbreit & Blair, 1997).

Not only is it necessary to show that function-based interventions can produce positive behavior change, it is equally important to show that such interventions have greater effects, are more efficient, or produce more durable generalized change than do non-function-based interventions that are systematically applied. Here the available data are even more limited and unclear. On the one hand, Reid and Nelson (2002) noted that the success of FBA-based interventions was impressive not only for the consistency of positive outcomes across studies but also that these very same target behaviors had been unresponsive to other interventions.

On the other hand, evidence that FBA interventions are not necessarily more effective than other standard behavioral interventions that are consistently applied is beginning to accrue. Schill, Kratochwill, and Elliot (1998) studied the effectiveness of behavioral consultation in resolving various behavior challenges of young children in Head Start programs using either functional assessment-based intervention or standardized behavior intervention packages. Although child behavior change scores were slightly greater for the functional assessment intervention group, this difference was not statistically significant. Overall, there were no significant differences between function-based and standard treatments in measures of treatment integrity. Consultee (teacher) satisfaction with the interventions was slightly, but not statistically, greater for the functional assessment group. Consultants felt that the functional assessment approach was more effective but that the standard behavior intervention package was more time-efficient. When actual time involved in the consultation was analyzed, no significant differences in the number of hours or days of consultation between the two approaches were found, while estimated financial costs were somewhat greater for the functional-based intervention approach (an average difference of approximately $26 of consultant time, materials, etc.). Clearly, additional systematic replications of this study comparing function- and non-function-based interventions delivered by both experts and by classroom personnel with direct measures of treatment integrity are needed.

In summary, although comparatively small, the existing empirical base for functional analysis and for function-based interventions has been quite positive in terms of being able to reliably identify one or more variables that occasion challenging behavior in students with EBD. That there are significant and continuing "holes" in this data base is apparent. There is a need for addi-

tional studies that (1) clearly link the intervention components to the assessed function of the challenging behavior, (2) either do not include or separate out other non-function based intervention components, (3) include additional measures of treatment integrity, time, and cost of the assessment and intervention process, and (4) empirically and systematically compare the effects of function-based interventions with other behavioral, non-function based interventions consistently applied.

TRAINING IN FUNCTIONAL ASSESSMENT TECHNOLOGY

In previous discussion, we have examined critically the accumulated research as it relates to the emergent technology of FBA and focused primarily on the complex and multifaceted process of behavioral assessment. It may seem that implementation of that technology in applied settings goes beyond the scope of the present discussion. However, federal legislation stipulates that, under certain conditions, a school-based IEP team must address student behavior that impedes the teaching–learning process via FBA. Accordingly, current knowledge of FBA has a direct bearing on the level of preparation of school personnel and the probability of a successful outcome. The mandate to transfer effective strategies from clinic to classroom interposes a new set of variables that likely influence both content and implementation— ranging from administrative policies and attributional assumptions regarding behavior to the willingness and ability of educators and others to work together to remediate those problems. Unfortunately, the literature is largely descriptive and as yet incomplete when it comes to the preparation of school-based teams to conduct an FBA.

Our review revealed little empirical consensus regarding what constitutes either the content knowledge or the skills necessary to successfully carry out the FBA process (Stichter, Shellady, Sealander, & Eigenberger, 2000; Quinn et al., 2001). While support for "one-shot" in-service programs seems unlikely, we found few studies on systematic approaches to the training of public school personnel. Most school-based studies have dealt with the challenging behavior of individual students under the auspices of university researchers or expert consultants (e.g., Kern, Childs, et al., 1994). Among the few studies conducted on training of school-based teams, Chandler, Dahlquist, Repp, and Feltz (1999) reported that, after receiving two 8-hour workshops, school-based FBA teams were able to decrease students' challenging behavior and increase both academic engagement and appropriate peer interactions. In contrast, Gable et al. (2003) found that about 40 hours of instruction was more effective. In addition, various authors report that it is useful if not essential to afford teams follow-up support. Previously trained teams have been given booster sessions and/or access to routine consultation. For example, Chandler et al. (1999) systematically faded in-class support across a 4-month period, while Gable et al. (2003) conducted follow-up assessment, periodically monitored the fidelity with which teams implemented the FBA process, and presented on-site booster training sessions to teams.

Our conceptual and empirical grasp of FBA in applied settings is essentially a "work in progress." In addition to an incomplete knowledge base, there are myriad pragmatic issues regarding the quality of instruction of school-based personnel. Problems range from the ability to integrate disparate skills to being able to suspend judgment regarding the motivation behind student behavior long enough to complete a thorough investigation that includes the context in which it occurs (Stichter et al., 2000). It is clear that what constitutes best-practice FBA does not yet equal its parts and that further investigation on its social validity is essential if research is to inform practice *and* vice versa.

SUMMARY, CONCLUSIONS, AND IMPLICATIONS

In looking critically at the accumulated research on FBA, it is tempting to refer to the old adage about the glass being half-empty or half-full. The "half empty" view is that, given the early and more recent history of FBA that we have outlined, it is both surprising and distressing that so little empirical progress has been accomplished with students with EBD. As is often the case, the ap-

plications of both assessment and intervention seem to have substantially exceeded our empirical knowledge. There is a critical lack of documentation of the technical adequacy of most FBA instruments and procedures as applied to students with EBD. The reliability and validity of virtually all of the major assessment instruments (interview protocols, behavior–situation rating scales, scatterplot, and direct observation procedures) mirrors the paucity of such studies with other populations but is even more profound when considering students with EBD. The severity of these empirical "holes" in our FBA knowledge regarding students with EBD is not new but has been repeatedly and distinctly articulated over the past 5 years (Fox et al., 1998; Heckaman et al., 2000; Lane et al., 1999; Nelson et al., 1999; Reid & Nelson, 2002; Sasso et al., 2001; Scott & Nelson, 1999). Even those studies in which FBA-based interventions have been shown to "work," there is a need to: (1) more clearly delineate the specific intervention variables responsible for behavior change (Sasso et al., 2001), (2) evaluate the durability and generality of that behavior change, and (3) document the relative effects and costs of FBA-based interventions as opposed to other standard behavioral interventions (Schill et al., 1998). The "half-empty" view might be succinctly summarized in the following way. Were FBA a drug, it is highly unlikely that regulatory agencies would allow it to be used on the scale to which it has been practiced since the basic and clinical trials research is so inadequate, especially for students with EBD.

There is, of course, a "half-full" view too. More FBA research with students with EBD is beginning to emerge. This research has begun to address critical questions for FBA in general and for students with EBD in particular. Research, for example, by Reed et al. (1997), Kinch et al. (2001), and Barton-Arwood et al. (2003) on the technical characteristics of interview and rating scale data have begun to fill the empirical holes and to help us understand how big some other holes are. Intervention research by Kern, Dunlap, Umbreit, their colleagues, and others (e.g., Blair, Umbreit, & Boss, 1999; Blair et al., 2000; Broussard & Northup, 1995, 1997; Dunlap et al., 1993; Kern, Childs, et al., 1994; Penno, Frank, & Wacker, 2000; Skinner et al., 2002; Umbreit & Blair, 1997) has shown that, despite inadequate technical knowledge, interventions based at least in part on FBA results can be effective in dealing with challenging behaviors of students with EBD. The task, now, is to increase research on the instruments, process, and interventions involved in FBA and to develop a data base that provides a firm foundation for the use or revision of these techniques, for training of personnel in their application, and for the behavioral-educational development of students with EBD.

To continue the analogy with which we began this section, "filling the glass" will be accomplished by pursuing an active, sequential, and extensive research agenda. The agenda expressed 2 years ago by Sasso et al. (2001) is still quite apt and can be succinctly summarized as follows:

1. Modify existing FBA instruments and procedures, and, where needed, develop new ones that better address the particular needs of students with EBD.
2. Conduct research and ensure the technical adequacy of current and future FBA instruments and procedures, with special attention to validating them with students with EBD.
3. Empirically evaluate the relative contributions of different functional assessment methods and instruments to the successful analysis of behavior function.
4. Further evaluate the effectiveness of functional assessment-based intervention packages for students with or at risk of having EBD.

This is an extensive, complicated, and ambitious research agenda, driven both by the relative paucity of data but also by the initial and scattered successes of prior research. It is, however, a necessary agenda. Until more of this research is accomplished, we are pressed to reiterate the cautions expressed by our colleagues, namely, that public policy may have exceeded our knowledge base when it comes to critical aspects of FBA in applied settings (Scott & Nelson, 1999). Over the past 20 years, we have witnessed remarkable progress in the education and treatment of students with EBD. Although the final chapter has yet to be written on the acceptability, practicality, or efficacy of FBA in the real-world context of schools and communities (e.g., Sugai, Horner, & Sprague, 1999), we feel strongly that FBA will play an important role in our efforts to better serve students. We believe its role is best advanced through the careful, systematic pursuit of applied research that began more than 40 years ago and that continues today.

REFERENCES

Akande, A. (1994). The motivation assessment profiles of low-functioning children. *Early Child Development and Care, 101,* 101–107.

Allen, K. E., Hart, B., Buell, J. S., Harris, F. R., & Wolf, M. M. (1964). Effects of social reinforcement on isolate behavior of a nursery school child. *Child Development, 35,* 511–518.

Baer, D. M., Wolf, M. M., & Risley, T. R. (1968). Some current dimensions of applied behavior analysis. *Journal of Applied Behavior Analysis, 1,* 91–97.

Bailey, J. S., & Pyles, D. A. M. (1989). Behavioral diagnostics. In E. Cipani (Ed.), *The treatment of severe behavior disorders: Behavior analysis approaches* (pp. 85–107). Washington, DC: American Association on Mental Retardation.

Bambara, L. M., & Knoster, T. (1998). Designing positive behavior support plans, *Innovations* (no. 13). Washington, DC: American Association on Mental Retardation.

Barton-Arwood, S. M., Wehby, J. H., Gunter, P. L., & Lane, K. L. (2003). Functional behavior assessment rating scales: Intrarater reliability with students with emotional or behavioral disorders. *Behavioral Disorders, 28,* 386–400.

Bihm, E. M., Kienlen, T. L., Ness, M. E., & Poindexter, A. R. (1991). Factor structure of the *Motivation Assessment Scale* for persons with mental retardation. *Psychological Reports, 68,* 1235–1238.

Bijou, S. W., Peterson, R. F., & Ault, M. H. (1968). A method to integrate descriptive and experimental field studies at the level of data and empirical concepts. *Journal of Applied Behavior Analysis, 1,* 175–191.

Blair, K. C., Umbreit, J., & Bos, C. S. (1999). Using functional assessment and children's preferences to improve the behavior of young children with behavioral disorders. *Behavioral Disorders, 24,* 151–166.

Blair, K. C., Umbreit, J., & Eck, S. (2000). Analysis of multiple variables related to a young child's aggressive behavior. *Journal of Positive Behavioral Interventions, 2,* 33–39.

Broussard, C. D., & Northup, J. (1995). An approach to functional assessment and analysis of disruptive behavior in regular education classrooms. *School Psychology Quarterly, 10,* 151–164

Broussard, C. D., & Northup, J. (1997). The use of functional analysis to develop peer interventions for disruptive classroom behavior. *School Psychology Quarterly, 12,* 65–76

Burke, M. D., Hagan-Burke, S., & Sugai, G. (2003).

The efficacy of function-based interventions for students with learning disabilities who exhibit escape-maintained problem behaviors: Preliminary results from a single-case experiment. *Learning Disability Quarterly, 26,* 15–25.

Carr, E. G., & Kemp, D. C. (1989). Functional equivalence of autistic leading and communicative pointing: Analysis and treatment. *Journal of Autism and Developmental Disorders, 19,* 561–578.

Chandler, L. K., Dahlquist, C. M., Repp, A. C., & Feltz, C. (1999). The effects of team-based functional assessment on the behavior of students in classroom settings. *Exceptional Children, 66,* 101–122.

Conroy, M. A., & Fox, J. J. (1994). Setting factors and challenging behaviors in the classroom: Incorporating contextual factors into effective intervention plans for children with aggressive behaviors. *Preventing School Failure, 38,* 29–34.

Conroy, M. A., Fox, J. J., Bucklin, A., & Good, W. B. (1996). An analysis of the reliability and stability of the *Motivation Assessment Scale* in assessing the challenging behaviors of children and youth with developmental disabilities. *Education and Training in Mental Retardation, 31,* 243–250.

Conroy, M. A., Fox, J. J., Crain, L., Jenkins, A., & Belcher, K. (1996). Evaluating the social and ecological validity of analog assessment procedures for challenging behaviors in young children. *Education and Treatment of Children, 19,* 233–256.

Crawford, J., Brockel, B., Schauss, S., & Miltenberger, R. G. (1992). A comparison of methods for the functional assessment of stereotypic behavior. *Journal of the Association for Persons with Severe Handicaps, 17,* 77–86.

Cunningham, E., & O'Neill, R. E. (2000). Comparison of results of functional assessment and analysis methods with young children with autism. *Education and Training in Mental Retardation and Developmental Disabilities, 35,* 406–414.

Demchak, M., & Bossert, K.W. (1996). *Assessing problem behaviors, innovations* (no. 4). Washington, DC: American Association on Mental Retardation.

Duker, P. C., & Sigafoos, J. (1998). The *Motivation Assessment Scale:* Reliability and construct validity across three topographies of behavior. *Research in Developmental Disabilities, 19,* 131–141.

Dunlap, G., Kern, L., dePerczel, M., Clarke, S., Wilson, D., Childs, K. E., White, R., & Falk, G. D. (1993). Functional analysis of classroom variables for students with emotional and behavioral disorders. *Behavioral Disorders, 18,* 275–291.

Dunlap, G., Kern-Dunlap, L., Clarke, S., & Robbins, F. R. (1991). Functional assessment, curricular revisions, and severe behavior problems. *Journal of Applied Behavior Analysis, 24,* 387–397.

Dunlap, G., & Kincaid, D. (2001).The widening world of functional assessment: Comments on four manuals and beyond. *Journal of Applied Behavior Analysis, 34,* 365–377.

Durand, V. M., & Crimmins, D. B. (1988). Identifying the variables maintaining self-injurious behavior. *Journal of Autism and Developmental Disorders, 18,* 99–117.

Durand, V. M., & Crimmins, D. B. (1992) *The Motivation Assessment Scale (MAS).* Topeka, KS: Monaco.

Ervin, R. A., DuPaul, G. J., Kern, L., & Friman, P. C. (1998). Classroom-based functional and adjunctive assessment: Proactive approaches to intervention selection for adolescents with attention deficit hyperactivity disorder. *Journal of Applied Behavior Analysis, 31,* 65–78.

Fox, J. J., & Conroy, M. A. (1995). Setting events and behavior problems in the classroom: An interbehavioral field analysis for research and practice. *Journal of Emotional and Behavioral Disorders, 3,* 130–140.

Fox, J. J., Conroy, M. A., & Heckaman, K. (1998). Research issues in functional assessment and intervention. *Behavioral Disorders, 24,* 26–33.

Gable, R. A., Butler, C. J., Walker-Bolton, I., Tonelson, S., Quinn, M. M., & Fox, J. J. (2003). Safe and effective schooling for all students: Putting into practice the disciplinary provisions of the 1997 IDEA, *Preventing School Failure, 47,* 74–78.

Gable, R. A., Hendrickson, J. M., & Sealander, K. (1998). Ecobehavioral observation: Ecobehavioral assessment to identify classroom correlates of students' learning and behavior problems. *Beyond Behavior, 8,* 25–27.

Gable, R. A., Quinn, M. M., Rutherford , R. B., Howell, K. W., Hoffman, C. C., & Butler, C. J. (2002). *Conducting functional behavioral assessment and developing positive behavioral intervention plans and supports: Promoting positive academic and behavioral outcomes for all students.* Washington, DC: Virginia Department of Education and the Center for Effective Collaboration and Practice/American Institutes for Research.

Gardner, W. I., Cole, C. L., Davidson, D. P., & Karan, O. C. (1986). Reducing aggression in individuals with developmental disabilities: An expanded stimulus control, assessment, and intervention model. *Education and Training of the Mentally Retarded, 21,* 3–12.

Girolami, P. A., & Scotti, J. R. (2001). Use of analog functional analysis in assessing the function of mealtime behavior problems. *Education and Training in Mental Retardation and Developmental Disabilities, 36,* 207–223.

Heckaman, K., Conroy, M. A., Fox, J. J., & Chait, A. (2000). Functional assessment-based intervention research on students with or at-risk for emotional and behavioral disorders. *Behavioral Disorders, 25,* 196–210.

Horner, R. H., & Day, H. M. (1991). The effects of response efficiency on functionally equivalent competing behaviors. *Journal of Applied Behavior Analysis, 24,* 719–732.

Horner, R. H, Sprague, J. R, O'Brien, M., & Heathfield, L. T. (1990). The role of response efficiency in the reduction of problem behaviors through functional equivalence training: A case study. *Journal of the Association for Persons with Severe Handicaps*, 15, 91–97.

Iwata, B., Dorsey, M., Slifer, K., Bauman, K., & Richman, G. (1982). Toward a functional analysis of self-injury. *Analysis and Intervention in Developmental Disabilities*, 3, 138–148.

Kahng, S. W., Iwata, B. A., Fischer, S. M., Page, T. J., Treadwell, K. R. H., Williams, D. E., & Smith, R. G. (1998). Temporal distributions of problem behavior based on scatter plot analysis. *Journal of Applied Behavior Analysis*, 31, 593–604.

Kearney, C. A. (1994). Interrater reliability of the *Motivation Assessment Scale*: Another, closer look. *Journal of the Association for Persons with Severe Handicaps*, 19, 139–142.

Kennedy, C. H., & Itkonen, T. (1993). Effects of setting events on the problem behavior of students with severe disabilities. *Journal of Applied Behavior Analysis*, 26, 321–327.

Kern, L., Childs, K. E., Dunlap, G., Clarke, S., & Falk, G. D. (1994). Using assessment-based curricular intervention to improve the classroom behavior of a student with emotional behavioral challenges. *Journal of Applied of Behavior Analysis*, 27, 7–19.

Kern, L., Dunlap, G., Clarke, S., & Childs, K. E. (1994). Student-assisted functional assessment interview, *Diagnostique*, 19, 29–39.

Kinch, C., Lewis-Palmer, T., Hagan-Burke, S., & Sugai, G. (2001). A comparison of teacher and student functional behavior assessment interview information from low-risk and high-risk classrooms. *Education and Treatment of Children*, 24, 480–494.

Lane, K. L., Umbreit, J., & Beebe-Frankenberger, M. E. (1999). Functional assessment research on students with or at risk for EBD: 1990 to present. *Journal of Positive Behavioral Interventions*, 1, 101–111.

Lerman, D.C., & Iwata, B.A. (1993). Descriptive and experimental analysis of variables maintaining self-injurious behavior. *Journal of Applied Behavior Analysis*, 26, 293–319.

Lewis, T. J., Scott, T. M., & Sugai, G. (1994). The *Problem Behavior Questionnaire*: A teacher-based instrument to develop functional hypotheses of problem behavior in general education classrooms. *Diagnostique*, 19, 103–115.

Lewis, T. J., & Sugai, G. (1996). Functional assessment of problem behavior: A pilot investigation of the comparative and interactive effects of teacher and peer social attention on students in general education settings. *School Psychology Quarterly*, 11, 1–19.

Matson, J. L., Bamburg, J. W., Cherry, K. E., & Paclawskyj, T. R. (1999). A validity study on the *Questions about Behavioral Function (QABF) Scale*: Predicting treatment success for self-injury, aggression, and stereotypies. *Research in Developmental Disabilities*, 30, 163–176.

Nelson, J. R., Mathur, S. R., & Rutherford, R. B. (1999). Has public policy exceeded our knowledge base?: A review of the functional behavioral assessment literature. *Behavioral Disorders*, 24, 169–179.

Nelson, J. R., Roberts, M. L., & Smith, D. J. (1998). *Conducting functional behavioral assessments: A practical guide*. Longmont, CO: Sopris West.

Newton, J. T., & Sturmey, P. (1991). The Motivation Assessment Scale: Inter-rater reliability and internal consistency in a British sample. *Journal of Mental Deficiency Research*, 35, 472–474.

O'Neill, R. E., Horner, R. H., Albin, R. W., Storey, K., Sprague, J. R., & Newton, J. S. (1997). *Functional analysis of problem behavior: A practical assessment guide* (2nd ed.). Pacific Grove, CA: Brooks/Cole.

O'Neill, R. E., & Johnson, J. W. (2000). A brief description of functional assessment procedures reported in *JASH* (1983–1999). *Journal of the Association of Persons with Severe Handicaps*, 25, 197–200.

O'Reilly, M. F. (1995). Functional analysis and treatment of escape-maintained aggression correlated with sleep deprivation. *Journal of Applied Behavior Analysis*, 28, 225–226.

Paclawskyj, T. R., Matson, J. L., Rush, K. S., Salls, Y., & Vollmer, T. R. (2000). *Questions about Behavioral Function (QABF)*: A behavioral checklist for functional assessment of aberrant behavior. *Research in Developmental Disabilities*, 21, 223–230.

Peck, J., Sasso, G. M., & Stambaugh, M. (1998). Functional analyses in the classroom: Gaining reliability without sacrificing validity. *Preventing School Failure*, 43, 14–16.

Penno, D. A., Frank, A. R., & Wacker, D. P. (2000). Instructional accommodations for adolescent students with severe emotional or behavioral disorders. *Behavior Disorders*, 25, 325–343.

Quinn, M. M., Gable, R. A., Fox, J. J., Rutherford, R. B., Van Acker, R., Conroy, M. A. (2001). Putting quality functional assessment into practice in schools: A research agenda on behalf of E/BD students. *Education and Treatment of Children*, 24, 261–275.

Reed, H., Thomas, E., Sprague, J. R., & Horner, R. H. (1997). The Student Guided Functional Assessment Interview: An analysis of student and teacher agreement. *Journal of Behavioral Education*, 7, 33–49.

Reid, R., & Nelson, J. R. (2002). The utility, acceptability, and practicality of functional behavioral assessment for students with high-incidence problem behaviors. *Remedial and Special Education*, 2, 15–23.

Risley, T. R. (1968). The effects and side effects of punishing the autistic behaviors of a deviant child. *Journal of Applied Behavior Analysis*, 1, 21–34.

Sasso, G., Conroy, M. A., Stichter, J., & Fox, J. J. (2001). Slowing down the bandwagon: The misapplication of functional behavior assessment for students with emotional and behavioral disorders. *Behavioral Disorders*, 26, 282–296.

Schill, M. T., Kratochwill, T. R., & Elliot, S. N. (1998). Functional assessment in behavioral consultation: A treatment utility study. *School Psychology Quarterly*, *13*, 116–140.

Scott, T. M., Desimone, C., Fowler, W., & Webb, E. (2000). Using functional assessment to develop interventions for challenging behaviors in the classroom: Three case studies. *Preventing School Failure*, *22*, 51–56.

Scott, T. M., Meers, D. T., & Nelson, C. M. (2000). Toward a consensus of functional behavioral assessment for students with mild disabilities in public school contexts: A national survey. *Education and Treatment of Children*, *23*, 265–285.

Scott, T. M., & Nelson, C. M. (1999). Functional behavioral assessment: Implications for training and staff development. *Behavioral Disorders*, *24*, 249–252.

Scott, T. M., & Sugai, G. (1994). The *Classroom Ecobehavioral Assessment Instrument*: A user-friendly method of assessing instructional behavioral relationships in the classroom. *Diagnostique*, *19*, 59–77.

Sigafoos, J., Kerr, M. M., & Roberts, D. (1994). Inter-rater reliability of the *Motivation Assessment Scale*: Failure to replicate with aggressive behavior. *Research in Developmental Disabilities*, *15*, 333–342.

Skinner, C. H., Belfiore, P. J., Mace, H. W., Williams-Wilson, S., Johns, G. A. (1997). Altering response topography to increase response efficiency and learning rates. *School Psychology Quarterly*, *12*, 54–64.

Skinner, C. H., Waterson, H. J., Bryant, D. R., Bryant, R. J., Collins, P. M., Hill, C. J., Tipton, M. F., Ragsdale, P., & Fox, J. J. (2002). Team problem solving based on research, functional behavioral assessment data, teacher acceptability, and Jim Carey's interview. *Proven Practices: Prevention and Remediation Solutions for Schools*, *4*, 56–64.

Slate, J. R., & Saudargas, R. A. (1986). Differences in the classroom behaviors of behaviorally disordered and regular class children. *Behavioral Disorders*, *12*, 45–53.

Stichter, J. P., Shellady, S. M., Sealander, K., & Eigenberger, M. (2000). Teaching what we do know: Preservice training and functional behavior assessment. *Preventing School Failure*, *44*, 142–146.

Sugai, G., Horner, R. H., & Sprague, J. R. (1999). Functional-assessment-based behavior support planning: Research to practice to research. *Behavioral Disorders*, *24*, 253–257.

Sugai, G., Lewis-Palmer, T., & Hagan, S. (1998). Using functional assessments to develop behavior support plans. *Preventing School Failure*, *43*, 6–14.

Symons, F. J., McDonald, L. M., & Wehby, J. H. (1998). Functional assessment and teacher collected data. *Education and Treatment of Children*, *21*, 135–159.

Thompson, S., & Emerson, E. (1995). Inter-informant agreement on the *Motivation Assessment Scale*: Another failure to replicate. *Mental Handicap Research*, *8*, 203–208.

Touchette, P. E., MacDonald, R. F., & Langer, S. N. (1985). Scatterplot for identifying stimulus control of problem behavior. *Journal of Applied Behavior Analysis*, *18*, 343–352.

Umbreit, J. (1995). Functional assessment and intervention in a regular classroom setting for the disruptive behavior of a student with attention deficit hyperactivity disorders. *Behavioral Disorders*, *20*, 267–278.

Umbreit, J. (1996). Functional analysis of disruptive behavior in an inclusive classroom. *Journal of Early Intervention*, *19*, 18–29.

Umbreit, J., & Blair, K. S. (1997). Using structural analysis to facilitate treatment of aggression and noncompliance in a young child at risk for behavioral disorders. *Behavioral Disorders*, *22*, 75–86.

Watson, T. S., & Steege, M. W. (2003). *Conducting school-based functional behavioral assessments: A practitioner's guide*. New York: Guilford Press.

White, O. R., & Haring, N. G. (1980). *Exceptional teaching* (2nd ed.) Columbus, OH: Merrill.

Yarbrough, S. C., & Carr, E. G. (2000). Some relationships between informant assessment and functional analysis of problem behavior. *American Journal on Mental Retardation*, *105*, 130–151.

Zarcone, J. R., Rodgers, T. A., Iwata, B. A., Rourke, D. A., & Dorsey, M. F. (1991). Reliability analysis of the Motivation Assessment Scale: A failure to replicate. *Research in Developmental Disabilities*, *12*, 349–360.

Zeilberger, J., Sampen, S. E, & Sloane, H. N., Jr. (1968). Modification of a child's problem behaviors in the home with the mother as therapist. *Journal of Applied Behavior Analysis*, *1*, 47–53.

Zimmerman, E. H., & Zimmerman, J. (1962). The alteration of behavior in a special classroom situation. *Journal of the Experimental Analysis of Behavior*, *5*, 59–60.

9

Psychiatric and Psychological Assessment of Emotional and Behavioral Disorders during School Mental Health Consultation

RICHARD E. MATTISON

The evaluation of a student for classification under the federal special education category of emotional disturbance (termed emotional and behavioral disorders [EBD] in this chapter) should include both psychiatric and psychological assessment through mental health consultation. The information produced by such clinical assessment (e.g., psychiatric diagnosis, level of severity, neurological risk factors, family stresses, and learning disorders) can assist school multidisciplinary teams in both their evaluation of a student for EBD services as well as in subsequent intervention planning. Such input can also inform school staffs about risk factors outside the classroom that they must consider during function behavioral analysis (FBA) for a student with EBD and subsequent development of a behavioral intervention plan (BIP). This chapter will *summarize research findings* from modern psychiatric and psychological assessment procedures, *analyze their relevance* for teachers of students classified as EBD (especially implications for classroom intervention), and *discuss future research directions*.

This chapter presents research results for special education students classified as EBD. The term EBD includes federal and state special education categories that have been used over time to designate this same group of special education children with emotional/behavioral problems, such as serious emotional disturbance (SED), behavioral disorders (BD), and the current federal category of emotional disturbance (ED). The chapter does not focus directly on another much larger group of children who are also commonly designated as EBD: children with emotional and behavioral disorders who have no special education classification and are referred to community mental health clinics or professionals, and are the 10% or more of the general population (in contrast to the 1% classified EBD) who have been the focus of most child psychiatric and psychological research. While clinical research findings established for this primary group of children are largely applicable to the EBD group, students with EBD do differ in significant ways from the general clinically referred group, such as type and severity of psychopathology, prevalence of learning disabilities (LD), and family background (Garland et al., 2001; Glassberg, Hooper, & Mattison, 1999; Mattison & Gamble, 1992; Silver et al., 1992). Thus, children who receive EBD services in school should be considered as a unique clinical population.

PSYCHIATRIC ASSESSMENT

Most research findings reported here have come from one of the largest and most comprehensive psychosocial study of students classified as EBD (its methodology has been extensively described in Mattison et al., 1986). The research design was based on a model for school psychiatric consultation proposed by Mattison (1993) where the consultant first reviews a student's school file before discussion with school staff members of their observations and questions. Next, a mental state interview is conducted with the student. Then, a parent is interviewed for the child's present and past problems and interventions, plus the student's medical/neurological history, developmental concerns, and family history (especially for stresses such as abuse and parent psychiatric illness) are collected. Established behavioral rating scales are completed by both teachers and parents to supplement basic psychoeducational testing results. The consultant then shares diagnoses, formulation of possible etiology, answers to questions, and initial treatment suggestions with the multidisciplinary team, and together they develop a practical intervention plan for both in and out of school. This clinical assessment is next discussed with family to address any questions or concerns, develop further intervention planning, and build collaboration between school staff and the child's family.

While this research was conducted in the 1980s (Mattison et al., 1986; Mattison, Morales, & Bauer, 1991, 1992, 1993), most of its results are quite likely still representative for students with EBD. Tables 9.1–9.4 present findings for the final numbers of the two groups of students ages 6–16 years who were consecutively evaluated for EBD services by multidisciplinary teams (including psychiatric consultation): 238 children who were evaluated and then recommended for EBD services by the teams, and 101 children who were evaluated for EBD services but were not classified and were then primarily

suggested for outpatient evaluation and/or treatment by community mental health professionals.

Psychiatric Disorders

Research Findings

The students with EBD showed a wide range of psychiatric diagnoses (Table 9.1) according to the third edition of the *Diagnostic and Statistical Manual of Mental Disorders* (DSM-III; American Psychiatric Association, 1980), including behavioral/externalizing disorders (attention deficit, conduct, and oppositional disorders) as well as emotional/internalizing disorders (depressive and anxiety disorders). The descending order of most common disorders was attention deficit disorders (hereafter termed ADHD to reflect its current usage in DSM-IV as attention-deficit/hyperactivity disorders), depressive disorders, and conduct disorders (all in the prevalence range of 36–43%). In addition, disorders commonly occurred comorbidly (over 50%), especially ADHD with either conduct or depressive disorders. Thus, although conduct disorder was found significantly more often in the students with EBD, it frequently was accompanied by a comorbid disorder.

Other more recent studies of similar students with differing methodologies have confirmed these results (Bussing, Zima, Belin, & Forness, 1998; Duncan, Forness, & Hartsough, 1995; Mattison, 2001a; McClure, Ferguson, Boodoosingh, Turgay, & Stavrakaki, 1989). That is, this additional research has also found that, although ADHD appears to be the most common disorder, a wide range of diagnoses is found and comorbidity is frequent. Teacher checklist ratings of psychopathology in students with EBD have also produced similar findings, i.e., the predominance of externalizing symptoms but also comorbid serious levels of internalizing symptoms (Mattison, Gadow, Sprafkin, & Nolan, 2002; Mattison & Gamble, 1992; McConaughy & Skiba, 1993).

Appropriately, severity appears more contributory to EBD placement than type of psychopathology. The mean Axis V (clinical) rating of 5.2 ("poor—marked impairment") for the students with EBD indicates the serious degree of psychopathology that im-

TABLE 9.1. Psychiatric Characteristics

Characteristic	Students classified EBD (N = 238)	Students not classified EBD (N = 101)
Most common DSM-III psychiatric disorders		
Attention deficit disorders	43.3%	47.5%
Conduct disorders	36.1%	9.9% ****
Oppositional disorder	9.7%	5.0%
Depressive disorders	39.9%	42.6%
Anxiety disorders	10.5%	20.8% **
Comorbid > 1 disorders	50.8%	37.6% *
Mean DSM-III Axis V rating	5.2 ±0	4.6 ± 0.8 ****
Current community mental health intervention		
Therapy	12.6%	14.8%
Medication	7.6%	10.9%
Neither	81.5%	77.2%
No treatment ever	48.7%	52.5%

*$p < .05$, **$p < .01$, ****$p < .0001$.

pacted school performance, and also significantly distinguished the EBD and non-EBD groups (Table 9.1). Comparison studies of EBD and non-EBD groups with teacher checklist ratings have also found significant higher levels of psychopathology in students with EBD (Mattison, Gadow, et al., 2002; Mattison & Gamble, 1992).

Despite their psychopathology, few students were receiving community treatment at the time of their evaluation for EBD services, and almost half had never received any treatment (Table 9.1). Unfortunately, other research has shown that, even after the start of EBD services, a high percentage (41%) of students continue not to receive any medication or therapy through community services (Mattison, 1999).

Analysis

This discussion of research findings for DSM disorders in students with EBD will focus on treatment implications, which is of primary importance for teachers of students with EBD. It will not summarize other accruing knowledge of DSM disorders that can help those teachers understand and plan for their students. Clinical diagnoses may help a teacher to understand the grouping of symptoms in a student, as well as its probable course and complications. For example, a student with a depressive disorder may also show agitation and poor attention, and remain vulnerable for a prolonged course with ongoing risk of suicidal behavior. Appropriate clinical knowledge of DSM disorders can also help teachers appreciate predisposing factors that commonly occur in specific disorders and potential etiological factors. For example, a student with an oppositional disorder may have been predisposed toward such a disorder secondary to chronic family chaos, but even earlier may have developed ADHD secondary to maternal substance abuse during pregnancy. For such information, the reader is referred to major textbooks for special educators, such as *Characteristics of Emotional and Behavioral Disorders of Children and Youth*, 8th Edition (Kauffman, 2004). Readers may also find the following important reviews interesting for their syntheses of contributions from major disciplines (genetics, neurobiology, developmental psychology, cognitive psychology, etc.) into current theories for externalizing disorders (Barkley, 1997; Hinshaw, 2002; Lahey, Waldman, & McBurnett, 1999; Moffitt, 1993).

Treatment studies of children with DSM psychiatric disorders have increasingly focused on short-term medication intervention. Simultaneously, the appropriate demands for evidence-based research require that specific treatments be shown to work not only in the controlled settings of clinical research studies (efficacy), but also in typical clinical settings, such as community mental health clinics (effectiveness) (Chambless & Hollon, 1998). As a result, short-term efficacy has been demonstrated for specific medications in two or more randomized controlled studies in youth in the treatment of disorders that are common in students with EBD: stimulants in ADHD (Greenhill, Halperin, & Abikoff, 1999), and selective serotonin reuptake inhibitors (SSRIs) in depressive disorder (Emslie et al., 2002) as well as anxiety disorders (Birmaher et al., 2003). Long-term efficacy and effectiveness must still be better proven. Less stringent evidence is available for the efficacy of medication for the aggression that is common in conduct disorders, although antipsychotics in particular continue to show promise (Schur et al., 2003). Thus, a high percentage of students with EBD would quite likely benefit from medication as one component of their treatment plan (Forness & Kavale, 2001).

However, while medication is a necessary part of intervention plans for many students with EBD, medicine alone will commonly not be sufficient for optimal stabilization of these students because of complicating factors, such as their frequent comorbidity (Jensen, Martin, & Cantwell, 1997). This point is demonstrated through a recent major treatment study of children with ADHD (MTA Cooperative Group, 1999). The efficacy for highly monitored medication management (primarily methylphenidate) in the treatment of children with ADHD was compared over 14 months with the efficacy for a sophisticated program of behavioral treatment, a combination of medication and the behavioral program, and routine community care (which was primarily a stimulant from a subject's own physician). For core ADHD symptoms, medication management and combined treatment were both significantly superior to behavior treatment alone or community intervention (but were not significantly different from each other). Thus, optimally monitored medication, either alone or in combined treatment, was necessary for reduction of ADHD symptoms. Secondary analyses have reconfirmed the efficacy of

medication for ADHD symptoms, but have begun to show that various comorbid combinations of ADHD plus another disorder also require behavioral treatment for optimal response (Jensen et al., 2001). Research paralleling the MTA design has now begun to compare SSRIs and cognitive behavioral treatment in children with depression; not surprisingly, in adults, characteristics of depressed patients appear to indicate which treatment modality or combination is optimal. Thus, combinations of treatments will likely be required for a large majority of students with EBD to produce the best response.

While medication research has predominated, important nonmedication research for the treatment of DSM disorders in children has evolved. In nonmedication research, particular attention has been paid to the production of manual-based therapies so that a specific treatment approach can be transferred to therapists in general treatment settings, a necessary step to achieve effectiveness. EBD teachers should especially be interested in these protocols because such well-described approaches may help teachers to develop comprehensive BIPs for many of their students, or even interventions that are universal in nature for even more therapeutic efficiency. Such protocols address the clusters of symptoms that are usually seen in disorders, rather than focus on single symptoms. They are well suited for adaptation by EBD teachers: they typically begin with education about the disorder, followed by subsequent cognitive (self-management) and behavioral components, and are designed as a series of lesson plans.

An important recent text presents and critiques the most currently well-developed protocols: *Evidence-Based Psychotherapies for Children and Adolescents* (Kazdin & Weisz, 2003). Noteworthy are specific treatment programs for depressive disorders (Adolescent Coping with Depression; Clarke, Lewinsohn, & Hops, 1990) and for anxiety disorders (Coping Cat; Kendall, 1990). Other important references have presented protocols for conduct disorders (Henggeler, Schoenwald, Borduin, Rowland, & Cunningham, 1998; Walker, Colvin, & Ramsey, 1995) and for ADHD (DuPaul & Stoner, 2003). In general, these protocols are in various stages of establishing proof of efficacy and effectiveness. Not all have school components, and few have been studied with students with EBD.

The treatment findings in Table 9.1 indicate another reality—despite an increasing array of effective treatments, obtaining mental health treatment in the community remains an issue. Indeed, this lack of mental health treatment for children with psychiatric disorders is a national problem (Burns et al., 1995). Thus, EBD teachers will need proactive support from team members to help students obtain treatment in the community to supplement the teachers' work in classrooms.

To summarize the implications of the increasing knowledge about the treatment of DSM disorders that occur in students with EBD, the above discussion emphasizes the necessity for EBD teachers to have a sufficient working knowledge of DSM disorders. They must be able to recognize these disorders in their students to alert parents of that possibility, so that families can then pursue community evaluation and treatment for the increasing number of interventions that are proving effective for such disorders, as noted above. Furthermore, this working knowledge must include awareness of both positive and negative responses to treatments so they can professionally correspond with community clinicians. Parents of students with EBD are often not good informants of their children's school response to treatment, and clinicians must depend on professional feedback from EBD teachers. Indeed, EBD teachers are uniquely well trained to conduct FBAs; to develop BIPs, however, they need to develop more understanding of medication trials, so they can not only observe for the effectiveness of a medication but also help pinpoint the dosage that provides a proper balance of improvement and minimal or no side effects. Such a working knowledge base is not unlike the equivalent knowledge base that teachers usually demonstrate to help parents and community professionals with students who have asthma, seizure disorders, or other chronic disorders that can affect school functioning. However, this knowledge must also be sophisticated enough to incorporate the evolving non-medication protocols that may be useful in the classroom. Consequently, teachers must increasingly stay informed of such research.

Future Research

The increased identification of DSM disorders as a research variable in the study of students with EBD would be an advantageous beginning. This requires development of instruments that can be practically used by teachers. Most research diagnoses of DSM disorders by other disciplines have used structured interviews of parents and/or children for epidemiological research and semistructured interviews for clinical research; similar instruments designed for use with teachers are still under development. These interviews may also not prove practical for special education research. A relatively new instrument, the teacher version of the Child Symptom Inventory—4 (CSI-4T; Gadow & Sprafkin, 1997, 1998), shows promise. This checklist screens for operational criteria of the major DSM disorders of children and adolescents by asking teachers to rate the frequency of each symptom. The CSI-4T has already been investigated in samples of students with EBD and has shown high reliability and validity (Mattison, Gadow, et al., 2002; Mattison, Gadow, Sprafkin, Nolan, & Schneider, 2003). Furthermore, since this instrument uses the operational criteria of the major DSM disorders, it can also function as a tool to educate EBD teachers about DSM disorders.

While the most common disorders will likely still appear, certain disorders have become better recognized since the results shown in Table 9.1 from work in the 1980s, e.g., bipolar disorder, Asperger's disorder, and posttraumatic stress disorder (PTSD), and may now show different patterns of prevalence. Comorbidity should be more carefully addressed, as evolving treatment strategies will focus on comorbid disorders. The severity of the disorders may well increase, particularly with the movement of children into the community out of hospitals and residential facilities. Treatment services should be reevaluated in light of new initiatives designed to reach such children and to better ascertain the breadth of services that these students receive in the community. Such knowledge of DSM disorders, their severity, and treatment options will help teacher trainers better understand how they must train new teachers for students with EBD.

Intervention studies of students with EBD have rarely addressed DSM disorders as a research variable to determine how influential an intrinsic factor such as a DSM disorder may be on the effect of the classroom intervention. The response of a child with serious temper outbursts to one behavioral intervention versus another may be affected by whether or not the child has conduct disorder, PTSD, Asperger's disorder, or major depressive disorder. Similarly, intervention studies in students with EBD too rarely identify noneducational treatments that children receive in addition to the specific classroom behavioral treatments. The effectiveness of behavioral interventions for students with EBD also remains uncertain. Consequently, future intervention research on students with EBD should address these important issues that could easily be affecting the outcomes of classroom interventions.

Most modern treatment research has not been school-based. Although we know the efficacy of various treatment approaches based on non-EBD research in the disciplines of child psychiatry and psychology, we know little about their effectiveness with students who have EBD. While we know the efficacy of specific treatments when children are treated without accompanying school intervention, we know little about their impact with the addition of school intervention, especially EBD programming. For example, most medication studies of non-ADHD disorders have not used teacher input for either diagnoses or outcome assessment (Mattison et al., 2003). The research communities of special education and of child psychiatry and psychology must undertake more meaningful collaborative research that will undoubtedly benefit both fields.

Family Stresses

Research Findings

Family stresses such as abuse and psychiatric illnesses in parents have rarely been studied in students with EBD. The results in Table 9.2 show that students with EBD encounter very high rates of family stresses in their lives, such as lower socioeconomic level, poorly educated mothers (42%), a biological parent who has a psychiatric disorder (82%), and the experience of either domestic, physical, and/or sexual abuse (60%). Indeed, these rates were significantly higher than the rates of family stresses for the comparison group of students who were subsequently referred to outpatient clinics (Table 9.2). The students with EBD also commonly experienced more than one of the listed stresses. Although specific psychiatric disorders could not always be determined for parents, substance abuse and/ or antisocial disorders were common in fathers and depressive disorders in mothers (Mattison et al., 1992).

TABLE 9.2. Demographic and Family Characteristics

Characteristic	Students classified EBD (N = 238)	Students not classified EBD (N = 101)
Demographics		
Mean age (years)	11.6 ± 3.0	11.2 ± 3.2
Male	86.5%	81.2%
Caucasian	87.4%	89.2%
Mean socioeconomic status (lowest = 7)	5.0 ± 1.4	4.3 ± 1.6 ***
Family stresses		
Mother with no GED/ high school degree	41.6%	20.4% ***
Abuse experience	60.4%	36.0% ****
Physical abuse	38.7%	14.0% ****
Parent with psychiatric disorder	81.8%	68.8% **

** $p < .01$, *** $p < .001$, **** $p < .0001$.

Analysis

The high prevalence of stresses in the family background of students with EBD is not surprising, because abuse and parental psychiatric illness are well-established etiological factors for child psychopathology. However, the types of stresses and their high prevalence have particular importance for special educators in their intervention planning for students with EBD.

Growing knowledge about family stresses and their impact on development can help teachers to better understand and teach students who experience such specific types of stresses as abuse. For example, children's reactions to abuse can be characterized from a neurodevelopmental viewpoint as hyperarousal and/or dissociative behaviors, which with persistent exposure can be "biologically wired" more permanently into the brain; thus, initial adaptive responses become maladaptive traits for a child (Perry, Pollard, Blakley, Baker, & Vigilante, 1995). Clearly, much of the clinical presentation in school of the many students with EBD whose history is most noteworthy for abuse experience may in large part be explained by the longitudinal effects of abuse experience. Cognitively, abuse may lead to actual neuronal loss in the brain with resultant decrease in IQ or specific neuropsychological skills (DeBellis, 2001). Intervention studies with abused children are limited, especially involving schools (Fantuzzo, Stevenson, Weiss, Hampton, & Noone, 1997). Nevertheless, results thus far suggest important general steps that teachers can provide for their students with EBD who have been abused (Cicchetti & Toth, 1995). They must first establish a positive, safe, and predictable classroom, and then identify the developmental lags or deviations most likely caused by the abuse that require more specific intervention planning.

Focus on parent and family psychopathology has allowed researchers to identify family contributions to the development of conduct disorders and antisocial behavior, which has helped to inform special education interventions (Walker et al., 1995). Similarly, family research is beginning to explain the development of specific behavioral and emotional patterns in children of parents with other psychiatric disorders. For example, when parents have depressive disorders, their children's subsequent emotions and behaviors may be affected by genetics, parenting problems, modeling, and/or caring for a psychiatrically ill parent (Beardslee, Versage, & Gladstone, 1998).

However, the high prevalence of family stresses has an even more basic implication for special educators—what is their role in addressing such stresses beyond mandatory reporting of abuse? Much of a teacher's work with students who have EBD involves behavioral and/or cognitive-behavioral management of behaviors and/or emotions that are not specific to school (i.e., they are generalized and problematic at both school and home). Consequently, successful generalization and maintenance are dependent on duplication and reinforcement in the home; Kazdin (2002) has discussed this issue in terms of contextual factors, or "moderators." Progress will be minimized when home atmospheres are conducive to abuse or where parental psychopathology continues to adversely affect a student. Indeed, research with youths who have chronic antisocial problems in the context of psychopathological families demonstrates the need for multisystemic involvement for effective intervention (Henggeler et al., 1998; Walker et al., 1995).

Thus, proactive assistance in helping families obtain community services appears to be a necessity, with emphasis on "proactive" However, the reality is that students with EBD commonly do not receive community treatment services, either at enrollment or during EBD programming. Thus, teachers of students with EBD must have support from a team social worker or psychologist who can both engage and assist parents—simple referrals for community services will not suffice. Then communication must be established with the community professional to ensure collaborative work to assure similar behavioral interventions at school and home.

Future Research

Students with EBD frequently come from complex backgrounds that include serious stresses. Research by other disciplines has begun to clarify the specific impact of such stresses on the behavioral and emotional development of children, and thereby shape the design and investigation of more specific intervention approaches. However, such research has rarely included schools; for example, abuse research remains compromised by a lack of school-based studies of abused children (Cicchetti & Toth, 1995; Fantuzzo et al., 1997). With the common occurrence of abuse and parental psychiatric disorder in students with EBD, special education is ideal for future research into the relationship of childhood stresses and school functioning, with particular attention to the common behavioral and emotional problems that teachers of students with EBD must address.

Such research might begin with a better understanding of the past and present stresses experienced by students with EBD through more comprehensive surveys of a wider range of childhood stresses and responses, using modern instrumentation such as that reviewed by Ohan, Myers, & Collett (2002). Additionally, Hyman and Perone (1998) advocate that such a survey should include unique school stressors experienced by current and prospective students with EBD. The association of specific stresses with serious school problems shown by students with EBD could be investigated by pairing such stress surveys with already established instruments that screen for critical behaviors in school (e.g., the Critical Events Index and the Adaptive and Maladaptive Behavior Rating Scales that are components of the *Systematic Screening for Behavior Disorders;* Walker & Severson, 1992).

The relationship between stresses and general school functioning (academic, behavioral, and social) of students with EBD who have experienced stresses should be examined. Specific symptoms of PTSD can be assessed with instruments such as those mentioned above. These measures can be used in conjunction with established instruments that evaluate academic functioning, behavioral/emotional psychopathology in school, and social skills.

Finally, school-based intervention studies centered on family stresses should be conducted. These studies should focus on students with EBD as subjects and on the EBD classroom as a primary intervention. Instruments described above could serve as objective measures both at baseline and follow-up. A naturalistic study of students just entering EBD programming could determine the impact on school functioning (and PTSD symptoms) of abused versus nonabused students using current treatment-as-exists (i.e., existent FBA/BIP intervention in the EBD classroom plus community services that families may obtain). A subsequent study could then measure the impact of more specific interventions directed toward family stresses, e.g., with multisystemic treatment (Henggeler et al., 1998).

Longitudinal Outcome

Research Findings

Intervention studies have generally not proven effective in producing long-term desirable outcomes for students with EBD. Annual government reports (although not based on cohorts) have repeatedly shown that students with EBD have the highest dropout rate (over 40%) for all categories of special education students, and, indeed, one of the highest dropout rates for any group of students in the nation. In a rare cohort study of students with EBD aged 8 to 18 years (Greenbaum et al., 1996), 43.1% dropped out of school over the course of 6 years. Mattison and Felix (1997) found that 58.9% of a cohort of secondary students with SED had left school after an average follow-up of 8 years. In the most extensive national follow-up study of special education students pre- and postgraduation, Wagner (1995) further demonstrated the guarded prognosis for students with EBD in terms of poor academic performance in high school, followed by a postgraduation period of limited advanced education, increased unemployment, and high arrest rates.

Although the educational prognosis for students with EBD is frequently not positive, many students do benefit from special education services and successfully finish their schooling despite their high risk for poor outcomes. Therefore, it is important to identify the characteristics for those students with EBD who are successful that make educational, community, and family-based services work for these at-risk students. Predictors of outcome for students with EBD had rarely been investigated until recently. Mattison, Spitznagel, and Felix (1998) followed up 151 students for an average of 8 years after their time of enrollment in EBD classes. Nearly half (75) had successfully graduated from high school or returned to non-EBD programming, while 76 had dropped out of school or had been transferred to more intensive placement. In descending order, a student was significantly more likely to be successful if he was younger, did not have the diagnosis of a conduct or oppositional disorder, had a verbal IQ that was not significantly lower than his or her performance IQ, and had a depressive or anxiety disorder. Importantly, the presence of abuse, parental psychiatric disorder, or the initial community treatment status was not predictive of poor educational success; that is, many students had successful school outcomes despite a background of stress. Similar findings were also found in a more recent 3-year follow-up study of students with EBD. Although the findings were based on a small sample size, the results indicated that negative outcome as measured by more restrictive placement, was significantly associated with delinquent psychopathology and lower verbal IQ (Mattison & Spitznagel, 2001).

Closer investigation of achievement progress in students with EBD also confirms the importance of enrollment academic skills. Students newly classified as EBD were followed over 3 years; their average IQ scores and low average achievement scores at enrollment were maintained at follow-up except for a significant decrease in written language skills (Mattison, Hooper, & Glassberg, 2002). This maintenance of academic functioning held true for both EBD/LD (learning disorders) and EBD/non-LD students.

Analysis

Pessimistic outcomes are not surprising since students with EBD are among the most psychiatrically ill children at school and in the community (Mattison & Gamble, 1992). Children with such clinical backgrounds are known to have a guarded educational prognosis (Greenbaum et al., 1996). Furthermore, the predictive characteristics noted above are consistent with the repeated findings that children with conduct disorders and low verbal IQs are very treatment-resistant and therefore also more vulnerable to poor outcomes (Moffitt, 1993).

Thus, the educational success in many students with EBD may be overlooked and underappreciated. Despite their status as the most at-risk children in their community, large numbers of children benefit from EBD services allowing them to eventually re-enter regular education programming and to graduate from high school. Those children with positive prognostic characteristics can do well despite their common stressful backgrounds. Importantly, the most powerful predictor was age—younger age increased the chance of success. This finding contrasts with the more common practice of delaying the initiation of EBD services for students (Duncan et al., 1995).

Future Research

An essential beginning is the simple recommendation for more large group longitudinal studies in order to gain a better understanding of the effectiveness of services for students with EBD. In addition, research should seek to identify characteristics of students who do and do not benefit from such programming. Currently, most longitudinal studies of students with EBD have used cases or small groups over short periods of follow-up. More cohorts of children need to be followed from the time they begin receiving services, and they should be followed for longer periods of time. Ideally, the studies should continue until cessation of services, or across important transition times such as from grade school to middle school or from EBD services to regular education programming. Most work has thus far focused on students with EBD at the end of their educational careers and has consequently not been very encouraging.

Longitudinal comparison studies should help us understand when children with emotional/behavioral disorders require EBD services, and at what level of intensity. The course of children referred to multidisciplinary teams for emotional/behavioral problems could be followed according to natural groupings to ascertain the accuracy of such referrals: only referred to community evaluation/services without school intervention, school intervention according to Section 504 guidelines, and classification as EBD. Future longitudinal research of students with EBD would also benefit from the development of more comprehensive, objective baselines. Tables 9.1–9.4 provide the outline of one model that might be improved, for example, with the addition of neurological risk factors such as maternal substance exposure during pregnancy. In particular, longitudinal studies should include important interim variables that can influence outcome, such as community mental health services and persistent or new family or environmental stresses.

Finally, outcomes need to be more extensively measured beyond general success or failure in school. Pre- and posttesting should be conducted on achievement tests, critical behaviors, and teacher ratings of student psychopathology. Annual rates of subject failure, absenteeism, and disciplinary actions should be ascertained (Mattison, 2000), as well as changes in group achievement tests at both the state and national levels. More positively, participation in school activities such as team sports and clubs should be assessed. Determination of success outside of school should also be obtained, for example, participation in age-appropriate civic activities and, more negatively, occurrence of critical events such as arrests, suicidal behavior, and substance abuse.

PSYCHOLOGICAL ASSESSMENT

McConaughy and Ritter (2002) have recommended a multidimensional approach as best practice for conducting psychological assessment of students with EBD. In addition to the assessment of cognitive ability and academic achievement, such an approach would include: clinical interviews with the student, interviews with parents and teachers, standardized behavioral rating scales completed by the student as well as by the parents and teachers, and direct observations in the school setting. Achenbach and McConaughy (2001) have discussed how one such integrated assessment, the Achenbach System of Empirically Based Assessment (Achenbach & Rescorla, 2001), can be used to help multidisciplinary teams and special education staff to objectively assess if a student is eligible for EBD programming, plan services, track the student's progress, and communicate with community professionals.

In addition to basic IQ and achievement testing, neuropsychological testing must now be considered because the definition of learning disorders is moving toward the identification and remediation of underlying cognitive deficits. Indeed, neuropsychological subtests have now become part of new versions of IQ-achievement batteries. Furthermore, as will be discussed below, learning disorders and neuropsychological deficits are emerging as important issues for students with EBD.

The following section will focus on findings for modern psychological assessment of students with EBD. Results will be presented for several components of the above best-practice model that have been investigated thus far, and thereby demonstrate its potential.

Learning Disorders

Research Findings

Studies consistently have shown that students with EBD have IQ scores in the low average range with lower verbal scores, as shown in Table 9.3. Past results for achievement scores have persistently demonstrated academic lags, often of two or more grade levels. Thus, Table 9.3 shows reading standard scores to be lower than predicted by IQ. Furthermore, 21% of the students newly classified as EBD are at least 1.5 standard deviations below the mean (and greater than the 9% that would be statistically expected).

Such academic lags may partially be accounted for by students with LD. Indeed, recent work using rigorous definitions of LD has shown that about half of students newly categorized as EBD have LD in reading, mathematics, and/or written language (Glassberg et al., 1999). This rate appears even higher (75%) in students who are not responding to EBD services (Mattison, 2001b). Furthermore, a 3-year follow-up study of a representative sample of the same students showed a marked persistence of LD (generally irrespective of achievement area or LD definition); students with LD and without LD were significantly likely to be defined by their original LD status (Mattison, Hooper, & Glassberg, 2002). Thus, students who were not originally defined as LD did not become LD over the subsequent 3

TABLE 9.3. Characteristics of Cognitive/Educational Testing

Characteristic	Students classified EBD	Students not classified EBD
Mean WISC-R IQ Scores	(N = 215)	(N = 95)
Verbal	94.2 ± 12.9	97.2 ± 14.2
Performance	98.3 ± 12.6	99.8 ± 15.3
Full Scale	95.7 ± 12.3	98.3 ± 14.3
Mean WRAT or WRAT-R	(N = 170)	(N = 73)
Reading Standard Score	91.1 ± 18.4	91.1 ± 21.9
Standard Score < 78 (9% expected)	20.6%	17.6%

years and continued to progress at their original rate of learning in terms of achievement standard scores. In those students who were initially defined as LD, their LD persisted and they continued to learn at their original LD rate.

One increasing emphasis in the study of LD is identification of underlying neuropsychological deficits. A recent study (Mattison, Hooper, & Carlson, in press) investigated neuropsychological deficits with the NEPSY (Korkman, Kirk, & Kemp, 1998) in elementary school students with EBD. Over half (54%) of the children scored at least two standard deviations below the mean on at least one of the four functional domains of the NEPSY, in particular Language and Attention/Executive Functions. While the NEPSY was not related to demographic or Teacher's Report Form (TRF; Achenbach, 1991b) scales of psychopathology, significant relationships were shown with achievement tests and neurological risk factors. For example, the Language subtests of Phonological Processing and Speeded Naming showed the highest significant correlations with reading performance, even after controlling for IQ. Overall, the worse that these students with EBD performed academically, the more likely they were to show neuropsychological deficits.

Other recent work has focused on differences in psychopathology for students with EBD who do or do not have comorbid LD. Interestingly, studies have found that psychopathology is *not* significantly different between students with EBD and students with EBD/LD (Handwerk & Marshall, 1998; Mattison, 2001b). Furthermore, another study has begun to show that addressing LD in students with EBD/LD produces a posi-tive impact on the degree of psychopathology in such comorbid students (Penno, Frank, & Wacker, 2000).

Analysis

This high prevalence rate of LD in students with EBD is consistent with the picture of poor academic performance and poor academic outcome in students with EBD (Wagner, 1995). The common occurrence of ADHD in students with EBD would also predict a high rate of LD. That is, Barkley (1998) has conservatively noted the prevalence of LD in children with ADHD as 8–39%, which might be expected to be higher in students with EBD and ADHD because of their increased school dysfunction. Finally, these students also showed well-established relationships between achievement areas and neuropsychological deficits, such as the association of a language deficit in phonological processing with reading dysfunction. Although the occurrence of language disorders has not been investigated in students with EBD, in addition to their increased risk due to lower verbal IQs, they also are at risk because of the common finding of language disorders in children with psychiatric disorders (40%; Cohen, Barwick, Horodezky, Vallance, & Im, 1998).

In addition to the importance of the high occurrence of LD in students with EBD to educators of these students, the nature of the relationship between LD and psychopathology is also of concern. That is, the academic performance of students with EBD may be more related to the presence of LD than to their psychopathology. Students with EBD have thus far not been distinguished in their psychopathology by the comorbid presence or absence of LD or of neuropsychological deficits. Over time, students who continue to receive EBD services for their serious psychopathology maintain their enrollment levels of standard scores whether or not they also have LD. This emerging finding would also be consistent with evidence from longitudinal studies of children without disabilities. That is, academic achievement is most affected by initial IQ and ADHD symptoms once conduct symptomology is controlled for; the ADHD effect on scholastic performance appears to be related to both behavioral and cognitive components of ADHD, especially working memory (Rapport, Scanlan, & Denney, 1999).

The common occurrence of LD in students with EBD leads to the question of how to teach such students. Gunter and Denny (1998) have reservations that teachers of students with EBD may not currently be sufficiently trained to accomplish this task. Although ideally both areas of disability should be addressed at the same time, commonly the approach is to first improve the behavior of a student with EBD/LD in order to get that student "ready to learn." However, recent work has begun to demonstrate that good academic instruction for students with EBD can lead to improvement in behavior (Penno et al., 2000).

Although LD appears to persist in students with EBD/LD, they do appear to grow at their enrollment rate. This maintenance of learning may be related to the direct teaching and coaching of academic skills that teachers of students with EBD can deliver in their classrooms, two general interventions that have been found to help students with LD (Swanson, Hoskyn, & Lee, 1999). Indeed, few protocols have been shown to be effective in remediating specific LD or neuropsychological deficits, and these mainly are limited to reading disorders. Thus, teachers of students with EBD may already know very useful general skills that can help to address learning disorders in their students until more effective protocols are developed.

Future Research

The more common use of LD status as a research variable may help in studies of students with EBD. The definition of LD could follow current recommendations for a cutoff percentile of low achievement rather than discrepancy with IQ, in addition to the identification of underlying neuropsychological deficits. Fortunately, new batteries combine achievement tests with cognitive assessment that includes more refined tests of neuropsychological skills.

An important starting point would be an epidemiological study to determine the occurrence of LD and neuropsychological deficits in students with EBD at all levels of intervention, using the students classified as having LD and/or language disorder for a comparison group. This study could replicate earlier work and expand our knowledge of existent neuropsychological deficits, in particular language and attentional disorders. Such a project would clarify whether the national movement away from IQ-achievement testing is wise. It would help teachers of students with EBD and their trainers further appreciate the range of LD that they must be prepared to remediate, as well as highlight neuropsychological deficits for which they must develop specific protocols.

The unclear interaction of LD and psychopathology could be elucidated in students with EBD. Most practically, what effects on achievement and behavior do specific teaching approaches have in students with well-defined EBD and LD—behavioral programming alone, LD remedial programming alone, or a combination? Also, how does the nature of the LD affect behavioral programming, for example, what is the effect of a language disorder on a BIP that requires a clear understanding by the student?

Finally, work cited above has begun to show that students with EBD/LD maintain their enrollment rate of learning. Does this finding represent a mixed response for such students—some LD improves, some plateaus, and some worsens? The definition of these potential subgroups will be important. EBD/LD students who plateau or worsen in their academic achievement, especially if related to intervention-resistant neuropsychological deficits, will quite likely require the teaching of alternative skills to acquire information and be productive. For example, a student who has a recalcitrant reading disorder may need to become increasingly skilled in the use of video aids to learn. Or he or she may require early exposure to vocational training, one intervention factor that appears to predict positive outcome for students with EBD (Rylance, 1997).

Empirical Measurement of Psychopathology

Research Findings

Standardized behavioral rating scales completed by teachers have provided objective results that describe the psychopathology of students classified as EBD in terms of dimensions, in contrast to the diagnostic categories of DSM. The instrument that has been used in such research most is the Teacher's Report Form (TRF; Achenbach, 1991b), along with its companion parent instrument, the Child Behavior Checklist (CBCL; Achenbach, 1991a).

Findings for the three broad scales of the TRF and the CBCL are shown in Table 9.4 for students with and without EBD who have served as the reference point for this chapter. It is important to note that the numbers of subjects for the TRF are reduced because before the TRF was available another teacher instrument was used. Most striking is the degree of total psychopathology for the students with EBD as rated by their teachers: the mean T score for Total Score was greater than 70 (two standard deviations). Between the two types of psychopathology, externalizing problems predominated but internalizing problems were in the clinical range ($T > 63$). Also, the dysfunction

for the students with EBD was global, that is, it presented not only at school but also at a serious level at home. Teacher scores were higher than parent scores, signifying more dysfunction at school; however, the general pattern was the same. Finally, for both measures, the students with EBD were significantly higher than the students without EBD on Externalizing and Total Score, although the ratings for the students without EBD group were within the clinical range in both environments.

These findings for the TRF have also been found for other groups of students with EBD (McConaughy, Mattison, & Peterson, 1994; Mattison, 2001b; Mattison & Spitznagel, 2001): Total Score that is near or above two standard deviations of deviance, Externalizing more severe than Internalizing (although both are in the clinical range), and teacher TRF ratings more severe than parent CBCL ratings. When the individual TRF scales in these studies are examined, problems with aggression and socialization are usually the highest. More specifically, McConaughy et al. (1994) found the following TRF scales were the most elevated (clinical range = $T > 67$ for narrow scales) for the sample of 366 students with EBD from three states: Aggressive Behavior ($T = 69.6$); Social Problems ($T = 68.4$); and Attention Problems ($T = 66.7$). Finally, in a comparison study of TRF ratings for boys with EBD ages 6–11 years (who were among the EBD group in Table 9.4) with same-age inpatient, outpatient, and general population comparison groups of boys from the same geographical region, the TRF ratings for the boys with EBD were the highest among all four

TABLE 9.4. Mean T Scores for the Teacher Report Form (TRF) and the Parent Child Behavior Checklist (CBCL)

	Students classified EBD	Students not classified EBD
TRF	($N = 116$)	($N = 51$)
Internalizing	65.3 ± 9.0	66.1 ± 8.3
Externalizing	74.1 ± 7.8	70.9 ± 8.1 *
Total Score	73.1 ± 6.6	70.9 ± 6.6 *
CBCL	($N = 210$)	($N = 93$)
Internalizing	65.3 ± 8.8	65.1 ± 7.8
Externalizing	70.6 ± 8.3	66.7 ± 8.6 ***
Total Score	70.2 ± 9.4	67.6 ± 8.4 *

* $p \leq .05$; *** $p < .001$.

groups and were significantly greater than both the outpatient and the general population groups (Mattison & Gamble, 1992).

The TRF has also been explored for its ability to distinguish characteristics of EBD from outpatient groups. Total Score most practically distinguished boys with EBD ages 6–11 years from same-age outpatient boys with the following accuracy values: 62.4% sensitivity, 85.5% specificity, and 76.7% overall correct classification (Mattison, Lynch, Kales, & Gamble, 1993). In addition, in a study of the TRF's ability to track change in students with EBD, significant TRF changes were found to accurately reflect subsequent multidisciplinary team decisions (that were blind to TRF scores) to decrease or increase the intensity of EBD services (Mattison & Spitznagel, 2001).

A more newly developed instrument, the teacher version of the Child Symptom Inventory—4 (CSI-4T; Gadow & Sprafkin, 1997, 1998) focuses on the objective rating of DSM-IV diagnostic criteria and has only recently appeared in research for students with EBD. The instrument has shown the following prevalence of DSM-IV disorders for a group of boys with EBD ages 6–12 years who were referred for psychiatric consultation: 64.2% ADHD, 64.2% oppositional defiant disorder, 41.5% conduct disorder, 20.8% depressive disorder, and 20.8% generalized anxiety disorder (Mattison, Gadow, et al., 2002). In the same study, the group with EBD had significantly higher symptom severity scores than a comparison group of same-age outpatient boys for 10 of the 12 CSI-4T symptom categories that were investigated. In a later study, CSI-4T ratings showed good convergence and divergence with TRF ratings in students with EBD, as well as with DSM-IV clinician diagnoses (Mattison et al., 2003).

Analysis

In students with EBD, the results for teacher ratings of standardized behavioral rating scales, primarily the TRF, are consistent with findings from DSM research that uses a different classification system for psychopathology (i.e., dimensional versus categorical). Although teacher checklists and DSM diagnoses have not been compared together for students with EBD, the checklist findings, like DSM studies, find: serious levels of dysfunction, the predomination of externalizing symptoms, and comorbidity as represented by clinically relevant levels of internalizing symptoms.

Thus, the TRF appears to represent the psychopathology of students with EBD. Most importantly, that representation is empirical and dimensional. These findings suggest that the TRF, as recommended by Achenbach and McConaughy (2001), would be a good tool for staff responsible for students with EBD to communicate with community professionals, to objectively track the progress of students with EBD, and to supplement and verify FBA and BIP data.

The usefulness of the TRF to predict outcomes for students with EBD requires further study. Scales of the CBCL have been shown to be helpful predictors across 6 years for important practical indicators of dysfunction, such as dropping out, substance abuse, police contacts, and suicidal behavior (Achenbach, Howell, McConaughy, & Stanger, 1998). The TRF may have similar predictive potential for important indicators of school outcome, such as absenteeism, subject failure, suspensions, retention, and dropping out. Furthermore, dimensions of psychopathology may have more predictive power than categorical psychiatric disorders (Fergusson & Horwood, 1995).

Future Research

A well-designed longitudinal study could begin to fulfill these purposes simultaneously. For example, the Achenbach battery, or at a minimum its parent, teacher, and child rating scales, could be administered to students as they are evaluated for EBD services for their first time by multidisciplinary teams. Scales of the two instruments could then be examined for their ability to correctly predict the teams' choice of EBD placement or no EBD placement.

The instruments could then be readministered annually for at least 2–3 years after baseline. The course of psychopathology could then be compared between the two groups (EBD and non-EBD), especially in students who appeared similar at enrollment. Students could be divided into the best and worse groups according to successful improvement in psychopathology, and baseline and interim predictive factors could then be identified.

Of particular importance in a study, as described above, would be relating the checklist empirical strengths to educational variables, that is, to understand the relationship between psychopathology and school variables as well as to determine how the checklists could objectively supplement school variables. Candidate school variables would be EBD services (such as level of placement plus daily amount of services), grade-point average, curriculum-based and achievement tests, absenteeism and tardiness, disciplinary referrals and suspensions, response to BIPs, and achievement of IEP goals.

CONCLUSIONS

Research findings from recent work in the psychiatric and psychological assessment of students with EBD have objectively verified what educators who teach students with EBD already know: they teach students who are among the most dysfunctional youths in their community. The prognosis for these students is jeopardized by factors that can mitigate their response to classroom interventions: global severity, high-intensity externalizing symptoms, comorbid psychiatric disorders, lack of treatment by community services, abuse experience, active parental psychiatric disorder, delayed referral, and co-occurrence of LD. Nevertheless, striking numbers of students with EBD progress despite the negative prognosis that their high-risk clinical profiles and backgrounds might predict.

Analysis of these findings begins to define what growing knowledge from other disciplines is relevant for EBD teachers, with inherent implications. Of greatest immediate relevance are findings for the treatment of DSM psychiatric disorders. Efficacious medication and nonmedication treatments are being established that will help these students. Therefore, EBD teachers must have sufficient clinical knowledge to recognize psychiatric disorders that have been matched with specific treatments and to help parents

and community professionals judge the clinical response of students to the treatments. Because of comorbidity, combined treatments often will be necessary. Therefore, teachers will require sufficient knowledge of nonmedication treatments that their students may receive in order to incorporate such protocols into their own BIPs and thereby not introduce conflicting approaches that may confuse the students. Teachers of students with EBD must also be able to recognize the LD of many of their students that may be intertwined with psychopathology. At the least, these students with EBD/LD will require the general interventions that teachers of students with EBD should already be skilled at implementing, and, with time, more targeted neuropsychological interventions that are gradually being developed. Finally, trainers of such teachers must assimilate this increasingly pertinent research from other disciplines into the basic and continuing training of such teachers to ensure their development into the unique clinician/teacher that is required by their special students and their schools (Forness & Kavale, 1991).

Future research will be especially demanding and challenging for special education researchers (Forness, Kavale, & Davanzo, 2002; Kauffman, 1996; Sugai, 1998). Much as child psychiatry has been experiencing in the past decade or two, special education researchers must demonstrate the efficacy and effectiveness of programming for large groups of students with EBD, or, as has already begun, students will be lost to ideology or cost cutting. They must more vigorously incorporate the scientific findings from other disciplines that are proving applicable to their students into their research. They must be prepared to assess the impact of noneducational treatments on their students in school and to collaborate in the design of school intervention programs to complement those treatments. Such collegiality cannot be overemphasized, as special education, child psychiatry, and child psychology researchers still too often conduct research on the same children without sufficient communication or awareness of how relevant their findings are for one another, and therefore for the children whom they study to improve their future.

ACKNOWLEDGMENT

I wish to acknowledge Stephanie H. McConaughy for her valuable comments.

REFERENCES

Achenbach, T. M. (1991a). *Manual for the Child Behavior Checklist/4–18 and 1991 Profile.* Burlington, VT: University of Vermont Department of Psychiatry.

Achenbach, T. M. (1991b). *Manual for the Teacher's Report Form and 1991 Profile.* Burlington, VT: University of Vermont Department of Psychiatry.

Achenbach, T. M., Howell, C. T., McConaughy, S. H., & Stanger, C. (1998). Six-year predictors of problems in a national sample: IV. Young adult signs of disturbance. *Journal of the American Academy of Child and Adolescent Psychiatry, 37,* 718–727.

Achenbach, T. M., & McConaughy, S. H. (2001). *School-based practitioners' guide for the Child Behavior Checklist and related forms* (2nd ed.). Burlington, VT: University of Vermont Research Center for Children, Youth, and Families.

Achenbach, T. M., & Rescorla, L. (2001). *Manual for the ASEBA school-age forms and profiles.* Burlington, VT: University of Vermont Research Center for Children, Youth, and Families.

American Psychiatric Association. (1980). *Diagnostic and statistical manual of mental disorders* (3rd ed.). Washington, DC: Author.

Barkley, R. A. (1997). Behavioral inhibition, sustained attention, and executive functions: Constructing a unifying theory of ADHD. *Psychological Bulletin, 121,* 65–94.

Barkley, R. A. (1998). *Attention-deficit hyperactivity disorder: A handbook for diagnosis and treatment* (2nd ed.). New York: Guilford Press.

Beardslee, W. R., Versage, E. M., & Gladstone, T. R. G. (1998). Children of affectively ill parents: A review of the past 10 years. *Journal of the American Academy of Child and Adolescent Psychiatry, 37,* 1134–1141.

Birmaher, B., Axelson, D. A., Monk, K., Kalas, C., Clark, D. B., Ehmann, M., Bridge, J., Heo, J., & Brent, D. A. (2003). Fluoxetine for the treatment of anxiety disorders. *Journal of the American Academy of Child and Adolescent Psychiatry, 42,* 415–423.

Burns, B. J., Costello, E. J., Angold, A., Tweed, D., Stangl, D., Farmer, E. M. Z., & Erkanli, A. (1995). Children's mental health service use across service sectors. *Health Affairs, 14,* 147–159.

Bussing, R., Zima, B. T., Belin, T. R., & Forness, S. R. (1998). Children who qualify for LD and SED programs: Do they differ in level of ADHD symptoms and comorbid psychiatric conditions? *Behavioral Disorders, 23,* 85–97.

Chambless, D. L., & Hollon, S. D. (1998). Defining empirically supported therapies. *Journal of Consulting and Clinical Psychology, 66,* 7–18.

Cicchetti, D., & Toth, S. L. (1995). A developmental psychopathology perspective on child abuse and neglect. *Journal of the American Academy of Child and Adolescent Psychiatry, 34,* 541–565.

Clarke, G., Lewinsohn, P., & Hops, H. (1990). *Adolescent coping with depression course: Leader's manual for adolescent groups.* Eugene, OR: Castalia.

Cohen, N. J., Barwick, M. A., Horodezky, N. B., Vallance, D. D., & Im, N. (1998). Language, achievement, and cognitive processing in psychiatrically disturbed children with previously identified and unsuspected language impairments. *Journal of Child Psychology and Psychiatry, 39,* 865–877.

DeBellis, M. D. (2001). Developmental traumatology: The psychobiological development of maltreated children and its implications for research, treatment, and policy. *Development and Psychopathology, 13,* 539–564.

Duncan, B. B. Forness, S. R., & Hartsough, C. (1995). Students identified as seriously emotionally disturbed in school-based day treatment: Cognitive, psychiatric, and special education characteristics. *Behavioral Disorders, 20,* 238–252.

DuPaul, G. J., & Stoner, G. (2003). *ADHD in the schools: Assessment and intervention strategies* (2nd ed.). New York: Guilford Press.

Emslie, G. J., Heiligenstein, J. H., Wagner, K. D., Hoog, S. L., Ernest, D. E., Brown, E., et al. (2002). Fluoxetine for acute treatment of depression in children and adolescents: A placebo-controlled, randomized clinical trial. *Journal of the American Academy of Child and Adolescent Psychiatry, 41,* 1205–1215.

Fantuzzo, J. W., Stevenson, H. C., Weiss, A. D., Hampton, V. R., & Noone, M. J. (1997). A partnership-directed school-based intervention for child physical abuse and neglect: Beyond mandatory reporting. *School Psychology Review, 26,* 298–313.

Fergusson, D. M., & Horwood, J. (1995). Predictive validity of categorically and dimensionally scored measures of disruptive childhood behaviors. *Journal of the American Academy of Child and Adolescent Psychiatry, 34,* 477–485.

Forness, S. R., & Kavale, K. A. (1991). School psychologists' roles and functions: Integration into the regular classroom. In G. Stoner, M. R. Shinn, & H. M. Walker (Eds.), *Intervention for achievement and behavior problems* (pp. 21–36). Silver Spring, MD: National Association of School Psychologists.

Forness, S. R., & Kavale, K. A. (2001). Ignoring the odds: Hazards of not adding the new medical model to special education decisions. *Behavioral Disorders, 26,* 269–281.

Forness, S. R., Kavale, K. A., & Davanzo, P. A. (2002). The new medical model: Interdisciplinary treatment and the limits of behaviorism. *Behavioral Disorders, 27,* 168–178.

Gadow, K. D., & Sprafkin, J. (1997). *Child Symptom*

Inventory-4 norms manual. Stony Brook, NY: Checkmate Plus.

Gadow, K. D., & Sprafkin, J. (1998). *Child Symptom Inventory-4 screening manual.* Stony Brook, NY: Checkmate Plus.

Garland, A. F., Hough, R. L., McCabe, K. M., Yeh, M., Wood, P. A., & Aarons, G. A. (2001). Prevalence of psychiatric disorders in youths across five sectors of care. *Journal of the American Academy of Child and Adolescent Psychiatry, 40,* 409–418.

Glassberg, L. A., Hooper, S. R., & Mattison, R. E. (1999). Prevalence of learning disorders at enrollment in special education students with behavioral disorders. *Behavioral Disorders, 25,* 9–21.

Greenbaum, P. E., Dedrick, R. F., Friedman, R. M., Kutash, K., Brown, E. C., Lardieri, S. P., & Pugh, A. M. (1996). National Adolescent and Child Treatment Study (NACTS): Outcomes for children with serious emotional and behavioral disturbance. *Journal of Emotional and Behavioral Disorders, 4,* 140–146.

Greenhill, L. L., Halperin, J. M., & Abikoff, H. (1999). Stimulant medications. *Journal of the American Academy of Child and Adolescent Psychiatry, 38,* 503–512.

Gunter, P. L., & Denny, R. K. (1998). Trends and issues in research regarding academic instruction of students with emotional and behavioral disorders. *Behavioral Disorders, 24,* 44–50.

Handwerk, M. L., & Marshall, R. M. (1998). Behavioral and emotional problems of students with learning disabilities, serious emotional disturbance, or both conditions. *Journal of Learning Disabilities, 31,* 327–338.

Henggeler, S. W., Schoenwald, S. K., Borduin, C. M., Rowland, M. D., & Cunningham, P. B. (1998). *Multisystemic treatment of antisocial behavior in children and adolescents.* New York: Guilford Press.

Hinshaw, S. P. (2002). Process, mechanism, and explanation related to externalizing behavior in developmental psychopathology. *Journal of Abnormal Child Psychology, 30,* 431–446.

Hyman, I. A., & Perone, D. C. (1998). The other side of school violence: Educator policies and practices that may contribute to student misbehavior. *Journal of School Psychology, 36,* 7–27.

Jensen, P. S., Hinshaw, S. P., Kraemer, H. C., Lenora, N., Newcorn, J. H., Abikoff, M. B., et al. (2001). ADHD comorbidity findings from the MTA study: Comparing comorbid groups. *Journal of the American Academy of Child and Adolescent Psychiatry, 40,* 147–158.

Jensen, P. S., Martin, D., & Cantwell, D. P. (1997). Comorbidity in ADHD: Implications for research, practice, and DSM-V. *Journal of the American Academy of Child and Adolescent Psychiatry, 36,* 1065–1079.

Kauffman, J. M. (1996). Research to practice issues. *Behavioral Disorders, 22,* 55–60.

Kauffman, J. M. (2004). *Characteristics of emotional and behavioral disorders of children and youth* (8th ed.). Upper Saddle River, NJ: Merrill/Prentice Hall.

Kazdin, A. E. (2002). The state of child and adolescent psychotherapy research. *Child and Adolescent Mental Health, 7,* 53–59.

Kazdin, A. E., & Weisz, J. R. (Eds.). (2003). *Evidence-based psychotherapies for children and adolescents.* New York: Guilford Press.

Kendall, P. C. (1990). *Coping cat workbook.* Ardmore, PA: Workbook.

Korkman, M., Kirk, U., & Kemp, S. (1998). *NEPSY: A developmental neuropsychological assessment.* San Antonio, TX: Psychological Corporation.

Lahey, B. B., Waldman, I. D., & McBurnett, K. (1999). Annotation: The development of antisocial behavior: An integrative causal model. *Journal of Child Psychology and Psychiatry, 40,* 669–682.

Mattison, R. E. (1993). A model for SED case evaluation. In G. K. Fritz, R. E. Mattison, B. Nurcombe, & A. Spirito (Eds.), *Child and adolescent mental health consultation in hospitals, schools, and courts* (pp. 109–129). Washington, D C: American Psychiatric Press.

Mattison, R. E. (1999). Use of psychotropic medications in special education students with serious emotional disturbance. *Journal of Child and Adolescent Psychopharmacology, 9,* 149–155.

Mattison, R. E. (2000). School consultation: A review of research on issues unique to the school environment. *Journal of the American Academy of Child and Adolescent Psychiatry, 39,* 402–413.

Mattison, R. E. (2001a). Consultation interactions between special education teachers and child psychiatrists. *Child and Adolescent Psychiatric Clinics of North America, 10,* 67–82.

Mattison, R. E. (2001b). Learning disabilities in special education students referred for psychiatric consultation. *Thalamus, 19,* 11–19.

Mattison, R. E., & Felix, B. C. (1997). The course of elementary and secondary school students with SED through their special education experience. *Journal of Emotional and Behavioral Disorders, 5,* 107–117.

Mattison, R. E., Gadow, K. D., Sprafkin, J., & Nolan, E. E. (2002). Discriminant validity of a DSM-IV-based teacher checklist: Comparison of regular and special education students. *Behavioral Disorders, 27,* 304–316.

Mattison, R. E., Gadow, K. D., Sprafkin, J., Nolan, E. E., & Schneider, J. (2003). A DSM-IV-referenced teacher rating scale for use in clinical management. *Journal of the American Academy of Child and Adolescent Psychiatry, 42,* 442–449.

Mattison, R. E., & Gamble, A. D. (1992). Severity of socially and emotionally disturbed boys' dysfunction at school and home: Comparison with psychiatric and general population boys. *Behavioral Disorders, 17,* 219–224.

Mattison, R. E., Hooper, S. R., & Carlson, G. A. (in press). Neuropsychological characteristics of special education students with serious emotional/behavioral disorders. *Behavioral Disorders.*

Mattison, R. E., Hooper, S. R., & Glassberg, L. A. (2002). Three-year course of learning disorders in special education students classified as behavioral disorder. *Journal of the American Academy of Child and Adolescent Psychiatry, 41,* 1454–1461.

Mattison, R. E., Humphrey, F. J., Kales, S. N., Handford, H. A., Finkenbinder, R. L., & Hernit, R. C. (1986). Psychiatric background and diagnoses of children evaluated for special class placement. *Journal of the American Academy of Child Psychiatry, 25,* 514–520.

Mattison, R. E., Lynch, J. C., Kales, H., & Gamble, A. D. (1993). Checklist identification of elementary schoolboys for clinical referral or evaluation of eligibility for special education. *Behavioral Disorders, 18,* 218–227.

Mattison, R. E., Morales, J., & Bauer, M. A. (1991). Elementary and secondary socially and/or emotionally disturbed girls: Characteristics and identification. *Journal of School Psychology, 29,* 121–134.

Mattison, R. E., Morales, J., & Bauer, M. A. (1992). Distinguishing characteristics of elementary schoolboys recommended for SED placement. *Behavioral Disorders, 17,* 107–114.

Mattison, R. E., Morales, J., & Bauer, M. A. (1993). Adolescent schoolboys in SED classes: Implications for child psychiatry. *Journal of the American Academy of Child and Adolescent Psychiatry, 32,* 1223–1228.

Mattison, R. E., & Spitznagel, E. L. (2001). Longitudinal use of the Teacher's Report Form in tracking outcome for students with SED. *Journal of Emotional and Behavioral Disorders, 9,* 86–93.

Mattison, R. E., Spitznagel, E. L., & Felix, B. C. (1998). Enrollment predictors of the special education outcome for students with SED. *Behavioral Disorders, 23,* 243–256.

McClure, G., Ferguson, H. B., Boodoosingh, L., Turgay, A., & Stavrakaki, C. (1989). The frequency and severity of psychiatric disorders in special education and psychiatric programs. *Behavioral Disorders, 14,* 117–126.

McConaughy, S. H., Mattison, R. E., & Peterson, R. L. (1994). Behavioral/emotional problems of children with serious emotional disturbances and learning disabilities. *School Psychology Review, 23,* 81–98.

McConaughy, S. H., & Ritter, D. (2002). Best practices in multidimensional assessment of emotional and behavioral disorders. In A. Thomas & J. Grimes (Eds.), *Best practices in school psychology IV* (pp. 1303–1320). Washington, DC: National Association of School Psychologists.

McConaughy, S. H., & Skiba, R. (1993). Comorbidity of externalizing and internalizing problems. *School Psychology Review, 22,* 421–436.

Moffitt, T. E. (1993). The neuropsychology of conduct disorder. *Development and Psychopathology, 5,* 135–151.

MTA Cooperative Group. (1999). A 14-month randomized clinical trial of treatment strategies for attention-deficit/hyperactivity disorder. *Archives of General Psychiatry, 56,* 1073–1086.

Ohan, J. L., Myers, K., & Collett, B. R. (2002). Ten-tear review of rating scales: IV. Scales assessing trauma and its effects. *Journal of the American Academy of Child Psychiatry, 41,* 1401–1422.

Penno, D. A., Frank, A. R., & Wacker, D. P. (2000). Instructional accommodations for adolescent students with severe emotional or behavioral disorders. *Behavioral Disorders, 25,* 325–343.

Perry, B. D., Pollard, R. A., Blakley, T. L., Baker, W. L., & Vigilante, D. (1995). Childhood trauma, the neurobiology of adaptation, and "use-dependent" development of the brain: How "states" become "traits." *Infant Mental Health Journal, 16,* 271–291.

Rapport, M. D., Scanlan, S. W., & Denney, C. B. (1999). Attention-deficit/hyperactivity disorder and scholastic achievement: A model of dual developmental pathways. *Journal of Child Psychology and Psychiatry, 40,* 1169–1183.

Rylance, B. J. (1997). Predictors of high school graduation or dropping out for youths with serious emotional disturbances. *Behavioral Disorders, 23,* 5–17.

Schur, S. B., Sikich, L., Findling, R. L., Malone, R. P., Crimson, M. L., Derivan, A., et al. (2003). Treatment recommendations for the use of antipsychotics for aggressive youth: Part I. A review. *Journal of the American Academy of Child and Adolescent Psychiatry, 42,* 132–144.

Silver, S. E., Duchnowski, A. J., Kutash, K., Friedman, R. M., Eisen, M., Prange, M. E., Brandenburg, N. A., & Greenbaum, P. E. (1992). A comparison of children with serious emotional disturbance served in residential and school settings. *Journal of Child and Family Studies, 1,* 43–59.

Sugai, G. (1998). Postmodernism and emotional and behavioral disorders: Distraction or advancement. *Behavioral Disorders, 23,* 171–177.

Swanson, H. L., Hoskyn, M., & Lee, C. (1999). *Interventions for students with learning disabilities: A meta-analysis of treatment outcomes.* New York: Guilford Press.

Wagner, M. M. (1995). Outcomes for youth with serious emotional disturbance in secondary school and early adulthood. *The Future of Children, 5,* 90–112.

Walker, H. M., Colvin, G., & Ramsey, E. (1995). *Antisocial behavior in school: Strategies and best practices.* New York: Brooks/Cole.

Walker, H. M., & Severson, H. H. (1992). *Systematic Screening for Behavioral Disorders: User's guide and administration manual.* Longmont, CO: Sopris West.

10

Curriculum-Based Measurement of Students with Emotional and Behavioral Disorders

Assessment for Data-Based Decision Making

KEITH J. HYATT *and* KENNETH W. HOWELL

In recent years, schools have come under increased pressure to be accountable for student learning and to justify their appropriations (Kane & Staiger, 2002; Marston & Magnusson, 1985). While accountability for student progress is certainly an important goal, many of the instruments currently used to measure student progress have limited instructional utility and may not be accurate indicators of student learning and achievement. The purpose of this chapter is to describe curriculum-based measurement (CBM) procedures as viable, instructionally relevant alternatives to the use of commercially prepared norm-referenced tests (NRTs). Before discussing CBM, a very brief overview of the use of NRTs will be given to help provide a basis for comparison of these two types of assessment strategies.

The 1983 report *A Nation at Risk*, by the National Commission on Excellence in Education, could be considered a major catalyst in the push toward academic excellence with student performance on standardized NRTs used as the basis for gauging student achievement. This report claimed that, when compared to other nations, our schools as a whole were woefully inadequate, and that if another nation had damaged our educational system in such a way, it would be con-sidered an act of war. While some (Berliner & Biddle, 1995; Bracey, 2002) have noted the inaccuracies in the comparison, the push toward the use of standardized norm-referenced testing within the "high stakes" framework of accountability will continue into the foreseeable future. In fact, the 2002 passage of the No Child Left Behind Act provided renewed pressure on schools to demonstrate their effectiveness or face negative consequences, including loss of funding. This increased focus on accountability has resulted in significant changes in school practices, with some states indexing teacher pay and school funding as well as possible school closure, to student performance on commercially prepared norm-referenced achievement tests (Kane & Staiger, 2002; Salvia & Ysseldyke, 2004).

While the results of these group-administered NRTs may provide a basis for describing a child's academic standing relative to peers on that particular test, they are of limited use in developing instructional interventions. Other problems with standardized norm-referenced instruments have also been well documented and include (1) that their emphasis on the reporting of relative standing prevents meaningful comparison between current and expected level of performance, (2) that they are insensitive to incremental changes in learning, and (3) that they are of little use in instructional planning because they are not tied directly to the curriculum (Blankenship, 1985; Good & Jefferson, 1998; Hargrove, Church, Yssel, & Koch, 2002). Despite these concerns, some test publishers maintain that their NRTs are curriculum-based. Since there is no national school curriculum and the tests aren't developed for a particular school or district, this statement is more of a marketing ploy than a fact. While group-administered achievement tests are being used to evaluate the effectiveness of a particular teacher or school, individually administered NRTs are commonly used by special educators in evaluating students and making instructional decisions. These instruments suffer the same inadequacies as the group-administered tests, such as insensitivity to change and lack of instructional utility. Still, students in many special education teacher-training programs are taught that individually administered normed achievement tests provide adequate pre- and postmeasures of student achievement and can be used to evaluate the effectiveness of programming and the attainment of individualized education program (IEP) goals and objectives.

Shinn (2002) noted that CBM and the problem-solving models that are associated with it are important and viable alternatives to the use of traditional norm-referenced measures in making instructional decisions. See Table 10.1 for a brief comparison of the attributes of commercially prepared NRTs with CBM assessment instruments. This table is based on one provided by Howell and Rueda (1996).

One of the most important things to realize about CBM is that it is not typically composed of a set of standardized stimulus materials (however, we will describe some options for using standardized stimulus materials). Rather, it is composed of sets of measurement procedures that can be applied in a standard fashion across a wide range of stimulus materials, including those selected from a student's own classroom. The standardized measurement procedures (sometimes referred to as "overlays" because the same systems can be imposed on a wide range of materials) are made up of rules for administration, scoring, and interpretation.

By following these rules the evaluator may tap into sets of decision rules including behavioral criteria that specify optimal levels of task performance and skill improvement over time. In addition many educational agencies have followed the procedures for developing local curriculum norms using the measurement overlays. For example, staffs at many schools have developed local CBM norms using whatever reading materials are in use within the school. These norms can be compared to other such databases, as well as to behavioral criteria established through research, because they are generated by following the set of measurement rules for scoring CBM oral reading samples that will be explained shortly.

Roberts, Marshall, Nelson, and Albers (2001) conducted a study using CBM within the context of functional behavioral assessment. However, with that exception, few research studies have directly discussed the use of CBM with students who have been identified as having a behavioral disorder. Plasencia-Peinado and Alvarado (2001) make a case that CBM may help reduce assessment bias among linguistically and culturally diverse students because the assessments focus on actual skills being taught, thereby minimizing inferences that may reflect bias. Similarly, McEvoy and Welker (2000) note that increased academic competence might minimize antisocial behavior, especially if literacy skills are improved, because reading can provide students with the opportunity to understand other points of view and to learn prosocial skills by providing students access to stories that have meaning in their own lives and that provide examples of effective use of strategies for dealing with challenging situations. Thus, accurate assessment of the academic skills of students may facilitate provision of effective services for students with behavioral disabilities by helping teachers select appropriate instructional materials. While CBM and the associated problem-solving procedures are not panaceas to current issues related to students with behavioral disorders, or any other group of students, they do provide educators with effective and easy-to-use tools for streamlining their instruction.

Complete coverage of CBM is beyond the scope of this chapter; however, we hope that the information provided here will give you

TABLE 10.1. A Comparison of Commercial NRTs with CBM

Attribute	Norm-referenced achievement tests	Curriculum-based measures
Structure	Traditional format; samples content across a wide range of levels; uses standard sets of stimulus tasks typically selected through item analysis; attempts to summarize standing within general domains such as "achievement" or "reading"; scores represent standing within norm sample.	Sample specific identifiable skills; use tasks drawn directly from the classroom (or representatives of those tasks); results are keyed to instructional objectives; make use of standard "overlay" procedures for scoring; often yield scores in the form of rate data; scores represent behavioral statements.
Use	Useful for comparing students to one another by way of the norming sample; cannot be readministered over a short time frame	Can be used to compare students to local norms; can be used to track student response to treatment; can be administered frequently
View of knowledge	Achievement is a stable trait indicated by performance on a sample of test items	Knowledge is indicated through the demonstration of skill mastery
Cost	Relatively expensive	Relatively inexpensive
Usefulness for individual planning	Limited utility for deciding what to teach and very little utility for deciding how to teach	High utility for deciding what to teach and, through repeated measurement, for deciding how to teach
Usefulness as group outcome measure	Norm-referenced measures recommended for program planning take far to long to administer to be useful for groups	Can be easily adapted to group use
Strengths	Long history of use; established reliability and validity	Aligned with curriculum; can be used for formative evaluation; correlate highly with norm-referenced measures
Weaknesses	Summative use only; limited instructional utility	If curriculum is flawed, CBM will be flawed; some concerns about limited "face" validity

the motivation to pursue more detailed information and implement the practices in your classroom or school (Gavois & Gickling, 2002; Good, Gruba, & Kaminski, 2002; Howell, Kurns, & Antil, 2002; Howell & Nolet, 2000; Shinn, 2002; Stewart & Kaminski, 2002). We will begin by defining CBM, differentiating summative from formative assessment, and then reviewing some key studies related to the validity and reliability of the measures. Since student learning and curricular characteristics vary considerably between elementary and secondary schools, we will discuss studies dealing with these populations separately. We will then describe one problem-solving procedure—curriculum-based Evaluation (CBE)—that is based on CBM, and follow that with an ex-

amination of how the CBM/CBE models might be used for social-behavioral concerns.

CBM AS A UNIQUE ASSESSMENT PROCEDURE

Assessment is the process of gathering information about a student through reviewing records, conducting interviews, observing behaviors, reviewing work samples, and testing (Heartland Area Education Agency 11, 1998; Howell & Nolet, 2000). All teachers make use of data sources such as teacher-made tests, homework assignments, projects, questioning, and publisher-prepared tests that accompany the curriculum. These assessments tend to be informal and are rarely administered in a standardized manner, so the reliability and validity of the data obtained are unknown (Deno, 1985). This is not meant to imply that the data are not useful, because they may provide important information, such as whether the student reads with correct inflection or differentiates fact from fiction. However, to best design instructional programs and assure that students are making adequate progress in the acquisition of basic skills, reliable and valid measurement procedures are required. This is where CBM comes into play. CBM has emerged as an alternative set of standardized assessment procedures that provide reliable and valid measures of student performance in basic skills (Deno, 1985). In addition to providing standardized frameworks for collecting data on students, CBM also allows for the more flexible and frequent data collection required in order to employ formative evaluation.

Assessments can be categorized as either summative or formative, each with its own purpose (Bloom, Madaus, & Hastings, 1981). Traditional classroom assessment practices tend to provide summative information. They are conducted after instruction has taken place and frequently take the form of end-of-unit tests, quizzes, or projects. This information typically provides the basis for determining content mastery and assigning grades. However, rather than waiting for the results of a summative assessment and re-teaching information that was not mastered, teachers can use formative tools to identify areas of skill deficiency and correct the errors before students develop the habit of providing incorrect responses. Formative assessment is conducted during instruction and can be helpful in determining *what*, as well as *how* to teach something. Because the assessment is conducted throughout the instructional process, it assists in determining how a student responds to intervention (Fuchs, 2003). If a student's progress is not satisfactory, the instructional method can be adjusted and followed up with additional formative assessment to determine the impact of instructional modifications on student learning. Thus, the use of formative assessment procedures is critical if teachers are to use effective instructional strategies to maximize student learning (Black & William, 1998).

In brief, CBM consists of a range of simple, standardized measurement procedures that teachers can use to monitor student progress in the curriculum. The procedures have been designed to be quickly administered, usually within 1 minute, and conducted on a repeated basis, once or twice weekly. Data obtained from these measures can be charted to provide a visual depiction of student learning (i.e., skill acquisition as documented through changes in behavior) as well as provide input on student attainment of IEP goals and objectives. This frequent measurement provides teachers with valid and reliable measures of student performance in basic skills that have been shown to be sensitive to incremental student growth. The sensitivity of the measures will allow teachers to make informed and timely instructional decisions regarding the effectiveness of a particular teaching strategy and student learning.

EXAMPLE CBM MEASURES

Following are basic descriptions of standard CBM procedures for reading, mathematics, and written expression. Of the six reading measures described, Oral Reading Fluency tends to be the most used indicator of decoding and comprehension with the highest levels of documented reliability and validity. Reading measures 4, 5, and 6 are rarely used, but they are described here to provide the reader with an understanding of the types of reading measures investigated.

Reading

1. *Oral Reading Fluency.* Students are provided with 300-word passages representative of those in their reading materials and read from these aloud for 1 minute. The number of words read correctly is tabulated and used to gauge reading proficiency (Howell & Nolet, 2000).

2. *Cloze.* Students are provided with a 300-word passage in which the first and last sentences are intact. On the remaining sentences, every fifth word is left blank and students provide the correct missing word, either orally or in writing, during a 1-minute timing. The number of correct words pro-

vided is used to determine reading proficiency (Deno, Mirkin, & Chiang, 1982).

3. *Maze*. This procedure is similar to Cloze. The first and last sentences of the passage are left intact, but rather than leaving every fifth word in the remaining sentences blank, students are required to select the correct word from a group of words provided. The number of words correctly selected from the selection in 1 minute is tabulated to describe reading skill (Howell & Nolet, 2000).

4. *Words in Isolation*. Students read from a list of high frequency words within 1 minute. The number of words read correctly in 1 minute is tabulated (Deno, Mirkin, & Chiang, 1982).

5. *Words in Context*. Students read from passages selected from grade-level materials. Every fifth word is underlined and students orally read the underlined words within 1 minute. The number of words read correctly is tabulated (Deno, Mirkin, & Chiang, 1982).

6. *Word Meaning*. Students are presented with 300-word passages with every fifth word underlined, and they supply the meaning of the underlined word. The number of correct word meanings provided in 1 minute is tabulated (Deno, Mirkin, & Chiang, 1982).

Mathematics

Students are provided with a set of problems taken from the actual curriculum with a representative sample of skills to be taught throughout the year. Students are given 3–5 minutes to complete as many problems as possible, and scoring is based on the number of digits written correctly (Shinn & Bamonto, 1998).

Written Expression

Students are provided with a story starter and given 1 minute to think about what to write. Then they write for 3 minutes, and the number of words written correctly, words spelled correctly, and/or correct word sequences is counted. (Howell & Nolet, 2000; Shinn & Bamonto, 1998).

Reliability and validity data for these procedures will be presented in the following review of studies. But first let's look at a quick snapshot of CBM use in a typical classroom.

Taking reading as an example, imagine that you are in a fourth-grade class where the teacher has placed students into different groups according to their skills. Every day the students do partner reading, and during that time the teacher moves around the class, taking 1-minute samples of oral reading from students. He works on a schedule so that each student reads to him three times a week, and the teacher and the students chart the scores on a graph. The samples are taken from a set of balanced reading passages, and the teacher reviews each student's progress at the end of the week to determine if the progress is adequate by comparing it to expected levels of growth. If not, he or she can make changes to the instruction the student is receiving or to the material from which the student is reading. Then, by continuing to collect the CBM data, the teacher can quickly determine if the changes made in the student's reading program were appropriate.

Now that we have covered the basics of CBM, we will describe some studies that have provided support for the reliability and validity of the measures at both the elementary and secondary levels. The majority of studies investigating CBM have been conducted at the elementary level. Selected studies that have investigated CBM in reading, mathematics, and written expression will be described.

ELEMENTARY-LEVEL STUDIES OF CBM

Reading

A majority of the research in CBM has been conducted in reading, perhaps because lack of reading skill is a leading cause of school failure (Hargrove, Church, Yssel, & Koch, 2002). Deno (1985) noted difficulties inherent in traditional norm-referenced measures of reading and recognized that CBM was a step toward addressing those concerns. Deno (1985) and Deno, Mirkin, and Chiang (1982) also noted, that if alternative measures were to be used by teachers to routinely monitor student progress in reading, the measures must be (1) reliable and valid, (2) simple and efficient, (3) easily understood, (4) inexpensive to implement, and (5) sensitive to change. CBM meets each of these criteria. The following summaries of research studies will provide information on these criteria and examples of how the procedures were implemented.

Deno, Mirkin, and Chiang (1982) conducted three studies that investigated the concurrent validity of five different CBM procedures. These five measures were chosen based on a review of research in the measurement of reading skills and because they appeared to be simple-to-develop measures of reading. These five measures were Words in Isolation, Words in Context, Oral Reading Fluency, Cloze, and Word Meaning.

To determine the degree of concurrent validity, students' performance on these CBM measures was compared to their performance on commercially prepared NRTs. The tests used were the reading comprehension subtest of the Stanford Diagnostic Reading Test and the word identification and word comprehension subtests of the Woodcock Reading Mastery Test.

In study 1, all measures were administered to 33 students in grades 1–5; 15 of the students had learning disabilities. On each of the five CBM tasks, students were given a 60-second time limit to complete the task. The correlations between Words in Isolation, Words in Context, and Oral Reading Fluency measures with the three NRTs were significant, with coefficients ranging from .73 to .91. The correlations between Cloze and Word Meaning measures with the NRTs were also significant, with coefficients ranging from .60 to .83. These values were particularly impressive given that the CBM measures were shorter, easier to score, and produced results of greater instructional utility.

The purpose of study 2 was to determine whether the grade level of the stimulus material and/or length of time the assessment was administered made a difference in the students' performance on CBM. Forty-five students from first through sixth grade participated in this study; 18 of the students had learning disabilities. The following changes were made in the CBM process: Words Aloud, Words in Isolation, and Oral Reading measures included stimulus selected from third-grade instructional materials and were administered in two 30-second and two 60-second tests. Cloze passages were the same, except every 10th word was left blank, and students were given 2 minutes to complete the test On the three read-aloud

tasks, the correlations between performance on the third-grade and sixth-grade measures were in the .80s and .90s. Similar correlations were found between performance on 30-second and 60-second measurements. Again, these results show that it is possible to generate useful information by having students work briefly from curriculum tasks and without resorting to time-consuming NRTs.

Study 3 was conducted to further investigate the findings in studies 1 and 2. Forty-three students without disabilities and 23 students with disabilities in the first through sixth grades participated in this study. A third-grade word list, a sixth-grade list, a 300-word third-grade reading passage, and a sixth-grade cloze passage were the administered. Additionally, different standardized instruments were used for comparison, including the phonetic analysis and reading comprehension subtests of the Stanford Diagnostic Reading Test (SDRT) and the reading comprehension subtest of the Peabody Individual Achievement Test (PIAT). Overall, student performance on all CBM instruments was highly correlated with the standardized measures. In fact, Oral Reading correlations with the Literal and Inferential Comprehension subtests (.78 and .80) on the standardized tests were higher than the correlations between Cloze and those measures (.67 and .71).

The results from these three studies indicate that student performance on the CBM procedures of Oral Reading Proficiency, Isolated Words, and Cloze all correlate strongly with the standardized norm-referenced reading tests. Thus, a student's performance on any of the three CBM measures would be a valid predictor of proficiency in both reading comprehension and decoding. Interestingly, scores on Cloze exercises, a technique frequently used to measure comprehension skills, actually had a stronger relationship with word recognition subtests on the NRTs than with the comprehension subtests. Overall, Oral Reading Proficiency scores correlated as high or higher than Cloze scores with NRT measures of reading comprehension. A second finding of this research was that correct performance was a more valid measure of reading skill than incorrect performance. So, rather than counting errors, teachers would be well advised to count accurate performance as a basis for judging student reading skill. However, since data on inaccurate performance is easy to collect during these assessments, it would make sense to collect that information, because it might help identify student skill deficiencies and guide instruction. A third finding of the study was that valid measures of student reading skill could be obtained through 1-minute measures of Oral Reading Proficiency, making this relatively simple, inexpensive, and quick measure a valuable tool in identifying reading skill. Finally, the researchers found that in most cases the difficulty of words to be read aloud did not impact validity of the measure. An exception to this finding would be if the student could not read any of the words at all.

In the studies described above, samples from the actual instructional material were used by the researchers to develop the CBM instruments. Fuchs and Deno (1994) reviewed the literature to determine whether CBM instruments must be based on the actual school materials. While using the actual materials provides teachers with belief that the measurements are accurate, the authors described studies reporting a mismatch between items on achievement tests and those found in school lessons. Since the difficulty level of different lessons can vary greatly, it is possible that a student may perform well in the actual curriculum being taught and yet perform poorly on the NRT. It is also possible that the NRT does not assess the same skills that are actually taught in the school. While these are concerns, they did note that research regarding the match or mismatch between curricula represented in lessons and NRTs is contradictory, with some finding a high degree of overlap particularly in mathematics. So, there is a question of whether student work samples must be taken from the student's actual lessons to ensure measurement validity and instructional utility of the information.

In their review, Fuchs and Deno found studies reporting that correlations between Oral Reading Fluency and NRTs were almost identical when materials from different basal series were used with the same group of students. They reported that teachers can use materials that are similar to those typically used in instruction as CBM and obtain valid results. They discussed the advantages

and disadvantages of sampling students' performance from the actual reading materials. The major advantage was face validity. However, there were several disadvantages to using the actual instructional materials. First, since the reading difficulty within a single book varies substantially, arbitrary selections of material could result in measurement error. For example, if an easy passage were picked for the Oral Reading Fluency stimulus, the student might receive an inflated score due solely to the passage selection. However, if the teacher uses reading stimuli that are controlled for difficulty, measurement error may be reduced. A second disadvantage to using the actual instructional materials relates to student familiarity with the reading selection. If the material was recently read or discussed in class, it is likely that a student's performance could be influenced. A third disadvantage is the use of highly controlled instructional material with limited phonetic or linguistic patterns. The student may perform well on a CBM from that material but perform poorly when assessed using text that contains more naturally occurring reading materials. In essence, it is possible to conduct instructionally useful assessment using standardized CBM procedures without measuring student performance on the actual instructional material as long as the content of the test passages is similar to that found in standard basal readers. This frees up teachers who may not have the time to develop CBM materials but can purchase commercially available CBM materials. It can also be useful for schools where there is not enough data to develop local norms for use in comparisons of students' performance.

Powell-Smith and Bradley-Klug (2001) noted that there were inconsistencies in the literature regarding the use of commercially prepared versus curriculum-based reading measures in CBM. They conducted a study to compare the performance of 36 second-grade students identified as low-performing readers on two different measures: CBM measures taken from a basal textbook and a commercially prepared CBM measure, the Test of Reading Fluency (TORF). The mean number of words read on the CBM taken from the basal (38.3) was lower than that obtained from the TORF (50.0) However, there was no significant difference in the average slopes of basal and TORF scores when comparing the number of words correct gained per week (2.69 and 2.41, respectively). The results indicate that student performance on the TORF was as accurate at monitoring student reading progress over time as was student performance on CBM materials developed directly from a basal. While it is possible to use commercially prepared CBM materials rather than developing samples from the traditional basals used in elementary schools, many teachers use literature-based basal materials as their instructional materials. Additional research investigated whether the measures were valid when used with these materials instead of the traditional basals that generally have a controlled vocabulary. Hintze, Shapiro, Conte, and Basile (1997) investigated whether there was a difference in the validity of oral reading measures when using the type of literature-based material frequently used in whole language instruction, including "authentic" reading material and literature-based basals. The study was conducted with 57 second-, third-, and fourth-grade students who received their primary instruction in literature-based basals supplemented with "authentic" reading materials. Three passages of at least 200 words were selected from first- through fifth-grade literature-based basals and from "authentic" collections, with these passages controlled for readability. Students read all 30 passages during two consecutive days, and the number of words read correctly was tabulated. For a criterion measure, each student was administered the Degree of Reading Power Test (DRP), which is a modified cloze procedure. This measure consisted of nonficition readings with seven deleted words and five selections to choose from. In isolation, each word would fit the sentence, but when considered in the context of the paragraph, only one word would work. Overall, the mean correlation for DRP and literature-based basal series was .655, and for the authentic trade book series and DRP the mean correlation was .665. Results of the study indicated that, regardless of the basal or "authentic" probes read by the students, both accurately predicted performance on the DRP. Therefore, it appears that CBM measures can be used effectively with "authentic" reading materials when the samples taken from the "authentic" sources

are controlled for readability level, to prevent students from being given extremely difficult passages that could result in errors in decision making.

Bradley-Klug, Shapiro, Lutz, and DuPaul (1998) also compared the performance of second- and fifth-grade students of average reading skill on CBM oral reading assessments drawn from a literature-based series and a traditional basal series. They reported that the mean number of words read correctly was lower on the literature-based probes than on probes taken from basal series. This was a common finding in the previous studies involving literature-based material; despite this fact, the measures described student progress in reading equally well.

In the final elementary reading study to be reviewed, Fuchs and Deno (1992) compared students' performance on two basal series that approached reading instruction from theoretically different perspectives. One series used an eclectic approach, while the other focused on comprehension and decoding skills. For all the difficulty levels of the two basals (ranging from preprimer through seventh grade), two 100-word passages, representative of the reading required at that level, were selected. The criterion measure was student performance on the passage comprehension subtest of the Woodcock Reading Mastery Test (WRMT). The correlations between CBM and WRMT ranged from .89 to .93 and were similar across grade levels and between reading series. Passage difficulty did not impact the validity of CBM measure, and the foci of the different reading approaches did not negatively impact the validity of CBM.

This summary of the research findings for CBM at the elementary level for reading indicates that Oral Reading Fluency measures were valid across grade levels and consistently represented the best measure of reading skill. Student performance on Oral Reading Fluency was highly correlated with both decoding and comprehension skills, was valid whether the instruction used traditional basals, literature-based basals, or authentic reading materials, and correlated highly with standardized norm-referenced measures of decoding and comprehension. Third-grade stimulus was acceptable across grade levels, and commercially available

CBM measures were valid indicators of reading skills. Thus, a large body of research consistently supports the validity of 1-minute CBM reading probes, particularly Oral Reading Fluency, in providing an accurate estimate of overall reading ability in both decoding and comprehension. In conclusion, it appears that the CBM measures yielded essentially the same information as the commercially prepared norm-referenced measures while taking only a fraction of the time to administer and using the student's own instruction materials. The reduced length of test administration alone would seem to be a major advantage for students with limited attention skills or tolerance for academic challenge.

Mathematics

In addition to providing valuable descriptors of reading progress, CBM can also be used to provide a reliable and valid index of student mastery of mathematics skills. To develop a CBM measurement for mathematics based on the actual curriculum, Fuchs, Fuchs, Hamlett, and Steckler (1991) noted that teachers must first identify every type of mathematics problem to be completed by the student during the course of the school year. Then, a short test that represents the content, including equal emphases on particular skill areas, must be developed. Parallel tests should also be developed to ensure that data collected through repeated student performance measures aren't affected by the practice effect. The tests should be administered once or twice a week, and scores should be assigned on the number of digits correct. This process does not indicate which skills the student has mastered; however, it does serve as an indicator of student proficiency in the math curriculum.

Fuchs, et al. (1991) noted that by graphing student performance on a set of CBM mathematics tests, the teacher could compare student growth rate to desired growth rate and modify instructional practices when the desired growth rate was not occurring. When changes in instructional strategy were made, they could be noted on the graph, so future tests could determine whether there was satisfactory change in student growth. Granted, developing a mathematics measure of this kind could take a considerable amount of time. However, the following studies, which describe the use of CBM mathematics measures, computer applications, and instructional support indicate that the time put into test development may be well spent.

Fuchs et al. (1991) investigated student learning in mathematics classes where the teachers were trained and used (1) CBM, (2) CBM with ExS, or (3) received no training, did not use CBM, and served as a control group. ExS was a computer program that provided CBM assessments, tracked and charted student performance, and provided the teacher with expert advice on teaching strategies, based on student performance on the CBM measures. The study involved 33 second- through eighth-grade teachers, each of whom chose two students who were low achievers in math and had been identified as having a mild disability to participate in the study. Students in the CBM and CBM with ExS groups were assessed twice weekly on parallel forms of a math CBM measure consisting of 25 questions each. First-grade students had 1 minute to complete the assessment, second- and third-grade students had 1.5 minutes, and students in grades 4–6, had 3, 4, and 5 minutes, respectively. Counting the number of correct digits and the number of problems that were correct determined the performance score. Teachers in the control group monitored student progress in the usual manner, which included standardized achievement tests, teacher-made tests, observations, daily work samples, and criterion-referenced tests.

Results indicate that CBM did result in more teacher-reported changes in instruction. However, CBM alone did not significantly improve student mathematics achievement, and student performance in the CBM-only group was similar to that of the control group. The teachers who used CBM tended to alter instruction by reteaching (generally using those methods that had previously failed) and by providing additional independent practice. In contrast, the teachers who used CBM with ExS and applied the recommended instructional strategies had students who showed significantly more growth in mathematics than students in either the CBM group or the control group. Thus, while monitoring student performance using CBM procedures is a critical factor in determining the effectiveness of instruction, it appears that some form of consultation or collaborative approach to providing efficient teaching strategies is necessary to improve student achievement.

In another study investigating the use of CBM and computer assisted programming in mathematics, Spicuzza et al. (2001) investigated whether using a commercially prepared basic skills mathematics program, Accelerated Mathematics (AM), as a supplement to a "conceptually based" curriculum that provided little instruction in basic math skills would positively impact student achievement. The subjects in this study included 137 fourth- and fifth-grade students in seven different classrooms and schools where teachers supplemented the core curriculum with AM. The AM program allowed teachers to monitor student progress and assign appropriate practice exercises. The results of the study indicated that the AM group demonstrated significantly more growth than the control group, regardless of grade level, when comparing their performance on the Northwest Achievement Level Mathematics Test, a norm-referenced instrument used in the district. Results on the second measurement used in the district, California's Standardized Testing And Reporting (STAR) Math exam, showed a different pattern. STAR Math is a standardized norm-referenced instrument, and all AM groups showed growth, but the most growth appeared in the middle and high groups. Interestingly, the low and high control groups actually scored lower than they did on the pretest.

Results from this study indicate that use of computer software that provides CBM and appropriate practice exercises in basic skills assists teachers in ensuring that their students acquired basic mathematics skills. This study added to the CBM literature and also to the position that the differentiation between conceptual skills (understanding) and basic skills (facts) is a "bogus dichotomy" (Wu, 1999). In fact, as Wu (1999) recognized, mathematics skills and understanding are intertwined, and students require instruction in both.

In summary, the mathematics studies reviewed indicate that CBM is an effective measure of student proficiency in mathematics. However, these studies also indicate that the use of a computer system that conducts CBM, analyzes skill deficiencies, provides additional practice, and recommends instructional interventions is effective in helping teachers implement instructional strategies that impact student learning.

Written Expression

Deno (1985) recognized that the criterion validity coefficients for CBM measures of written expression were similar to those obtained with CBM measures for reading. In contrast, Fewster and MacMillan (2002) reported that studies have indicated that the reliability and validity coefficients for written expression CBMs were lower but still high enough to make them useful measures. A standard method for conducting CBM for written expression is to provide students with a story starter and give them 3 minutes to write a story. The story is then analyzed to determine the number of words written correctly, spelled correctly, and/or words in correct sequence. Unlike Oral Reading Fluency, this procedure can be conducted with the entire class at one time.

Naquin & Slider (2002) collected 3-minute writing samples 2 days in a row from 179 third- and fourth-grade students. They then scored these samples using 19 separate variables, including total words written and words written in correct sequence. The authors concluded that, while words in correct sequence is a good indicator of skill at written expression, another index, correct punctuation, was also a good indicator of overall writing quality.

SECONDARY-LEVEL STUDIES OF CBM

Earlier discussion has demonstrated that CBM procedures are reliable and valid indicators of the basic skill acquisition of elementary-age students. In this section, the use of CBM at the secondary level will be briefly described.

It is well known that reading tasks change considerably as students move from elementary school, where the focus is on developing basic skills, to the secondary school, where the assumption is that students have the basic skills and the instructional focus changes to obtaining information from content-specific text, such as science and history books. Jenkins and Jewell (1993) indicated that reading aloud from text might be a less sensitive measure of students' skills as they get older, possibly due to the differences in reading tasks in the advanced grades.

Espin and Deno (1993) investigated the predictive power of reading from content text on a variety of school tasks including grade-point average and performance on a standardized achievement test among a group of 121 tenth-grade students. They coined the term "Text-Based Measurement" (TBM), as distinguished from CBM, because the reading tasks required were clearly different than most CBM measures used with elementary students. In this study, secondary students had taken the Tests of Achievement Proficiency (TAP), a commercially prepared norm-referenced test, in fall and completed the TBM in spring.

Three TBM tasks were conducted in both English and science content areas. First, students read for 1 minute from a text passage. In the second TBM, students completed a study task where they were given a passage from a text along with 25 multiple-choice questions to answer as they read. Third, they read again for 1 minute from a text passage. Their performance on Oral Reading Fluency assessments and the reading subtest of the TAP was compared to grade-point average (GPA) and performance on the nonreading subtests of the TAP. For all students, there was a significant, yet moderate, correlation between measures. For the English TBM, correlations ranged from .32 to .50, the science TBM correlations ranged from .37 to .53, and for the TAP reading subtest the correlations ranged from .56 to .86.

Next, they compared the performance of students whose GPA was at or below the 20th percentile with those whose GPA was at or above the 80th percentile to determine whether Oral Reading Fluency scores provided different predictive power based on student achievement level. For GPA, correlations between low-achieving students and Oral Reading Fluency were in the low to moderate range but higher than the correlations for high-achieving students. Correlations between Oral Reading Fluency and TAP subtests were higher for low-achieving students than for the high-achieving students

in all areas. The relationships between Oral Reading Fluency scores and GPA were not as high as the correlations between Oral Reading Fluency and norm-referenced test scores; however, they were significant and indicated that Oral Reading Fluency scores from content area texts can predict academic success at the secondary level, particularly among students with limited reading skills.

As a follow-up to the Espin and Deno (1993) study, Fewster and MacMillan (2002) evaluated the predictive validity of written expression and Oral Reading Fluency scores of 465 sixth- and seventh-grade students on their academic performance in grades 8, 9, and 10. Students completed 1-minute Oral Reading Fluency probes on six short passages taken from grade-level material in the approved curriculum to obtain Words Read Correctly (WRC). The writing probes consisted of six story starters. Each student was given a story starter, 1 minute to think and 3 minutes to write. The writing measure was scored by total number of Words Spelled Correctly (WSC). Two years later, they reviewed student records to determine whether these measures were predictive of placement (special education, remedial, general, honors). Grades were converted to percentages when necessary and were available for all but students enrolled in special education. The grades received in English and social studies were significantly correlated with elementary (grades 6 and 7) CBM scores. Correlations between WRC and English grades ranged from .40 at tenth grade to .58 at eighth grade, and for social studies grades the correlations ranged from .38 at tenth grade to .49 at eighth grade. Correlations between WSC and English grades were generally lower and ranged from .41 at tenth grade to .50 at eighth grade. Correlations between social studies grades and WSC were the lowest, ranging from .31 at tenth grade to .36 at eighth grade. Oral Reading Fluency scores tended to have a higher correlation than WSC, and both measures correlated more highly with English than social studies. When scores from students in special education and remedial placements were combined, both CBM measures reliably predicted group placement into the special education/remedial, general, or honors programs.

The results of secondary school studies provide additional confirmation to the validity of CBM measures; however, the measures don't appear to be as strong as at the elementary level. This may be related to the differences in task and learning demands between elementary and secondary settings. While the studies reported here utilized secondary students, they did not tend to focus on basic skills such as reading and written expression. Few studies can be located which include content of secondary curriculum. As noted by Fewster and MacMillan (2002), this continues to be an area that may benefit from further research. (See Espin & Tindal, 1998, for a detailed review of studies conducted at the secondary level.)

SUMMARY OF CBM

Thus far, we have discussed the methods of conducting CBM in different skill areas, the validity of CBM, and the use of CBM at the elementary and secondary level. While CBM has been shown to be an efficient, inexpensive, easy-to-administer and sensitive measure of student proficiency in basic academics, it also has been shown to be useful in predicting academic success at the secondary level. However, the results from CBM do not necessarily tell teachers "what" to teach. For example, while Oral Reading Fluency is an excellent index for screening to recognize students having difficulty, the scores don't tell whether a student understands inferences, understands the value of skimming or scanning, or knows how to identify a topic sentence. To determine the exact skills in which a student needs instruction, a problem-solving model must be implemented. This need can be addressed using Curriculum-Based Evaluation (CBE). Proper instructional decision making is critical, especially when recognizing that students with disabilities are already behind their peers academically and require effective instructional activities to enhance their learning. If they are to catch up with their peers academically, then they must learn more during a single school year; otherwise, they will remain in a skill deficit position. Simply put, we don't have time to use ineffective instructional methods and just hope for the best. While there is considerable research to support the efficacy of computer applications, the use of computers in determining what to teach is still only an area of promising research (Fuchs, 1998).

CBE MODEL

The following brief description of CBE is based on the work of Howell and his colleagues (Howell, Kurns, & Antil, 2002; Howell & Nolet, 2000). CBE operates under the relatively simple assumption "If a student can't do something, then it is because the student doesn't know how." That is to say, the unsuccessful student must be missing essential knowledge of the task or its subtasks. From this frame of reference, a series of "If . . . then" statements can be constructed based on a task analysis of the curriculum. A sample of these questions is shown in Table 10.2.

Before making instructional decisions within the CBE model, teachers must be familiar with the content and the skill requirements to complete curricular objectives. Thus, one focus of CBE is identifying the prerequisite skills that the student must master to succeed. These learning objectives are identified by conducting a task analysis of the major outcomes in the curriculum (Bateman & Herr, 2003). Since academic behavior will be measured, the task analysis should be written in clearly observable behavioral terms. In other words, they should pass the "stranger test" (Kaplan, 1995). Simply stated, this test asks if someone who was not involved in the development of the curriculum can read and understand the behavioral objectives and the task analysis.

Once the objectives have been identified, performance criteria and proficiency should be determined. Howell and Nolet (2000) identified three levels of proficiency: accuracy, mastery, and automaticity. Accuracy is simply how well a student can perform a particular task. Mastery or fluency is a higher level of proficiency that requires a student to complete a task quickly and accurately. Finally, automaticity is the skill to quickly apply the skills in a variety of novel situations. The automatic performance of skills depends on the student's accuracy and

TABLE 10.2. Sample "If . . . Then" Statements to Guide Evaluation in Basic Computation Facts

If . . .	Then . . .
The student is accurate and fluent	Discontinue
Written work is accurate but slow	Check to see if oral responses are at rate
If oral responses are at rate	Check handwriting fluency
If oral responses are not at rate	Teach math facts
If the student is inaccurate	Check accuracy in an untimed format
If accuracy improves	Emphasize fluency
If accuracy does not improve	Emphasize accuracy

mastery of the skill. The importance of addressing these areas can be demonstrated through a simple reading example. Imagine that a student is reading at a slow rate as indicated by performance on a test of Oral Reading Fluency even though he or she does so at a high level of accuracy. This slow rate may pose a problem as reading assignments get longer—the student may simply not have the time to read assignments and thereby be falling behind academically. While there could be several possible reasons for this type of performance, you might hypothesize that the student has the basic decoding skills but does not apply them fluently. It is this hypothesis that the evaluator would attempt to confirm or reject as he or she searches for an explanation for the accurate but slow reading rate. However, to pursue this hypothesis one must have some idea about what is—or is not—an acceptable level of reading fluency.

Acceptable levels of proficiency can be determined by reviewing research, by developing local norms at the grade, school, or district level, or identifying appropriate goals and objectives in the IEP. (Previously, we discussed the drawbacks of commercially prepared NRTs, but this does not mean that NRTs have no value. Rather, it means that the value of NRTs varies by test and normative group, and locally developed norm-referenced CBM measures may provide more pertinent information for instructional and special education eligibility decision making than the commercially prepared instruments. For a discussion on the development of local norms, see Stewart and Kaminski (2002).

In addition to identifying the levels of pro-

ficiency, a task analysis can be conducted to identify the specific skills that must be mastered in order to perform the objective. In the example above, it may be that the student does not use basic decoding skills fluently and is missing key skills identified through a task analysis of fluent decoding. Instruction could be developed that focuses on the target decoding skills, and the student's progress could be monitored. If skills do not improve, then a different intervention strategy should be developed and implemented. If skill growth is acceptable, then the current instructional strategy should continue until the student has the prerequisite skill required for successful completion of the next academic task identified in the task analysis. It is possible that, for this student, remediation of decoding skill deficits may generalize to other areas in the reading program. That is, more fluent reading may allow for completion of assignments and participation in classroom discussions. CBE uses CBM results as indicators of academic performance but provides a model for diagnosing exactly which skills require further instruction. The following five-step process for conducting CBE is an abbreviated version of that provided by Howell and Nolet (2002).

Step 1: Define Your Purpose

In this step of the decision making process, the teacher must decide why the assessment is being conducted and what type of decision will be based on the results. For example, is the assessment being conducted as a screening to identify possible areas of academic concern, as a specific diagnostic assessment to identify areas requiring remediation, or as a monitoring technique to ensure that the student has maintained learned skills? If screening is desired, a broad-based survey level assessment should be conducted. If the screening indicates a need for further assessment, then a specific diagnostic assessment should be conducted to identify skill deficiencies.

Step 2: Define What Is to Be Measured

Identify exactly what curricular items or skills are to be measured. This can be facilitated by developing a table of specifications, which is an analysis of the skills required by the curriculum. The skills should be described in behavioral terms so that they are made measurable.

Step 3: Devise a Way to Make the Skills in Step 2 Observable

Once the skills are identified, develop a measurement task that will require the student to display the skill(s) identified in step 2. The specific diagnostic measure would be administered only if concerns were identified in the survey assessment and would be a specific measurement designed to identify those prerequisite skills in which a student may have deficiencies.

Step 4: Conduct Assessment

Essentially, this step requires that the assessment be conducted in the standard CBM manner, with the examiner using effective strategies for ensuring accurate results. Some things to consider when conducting the assessment are (1) having all material ready, (2) knowing exactly how to conduct the assessment, (3) developing rapport with the student, (4) observing student behavior during the assessment, and (5) limiting feedback that will indicate to the student how he or she performed on a particular item. In this respect, the implementation of CBE is no different than any other evaluation scheme.

Step 5: Use the CBE Process of Inquiry

As the assessment is being conducted, the information must be used to develop hypotheses regarding student performance and to develop instructional strategies. There are 5 stages in the CBE process of inquiry.

• *Stage 1: Fact finding.* In this stage, you identify what the student actually does. This information may come from many sources, including portfolio assessment, record reviews, and interviews, as well as broadbased or survey CBM.

• *Stage 2: Assumed causes for the problem(s) are developed.* In this stage, the student's performance is analyzed to try to determine what skills the student may, or may not, be missing. Depending on how well the curriculum has been task analyzed, this task may be relatively simple.

• *Stage 3: Validate.* In this stage, the hypotheses in stage 2 are tested. More specific CBM measures are administered, for example, if it is suspected that the student had trouble adding, a measurement could be administered to determine the level of his or her skill in that area.

• *Stage 4: Summative decision making.* In this step, information is used to describe the student's present levels of performance. This provides a record of what the student can and can't do as related to the task.

• *Stage 5: Formative decision making.* During instruction, repeated measures are conducted and the data visually displayed to track student performance. This information is used to determine whether strategies are having the desired effects and to ensure that students maintain newly learned skills.

In summary, the CBE procedure provides a structured approach to making instructional decisions based on student performance of the skills required by the task or in the curriculum. Since it makes use of repeated measures of student performance, it provides an opportunity to determine whether the instructional program is producing the desired outcomes. This is a critical determination because students, especially those with disabilities, require the most effective instruction to avoid falling further behind their peers. Due to the sensitivity of the data collection procedure, the use of CBE may prevent teachers from discontinuing interventions that are making a change in student performance or from continuing interventions that are really having no effect on the targeted behaviors.

IMPLICATIONS FOR STUDENTS WITH BEHAVIORAL DISABILITIES

As noted earlier, there is a relative absence of information on the use of CBM specifically with students with behavioral disabilities. However, given that students with behavioral disabilities exhibit academic skill deficits that require special education services, it is reasonable to assume that CBM and CBE procedures would be appropriate for use with this group of students. If students are provided with effective instruction that provides them with a sense of accomplishment and helps narrow the performance gap between them and their peers, it is likely that fewer disruptive incidents stemming from failure or frustration will occur.

CBM is difficult to conduct within the area of social skills. Part of the difficulty is related to the variability of acceptable social behaviors and the associated lack of a specific curriculum. The variability of acceptable social behaviors means that different behaviors may be acceptable, depending on the locale and social situation. This may represent a strength of using CBM when teaching social skills rather than just relying on published curricula. For example, in some parts of the country, it would be common to hear people greet each other with the word "howdy" while in other parts of the country use of "howdy" in a greeting would be considered unusual. It certainly wouldn't be good practice to teach the student to greet others by saying "howdy" when peers use different terms. This simple digression from the standards of the group could set the student up for taunting and teasing.

The lack of a specific curriculum is also related to the idea of socially acceptable behaviors, or social validity. While there are commercially prepared social skill curricula available, they cannot cover the vast array of skills needed to interact in all situations. While they may provide users with task analyses of certain behaviors as well as instructional and motivational strategies, they can cover only a limited number of behaviors.

Academic skills, such as math, can often be task analyzed and sequenced, but it is hard to argue that there is a specified sequence of social skills and a linear progression of these skills that applies to all persons. While one could make the case that an understanding of 1:1 correspondence is a prerequisite skill for addition, one could not make the same case for most social skills, because social skills are not necessarily hierarchical in nature. For example, "greeting someone" is not a prerequisite for "saying goodbye to someone." However, a task analysis may reveal that there are prerequisite skills for greeting a person, even though those skills may vary by setting or person. So, while 1 + 1 = 2 in all situations and is easily task analyzed, "greeting someone" can be a much more complex skill to analyze and teach. In addition, one must always consider the cultural acceptability of different social behaviors. In the past, "making eye contact" was commonly identified as an area for social skills training; however, researchers have recognized that the use of "eye contact" is governed by cultural values and tradition, thus affecting the social validity of the behavior and the likelihood or wisdom of changing that behavior if it is considered inappropriate in the child's culture.

One aspect of CBM, formative evaluation, should be quite familiar to researchers and practitioners working in the field of behavioral disorders. These professionals have a long history of taking repeated samples of student behavior and recording those samples across time in visual displays. Therefore concepts such as highly focused measurement and formative evaluation are not new to most of the readers of this chapter. So, even though there is still much work to be done in the area of specifying social skills curriculum, it is already clear that one must be able to measure a student's level of social skill performance against some standard of acceptable performance. Because this is a concept that is more familiar to many who work with behavioral content than it is to some who work with mathematics computation or reading the step to implementing CBE may not be as large as it seems.

If a curriculum is available that covers a particular set of social skills in a culturally acceptable manner, then it may provide a task analysis of the skills as well as teaching strategies. If not, then the teacher would be required to conduct the task analysis. Following a task analysis, the teacher could compare the student's performance with that of the peer and determine whether the student was exhibiting a skill deficit (does not know the steps) or a performance deficit (will not perform under the current conditions). Based on this information, the CBE process could be used to identify what to teach. Remember, CBE assumes that a student does not perform a skill because he or she does not have the skills needed to perform it. These include the skills required to deal with particular social situations and reinforcement schedules. Using the CBE process, teachers could develop some reasonable hypotheses for a behavior, by developing a set of "If . . . then" statements. This process is entirely compatible with the process of functional behavioral assessment (O'Neil, Horner, Sprague, Storey, & Newton, 1997).

SOME FINAL THOUGHTS

Curriculum-based evaluation and measurement offers an alternative to traditional test-based evaluation systems that goes well beyond the replacement of NRTs with alternative measures. Shinn (2002) and Shinn and Bamonto (1998) characterized CBM as Dynamic Indicators of Basic Skills (DIBS). The term "Dynamic" indicated that CBM procedures provided measures that were sensitive to changes in student performance. Since the procedures required frequent, repeated measures of student performance, they could help determine whether a particular instructional intervention actually resulted in improved student performance, and when used within a problem-solving approach, could help guide instruction. The term "Indicators" referred to the ability of the measures to describe academic "vital signs" and was described as an "educational thermometer." The use of this thermometer could help determine whether there was a problem, the severity of the problem, the intervention goals, whether the intervention was effective, and when the intervention was no longer needed. Finally, the "Basic Skills" in DIBS indicated that CBM procedures were

typically designed to measure basic skills. Just as a thermometer is a relatively quick way of screening and monitoring a person's health, CBM procedures are quick assessment techniques that screen and monitor students' acquisition of basic skills.

CBM can also assist in meeting the legal requirement that children with disabilities have access to, and make progress in, the general education curriculum because it provides a framework for reliable and valid measurements. Additionally, regulations and best practices require that teachers report student progress in the general education curriculum and identify how the child's disability impacts access/progress in the general education curriculum. CBM certainly provides a more accurate description of these conditions when compared to those "gleaned" from commercially prepared NRTs that are not based on the actual curriculum taught in the schools. Results from CBM can also be used to help develop educationally relevant IEP goals and objectives as well as provide critical information during the screening and eligibility processes (Bateman & Herr, 2003; Fewster & MacMillan, 2002; Hargrove, Church, Yssel, & Koch, 2002; Shinn, 2002). In addition, CBM is probably the only currently available measurement technology that is sufficiently sensitive to instruction to allow the tracking of student responses to intervention. The ability to document reactions to interventions is at the heart of recent calls for modifications in the evaluation algorithm employed when making entitlement decisions for special education (Vaughn & Fuchs, 2003).

While CBM data can be used when making numerous decisions that impact student learning, conducting CBM is surprisingly simple. The data are available for immediate analysis, have high levels of reliability and validity, and can provide for continuous monitoring of student progress. In spite of CBM's strengths, the lack of acceptance of the face validity of the measures appears to have impeded their use (Foegen, Espin, Allinder, & Markell, 2001). In essence, despite research support, many teachers simply do not believe that knowing the number of words correctly read aloud in 1 minute is a reliable measure of reading skill, particularly reading comprehension.

Other reasons for not adopting CBM include: (1) teacher perceived lack of time, (2) lack of training, and (3) faulty beliefs about the validity of CBM (Foegen et al., 2001; Yell, Deno, & Marston, 1992). This means that educators who understand the procedures may need to be the catalyst for increasing the use of CBM procedures at the local level. The information contained in this chapter should provide essential background for accomplishing this task.

As school accountability continues to make headlines, generate debate, and foster legal challenges to the public school system, educators will be called upon to justify their practices. In addition to responsibility to the taxpayers, educators have an even higher level of responsibility to the students they serve. Through the use of reliable and valid formative measures, such as CBM, and a data-driven decision making process, such as CBE, educators will be best prepared to meet current and unforeseen challenges. The technical adequacy of CBM in the basic skills areas has been well documented; however, a few challenges remain: (1) increase the use of CBM in the schools, (2) implement a thoughtful CBE program, and (3) develop a way to incorporate CBM into the behavioral area. Functional behavioral assessment (discussed in Chapter 8, this volume) is one strategy that could be used in conjunction with the CBM/CBE procedures to advance these goals.

REFERENCES

Bateman, B. D., & Herr, C. M. (2003). *Writing measurable IEP goals and objectives*. Verona, WI: IEP Resources.

Berliner, D. C., & Biddle, B. J. (1995). *The manufactured crisis: Myths, fraud, and the attack on America's public schools*. New York: Addison Wesley.

Black, P., & William, D. (1998). Inside the black box: Raising standards through classroom assessment. *Phi Delta Kappan, 80*, 139–148.

Blankenship, C. S. (1985). Using curriculum-based assessment data to make instructional decisions. *Exceptional Children, 52*, 233–238.

Bloom, B. S., Madaus, G. F., & Hastings, J. T. (1981). *Evaluation to improve learning*. New York: McGraw-Hill.

Bracey, G. W. (2002). *The war against America's public schools: Privatizing schools, commercializing education*. Boston: Allyn & Bacon.

Bradley-Klug, K. L., Shapiro, E. S., Lutz, J. G., &

DuPaul, G. J. (1998). Evaluation of oral reading rate as a curriculum-based measure within literature-based curriculum. *Journal of School Psychology, 36*, 183–197.

Deno, S. L. (1985). Curriculum-based measurement: The emerging alternative. *Exceptional Children, 52*, 219–232.

Deno, S. L., Mirkin, P. K., & Chiang, B. (1982). Identifying valid measures of reading, *Exceptional Children, 49*, 36–45.

Espin, C. A., & Deno, S. L. (1993). Performance in reading from content area text as an indicator of achievement. *Remedial and Special Education, 14*, 47–59.

Espin, C. A., & Tindal, G. (1998). Curriculum-based measurement for secondary students. In M. R. Shinn (Ed.), *Advanced applications of curriculum-based measurement* (pp. 214–253). New York: Guilford Press.

Fewster, S., & MacMillan, P. D. (2002). School-based evidence for the validity of curriculum-based measurement of reading and writing. *Remedial and Special Education, 23*, 149–156.

Foegen, A., Espin, C. A., Allinder, R. M., & Markell, M. A. (2001). Translating research into practice: Preservice teachers' beliefs about curriculum-based measurement. *The Journal of Special Education, 34*, 226–236.

Fuchs, L. S. (1998). Computer applications to address implementation difficulties associated with curriculum-based measurement. In M. R. Shinn (Ed.), *Advanced applications of curriculum-based measurement* (pp. 89–112). New York: Guilford Press.

Fuchs, L. S. (2003). Assessing intervention responsiveness: Conceptual and technical issues. *Learning Disabilities Research and Practice, 18*, 172–186.

Fuchs, L. S., & Deno. S. L. (1992). Effects of curriculum within curriculum-based measurement. *Exceptional Children, 58*, 232–243.

Fuchs, L. S., & Deno. S. L. (1994). Must instructionally useful performance assessment be based in the curriculum? *Exceptional Children, 61*, 15–24.

Fuchs, L. S., Fuchs, D., Hamlett, C. L., & Stecker, P. M. (1991). Effects of curriculum-based measurement and consultation on teacher planning and student achievement in mathematics operations. *American Educational Research Journal, 28*, 617–641.

Gavois, T. A., & Glicking, E. E. (2002). Best practices in curriculum-based assessment. In A. Thomas & J. Grimes (Eds.), *Best practices in school psychology* (Vol. 1, pp. 885–898). Bethesda, MD: National Association of School Psychologists.

Good, R. H., Gruba, J., & Kaminski, R. A. (2002). Best practices in using dynamic indicators of basic early literacy skills (DIBELS) in an outcomes-driven model. In A. Thomas & J. Grimes (Eds.), *Best practices in school psychology* (Vol. 1, pp. 699–720). Bethesda, MD: National Association of School Psychologists.

Good, R. H., III, & Jefferson, G. (1998). Contemporary perspectives on curriculum-based measurement. In M. R. Shinn (Ed.), *Advanced applications of curriculum-based measurement* (pp. 61–88). New York: Guilford Press.

Hargrove, L. J., Church, K. L., Yssel, N., & Koch, K. (2002). Curriculum-based assessment: Reading and state academic standards. *Preventing School Failure, 46,* 148–151.

Heartland Area Education Agency 11. (1998). *Technical Manual: Academic and social/behavior problem decision making.* Johnston, IA: Author.

Hintze, J. M., Shapiro, E. S., Conte, K. L., & Basile, I. M. (1997). Oral reading fluency and authentic reading material: Criterion validity of the technical features of CBM survey-level assessment. *School Psychology Review, 26,* 535–553.

Howell, K. W., Kurns, S., & Antil, L. (2002). Best practices in curriculum-based evaluation. In A. Thomas & J. Grimes (Eds.), *Best practices in school psychology* (Vol. 1, pp. 753–772). Bethesda, MD: National Association of School Psychologists.

Howell, K. W., & Nolet, V. (2000). *Curriculum-based evaluation: Teaching and decision making* (3rd ed.). Belmont, CA: Wadsworth/Thomson Learning.

Howell, K. W., & Rueda, R. (1996). Achievement testing with culturally and linguistically diverse students. In L. A. Suzuki, P. J. Meller & J. G. Pontertotto (Eds.), *Handbook of multicultural assessment* (pp. 253–290). San Francisco: Jossey-Bass.

Jenkins, J. R., & Jewell, M. (1993). Examining the validity of two measures of formative teaching: Reading aloud and maze. *Exceptional Children, 59,* 421–432.

Kane, T. J., & Staiger, D. O. (2002). The promise and pitfalls of using imprecise school accountability measures. *Journal of Economic Perspectives, 16*(4), 91–114.

Kaplan, J. S. (1995). *Beyond behavior modification* (3rd ed.). Austin, TX: Pro-Ed.

Marston, D., & Magnusson, D. (1985). Implementing curriculum-based measurement in special and regular education settings. *Exceptional Children, 52,* 266–276.

McEvoy, A., & Welker, R. (2000). Antisocial behavior, academic failure, and school climate: A critical review. *Journal of Emotional and Behavioral Disorders, 8,* 130–140.

National Commission on Excellence in Education. (1983, April). *A nation at risk: The imperative for educational reform.* Retrieved May 20, 2003, from *http://www.ed.gov/pubs/NatAtRisk/title.html.*

Naquin, G. M., & Slider, N. J. (2002). Moving beyond total words written: The reliability, criterion validity, and time cost of alternative measures for curriculum-based measurement in writing. *School Psychology Review, 31,* 477–497.

O'Neil, R., Horner, R., Sprague, R., Storey, K., & Newton, J. (1997). *Functional assessment of problem behavior: A practical guide* (2nd ed.) Pacific Grove, CA: Brooks/Cole.

Plasencia-Peinado, J., & Alvarado, J. L. (2001). Assessing students with emotional and behavioral disorders using curriculum-based measurement. *Assessment for Effective Intervention, 26,* 59–66.

Powell-Smith, K. A., & Bradley-Klug, K. L. (2001). Another look at the "c" in CBM: Does it really matter if curriculum-based measurement reading probes are curriculum based? *Psychology in the Schools, 38,* 299–312.

Roberts, M. L., Marshall, J., Nelson, R. & Albers, C. (2001). Curriculum-based assessment procedures embedded within functional behavioral assessments: Identifying escape-motivated behaviors in a general education classroom. *The School Psychology Review, 30,* 64–77.

Salvia, J., & Ysseldyke, J. E. (2004). *Assessment in special and inclusive education* (9th ed.). New York: Houghton Mifflin.

Shinn, M. R. (2002). Best practices in using curriculum-based measurement in a problem-solving model. In A. Thomas & J. Grimes (Eds.), *Best practices in school psychology* (Vol. 1, pp. 671–698). Bethesda, MD: National Association of School Psychologists.

Shinn, M. R., & Bamonto, S. (1998). Advanced applications of curriculum-based measurement: "Big ideas" and avoiding confusion. In M. R. Shinn (Ed.), *Advanced applications of curriculum-based measurement* (pp. 1–32). New York: Guilford Press.

Spicuzza, R., Ysseldyke, J., Lemkuil, A., Kosciolek, S., Boys, C., & Teeluchsingh, E. (2001). Effects of curriculum-based monitoring on classroom instruction and math achievement. *Journal of School Psychology, 39,* 521–542.

Stewart, L. H., & Kaminski, R. (2002). Best practices in developing local norms for academic problem solving. In A. Thomas & J. Grimes (Eds.), *Best practices in school psychology* (Vol. 1, pp. 737–752). Bethesda, MD: National Association of School Psychologists.

Vaughn, S., & Fuchs, L. S. (2003). Redefining learning disabilities as inadequate response to instruction: The promise and potential problems. *Learning Disabilities Research and Practice, 18,* 137–146.

Wu, H. (1999). Basic skills versus conceptual understanding: A bogus dichotomy in mathematics education. *American Educator, 27*(3), 14–52.

Yell, M. L., Deno, S. L., & Marston, D. B. (1992). Barriers to implementing curriculum-based measurement. *Diagnostique, 18,* 99–112.

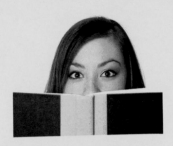

Avoid Fines!

Items should be **returned** on or before the last date on the label or renewed (see overleaf)

Term-time opening hours:

08:30am - 6.00pm
Tuesday, Wednesday & Thursday

08:30am – 4.30pm

Monday & Friday

Fines:

7 Day & Standard loan:

20p per item per day then after 4 days overdue:

50p per item per day

1 & 3 Day loans:

£1 per item per day

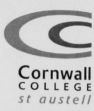

Cornwall
C O L L E G E
st austell

Renewing:
To renew items, please contact the Learning Centre

 In person
with your ID Card

 By phone on
01726 226787

 By e-mail
staustell.learningcentre@
cornwall.ac.uk

 Online @
http://
webopac.cornwall.ac.uk/

or via this QR code:

Log-in with your ID number to renew your items online

11

Early Identification and Prevention of Emotional and Behavioral Disorders

MAUREEN A. CONROY, JO M. HENDRICKSON, *and* PEGGY P. HESTER

Prevention of emotional and behavioral disorders seems to be everyone's rhetorical darling, but I have come to the sad conclusion that most of our talk about prevention is of little substance. We often find ways to avoid taking primary or secondary preventive action, regardless of our acknowledgment that such prevention is a good idea. Other concerns take precedence, and as a result we are most successful in preventing prevention itself.

—JAMES KAUFFMAN (1999, p. 448)

The prevention of problem behaviors, antisocial behaviors, school violence, and educational failure receives a great deal of publicity and often takes center stage in the political arena as well as the national media. The *Twenty-Third Annual Report to Congress* (2001) substantiates this national concern, with statistics showing a trend of increasing numbers of school-age children at risk for or identified as having emotional and behavioral disorders (EBD). Research offers solid evidence that the majority of severe and chronic problem behaviors demonstrated by school-age children and adolescents emanate from behavior patterns established during the early childhood years (e.g., Campbell & Ewing, 1990; Patterson, Capaldi, & Bank, 1989; Webster-Stratton, 2000). Unfortunately, current identification and intervention policies and practices are *reactive*, targeting children once *significant* behavior problems are well established and

more difficult to impact. As a result of these flawed policies and practices, children are labeled EBD and given diagnoses such as conduct disorder when *proactive* identification of and intervention with those same youngsters earlier in life might have prevented the development of EBD. We concur with leaders in the field who argue eloquently for the vital need to focus our attention and resources on children who are at risk for EBD—especially young children with significant behavior problems (Kauffman, 1999; Shonkoff & Phillips, 2000). In this chapter we address this imperative by providing a synthesis of key aspects of the early identification, prevention, and intervention literature pertaining to EBD in young children. The following four areas are discussed: (1) prevalence of EBD in young children, (2) current identification and service delivery policies and practices, (3) evidence-based intervention practices, and (4) implications for future research and practice.

PREVALENCE OF EBD IN YOUNG CHILDREN

There is an alarming increase in the number of young children with problem behaviors in early childhood settings (Briggs-Gowen, Carter, & Skuban, 2001; Kaiser, Cai, Hancock, & Foster, 2002). Accumulated evidence suggests that problem behaviors may originate in young children as early as the toddler years and often persist over time into adolescence and adulthood (Briggs-Gowen et al., 2001). Although limited normative data are available regarding the prevalence of emotional and behavioral problems in 1- to 2-year-olds, Briggs-Gowan and colleagues (2001) note that rates of emotional and behavioral problems in 2-year-olds range from 12% to 16%, with one-third of those toddlers demonstrating a significant delay in social-emotional competence. In addition, Mathiesen and Sanson (2000) indicate that 37% of 18-month-olds who demonstrate emotional and behavioral problems continue to exhibit troubling behaviors 1 year later. Similarly, Lavigne et al. (1998) report that over 50% of 2- to 3-year-olds with psychiatric disorders continue to demonstrate psychiatric characteristics 1–2 years later. Webster-Stratton (1997) concludes that 7–25% of all preschool-age children demonstrate significant problematic behavior, and Jones-Harden and colleagues (2000) report that 24% of the children in Head Start have externalizing behavior problems (e.g., overt, acting out, disruptive behaviors) in the clinical or borderline range, and 6.5% have internalizing behavior problems (e.g., covert, withdrawn behaviors).

Unfortunately, the prevalence rate of EBD increases markedly based on children's exposure to multiple risk factors. For example, Kaiser and her colleagues indicate that as many as 21–33% of the children served in Head Start demonstrate significant problem behaviors (Kaiser et al., 2002). When followed longitudinally, Forness and his colleagues (1998) determined that many children displaying significant problem behaviors in early childhood were at high risk for school failure and later being identified as

EBD. Campbell (1994) notes that preschool-age children who demonstrate significant problem behaviors have a 50% chance of demonstrating continued problems such as peer rejection, drug abuse, depression, juvenile delinquency, and school dropout during their adolescent years. Indeed, many of these high-risk children are likely to have problems well into adulthood (Kazdin, 1993). Without early identification and proactive prevention of young children at risk for the development of EBD, problem behavior patterns are very likely to continue to develop (Del'Homme, Kasari, Forness, & Bagley, 1996) and lead to long-term, chronic, and disabling conditions (Patterson, Reid, & Dishion, 1992). Given the alarming statistics, early identification of at-risk young children and the realization of proactive preventative services are more pressing needs than ever.

CURRENT IDENTIFICATION AND SERVICE DELIVERY POLICIES AND PRACTICES

Multiple and complex factors combine to impinge negatively on the early identification of young children with emotional and behavioral problems and the delivery of efficacious intervention strategies. In addition to the lack of a federal definition that is sensitive to the unique characteristics of young children, we briefly discuss factors that negatively affect prevention services—factors such as eligibility criteria, entry into available programs/service systems, lack of universal screening, and the lack of a coordinated, comprehensive service delivery system (Brown et al., 1996; Conroy, Brown, & Brown, 1998).

Currently, multiple entry points and multiple service delivery options are available to proactively identify and provide services for young children at risk for or with EBD (for a review of service delivery systems, see Smith & Fox, 2003). These systems and services range from privately funded, clinic-based mental health programs that target specific populations such as children with attention-deficit disorders to publicly funded community- and school-based early intervention programs serving a range of children with varying abilities and needs. Since the development of EBD is linked to a number of child and environmental risk factors (Conduct Problems Prevention Research Group [CPRRG], 1992), often there is no single entry point for identification or service delivery. One common point of identification and entry into services is through existing community-based child care programs and federally funded programs targeting children with identified disabilities, or programs such as Head Start serving children who live in poverty (Smith & Fox, 2003). However, children and families are just as likely to be referred by medical professionals (e.g., private pediatricians, public health centers) or, unfortunately, not be identified at all (Smith & Fox, 2003).

Although there are a wide variety of available services and programs to address the needs of young children at risk for or with EBD, there are a number of factors that impede young children's access to these services, resulting in considerable delays in the identification and provision of services. For the most part, access to services usually is based on a program's eligibility criteria rather than on the needs of children and families. Thus, proactive and systematic identification of high-risk children with specific needs matched to services seldom occurs. For example, in order for children to attend Head Start, families must demonstrate a substantial level of financial need or meet Head Start criteria as a child with a disability. Young children served by programs funded through the Individuals with Disabilities Education Act (IDEA) must meet the local education agency criteria for having a developmental delay or an identified disability that impacts their ability to learn. Other programs, generally speaking, have even more restrictive eligibility requirements and may only serve children who have a specific diagnosis such as conduct disorder (e.g., Webster-Stratton & Hammond, 1997).

Service delivery systems that have eligibility criteria that exclude participation of all children who may benefit limit children's access to primary services, and, as a result, children are less likely to receive preventative services. In many community programs, for example, preschoolers with behavior problems are not eligible for services unless they have additional cognitive, language, or social delays (Bryant, Vizzard, Willoughby, & Kupersmidt, 1999). Due to these and other limitations and biases in the current service systems, procedures for identifying young children with EBD are more often than not *reactive* in nature. Consequently, an unacceptably large percentage of needy children do not meet a program's eligibility criteria and end up "falling through the cracks" (Conroy et al., 1998). Not receiving primary prevention services early in life, only to be identified later for tertiary services, after the child's EBD patterns of behavior are fully developed and entrenched across environments and people, is devastating for these young children and families.

A related factor that hinders young children's identification and access to intervention is the lack of a universal, systematic, comprehensive screening program. Although many researchers have discussed the need for early identification and primary prevention services (e.g., see Kauffman, 1999, for a discussion) and models have been proposed in the literature (e.g., Forness, Kavale, MacMillan, Asarnow, & Duncan, 1996), for the most part, proactive identification and prevention models are not being implemented on a wide-scale basis (Smith & Fox, 2003). If we are to identify children at a young age and provide preventative services, we need to implement large-scale systematic, comprehensive screening programs that will detect children who are at a heightened risk for developing EBD (Kamps, Kravits, Stolze, & Swaggart, 1999). To date, little research exists on the effectiveness of systems of identification or on systems of service for young children at risk for or with EBD. Clearly, the need to further develop, implement, and research systems that effectively screen for, identify, and provide intervention for these young children and their families should be a high priority nationally and locally.

BASIC TOOLS OF EARLY IDENTIFICATION

It seems reasonable to assume that a proactive system of early detection and identification of young children at risk for or with EBD is the first step toward prevention. Similar to the identification of other disabilities, early identification of EBD should include multiple sources of data (Patterson et al., 1992). To obtain accurate information to be used in identification of children at risk for EBD, indirect, direct, and multimodal approaches are recommended. Of these, we wish to stress the important role and value of direct observation of children in multiple contexts interacting with others in natural settings (Feil, Severson, & Walker, 1998).

Indirect Measures

Although a number of indirect measures are available to assist in early identification of EBD, we will focus only on several of the most widely used tools, including the Early Screening Profile (ESP; Walker, Severson, & Feil, 1995), the Social Skills Rating Scale (SSRS; Gresham & Elliot, 1990), and the Child Behavior Checklist (CBCL; Achenbach, 1991, 1997).

The Early Screening Profile (Walker et al., 1995) is a multigated screening tool that assists in identifying children 3–5 years old who display externalizing and/or internalizing behavior and are at high risk for the development of EBD. The ESP includes three stages. In completing stage 1, the early childhood practitioner is asked to rank the top five children in the classroom who are demonstrating externalizing and internalizing problem behaviors. Stage 2 requires the early childhood practitioner to complete five checklists, including the *Critical Events Index (CEI)*, *Adaptive Behavior Scale*, *Maladaptive Behavior Scale*, *Aggressive Behavior Scale*, and *Social Interaction Scale* on each of the children identified in stage 1. These checklists provide more detailed information by examining the frequency and intensity of the externalizing or internalizing behaviors demonstrated by target children. However, stage 2 requires additional teacher time to complete checklists on each child. Data on target children obtained in stage 2 are then compared to a normative sample of children of the same age and gender. The children who are identified in stage 2 as high-risk are evaluated in stage 3. Stage 3 includes direct observational measures of the target children's behavior in academically related and social settings. Data gathered and calculated for the target children at stage 3 are compared to data of children of the same age and gender; a standardized score is obtained.

The ESP provides a strategy for identifying young children who are at high risk for the development of EBD and in need of preventative intervention techniques. The efficacy and utility of the ESP has been extensively researched and empirically validated (see Feil & Becker, 1994; Feil et al., 1998; Feil, Walker, Severson, 1995; Feil, Walker, Severson, & Ball, 2000), and it is recommended as a universal screening device to identify children who are at heightened risk for the development of EBD.

A more in-depth identification tool that focuses on social skills development is the Social Skills Rating Scale (Gresham & Elliott, 1990). The SSRS has both a teacher (SSRS-T) and parent (SSRS-P) rating form for identifying high-risk children ages 3–8 years old. The SSRS examines both social and behavioral skill deficits in such categories as cooperation, social initiations, and aggression. The rating scale uses a Likert scale from 0 to 2 (0 indicating never and 2 indicating very often), and a standardized score is obtained. The SSRS score can be used as one measure in the identification of young children at high risk for the development of EBD.

Finally, the Child Behavior Checklist (Achenbach, 1991, 1997) is one of the most widely used instruments for identifying young children with or at risk for EBD. Extensive research supports its reliability and validity (see Achenbach, 1991). The CBCL is appropriate for use with children ranging in ages from 2 to 18 years old, and it differentiates children who demonstrate clinically significant problem behaviors from those who do not. The CBCL is a checklist that can be self-administered or administered by an interviewer; parents and teachers typically complete it. When completing the CBCL, informants rate children's behaviors using a 3-point Likert scale ranging from "not true" to "often true." The CBCL consists of 118 items that evaluate target children's behavior problems and 20 social competency items that evaluate children's adaptive behaviors. As with the other instruments, a score from the CBCL should serve as one measure in the identification process.

Direct Measures

In many ways, the most vital component of the process of identifying children at risk for or with EBD is direct observation of child behavior within natural settings. Such observations allow for an evaluation of the frequency, intensity, and topography of the behaviors as well as the impact of environmental factors on the occurrence of the behaviors. Although several direct observation instruments are commercially available to employ in the observation of children, the most commonly used method is an antecedent–behavior–consequence analysis (A–B–C) that was developed many years ago (Bijou, Peterson, & Ault, 1968). The A–B–C is a direct measure that involves careful observation and recording of events that occur prior to and following the target behavior(s). When the measure is repeated over time, the trained observer is able to identify "patterns" that surround the behavior. In turn, these behavior patterns assist in identifying factors that are contributing to and are maintaining the target behavior. Although an A–B–C assessment does not identify the "cause" of a problem behavior, the technique provides critical information that can directly be used to enhance the appropriateness and efficacy of an intervention strategy. In addition, an A–B–C assessment can be used to help differentiate patterns of behavior across settings, tasks, or activities, and between individuals. (For a more complete description of A–B–C analysis, see Kerr & Nelson, 2002.)

Multimodal Approaches

Clearly, no single approach will suffice in the identification of young children at risk for EBD. Many researchers have suggested that early identification should begin with the implementation of universal screening procedures, such as the Early Screening Profile (see Kaiser et al., 2002; Serna, Nielsen, Lambros, & Forness, 2000). Implementing a universal screening procedure such as the multigated ESP is a proactive, cost-effective method for identifying high-risk children. Following the universal screening of a cohort of young children, a comprehensive evaluation across caretakers, peers, and settings is recommended. This comprehensive evaluation should use a multimodal approach and include the direct and indirect standardized measures described earlier. We are confident that, with comprehensive evaluation procedures in place, practitioners can reliably identify children who need proactive and preventative interventions to minimize the risk of the development of EBD.

RESEARCH-BASED INTERVENTIONS FOR YOUNG CHILDREN WITH EBD

A host of programs have been developed to respond to the prevention and intervention needs of young children with or at risk for EBD. Our goal in this section is to highlight several model programs, including (1) the Regional Intervention Program, (2) Incredible Years, (3) First Step to Success, and (4) the Fast Track Project. Each of these programs targets young children who demonstrate significant problem behaviors, and each emphasizes preventative practices. In addition, each of these programs has rigorous evidence demonstrating its effectiveness, durability, and utility. We provide a description of the program, followed by a brief overview of the research evidence.

Regional Intervention Program

The Regional Intervention Program (RIP) is a time-tested, data-based, parent-implemented early intervention program that provides comprehensive services to parents and children under the age of 60 months who are at risk for the development of EBD (Ora, 1972). The children and families served by RIP exhibit a wide range of presenting problems, from severe developmental delays to mild behavior disorders; however, young children with moderate to severe behavioral disorders constitute the largest group of participants in RIP (Timm, 1993).

All of the RIP children who demonstrate problem behaviors (and their families) are provided direct intervention and training through the *Behavior Management Module*. The Behavior Management Module is designed to teach parents new ways of interacting with their children to decrease problem behaviors. Parents and children participate in individual play sessions that proceed through five phases—baseline, intervention, reversal, intervention, and follow-up. The baseline phase consists of three to five sessions in which the current levels of child and adult behavior are assessed. During the first intervention, parents are taught to apply the principles of differential reinforcement to reduce problem behaviors while interacting with their children. This phase helps parents understand the relationship between their behavior and their child's behavior. Following intervention, a reversal phase is instituted; parents are instructed to stop using differential reinforcement and are provided an opportunity to observe the effects of withdrawing the intervention on the child's behavior. Next, the intervention is reinstated and supplemented with individual programming to solve behavior problems the parents or child's teacher may have outside of RIP. Finally, a follow-up phase is instituted in which sessions at RIP are systematically faded.

Ten factors constitute parent training at the RIP. These factors have been shown to be critical to the program's long-term effectiveness.

1. RIP focuses on early intervention for children 5 years old or younger. Targeting problem behaviors for intervention at an early age appears to thwart the development of further behavioral problems (Strain & Timm, 2001).
2. RIP emphasizes treating problem behaviors rather than diagnostic labels. Parents do not need a referral to enroll in RIP, nor do children need a diagnosis. This admission policy helps children who have behavioral issues that are not at clinically significant level.
3. RIP offers ongoing year-round enrollment. Parents do not have to wait to enroll themselves (i.e., no residency requirement) or qualify their children (i.e., no evaluation requirement).
4. RIP's parent implementation feature is central to its success (Hester, 1977; Timm, 1993). While many early intervention programs emphasize parent involvement, in RIP parents assume key roles and responsibilities in program implementation. Simply put, without parents there is no program. By way of example, veteran parents in RIP are directly responsible for clinical and management functions generally reserved for professionals in other service agencies. With the exception of three resource members of the staff who hold masters'

degrees in special education or a related discipline, parents run and manage the day-to-day operation of RIP. Parents are responsible for conducting behavior management sessions with new parents, collecting data on child and parent progress, implementing programs in the classroom for individuals and groups of children, conducting intake interviews with prospective parents and follow-up sessions after families have completed the program, and implementing and monitoring intervention programs to remediate problem behaviors at home, in the community, and at school. Although parents are the primary interventionists, RIP has a resource person assigned to each parent–child dyad. This person is responsible for coordinating all services necessary to meet the family's needs and acts as a case manager for issues related to different aspects of referral and treatment.

5. RIP's data-based interventions are a critical component. Many service delivery systems and intervention programs purport to be data-based; however, in RIP, all programming decisions related to parent–child interaction sessions as well as decisions regarding classroom behavior, home interventions, or interventions in community classrooms are based on analysis of reliably collected and graphed data.
6. RIP has a unique payback component. Rather than charging fees, family members (typically the mothers) agree to participate in the program by working with their children and other families during the active treatment period. Parents provide services and training for new families after the work with their child is complete. This arrangement not only provides personnel to manage the daily operation of RIP but also serves to strengthen the skills learned by parents in their individual sessions by generalizing those skills across settings, with other children and families, and over time. Moreover, the acts of teaching and supporting novice parents reinforce and solidify the skills of the veteran parents.
7. RIP creates a support network for families through parent involvement, commitment, and interactions with one an-

other. This network operates in a functional manner on- and off-site as well as across time and settings. The active involvement and leadership of parents also helps connect parents to services as the child progresses and reaches various developmental milestones.

8. RIP conducts follow-up interviews (every 6 months) once families and children complete the intervention and payback period. These may be in the form of a follow-up session at RIP, a phone call consultation, or a face-to-face meeting with the parents. In the process, the need for new transitional services and support for children who are moving to other settings may become apparent. Transition assistance in the form of booster training, consultation, and referral occur naturally at this time.

9. RIP includes a systematic management and program evaluation tool that ensures that the program is accountable to its clients, funding sources, and resource personnel. Such a tool provides RIP measures of treatment integrity and assists in program refinement.

10. RIP has been successfully replicated nationally and internationally, testifying to the robustness and feasibility of the model. Replication is a high and necessary standard of a program's ultimate feasibility, utility, and durability.

Each of the components of RIP has been identified singularly and in combination as essential in early intervention programs for the prevention of EBD. Because of the unique nature of the types of services provided through RIP, it is not easy to isolate the most salient components that contribute to its success. It is likely that the interaction of multiple programmatic features contribute to the positive longitudinal outcomes associated with RIP.

Two studies (Strain, Steele, Ellis, & Timm, 1982; Strain & Timm, 2001) examine the long-term effects of the behavior skills training of RIP parents and children. The results, based on direct observational assessments in school and home settings, indicate long-term maintenance of intervention gains and highly acceptable ratings of consumer satisfaction of intervention strategies. The first study consisted of 40 families who were 3–9

years posttreatment (Strain et al., 1982). Results showed that parent behavior in the home setting was consistent with the skills parents learned at RIP and that during parent–child interactions in the home former RIP children were overwhelmingly positive and complied with parent requests. In addition, Strain and colleagues found no significant differences in classroom teachers' commands, negative feedback, and positive reinforcement when the teachers' attention was directed toward former RIP children or randomly selected peers.

The second study (Strain & Timm, 2001), based on direct observation assessments in the school and home settings, recruited 23 different families that were 3–9 years posttreatment. Results replicate the findings of the previous study with families who had received treatment from an entirely different intervention staff. Another aspect of this follow-up study included the use of a rating scale to evaluate the employment status, educational history, and problem behavior history of former RIP children. These former RIP children indicate long-term treatment gains and rated RIP intervention strategies as highly acceptable. Moreover, cumulative data obtained from 1,300 RIP families indicated the short-term efficacy of treatment effects for parents with diverse demographic backgrounds. Strain and Timm (2001) hypothesize that the parents continued the use of the skills due to the acceptability and usefulness of the learned behavioral strategies demonstrated over time.

In summary, RIP has an extensive database documenting its effectiveness over time and populations. The research indicates that hands-on training with parents in behavioral principles (to change their interaction patterns with their children) appears to have positive long-term implications, reducing factors related to the development of EBD.

Incredible Years

Incredible Years is an empirically validated intervention program targeting children ages 3–12 who are at risk for or have a conduct disorder (Webster-Stratton, Reid, & Hammond, 2001). Incredible Years is designed to promote social competence while preventing and treating conduct problems and aggression through an intensive training program targeting parents, teachers, and children. As described by Webster-Stratton and her colleagues (2001), the three objectives of Incredible Years are (1) to promote social competencies, (2) to promote parent competencies and strengthen families, and (3) to promote teacher competencies and strengthen home–school connections. There are several training components of the Incredible Years program for different ages and populations (e.g., Basic, Advanced, School-Age, Supporting Your Child's Education). The Basic and Advanced parent training series each lasts approximately 12 weeks and involves group discussions with 12–14 parents and a group leader. Discussions are used to review various situations depicting children's prosocial and problem behaviors and adult responses to the behaviors. Parents are taught skills such as interactive play, reinforcement, appropriate use of time out, and skills for ignoring problem behaviors. Videotape modeling is used to illustrate techniques for fostering appropriate behaviors and decreasing problem behaviors in children. A collaborative approach to training is emphasized by including parents in group discussions, problem-solving strategies, and supports. The Advanced training program supplements the Basic training by addressing family risk factors, such as marital problems, depression, and lack of social support systems.

The teacher training series of the Incredible Years is modeled in a manner similar to the parent training series. Teachers are taught concepts such as providing teacher attention and praise, using reinforcement to motivate children to engage in appropriate behaviors as well as preventing problem behaviors, building positive social relationships with children, and developing social skills and problem-solving skills in the classroom. Similar to the parent training approach, teachers meet in a group and discuss videotape vignettes.

The third component of the Incredible Years program is a child intervention program called *Dina Dinosaur Social Skills and Problem Solving Curriculum* (see Webster-Stratton & Hammond, 1997). The curriculum is coordinated with the parent and teacher training programs; it teaches children social competence, peer interaction skills, and conflict resolution strategies, and

it is coordinated with the parent and teacher training programs. Once again, videotape modeling is used to teach and reinforce skills. Puppets are used to help illustrate and provide appropriate social skill models. One of the benefits of the Incredible Years program is that the procedures and products needed for implementation are standardized, assuring a high level of consistency in application, fidelity of implementation, and replicability (Webster-Stratton et al., 2001).

The Incredible Years training series has an extensive research base that documents its effectiveness and utility in addressing conduct disorders in young children (Gross et al., 2003; Webster-Stratton, 1998; Webster-Stratton et al., 2001). The Basic program has been examined across a series of studies indicating improvement in parent–child interactions, a reduction in inappropriate disciplinary strategies, and a reduction in conduct problems (see Webster-Stratton, 1984; Webster-Stratton, 1989; Webster-Stratton, Hollinsworth, & Kolpachoff, 1989). The Advanced program has been demonstrated to improve parents' problem-solving and communication skills as well as increasing social and problem-solving skills of children at home (Webster-Stratton, 1990).

As noted, a number of studies were conducted to examine the effectiveness of the Incredible Years program. In 1998, Webster-Stratton investigated the effectiveness of the parent training component with 394 mothers whose children were enrolled in Head Start. Using a controlled, randomized design, nine Head Start centers were assigned to an experimental or a control condition. In the experimental condition, parents, teachers, and family service providers were provided training in the Basic program, as described above. The results indicate a significant decrease in negative parenting styles and an increase in positive discipline strategies in the experimental group in comparison to the control group. In addition, the teachers report that parents in the experimental group were more involved in their children's education. Finally, the children in the experimental group demonstrated increased positive affect and less problem behaviors. Follow-up was conducted after a year, and the results were maintained.

In another study, Gross and colleagues (2003) examine the effectiveness of the Basic training program in child care centers serving low-income parents who were ethnically diverse. Eleven centers were randomly assigned to one of the following conditions: (1) parent and teacher training, (2) parent training only, (3) teacher training only, and (4) wait list control group. The target children in the study ranged in age from 2 to 3 years old. Gross et al. report significant gains in parents' self-efficacy and positive discipline practices in both the parent training only and parent and teacher training groups. In addition, the toddlers whose parents received treatment demonstrated a decrease in problem behaviors, which was still maintained a year later.

In a third study, Webster-Stratton et al. (2001) examine the effectiveness of the parent and teacher training program as a preventative program for 4-year-old children enrolled in Head Start. Thirty-four classrooms were randomly assigned to experimental and control conditions. Following intervention, the mothers who received intervention demonstrated lower negative parenting styles in comparison to the control group mothers. In addition, the parent–teacher bond was significantly higher in the experimental group, and the children in the experimental group demonstrated significantly fewer conduct problems at school. Finally, the experimental group teachers demonstrated improved classroom management skills. Again, after a year, the effects of the experimental group were maintained for the parents and children.

In summary, Incredible Years is an early intervention program that research has documented as highly effective in reducing behaviors related to the development of EBD in young children. In addition, the research indicates that the Incredible Years program has been successful in remediating coercive parenting interaction and discipline styles as well as improving the teacher–child interaction and parent–teacher bond. Finally, it appears from the results that Incredible Years is not only effective but also durable over time.

First Step to Success

First Step to Success (Walker et al., 1998) is an early intervention program for kindergarten-age children who are at risk for develop-

ing EBD. First Step to Success is composed of three levels of intervention. The first level is screening children in kindergarten to identify those children at heightened risk for development of EBD. For a screening tool, the Early Screening Profile (Feil et al., 1995), described earlier, is used to identify children in the classroom who may benefit from intervention. The second level of the First Step to Success program provides instruction to teachers and facilitates teaching targeted children and peers strategies for promoting social-behavioral skills. The third and final level is a home-based component that provides families of targeted children strategies for facilitating children's success in school. First Step to Success is a very intensive program that lasts approximately 3 months. A brief overview of program components and the research conducted evaluating the efficacy and durability of the program follow.

The school-based intervention of First Step to Success is designed to teach children appropriate academically related skills and social skills while interfacing with the existing classroom curriculum. Children identified through screening are targeted for intervention that addresses their specific problem behaviors. Behavioral goals are developed for each child, and each child is provided reinforcement for meeting appropriate behavior goals. First Step to Success uses a consultant training model. In the beginning, the consultant implements the intervention, gradually fading into a supervisory role as the teacher learns how to implement the program. Following an intervention phase, a maintenance phase occurs in which the teacher, consultant, and parent work together to improve the child's appropriate behavior.

The home-based component is very intensive. First Step consultants make weekly home visits, teaching parents intervention strategies for managing their children's problem behaviors. Again, parents are taught strategies for reinforcing appropriate behaviors as well as strategies for developing their children's problem-solving and social skills. Six specific skills are targeted in the home-based program: (1) communication and sharing, (2) cooperation, (3) limit setting, (4) problem solving, (5) friendship making, and (6) developing confidence.

A number of comprehensive studies have

been conducted evaluating the effectiveness of the First Step to Success program. Walker and colleagues (1998) report the results of a 4-year study designed to evaluate the home and school components of the First Step to Success program. Their investigation included 46 kindergartners identified as "high-risk" through the screening process. A randomized, experimental, wait-list control group design was utilized to evaluate the effects of the intervention components. The results indicate that the target children's problem behaviors decreased significantly (i.e., aggressive behaviors were indicated to be within the normal range as measured by the CBCL) and their academically engaged time increased to within the normal range. Children's adaptive increased and maladaptive behavior also improved slightly. Follow-up investigations indicated that children's behavioral improvement was maintained for several years.

In another investigation, Golly and colleagues conducted a replication of previous research and extended the research by examining the social validity of the First Step to Success program (Golly, Stiller, & Walker, 1998). Twenty kindergarten-age students from 10 schools were included in the study. As found in previous research, the results indicated that academic engagement and adaptive skills increased while maladaptive and aggressive behaviors decreased. Additional data collected indicated that the training was rated highly by the teachers, and approximately half of them continued to implement the program subsequent to training.

In a recent investigation, Golly and colleagues (Golly, Sprague, Walker, Beard, & Gorham, 2000) conducted an in-depth investigation of the First Step to Success with two sets of twins attending kindergarten. Over time, they examined specific problem behaviors including noncompliance, inappropriate touching, out of seat, talking out, and academic engaged time. Using a single-subject multiple baseline design across participants, the results indicated substantial increases in appropriate behaviors across all four participants.

In summary, there is ample evidence to support the positive effects of the First Step to Success early intervention program. As the research indicates, the First Step to Success program has been implemented across a number of children and classrooms, resulting in positive gains. In addition, it appears that these positive results maintain for a period of time, and some teachers are likely to continue to implement the intervention following training.

Fast Track Project

The Fast Track Project (Conduct Problems Prevention Research Group [CPPGR], 1992, 2000, 2002) is a multisite, multicomponent prevention intervention for young children who are at risk for the development of conduct problems. The theoretical principles and clinical strategies utilized in the Fast Track Project are predicated on a biopsychosocial model of the development of chronic conduct problems in adolescence (Dodge & Pettit, 2003). The theory posits that the multiplicity of reciprocal influences among biological dispositions, contexts, and life experiences serve to exacerbate or diminish antisocial development over time. This developmental model proposes that proximal changes in parenting, school success, and social cognition are correlated to distal changes in antisocial outcomes (CPPRG, 2002). The primary aims of the Fast Track Project (CPPRG, 2000) are to develop, implement, and evaluate an intervention to prevent conduct problems in children as they move from early childhood into adolescence.

The Fast Track Project (CPPRG, 1992, 2000, 2002) provides for multistage screening of all kindergarten children and has been implemented in four diverse geographical sites selected as high-risk based on neighborhood crime and poverty statistics. Teacher and parent ratings of problem behavior were combined to identify high-risk children, whose mean age is 6.5 years (SD = 0.48). The Fast Track intervention is implemented in two phases—an elementary school phase and an adolescent phase. Both phases of intervention include universal and specifically indicated interventions (according to criterion-referenced assessments) to promote competency development in parents, teachers, and children. For the purposes of this chapter, we will focus on the elementary school phase.

The elementary school phase of the Fast Track Project includes universal prevention at the school level, standard prevention support services to high-risk families, and individualized prevention support for children and families as needed. This phase focuses on parenting, child problem-solving and emotional coping skills, peer relations, classroom atmosphere and curriculum, academic achievement with a focus on reading, and home–school relations.

Extensive research has been conducted on the Fast Track Program. Various assessment procedures have been used to evaluate change, including rating scales, interviews, peer nominations, and direct observations in homes and schools. Outcome measures have been obtained on children's aggressive-disruptive behaviors, social cognition and reading skills, peer relations and social competence, and parenting behaviors.

Four-year outcomes are reported on target children's behaviors, including aggressive and oppositional behavior at home, social preference, association with deviant peers, and teacher-reported child behavior change. Findings indicate a modest positive effect on parent reports of aggressive behavior, peer social preference, association with deviant peers, and teacher ratings of social and academic competence (CPPRG, 2002).

The Fast Track Project has been applauded as an impressive prevention and intervention project (Prinz, 2002) and as a landmark in the fields of child psychopathology research and prevention science (Hinshaw, 2002). It is a complex model, with each component theoretically driven (CPPRG, 1992, 2002; Prinz, 2002). Yet, the Fast Track Project is not without its controversies and questions (Hinshaw, 2002; Prinz, 2002). It is a model that is not easily replicated with individual children, and the complexity of the intervention makes it difficult to identify the most salient aspects of its effectiveness (Hester, Baltodano, Gable, Tonelson, & Hendrickson, 2003; Hinshaw, 2002; Prinz, 2002). In any intervention of large magnitude, the occurrence of false positives in the identification of children at high risk is increased. As Hinshaw (2002) points out in his review of this research, early results may not predict adolescent outcomes, as the complexity of the intervention is a liability when attempting to isolate causal processes underlying children's behavior change.

Summary and Synthesis of Evidence-Based Practices

Although a number of other worthy early intervention projects exist, due to space constraints, we have limited our chapter to only four empirically supported early intervention programs serving young children with or at risk for EBD. All of these programs have credible evidence as to their effectiveness and durability for remediating behavioral deficits in children, 6 years and under. We remind the reader that this is not an exhaustive review, and we encourage examination of other successful early intervention programs such as KidTalk (Kaiser, Hancock, & Hester, 1998) and Parent Training Interaction Therapy (PCIT; Eyberg, Boggs, & Algina, 1995). The projects discussed in this chapter have a number of features worth reiterating. First, as illustrated in this chapter, early intervention is key. Next, these successful programs each provided for training that (1) directly and systematically teaches parents new techniques for addressing their children's problem behaviors and (2) directly teaches parents how to work collaboratively with and within the school. The four programs reviewed specifically focus on changing adult–child interactions and working directly with the parents to reduce or eliminate coercive interactional patterns. Behavioral principles appear to be the bedrock of this training. Across programs, training occurred in relatively short but intense periods of time and was accomplished in small groups or 1:1 instruction. These formats allow for individual feedback and provide a mechanism for ongoing support. Successful programs provide direct intervention to children as well as services and supports to address the broader needs of families. While universal screening was a component of only two of the four programs reviewed (e.g., First Step to Success and Fast Track), universal screening is recommended and holds great promise as a cost-effective strategy for early identification.

RECOMMENDATIONS FOR FUTURE RESEARCH AND PRACTICE

The research and practice agenda of early intervention programs for EBD often are or appear to be at odds with one another. This is a natural tension that must be surmounted if the scientific basis for early identification and prevention of EBD is to advance. Research and the scientific method, for example, rely on procedural consistency and adherence to preestablished protocols within which confounding variables are minimized or eliminated so that results can be attributed to treatment. Practice, on the other hand, is obligated to be responsive to the individual client within the constraints of the social service, community, and educational agencies that provide funding. Practice is frequently driven by the expertise, flexibility, and creativity of the service provider, and the idiosyncratic process may be more immediately rewarding than a standardized approach. With this in mind, we use this section to offer suggestions to improve research and practice in the prevention of EBD in young children. We recognize that often it is easier to identify the shortcomings of research and practice than to make cogent, tenable recommendations; we will strive for balance in this regard.

Specifying precisely what constitutes a quality program of early intervention for children with or at risk for EBD is not simple (Bailey, Aytch, Odom, Symons, & Wolery, 1999). Most experts (e.g., Hamblin-Wilson & Thurman, 1990; Hester & Kaiser, 1998; Hester et al., 2003; Rule, Fietchtl, & Innocenti, 1990; Rous, Hemmeter, & Schuster, 1994) agree that prevention of EBD requires intervention across multiple environments by multiple agents over time, with continued intervention, support, and transition services as children reach developmental milestones and advance to new settings with new expectations. Child characteristics, parent characteristics, the interaction patterns between the parent and child, and how that relationship is influenced by economic, cultural, and social circumstances all affect children's development and thus must be taken into account in program development (CPPRG, 1992). The long-term efficacy of the intervention process appears to be dependent largely on its continuity and consistency across persons, across settings, and over time. Putting these elements of intervention into place is not an easy undertaking. As researchers, theorists, and practitio-

ners, our mission is to identify efficacious, replicable strategies that lead to prevention and remediation of EBD in young children. We have learned and must remember that neither the so-called problem nor its solution resides solely in the child. That is, our focus should never be exclusively on the child's behavioral excesses or deficits; unequivocally, we can conclude that the dependent variable(s) of interest as well as the independent treatment variable(s) are more complex than child behavior change. At a minimum we must be concerned with assessing and impacting the interface between behavior and environment.

Kauffman (1999) contends that for early intervention is to be successful it is imperative that we provide young at-risk children with environments that both directly teach and actively support adaptive behaviors. This recommendation implies that we focus our efforts on modifying environments, not children. Our examination of four successful early intervention programs underscores the importance of environment on child short- and long-term outcomes. We can readily ascertain that, in research and practice, effective intervention is multidimensional and takes into account child characteristics as well as the characteristics and cultural expectations of the settings in which they live and learn.

In the remainder of this section we delineate six key issues researchers in early preventative intervention must continue to address. These issues are discussed in greater detail by Hester et al. (2003). As a preface, however, we should point out that, although we have not emphasized the fact that children, families, and neighborhoods have many strengths and that often these strengths are ignored in the research literature or understated in practice, they are in fact the basis upon which good intervention programming takes place. The mandate to do no harm is in part fulfilled when the interventionist clearly identifies, articulates, and builds upon the strengths of the child, family, and community. Relatedly, individuals and groups of individuals have preferences, and it is equally important that these preferences are voiced, recognized, and accounted for in the development of intervention plans and programs.

Participant Characteristics and Selection Criteria

As evidenced in our review of programs, no standard definition and no objective criteria for identifying EBD in young children exist. This dilemma is further compounded by wide variability in the instrumentation used by researchers and practitioners to identify children at risk for EBD. To obtain accurate, generalizable results, it is essential that we develop standardized terminology, objective criteria, and valid, reliable instrumentation (August, Realmuto, Crosby, & MacDonald, 1995). These tasks and related issues are clearly within the mission of our institutions of higher education and professional organizations as well as local and national government educational leadership agencies.

In addition to the above issues, research reveals that parents and teachers do not identify the same children as high-risk (Kaiser et al., 2002; Offord et al., 1996). Unfortunately, many researchers continue to rely exclusively on informant-based data, and this can be problematic. Informant-based assessment is indeed more efficient and cost-effective than direct observation; however, direct observation is by far more reliable (Bailey et al., 1998) and should not be omitted in favor of indirect measures.

Also noteworthy is the fact that many programs do not target prevention and intervention services until children are at least 5 years old. The earlier intervention begins, the more effective it will be (Kamps & Tankersley, 1996; Kauffman, 1999) and the less likely that secondary complications will arise (e.g., Guralnick & Bennett, 1987). If we are to prevent EBD, then we need to begin as early as problematic behavior patterns are observed. A standard definition and objective criteria would help to identify children at-risk for EBD and contribute immensely to our ability to conduct research that can be aggregated as well as disaggregated for analysis purposes.

Types of Measures

Measurement is the backbone of behavioral science, and our ability to determine the effectiveness of any educational intervention relies on proper measurement. Unfortu-

nately, the most common method of identifying the severity of specific problem behaviors in young children is the use of adult informant(s) (e.g., parent, teacher, child care provider) and indirect measurement tools that often have poor reliability and validity. Further compounding the measurement problem is the common practice of using a single informant. Since EBD is defined by the occurrence of problematic behavior over settings and time, using a single informant on an indirect measure may not provide an accurate representation of the child's behavioral characteristics. In short, for correct interpretations of data and sound decision making, it is critical that sensitive and accurate measures be used in research and practice targeting young children at risk for or with EBD.

Type and Length of Intervention

Few would contest the sentiment that multidimensional intervention is essential for successful early intervention/prevention programming (see CPPRG, 2000; Dodge, 1993; Kaiser & Hester, 1997). The origins of behavior problems in adolescence and adulthood appear to be linked to behavioral problems in childhood. Behavioral issues often arise early in the lives of children and can persist for decades without intervention. The evidence-based programs we present in this chapter all provide intense but relatively brief treatments. Although follow-up data were collected indicating that much of the progress made by the children and caregivers was maintained, with the exception of the Regional Intervention Program follow-up outcome evaluations and needs assessments are not common in the literature. Furthermore, research is lacking that evaluates the effectiveness of the current continuum of services for children at risk for EBD.

Treatment Effects and Fidelity

Implementation itself poses challenges to researchers and practitioners. Recruitment and retention of participants (Hester & Kaiser, 1998; Ikeda, Simon, & Swahn, 2001) becomes more challenging with multicomponent and comprehensive interventions.

Monitoring and maintaining treatment fidelity is a critical component made more difficult as the complexity of interventions increases. Evidence of treatment fidelity gives one confidence in the interpretation of results. Written intervention protocols, fidelity checklists that align with intervention components, and well-trained and supervised intervention agents to promote consistency in intervention implementation over time are integral to quality programs (Dumas, Lynch, Laughlin, Smith, & Prinz, 2001). Ultimately, it is the researchers' responsibility to demonstrate that their interventions were implemented with integrity.

Social Validity

The need for measuring social validity, that is, consumer satisfaction, can be argued as supercilious or of great importance. Although an intervention may be difficult and disliked, it may be effective. However, in education effectiveness is not the ultimate standard for research or practice. For both researchers and practitioners in early intervention and prevention of EBD, there are pragmatic reasons to assess the social validity of a program and its components. Effective programs are likely to be multidimensional and complex to implement. Participant involvement across time and settings is essential. Therefore, it is critical that the services are highly acceptable to and viewed positively by program participants. Attrition and retention will undermine theoretically sublime (but pragmatically intrusive or misunderstood) treatment programs. Of the programs we reviewed, social validity was typically examined as an afterthought. Clearly there is a need for future research to include social validity measures—if only to determine factors that may have lessened positive outcomes. Social validity information not only can provide insight into issues of participant attrition and retention but also can inform our strategies for recruiting future participants and refining our programs to more effectively meet participant needs (McNaughton, 1994). Needless to say, policymakers and funding agencies are deeply concerned about the relationship between program effectiveness and consumer satisfaction (Wolery, 1987).

Longitudinal Assessment

It is self-evident that the outcomes and impact of early intervention on young children at risk for EBD can only be understood when treatment effects are monitored over time. Historically, many factors have limited the quantity and quality of longitudinal data collection. However, the importance of considering longitudinal trends and effects cannot be overstated when policymakers and those in leadership positions prioritize and allocate limited resources.

SUMMARY

In this chapter we reviewed the prevalence and characteristics of EBD in young children, current identification and service delivery policies and practices, basic tools of early identification, research-based interventions, and recommendations for future research and practice. The literature presented documents the power of preventative intervention in the short- and long-term outcomes of children at risk for and with EBD. Although much work remains to improve existing programs and further the scientific study of these programs and their components, a primary goal at this point should be to encourage and enable the wide application of quality early intervention practices with the objective of preventing emotional and behavioral disorders in young children.

ACKNOWLEDGMENTS

Development of this chapter was partially supported with funding from the U.S. Department of Education, Office of Special Education Programs, Center on Evidence-Based Practices: Young Children with Challenging Behavior (Grant No. H324Z010001), and the U.S. Department of Education, Office of Special Education Programs, Earn as You Learn Behavior Disorders Master Teacher Preparation Program (Grant No. H325H000108). The opinions expressed by the authors are not necessarily reflective of the position of or endorsed by the U.S. Department of Education.

REFERENCES

Achenbach, T. (1991). *The Child Behavior Checklist: Manual for the teacher's report form.* Burlington: University of Vermont, Department of Psychiatry.

Achenbach, T. (1997). Guide for the caregiver-teacher report form for ages 2–5. Burlington: University of Vermont, Department of Psychiatry.

August, G. J., Realmuto, G. M., Crosby, R. D., & Mac-Donald, A.W. (1995). Community-based multiple-gate screening of children at risk for conduct disorder. *Journal of Abnormal Child Psychology, 23,* 521–544.

Bailey, D. B., Aytch, L. S., Odom, S. L., Symons, F., & Wolery, M. (1999). Early intervention as we know it. *Mental Retardation and Developmental Disabilities, 5,* 11–20.

Bailey, D. B., McWilliam, R. A., Darkes, L. A., Hebbeler, K., Simeonsson, R. J., Spiker, D., & Wagner, M. (1998). Family outcomes in early intervention: A framework for program evaluation and efficacy research. *Exceptional Children, 64,* 313–329.

Bijou, S. W., Peterson, R. F., & Ault, M. H. (1968). A method to integrate descriptive and experimental field studies at the level of data and empirical concepts. *Journal of Applied Behavior Analysis, 1,* 175–191.

Briggs-Gowen, M. J., Carter, A. S., & Skuban, E. M. (2001). Prevalence of social-emotional and behavioral problems in a community sample of 1- and 2-year-old children. *Journal of American Academy of Child and Adolescent Psychiatry, 40,* 811–819.

Brown, W., Conroy, M. A., Fox, J. J., Wehby, J. H., Davis, C. A., & McEvoy, M. A. (1996). *Early intervention for young children at risk for emotional/behavioral disorders: Implications for policy and practice.* Reston: VA: Council for Children with Behavioral Disorders.

Bryant, D. M., Vizzard, L. H., Willoughby, M., & Kupersmidt, J. (1999). A review of interventions for preschoolers with aggressive and disruptive behavior. *Early Education and Development, 10,* 47–68.

Campbell, S. B. (1994). Behavior problems in preschool children: A review of recent research. *Journal of Child Psychology and Psychiatry, 36,* 113–149.

Campbell, S. B., & Ewing, L. J. (1990). Follow-up of hard-to-manage preschoolers: Adjustment at age 9 and predictors of continuing symptoms. *Journal of Child Psychology and Psychiatry and Applied Disciplines, 31,* 871–889.

Conduct Problems Prevention Research Group. (1992). A developmental and clinical model for the prevention of conduct disorder: The FAST Track Program. Special Issue: Developmental Approaches to Prevention and Intervention. *Developmental Psychopathology, 4,* 509–527.

Conduct Problems Prevention Research Group. (2000). Merging universal and indicated prevention programs: The Fast Track Model. *Addictive Behaviors, 25,* 913–927.

Conduct Problems Prevention Research Group. (2002). Evaluation of the first 3 years of the Fast Track prevention trial with children at high risk for adolescent conduct problems. *Journal of Abnormal Child Psychology, 30,* 19–36.

Conroy, M., Brown, W. H., & Brown, W. (1998, July). Serving young children with emotional and behavioral challenges in early childhood programs: Policy and research issues. Paper presented at the Head Start 4th National Research Conference, Washington, DC.

Del'Homme, M.A., Kasari, C., Forness, S. R., & Bagley, R. (1996). Prereferral intervention and children at risk for emotional or behavioral disorders. *Education and Treatment of Children, 19,* 272–285.

Dodge, K. A. (1993). The future of research on the treatment of conduct disorder. *Development and Psychopathology, 5,* 311–319.

Dodge, K A., & Pettit, G.S. (2003). A biopsychological model of the development of chronic conduct problems in adolescence. *Developmental Psychology, 39,* 349–371.

Dumas, J. E., Lynch, A. M., Laughlin, J. E., Smith, E. P., & Prinz, R. J. (2001). Promoting intervention fidelity: Conceptual issues, methods, and preliminary results from the Early Alliance prevention trial. *American Journal of Preventive Medicine, 20*(1), 38–47.

Eyberg, S. M., Boggs, S. R., & Algina, J. (1995). Parent–child interaction therapy: A psychosocial model for the treatment of young children with conduct problem behavior and their families. *Psychopharmacology Bulletin, 31,* 83–91.

Feil, E. G., & Becker, W. C. (1994) Investigation of a multiple-gated screening system for preschool behavior problems. *Behavioral Disorders, 19,* 44–55.

Feil, E. G., Severson, H. H., & Walker, H. M. (1998). Screening for emotional and behavioral delays: The early screening project. *Journal of Early Intervention, 21,* 252–266.

Feil, E. G., Walker, H. M., & Severson, H. H. (1995). Young children with behavior problems: Research and development of the early screening project. *Journal of Emotional and Behavioral Disorders, 3,* 194–202.

Feil, E. G., Walker, H. M., Severson, H. H., & Ball, A. (2000). Proactive screening for emotional/behavioral concerns in Head Start preschools: Promising practices and challenges in applied research. *Behavioral Disorders, 26,* 13–25.

Forness, S. R., Kavale, K. A., MacMillan, D. L., Asarnow, J. R., & Duncan, B. B. (1996). Early detection and prevention of emotional and behavioral disorders: Developmental aspects of systems of care. *Behavioral Disorders, 21,* 226–240.

Forness, S. R., Ramey, S. L., Ramey, C. T., Hsu, C., Brezausek, C. M., MacMillan, D. L., Kavale, K. A., & Zima, B. T. (1998). Head Start children finishing first grade: Preliminary data on school identification of children at risk for special education. *Behavioral Disorders*, 23, 111–124.

Golly, A. M., Sprague, J., Walker, H. M., Beard, K., & Gorham, G. (2000). The First Step to Success Program: An analysis of outcomes with identical twins across multiple baselines. *Behavioral Disorders*, 25, 170–182.

Golly, A. M., Stiller, B., & Walker, H. M. (1998). First Step to Success: Replication and social validation of an early intervention program. *Journal of Emotional and Behavioral Disorders*, 6, 243–249.

Gresham, F. M., & Elliot, S. N. (1990). *The Social Skills Rating System (*SSRS). Circle Pines, MN: American Guidance Service.

Gross, D., Fogg, L., Webster-Stratton, C., Garvey, C., Julion, W., & Grady, J. (2003). Parent training of toddlers in day care in low-income urban communities. *Journal of Consulting and Clinical Psychology*, 71, 261–278.

Guralnick, M. J., & Bennett, F. C. (1987). *The effectiveness of early intervention for at-risk and handicapped children.* New York: Academic Press.

Hamblin-Wilson, C., & Thurman, S. K. (1990). The transition from early intervention to kindergarten: Parental satisfaction and involvement. *Journal of Early Intervention*, 14, 55–61.

Hester, P. P. (1977). Evaluation and accountability in a parent-implemented early intervention service. *Community Mental Health Journal*, 13, 261–267.

Hester, P. P., Baltodano, H. M., Gable, R. A., Tonelson, S. W., & Hendrickson, J. M. (2003). Early intervention with children at risk for emotional/behavioral disorders: A critical examination of research methodology and practices. *Education and Treatment of Children*, 26, 362–381.

Hester, P. P., & Kaiser, A. P. (1998). Early intervention for the prevention of conduct disorder: Research issues in early identification, implementation, and interpretation of treatment outcome. *Behavioral Disorders*, 24, 57–65.

Hinshaw, S. P. (2002). Prevention/intervention trials and developmental theory: Commentary on the Fast Track special section. *Journal of Abnormal Child Psychology*, 30, 53–59.

Ikeda, R. M., Simon, T. R., & Swahn, M. (2001). The prevention of youth violence: The rationale for and characteristics of four evaluation projects. *American Journal of Preventive Medicine*, 20(1), 15–21.

Jones-Harden, B., Winslow, M. B., Kendziora, K. T., Shahinfar, A., Rubin, K. J., Fox, N.A., Crowley, M. J., & Zahn-Waxler, C. (2000). Externalizing problems in Head Start children: An ecological exploration. *Early Education and Development*, 11, 357–385.

Kaiser, A. P., Cai, X., Hancock, T. B., & Foster, E. M. (2002). Teacher-reported behavior problems and language delays in boys and girls enrolled in Head Start. *Behavioral Disorders*, 28, 23–29.

Kaiser A. P., Hancock. T. B., & Hester, P. P. (1998). Par-

ents as co-interventionists: Research on applications of naturalistic language teaching procedures. *Infants and Young Children*, 10, 1–11.

Kaiser, A. P., & Hester, P. P. (1997). Prevention of conduct disorder through early intervention: A social-communicative perspective. *Behavioral Disorders*, 22, 117–130.

Kamps, D. M., Kravits, T., Stolze, J., & Swaggart, B. (1999). Prevention strategies for at-risk students and students with EBD in urban elementary schools. *Journal of Emotional and Behavioral Disorders*, 7, 178–188.

Kamps, D. M., & Tankersley, M. (1996). Prevention of behavioral and conduct disorders: Trends and research issues. *Behavioral Disorders*, 22, 41–48.

Kauffman, J. M. (1999). How we prevent the prevention of emotional and behavioral disorders. *Exceptional Children*, 65, 448–468.

Kazdin, A. E. (1993). Treatment of conduct disorder: Progress and directions in psychotherapy research. *Development and Psychopathology*, 5, 277–310.

Kerr, M. M., & Nelson, C. M. (2002). *Strategies for addressing behavior problems in the classroom* (4th ed.). Columbus, OH: Merrill/Prentice Hall.

Lavigne, J. V., Arend, R., Rosenbaum, D., Binns, H. J., Christoffel, K. K., & Gibbons, R. D. (1998). Psychiatric disorders with onset in the preschool years: Stability and diagnosis. *Journal of American Academy of Child and Adolescent Psychiatry*, 37, 1246–1254.

Mathiesen, K. S., & Sanson, A. (2000). Dimensions of early childhood behavior problems: Stability and predictors of change from 18 to 30 months. *Journal of Abnormal Child Psychology*, 28, 15–31.

McNaughton, D. (1994). Measuring parent satisfaction with early childhood intervention programs: Current practice, problems, and future perspectives. *Topics in Early Childhood Special Education*, 14, 26–48.

Offord, D. R., Boyle, M. H., Racine, Y., Szatmari, P., Fleming, J. E., Sanford, M., & Lipman, E. L. (1996). Integrating assessment data from multiple informants. *Journal of the American Academy of Child and Adolescent Psychiatry*, 35, 1078–1085.

Ora, J. P. (1972). The involvement and training of parent- and citizen-workers in early education for the handicapped and their implications. In J. B. Jordan & R. F. Daily (Eds.), *Not all little wagons are red* (pp. 66–76). Washington, DC: Council for Exceptional Children.

Patterson, G. R., Capaldi, D., & Bank, L. (1989). An early starter model for predicting delinquency. In D. J. Pepler & K. H. Rubin (Eds.), *The development and treatment of childhood aggression* (pp. 139–168). Hillsdale, NJ: Erlbaum.

Patterson, G. R., Reid, J. B., & Dishion, T. J. (1992). *Antisocial boys.* Eugene, OR: Castalia.

Prinz, R. J. (2002). The Fast Track Project: A seminal intervention efficacy trail. *Journal of Abnormal Child Psychology*, 30, 53–59.

Rous, B., Hemmester, M. L., & Schuster, J. (1994). Sequence transition to education in the public schools:

A systems approach to transition planning. *Topics in Early Childhood Special Education, 14,* 374–393.

Rule, S., Fietchtl, B., & Innocenti, M. (1990). Preparation for transition to mainstreamed post-preschool environments: Development of a survival skills curriculum. *Topics in Early Childhood Special Education, 9,* 78–90.

Serna, L., Nielsen, E., Lambros, K., & Forness, S. R. (2000). Primary prevention with children at risk for emotional and behavioral disorders: Data on a universal intervention for Head Start classrooms. *Behavioral Disorders, 26,* 70–84.

Shonkoff, J. P., & Phillips, D. A. (Eds.). (2000). *From neurons to neighborhoods: The science of early development.* Washington, DC: National Academy Press.

Smith, B. J., & Fox, L. (2003). *Systems of service delivery: A synthesis of evidence relevant to young children at risk of or who have challenging behavior.* Denver, CO: Center for Evidence-based Practice: Young Children with Challenging Behaviors.

Strain, P. S., Steele, P., Ellis, T., & Timm, M. A. (1982). Long-term effects of oppositional child treatment with mothers as therapists and therapist trainers. *Journal of Applied Behavior Analysis, 15,* 163–169.

Strain, P. S., & Timm, M. A. (2001). Remediation and prevention of aggression: An evaluation of the Regional Intervention Program over a quarter century. *Behavioral Disorders, 26,* 297–313.

Timm, M. A. (1993). The Regional Intervention Program. *Behavioral Disorders, 19,* 34–43.

Twenty-Third Annual Report to Congress. (2001). Washington, DC: Office of Special Education Programs.

Walker, H. M., Kavanagh, K., Stiller, B., Golly, A., Severson, H. H., & Feil, E. G. (1998). First Step to Success: An early intervention approach for preventing school antisocial behavior. *Journal of Emotional and Behavioral Disorders, 6,* 66–80.

Walker, H. M., Severson, H. H., & Feil, E. G. (1995). *The Early Screening Project: A proven child-find process.* Longmont, CO: Sopris West.

Webster-Stratton, C. (1984). Randomized trial of two parent training programs for families with conduct-disordered children. *Journal of Consulting and Clinical Psychology, 52,* 666–678.

Webster-Stratton, C. (1989). Systematic comparison of consumer satisfaction of three cost-effective parent training programs for conduct problem children. *Behavior Therapy, 20,* 103–115.

Webster-Stratton, C. (1990). Enhancing the effectiveness of self-administered videotape parent training for families with conduct-problem children. *Journal of Abnormal Child Psychology, 18,* 479–492.

Webster-Stratton, C. (1997). Early intervention for families of preschool children with conduct problems. In M. J. Gurlanick (Ed.), *The effectiveness of early intervention* (pp. 429–454). Baltimore: Brookes.

Webster-Stratton, C. (1998). Preventing conduct problems in Head Start children strengthening parenting competencies. *Journal of Consulting and Clinical Psychology, 66,* 715–730.

Webster-Stratton, C. (2000). Oppositional-defiant and conduct-disordered children. In M. Hersen & R. T. Ammerman (Eds.), *Advanced abnormal child psychology* (2nd ed., pp. 387–412). Mahwah, NJ: Erlbaum.

Webster-Stratton, C., & Hammond, M. (1997). Treating children with early-onset conduct problems: A comparison of child and parent training interventions. *Journal of Consulting and Clinical Psychology, 65,* 93–109.

Webster-Stratton, C., Hollinsworth, T., & Kolpachoff, M. (1989). The long-term effectiveness and clinical significance of three cost-effective training programs of families with conduct problem children. *Journal of Consulting and Clinical Psychology, 57,* 550–553.

Webster-Stratton, C., Reid, M. J., & Hammond, M. (2001). Preventing conduct problems, promoting social competence: A parent and teacher training partnership in Head Start. *Journal of Clinical Child Psychology, 30,* 283–302.

Wolery, M. (1987). Program evaluation at the local level: Recommendations for improving services. *Topics in Early Childhood Special Education, 7,* 111–123.

12

Accountability and Assessment for Students with Emotional and Behavioral Disorders

JAMES G. SHRINER *and* JOSEPH H. WEHBY

Over the past several years, there has been a movement toward the participation of students with disabilities in large-scale assessments. This movement is a direct result of the expectations of higher levels of student achievement by politicians and the public at large. In response to recently passed legislation, including the Individuals with Disabilities Education Act Amendments of 1997 (IDEA; 1997) and the No Child Left Behind Act of 2001 (NCLB; 2002), all states have developed guidelines for increasing the participation of students with disabilities in high-stakes assessments. However, as with significant change at any level, there have been a number of concerns raised regarding the shift toward performance on a statewide achievement measure as the primary educational evaluation tool. These concerns include the influence of test scores on the graduation rates of students with disabilities and the degree to which special education services will be evaluated on the basis of student performance on these assessments, as well as the degree to which different states have different guidelines for test participation and for test accommodations (DeStefano, Shriner, & Lloyd, 2001).

Perhaps the concerns associated with the inclusion of students with disabilities into large-scale assessments may be most apparent for students identified as having emotional and behavioral disorders (EBD). These students, primarily categorized as having emotional disturbance (ED) under IDEA provisions, have the poorest academic outcomes when compared to students with other high incidence disabilities like learning disabilities. Between 13 and 14% of students with EBD receive services in separate facilities, including alternative schools (U.S. Department of Education, 2000, 2001). Students attending alternative schools often are at increased risk for dropout and exhibit academic and/or behavior problems of varying degrees (Lehr & Lange, 2003). In addition, students identified as EBD show high rates of absenteeism, low grade-point averages, and increased course failure (National Longitudinal Transition Study-2, 2003). It has been speculated that the poor academic outcomes for students with EBD are tied to a number of issues, including behavior problems that interfere with teaching, lack of quality instruction in classrooms for students with EBD, and the poor preparation in the area of academics for teachers of this population of students (Wehby, Lane, & Falk, 2003). Regardless of the reason, it appears that students with EBD are ill equipped to participate in the large-scale assessments required by states for educational advancement.

Unfortunately, little is known about the

performance and participation of students with EBD in the assessment process. The purpose of this chapter is to identify what is and is not known about this area of research. Specifically, we will (1) overview the broad issues of assessment and accountability in the area of special education, (2) identify the types of test accommodations that are available to students with EBD, (3) overview the literature regarding the participation and performance of students with EBD in state assessments, and (4) identify areas of future research in the area of assessment for this population.

ASSESSMENT AND ACCOUNTABILITY

Assessment refers to the process of administering tests and collecting other information for the purpose of making decisions about individuals and/or groups (Salvia & Ysseldyke, 2001). Accountability is a much broader process of data collection and use in determining the relative success or failure of students, schools, districts, states, and the nation (Education Commission of the States, 2000). Accountability efforts are most visible in the public reporting and comparison of assessment results and other information resulting in the determination of rewards and consequences. As mandated in the reauthorization of IDEA, states and districts must include students with disabilities in their assessments. States also are required to report on the performance of students with disabilities, both aggregated and disaggregated. However, required participation in assessment does not equate with inclusion in the accountability system of a school district or state. In fact, IDEA does not specifically require that the state assessment scores of students with disabilities be incorporated into system accountability. NCLB, however, represents a significant improvement over past practices in which students with disabilities were, perhaps, included in assessments but excluded from the overall accountability system. As a result of NCLB, many states and districts must not only consider the performance of the overall school but also broaden their systems to include a defined set of student subgroups (i.e., students with disabilities, limited English proficiency, low socioeconomic, and ethnicity). Because districts are most likely to offer assistance to students, including those with disabilities, in schools where assessment results are reported *and* used for accountability purposes, NCLB was "motivated by a . . . desire to improve the education [and achievement] of the nation's youth" (Linn, Baker, & Betebenner, 2002, p. 14).

PARTICIPATION IN ASSESSMENT

IDEA regulations regarding the participation and accommodation of students with disabilities emphasize the role of the individualized education program (IEP). According to the regulations, the IEP must include "a statement of any individual modifications in the administration of State or district-wide assessments of student achievement that are needed in order for the child to participate in the assessment; and if the IEP team determines that the child will not participate in a particular . . . assessment of student achievement, a statement of why that assessment is not appropriate for the child; and how the child will be assessed" (IDEA Regulations, 1998). However, nothing in the law states that the process of including students with disabilities in large-scale assessment must differ from what occurs for the general school population. Assessment participation of students with disabilities may occur in the same way it does for students without disabilities; many students with disabilities take the same tests under the same circumstances as their nondisabled peers. Also, a student may participate in state or district assessment by taking the same tests with accommodations if needed. Finally, if participation in an assessment is not appropriate, even with accommodations, an alternate assessment developed to measure a student's progress must be developed and used. As such, the IEP team is responsible for deciding how, not if, a student with disabilities is part of the assessment system. Table 12.1 is a summary of possible assessment scenarios under IDEA. Based on a set of assessment scenarios originally presented by Rouse, Shriner, and Danielson (2000), the table shows assessment strategies in which IEP teams must document a student's (1) degree of access to the general curriculum in each content area, (2) need for reasonable accommodations in

TABLE 12.1 Strategies for Large-Scale Assessment by Content Area and Accommodation Need

Student's instructional plan relative to standards	Accommodation need: Regular assessment(s)	Assessment strategy: Participation and accommodation
1. General education curriculum—All areas	1. None	1. Participation—*Full* Accommodation—*None*
2. General education curriculum—All areas	2. Needed for some areas	2. Participation—*Full* Accommodation—*Partial*
3. General education curriculum—All areas	3. Needed for all areas	3. Participation—*Full* Accommodation—*Full*
4. General education curriculum—Some areas Significantly modified curriculum—Some areas	4. Needed for some areas (i.e., general education) Not valid/helpful for other areas	4. Participation—*Partial* (i.e., some area(s) tested by *Alternate Assessment*) Accommodation—*Partial or Full*
5. Significantly modified curriculum—All areas	5. Not valid/helpful for all areas	5. Participation—*Alternate Assessment* Accommodation—*None*

testing, and (3) level of participation and accommodation strategies (*full*, *partial*, or *none*) that are most likely to portray the student's knowledge and skills as accurately as possible.

ACCOMMODATIONS AND MODIFICATIONS IN ASSESSMENT

Increased attention also has been focused on the issue of provision of accommodations to students with disabilities in national, state, and districtwide testing programs. For the purposes of this chapter, an important distinction between the terms "accommodation" and "modification" needs to be made (Tindal, Heath, Hollenbeck, Almond, & Harniss, 1998; Tindal, Hollenbeck, Heath, & Almond, 1997). *Accommodations* are changes in the normal testing procedure that allow a student with disabilities to take part in state- or districtwide assessment. Accommodated assessments are intended to level the playing field so that a student with a disability may demonstrate performance relative to the same goals on an assessment. Usually the term accommodation is used when the student is taking the same general test under different circumstances. By contrast, the term *modification* refers to a change in the test content that makes the test substantially different from its original form. Modifications include deletions of test items

or test sections, or substituted items and/or assessment tasks. As such, modifications are more likely to change what a test measures.

One common type of test modification is the administration of easier test forms intended for younger children ("out-of-level testing") (Thurlow, Elliott, & Ysseldyke, 1998). It should be noted that, though allowable under certain circumstances under NCLB , out-of-level testing is not considered to be best practice as a strategy, largely because of the suspect validity of inferences made based on scores obtained with this method of assessment (Thurlow, 2002).

TYPES OF ACCOMMODATIONS

Accommodations for testing are quite numerous and varied. Technological advances continue to expand the types of accommodations that might be considered. Generally, however, most accommodations in use fall into four broad categories (Thurlow, Scott, & Ysseldyke, 1995; Thurlow et al., 1998). Examples of changes in *setting* include administration in a test carrel or a separate room, or may consist of individual or small-group administrations. Some students with physical disabilities may be administered an assessment in a standard setting with some form of physical accommodation (e.g., a special desk or lighting) but with no other change to the environment or test. Changes in *timing* include offering extra time within a given testing session, alternating lengths of test sessions, and breaking test sessions into smaller time blocks. Changes in *presentation* format include large print or Braille forms for students with visual impairments, or manually signed questions for students with hearing impairments. Versions of a test delivered either by audiotape or computer for students with reading disabilities are considered presentation accommodations as well. Finally, changes in *response mode* might include use of a scribe or computer-assisted responses and dictation of responses into a tape recorder. Additionally, a student might be permitted to use some sort of template to keep track of test questions and answers or be permitted to write answers in his or her test book.

For students with EBD, these groups of accommodations might be categorized into two main types: those that focus primarily on an *academic* need (e.g., reading aloud) and those that address a *social/behavioral* need (e.g., praise and prompting for on-task behavior during testing). To date, however, this delineation and terminology have not been used in discussions or investigations of accommodations and their importance in testing students with EBD.

RESEARCH ON PARTICIPATION AND ACCOMMODATION

Issues Examined: Participation, Accommodation, and Score Validity

In the late 1990s, public policy at both the national and state levels regarding the inclusion of students with disabilities in assessment systems outpaced research and practice by several years (Rouse et al., 2000). Thurlow et al. (1998) emphasized that, while the use of assessment accommodations was a viable way to increase the participation of students with disabilities, the effects of accommodations on test results were primarily *opinion-based* at that time. As a result, a significant research effort was undertaken to examine policies, perceptions, and decision making regarding participation, accommodation effects, and test validity issues. Most of this work has addressed questions of the "appropriateness" of participation and accommodations from legal and technical per-

spectives. The educative value of inclusion in assessment and accountability systems has been addressed as well. The literature base in this area for all students with disabilities is emerging, and the need for sound research remains strong. There are, however, several very thorough and excellent reviews of legal and research issues as well as general testing accommodations that we recommend to the readers of this chapter (e.g., Pitoniak, & Royer, 2001; Thompson, Blount, & Thurlow, 2002; Thurlow et al., 2000; Tindal & Fuchs, 1999).

With respect to students with EBD, the essence of the research agenda applies. Some research in this area has been directed toward the attitudes of educators toward test accommodations for students with disabilities (including those with EBD), as well as some work on the degree to which students with EBD have participated in the high-stakes assessments required by states and local school districts. The next major section of this chapter will address these two areas. Preceding this section will be a description of how articles and reports for these areas were gathered.

Search Procedures

Our charge for this chapter was to summarize and critique the research on assessment and accountability for students with EBD. We wish to clarify again that by "assessment" we mean those tests and measures of educational results that are part of states' and districts' accountability systems. We did not intend to address assessment for the purposes of diagnosis, classification, eligibility for service, or routine progress measurement. Thus, although our initial literature search parameters were intentionally broad, we limited our review to those manuscripts and reports that addressed assessment from an educational reform and accountability perspective.

Four indexes (Digital Dissertations, ERIC, Education Abstracts, and PsycInfo) were searched for studies using certain keywords that were varied contingently to match to those databases. Primary search terms included the following and/or combinations thereof: test changes, assessment, accommodation, adaptation, modification, state testing, large-scale assessment, high-stakes assessment, emotional disturbance, behavior disorders, disabilities, special education. In addition, the National Center on Educational Outcomes (NCEO) has maintained a database of assessment and accommodation research. Thus, the first author contacted NCEO for assistance with its searchable database of published and unpublished documents related to standards, assessment accountability, and reform (*http://education. umn.edu/NCEO/AccomStudies.html*). To ensure that published empirical studies inclusive of students with EBD were identified (and in which those students could be identified), NCEO staff assisted with a replication of the online database search (M. Thurlow, personal communication, January 20, 2003).

As a result, 48 studies, published through December 2002, were identified. However, many of these studies were found not to describe the subjects in enough detail to ensure that students with EBD were included *and* identified in the data and analyses. Thus, of those 48 studies, only 11 were selected for review. We included those studies we believed represented the major research issues within the assessment and accountability environment (e.g., participation and accommodation) and which are indicative of the more broad-based literature reviewed by the authors mentioned earlier. As such, some studies that were examined address instructional and testing accommodations and include students other than those with EBD. For example, one study (Simpson, Griswold, & Smith-Myles, 1999) was selected largely because it was among the first to focus on participation and accommodation within high-stakes tests for students who show some level of disordered behavior. After the formal search was conducted, the NCEO database was monitored. One study (Gagnon, McLaughlin, & Leone, 2003) was subsequently added to the review.

Studies of the Perceptions of Professionals Regarding Assessment Issues and Decisions

The perceptions of teachers and district-level personnel regarding the use of accommodations have been documented largely through the use of surveys and questionnaires. Some studies were conducted prior to the 1997 reauthorization of IDEA and thus precede

the beginning of the most current wave of general curricular access, assessment, and accountability reforms. For example, Gajria, Salend, and Hemrick (1994) surveyed 64 general education teachers about both the degree of difficulty and effectiveness of implementing over 30 individual accommodations for students with disabilities. Respondents thought more favorably about accommodations that were effective and easy to use. Jayanthi, Epstein, Polloway, and Bursuck (1996) collected survey responses from a nationally representative sample of 401 general education teachers (228 elementary school, 81 middle school, 76 secondary school, 16 cross level). Teachers were presented with 24 specific accommodations and were asked questions about the responsibility for making accommodations, the accommodations' use and helpfulness, the ease of making each accommodation, and the relative fairness of the accommodations for use with students with disabilities.

Jayanthi et al. (1996) found that about 47% of general education teachers thought it was their responsibility to make test accommodations, with about 36% indicating accommodations were a joint responsibility with the special education teachers. Elementary teachers were more likely than both middle school and high school teachers to offer several accommodations, most notably, *reading test items, simplifying wording of items, allowing oral instead of written answers, testing in small groups, and reducing test content*. In addition, elementary teachers thought *giving help with directions, reading test items, allowing oral instead of written answers, and testing in small group* were more helpful than did their colleagues who taught older students. The accommodations that were identified to be the most helpful to students were thought to be among those most difficult to offer (e.g., *reading test items*). Finally, most teachers thought it was unfair to make accommodations only for students with disabilities, citing a high degree of need among other student groups.

With the reauthorization of IDEA in 1997, students with disabilities were to participate in state- and districtwide assessment systems, with the individual student's degree of access to the general curriculum as a key consideration for deciding the appropriate assessment strategy (Rouse et al., 2000; Yell & Shriner, 1997). Whereas inclusion of students with disabilities in such tests had received increasing attention prior to this time (cf. Elliott, Erikson, Thurlow, & Shriner, 2000), IDEA forced states and districts to reexamine their complete assessment systems and caused educators to thoroughly evaluate their beliefs and decision making, including all students in large-scale assessments.

In an initial study of the perceptions of educators, Simpson et al. (1999) surveyed educators about the inclusion of students with varying levels (mild, moderate, severe) of autism-related disorders in districtwide assessment. The authors presented 133 special education teachers with descriptions of three students and then asked them to rate their willingness to include each student in testing. In addition, respondents were to recommend the accommodations that should be used by each student by indicating whether an accommodation was "minimally necessary or not necessary" (Simpson et al., 1999, p. 213). It should be noted that accommodation recommendations were generic and not based upon a specific content area test (e.g., reading).

Results were reported for both participation and accommodation recommendations. As expected, the vast majority of respondents (84.5%) thought that the student with mild autism could be appropriately recommended for participation in district-wide assessment. Lesser percentages of respondents thought participation was appropriate for the students with moderate (54.9%) and severe (8.3%) autism-related disorders. Most educators (> 50% for all students) thought that the students should only be responsible for taking those portions of the test for which they had received appropriate instructional preparation. This recommendation matches the "partial participation" option shown in Table 12.1.

Recommendations for necessary *presentation* accommodations emphasized intense, personal support for the students, with over 60% of respondents indicating that all three student types needed help with directions (oral reading, repetition, interpretation) and paraphrasing or rephrasing of test items. Simpson et al. (1999) listed *test format* accommodations separately and reported that most respondents suggested giving the students tests that both looked familiar to them and omitted extraneous information. *Response* accommodations recommended most often for all three students included use of a computer or keyboard, writing on the test booklet, and oral responding. In addition, for the students with moderate and severe autism, many respondents recommended tape recording answers (69% and 82%, respectively) or pointing to answers (68% and 82%).

Setting accommodation recommendations reflected that a highly individualized approach to assessment was needed for student participation. On average, over 70% of respondents thought the students should be assessed by a special educator in a separate setting and given verbal and/or physical praise and prompting during testing. Finally, *timing* accommodations were pervasive, with no fewer than 50% of respondents suggesting each of the possible accommodations that were listed (e.g., extra time, frequent breaks, cessation of testing at educators' discretion). Simpson et al. (1999) concluded that the participation of students with autism-related disorders in large-scale assessment was deemed important by the surveyed teachers and that most educators were cautious in recommending participation strategies and concerned about the degree to which recommended accommodations would result in an unfair advantage for any student.

Summary on Perceptions

Teachers and other IEP team members report that they are generally more confident about accommodation decisions than they are about student participation in high-stakes assessment (DeStefano et al., 2001). This difference might be due, in part, to the amount of "practice" teachers have had in making such decisions—accommodations are provided routinely in school settings, but end-of-year testing decisions and options have been changing in recent years. For example, participation in an alternate assessment of achievement in one or more content areas, as is now an option that must be considered, was not a concern prior to IDEA, in 1997. Despite the limited experience with accommodation decisions, from these studies it appears that teachers are willing to make accommodations for students with disabilities, including those students with EBD. However, it is important to note that there were some caveats associated with this willingness. First, teachers were willing to make accommodations as long as these changes were easy to incorporate within the test conditions. In fact, teachers reported that accommodations were a necessary part of the assessment process. In addition, it seemed as though some of the respondents believed that accommodations should be available to some students without disabilities, as well. However, the ease of implementing accommodations seemed to be an important finding in this work. As noted above, reading test items to students was rated as effective, yet difficult to implement. So, while it appears that educators are generally supportive of providing support during assessment situations, there is a limit to the level of support that they are willing or able to provide.

Studies of Student Participation

When the issues of high academic standards and standards-referenced assessments first gained national attention, students with disabilities were largely not part of the assessment/accountability equation. Only a few states had formal test participation policies and most states estimated that less than 10% of students with disabilities participated in state assessments (Shriner, Spande, & Thurlow, 1994). A decade later, state policies for participation are more specific and offer more options for student participation. In addition, for the first time in NCEO's investigations, state policies included *student emotional anxiety* as a valid reason for students *not* to participate in state assessments (Thurlow, Lazarus, Thompson, & Robey, 2002).

Participation of students with disabilities still is not a consistent and routine practice nationwide. Although improving overall, some states' participation rates remain unreliable, mostly because of variability in methods used to count those students with disabilities within testing programs. Thompson and Thurlow (2001) comment that changes in state-level data, while positive, may mask the experiences of students with disabilities at the local level. Also, significant variability

in local implementation of participation decisions has implications in light of the increased attention to be focused on school-level accountability required by NCLB. Therefore, careful application of participation rules will be the responsibility of local assessment personnel, as the percentage of students with disabilities who participate in the assessments will be a key indicator in the overall accountability system.

Studies with Students with Emotional/Behavioral Disorders: Disaggregated Results

As previously mentioned, while the data regarding accountability and participation are somewhat sparse for the disability population in general, it is particularly limited in the area of EBD. However, two recent investigations have reported some data in this area.

As part of an effort to explore the role of the IEPs of students with EBD in the implementation of the educational aims of assessment and accountability systems, Shriner and Wehby (2002) examined the participation and accommodation decisions that were specific to students with EBD. Data for those students with a school-identified disability of EBD were extracted from a larger study (cf. DeStefano et al., 2001; Shriner & DeStefano, 2001) that examined the effects of a year-long professional development effort to enhance IEP team decision making about curricular access and large-scale assessment. Of primary interest were the observed patterns about the degree to which the IEP meetings and procedures were used to document decisions about a student's participation and accommodation in the general curriculum and state testing programs, and the extent to which participation and accommodation decisions documented on the IEP accurately reflected student experiences during state testing (DeStefano et al., 2001).

Data collection for the larger study took place in three school districts (urban, suburban, and rural) and included students in grades 3–10 (see DeStefano et al., 2001, for detailed demographics). An examination of each student's IEP for information relating to the statements required by IDEA was conducted. Information on students' IEPs about the nature of the instructional curriculum, instructional accommodations, accommodations used for classroom assessment, the participation strategy intended for the student, and the number and type of accommodation(s) planned on the state assessment were recorded. In addition, the students' teachers completed a survey that primarily assessed the extent to which each student participated in the state assessment, the instructional accommodations students received routinely, and the accommodations actually received during the state assessment. The survey was completed during the state assessment period in spring 1999 and again in spring 2000. IEPs that were in effect for each session were matched to the survey for that academic year. Cross-tabulations and kappa statistics were used to examine the relationship between participation and accommodation decisions documented on the IEP and those actually experienced by students during testing. For the subsample used by Shriner and Wehby (2002), all students with EBD as a primary disability and those for whom EBD was listed as a secondary disability for the study's duration were examined as a group, with 65 students initially included in year 1 and 102 in year 2. Given the findings from previous studies (DeStefano et al., 2001; Espin, Deno, & Albayrak-Kaymak, 1998; Shriner & DeStefano, 2001) that reading is often the most carefully documented content area, reading was chosen as the content area of interest for this group. Even so, about one out of three IEPs was found to be lacking in information related to either the degree of curricular access or assessment participation; thus, only those students within a year for whom a complete data set existed from both the IEP and teacher survey were included in the analyses (year 1, $N = 46$; year 2, $N = 65$). Keeping in mind that these data are summarized across schools and grades, results for this small sample of students with EBD provide a very preliminary description of their experiences in large-scale assessment and accountability systems. The strategies for assessment included in Table 12.1 were used as a basis for the description.

Participation and Accommodation

In year 1, 18% of IEPs indicated that the students' instruction was primarily within the general curriculum, whereas 31% of students had this focus in year 2. Approximately half of the students' IEPs indicated a highly modified curricular focus to be appropriate for their instruction. Participation totals for year 1 showed that about 74% of the students took all parts of the state test either without accommodations (38%) or with accommodations for all parts (34%). Only 3% of the students considered during year 1 had IEPs that indicated the intention of using either partial assessment or the alternate assessment. Nearly a quarter of the students' IEPs had no planned participation and accommodation scenarios.

For year 2, 94% of the students took the entire state assessment. About one-third of students received no accommodations, and half of them had accommodations on all parts of the test. Partial participation in the state test was indicated on 7% of the IEPs in year 2. Alternate assessment was not documented as a planned primary option for any of the students. Most notably, only 3% of students' IEPs were void of assessment plans, down over 20% from year 1.

Across years, instructional accommodations (i.e., *scheduling, setting, presentation,* and *response*) documented on IEPs remained fairly steady for *scheduling* (30%) and *response* (40%), but showed a drop in *setting* (62% vs. 40%) and *presentation* (72% vs. 45%). Planned assessment accommodations, however, were found to be higher in all groups from year 1 to year 2. On average, about 25% of students were to receive accommodations in year 1. By contrast, 40% were to receive assessment accommodations in year 2. The biggest increase was in *response* accommodations, up from 6% in year 1 to 25% in year 2.

Relation between IEP Decisions and Participation in State Assessment

Kappa coefficients (Table 12.2) were generated to describe the degree to which students' IEPs reflected their actual participation and accommodation scenarios in state assessment as recorded by the school at the time of testing (cf. DeStefano et al., 2001). For participation, kappa values were low in both years (year 1 = .14; year 2 = .20), reflecting that some students' IEPs did not reflect their actual assessment participation.

TABLE 12.2. Kappa Coefficients' Agreement of IEP-Documented Accommodations and State Assessment Accommodations

| Accommodation | Year | Kappa | Disagreements | Discrepancies | |
				+IEP–TEST[a]	–IEP+TEST[b]
Scheduling	1	.74	6	4	2
	2	.53	15	9	6
Setting	1	.50	12	2	10
	2	.29	24	5	19
Presentation	1	.19	16	6	10
	2	.09	28	25	3
Response	1	−.03	16	3	13
	2	.03	15	14	1

[a] Accommodation indicated on IEP but not used during state testing.

[b] Accommodation not indicated on IEP but was used during state testing.

However, no clear pattern of representation was noticed either across years or for participation strategy. Of the 19 observed discrepancies, 11 were cases in which a student's IEP indicated planned participation that, in fact, did not occur.

Examination of agreement between planned and provided accommodations was analyzed by the four major accommodation categories in both years. The major accommodation categories and the IEP–Test discrepancies for both years are shown in Table 12.2. For *scheduling* accommodations, there was relatively high agreement in year 1 (kappa = .74) and moderate agreement in year 2 (kappa = .53). Moderate agreement was found for *setting* in year 1 (kappa = .50), and low-moderate agreement for year 2 (kappa = .29). Minimal agreement was observed also for *presentation* across years (kappa = .19 and .09), with the weakest agreement between IEPs and actual assessment noted for response accommodations (kappa = −.03 and .03, respectively). Across all students, IEPs tended to underrepresent overall accommodations, meaning that students often received accommodations during end-of-year testing that they had not used during the school year nor were intended to have at test time. However, in year 2, IEPs tended to markedly overrepresent both *presentation* and *response* accommodations. In these cases, students' IEPs indicated that they were supposed to receive accommodations during testing; however, no accommo-

dation was reportedly used during state assessment.

In a second study, Gagnon et al. (2003) examined assessment and accountability issues with specific attention to the experiences of students with EBD. They present the results of a national survey of principals (N = 271) and elementary teachers (N = 229) from 480-day treatment and residential facilities serving children with EBD. Respondents were queried about student participation, accommodation use, and accountability aims. Expecting to find differences of perceptions about these issues between the administrators and teachers, Gagnon et al. (2003) instead found no responses that were statistically different. This finding was interpreted to mean that both groups were "on the same page" (p. 9) and as evidence of the representativeness of their data regarding assessment and accountability policies for students served in these types of programs.

Most principals (N = 167) and teachers (N = 131) said their schools were relying on state and local assessments for their accountability efforts, and that the main purposes of their efforts were to adjust instructional and curricular resources. About 65% of principals and 59% of teachers reported that at least 80% of students participated in these assessments. Still, the finding that about one of five respondents said less than half of the students they served participated in assessments concerned these authors. Chi-square analysis revealed student participation to be more likely if the school enrolled children from within a single district or state than if it served students from multiple districts or states.

Over 80% of both principals and teachers reported a set policy (often based upon that used in the state where the school was located) regarding the use of assessment accommodations. Almost all remaining respondents said their schools did not offer accommodations during assessments—a "disconcerting [finding, given] federal mandates that require appropriate accommodations" (Gagnon et al., 2003, p. 14).

These authors reported on educators' perceptions of the experiences of students with EBD in assessment and accountability systems. The key issues of participation and accommodation are thoroughly described. The relationship these observations had to the plans and services detailed in these students' IEPs, however, was not examined.

Studies with Students with EBD: Aggregate Results

In addition to the above studies, there were several studies identified that included students with EBD with a larger sample of students with disabilities; however, the data for students with EBD were not analyzed separately. While not ideal, we believe that the studies do shed some additional light into the area of accountability and test participation for this student population.

Marquart (2000) examined the effect of providing extended time on a mathematics portion of the Terra Nova. She tested 69 middle school students who were divided into three groups: those with disabilities, those at risk for school problems in mathematics, and those thought to be performing at grade level. She examined both student performance and their reactions to testing. Marquart found no significant differences in the performance of students with disabilities, students at risk, and students functioning at or above grade level on the standard versus the extended time conditions. There was no significant difference in the effect sizes for the accommodation among the three student groups. Student reactions to the test were more positive when they were given extra time rather than the standard

time to complete the test. Across groups, students felt less stressed, more motivated, and thought they performed better when extended time was allowed.

Schulte, Elliott, and Kratochwill (2000) investigated the views educators had regarding the accommodations that should be offered to students with various degrees of disability. Using a survey containing vignettes, respondents were asked to rate the usefulness of a series of accommodations provided on a checklist. These authors found that teachers recommended that students receive "packages" of accommodations and rarely recommend that a single accommodation to be used during testing. In addition, educators reported that accommodations were needed more often for performance assessments than for multiple-choice tests for students with more significant disabilities.

In one of the few experimental studies in this area, Elliott, Kratochwill, and McKevitt (2001) used an alternating treatments design to investigate the accommodations used by students with disabilities ($N = 41$, 3 of whom were identified as having EBD) and students without disabilities ($N = 59$) on performance assessments in mathematics and science. In this study, student performance was compared under three conditions: no accommodation, standard accommodations (i.e., extra time, assistance with and reading of directions/materials, and verbal encouragement), and teacher-recommended accommodation(s) based on IEP and instructional information. The use of the alternating treatments design made possible both between-group comparisons and within-individual comparisons. Given performance-based assessment items, the average calculated effect size when comparing accommodated and nonaccommodated conditions for students with disabilities was .83. Thus, the performance of students with disabilities under individualized accommodation conditions on this type of test item was very similar to that of their nondisabled peers. Additionally, for more than 75% of students with disabilities, testing accommodation packages and those suggested by students' IEP teams had a moderate to large effect on test scores, and test scores for 55% of students without disabilities also showed a similar effect. The effects of recommended accommodations were not positive for a small number of students.

Using analyses of extant data, Koretz (1997) and Koretz and Hamilton (2000) examined the inclusion of students with disabilities in the Kentucky statewide assessment Kentucky Instructional Results Information System (KIRIS). Additionally, the types of assessment accommodations offered and the performance of students with disabilities on multiple-choice and open-response items were examined as a function of the accommodations received. Students with EBD were included in both studies; however, the more elucidating results specific to this group were presented in the earlier report (Koretz, 1997).

Overall, students with disabilities received a variety of accommodations that were permitted and that were determined to be appropriate based on their individual needs. Accommodations that were most prevalent included dictation, oral presentation, paraphrasing, and assistance with spelling. As in the Schulte et al. (2000) study, students with disabilities most often received combinations of these accommodations. In general, students received a greater number of accommodations in elementary school (grade 4) than in junior (grade 8) or senior (grade 11) high grades. Over 80% of students with disabilities in grade 4 were awarded at least one accommodation, with two out of three receiving multiple accommodations. For students with EBD who are accommodated, the same pattern is reported. Of interest, however, is the finding that *more* students with EBD participated *without* accommodations when compared with students with learning disabilities or mental retardation. In grade 4, for example, 28% of students with EBD participated without accommodations, compared to 8% of students with learning disabilities and 9% of students with mental retardation. Just over 50% of students with EBD are reported to have participated without accommodations in both grades 8 and 11, whereas approximately 30% of students with learning disabilities and 25% of students with mental retardation were not accommodated in those grades.

Also, Koretz (1997) included limited category-specific performance test data in his arguments that the inappropriate use of accommodations (particularly dictation) may lead to unreliable and unusually high scores on certain mathematics and science assessments for elementary students with learning disabilities or mental retardation. In some instances, students with learning disabilities scored between 0.2 and 0.5 standard deviations above the mean of students without disabilities (mathematics and science). Students with EBD, as a group, always scored more than 0.5 standard deviations below the mean obtained by same-grade students without disabilities, with greater deficits observed in grades 8 and 11.

For open response item formats, item-test correlations were no different for students with disabilities (with or without accommodations) than for students without disabilities, and differential item functioning (DIF) was relatively infrequent in some subject areas. There were several cases of notable differential item functioning shown by students receiving accommodations, mainly in mathematics.

In a study of student perceptions and comfort with test adjustments, Kosciolek and Ysseldyke (2000) examined the impact of a read-aloud recording on a test of reading comprehension. Using a counterbalanced design, students in general education ($N = 17$) and in special education ($N = 15$; 4 were receiving services under the category EBD) were given two equivalent forms of the comprehension test of the California Achievement Tests, Fifth Edition (CAT/5) Survey Version. Each student took one form of the test under standard procedures and the other form of the test with the read-aloud accommodation. The read-aloud was presented via audiotape controlled by the student. Students were then asked to state which condition they preferred and why they felt that way.

These authors reported that students without disabilities outperformed those with disabilities on both the accommodated and nonaccommodated test versions. On average, general education students' scores improved only slightly when using accommodations, whereas the scores of the students with disabilities as a group improved about one-half of a standard deviation. Still, this gain was not found to be statistically significant ($p < .06$). Kosciolek and Ysseldyke (2000) attribute the lack of significance to the small sample size of the group and assert that with a "reasonably larger sample size for both groups, the difference in the effect of the accommodation for students by group may reach significance" (p. 16).

Finally, for examining levels of student perception of the accommodation, qualitative data were gathered and analyzed. Students in general education preferred to take the test without accommodations, indicating that the read-aloud slowed them down. Students with disabilities, by contrast, preferred the accommodated test version, largely because of a perceived reduction in the difficulty of the tasks.

Summary of Literature on Accommodations and Participation

Given the limited body of research on actual types of accommodations implemented and the degree of participation for students with EBD in state assessments, any conclusions from this literature must be viewed as tentative. However, a few themes emerge. As reported in the Shriner and Wehby (2002) and Gagnon et al. (2003) studies, a large percentage of the EBD participants took part in the statewide assessments offered by local districts. However, from these data, it did not appear that these students were being offered accommodations on a consistent basis. The finding that a number of students were not offered accommodations that were a part of their IEP highlights this trend. Koretz (1997) reported that a higher percentage of students with EBD participated in state assessments without accommodations when compared to other disability groups. Taken together, it appears that, while students with EBD are participating in assessments, they are doing so with little support in terms of accommodations. This finding is particularly troublesome given the findings that when accommodations are provided, students tend to perform at higher levels and are less stressed by the assessment process.

FUTURE ISSUES FOR RESEARCH

Perceptions of Educators

As we go forward in this time of advances and challenges in states' and districts' efforts to include students with disabilities in their assessment and accountability systems, we would be misguided in planning research and evaluation agendas without due consid-eration of the perceptions, attitudes, and practices of teachers. Thurlow (2002) reminds us that the politics and rhetoric surrounding assessment/accountability discussions ultimately acknowledge that high expectations for teachers and students and the extent to which students experience success in these systems both remain in the hands of teachers. Researchers should heed that advice as well, we believe.

We know to date that teachers as a group believe that students with EBD should be afforded the opportunity to participate in a meaningful way in assessment and accountability systems. Teachers also view accommodation needs and strategies to be real and valid, and in most cases they see merit to providing helpful accommodations to *all* students. We know also that instructional and assessment accommodations are more likely offered to students in lower grades than to those in higher grades (Belinski, Ysseldyke, Bolt, Freidebach, & Freidebach, 2001; Jayanthi et al., 1996; Koretz, 1997), and research specific to the use of some accommodations during *instruction* is associated with reductions in problem behavior (Penno, Frank, & Wacker, 2000). We do not know the extent to which these views hold specifically to students with EBD who are showing *significant* academic and behavioral problems. Nor do we know if the attitudes of teachers toward accommodation usage changes as a function of students' age and severity of behavioral disability. Because over the past few years concern about student anxiety has appeared in state policies as a legitimate reason for exclusion/excusal from testing (Thurlow et al., 2002), we cannot clearly describe the extent to which educators consider the implementation of behavioral accommodations as good practice in testing scenarios. For example, one might envision the IEP and behavior plan of a student with extreme difficulty in controlling his or her verbal outbursts when frustrated or anxious as requiring the use of a praise/point system or a token economy in both general education and special education classrooms. Knowing that such a system is targeted to enhance behavioral performance and not academic performance, to what extent would an IEP team support its implementation during end-of-year high-stakes testing? How would assessment coordinators in districts perceive these plans? Can and should they be offered? These questions must be answered before we can determine the extent to which educators will wholly support the full range of accommodations for students with EBD.

Participation, Accommodation, and Results

As we have suggested, research about students with EBD in assessment and accountability systems has not been a primary area of inquiry; yet, this work remains relevant, as they will be part of the activities in states, districts, and schools. Simply put, for those interested in the experiences of these students, the picture is far from complete. As we plan what research to pursue, we should be aware of the current status of students with EBD in the present. Using the descriptors in Table 12.1 as a reference point, we think it may be informative to fully explain the patterns of participation in the general curriculum, and in assessments, with attention to the unique instructional and accommodation needs of students. The literature allows us to answer several questions about what educators are recommending for many students. First, do teachers find accommodation strategies acceptable? We think they do. Second, given that teachers are willing to use accommodations to support participation, can they identify valid and reasonable accommodations for students with learning and behavioral needs? We think that teachers are fairly good judges of their students' needs and that their decision making can be enhanced with tools such as the Dynamic Assessment of Test Accommodations (DATA; Fuchs et al., 2000)—a software and decision-making package that can be used to compare anticipated and actual effects of accommodations on student test performance. However, for the third main question—to what extent do teachers use planned accommodations and implement them with fidelity, and does this usage translate to assessment practice?—we honestly do not know the answer. The picture of these experiences is, quite possibly, the most incomplete of all. In examining the data for students with EBD from the DeStefano et al. (2001) and Shriner and Wehby (2002) studies, we were extremely conservative in our decisions regarding which student records to include in their analyses. We eliminated over 45% of potential students from the subject pool because of missing or incomplete IEPs or student records pertaining to assessment participation. Is this an artifact of sloppy data collection? Perhaps. But, the alarming number of student records from which participation and accommodation documentation was missing illustrates that, for whatever reason, decisions about high-stakes and large-scale assessment were not among the higher priorities for educators planning for students with EBD.

Finally, we must raise issues of the technical characteristics in the design of assessments that are being investigated in an effort to include the widest possible range of students in the increasing number of high-stakes tests. The goal of such work is to develop tests that ascertain students' construct-relevant knowledge and skill while minimizing the effect of disabilities and other interferences (Rose, 2001). By developing tests from the outset from a universal design perspective, the need for accommodations during assessment should be reduced, thereby making the test more accessible (increasing participation options) and rendering the testing situation less complex to manage (improving teacher perception of the task).

The degree to which the learning and behavioral characteristics of students with EBD are affected by universally designed assessments may be worthy of focused investigation. Some work is under way (e.g., Thompson, 2002), and although students with EBD are not primary subjects in these efforts, the research examines attention-related behaviors of examinees under differing testing situations (e.g., timed versus untimed; reduced print per page). There is initial anecdotal and student self-report evidence from this work that the reduced readability demands of some universally designed assessments are an important stress reduction strategy that enables students to "better remember what they were taught and to think better during the test" (C. Johnstone, personal communication, July, 10, 2003).

SUMMARY

From this brief review, it is clear that there is much work to be done before we can make some definitive statements regarding the successful participation in high-stakes assessments for students with EBD. However, we believe that much of this work may be premature given the current state of academic instruction delivered to students with EBD. There is a strong body of evidence to suggest that students with EBD receive little high-quality instruction on an ongoing basis (e.g., Steinberg & Knitzer, 1992; Wehby, Symons, Canale, & Go, 1998; Wehby, Symons, & Shores, 1995). In addition, there is a lack of research to guide practice in this area (Coleman & Vaughn, 2000; Mooney, Epstein, Reid, & Nelson, 2003). While there are a number of issues that may help explain the lack of instruction (and research on instruction) for students with EBD, the fact is that under current conditions students with EBD are ill prepared to meet the academic standards demanded by local school districts. Thus, while the field of EBD pursues additional answers in the areas of assessment and accountability for this population, this work will have only limited impact until improvements can be made in classrooms regarding the delivery of high-quality, empirically valid instruction.

ACKNOWLEDGMENTS

Preparation of this chapter was supported, in part, by a grant (No. H325N020081) from the U.S. Department of Education, Office of Special Education and Rehabilitative Services, Office of Special Education Programs, awarded to James G. Shriner. Opinions expressed herein do not necessarily reflect those of the U.S. Department of Education or Offices within it.

REFERENCES

Bielinski, J., Ysseldyke, J., Bolt, S., Freidebach, M., & Freidebach, J. (2001). Prevalence of accommodations for students with disabilities participating in a statewide testing program. *Assessment for Effective Intervention, 26*(2), 21–28.

Coleman, M., & Vaughn, S. (2000). Reading interventions for students with emotional/ behavioral disorders. *Behavioral Disorders, 25,* 93–104.

DeStefano, L., Shriner, J. G., & Lloyd C. (2001). Teacher decision making in participation of students with disabilities in large-scale assessment. *Exceptional Children, 68,* 7–22.

Education Commission of the States. (2000). *Results matter: The new approach to accountability* (Accountability Brief, Vol. 2, No. 1). Denver, CO: Author.

Elliott, J., Erickson, R., Thurlow, M. L., & Shriner, J. G. (2000). State-level accountability for the performance of students with disabilities: Five years of change? *Journal of Special Education, 34,* 39–47.

Elliott, S. N., Kratochwill, T. R., & McKevitt, B. (2001). Experimental analysis of the effects of testing accommodations on the scores of students with and without disabilities. *Journal of School Psychology, 39,* 3–24.

Espin, C. A., Deno, S. L., & Albayrak-Kaymak, D. (1998). Individualized education programs in resource and inclusive settings: How individualized are they? *Journal of Special Education, 38,* 164–174.

Fuchs, L. S., Fuchs D., Eaton, S. B., Hamlett, C., Binkley, E., & Crouch, R. (2000). Using objective data sources to enhance teacher judgments about test accommodations. *Exceptional Children, 67,* 67–81.

Gagnon, J. C., McLaughlin, M. J., & Leone, P. E. (2003). *Educational accountability in day treatment and residential schools for students with emotional and behavioral disorders: Report on a national survey* (Issue Brief No. 3). College Park, MD: University of Maryland, Educational Policy Reform Research Institute.

Gajria, M., Salend, S. J., & Hemrick, M. A. (1994). Teacher acceptability of testing modifications mainstreamed students. *Learning Disabilities Research and Practice, 9,* 236–243.

Individuals with Disabilities Education Act Amendments of 1997, Pub. L. No. 105-17, 37 Stat. 111. (1997).

Individuals with Disabilities Education Act of 1997 Regulations, 34 C. F. R. § 300.347(5)(i)–(ii). (1998).

Jayanthi, M., Epstein, M. H., Polloway, E. A., & Bursuck, W. D. (1996). A national survey of general education teachers' perceptions of testing adaptations. *The Journal of Special Education, 30,* 99–115.

Koretz, D. (1997). *Assessment of students with disabilities in Kentucky* (CSE Technical Report No. 431). Los Angeles, CA: Center for Research on Standards and Student Testing.

Koretz, D., & Hamilton, L. (2000). Assessment of students with disabilities in Kentucky: Inclusion student performance and validity. *Educational Evaluation and Policy, 22,* 255–272.

Kosciolek, S., & Ysseldyke, J. E. (2000). *Effects of a reading accommodation on the validity of a reading test* (Technical Report 28). Minneapolis, MN: University of Minnesota, National Center on Educational Outcomes. Retrieved February 6, 2003, from *http://education.umn.edu/NCEO/OnlinePubs/Technical28.htm.*

Lehr, C., & Lange, C. (2003). *Alternative schools and the students they serve: Perceptions of state directors of special education* (Policy Research Brief No. 14). Minneapolis, MN: University of Minnesota, Institute on Community Integration.

Linn, R. L., Baker, E. L., & Betebenner, D. W. (2002). Accountability systems: Implications of requirements of the No Child Left Behind Act of 2001. *Educational Researcher, 31*(6), 3–16.

Marquart, A. M. (2000). *The use of extended time as an accommodation on a standardized mathematics test: An investigation of effects on scores and perceived consequences for students with various skill levels.* Madison: University of Wisconsin, Wisconsin Center for Education Research.

Mooney, P., Epstein, M. H., Reid, R., & Nelson, J. R. (2003). Status and trends of academic research for students with emotional disturbance. *Remedial and Special Education, 24,* 273–287.

No Child Left Behind Act of 2001, Pub. L. No. 107-110, 115 Stat. 1425 (2002).

Penno, D. A., Frank, A., & Wacker, D. P. (2000). Instructional accommodations for adolescent students with severe emotional and behavioral disorders. *Behavioral Disorders, 25,* 325–343.

Pitoniak, M. J., & Royer, J. M. (2001). Testing accommodations for examinees with disabilities: A review of psychometric, legal, and social policy issues. *Review of Educational Research, 71,* 53–104.

Rose, D. (2001). Universal design for learning. *Journal of Special Education Technology, 16,* 64–67.

Rouse, M., Shriner, J. G., & Danielson, L. (2000). National assessment and special education in the United States and England and Wales. In M. McLaughlin & M. Rouse (Eds.), *Special education and school reform in the United States and Britain* (pp. 66–97). London: Routledge.

Salvia, J., & Ysseldyke, J. E. (2001). *Assessment* (8th ed.). Boston: Houghton Mifflin.

Schulte, A. G., Elliott, S. N., & Kratochwill, T. R. (2000). Educators' perceptions and documentation of test accommodations for students with disabilities. *Special Services in the Schools, 16,* 35–56.

Shriner, J. G., & DeStefano, L. (2001). Participation in statewide assessments: view of district level personnel. *Assessment for Effective Intervention, 26,* 9–16.

Shriner, J. G., Spande, G., & Thurlow, M. L. (1994). *State special education outcomes 1993.* Minneapolis: University of Minnesota, National Center on Education Outcomes.

Shriner, J. G., & Wehby, J. H. (2002, November). *Assessment and accountability for students with emotional/behavioral disorders: Some data and some issues.* Paper presented at the 26th Annual Conference on Severe Behavior Disorders of Children and Youth (Teacher Educators for Children with Behavioral Disorders), Tempe, AZ.

Simpson, R. L., Griswold, D. E., & Smith-Myles, B. (1999). Educators' assessment accommodation preferences for students with autism. *Focus on Autism and Other Developmental Disabilities, 14,* 212–219.

Steinberg, Z., & Knitzer, J. (1992). Classrooms for emotionally and behaviorally disturbed students: Facing the challenge. *Behavioral Disorders, 17,* 145–156.

Thompson, S. L. (2002). *Development Techniques for Universally Designed Assessments.* Minneapolis, MN: University of Minnesota, Institute on Community Integration.

Thompson, S. L., Blount, A., & Thurlow, M. L. (2002). *A summary of research on the effects of test accommodations: 1999 through 2001* (Technical Report 34). Minneapolis, MN: University of Minnesota, National Center on Educational Outcomes.

Thompson, S. L., & Thurlow, M. L. (2001). *2001 State special education outcomes: A report on state activities at the beginning of a new decade.* Minneapolis, MN: University of Minnesota, National Center on Educational Outcomes.

Thurlow, M. L. (2002, July). *Accountability: A national perspective.* Paper presented at the OSEP Research Project Directors' Conference. U.S. Department of Education, Office of Special Education Programs, Washington, DC.

Thurlow, M. L., Elliott, J. L., & Ysseldyke, J. E. (1998). *Testing students with disabilities: Practical strategies for complying with district and state requirements.* New York: Corwin Press.

Thurlow, M. L., Lazarus, S., Thompson, S. L., & Robey, J. (2002). *2001 state policies on assessment participation and accommodations* (Synthesis Report 46). Minneapolis, MN: University of Minnesota, National Center on Educational Outcomes.

Thurlow, M. L., McGrew, K. S., Tindal, G., Thompson, S. L., Ysseldyke, J. E., & Elliott, J. L. (2000). *Assessment accommodations research: Considerations for design and analysis* (Technical Report 26). Minneapolis, MN: University of Minnesota, National Center on Educational Outcomes.

Thurlow, M. L., Scott, D., & Ysseldyke, J. E. (1995). *A compilation of states' guidelines for accommodations in assessment for students with disabilities* (Synthesis Report No. 18). Minneapolis, MN: University of Minnesota, National Center on Educational Outcomes.

Tindal, G., & Fuchs, L. S. (1999). *A summary of research on testing accommodations: What we know so far.* Lexington, KY: University of Kentucky Mid-South Regional Resource Center.

Tindal, G., Heath, B., Hollenbeck, K., Almond, P., & Harniss, M. (1998). Accommodating students with disabilities on large-scale tests: An experimental study. *Exceptional Children, 64,* 439–450.

Tindal, G., Hollenbeck, K., Heath, B., & Almond, P. (1997). *The effect of using computers as an accommodation in a statewide writing test* (Technical Research Report). Eugene, OR: Behavioral Research and Teaching.

U.S. Department of Education (2000). *Twenty-second annual report to Congress on the implementation of the Individuals with Disabilities Education Act.* Washington, DC: Author.

U.S. Department of Education (2001). *Twenty-third annual report to Congress on the implementation of* the *Individuals with Disabilities Education Act*. Washington, DC: Author.

Wehby, J. H., Lane, K. L., & Falk, K. F. (2003). Academic instruction for students with emotional and behavioral disorders. *Journal of Emotional and Behavioral Disorders, 11,* 194–197.

Wehby, J. H., Symons, F. M., Canale, J., & Go, F. (1998). Teaching practices in classrooms for students with emotional and behavioral disorders: Discrepancies between recommendations and observations. *Behavioral Disorders, 24,* 52–57.

Wehby, J. H., Symons, F., & Shores, R. E. (1995). A descriptive analysis of aggressive behavior in classrooms for students with emotional and behavioral disorders. *Behavioral Disorders, 20,* 87–105.

Yell, M. L., & Shriner, J. G., (1997). The IDEA Amendments of 1997: Implications for special and general education teachers, administrators, and teacher trainers. *Focus on Exceptional Children, 30*(1), 1–20.

PART III

CHARACTERISTICS OF EMOTIONAL AND BEHAVIORAL DISORDERS

Introduction

STEVEN R. FORNESS

In its narrowest definition, the field of "behavioral disorders" refers to special education for children with a range of emotional or behavioral disorders. Thus, its professional journal is *Behavioral Disorders*, and its professional association is the Council for Children with Behavioral Disorders, a division of the Council for Exceptional Children, the primary special education professional association. In its broadest definition, however, both the journal and the association also focus on other children with emotional or behavioral disorders, including both externalizing and internalizing disorders, delinquent behaviors, and autistic spectrum disorders, across the entire span of childhood and adolescence, without regard to their special education eligibility. In this sense, the field encompasses primary prevention of such disorders, schoolwide behavioral programs, prereferral intervention, and related programs, including, of course, special education and other school-related mental health, child welfare, or juvenile justice programs.

The disparity in these two definitions is nowhere near as evident as in the respective prevalence differences between the broad and narrow interpretations of this field. The eligibility of children in the special education category of emotional disturbance is a scant 0.94% of school enrollment, with autism another 0.16% (U.S. Department of Education, 2002), while review of 52 epidemiology studies of children with emotional or behavioral disorders suggests a mean prevalence of 10.2% for preschoolers, 13.2% for elementary children, and 16.5% for adolescents (Roberts, Attkisson, & Rosenblatt, 1998). Such an enormous disparity can be at least partially resolved by further research on the types of emotional or behavioral disorders of children that are referred to and/or identified as eligible for special education.

The four major types of disorders that have traditionally been most studied in this regard, at least in special education, are exemplified in the four chapters in this section on externalizing behaviors (Chapter 13, by Michael J. Furlong, Gale M. Morrison, and Shane R. Jimerson), internalizing behaviors (Chapter 14, by Frank M. Gresham and Lee Kern), youth delinquency (Chapter 15, by C. Michael Nelson, Peter E. Leone, and Robert B. Rutherford Jr.), and autistic spectrum disorders (Chapter 16, by Dwight P. Sweeney and Charles D. Hoffman). While it is an obvious oversimplification to summarize the conclusions of these authors in regard to special education eligibility, it is not too far off the mark to conclude from their reviews that children with externalizing behaviors are more likely than children with internalizing behaviors to be referred for special education, that youth delinquency is likely to divert children from special education into the child welfare or juvenile justice systems, and that eligibility of children with autistic spectrum disorders has increased dramatically in the past few years with the advent of special education and related services designated for such children. These four chapters, however, also provide a comprehensive review of other related issues including the subtypes within each of these four behavioral disorders, the school context of the identification, and treatments or programs for each that form the primary evidence base for school intervention.

The purpose of this brief introduction is to raise other selected research issues not systematically covered in these four chapters. These include (1) the special education identification of children with such disorders in categories other than emotional disturbance or autism, (2) the potential use of psychiatric diagnoses to identify children in need of services, (3) the dilemma of comorbidity in identification and intervention, and (4) the role of special education for children with emotional or behavioral disorders in the larger context of mental health treatment.

IDENTIFICATION IN OTHER CATEGORIES OF SPECIAL EDUCATION

Although emotional disturbance (ED) and autism are considered the primary special education categories for children with emotional or behavioral disorders, there is some evidence that significant numbers of children with such disorders may be found in other special education categories. This misidentification, as opposed to underidentification, of children with emotional or behavioral disorders has not been a primary focus of research in the field of behavioral disorders, but it is nonetheless a potentially productive research area.

The U.S. Department of Education (2002) has recently underlined the seriousness of this issue by devoting a special section of their annual report on the Individuals with Disabilities Education Act (IDEA) to a description of social adaptation and problem behaviors of elementary and middle school students receiving special education. In this section, they detail selected findings from their Special Education Elementary Longitudinal Study (SEELS) based on social skills and problem behavior ratings obtained from a total of 4,541 teachers and 4,466 parents of children (ages 6–12) in 12 categories of special education. Across *all* special education categories, nearly 40% of children were rated by teachers as "easily distracted" on a frequent basis, 25% as "acting impulsively," and 7–10% as depressed or lonely. As expected, social skill impairments and problem behaviors were greatest in the ED and autism categories. Children in other categories such as mental retardation and other health impairments, however, also had substantial impairments in social skills; and children in the categories of other health impairments and traumatic brain injury had substantial levels of problem behaviors. Children in the categories of learning disabilities and other health impairments tended to be suspended or expelled for disciplinary reasons in substantial numbers, though somewhat less so than children in the ED category.

In a similar vein, Redden, Forness, and their colleagues (1999, 2002) followed over 4,000 Head Start children until the end of third grade in terms of their risk for emotional or behavioral disorders as well as subsequent eligibility of at-risk children for special education. In contrast to the first study, risk was established using a diagnostic analog of clinical cutoff points, both for symptoms of emotional or behavioral disorders and for concurrent impairment in either social skills and/or academic performance, as measured for each child on individual testing and teacher ratings at the end of third grade. Testing and teacher ratings were done independently of local schools by trained research staff. Although nearly 17% of children met clinical cutoffs for concurrent symptoms *and* impairment by the end of third grade, only 24% of children diagnosed in this way were found eligible for special education by their schools. Children meeting cutoffs for emotional or behavioral disorders were, however, *five* times more likely to be identified in the learning disorder (LD) or speech and language impairment category (if they were found eligible) than they were in the ED category. This was despite the fact that possible comorbid learning or speech and language disorders were first *ruled out* through testing or teacher ratings prior to these children being diagnosed at risk for emotional or behavioral disorders.

In the above studies, it seems clear that more children with emotional or behavioral disorders may currently be identified in *other* special education categories than they are in the typical categories of ED or autism. Very few studies have been done on children, furthermore, with attention-deficit/hyperactivity disorder (ADHD) who have been identified in the category of other health impairments (OHI), as compared with those identified in the ED or LD category, despite the fact that possibly more than half the OHI category is now made up of children with ADHD (Forness & Kavale, 2002). Several unanswered research questions suggest themselves, including types of emotional or behavioral disorders that are served in special education inside versus outside the traditional categories of ED or autism, whether school interventions differ for such children depending on such identification, the likelihood of referrals for community mental health services for each, and the training of special education teachers to manage or care for children with emotional or behavioral disorders who are *not* identified in the ED or autism categories.

USING PSYCHIATRIC DIAGNOSES IN SPECIAL EDUCATION

As noted above, the term "behavioral disorders" is used as an all-encompassing term in the field of special education, denoting both externalizing and internalizing problems along with autism and delinquency. It is ironic that the same term, sometimes preceded by the term "disruptive," is used by psychiatrists and other mental health professionals to denote only oppositional defiant disorders, conduct disorders, or ADHD (American Psychiatric Association, 2000). This disparity is emblematic of differences in purpose of diagnosis and theoretical orientation between the two fields. Gresham and Kern discuss these differences and critique the diagnostic system used by mental health professionals, known as DSM-IV (fourth edition of the *Diagnostic and Statistical Manual of Mental Disorders*). Their criticisms include the fact that DSM-IV focuses on "within-person" problems, includes symptoms that are difficult to operationalize, has significant weaknesses in reliability, and lacks treatment validity.

These criticisms were probably much more relevant some years ago. Recent research, however, has established that most serious emotional or behavioral disorders are indeed primarily "within-person" problems, as genetic and brain-imaging findings have now largely established (Hyman 2002, 2003; Pennington, 2002). While environmental or external influences are important, they are nowhere nearly as significant in the genesis of psychopathology as most behaviorists once thought. While some psychiatric symptoms are difficult to operationalize, thus leading to problems in reliability, these problems are not insurmountable and are probably no less troublesome psychometrically than factorially based measures for the purpose of diagnosis or treatment. Recent advances in the development of psychiatric rating scales and structured psychiatric interviews have largely begun to address these issues (Brooks & Kutcher, 2003; Collett, Ohan, & Myers, 2003a, 2003b; McClellan & Werry, 2000; Myers & Winters, 2002a, 2002b). That similar reliability problems also occur in the existing field of behavior disorders is nowhere more evident than in the state-by-state variation on children identified in the ED category. While it is perhaps somewhat gratuitous to use this example in this context, identification currently ranges from 0.10% in Arkansas to 2.09% in the District of Columbia (U.S. Department of Education, 2002). Even applying multisource, multi-informant measures to relatively large samples of children at risk for emotional or behavioral disorders results in interrater reliability rates no better than those that Gresham and Kern decry for DSM-IV and/or produces widely varying types of children in terms of ethnicity and gender (Cluett et al., 1998; Serna, Nielsen, Mattern, Schau, & Forness, 2002). As to the criticism that DSM-IV lacks treatment validity, one need look no further for refutation than recent impressive large-scale multicenter trials for treatment of ADHD, depression, and anxiety disorders, some of which include direct comparisons of behavioral or cognitive-behavioral interventions versus psychopharmacologic treatment (Burns, Hoagwood, & Mrazek, 1999; Wasserman, Ko, & Jensen, 2001; Kazdin & Weisz, 2003).

Even if Gresham and Kern's criticisms were substantially correct, the fact remains that DSM-IV remains, for the foreseeable future, the gold standard for psychiatric and psychological diagnosis and treatment in the larger field of mental health. The point has also been made that referrals for psychopharmacological treatment in particular, not to mention its research base, depend significantly on establishing possible presence of a DSM-IV diagnosis and that the potential for such treatment may match or exceed that for school behavioral treatments (Forness & Kavale, 2001; Forness, Kavale, & Davanzo, 2002). A widely accepted school definition for emotional or behavioral disorders, intended to replace the current federal ED definition, indeed lists examples of DSM-IV diagnoses that could qualify a child as eligible for special education but does so with the understanding that *school* functioning is also impaired (Forness & Kavale, 2000). This was done primarily to *facilitate* referrals to mental health systems outside of the school, not to dictate special education interventions or programs.

Thus, it seems clear that the time has now come for the field of behavioral disorders to begin using DSM-IV as a supplemental if not primary diagnostic system for special education and related mental health services. Both Furlong, Morrison, and Jimerson (in Chapter 13, this volume) and Gresham and Kern (Chapter 14) in fact use DSM-IV diagnoses as primary exemplars of externalizing and internalizing disorders, respectively; and Forness, Walker, and Kavale (2003) provide a primer for teachers regarding these diagnoses. Forness, Kavale, Sweeney, and Crenshaw (1999) review the impressive evidence for efficacy of psychopharmacological treatments for various DSM-IV diagnoses and also provide guidelines for collaboration between teachers and prescribing psychiatrists. Mutual benefits would therefore seem to accrue to both special education and mental health with use of DSM-IV diagnoses in this regard.

THE DILEMMA OF COMORBIDITY

Despite the potential usefulness of DSM-IV diagnoses, the fact remains that comorbidity, the co-occurrence of two or more disorders in one child, renders both diagnosis and treatment much more complex in both special education and mental health. In actual fact, comorbidity seems to be the norm in children referred for mental health services including special education (Angold, Costello, & Erklani, 1999). Failure to detect such comorbidity in school settings may in fact lead not only to mistakes in choice of intervention but also to problems in prioritizing referral opportunities for psychiatric treatment outside of school settings. Development of a relatively simple rating scale to screen for such mixed disorders in young school children is in fact currently under way (Walker, Severson, Feil, Stieber, & Forness, 2003). By not attending to possible comorbid diagnoses, special educators and related school professionals may not only be potentially mismanaging treatment resources but also be missing critical opportunities for determining the most effective treatment, especially since comorbid disorders are apt to be the most treatment-resistant.

A prime example comes from the national multimodal treatment of ADHD (MTA) study (Jensen et al., 2001). Children in this study with only an ADHD diagnosis responded quite well to stimulant medication *only*. Children with ADHD and a comorbid diagnosis of anxiety disorder responded equally well to either stimulant medication *or* to home-school behavioral interventions. Children with ADHD and conduct or oppositional defiant disorder responded well only to a *combination* of both treatments. Children with ADHD and both anxiety and conduct disorders responded only *partially* to combination treatment and clearly needed additional treatment or modifications of their existing interventions.

Another instructive example is contained in a series of studies on children with disruptive disorders who also have comorbid depression or anxiety disorders. In sequential behavioral observations of adult–child interactions, children with such a mixed pattern were often significantly less likely to pursue adaptive responses and much more likely to revert to impulsive responding without regard to consequences of their actions than children with just disruptive behavior disorders (Granic & Lamey, 2002). They simply did not respond to traditionally effective behavioral approaches. Both prospective and retrospective follow-up of children with mixed disorders also suggested very different developmental patterns of adjustment, with implications for differential treatment involving much more emphasis on cognitive-behavioral and emotional-regulation approaches than needed for children with simple disruptive behavioral disorders (Capaldi & Stoolmiller, 1999; Jaffee, Moffitt, Caspi, Taylor, & Arseneault, 2002). Children with such mixed disorders (externalizing *and* internalizing) also demonstrated very different patterns of perturbation on neuroimaging in the anterior cingulate gyrus (governing some aspects of emotion or motivation) and the orbitofrontal cortex (governing some aspects of impulse control) than children with "pure" externalizing disorders (Luu, Collins, & Tucker, 2000).

Comorbidity thus represents a significant and largely unaddressed research issue in the field of behavioral disorders. That children with comorbid disorders represent those most likely to be treatment-resistant makes this issue even more compelling (Connor et al., 2003; Marmorstein & Iacono, 2003; Talbott & Fleming, 2003). Comorbidity is also more likely to be missed in diagnosis and not considered in treatment if DSM-IV is not used. A promising diagnostic rating measure based on DSM-IV has been shown to be potentially helpful for classroom use in this regard (Mattison, Gadow, Sprafkin, Nolan, & Schneider, 2003).

SPECIAL EDUCATION AS A MENTAL HEALTH TREATMENT

The preceding research issues—(1) misidentification of children with emotional or behavioral disorders, (2) use of DSM-IV diagnoses in special education and related services, and (3) implications of comorbidity for diagnosis and intervention—are, in the final analysis, all components of the last issue. This has to do with the context of special education for children with emotional or behavioral disorders in the larger field of child mental health. Hoagwood and Johnson (2003) have noted that schools are by far the largest provider of mental health services for children and adolescents in the United States. It can be argued that the professions of special education and school psychology are, in turn, the two most knowledgeable and effective providers of mental health services in schools.

There is considerable evidence, on the other hand, that mental health professionals remain largely unaware and/or unappreciative of the expertise of special educators and, to a lesser extent, school psychologists. The most telling evidence of this lack of appreciation—one might even use the term "lack of *respect*"—is that neither special education nor school psychology were significantly represented in the two arguably most important national child mental health conferences in the past 5 years. Only *one* special education or school psychology research presentation was included among the more than 24 research presentations in the National Institute of Health Consensus Development Conference on ADHD (Forness & Kavale, 2002), and only *two* such presentations were included in the 22 primary presentations in the U.S. Surgeon General's Conference on Children's Mental Health (Forness, 2000; Lewis, 2000). This, in spite of the fact that special education and school psychology probably serve not only the largest numbers of children with mental health disorders but also ostensibly spend the most contact hours with such children.

As has been noted elsewhere (Forness, 2003), modern special education for children with emotional or behavioral disorders has been largely dominated by a behaviorist perspective since its inception as an academic discipline. This has led to an emphasis on behavioral analysis as its primary approach and even to an overreliance on single-subject methodology in its research base (Mooney, Epstein, Reid, & Nelson, 2003). As noted above, this has in turn led to a continuing reluctance by special educators to embrace DSM-IV diagnoses and psychopharmacological treatments. Single-subject research studies, while important, are less than convincing when it comes to acceptance in the larger field of mental health that largely emphasizes clinical trials as the current standard for its evidence base. Hill Walker's analogy (personal communication, September 2003) is that a single-subject study will secure a Saturday night date but that, if one wants to get invited to the big prom, a group-controlled experimental-design study is indispensable (this statement is, of course, intended to be gender-neutral).

It seems inevitable that special education for children with emotional or behavioral disorders will not secure the necessary respect or influence it deserves as a field unless and until it addresses the foregoing research issues as part of its research base. Its future evidence-based practice must begin to depend more fully on collaborative research efforts using DSM-IV diagnoses, adjunctive psychopharmacological treatments, and clinical trials. In such a way both special education *and* mental health may be better served.

REFERENCES

American Psychiatric Association. (2000). *Diagnostic and statistical manual of mental disorders* (4th ed., text rev.). Washington, DC: Author.

Angold, A., Costello, E. J., & Erkanli, A. (1999). Comorbidity. *Journal of Child Psychology and Psychiatry, 40,* 57–87.

Brooks, S. W., & Kutcher, T. (2003). Diagnosis and measurement of anxiety disorders in adolescents: A review of commonly used instruments. *Journal of Child and Adolescent Psychopharmocology, 13,* 351–400.

Burns, B. J., Hoagwood, K. S., & Mrazek, P. H. (1999). Effective treatment for mental disorders in children and adolescents. *Clinical Child and Family Psychology Review, 2,* 199–254.

Capaldi, D. M., & Stoolmiller, M. (1999). Co-occurrence of conduct problems and depressive symptoms in early adolescent boys: III. Prediction to young-adult adjustment. *Developmental Psychopathology, 11,* 59–84.

Cluett, S. E., Forness, S. R., Ramey, S. L., Ramey, C. E., Hsu, C., Kavale, K. A., & Gresham, F. M. (1998). Consequences of differential diagnostic criteria on identification rates of children with emotional or behavioral disorders. *Journal of Emotional and Behavioral Disorders, 6,* 130–140.

Collett, B. R., Ohan, J. L., & Myers, K. M. (2003a). Ten-year review of rating scales: V. Scales assessing attention deficit hyperactivity disorder. *Journal of the American Academy of Child and Adolescent Psychiatry, 42,* 1015–1037.

Collett, B. R., Ohan, J. L., & Myers, K. M. (2003b). Ten-year review of rating scales: VI. Scales assessing externalizing behaviors. *Journal of the American Academy of Child and Adolescent Psychiatry, 42,* 1143–1170.

Connor, D. F., Edwards, G., Fletcher, K. E., Baird, J., Barkley, R. A., & Steingard, R. J. (2003). Correlates of comorbid psychopathology in children with ADHD. *Journal of the American Academy of Child and Adolescent Psychiatry, 42,* 193–200.

Forness, S. R. (2000). Schools and identification of mental health needs. In U.S. Public Health Service, *Report of the Surgeon General's conference on children's mental health* (pp. 22–23). Washington, DC: Author.

Forness, S. R. (2003). Barriers to evidence-based treatment: Developmental psychopathology and the interdisciplinary disconnect in school mental health practice. *Journal of School Psychology, 41,* 61–67.

Forness, S. R., & Kavale, K. A. (2000). Emotional or behavioral disorders: Background and current status of the EBD terminology and definition. *Behavioral Disorders, 25,* 264–269.

Forness, S. R., & Kavale, K. A. (2001). Ignoring the odds: Hazards of not adding the medical model to special education decisions. *Behavioral Disorders, 26,* 269–281.

Forness, S. R., & Kavale, K. A. (2002). Impact of ADHD on school systems. In P. S. Jensen & J. R. Cooper (Eds.). *Attention deficit hyperactivity disorder: State of the science; best practices* (pp. 24:1–20). Kingston, NJ: Civic Research Institute.

Forness, S. R., Kavale, K. A., & Davanzo, P. A. (2002). The new medical model: Interdisciplinary treatment and the limits of behaviorism. *Behavioral Disorders, 27,* 168–178.

Forness, S. R., Kavale, K. A., Sweeney, D. P., & Crenshaw, T. M. (1999). The future of research and practice in behavioral disorders: Psychopharmacology and its school treatment implications. *Behavioral Disorders, 24,* 305–318.

Forness, S. R., Walker, H. M., & Kavale, K. A. (2003). Psychiatric disorders and treatments: A primer for teachers. *Teaching Exceptional Children, 36*(2), 42–49.

Granic, I., & Lamey, A. V. (2002). Combining dynamic systems and multivariate analyses to compare the mother–child interactions of externalizing subtypes. *Journal of Abnormal Child Psychology, 30,* 265–283.

Hoagwood, K., & Johnson, J. (2003). School psychology: A public health framework: I. From evidence-based practices to evidence-based policies. *Journal of School Psychology, 41,* 1–22.

Hyman, S. E. (2002). Neuroscience, genetics, and the future of psychiatric diagnosis. *Psychopathology, 35*(2–3), 139–144.

Hyman, S. E. (2003). Psychiatry: Diagnosing disorders. *Scientific American, 289*(3), 96–103.

Jaffee, S. R., Moffitt, T. E., Caspi, A., Taylor, A., & Arseneault, L. (2002). Influence of adult domestic violence on children's internalizing and externalizing problems: An environmentally informative twin study. *Journal of the American Academy of Child and Adolescent Psychiatry, 41,* 1095–1103.

Jensen, P. S., Hinshaw, S. P., Kraemer, H. C., Lenora, N., Newcorn, J. H., Abikoff, H B., March, J. S., Arnold, L. E., Cantwell, D. P., Conners, C. K., Elliott, G. R., Greenhill, L. L., Hechtman, L., Hoza, B., Pelham, W. E., Severe, J. B., Swanson, J. M., Wells, K. C., Wigal, T., & Vitiello, B. (2001). ADHD comorbidity findings from the MTA study: Comparing comorbid subgroups. *Journal of the American Academy of Child and Adolescent Psychiatry, 40,* 147–158.

Kazdin, A. E., & Weisz, J. R. (Eds.). (2003). *Evidence-based psychotherapies for children and adolescents.* New York: Guilford Press.

Lewis, T. (2000). Prevention, early intervention, and community-based services. In U.S. Public Health Service, *Report of the Surgeon General's conference on children's mental health* (pp. 36–37). Washington, DC: Author.

Luu, P., Collins, P., & Tucker, D. M. (2000). Mood, personality, and self-monitoring: Negative affect and emotionality in relation to frontal lobe mechanisms of error monitoring. *Journal of Experimental Psychology: General, 129,* 43–60.

Marmorstein, N. R., & Iacono, W. G. (2003). Major depression and conduct disorder in a twin sample: Gender, functioning, and risk for future psychopathology. *Journal of the American Academy of Child and Adolescent Psychiatry, 42,* 225–233.

Mattison, R. E., Gadow, K. D., Sprafkin, J., Nolan, E. E., & Schneider, J. (2003). A *DSM-IV-*referenced teacher rating scale for use in clinical management. *Journal of the American Academy of Child and Adolescent Psychiatry, 42,* 442–449.

McClellan, J. M., & Werry, J. S. (2000). Introduction to special section: Research psychiatric diagnostic interviews for children and adolescents. *Journal of the American Academy of Child and Adolescent Psychiatry, 39,* 19–99.

Mooney, P., Epstein, M. H., Reid, R., & Nelson, J. R. (2003). Status of and trends in academic intervention research for students with emotional disturbance. *Remedial and Special Education, 24,* 273–287.

Myers, K., & Winters, N. C. (2002a). Ten-year review of rating scales: I. Overview of scale functioning, psychometric properties, and selection. *Journal of the American Academy of Child and Adolescent Psychiatry, 41,* 114–122.

Myers, K., & Winters, N. C. (2002b). Ten-year review of rating scales: II. Scales for internalizing disorders. *Journal of the American Academy of Child and Adolescent Psychiatry, 41,* 634–659.

Pennington, B. F. (2002). *The development of psychopathology: Nature and nurture.* New York: Guilford Press.

Redden, S. C., Forness, S. R., Ramey, S. L., Ramey, C. T., & Brezausek, C. M. (2002). Mental health and special education outcomes of Head Start children followed into elementary school. *National Head Start Association Dialog: A Research-to-Practice Journal for the Early Intervention Field, 6,* 87–110.

Redden, S. C., Forness, S. R., Ramey, S. L., Ramey, C. T., Zima, B. T., Brezausek, C. M., & Kavale, K. A. (1999). Head Start children at third grade: Preliminary special education identification and placement of children with emotional, learning, or related disabilities. *Journal of Child and Family Studies, 8,* 285–303.

Roberts, R. E., Attkisson, C. A., & Rosenblatt, A. (1998). Prevalence of psychopathology among children and adolescents. *American Journal of Psychiatry, 155,* 715–725.

Serna, L., Nielsen, E., Mattern, N., Schau, C., & Forness, S. R. (2002). Use of different measures to identify preschoolers at risk for emotional or behavioral disorders: Impact on gender and ethnicity. *Education and Treatment of Children, 25,* 415–437.

Talbott, E., & Fleming, J. (2003). The role of social contexts and special education in the mental health problems of urban adolescents. *Journal of Special Education, 37,* 111–123.

U.S. Department of Education (2002). *Twenty-fourth annual report to Congress on the implementation of the Individuals with Disabilities Education Act.* Washington, DC: Author.

Walker, H. M., Severson, H., Feil, E. G., Stieber, S., & Forness, S. R. (2003). *Ratings of Internalizing and Severely Challenging Behavior (RISC-B): Scale development procedures and initial results.* Eugene, OR: College of Education, University of Oregon.

Wasserman, G. A., Ko, S. J., & Jensen, P. S. (2001). Columbia guidelines for child and adolescent mental health referral. *Emotional and Behavioral Disorders in Youth, 2,* 9–14, 23.

13

Externalizing Behaviors of Aggression and Violence and the School Context

MICHAEL J. FURLONG, GALE M. MORRISON,
and SHANE R. JIMERSON

Not all youths who commit acts of aggression or violence have an externalizing disorder, but many youths with a diagnosable externalizing disorder (particularly conduct disorders) are at increased risk of aggressive behavior (Connor, 2002). A dramatic increase in youth violence during the early 1990s, and increasing recognition that the mental health needs of youths involved with the juvenile authorities were being unmet (Dwyer, Osher, & Warger, 1998), led to a heightened concern about the link between externalizing disorders and violence. This concern grew out of the awareness that in the United States violent acts committed by (and to) youths were a major public health problem, with these acts accounting for 40% of all deaths among teenagers (Snyder, 2000). Firearms are, in fact, the second leading cause of death among all youths ages 15–19 and the leading cause for African American males (Snyder, 2000). During the late 1990s, this trend began to reverse, and by 2000 there was a 64.2% decrease in the number of homicides committed by youths ages 14–17 since the historic high in 1994. The rate of youth homicides per 100,000 was actually near its lowest point in 2000

(see Figure 13.1; Bureau of Justice Statistics, 2001). Similar decreases were noted in other categories of violent crimes committed by youths (e.g., aggravated and simple assaults; Bureau of Justice Statistics, 2001).

Despite the promising reversal in serious violent acts by youths, other less serious but harmful aggression continues to occur with increasing attention being given to their incidence in school contexts. The 2001 administration of the Youth Risk Behavior Surveillance Survey (YRBS; Grunbaum et al., 2002) found that 10.3% of males and 1.3% of females (in grades 9–12) nationwide reported they had carried a gun during the past 30 days. In addition, 43.2% of males and 23.9% of females indicated they had been in a physical fight in the past year. Similar patterns were found when youths were asked about aggression-related behaviors on school campuses. Among males, 10.2% reported carrying a weapon (gun, knife, or club) to school in the past month, compared to 6.5% of females. School fighting (in the past 12 months) was reported by 18.0% of males and 7.2% of females. The rates of antisocial behavior reported in the 2001 YRBS were lower than in previous years but, nonethe-

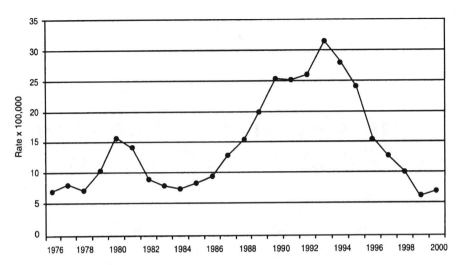

FIGURE 13.1. Homicides committed by youths ages 14–17, 1976–2000, rate per 100,000 population. Data from Bureau of Justice Statistics (2001).

less, continue to show the high incidence of antisocial and aggression-related behaviors among American adolescents. In addition, although less than 1% of all homicides among school-age children (5–19 years of age) occur in or around school grounds or on the way to and from school, in raw numbers this included more than 220 deaths between July 1, 1994, and June 30, 1999 (Anderson et al., 2001; note that in 2001–2003 there were only 10 school-associated deaths). Although these events are not the most pressing youth violence problem on a day-to-day basis, they have resulted in increased attention by educators to the origins and occurrence of externalizing disorders among students.

This chapter focuses specifically on those externalizing disorders that have a primary element of aggressive or violent behavior. We will begin by presenting an overview of aggressive diagnostic patterns as embodied in the DSM-IV and the Individuals with Disabilities Education Act (IDEA). We then turn to a discussion of research-derived models of how externalizing disorders involving aggressive behavior emerge from the developmental process. The third section of the chapter focuses on the important context of the school as it relates to youth aggression and violence. Here, school system factors may exacerbate the development of aggression or serve as a buffer or have a protective

influence. We conclude with a focus on future research needs for aggressive externalizing disorders.

DIAGNOSTIC AND DEVELOPMENTAL PATTERNS OF AGGRESSION AND VIOLENCE

Two externalizing disorders for which aggression and violence are central concerns are conduct disorder and attention-deficit/hyperactivity disorder (ADHD). Behaviors associated with conduct disorder constitute the most frequent bases for referral of children and adolescents for psychological and psychiatric problems, criminal behaviors, and social maladjustment (Doll, 1996; Kazdin, 1995, 1997). Conduct disorder, in particular, encompasses a range of chronic antisocial behaviors that typically begin in early childhood and extends into adulthood (Moffitt, Caspi, Rutter, & Silva, 2001; Robins & Ratcliff, 1979).

Within the school context, children who exhibit these problematic behaviors usually present challenges in the traditional classroom environment, and such behaviors often result in poor academic performance. Children manifesting behavioral problems may have learning disabilities and sometimes previously are diagnosed with attention-deficit/hyperactivity disorder. Research also indicates that antisocial behavior is related to truancy and dropout rates (Rumberger, 1987). Additional concurrent deleterious experiences include alcohol and substance abuse. Behaviors associated with conduct disorder constitute the most frequent bases for referral of children and adolescents for psychological and psychiatric problems, criminal behaviors, and social maladjustment (Kazdin, 1995). In addition, research has shown that the characteristics of this disorder can be passed on across generations, forming a cyclical pattern (Kazdin, 1995). Therefore, the knowledge and research pertaining to this childhood disorder can serve as a useful tool to clinicians, professionals, teachers, and the community.

DSM-IV-TR Criteria of Conduct Disorder

Children with conduct disorder diagnosis may vary in symptoms and behaviors. The following are a list of symptoms relevant to this particular disorder according to the *Diagnostic and Statistical Manual of Mental Disorders* (American Psychiatric Association, 2000, pp. 98–99); criteria with references to aggression are **shown in bold**:

1. A repetitive and persistent pattern in which the rights of others or societal norms or rules are violated, as manifested by the presence of at least three of the following criteria in the past 12 months (with at least one criterion present in the past 6 months).
2. *Aggression to people and animals*, for example, **bullying, threatening,** or intimidating others, initiating **physical fights, using a weapon** that can cause serious physical harm to others (e.g., a bat, brick, broken bottle, knife, gun), being **physically cruel** to people or animals, or has stolen while confronting a victim (e.g., **mugging, purse snatching, extortion, armed robbery**), has **forced someone into sexual activity**).
3. *Destruction of property*, such as deliberately engaged in **fire setting** with the intention of causing serious damage, or has deliberately **destroyed others' property** (other than by fire setting).
4. *Deceitfulness or theft*, for instance, has broken into someone else's house, building, or car, often lies to obtain goods or

favors or to avoid obligations (i.e., "cons" others), or has stolen items of nontrivial value without confronting a victim (e.g., shoplifting, but without breaking and entering; forgery).
5. *Serious violation of rules such as* staying out at night despite parental prohibitions (beginning before age 13 years), running away from home overnight (at least twice while living in parental or parental surrogate home or once without returning for a lengthy period), or is often truant from school (beginning before age 13 years).

There is a "childhood-onset type" wherein onset of at least one criterion characteristic of conduct disorder occurs prior to age 10 years, and also "adolescent-onset type," which occurs when there is an absence of any criteria characteristic of conduct disorder prior to age 10 years. Prevalence of conduct disorder is estimated at about 2% for girls with an onset typically between 14 and 16 years old and 9% in boys with onset generally before age 10 years (Russo & Beidel, 1994). Conduct disorders differ from other childhood challenges due to the antisocial behavior, the chronicity of such behavior, as well as the impairment of functioning of those exhibiting such behaviors. Although it is it possible for a youth to be given a diagnosis of conduct disorder without a record of overt physical aggression, the symptoms are heavily loaded with this class of behaviors.

Diagnosis of Attention-Deficit/Hyperactivity Disorder

Attention-deficit/hyperactivity disorder is the most commonly diagnosed behavioral disorder during childhood (Tannock & Schachar, 1996). The symptoms of this disorder are closely tied to behavioral difficulties. ADHD includes a heterogeneous array of symptoms, which overlaps markedly with oppositional defiant disorder, conduct disorder, affective disorders such as depression, anxiety, learning disabilities, and communication disorders. DSM-IV-TR includes multiple subtypes of ADHD—inattentive, hyperactive/impulsive, and combined type—and specifies a range of diagnostic criteria. The most common age for diagnosis is between the ages of 7 and 9, although symptoms may be apparent before the age of 3. The number of boys diagnosed with ADHD outnumbers girls by at least 4 to 1. Comorbidity of ADHD with conduct disorder (50%), oppositional-defiant behavior, anxiety disorders, speech and language disorders (78%), and learning disabilities (LD) (40–70%) is extremely high (Mayes, Calhoun, & Crowell, 2000).

Externalizing Disorders and Comorbidity

Youths meeting the criteria for conduct disorder classification often present symptoms of attention-deficit/hyperactivity disorder, oppositional defiant disorder, and anxiety disorders. As highlighted in a review of epidemiological studies by Russo and Beidel (1994), there is significant comorbidity between anxiety disorders, externalizing disorders, and depression. In fact, the DSM-IV-TR includes aggression as a childhood criterion for the diagnosis of depression. As Achenbach (1998) has previously argued, often it is more important to understand the individual's developmental history and constellation of behaviors, as there is a great degree of overlap among youths that are identified as having a conduct disorder and other conditions.

Early Onset versus Adolescent Onset of Externalizing Behaviors

Moffitt and Caspi (2001) provide a comprehensive summary of childhood predictors that differentiate life-course persistent and adolescence-limited antisocial pathways. This study provides a comparison of childhood risk factors of males and females exhibiting childhood-onset and adolescent-onset antisocial behavior, using data from the Dunedin, New Zealand, longitudinal study. The outcomes associated with early-onset are much more deleterious relative to those youths who initiate behavior problems during adolescence. Some have argued that this may not be accurate among females (Frick, 1998); however, there have been few systematic comparisons of developmental trajectories by gender (Kratzer & Hodgins, 1999; Mazerolle, Brame, Paternoster, Piquero, & Dean, 2000). Results of

the Moffitt and Caspi (2001) study indicate that both males and females, with childhood-onset delinquency had childhoods of inadequate parenting, neurocognitive problems, behavior problems, whereas adolescent-onset delinquents did not have these pathological backgrounds (Burke, Lahey, Loeber, & Rathouz, 2002). Likewise, attention or hyperactivity problems during elementary school have a cumulative deleterious impact on peer relations and academic performance. Considering the developmental trajectories of children displaying behavior problems indicating early aggressive behaviors characteristic of life-course persisters (Burke et al., 2002; Stanger, Achenbach, & Verhulst, 1997), it is especially important to provide appropriate early interventions to address both behavioral and underlying emotional problems.

Individuals with Disabilities Education Act and Emotional Disturbance

The Individuals with Disabilities Education Act (IDEA; Public Law 101-476) defines emotional disturbance as a condition exhibiting one or more of the following characteristics over a long period of time and to a marked degree that adversely affects educational performance: (1) an inability to learn that cannot be explained by intellectual, sensory, or health factors; (2) an inability to build or maintain satisfactory interpersonal relationships with peers and teachers; (3) inappropriate types of behavior or feelings under normal circumstances; (4) a general pervasive mood of unhappiness or depression; or (5) a tendency to develop physical symptoms or fears associated with personal or school problems (U.S. Department of Education, 1999). IDEA *does not* apply to children who are socially maladjusted, unless it is determined that they have an emotional disturbance. Often conduct disorder falls into the emotional disturbance category, whereas attention deficit disorder is discussed in the IDEA regulations as other health impairment. As characteristics of conduct disorder, emotional disturbance, and attention deficit disorder often are interrelated, the distinctions become blurred and these definitions continue to evolve (Forness & Kavale, 2000).

Educational Considerations

It is the responsibility of school-based professionals to determine whether a child needs special education and related services as a result of having an emotional or behavioral disorder. Significant emotional and behavioral problems may interfere with students' academic progress and for some youths require additional support and assistance to participate in general education classrooms. School psychologists and other school-based professionals may provide valuable professional contributions to facilitate the success of students with emotional or behavioral problems (Center for Mental Health in the Schools at UCLA, 1999).

It is always good educational practice for school child study teams to focus on addressing behavioral problems of children with disabilities in order to enhance their success in the classroom. In particular, (1) the team should explore the need for strategies and support systems to address any behavior that may impede the learning of the child with the disability or the learning of his or her peers; and (2) states shall address the needs of inservice and preservice personnel (including professionals and paraprofessionals who provide special education, general education, related services, or early intervention services) as they relate to developing and implementing positive intervention strategies. Intervention plans emphasizing skills students need in order to behave in a more appropriate manner, or plans providing motivation to conform to required standards, are generally more effective than plans that simply serve to control behavior (Hinshaw, 1996, 2000). Such plans often include positive strategies, program or curricular modifications, and supplementary support to address the problem behaviors.

Analysis of U.S. Department of Education national survey data found that school districts' sociodemographic characteristics were strongly associated with the proportion of students identified as having emotional disturbance (ED; Coutinho, Oswald, & Forness, 2002). Results also indicated a clear association between ethnicity/gender and the likelihood of being identified as having ED, even after accounting for sociodemographic effects.

PATHWAYS TO AGGRESSION IN EXTERNALIZING DISORDERS

The development of schemas to organize research and practice for youths with externalizing disorders is an essential ongoing process. In addition, researchers have recognized that aggression emerges from an interaction between the individual youths and the social contexts in which they develop. Recent theories have suggested that there is not one single developmental trajectory that leads to long-term antisocial and aggressive behavior but that it evolves through periods of quiescence and more dynamic increases (Patterson & Yoerger, 2002). In addition, consensus has not been reached among researchers even on the fundamental issue of how to best classify subtypes of aggressive behavior patterns. Although various subtypes have been proffered (e.g., instrumental–hostile; predatory–affective, and offensive–defensive), Connor (2002) suggests that the distinctions between *overt* (observable behaviors such as fighting) versus *covert* (more hidden behaviors such as vandalism), and the *reactive* (angry defensive responses) versus *proactive* (purposeful goal-directed acts) subtypes have the strongest internal and external validation. Development-based models of the how antisocial and aggressive behavior patterns emerge (whether in overt behavior, covert behavior, or both) in children and adolescents have focused on the family, the peer group, and the school as the primary settings in which aggression is modeled and learned. This next section provides a brief overview of the predominant research-based perspectives about the emergence of aggressive behavior in youths with externalizing disorders.

Multiple Factors, Differing Theoretical Perspectives

Social Learning Model

The social learning model emphasizes the importance of multiple proximal factors related to aggression, particularly antecedents and consequences of behaviors occurring in daily social exchanges between children, siblings, and parents within dysfunctional families (Patterson, Capaldi, & Bank, 1991; Patterson & Yoerger, 2002). Youths begin to learn aggressive behaviors through these everyday social exchanges between family members, as well as through such parenting styles that include inconsistent discipline and negative and positive reinforcement of antisocial behaviors and cognitions. Furthermore, the family environment and interactions of aggressive youth are characterized by coercion, typified by a family member using physical or verbal aggression to stop another family member from aggravating him or her or from interfering with his or her goals. These coercive behaviors become cyclical and reinforced such that children do not comply with their parents' requests; parents make harsher demands; children's noncompliance becomes more escalated; and parents give in to their child's noncompliance. Thus, parents of aggressive children do not model prosocial and appropriate problem-solving behaviors and instead actually teach aggressive behaviors.

In addition to the relationship between harsh discipline and children's aggression, such qualities of parent–child relations as lack of warmth with a primary caregiver (Doll & Lyon, 1998) can also contribute to children's aggression. Another possible factor leading to poor parenting and parent–child relationships include family life stressors related to socioeconomic disadvantage. Parents of children with conduct problems reported a greater degree of stress than parents of typically developing children (Webster-Stratton, 1990). The stressors, in turn, further impact their parenting styles.

Social Information-Processing Model

The social information-processing theory focuses on the cognitive role in social adjustment (Crick & Dodge, 1994) in that social cognitive skills, deficits, and biases are learned through the same social learning processes as noncompliance and coercive behavior. This theory differs from the social learning theory in that the latter speculates that it is the student's own social cognitions that account for various antisocial behaviors rather than the external modeling and reinforcement of behaviors (Dodge, Price, Bachorowski, & Newman, 1990).

Dodge's developmental model of social information processing (Dodge & Crick, 1994) has been studied extensively. Six pro-

cessing steps elucidate the types of information a student retrieves from memory and how the information is interpreted. The first two steps are encoding and interpreting social cues, in which the student reads specific cues in the situation. Here, the student may compare the immediate situation cues to those already stored in memory, analyze the potential problem and why the problem exists, infer what others might be thinking or intending to do, compare the present social exchange with the previous one, and consider the importance of the exchange to the self and the peer. Researchers (Dodge & Tomlin, 1987; Slaby & Guerra, 1988) found that habitually aggressive children tend to concentrate more on hostile or aversive social cues, have memory difficulties that interfere with their ability to process social information, and interpret cues from their existing aggressive schema.

The third step is determining goals in a given situation. Children determine their personal goals or desired outcomes for a given situation, based on their previous experiences and preexisting cognitive scripts (Crick & Dodge, 1994). Aggressive children, although desiring to be socially accepted, seek goals such as getting what they want and retaliating against those who present obstacles to those goals (Erdley & Asher, 1998; Slaby & Guerra, 1988).

The next step in the model is constructing a response. With aggressive children, alternative behavioral or emotional responses are drawn from memory and past experiences but, when confronted with novel situations, form new alternative responses. Slaby and Guerra (1988) found that aggressive children tend to generate fewer prosocial alternative solutions, compared to socially adjusted children. Specifically, these responses tended to be more atypical, maladaptive, and aggressive (Rubin, Bream, & Rose-Krasnor, 1991), with the latter viewed as socially acceptable and not immoral (Boldizar, Perry, & Perry, 1989; Crick & Ladd, 1990).

The fifth step of the social information-processing model is response–decision. This refers to the process by which the individual evaluates the alternative responses. Aggressive children tend to consider immediate egotistical gains when using moral reasoning rather than considering others' needs or long-term consequences. Research shows that ag-

gressive children believe their aggressive behaviors will indeed "work" and that their
choices will lead to more favorable outcomes than prosocial alternatives (Quiggle,
Garber, Panak, & Dodge, 1992).

The final step of the model is enacting, or
committing an aggressive act. Deficits at this
step are apparent when a student is aware of
the prosocial act, yet is unable or unwilling
to perform this act because he or she performs the very first alternative that comes to
mind.

Cognitive-Neoassociationistic Model

Cognitive-neoassociationistic theory (Berkowitz, 1989, 1990a, 1990b) is comparable
to the social information-processing model,
particularly its emphasis on social cognition.
Aggressive behavior is a result of both negative affect and environmental stimuli. Therefore, negative affect may trigger ideas, memories, and reactions associated with anger
and aggression. Relative to the school setting, the cognitive-neoassociationistic theory
highlights the importance of school climate
and the relationships between students and
teachers. Thus, for example, recent research
has explored the link between students' perceptions of campus bullying and school staff
responses to it. Students often report that, in
their view, staff do not systematically respond to bullying when it occurs, even when
they have witnessed it. In such circumstances, Unnever and Cornell (2003) have
referred to this as the "culture of bullying."
At schools where staff members do not consistently respond to bullying, they may send
an unintended message to students that bullying is tolerated. As might be expected,
schools with such a climate are more prone
to bullying, and, of course, the more frequently bullying occurs, the more numerous
are the context cues to trigger future aggressive bullying incidents.

"Life-Course-Persistent" and "Adolescent-Limited" Models of Aggression

There is a small group of youths who continue their aggressive behaviors from childhood through adolescence and are considered "life-course-persistent." A larger group
of youths commit their one and only crime
between the ages of 14 and 17 and are

considered "adolescent-limited" aggressors
(Moffitt, 1993a). Moffitt (1993a) argues
that social learning, social information processing, and emotion-based theories do not
explain or differentiate those who are life-
course-persistent or adolescent-limited aggressors and, instead, proposes two theories
that account for such differences in etiology,
developmental course, prognosis, and pa-
thology or normality.

Life-Course-Persistent Aggressors. Moffitt and colleagues (Caspi & Moffitt, 1995;
Moffitt, 1993a, 1993b) argue that, based on
research from neuropsychology, temperament, attention-deficit/hyperactivity disorder,
chronic aggression begins with neurological
impairment. Such sources of neurological
impairment as genetics, maternal drug
abuse, exposure to toxic agents, brain injury,
poor nutrition, lack of stimulation or affec-
tion, and child abuse have been associated
with children's antisocial behavior. However, neurological effects are not viewed as
deterministic. Instead, research has demonstrated the malleability in neuropsychological functioning and how neurological and
environmental factors interact in determining aggression. The main role of neuropsychological impairment in influencing the development of aggression is its effects on
language-based verbal skills and executive
functions of the brain (Moffitt, 1990). A deficiency in these areas can lead to poor academics, poor social-information processing,
impulsive behavior, a restricted behavioral
repertoire, social rejection, and poor self-
concept—thus, furthering the continuity in
aggressive behaviors. These deficits can also
place the child at risk for more negative outcomes, such as substance abuse, school
dropout, and gang membership. Together,
these factors contribute to the development
and maintenance of life-course-persistent aggression.

Adolescent-Limited Aggressors. The adolescents who engage in antisocial behaviors
between early adolescence and young adulthood tend to commit crimes less violent than
those of the life-course-persistent aggressors.
Such crimes include fighting, theft, vandalism, and drug use. Although Moffitt (1993a)
argues that neither social learning nor social
information-processing models explain the

sudden onset and discontinuity of aggressive behaviors in adolescence, her model agrees that reinforcement and punishment contingencies contribute to adolescent-limited aggression. Adolescents' desires to gain adult status lead them to seek less constructive or antisocial ways by committing aggressive acts. Thus, it is the adolescent's quest for maturity and autonomy that serves as a primary factor of aggression (Moffitt, 1993a).

Research examining the emergence of externalizing behavior disorders involving aggressive behavior has suggested that there are multiple pathways and that the meaning and stability of the aggression is different, depending on the age at which the behavior first emerges (Connor, 2002). Of great concern to educators is to better understand how to recognize and respond to those youths who show early signs of externalizing behavior symptoms and to respond with prevention efforts to deflect these youths from what can be a long-term pattern of aggression (Patterson & Yoerger, 2002).

SCHOOL AS A CRITICAL CONTEXT FOR AGGRESSION AND VIOLENCE

Much of what we know about child and adolescent aggressive and violent behavior comes to us from the context of schools. The boundaries for aggressive and violent behavior are often first met within classroom, peer, or schoolwide contexts where the behavior goes beyond a norm for acceptable behavior. Schools are also the most likely venue for intervention for aggressive or violent behavior. As such, in order to fully understand the development of child and adolescent aggression and violence, a complete understanding of how these behaviors interact within school systems is necessary. The focus of this section is on ways schools react to aggressive and violent behavior and how these reactions help to reduce or exacerbate the behavior.

Two sources for how schools react to aggressive or violent behavior are the disciplinary system and the systems for identification and education for students with disabilities. The externalizing behaviors of aggression and violence are most likely seen within the special education category of emotional disturbance (ED). However, many states use the narrow definition of ED (as opposed to EBD, emotional and behavioral disorder; see Cullinan, Chapter 3, this volume) and exclude students who may be exhibiting aggressive or antisocial behavior and therefore are considered socially maladjusted (Forness & Kavale, 2000). In this case, students who are considered by schools to be socially maladjusted are more likely to be seen on the lists for school exclusion, i.e., suspension and expulsion. Students who have learning disabilities (LD) and who also exhibit antisocial or aggressive behavior are likely to be served under the LD category unless the behavior becomes a primary focus for school intervention, in which case they are at risk for being determined "ineligible" under IDEA categories (Morrison & D'Incau, 2000). Because of the conflicting attitudes about serving students who might be considered socially maladjusted in special education, the focus here is on the disciplinary system as one of the primary school responses to aggressive and violent behavior.

The school disciplinary system consists of office referrals, suspensions, and expulsions as outcomes or consequences for behavior that breaks school rules. The behaviors punished by these mechanisms get progressively worse; i.e., an office referral may result from pushing or shoving behavior, whereas suspension and expulsion are used for state-defined rule-breaking behaviors. For example, aggressive and violent behavior such as weapon use or possession, fighting, vandalism, sexual harassment, stealing are typically included in state education codes as suspendable offenses (Civil Rights Project, 2000). In the case of weapon use or possession, mandatory recommendation for expulsion may be required (e.g., California Education Code, 1994). Zero-tolerance policies have led to variations in how strictly and comprehensively these codes are applied, sometimes leading to a rigidity in implementation that ignores extenuating circumstances related to the offense, leading Morrison and D'Incau (1997) to refer to recent practice in disciplinary processes as the "web of zero tolerance."

To what extent do students with behavior or aggression problems get caught in the "web of zero tolerance?" First, physical fights and aggression are the most common reasons for suspension (Costenbader &

Markson, 1994; Skiba, Peterson, & Williams, 1997). Students who engage in harassment, bullying, or other aggressive behavior are at greater risk for being caught in a disciplinary action (Tobin, Sugai, & Colvin, 1996). With regard to disabilities that might co-occur with aggressive behavior, even given the protections that have been provided through IDEA, Leone, Mayer, Malmgren, and Meisel (2000) reviewed data from a number of state and national databases and found that students with disabilities represent about 20% of all students suspended, although their representation in the overall school population is around 11%.

Although these figures give the impression that a major school reaction to students with aggressive or antisocial behavior is through school disciplinary processes, they do not supply a comprehensive picture of the day-to-day interactions among students, peers, teachers, and school administrators that help shape the ongoing school behavior of these students. Caspi, Elder, and Bem (1988) note that, once a child or adolescent engages in antisocial, deviant behaviors, the reactions of school officials, teachers, parents, and others may or may not facilitate positive outcomes. The paradigm of developmental psychopathology provides a model for exploring the complex, multifaceted issues that impact students as they move through their school years. Sroufe and Rutter (1984) define developmental psychopathology as the "study of the origins and course of individual patterns of behavioral maladaptation" (p. 18). This conceptualization has relevance to the discussion of school discipline in that the developmental perspective views the onset, course, and outcome of problematic behaviors across the developmental span from a broad perspective and examines the context in which these behaviors occur. This perspective contrasts to the special education system, where eligibility is considered at discreet points in time (mandated assessments taking place at least every 3 years).

In recognition that behavior interacts with critical contexts across time, we examine the likely impacts of these contexts on students who struggle with behavioral issues of aggression and antisocial behavior. These contexts provide opportunities to improve behavior or lead to continued misbehavior; thus, we highlight protective and risk factors associated with each context (Masten, Best, & Garmezy, 1990). Observations collected in the context of research on school discipline funded by the U.S. Department of Education, Office of Special Education Programs, will be used as examples for each area (Morrison, 2003).

Individual Characteristics Associated with Aggressive and Violent Behavior at School

First, it is important to identify the behaviors and individual characteristics that are likely to get students into trouble in various school contexts. Students who act out at school often show early signs of aggression and difficult temperament (Loeber, 1990; Moffitt, 1993b; Tubman & Windle, 1995). They may show deficits in social skills such as awkward initiation of social interactions, poor perspective taking, and deficits in conflict resolution (Coie, Dodge, & Kupersmidt, 1990; Walker, Colvin, & Ramsey, 1995). Behavioral impulsivity also is a strong predictor of antisocial behavior in the preadolescent years (White, Moffitt, Earls, Robins, & Silva, 1990). McFadden, Marsh, Price, and Hwang (1992) noted that students with disabilities differed from their nondisabled classmates, with a higher incidence of office referrals for "bothering others" and "unacceptable physical contact." School failure is a strong correlate of later psychological disturbance and delinquency (Cernkovich & Giordano, 1992; Gold & Osgood, 1992; Hawkins & Lishner, 1987; Roff, Sells, & Golden, 1972; Walker et al., 1995). In general, aggressive or violent behavior may result from a combination of traumatic experiences, a history of poor behavior control, and heightened negative emotions (Shields, Cicchetti, & Ryan, 1994). These latter characteristics point to the importance of considering the contexts within school that are likely to trigger aggressive actions.

On the other hand, resilience factors that could counterbalance some of the above deficits include constitutional dispositions (sociability, problem-solving ability, planning ability, and internal locus of control) that help the child establish relationships with parents, teachers, and other critical adults, and an ability to make positive life-course decisions (Clarke & Clarke, 1994). Within the individual and behavioral domains, critical variables include the students' perceptions of their self-control, cooperation, self-efficacy, and social problem solving. Personal control and cooperation were significant protective factors (Jessor, Van Den Bos, Vanderryn, Costa, & Turbin, 1995), while self-efficacy was suggested by the foundational research of Garmezy, Rutter and Werner (Garmezy, Masten, & Tellegen, 1984; Rutter, 1979; Werner & Smith, 1982). Elias and Branden (1988) have identified problem-solving skills as important in maintaining positive coping in the face of stressful situations.

Some examples of how these characteristics play out in a school setting with regard to students who get referred out of the classroom are displayed in Table 13.1. An important dimension not noted previously is the aspect of negotiating the school environment. One of the reasons that students with the characteristics described above find themselves involved in the disciplinary systems is that they experience difficulty in negotiating the demands, rules, and norms of the school context with regard to being a student. They may use disrespectful language with the teacher or may lack the verbal skills to explain their way out of an offense committed on campus.

TABLE 13.1 Individual Risk and Protective Factors

Protective	Risk
Sociability and temperament	
Friendly, quiet, respectful	Annoying
Sociability noted as a positive in early years	Early sociability not curbed as behavior expectations change; too talkative, gets in trouble for talking in class and not editing language
Can sit still and listen	Distractible and distracting to other students
Cognitive ability	
"With it"	Not "with it" enough to stay out of trouble or talk self out of trouble; verbal skills are limited (especially in children with learning disabilities)
Perspective taking	
Sensitive to others	Doesn't understand impact of behavior on others
Student is aware of reason for discipline	Cannot articulate why he or she is being disciplined
Ability to reflect on present and future	
Thinks about future; has ideas about what he or she wants to do	Lives for the present
Individual approach to conflict resolution/problem solving	
Talks it out	Fighting is response for conflict resolution, standing up for friends, making a point
Resources to persist in the face of academic failure or discipline setback	Student gives up
Negotiating the school environment	
None	Second language issue is evident in ability to process academic and institutional information
Seen as trying hard and making an effort	Student communication style is disrespectful

Peer Influences Associated with Aggressive and Violent Behavior at School

The power of social or peer affiliations in the trajectory toward delinquent behavior is described by Cairnes and Cairnes (1994). They note that peer social clusters are highly influential and supporting of behaviors considered "normative" for the group. Individuals carry the personal impact of these peer associations forward, even after their group affiliation changes. Research has found that peer social networks can influence negative behaviors such as aggression, bullying, and ostracism (Rodkin, Farmer, Pearl, & Van Acker, 2000). However, they can also influence positive behaviors in the academic and social realms. Specifically, a prosocial peer group that provides social support can play a stress-buffering function (Clarke & Clarke, 1994; Dubow & Tisak, 1989). Specific examples of peer risk and protective factors are listed in Table 13.2.

The Classroom Context for Aggression and Misbehavior

The classroom is one of the main contexts where a student's behavior comes into conflict with the rules and norms of the school. The skills of the teacher to handle misbehavior and encourage positive behavior are critical setting characteristics for student behavior (Osher et al., 2004; Scott, Nelson, & Liaupsin, 2001; Stage, 1997). Some of the risk factors for students who struggle with behavior issues in the classroom include a teacher who has few strategies for addressing developmental lags (La Paro, Pianta, & Cox, 2000) and an increase of negative attention that works against the establishment of a positive relationship (Blankemeyer, Flannery, & Vazsonyi, 2002; Reinke & Herman, 2002). Research indicates that students with EBD are less likely to be called on in classroom discussions (Sutherland & Wehby, 2001) and receive less positive reinforcement for providing correct answers (Gable, Hendrickson, Tonelson, & Van Acker, 2002).

Teachers vary in their ability to handle student misbehavior in their classroom. In one investigation at the middle school level, two-thirds of all disciplinary referrals came from 25% of the school's teachers (Skiba et al., 1997). Classrooms that are characterized by low rates of academic engagement, praise, and reinforcement and high rates of reprimands are associated with high rates of misbehavior, setting up a cycle of negative student–teacher interactions (Farmer, Farmer, & Gut, 1999; Reinke & Herman, 2002). Osher et al. (2004) refer to these characteristics as "warning signs" for unsafe classrooms.

In contrast, teacher management strategies, effective instructional techniques (e.g., classwide peer tutoring), early intervention for students with learning problems, and positive teacher–student relationships are critical components for keeping students in the classroom or avoiding the necessity of excluding them for disciplinary reasons (Reinke & Herman, 2002; Scott et al., 2001). Effective instruction and positive student–teacher relationships should be accompanied

TABLE 13.2. Peer Risk and Protective Factors

Protective	Risk
Student helps with younger students at school	Student "runs with" other troubling kids—they plan trouble together
Student is part of after-school program where he or she does homework with peers	Student is teased
None	Student is part of culture of "play fighting"
Student thinks he or she has friends	Those friends are "not really" friends
Student is able to separate him- or herself from negative behavior of peers	Student has few boundaries with friends; will get swept into negative activities of peers—student is a follower
Student moves to another school; establishes more positive group of friends	Student hangs out with older peers

by opportunities for students to be involved in activities to promote the development of desired social and emotional skills (Skiba & Peterson, 2003). Table 13.3 lists examples of the risk and protective factors in classrooms for children who are aggressive or who misbehave.

Schoolwide Context for Aggressive and Violent Behavior

A rich line of research and professional practice has been published on school effectiveness and school reform (Levine & Lezotte, 1990; Reynolds, Teddlie, Creemers, Scheerens, & Townsend, 2000). Information from this research informs us about how schoolwide practices can help or harm students who are at risk for behavior problems. One sign of an ineffective school is a disorderly school environment with vague rules and expectations; this situation is likely to place students at risk who are especially in need of clear expectations and structure (Gottfredson, 1989). A disorderly school environment is associated with high suspension and expulsion rates (Civil Rights Project, 2000). McEvoy and Welker (2000) note that schools that have low academic achievement and high antisocial behavior often rely on suspension and expulsion as a preferred method of maintaining control. "Get-tough" school expulsion policies place a student who is struggling with behavior and compliance issues at risk for school exclusion (Morrison et al., 2001), school exclusion being a policy that virtually lacks evidence about its effectiveness (Skiba & Peterson, 2000). Mayer and Leone (1999) have found that ambiguous sanctions, punitive teacher attitudes, poor high school teacher–administrator cooperation, and use of physical restrictions (metal detectors, high fencing, etc.) can increase rates of problem behavior as well as alienate students.

Rates of suspension are influenced by a variety of other school factors. Schools with higher rates of suspension have been reported to have higher student–teacher ratios, negative teacher attitudes and low expectations of students, and a lower level of academic quality (Ostroff, 1992; Wu, Pink, Crain, & Moles, 1982). School personnel spend more time on discipline-related matters and pay significantly less attention to issues of school climate (Bickel & Qualls, 1980). As a result of such interactions, adults and student relationships are often further fractured in the process of these disciplinary actions, leading to a negative cycle.

In contrast, a protective school environment for these students would be one where there are (1) effective schoolwide discipline practices that include a clear statement of rules and expectations, and consistently communicated and applied consequences for rule-breaking behavior; (2) concrete efforts to teach students appropriate behavior; and (3) positive consequences available for positive behavior (Sugai & Horner, 1999). Characteristics of programs that contribute to the development and enhancement of positive

TABLE 13.3. Classroom Risk and Protective Factors

Protective	Risk
Teacher as encourager, champion—is flexible with level of activity allowed	Teacher has narrow norms for behavior—won't "explain" (or re-explain) material
Students take threat of retention seriously and "get with it"—start doing their work	Retention is being enforced
Work noncompletion is addressed through additional supports	Academic press makes "work" noncompletion a discipline issue
Every student given a chance to contribute/shine	Opportunities for awards/rewards only for high achievers
Long-term substitutes are available who know students and can handle misbehavior	Academic school reform and teacher release leads to problems with substitutes
Behavior plan is effectively implemented	Behavior plans are not part of IEP; socioemotional assessments not considered

behavior include the use of multiple strategies to reduce negative behavior and support positive behavior; early intervention; targeting students with specific needs; building a positive school climate; and the involvement of families, students, and the community (Flay, Allred, & Ordway, 2001; Skiba & Peterson, 2000).

Support from the leadership of the school is critical in creating and maintaining the school-level characteristics in support of positive behavior (Safran & Oswald, 2003). Teachers need the support of school administrators through consistent disciplinary practice and technical assistance provided for classroom management in order to keep problematic students in their classrooms (Cheney, Osher, & Caesar, 2002). Administrators can also provide leadership through use of continuous data analysis to examine disciplinary office referrals (number, type of offense, who refers, who offends) to provide insight into patterns of problem behavior and situations/interactions that result in disciplinary referrals (Sugai, Sprague, Horner, & Walker, 2000).

School–Family Relationships

An important component of a protective school environment is the constructive involvement of parents in the education of their children and in the determination of the overall school mission and function (Henderson & Berla, 1996). Communication and cooperation between families and schools is particularly difficult when there are barriers of race, ethnicity, language, and social class (Osher, 2000) and when families and schools do not perceive each other as having the same goals for their individual child/student (Bryk & Schneider, 2002). When behavior is an issue, it is particularly important to have an open and positive communication between parents and school officials. This is particularly difficult because behavior problems at school require that information about the negative behavior of the child be communicated.

Home–school collaboration is particularly important when a student is showing aggressive and/or antisocial behavior. The nature of interactions between parents and students in this regard is bound to be adversarial. Disparities between school and home expectations undermine attempts to improve students' behavior; therefore, enhanced communication between school and home is particularly important (Dorries, 2002; Henggeler & Hoyt, 2001). Where children's behavior is excessive or dangerous, parents, school officials, and community agencies work together to support the child and family in receiving appropriate assessment and targeted intervention. Table 13.4 lists examples of the family and school risk and protective factors for children who are aggressive or who misbehave.

SUMMARY

In this chapter we have highlighted the importance of making explicit linkages between schooling practices and (1) having access to a social setting in which to systematically screen for youths with such behavioral patterns and (2) to intervene as early as possible. School is the primary nonhome social context in which youths' behavior can be objectively and intensively observed. It is also the context in which focused social and academic performance is expected and evaluated. Youths whose developmental histories have increased their risk of engaging in antisocial aggressive behavior will typically have behavior and performance patterns showing their struggles in the student role. Research focusing on the interface of antisocial developmental patterns and the schooling process has the potential to support screening, prevention, and intervention efforts.

In commenting on the observation that the incidence of overt antisocial behaviors, as rated by mothers and teachers, shows no increases (and some declines) from ages 2 through 12, Patterson and Yoerger (2002) suggest that this is a "quiescent" phase when considered as part of a developmental trajectory. They go on to state:

> It should be noted, however, that there is an important sense in which the problem child may be said to be getting worse during the quiescent period. With each passing year in the coercion process, the child's arrested socialization becomes increasingly apparent. For example, academic difficulties become apparent by the 2nd or 3rd grade, and rejection by normal

TABLE 13.4. School and Family Risk and Protective Factors

Protective	Risk
"Discipline" is seen as a learning opportunity for the child and a chance for the school to offer help	Zero-tolerance criteria vary from school to school (e.g., for inappropriate language, for not being "ready" for class)
Multiple services and supports are available	Support services not available to students with behavioral challenges
Student acts as office helper when tolerance for class (and teacher's for him or her) has been exhausted	Students do a lot of "office sitting" for not being ready for class—in the meantime they are missing class content (culture of "office sitting" develops)
After-school and playground staff act as a supportive adult resource for students ("janitor as the secret weapon")	Playground is supervised by nonteaching staff . . . often without training in conflict resolution
School makes a commitment to meet the child's needs at school	Students are passed from school to school
Full school staff participates in training on schoolwide positive behavior support. Staff has common language for behavior expectations and rule violation consequences	Standards for behavior and consequences for rule violations are not clear or consistent
Principal sets the tone for respectful communication, expects staff to model respectful communication	Office staff members are disrespectful to "office sitting" students
Data are collected and analyzed	Data system is not in place
School staff members are bilingual and perceived as approachable by monolingual (Spanish) parents	Few bilingual staff members are available
Office staff is welcoming	Office staff is not welcoming
Parents reinforce importance of schoolwork	Parents busy working; little talk about school
Parents advocate for student at school; mediate the schooling process (special education services and after-school programs)	Parents play passive backseat role to educators; students doing their own "mediation" (parents have to ask students during interview) or parents are confrontational with school officials
Siblings act as "translators" of school expectation and knowledge	Home language and culture is very different from that of school
Parents support school in their discipline efforts	Parents support aggressive problem-solving style
Parents attend conference and are seen as supportive	Perception of parental nonsupport is seen as a risk factor by school personnel

peers is evident within a few weeks of school entrance. The clear signs of social incompetence and failure plus the warning signs provided by juvenile forms of aggression lead responsible adults to begin referring the child for testing and special classroom placement. (p. 149)

This observation that at least some youths show early signs of aggressive and antisocial behaviors but that the rate of its acceleration is slow prior to adolescence should be a primary topic of future research and encourage increasing research–school collaborations.

Even as researchers more closely examine the place of schools in the development of antisocial behavior, they will need to continue to take steps to refine the developmental models associated with antisocial behavior and aggression, as discussed in the chapter. Tolan and Gorman-Smith (2002) recently argued that researchers' understanding of the multiple pathways that lead to antisocial behavior is incomplete. They suggest that the prominence given to the age of onset of delinquency needs to be further scrutinized due to evidence that some youths engage in low-level delinquency over time, some in chronic serious delinquency, and others escalate behaviors starting later in life (Tolan & Gorman-Smith, 2002). As this research proceeds, it will be important to enhance the linkages between research and the clinical definitions of externalizing disorders of youths.

We close with the thought that, although recent commentaries on youth violence continue to refer to a growing youth violence problem (e.g., Fields & McNamara, 2002), this has not been supported by official and self-reported youth violence. One of the most intriguing future research topics related to antisocial behavior and aggression is what factors have contributed to the recent sizable decreases in youth homicide and other violent crimes. Despite concerns that programs to prevent youth violence may not be as effective or scientific as claimed (Gorman, 2003), communities and schools have quietly seen reductions in youth violence. With youth homicide near historical low rates, researchers may want to turn more attention to better understand what has contributed to this decline and to gain more knowledge of those factors that deflect youths from antisocial developmental trajectories (Tolan & Gorman-Smith, 2002).

ACKNOWLEDGMENTS

Work on this chapter was supported by the Don and Maryilyn Gevirtz Fund for Excellence and *Turning Point Effects for Students with and without Disabilities Who Are Involved in School Disciplinary Actions*, a grant awarded to Gale Morrison by the U.S. Department of Education, Office of Special Education Programs, Award No. H324C000072.

REFERENCES

Achenbach, T. (1998). Diagnosis, assessment, taxonomy, and case formulations. In T. Ollendick & M. Hersen (Eds.), *Handbook of child psychopathology* (3rd ed., pp. 63–87). New York: Plenum.

American Psychiatric Association. (2000). *Diagnostic and Statistical Manual of Mental Disorders* (4th ed., text rev.). Washington, DC: Author.

Anderson, M., Kaufman, J., Simon, T. R., Barrios, L., Paulozzi, L., Ryan, G., Hammond, R., Modzeleski, W., Feucht, T., & Potter, L., (2001). *Journal of the American Medical Association, 286,* 2695–2702.

Berkowitz, L. (1989). Situational influences on aggression. In J. Groebel & R. A. Hinde (Eds.), *Aggression and war: Their biological and social bases* (pp. 91–100). Thousand Oaks, CA: Sage.

Berkowitz, L. (1990a). On the formation and regulation of anger and aggression: A cognitive-neoassociationistic analysis. *American Psychologist, 45,* 494–503.

Berkowitz, L. (1990b). Biological roots: Are humans inherently violent? In B. Glad (Ed.), *Psychological dimensions of war* (pp. 24–40). Thousand Oaks, CA: Sage.

Bickel, F., & Qualls, R. (1980). The impact of school climate on suspension rates in the Jefferson County Public Schools. *The Urban Review, 12,* 79–86.

Blankemeyer, M., Flannery, D. J., & Vazsonyi, A. T. (2002). The role of aggression and social competence in children's perceptions of the child–teacher relationship. *Psychology in the Schools, 39,* 293–304.

Boldizar, J. P., Perry, D. G., & Perry, L. C. (1989). Outcome values and aggression. *Child Development, 60,* 571–579.

Bryk, A. S., & Schneider, B. (2002). *Trust in schools: A core resource for improvement.* New York: Sage.

Bureau of Justice Statistics. (2001). *Homicide trends in the United States 1976–2000.* Retrieved July 1, 2003, from *www.ojp.usdoj.gov/bjs/homicide.*

Burke, J., Lahey, B. B., Loeber, R., & Rathouz, P. J. (2002). Adolescent outcomes of childhood conduct disorder among clinic-referred boys: Predictors of improvement. *Journal of Abnormal Child Psychology, 30,* 333–348.

Cairnes, R. B., & Cairnes, B. D. (1994). *Lifelines and risks: Pathways of youth of our time.* Cambridge, UK: Cambridge University Press.

California Education Code. (1994). Chapter 6, Article 1, Sections 48900-48926.

Caspi, A., Elder, G. H., & Bem, D. (1988). Moving against the world: Life course patterns of explosive children. *Developmental Psychopathology, 24,* 824–831.

Caspi, A., & Moffitt, T. E. (1995). The continuity of maladaptive behavior: From description to explanation in the study of antisocial behavior. In D. Cicchetti & D. Cohen (Eds.), *Developmental psychopathology* (Vol. 2, pp. 472–511). New York: Wiley.

Center for Mental Health in Schools at UCLA. (1999). *An introductory packet on conduct and behavior problems related to school aged youth.* Los Angeles: Author.

Cernkovich, S. A., & Giordano, P. G. (1992). School bonding, race, and delinquency. *Criminology, 30,* 261–290.

Cheney, D., Osher , T. W., & Caesar , M. (2002). Providing ongoing skill development and support for educators and parents of students with emotional and behavioral disabilities. *Journal of Child and Family Studies, 11,* 79–90.

Civil Rights Project. (2000). *Opportunities suspended: The devastating consequences of zero tolerance and school discipline policies.* Cambridge, MA: Harvard University.

Clarke, A. M., & Clarke, A. D. B. (1994). Individual differences as risk factors: Development, birth weight, and chronic illness. In W. B. Carey & S. C. McDevitt (Eds.), *Prevention and early intervention: Individual differences as risk factors for the mental health of children* (pp. 83–91). New York: Brunner/Mazel.

Coie, J. D., Dodge, K. A., & Kupersmidt, J. B. (Eds.). (1990). *Peer group behavior and social status.* New York: Cambridge University Press.

Connor, D. F. (2002). *Aggression and antisocial behavior in children and adolescents: Research and treatment.* New York: Guilford Press.

Costenbader, V. K., & Markson, S. (1994). School suspension: A survey of current policies and practices. *NASSP Bulletin, 78,* 103–107.

Coutinho, M. J., Oswald, D. P., & Forness, S. R. (2002). Gender and sociodemographic factors and the disproportionate identification of culturally and linguistically diverse students with emotional disturbance. *Behavioral Disorders, 27,* 109–125.

Crick, N. R., & Dodge, K. A. (1994). A review and reformulation of social information-processing mechanisms in children's social adjustment. *Psychological Bulletin, 115,* 74–101.

Crick, N. R., & Ladd, G. W. (1990). Children's perceptions of the outcomes of social strategies: Do the ends justify being mean? *Developmental Psychology, 26,* 612–620.

Dodge, K. A., Price, J. M., Bachorowski, J., & Newman, J. P. (1990). Hostile attributional biases in severely aggressive adolescents. *Journal of Abnormal Psychology, 99,* 385–392.

Dodge, K. A., & Tomlin, A. M. (1987). Utilization of self-schemas as a mechanism of interpetational bias in aggressive children. *Social Cognition, 5,* 280–300.

Doll, B. (1996). Prevalence of psychiatric disorders in children and youth: An agenda for advocacy by school psychology. *School Psychology Quarterly, 11,* 20–47.

Doll, B., & Lyon, M. A. (1998). Risk and resilience: Implications for the delivery of educational and mental health services in schools. *School Psychology Review, 27,* 348–363.

Dorries, D. (2002). Creating home–school connections: Opportunities and barriers. In G. McAuliffe (Ed.), *Working with troubled youth in schools: A guide for all school staff* (pp. 49–60). Westport: CT: Bergin & Garvey.

Dubow, E. F., & Tisak, J. (1989). The relation between stressful life events and adjustment in elementary school children: The role of social support and social problem-solving skills. *Child Development, 60,* 1412–1423.

Dwyer, K., Osher, D., & Warger, C. (1998). *Early warning timely response: A guide to safe schools.*

Washington, DC: U.S. Department of Education. Retrieved July 1, 2003, from *www.air-dc.org/cecp/guide/annotated.htm.*

Elias, M. J., & Branden, L. R. (1988). Primary prevention of behavioral and emotional problems in school-aged populations. *School Psychology Review, 17,* 581–592.

Erdley, C. A., & Asher, S. R. (1998). Linkages between children's beliefs about the legitimacy of aggression and their behavior. *Social Development, 7,* 321–339.

Farmer, T. W., Farmer, E. M. Z., & Gut, D. M. (1999). Implications for social development research for school-based interventions for aggressive youth with EBD. *Journal of Emotional and Behavioral Disorders, 7,* 130–136.

Fields, S. A., & McNamara, J. R. (2002). The prevention of child and adolescent violence: A review. *Aggression and Violent Behavior, 8,* 61–91.

Flay, B. R., Allred, C. G., & Ordway, N. (2001). Effects of the Positive Action Program on achievement and discipline: Two matched-control comparisons. *Prevention Science, 2*(2), 71–89.

Forness, S. R., & Kavale, K. A. (2000). Emotional or behavioral disorders: Background and current status of the E/BD terminology and definition. *Behavioral Disorders, 25,* 264–269.

Frick, P. J. (1998). *Conduct disorders and severe antisocial behavior.* New York: Plenum.

Gable, R. A., Hendrickson, J. M., Tonelson, S. W., & Van Acker, R. (2002). Integrating academic and nonacademic instruction for students with emotional/behavioral disorders. *Education and Treatment of Children, 25,* 459–475.

Garmezy, N., Masten, A. S., & Tellegen, A. (1984). The study of stress and competence in children: A building block for developmental psychopathology. *Child Development, 55,* 97–111.

Gold, M., & Osgood, D. (1992). *Personality and peer influence in juvenile corrections.* Westport, CN: Greenwood.

Gorman, D. M. (2003). Alcohol & drug abuse: The best of practices, the worst of practices: The making of science-based primary prevention programs. *Psychiatric Services, 54,* 1087–1089

Gottfredson, D. G. (1989). *Reducing disorderly behavior in middle schools.* Baltimore, MD: Center for Research on Elementary and Middle Schools.

Grunbaum, J., Kann, L., Kinchen, S. A., Williams, B., Ross, J. G., Lowrey, R., & Kolbe, L. (2002, June 28). Youth risk behavior surveillance—United States, 2001: Surveillance summaries. *Morbidity and Mortality Weekly Report, 51*(SS04), 1–64.

Hawkins, J. D., & Lishner, D. (1987). Etiology and prevention of antisocial behavior in children and adolescents. In D. H. Crowell, I. M. E. Clifford, & R. O. Donnell (Eds.), *Childhood aggression and violence: Sources of influence, prevention, and control. Applied clinical Psychology* (pp. 263–282). New York: Plenum.

Henderson, A. T., & Berla, N. (1996). *A new generation of evidence: The family is critical to student achievement. Washington, DC: Center for Law and Education.

Henggeler, S. W., & Hoyt, S. W. (2001). Multisystemic therapy with serious juvenile offenders and their families. In J. M. Richman & M. W. Fraser (Eds.), The context of youth violence (pp. 115–132). Westport, CT: Praeger.

Hinshaw, S. P. (1996). Enhancing social competence: Integrating self-management strategies with behavioral procedures for children with ADHD. In E. D. Hibbs & P. S. Jensen (Eds.), Child and adolescent disorders: Empirically based strategies for clinical practice (pp. 285–310). Washington, DC: American Psychological Association.

Hinshaw, S. P. (2000). Attention-deficit/hyperactivity disorder: The search for viable treatments. In P. C. Kendall (Ed.), Child and adolescent therapy: Cognitive-behavioral procedures (2nd ed., pp. 88–128). New York: Guilford Press.

Jessor, R., Van Den Bos, J., Vanderryn, J., Costa, F. M., & Turbin, M. S. (1995). Protective factors in adolescent problem behavior: Moderator effects and developmental change. Developmental Psychology, 31, 923–933.

Kazdin, A. E. (1995). Risk factors, onset, and course of dysfunction. In Conduct disorders in childhood and adolescence (2nd ed., pp. 50–74). Thousand Oaks, CA: Sage.

Kazdin, A. E. (1997). Practitioner Review: Psychosocial treatments for conduct disorder in children. Journal of Child Psychology and Psychiatry, 38, 161–178.

Kratzer, L., & Hodgins, S. (1999). A typology of offenders: A test of Moffitt's theory among males and females from childhood to age 30. Developmental Psychology, 29, 19–30.

La Paro, K. M., Pianta, R. C. , & Cox, M. (2000). Teachers' reported transition practices for children transitioning into kindergarten and first grade. Exceptional Children, 67, 7–20.

Leone, P. E., Mayer, M., Malmgren, K., & Meisel, S. M. (2000). School violence and disruption: Rhetoric, reality, and reasonable balance. Focus on Exceptional Children, 33, 1–20.

Levine, D. U., & Lezotte, L. W. (1990). Unusually effective schools: A review and analysis of unusually effective schools. Madison, WI: National Center for Effective Schools Research and Development.

Loeber, R. (1990). Developmental and risk factors of juvenile antisocial behavior and delinquency. Clinical Psychology Review, 10, 1–41.

Masten, A. S., Best, K. M., & Garmezy, N. (1990). Resilience and development: Contributions from the study of children who overcome adversity. Development and Psychopathology, 2, 425–444.

Mayer, M. J., & Leone, P. E. (1999). A structural analysis of school violence and disruption: Implications for creating safer schools. Education and Treatment of Children, 22, 333–356.

Mayes, S. D., Calhoun, S. L., & Crowell, E. W. (2000).

Learning disabilities and ADHD: Overlapping spectrum disorders. Journal of Learning Disabilities, 33, 417–424.

Mazerolle, P., Brame, R., Paternoster, R., Piquero, A., & Dean, C. (2000). Onset age, persistence, and offending versatility: Comparisons across gender. Criminology, 38, 1143–1172.

McEvoy, A., & Welker, R. (2000). Antisocial behavior, academic failure, and school climate: A critical review. Journal of Emotional and Behavioral Disorders, 8, 130–140.

McFadden, A. C., Marsh, G. E., Price, B. J., & Hwang, Y. (1992). A study of race and gender bias in the punishment of handicapped school children. Urban Review, 24, 239–251.

Moffitt, T. E. (1990). The neuropsychology of juvenile delinquency: A critical review. In M. Tonry & N. Morris (Eds.), Crime and justice: A review of research (Vol. 12, pp. 99–169). Chicago: University of Chicago Press.

Moffitt, T. E. (1993a). Adolescence-limited and life-course persistent antisocial behavior: A developmental taxonomy. Psychological Review, 100, 674–701.

Moffitt, T. E. (1993b). The neuropsychology of conduct disorder. Development and Psychopathology, 5, 135–151.

Moffitt, T. E., & Caspi, A. (2001). Childhood predictors differentiate life-course persistent and adolescence-limited antisocial pathways among males and females. Development and Psychopathology, 13, 355–375.

Moffitt, T. E., Caspi, A., Rutter, M., & Silva, P. A. (2001). Sex difference in antisocial behaviour: Conduct disorder, delinquency, and violence in the Dunedin longitudinal study. New York: Cambridge University Press.

Morrison, G. M. (2003). Turning point effects for students with and without disabilities who are involved in school disciplinary actions. U.S. Department of Education, Office of Special Education Programs, Award No. H324C000072.

Morrison, G. M., Anthony, S., Storino, M., Cheng, J., Furlong, M. J., & Morrison, R. L. (2001). School expulsion as a process and an event: Before and after effects on children at-risk for school discipline. New Directions for Youth Development: Theory, Practice, Research, 92, 45–72.

Morrison, G. M., & D'Incau, B. (1997). The web of zero-tolerance: Characteristics of students who are recommended for expulsion from school. Education and Treatment of Children, 20, 316–335.

Morrison, G. M., & D'Incau, B. (2000). Developmental and service trajectories of students with disabilities recommended for expulsion from school. Exceptional Children, 66, 257–272.

Osher, D. (Ed.). (2000). Breaking the cultural disconnect: Working with families to improve outcomes for students placed at risk of school failure. Miami: Florida International University.

Osher, D., Van Acker, R., Morrison, G., Gable, R. A., Dwyer, K., & Quinn, M. M. (2004). Warning signs of problems in schools: Ecological perspectives and effective practices for combating school aggression and violence. *Journal of School Violence, 3*(2-3), 13–37.

Ostroff, C. (1992). The relationship between satisfaction, attitudes and performance: An organizational level analysis. *Journal of Applied Psychology, 77,* 963–974.

Patterson, G. R., Capaldi, D., & Bank, L. (1991). An early starter model for predicting delinquency. In D. J. Pepler & K. H. Rubin (Eds.), *The development and treatment of childhood aggression* (pp. 139–168). Hillsdale, NJ: Erlbaum.

Patterson, G. R., & Yoerger, K. (2002). A developmental model for early- and late-onset delinquency. In J. B. Reid, G. R. Patterson, & J. Snyder (Eds.), *Antisocial behavior in children and adolescents: A development analysis and model for intervention* (pp. 147–172). Washington, DC: American Psychological Association.

Quiggle, N. L., Garber, J., Panak, W. F., & Dodge, K. A. (1992). Social information processing in aggressive and depressed children. *Child Development, 63,* 1305–1320.

Reinke, W. M., & Herman, K. C. (2002). Creating school environments that deter antisocial behaviors in youth. *Psychology in the Schools, 39,* 549–560.

Reynolds, D., Teddlie, C., Creemers, B., Scheerens, J., & Townsend, T. (2000). An introduction to school effectiveness research. In C. Teddlie & D. Reynolds (Eds.), *The international handbook of school effectiveness research* (pp. 3–25). London: Falmer.

Robins, L., & Ratcliff, K. (1979). Risk factors in the continuation of childhood antisocial behavior into adulthood. *International Journal of Mental Health, 7,* 96–116.

Rodkin, P., Farmer, T. W., Pearl, R., & Van Acker, R. (2000). Heterogeneity of popular boys: Antisocial and prosocial configurations. *Developmental Psychology, 36,* 14–24.

Roff, M., Sells, S. B., & Golden, M. M. (1972). *Social adjustment and personality development in children*: Minneapolis, MN: University of Minnesota Press.

Rubin, K. H., Bream, L. A., & Rose-Krasnor, L. (1991). Social problem solving and aggression in childhood. In D. J. Pepler & K. H. Rubin (Eds.), *The development and treatment of childhood aggression* (pp. 219–248). Hillsdale, NJ: Erlbaum.

Rumberger, R. W. (1987). High school dropouts: A review of issues and evidence. *Review of Educational Research, 57,* 101–121.

Russo, M. F., & Beidel, D. C. (1994). Comorbidity of childhood anxiety and externalizing disorders: Prevalence, associated characteristics, and validation issues. *Clinical Psychology Review, 14,* 199–221.

Rutter, M. (Ed.). (1979). *Protective factors in children's responses to stress and disadvantage.* Hanover, NH: University Press of New England.

Safran, S., & Oswald, K. (2003). Positive behavior supports: Can schools reshape disciplinary practices? *Exceptional Children, 69,* 361–373.

Scott, T., Nelson, C. M., & Liaupsin, C. J. (2001). Effective instruction: The forgotten component in preventing school violence. *Education and Treatment of Children, 24,* 309–322.

Shields, A. M., Cicchetti, D., & Ryan, R. M. (1994). The development of emotional and behavioral self-regulation and social competence among maltreated school-age children. *Development and Psychopathology, 6,* 57–75.

Skiba, R. J., & Peterson, R. (2000). School discipline at a crossroads: From zero tolerance to early response. *Exceptional Children, 66,* 335–346.

Skiba, R. J., & Peterson, R. (2003). Teaching the social curriculum: School Discipline as instruction. *Preventing School Failure, 47,* 66–73.

Skiba, R. J., Peterson, R. L., & Williams, T. (1997). Office referrals and suspension: Disciplinary intervention in middle schools. *Education and Treatment of Children, 20,* 295–315.

Slaby, R. G., & Guerra, N. G. (1988). Cognitive mediators of aggression in adolescent offenders: I. Assessment. *Developmental Psychology, 24,* 580–588.

Snyder, H. S. (2000). *Juvenile arrests.* Washington, DC: U.S. Department of Justice, Office of Justice Programs, Office of Juvenile Justice and Delinquency Prevention.

Sroufe, L. A., & Rutter, M. (1984). The domain of developmental psychopathology. *Child Development, 55,* 17–29.

Stage, S. A. (1997). A preliminary investigation of the relationship between in-school suspension and the disruptive classroom behavior of students with behavior disorders. *Behavioral Disorders, 23,* 57–76.

Stanger, C., Achenbach, T., & Verhulst, F. C. (1997). Accelerated longitudinal comparisons of aggressive versus delinquent syndromes. *Development and Psychopathology, 9,* 43–58.

Sugai, G., & Horner, R. (1999). Discipline and behavioral support: Practices, pitfalls, and promises. *Effective School Practices, 17,* 10–22.

Sugai, G., Sprague, J. R., Horner, R. H., & Walker, H. M. (2000). Preventing school violence: The use of office discipline referrals to assess and monitor schoolwide discipline interventions. *Journal of Emotional and Behavioral Disorders, 8,* 94–101.

Sutherland, K., & Wehby, J. H. (2001). Exploring the relationship between increased opportunities to respond to academic requests and the academic and behavioral outcomes of students with EBD. *Remedial and Special Education, 22,* 113–121.

Tannock, R., & Schachar R. (1996). Executive dysfunction as an underlying mechanism of behavior and language problems in attention deficit hyperactivity disorder. In J. H. Beitchman, N. Cohen, M. M. Konstantareas, & R. Tannock (Eds.), *Language, learning, and behavior disorders: Developmental, biological, and clinical perspectives* (pp. 128–155). New York: Cambridge University Press.

Tobin, T., Sugai, G., & Colvin, G. (1996). Patterns in middle school discipline records. *Journal of Emotional and Behavioral Disorders, 4,* 82–94.

Tolan, P. H., & Gorman-Smith, D. (2002). What violence prevention research can tell us about developmental psychopathology. *Development and Psychopathology, 14,* 713–729.

Tubman, J. G., & Windle, M. (1995). Continuity of difficult temperament in adolescence: Relations with depression, life events, family support, and substance use across a one-year period. *Journal of Youth and Adolescence, 24,* 133–153.

Unnever, J. D., & Cornell, D. G. (2003). The culture of bullying in middle school. *Journal of School Violence, 2,* 5–27.

U.S. Department of Education. (1999). Assistance to states for the education of children with disabilities and the early intervention program for infants and toddlers with disabilities: Final regulations. *Federal Register, 64*(48), 12406–12672.

Walker, H. M., Colvin, G., & Ramsey, E. (1995). *Antisocial behavior in school: Strategies and best practices.* Pacific Grove, CA: Brooks/Cole.

Webster-Stratton, C. (1990). Long-term follow-up of families with young conduct problem children: From preschool to grade school. *Journal of Clinical Child Psychology, 19,* 144–149.

Werner, E., & Smith, R. S. (1982). *Vulnerable but invincible: A longitudinal study of resilient children and youth.* New York: McGraw-Hill.

White, J. L., Moffitt, T. E., Earls, F., Robins, L., & Silva, P. A. (1990). How early can we tell? Predictors of childhood conduct disorder and adolescent delinquency. *Criminology, 28,* 507–533.

Wu, S. C., Pink, W. T., Crain, R. L., & Moles, O. (1982). Student suspension: A critical reappraisal. *The Urban Review, 14,* 245–303.

14

Internalizing Behavior Problems in Children and Adolescents

FRANK M. GRESHAM *and* LEE KERN

Childhood and adolescent behavior problems can be classified dichotomously as being either *externalizing behaviors* or *internalizing behaviors* (Achenbach, 1982, 1991; Cicchetti & Toth, 1991). Externalizing behavior patterns are directed outwardly toward the social environment and can be characterized as an undercontrolled and outer-directed mode of responding. Examples of these behaviors include aggression, disruption, opposition/defiance, and impulsivity/hyperactivity (see Furlong, Morrison, & Jimerson, Chapter 13, this volume). In contrast, internalizing behavior patterns are behaviors that are directed inwardly toward the individual and represent an overcontrolled and inner-directed pattern of behavior. Examples of these behaviors include social withdrawal, depression/dysthymia, anxiety, somatization problems, obsessive–compulsive behaviors, and selective mutism.

Unlike externalizing behaviors, which are overt and obvious to others in the social environment, internalizing behaviors are subtle and often go unnoticed by others in a child's social environment, particularly classrooms. Algozzine (1977) characterized externalizing behaviors as "disturbing" to others in the social environment and internalizing behaviors as "disturbing" to the individual. As such, internalizing behaviors present unique challenges in referral, assessment, and intervention practices in school settings because

of the covert and nonintrusive nature of these kinds of behaviors. In school settings, teachers typically under-refer students with internalizing behavior problems, compared to students with externalizing behavior patterns (Kauffman, 2001; Walker & Severson, 1992).

MODEL BEHAVIOR PROFILE AND REFERRAL OF INTERNALIZING PROBLEMS

General education teachers are the primary source of referrals to either prereferral intervention and/or special education placement teams in schools. Students who are at risk for and who subsequently are referred for emotional and behavioral disorders (EBD) often fail to meet teachers' social behavior standards for the classroom and exceed teachers' tolerance limits for student social behavior (Hersh & Walker, 1983; Walker, Ramsey, & Gresham, 2004). This occurs despite the current federal definition of emotional disturbance being skewed toward internalizing rather than externalizing behavior problems. Teachers' social behavior standards are based on students' social behaviors that are valued by teachers because they create quieter and more manageable classroom environments with fewer discipline problems and greater learning rates

(Brophy, 1986; Colvin, Kame'enui, & Sugai, 1993; Sugai, Horner, & Gresham, 2002; Walker et al., 2004). Hersh and Walker (1983) have referred to this as the *model behavior profile* expected by most teachers. Teachers' tolerance for maladaptive behavior represents the degree to which teachers will tolerate or otherwise accommodate inappropriate behaviors in their classrooms (Gresham & Noell, 1999; Hersh & Walker, 1983).

The least tolerated behaviors among teachers are those that challenge the teacher's authority and ability to effectively manage the classroom. In almost every case, these behaviors are externalizing (noncompliance, aggression, disruption) rather than internalizing (social withdrawal, anxiety, depression) behavior patterns. Students who have a high probability of being referred for assessment, intervention, and/or placement are those who exhibit a pattern of behavior that reflects a poor fit or mismatch between teachers' expectations for appropriate academic and social behaviors and that exceeds teachers' tolerance limits for maladaptive behavior. As such, students with internalizing behaviors are rarely referred to prereferral intervention teams or placed in special education under the label of emotionally disturbed (ED) (Kauffman, 2001; Walker, Reavis, Rhode, & Jenson, 1985).

PURPOSE OF THE PRESENT CHAPTER

In this chapter, we review the characteristics of internalizing disorders and describe various clinical and empirical classification systems for internalizing behavior problems. We begin the topic of classification with a brief overview and critique of the current definition of emotional disturbance specified in the Individuals with Disabilities Education Act (IDEA). Subsequently, we review the fourth edition of the *Diagnostic and Statistical Manual of Mental Disorders* (DSM-IV; American Psychiatric Association, 1994) and critique it on the basis of its medical model orientation, psychometric concerns, and the absence of treatment validity. Empirical classification systems using various multi-informant rating scales will be reviewed briefly along with validated screening systems for the identification of internalizing

behavior problems. The chapter concludes with a review of evidence-based intervention approaches for internalizing behavior problems.

CLASSIFICATION OF INTERNALIZING BEHAVIOR PROBLEMS

IDEA Definition of Emotional Disturbance

The definition of "emotional disturbance" specified in the Individuals with Disabilities Education Act characterizes the disorder as:

(i) . . . a condition exhibiting one or more of the following characteristics over a long period of time and to a marked degree which adversely affects school performance: (a) an inability to learn which cannot be explained by intellectual, sensory, or health factors; (b) an inability to build or maintain satisfactory relationships with peers and teachers; (c) inappropriate types of behaviors or feelings under normal circumstances; (d) a general pervasive mood of unhappiness or depression; or (e) a tendency to develop physical symptoms or fears associated with personal or school problems.
(ii) The term includes children who are schizophrenic. The term does not include children who are socially maladjusted, unless it is determined that they also are emotionally disturbed.

To qualify for special education and related services, a student must exhibit at least one of the five criteria and is required to meet the three *limiting criteria* of severity ("to a marked degree"), duration ("for a long period of time"), and impact on school performance ("adversely affects educational performance") (Gresham, 1999). Forness and Knitzer (1992) suggested that these limiting criteria are highly subjective, nebulous, and difficult to operationalize.

It should be noted that the current ED definition is biased toward internalizing behavior problems and against externalizing behavior problems. For example, four of the five ED criteria could be interpreted as internalizing behavior problems (difficulty in interpersonal relationships, inappropriate behaviors or feelings, unhappiness or depression, and physical symptoms and fears). In fact, the so-called *social maladjustment* exclusion clause has been interpreted by and used by some to exclude any child from ED services who exhibits characteristics of oppositional-defiant or conduct disorders (Forness & Knitzer, 1992; Kauffman, 2001; Merrell, 1999; Skiba & Grizzle, 1992).

A detailed critique of the current ED definition is beyond the scope of the present chapter, however, some points should be made with respect to the difficulties this definition creates for school professionals. First, Kauffman (2001) suggested that the phrase "adversely affects educational performance" is redundant with the phrase "an inability to learn," particularly if the former phrase was intended to connote *academic achievement or performance* rather than a broader meaning of personal, social, or vocational performance. Second, some children who exhibit characteristics of anxiety disorders or depression also manifest adequate academic achievement. Based on the current ED definition, these children should be excluded from ED services because their disorders do not adversely affect educational performance. Consequently, their mental health needs will be left unmet. Third, most children are considered socially maladjusted based on their inability to build or maintain satisfactory interpersonal relationships (criterion "b") and their tendency to exhibit inappropriate behaviors or feelings under normal circumstances (criterion "c") (Kauffman, 2001). Finally, the ED definition ignores the well-established finding that psychological disorders in children and adolescents often co-occur, a condition known as *comorbidity* (see Mattison, Chapter 9, this volume).

DSM-IV

DSM-IV (American Psychiatric Association, 1994) is the most commonly used diagnostic classification system for psychopathology in the United States and Canada. It uses a multiaxial classification system in which individuals are classified on five dimensions or axes. These axes are Axis I: Clinical Disorders (excluding mental retardation); Axis II: Personality Disorders and Mental Retardation; Axis III: General Medical Conditions; Axis IV: Psychosocial and Environmental Problems that exacerbate mental disorders; and Axis V: Global Assessment of Functioning. All internalizing disorders for children and adolescents are coded on Axis I. Table 14.1 shows the internalizing disorders and their respective descriptions found in DSM-IV.

Although highly valued among most psychiatrists and clinical psychologists, it is questionable that DSM-IV is particularly useful or relevant in establishing ED eligibility or, more importantly, in informing interventions for students exhibiting emotional and behavioral problems in school settings (Gresham, 1999; Gresham & Gansle, 1992). We will not present a comprehensive critique of the DSM-IV in this chapter; however, readers should be aware of some of the major conceptual and psychometric issues involved in using the DSM-IV. More comprehensive treatments of this topic can be found in special issues of the *Journal of Consulting and Clinical Psychology* (Vol. 64, No. 6, 1996) and the *School Psychology Review* (Vol. 25, No. 3, 1996) and in Mattison, Chapter 9, this volume.

Criticisms of the DSM System

Gresham and Gansle (1992) identified four major difficulties in using the DSM system in school systems to qualify students for services under the ED label in schools. First, the DSM is based on a medical model view of human behavior in which disorders are considered to be "within-person" problems. Terminology in DSM such as "symptoms," "signs," "syndromes," and "diseases" are characteristic of the terminology used in physical medicine to diagnose medical conditions. While valuable in physical medicine, the use of a medical model in psychiatry and psychology is problematic because the etiologies, or causes, of most emotional and behavioral problems simply are unknown (Carson, 1996; Follette & Houts, 1996). Moreover, there is little relationship between the diagnostic category assigned in DSM-IV and appropriate interventions based on that diagnostic category.

Second, the DSM system uses a structural or descriptive approach to behavior rather than a functional approach (Gresham & Gansle, 1992). A structural approach focuses on *what* the person does or feels (low energy or fatigue, feels hopeless) rather than *why* (function) the person behaves or feels in certain ways (see Scotti, Morris, McNeil, &

TABLE 14.1. Internalizing Disorders Described in DSM-IV

Disorder	Description
Separation anxiety disorder	Excessive anxiety concerning separation from home or those to whom person is attached.
Selective mutism	Persistent failure to speak in specific social situations (e.g., school, with playmates) where speaking is expected, despite speaking in other situations.
Reactive attachment disorder of infancy or early childhood	Markedly disturbed and developmentally inappropriate social relatedness in most contexts that begins before 5 years of age
Major depressive disorder	Depressed mood or the loss of interest or pleasure in nearly all activities. In children and adolescents, the mood may be irritable rather than sad.
Dysthymic disorder	Chronically depressed mood that occurs for most of the day more days than not for a minimum duration of 1 year. In children, the mood may be irritable rather than depressed.
Obsessive–compulsive disorder	Recurrent obsessions or compulsions that are severe enough to be time-consuming or cause marked distress or significant impairment.
Specific phobia	Marked and persistent fear of clearly discernible, circumscribed objects or situations. Exposure to the phobic stimulus almost invariably provokes an immediate anxiety response. Types include: animal, natural environment, blood–injection–injury, and situational types.
Social phobia	Marked and persistent fear of social or performance situations in which embarrassment may occur.
Posttraumatic stress disorder	Development of characteristic symptoms following exposure to an extreme traumatic stressor involving direct personal experience of an event that involves actual threat or threatened death, injury, or threat to the physical integrity of another person.
Generalized anxiety disorder	Excessive anxiety and worry occurring more days than not for a period of at least 6 months, about a number of events or activities.
Somatization disorder	Pattern of recurring, multiple, clinically significant somatic complaints.
Adjustment disorder	Development of clinically significant emotional or behavioral symptoms in response to an identifiable psychosocial stressor or stressors. Can be with depressed mood, with anxiety, with mixed anxiety and depressed mood, with disturbance of conduct, with mixed disturbance of emotions and conduct.
Anorexia nervosa	Refusal to maintain a minimally normal body weight, is intensely afraid of gaining weight, and exhibits a significant disturbance in the perception of the shape and size of his or her body.
Bulimia nervosa	Binge eating and inappropriate compensatory methods to prevent weight gain.

Note. Data from American Psychiatric Association (1994).

Hawkins, 1996). Descriptive accounts of behavior used in DSM-IV do not identify important, identifiable, or controllable environmental events that can be used in designing interventions. For example, an individual with a diagnosis of major depressive disorder may frequently express feelings of hopelessness, low self-esteem, and low energy to friends and family. Many of these verbalizations might be maintained by social attention from family and friends and thus would be strengthened by continued attention. In other cases, behaviors characteristic of depression such as school refusal, social withdrawal, and low physical activity might be maintained by escape or avoidance of aversive social situations (see Watson & Robinson, 1998, for a complete discussion).

Third, the DSM system has significant weaknesses in terms of reliability issues. Reliability in the DSM can refer to the agreement between two clinicians in assigning a particular diagnosis to the same individual. It can also refer to the stability of these clinicians' diagnoses over time. Past research with the current and earlier versions of the DSM has shown it to have poor interclinician agreements for most Axis I disorders with children and adolescents. Using the kappa statistic (which corrects for change agreements), the average interclinician agreement rates for various editions of the DSM system (childhood and adolescent disorders) are in the .50–.60 range (Achenbach, 1982; Atkins, McKernal, McKay, Talbott, & Arvanitis, 1996; Eysenck, Wakefield, & Friedman, 1983; Gresham & Gansle, 1992; Lahey et al., 1994; Werry, Methuen, Fitzpatrick, & Dixon, 1983). This is considered quite low and underscores the limitations in using it to diagnose an emotional disorder.

Finally, perhaps the greatest weakness of the DSM system is the absence of treatment validity. Treatment validity refers to the extent to which an assessment or classification system is effective in treatment planning and contributes to beneficial treatment outcomes (Hayes, Nelson, & Jarrett, 1987). It is often assumed in the DSM-IV that, once a diagnosis is assigned, appropriate treatments can be planned and implemented based on that diagnosis and that certain diagnoses dictate different treatments (Gresham, 1999). To date, there is little empirical evidence that the DSM system has treatment validity for the majority of Axis I disorders for children and adolescents. The structural/descriptive nature of the DSM system is antithetical to a functional approach to assessment and intervention planning.

Empirical Classification Systems

Unlike clinical classification systems for childhood and adolescent psychopathology (e.g., the DSM-IV), empirical classification systems employ more objective statistical procedures to identify clusters of behavior difficulties. Empirical classification systems typically employ factor analyses of teacher and parent rating scales to derive behavioral domains or clusters. Various numbers and types of behavioral dimensions are influenced by variables such as the nature of the sample, the informant providing the ratings, the item content of the rating scale, and the type of factor analysis used (Gresham, 1999).

Empirical classification systems differ from systems such as the DSM-IV on the basis of several factors, including (1) the behaviors are quantitatively scored rather than being coded either present or absent, (2) diagnoses are derived from empirically based quantitative data rather than subjective judgment, (3) the degree of psychopathology is based on cut scores that are stratified by age and gender, and (4) comparisons and correlations are made among different raters (e.g., parents, teachers, students) (see Achenbach & McConaughy, 1997, and McConaughy & Ritter, 2002, for comprehensive discussions of these issues).

Empirical classification systems are advantageous because they use objective criteria to identify which behaviors belong to a certain class or dimension of psychopathology. The objective criteria are based on the extent to which certain behaviors correlate with each other, thereby forming a factor (category of psychopathology). These resulting categories can be profiled using a normative database for each individual to target specific areas of concern. Research strongly supports both the reliability and validity of empirical classification systems for classifying child and adolescent psychopathology (Gresham, 1999; Merrell, 1999).

Table 14.2 presents two of the most popular empirical classification systems for child and adolescent psychopathology: (1) the *Achenbach System of Empirically Based Assessment* (ASEBA; Achenbach, 1991) and (2) the *Behavior Assessment System for Children* (BASC; Reynolds & Kamphaus, 1992). Note that we have included only the internalizing disorders from the ASEBA and BASC systems for the purposes of this chapter. Readers should also note the similarity in the domains or clusters of psychopathology in these two systems. Table 14.2 also shows specific measures of internalizing problems such as depression (Kovacs, 1991; Reynolds, 1989), anxiety (Reynolds & Richman, 1985; Spielberger, 1973), and negative affectivity (Merrell & Walters, 1998) that have been shown to be useful in identifying children and adolescents for these difficulties

TABLE 14.2. Comprehensive and Specific Rating Scales for Internalizing Problems

Achenbach System of Empirically Based Assessment

CBCL	TRF	YSR
Anxious/Depressed	Anxious/Depressed	Anxious/Depressed
Somatic Complaints	Somatic Complaints	Somatic Complaints
Withdrawn	Withdrawn	Withdrawn
Total Internalizing	Total Internalizing	Total Internalizing

Behavior Assessment System for Children

TRS	PRS	SRP
Anxiety	Anxiety	Anxiety
Depression	Depression	Depression
Somatization	Somatization	Somatization
Internalizing Problems	Internalizing Problems	Emotional Symptoms Index

Specific self-report measures of internalizing problems

Scale	Description
Children's Depression Inventory	Measure of depressive symptoms for children and adolescents, ages 6–17 years
Internalizing Symptoms Scale for Children	Measure of negative affect/general distress and positive affect for children in grades 3–6
Revised Manifest Anxiety Scale	Measure of trait anxiety for children and adolescents, ages 6–17 years
Reynolds Child Depression Scale	Measure of depressive symptoms for children, ages 8–12 years
State–Trait Anxiety Scale for Children	Measure of state anxiety and trait anxiety in children, ages 9–12 years

Note. TRF, Teacher Rating Form; CBCL, Child Behavior Checklist; YSR, Youth Self-Report; TRS, Teacher Report Scale; PRS, Parent Report Scale; SRP, Self-Report of Personality.

(see Merrell, 1999, for an in-depth discussion).

The primary advantage of empirical classification systems is that dimensions of behavior can be quantified and compared to a representative normative sample to define the level or degrees of psychopathology (typically > 98th percentile). The DSM-IV, on the other hand, is much more subjective and suffers from rather serious problems in interclinician agreement with respect to specific diagnoses. Empirical classification systems have known indices of reliability and validity that are specific to informants (parents, teachers, and students), age level (early childhood, childhood, and adolescence), and gender. Like the DSM-IV, empirical classification systems also suffer from an absence of treatment validity evidence. Although these systems can quantify significant areas of concern, they do not yield the required information for designing appropriate evidence-based interventions (Gresham, 1999; McConaughy & Ritter, 2002). Also, like the DSM-IV, empirical classification systems are based on informants' judgments rather than objective criteria, which are operationalized by ratings of behavior frequency that are quantified on Likert-type scales.

SCREENING AND ASSESSMENT OF INTERNALIZING BEHAVIOR PROBLEMS

As mentioned earlier, students with internalizing behavior problems tend to be under-identified in school settings simply because their behavior patterns are not particularly disturbing to others in their social environment. That is, many of these students might be termed *false negatives* (i.e., students identified as *not* having problems when in fact they do). Despite this tendency not to identify these students, it is clear that many of them may have difficulties in the areas of anxiety, depression, and/or affect that may portend rather serious proximal and distal outcomes. As such, it is important to proactively identify these students early on to have the best chance at reversing this potentially serious behavior pattern.

The general education classroom teacher represents the primary link between students who exhibit problematic behavior and their access to appropriate school-based services. Teachers are an invaluable resource with the potential to assist in the referral and evaluation of students who may be in need of more specialized interventions for internalizing behavior problems (Severson & Walker, 2002). Exclusive reliance on unstructured teacher referrals will result in continued over-identification of externalizing behavior problems and underidentification of internalizing behavior problems (Severson & Walker, 2002; Walker & Shinn, 2002). Based on this, the use of systematic, structured screening of students for internalizing behavior problems is advocated. When teacher judgments are structured and solicited in the right context, they can be highly accurate and useful for identifying this group of students (Walker & Severson, 1992).

Systematic Screening for Behavior Disorders (SSBD)

The SSBD is a multiple-gating screening procedure that has proven useful in identifying students at risk for emotional and behavioral disorders in grades 1–6 (Walker & Severson, 1992). The SSBD uses a systematic and structured set of assessment procedures that is teacher-driven and involves a series of progressively more expensive and precise assessments or gates. It employs teacher nominations, teacher ratings, and direct observations of classroom and playground behavior. Although the SSBD is intended to identify both students with externalizing and internalizing behavior patterns, we focus on the latter for purposes of this chapter. Teachers

are asked to rank-order all students in their classrooms meeting the definition of an internalizing behavior pattern, using the following description from the SSBD manual (Walker & Severson, 1992):

> Internalizing refers to all behavior problems that are directed inwardly (i.e., away from the external social environment) and that represent problems with self. Internalizing behavior problems are often self-imposed and frequently involve behavioral deficits and patterns of social avoidance. Examples of internalizing behavior problems include: having low or restricted activity levels, not talking with other children, being shy, timid or unassertive, avoiding or withdrawing from social situations, preferring to spend time alone, acting in a fearful manner, not participating in games and activities, being unresponsive to social initiations by others, and not standing up for oneself. (p. 9)

Based on this rank ordering, teachers are requested to select the three highest-ranked students meeting the above definition of internalizing problems (i.e., they pass gate 1). These three students move on to gate 2, in which they are rated on a behavior rating scale and behavior checklist. Students exceeding normative criteria on these two instruments move on to gate 3, which involves direct observations of students in the classroom and on the playground. If these students exceed normative criteria on these assessments, they may be referred to a student study team for further assessment/intervention services.

The SSBD is an extremely well conceptualized and validated system for early identification of students with emotional and behavioral difficulties. It is particularly useful for proactive identification of students with internalizing problems because these students often go unnoticed and unreferred by teachers. Experts in the field of behavior disorders have reviewed the SSBD favorably because of its systematic and comprehensive screening of behavior problems within general education settings (Forness, Kavale, MacMillan, Asarnow, & Duncan, 1996; Gresham, Lane, & Lambros, 2002; Kauffman, 1999; Severson & Walker, 2002). A downward extension of the SSBD, the Early Screening Project (Walker, Severson, & Feil,

1995) is available for students 3–6 years of age.

Multimodal Behavioral Assessment

Behavioral assessment of internalizing behavior problems should be based on multi-source, multi-informant sources of information (Gresham & Lambros, 1998; Kratochwill & Shapiro, 2000). First proposed by Cone (1978) and later expanded by Gresham and Lambros (1998), the concept of a Behavioral Assessment Grid (BAG) is a useful heuristic that is based on the concurrent consideration of six aspects of behavioral assessment: (1) the nature of behavior problems (excesses, deficits, situational inappropriateness), (2) the dimensions of behavior assessed (frequency, temporality, intensity, permanent products), (3) the system through which behavior is expressed (cognitive-verbal, overt-motoric, physiological-emotional), (4) methods used to assess behavior (direct or indirect), (5) quality of assessment information (reliability, validity), and (6) social validity (significance, acceptability, importance).

We previously described the use of teacher, parent, and self-report measures for internalizing problems in the section describing empirical classification systems (see Table 14.2). The ASEBA and BASC systems assess the major categories of internalizing behavior problems and are used extensively in behavioral assessment. Given the space constraints of this chapter, we will not discuss behavioral assessment procedures in detail. Comprehensive and complete discussions of behavioral assessment procedures can be found in the excellent texts by Merrell (1999), (Chapters 7 and 8, this volume), and Shapiro and Kratochwill (2000).

MAJOR INTERNALIZING DISORDERS

In this section, we describe the major internalizing disorders of childhood and adolescence. These disorders are classified into three superordinate categories: anxiety-related disorders, depressive disorders, and problems in peer relationships. Consistent with Table 14.1, we rely primarily on the DSM-IV labels and descriptions for these

disorders with the realization that this system of classification has some drawbacks that we have previously noted.

Anxiety-Related Disorders

Behavioral, emotional, and physiological responses to anxiety-provoking stimuli most certainly serve an adaptive function in humans because they lead to the avoidance of certain environmental events. When these responses occur in disproportion to the nature of the anxiety-provoking stimuli and interfere with everyday functioning, they become debilitating and can no longer be considered adaptive (Hintze, 2002; Kendall & Ronan, 1990).

Two behavioral models are frequently used to conceptualize the acquisition, maintenance, and elimination of anxiety disorders. The first model is based on principles of respondent (classical) conditioning in which anxiety of fear is acquired and maintained by the pairing of an unconditioned stimulus (UCS) with a conditioned stimulus (CS). Repeated pairing of the UCS with the CS results in the CS alone being responsible for eliciting an anxiety response. The second model is based on principles of operant conditioning in which anxiety responses can be either positively or negatively reinforced by agents in the child's social environment (e.g., teachers, parents, or peers) (Hintze, 2002).

A third model based on a cognitive-behavioral theory suggests that anxiety responses are developed and maintained by cognitive distortions of environmental stimuli that contain themes of danger to self and/or the family (Beck, 1976; Hintze, 2002). According to Beck (1976), in an anxiety disorder, anxiety and its behavioral manifestation (e.g., social withdrawal) result from distorted cognitive excesses or deficits (Beck, 1976). In the sections below, we briefly describe the major anxiety-related disorders of childhood and adolescence.

Separation Anxiety Disorder

The fundamental feature of this disorder is excessive anxiety concerning separation from the home or from those to whom the person is attached (American Psychiatric Association, 1994). According to DSM-IV, this condition must have been present for at least 4 weeks and cause distress or impairment in social, academic, or other important areas of functioning. The disorder can have an early onset (before 6 years of age) but can occur anytime prior to 18 years of age. Prevalence estimates are around 4% in children and young adolescents.

Selective Mutism

This disorder entails the persistent failure to speak in specific social situations where speaking is expected. Typically, selective mutism occurs in school settings, and it interferes with educational achievement because speaking is expected in school settings in response to instructional requests and directives. It is often associated with excessive shyness, fear of social embarrassment, social isolation and withdrawal, compulsive behaviors, and negativism (American Psychiatric Association, 1994). Selective mutism typically occurs before 5 years of age and is slightly more common in females than in males. It is rare, as it occurs in less than 1% of the school-age population and usually lasts only a few months (American Psychiatric Association, 1994).

Obsessive-Compulsive Disorder

This disorder reflects recurrent obsessions (ideas, thoughts, impulses, images) or compulsions (behaviors or mental acts) that are severe enough to be time-consuming or cause marked distress or impairment (American Psychiatric Association, 1994). The most frequent obsessions involve thoughts about contamination, repeated doubts, a need to have things in a certain order, or aggressive impulses or images. The most common compulsions involve repetitive behaviors such as hand washing, ordering, checking, or mental acts such as praying, counting, or repeating words silently.

In children, obsessions and compulsions are similar to those of adults. Typically, parents rather than teachers identify the behaviors since children do not usually perform ritualistic behaviors in front of teachers or peers (American Psychiatric Association,

1994). Obsessive–compulsive disorder is equally prevalent in males and females and appears to have a prevalence rate of between 1 and 2%.

Posttraumatic Stress Disorder

The essential characteristic of posttraumatic stress disorder (PTSD) is the emergence of behavioral symptoms following exposure to an extreme traumatic stressor involving direct personal experience of an event that involves threat of serious injury or death (American Psychiatric Association, 1994). It can also occur in response to serious injury or death to a family member or close friend. The typical response involves intense fear, helplessness, horror, and agitation/disorganization.

Younger children may have nightmares several weeks after exposure to the traumatic event that may involve themes about monsters, rescuing others, or threats to themselves. Children may also exhibit physical symptoms such as stomachaches and headaches. Symptoms of PTSD typically occur within 3 months of exposure to the severe stressor.

Mood Disorders

Disturbances in mood (also known as affective disorders) include a variety of behavioral characteristics and include major depressive disorder, dysthymia, bipolar disorders, and cyclothymic disorder (American Psychiatric Association, 1994). It is sometimes difficult to differentiate depressive disorders from anxiety disorders because of shared characteristics of the disorders and poor discrimination of these two disorders on standardized measures (Watson & Robinson, 1998). In general, depressed children and adolescents are more likely to demonstrate an overall decrease in activity levels, whereas individuals with anxiety disorders are likely to show increases in activity levels in the form of escape or avoidance behaviors (Watson & Robinson, 1998). The following sections focus on two mood disorders of depression and dysthymia. We also include a discussion of suicidal behavior in children and adolescents, given that most suicides and suicide attempts are committed by individuals with a history of major affective disorders (Brent & Perper, 1995; U.S. Department of Health and Human Services, 1999).

Major Depressive Disorder

The key feature of major depressive disorder is a course of behavior that is characterized by one or more major depressive episodes. A major depressive episode involves either a depressed mood or the loss of interest in nearly all activities (American Psychiatric Association, 1994). Children are more likely to show irritability in mood rather than a sad affect. Depression frequently involves the following: changes in appetite, weight, and/or sleeping patterns, decreased energy (psychomotor retardation), irritability (in children), feelings of worthlessness, hopelessness, or helplessness, guilt, poor concentration, and/or suicidal ideation, plans, or attempts (to be discussed later). These characteristics must persist for most of the day, nearly every day, for at least 2 consecutive weeks (American Psychiatric Association, 1994).

Major depressive disorder frequently co-occurs with other disorders such as anxiety disorders (e.g., separation anxiety disorder, obsessive–compulsive disorder) and disruptive behavior disorders (e.g., conduct disorder, attention-deficit/hyperactivity disorder). In children, major depressive disorder is characterized by social withdrawal, irritability, and somatic complaints. In adolescence, this pattern changes to psychomotor retardation, hypersomnia, and delusional thought patterns (American Psychiatric Association, 1994).

Dysthymic Disorder

Dysthymic disorder in children refers to a chronically depressed mood that occurs most of the day more days than not, and for a period of 1 year or more. Like depression, children may experience an irritable mood rather than a sad affect. Dysthymia also is characterized by poor appetite or overeating, insomnia or hypersomnia, low energy, low self-esteem, and poor concentration. Children and adolescents with this disorder are typically irritable, cranky, and have poor social skills.

The major difference between dysthymic disorder and major depressive disorder is based on the *chronicity* and *severity* of the symptoms. Dysthymia is chronic (may last several years), and the depressive symptoms are less severe. Sometimes it is difficult to distinguish the mood disturbance in dysthymia from the individual's typical or usual way of functioning.

Suicidal Behavior

Suicide is the third leading cause of death for adolescents and young adults (ages 15–24) and the fourth leading cause of death for children 10–14 years of age (Hoyert, Konanek, & Murphy, 1999). The American Association of Suicidology (1996) reports that male adolescents (ages 15–19 years) are over four times more likely to commit suicide than their female counterparts. This ratio, however, is smallest in the age group of elementary/middle school students (ages 10–14 years) with a figure of 2.7:1 male-to-female suicide ratio.

Poland and Lieberman (2002) report that suicide is much more common in children and adolescents diagnosed with an affective disorder, particularly depression. Moreover, suicide victims are much more likely to have a comorbid diagnosis of conduct disorder or drug/alcohol abuse (in adolescents) (Anderson & McGee, 1994). Although children will not typically self-refer, Poland and Lieberman (2002) indicated that they do show warning signs of suicidal intent such as threats ("I want to die"), plan/method/access (behaviors rather than thoughts), previous attempts, making final arrangements (giving away valued possessions), depression (feelings of helplessness and hopelessness), and sudden changes in behavior or personality.

Children and youth with internalizing problems, particularly depression coexisting with other disorders, are much more likely to commit suicide than individuals with other types of emotional or behavioral difficulties. Poland and Lieberman (2002) present an extremely useful and practitioner-friendly guide to suicide risk identification, intervention, and postvention guidelines for school professionals working with students with or at risk for emotional behavioral disorders.

INTERVENTION APPROACHES FOR INTERNALIZING BEHAVIOR PROBLEMS

To date, much of the special education research in the area of internalizing problems has focused on classification and assessment rather than intervention practices. The same is not true, however, of the research literature in the clinical child and school psychology literatures (Kendall & Morris, 1991; Kratochwill & Morris, 1993; Morris, Shah, & Morris, 2002). These literatures amply document intervention approaches that effectively reduce behaviors associated with internalizing difficulties. It should be noted, however, that there is a dearth of control comparison studies that contrast more than one treatment procedure in randomized internally valid group experimental designs (Morris et al., 2002). The following section describes empirically validated intervention approaches for behaviors associated with internalizing disorders. Table 14.3 provides an overview of these approaches along with common applications described in the literature.

Systematic Desensitization

Originally developed by Wolpe (1958), systematic desensitization has been applied primarily with anxiety-related problems. This intervention approach is based on the premise that anxiety responses are the result of learning through respondent (classical) conditioning that occurs when a neutral environmental stimulus (e.g., animal) is paired with a painful or aversive stimulus (e.g., parent screaming, loud noise). Systematic desensitization works to methodically countercondition this relationship by teaching a response that is incompatible with anxiety, such as relaxation, while simultaneously presenting variants of the anxiety-provoking stimulus in gradually increasing intensity. This process is termed "reciprocal inhibition" because relaxation will inhibit an anxiety response. Eventually, the individual is able to induce a deeply relaxed state, making it impossible to experience anxiety.

The procedure of systematic desensitization is carried out in three phases. The first phase is relaxation training. This involves progressive deep muscle relaxation. Exercises consist of successively tensing and then relaxing a specific muscle group. For example, 5–10 seconds of tensing may precede 15–30 seconds of relaxation. Tensing and relaxing usually begins with muscles at the top of the body, ending with those at the bottom of the body. A typical sequence would be (1) head and neck, (2) hands, arms, and shoulders, (3) back, stomach, and hips, and (4) legs and feet. This muscle relaxation is often accompanied by deep-breathing training and instruction in self-vocalizations (e.g., singing) that are incompatible with anxiety-producing vocalizations.

In the second phase of systematic desensitization, the individual constructs an anxiety hierarchy. Anxiety-producing stimuli are arranged in order from least anxiety-producing to most anxiety-producing. For example, MacDonald (1975) developed a hierarchy consisting of 37 stimuli for an 11-year-old boy who exhibited an extreme fear of dogs. At the low end of hierarchy, the boy was to imagine himself on his front porch with his father seeing a beagle down the street, minding his own business. At the high end of the hierarchy, the boy imagined himself playing

TABLE 14.3. Intervention Approaches for Internalizing Disorders

Strategy	Common applications
Systematic desensitization	Anxiety-related problems
Exposure-based intervention	Anxiety-related problems Obsessive–compulsive disorders
Modeling	Anxiety-related problems Social withdrawal
Cognitive-behavioral intervention	Anxiety-related problems
Antecedent- and consequence-based interventions	Anxiety-related problems Social withdrawal
Social skills training	Social withdrawal

outside alone and looking up to see an unfamiliar collie running down his driveway.

During the third phase of systematic desensitization, relaxation training is paired with presentation of each stimulus on the anxiety hierarchy. Once the individual is fully relaxed, anxiety-producing stimuli are gradually introduced, beginning with the least anxiety-producing and concluding with the most anxiety-producing. The stimuli can be introduced either *in vivo* or through imagery. During *in vivo* desensitization, the actual item of fear is presented. An example of *in vivo* desensitization for an individual with test anxiety would be presentation of actual test materials, such as a pencil, test booklet, and scan sheet. An alternative to actually presenting anxiety-producing stimuli is imaginal desensitization, whereby the individual produces clear images of the stimuli. In this case, the individual would be asked to visualize herself sitting at her desk with a pencil, test booklet, and scan sheet in front of her. If at any point during presentation or visualization the individual experiences feelings of anxiety, the image or item is removed and the process reverts to a lesser anxiety-provoking stimulus. Ideally, progression through the hierarchy should occur in the absence of feelings of anxiety.

Taylor (1972) described the successful application of systematic desensitization with a 15-year-old young girl who experienced an excessive need to urinate during school and school-related activities. Using imaginal desensitization, she was taught relaxation while visualizing hierarchies related to riding the bus, being present in areas of the school, and engaging in classroom activities. The intervention was implemented over the summer, during five 1-hour sessions, and resulted in a typical frequency of urination the following school year.

Systematic desensitization has been widely applied to reduce a range of anxieties in children, including school phobia, test anxiety, fear of public speaking, fear of water, nyctophobia, acrophobia, fear of weight gain, and fear of animals. However, a few caveats should be noted when using this procedure. First, a successful outcome requires that an individual is capable of attaining a state of relaxation. For individuals incapable of achieving such a state, this intervention is not recommended. In addition, it is often

difficult to teach relaxation techniques to young children. To address this problem, scripts are available that are short, focus on just a few muscle groups, and incorporate components that are appealing to that age group (e.g., Koeppen, 1974).

A second caution is that young children may have limited ability to visualize anxiety-producing items or situations because of their developmental status. Some recommend avoiding imaginal desensitization with individuals younger than 9 years of age (e.g., Morris & Kratochwill, 1998). With this age group, *in vivo* desensitization is likely to be more effective.

Finally, it is strongly recommended to explicitly program for generalization. Systematic desensitization is generally carried out in a clinical setting. Exposure to anxiety-producing stimuli and learning to generate responses to overcome associated feelings of fear may be very different in a safe and supportive clinical environment than in naturalistic settings. To assure generalization, systematic desensitization procedures must be extended to the natural environment by introducing and training on stimuli as they naturally occur.

Exposure-Based Interventions

Exposure-based interventions are generally used with anxiety disorders or obsessive–compulsive disorders (Hintze, 2002; Laurent & Potter, 1998). These types of interventions operate on the principle of extinction. Extinction is a process in which reinforcement for a behavior is discontinued. In the context of anxiety-producing situations, it is presumed that anxious behaviors such as trembling, crying, or running away ultimately result in avoidance or escape from the anxiety-producing stimulus. Similarly, it is assumed that obsessive–compulsive behaviors function to avoid a presumed negative consequence if the behavior were not repeatedly performed. Applying extinction means discontinuing or preventing those avoidance or escape behaviors that were previously reinforced. Once the individual learns that the behaviors no longer produce avoidance or escape, the behaviors cease.

Unlike systematic desensitization, exposure-based techniques immediately introduce the individual to the most anxiety-producing stimulus along the anxiety hierarchy. The rationale is to occasion behaviors that can be exposed to extinction. That is, a situation is set up so that behaviors occur that are no longer reinforced through escape or avoidance.

A common form of this type of intervention is flooding. As with systematic desensitization, the anxiety-producing stimulus is presented either *in vivo* or through imagery. Likewise, for obsessive–compulsive disorder, the individual is exposed to or imagines the consequences of not ritualistically performing a behavior. Anxiety or ritualistic responses that occur in the presence of the *in vivo* or visualized stimulus are blocked or ignored. In some cases, individuals are asked to report the amount of anxiety or discomfort they experience corresponding to some type of rating scale. Intervention continues until self-reported anxiety or discomfort is low.

Another variation of exposure-based intervention is to establish a hierarchy of behaviors that the individual performs, which result in gradually increased contact with the anxiety-producing stimulus. The behaviors are generally denoted through a task analysis. For example, the first step of exposure in a task analysis for an individual with a phobia of insects might be to sit in a chair with a spider placed across the room. Each step of the task analysis would involve moving the spider gradually closer to the individual until it is within very close proximity.

Houlihaun, Schwartz, Miltenberger, and Heuton (1993) successfully demonstrated the application of flooding with a young man experiencing extreme anxiety associated with balloon popping. The individual reported that he avoided situations where balloons might be present. Clinical assessments indicated that he was unable to be within 4 feet of a balloon without experiencing intense fear and anxiety. The flooding intervention consisted of popping hundreds of balloons, with his participation, during sessions conducted across consecutive days. After 3 days of intervention, no avoidance behaviors were observed, and he reported almost no feelings of fear or anxiety.

Several cautions should be noted when considering this procedure. First, because this technique requires exposure to stimuli considered extremely offensive and associated with unpleasant and uncomfortable reactions, it is considered to be a quite aversive procedure. Consequently, parents and professionals may consider it objectionable. Less intrusive interventions should be attempted prior to considering this type of more intrusive intervention. In addition, as with other interventions primarily applied in clinical settings, it is critical that positive outcomes generalize to natural settings. This requires application or extension of the procedures across naturally occurring stimuli.

Modeling

Used primarily to treat anxiety disorders, modeling is based on social learning theory developed by Bandura (1969). According to social learning theory, behavior can be learned through observation of others. In the same way that fears can be learned vicariously, modeling is used as an intervention to decrease those fears by observing another (or, in recent applications, oneself) engage in a nonfearful response to stimuli that are the subject of fear.

Certain pretreatment criteria are required for modeling interventions to be successful (Bandura, 1977). First, the target individual must be able to attend to relevant dimensions of the modeling situation. Second, the individual must be able to retain what he or she has observed during the modeling situation. Third, the individual must be capable of motorically mimicking what was observed. Finally, the individual must be motivated to engage in the observed behavior.

Implementation of a modeling intervention begins by identifying an individual who will serve as a model. This often is a parent, teacher, peer, therapist, or even oneself. The model then engages in nonfearful behavior in the presence of a stimulus (e.g., dog) that is feared or avoided by the target individual. The individual watches the model engage in the nonfearful behavior, either live or via videotape. The individual is then encouraged to replicate the observed behavior. Feedback is provided and successful imitation is rewarded.

In an interesting application of self-modeling, Kehle, Owen, and Cressy (1990) demonstrated the complete remediation of selective mutism in a 6-year-old boy. Vocalizations were completely absent at school. To begin the intervention, his mother was brought to school and instructed to ask him nine simple questions (e.g., "What is your favorite flavor of ice cream?"), encouraging him to provide elaborate responses. Questioning took place while the boy and his mother were alone in a classroom, and the session was videotaped. Subsequently, the boy's teacher asked him identical questions in the presence of his classmates, which elicited no response. This session also was videotaped. The two tapes were edited so that the boy could observe himself answering teacher questions in the presence of his classmates. Following only seven intervention sessions lasting approximately 5 minutes each, the boy's responses to the teacher's questions increased to 100%. Interactions also generalized to peers as well and maintained after 7 months.

Although research supports modeling as an effective intervention, as with exposure-based interventions, the presence of highly feared stimuli may produce high levels of fear and anxiety. Variations, such as the videotaped self-observation used by Kehle et al. (1990), may offer a less intrusive alternative. In addition, because modeling is generally implemented in a clinical or analogue setting, it is critical to include strategies to assure that intervention results generalize to natural settings.

Cognitive-Behavioral Interventions

Cognitive-behavioral interventions rest on the belief that an individual's response to the environment involves a process that is cognitively mediated. Thus, behavior depends on thoughts and how they are cognitively processed. An assumption of cognitive-behavioral interventions is that changes in thought and cognitive processes will lead to changes in behavior. As such, this calls for the ability to regulate one's own behavior.

Implementation of cognitive-behavioral strategies usually occurs in four phases (Kendall et al., 1992). The first phase entails identifying occurrences of the problem. For example, in the case of anxiety disorder, one would be taught to recognize feelings of anxiety and related physical reactions. Identification of anxious feelings may be facilitated through discussion and/or self-recording of those feelings. After the individual learns to identify occurrences of the prob-

lem, the next step is to assist the individual in developing an alternative strategy when confronted with the problem-producing situation. This usually involves self-talk or self-statements that function to reduce the unwanted feelings and physical symptoms. The final step is to self-evaluate initiation of adaptive responses and self-reward for success and partial success.

In a study by Kane and Kendall (1989), four children diagnosed with overanxious disorder were successfully treated using a cognitive-behavioral intervention. The intervention consisted of four components: (1) teaching the children to recognize anxious feelings and somatic reactions; (2) identifying unrealistic or negative thoughts that occurred during anxiety-provoking situations; (3) generating a coping plan, including replacing anxious self-talk with coping self-talk and determining effective coping actions; and (4) evaluating the success of the strategy and self-reinforcing when appropriate. The intervention resulted in significant reductions in anxiety, measured by standardized assessments.

A concern noted with the cognitive-behavioral approach is the lack of a procedure for measuring cognitive changes. This has led some to argue that the reward component alone may be responsible for the effectiveness of the procedure, rather than cognitive changes. Although empirical research supports this method of intervention, particularly for fear or anxiety, it is far less researched than other methods, such as systematic desensitization, modeling, and contingency management procedures (Morris et al., 2002). As with other intervention approaches, programming for generalization is crucial. Parent involvement and homework assignments have been shown to enhance generalization (e.g., March & Mulle, 1995).

Antecedent- and Consequence-Based Strategies

Antecedent- and consequence-based strategies are derived from the principles of operant psychology developed by Skinner (1953). These principles, known as the 3-term contingency, recognize the relationship between behavior and the environment. The 3-term contingency refers to the interrelationship between antecedents, behaviors, and their consequences (A–B–C). Environmental events can either encourage or discourage occurrences of a behavior. As such, internalizing behaviors exist as a result of learning that has been shaped and reinforced through environmental processes and contingencies. Intervention seeks to change the environmental events that have and continue to promote the behavior, both by teaching alternative behaviors and by arranging for reinforcement to occur for adaptive behavior rather than maladaptive behavior.

In the case of antecedent-based approaches, environmental events that occur just prior to problem behavior are modified in some way to encourage desirable behavior and prevent or decrease the likelihood of undesirable behavior occurring. Two antecedent approaches commonly used for internalizing disorders are shaping and stimulus fading. The process of shaping entails reinforcing behavior in forms that gradually resemble the desired end behavior. Reinforcement occurs in steps (known as successive approximations to the terminal behavior) and is provided only as behavior successively moves toward the end goal.

Luiselli (1978) illustrated the use of shaping to eliminate a 7-year-old boy's fear of riding the school bus. Intervention began with the boy's mother seated next to him on a parked bus for 2 minutes while simultaneously delivering praise for appropriate bus riding. The next day resembled the first day, but halfway through the "bus ride" his mother stood outside the bus, just below his window. Praise was delivered for appropriate behavior. On the third day, his mother and therapist placed him on the bus, but his mother did not sit with him. The following day his mother remained in the car while the therapist alone placed him on the bus. On day 5, the therapist walked him to the bus, where his mother was already seated. After receiving edible reinforcement, the threesome rode the bus to school together. The next and final day of treatment, the boy was placed on the bus by his mother, but rode alone. This shaping process resulted in the boy's continued successful and independent bus riding.

Stimulus fading involves systematically introducing variants of the objectionable stimulus. When applied to internalizing problems, an individual is exposed to an avoided stimulus in a gradual and systematic way so that aversive feelings and behaviors associated with the original stimulus are avoided. Watson and Kramer (1992) used stimulus fading as part of an intervention package to increase the frequency of speech exhibited by Tim, a 9-year-old boy with selective mutism. In Tim's class, there was one peer with whom he regularly spoke. Tim was paired with this classmate. During class, other students were gradually moved closer to Tim and added to his group. This continued until eventually the entire class of students became a part of Tim's group. The number of classmates Tim spoke to gradually increased.

Consequence approaches are based on research showing that behavior that is reinforced will continue to occur, while behavior that is not reinforced will discontinue or extinguish. Thus, consequence-based interventions manipulate contingencies that follow behavior. In the case of internalizing disorders, the processes of positive reinforcement and extinction are commonly applied. Positive reinforcement is defined as an event or activity presented just after a behavior that results in an increase in that behavior. When applied to internalizing behaviors, positive reinforcement is delivered for behavior that is incompatible with undesirable behavior. For example, a social initiation toward a peer by a socially withdrawn child would generate praise or a reward.

In the case of occurrences of unwanted behavior, extinction is applied. Extinction is a consequence procedure that involves discontinuing reinforcement following the unwanted behavior. It is often the case that behavior continues because it is inadvertently rewarded in some way. Take, for example, an individual who experiences test anxiety. A teacher may respond in a number of different ways in the attempt to reduce behaviors indicating fear. He or she may sit with the student during the test, providing encouragement and assistance, allow the student to complete the test at home, or offer an alternative assignment (e.g., writing a paper). Although well intentioned, each of these consequences reinforces the fearful behaviors by allowing the student to escape various aspects of the testing situation, or even avoid it altogether. By removing these responses, the individual learns that reinforcement (i.e., escape) is no longer forth-coming, and the behaviors eventually disap-pear.

One objectionable side effect of extinc-tion, referred to as an extinction burst, is that the behavior sometimes increases prior to decreasing. This happens when an indi-vidual accelerates the rate of behavior in an effort to obtain reinforcement that occurred previously. In the case of behaviors that are detrimental to an individual's well-being, this strategy may not be advised. When us-ing extinction, it also is recommended that it be used in conjunction with other approaches, such as antecedent-based strategies or sys-tematic desensitization and/or consequence-based approaches such as differential rein-forcement of incompatible behavior (DRI).

Social Skills Training

Interventions that train social skills are com-mon for internalizing disorders, particularly problems with peer relations, such as social withdrawal. Social skills interventions are based on the presumption that individuals who experience peer relation problems of an internalizing nature either (1) lack the skills necessary for adequate interrelations, (2) possess social skills but are unable to employ them when needed, or (3) are unable to emit social skills in a fluent manner (Gresham, 2002). The nature of social skills training differs, depending on which of these sources accounts for the social skill problem.

In addition to peer relation problems, so-cial skills interventions also have been used with individuals experiencing depressive symp-toms. The rationale underlying this mode of treatment stems from operant theory and is indirectly supported by the established co-occurrence of depressive symptoms and poor social relations (e.g., Matson, 1989). The presumption is that social skill deficits result in a limited amount of reinforcement from others, which then leads to the devel-opment of depression (Lewinsohn, 1974; Watson & Robinson, 1998). Three possible sources of diminished reinforcement have been described. First, an individual may lack the skills to engage in prosocial behaviors that generally result in reinforcement. Sec-ond, others may avoid interactions with an individual who exhibits asocial or antisocial behaviors. Third, an individual may be un-

able to reinforce others, reducing the rate of mutual reinforcement.

For the most part, social skills interven-tions rely on various configurations of in-struction, modeling, and/or role play. Copi-ous variations of social skills interventions have been described in the literature. Many involve peers as change agents rather than adults as instructors, which may enhance generalization. Recent permutations include self-observation via videotape, along with instruction, to increase social interactions among withdrawn children (e.g., Falk, Dun-lap, & Kern, 1996).

Miller and Cole (1998) demonstrated the effectiveness of social skills training with Ryan, an adolescent with comorbid depres-sion and conduct disorder. The social skills intervention began with descriptions of a problematic scenario. Ryan was asked to respond to the scenario. Appropriate re-sponses were praised while feedback was provided for inappropriate responses, along with a model of an appropriate response. The scenario was repeated until an appro-priate response occurred. Intervention con-tinued until appropriate responses occurred across 10 different scenarios. This was repli-cated across three behaviors, including giv-ing compliments, offering help, and appro-priately responding to teasing. Each of these behaviors was greatly increased as a result of the social skills training.

CONSIDERATIONS FOR INTERVENTION SELECTION AND USE

Although the intervention approaches de-scribed above benefit from empirical support, a fundamental concern pertains to generalization. Very few research studies de-scribe applications of the interventions ap-plied in natural contexts. Equally concern-ing is the absence of data supporting generalized effects of the intervention from clinical or analog settings to typical every-day environments. For the most part, when present, information about generalization is limited to anecdotal accounts.

A second concern is that the research predominantly describes interventions im-plemented by researchers or clinicians in specialized settings (e.g., outpatient hospital clinics). This type of service is typically not available to most school children. An unanswered question is whether typical school personnel can implement these interventions successfully. Further, the training required to do so remains unspecified.

Finally, notably absent is information pertaining to the match between child characteristics and intervention effectiveness. The etiology as well as the variables that predict and play a role in occurrences of any given internalizing problem (e.g., depression) differ greatly across individuals. Thus, it is reasonable to assume that intervention effectiveness will likewise differ, depending on its match to variables that contribute to and sustain the behavior. A few studies provide preliminary support for such an approach. For example, Kearney and Silverman (1999) demonstrated the effectiveness of intervention based on functional assessment information for students with school refusal behavior. Additional research is warranted in this area.

CONCLUSION

This chapter has reviewed the major assessment, classification, and intervention issues for children with internalizing behavior patterns. We provided a description and critical review of DSM-IV, the most commonly used classification system for emotional and behavioral disorders for children and adolescents. Despite its widespread popularity among psychiatrists and clinical psychologists, we pointed out several concerns with its use in school settings. Among these concerns is its medical model orientation that favors a within-child conceptualization of behavior problems rather than a person–environmental fit explanation, its questionable reliability, and the absence of treatment validity.

We concluded that empirical screening and assessment systems had several advantages over the DSM approach, particularly their objective/statistical criteria for assigning specific behaviors to clusters of behavior problems, their superior reliability and validity evidence, and the use of multiple informants to assess behavior. The use of teacher nominations and ratings in early identification screening systems such as the SSBD (Walker & Severson, 1992) and the ESP

(Walker et al., 1995) was viewed as especially advantageous.

Finally, we reviewed a number of evidence-based intervention procedures for child and adolescent internalizing problems. Some of these (e.g., systematic desensitization, exposure-based treatments, and antecedent-consequent-based strategies) have more evidence for their efficacy than other techniques (e.g., cognitive-behavior therapy). However, these interventions come with limitations, including a lack of empirical data supporting generalization and the need for highly trained personnel for implementation.

REFERENCES

Achenbach, T. (1982). *Developmental psychopathology* (2nd ed.). New York: Wiley.

Achenbach, T. (1991). *Integrative guide for the 1991 CBCL/4-18, YSR, and TRF profiles.* Burlington, VT: University of Vermont, Department of Psychiatry.

Achenbach, T., & McConaughy, S. (1997). *Empirically based assessment of child and adolescent psychopathology: Practical applications.* Thousand Oaks, CA: Sage.

Algozzine, R. (1977). The emotionally disturbed child: Disturbed or disturbing? *Journal of Abnormal Child Psychology, 5,* 205–211.

American Association of Suicidology (1996). Youth suicide by firearms task force. Available at *http://www.suicidology.org/youthsuicidetaskforce.htm.*

American Psychiatric Association. (1994). *Diagnostic and statistical manual of mental disorders* (4th ed.). Washington, DC: Author.

Anderson, J., & McGee, R. (1994). Comorbidity of depression in children and adolescents. In W. Reynolds & H. Johnson (Eds.), *Handbook of depression in children and adolescents* (pp. 581–601). New York: Plenum.

Atkins, M., McKernal, M., McKay, M., Talbott, E., & Arvanitis, P. (1996). DSM-IV diagnosis of conduct disorder and oppositional defiant disorder: Implications and guidelines for school psychologists. *School Psychology Review, 25,* 274–283.

Bandura, A. (1969). *Principles of behavior modification.* New York: Holt.

Bandura, A. (1977). *Social learning theory.* Englewood Cliffs, NJ: Prentice Hall.

Beck, A. (1976). *Cognitive therapy and emotional disorder.* New York: International Universities Press.

Brent, D., & Perper, J. (1995). Research in adolescent suicide: Implications for training, service delivery, and public policy. *Suicide and Life-Threatening Behavior, 25,* 222–230.

Brophy, J. (1986). Classroom management techniques. *Education and Urban Society, 18*, 182–194.

Carson, R. (1996). Aristotle, Galileo, and the DSM taxonomy: The case of schizophrenia. *Journal of Consulting and Clinical Psychology, 64*, 1133–1339.

Cicchetti, D., & Toth, S. (1991). A developmental perspective on internalizing and externalizing disorders. In D. Cicchetti & S. Toth (Eds.), *Internalizing and externalizing expressions of dysfunction* (pp. 1–19). Hillsdale, NJ: Erlbaum.

Colvin, G., Kame'enui, E. J., & Sugai, G. (1993). Schoolwide discipline and classroom management: Reconceptualizing the integration and management of students with behavior problems in general education. *Education and Treatment of Children, 11*, 361–381.

Cone, J. (1978). The behavioral assessment grid (BAG): A conceptual framework and taxonomy. *Behavior Therapy, 9*, 882–888.

Eysenck, H., Wakefield, J., & Friedman, A. (1983). Diagnosis and clinical assessment: The DSM-III. *Annual Review of Psychology, 34*, 42474–42518.

Falk, G., Dunlap, G., & Kern, L. (1996). An analysis of self-evaluation and videotape feedback for improving the peer interactions of students with externalizing and internalizing behavioral challenges. *Behavioral Disorders, 21*, 261–276.

Follette, W., & Houts, A. (1996). Models of scientific progress and the role of theory in taxonomy: A case study of the DSM. *Journal of Consulting and Clinical Psychology, 64*, 1120–1132.

Forness, S. R., Kavale, K. A., MacMillan, D. M., Asarnow, J., & Duncan, B. (1996). Early detection and prevention of emotional or behavioral disorders: Developmental aspects of systems of care. *Behavioral Disorders, 23*, 226–240.

Forness, S. R., & Knitzer, J. (1992). A new proposed definition and terminology to replace "Serious Emotional Disturbance" in Individuals with Disabilities Education Act. *School Psychology Review, 21*, 12–20.

Gresham, F. M. (1999). Noncategorical approaches to K–12 emotional and behavioral difficulties. In D. Reschly, D. Tilly, & J. Grimes (Eds.), *Special education in transition: Functional assessment and non-categorical programming* (pp. 107–137). Longmont, CO: Sopris West.

Gresham, F. M. (2002). Teaching social skills to high-risk children and youth: Preventative and remedial strategies. In M. Shinn, H. Wallace, & G. Stone (Eds.), *Interventions for academic and behavior problems II* (pp. 403–432). Bethesda, MD: National Association of School Psychologists.

Gresham, F. M., & Gansle, K. (1992). Misguided assumptions in DSM-III-R: Implications for school psychological practice. *School Psychology Quarterly, 7*, 79–95.

Gresham, F. M., & Lambros, K. (1998). Behavioral and functional assessment. In T. S. Watson & F. M. Gresham (Eds.), *Handbook of child behavior therapy* (pp. 3–22). New York: Plenum.

Gresham, F. M., Lane, K. L., & Lambros, K. (2002). Children with conduct and hyperactivity–impulsivity–attention problems: Identification, assessment, and intervention. In K. L. Lane, F. M. Gresham, & T. E. O'Shaughnessy (Eds.), *Interventions for children with or at-risk for emotional and behavioral disorders* (pp. 210–222). Boston: Allyn & Bacon.

Gresham, F. M., & Noell, G. H. (1999). Functional analysis assessment as a cornerstone for noncategorical special education. In D Reschly, D. Tilly, & J. Grimes (Eds.), *Special education in transition: Functional assessment and noncategorical programming* (pp. 49–79). Longmont, CO: Sopris West.

Hayes, S., Nelson, R., & Jarrett, R. (1987). The treatment utility of assessment: A functional approach to evaluating assessment quality. *American Psychologist, 42*, 963–974.

Hersh, R., & Walker, H. M. (1983). Great expectations: Making schools effective for all students. *Policy Studies Review, 2*, 147–188.

Hintze, J. (2002). Interventions for fears and anxiety problems. In M. Shinn, H. M.Walker, & G. Stoner (Eds.), *Interventions for academic and behavior problems: Preventive and remedial approaches* (2nd ed., pp. 939–960). Bethesda, MD: National Association of School Psychologists.

Houlihan, D., Schwartz, C., Miltenberger, R., & Heuton, E. (1993). The rapid treatment of a young man's balloon (noise) phobia using in vivo flooding. *Journal of Behavior Therapy and Experimental Psychiatry, 24*, 233–240.

Hoyert, D., Konanek, K., & Murphy, S. (1999). Deaths: Final data for 1997. In *National Vital Statistics Report, 47* (DHHS Publication No. [PHS] 99-1120). Hyattsville, MD: National Center for Health Statistics.

Kane, M. T., & Kendall, P. C. (1989). Anxiety disorders in children: A multiple-baseline evaluation of a cognitive-behavioral treatment. *Behavior Therapy, 20*, 499–508.

Kauffman, J. M. (1999). How we prevent the prevention of emotional and behavioral disorders. *Exceptional Children, 65*, 448–468.

Kauffman, J. M. (2001). *Characteristics of emotional and behavioral disorders of children and youth* (7th ed.). Upper Saddle, NJ: Merrill/Prentice Hall.

Kearney, C. A., & Silverman, W. (1999). Functionally-based prescriptive and non-prescriptive treatment for children and adolescents with school refusal behavior. *Behavior Therapy, 30*, 673–695.

Kehle, T. J., Owen, S. V., & Cressy, E. T. (1990). The use of self-modeling as an intervention in school psychology: A case study of an elective mute. *School Psychology Review, 19*, 115–121.

Kendall, P. C., Chansky, T. E., Kane, M. T., Kim, R. S., Kortlander, E., Ronan, K. R., et al. (1992). *Anxiety disorders in youth: Cognitive-behavioral interventions*. Needham Heights, MA: Allyn & Bacon.

Kendall, P. C., & Morris, R. (1991). Child therapy: Issues and recommendations. *Journal of Consulting and Clinical Psychology, 59,* 777–784.

Kendall, P. C., & Ronan, K. (1990). Assessment of children's anxieties, fears, and phobias: Cognitive-behavioral models and methods. In C. Reynolds & R. Kamphaus (Eds.), *Handbook of psychological and educational assessment of children* (pp. 223–244). New York: Guilford Press.

Koeppen, A. S. (1974). Relaxation training for children. *Elementary School Guidance and Counseling, 9,* 14–21.

Kovacs, M. (1991). *The children's depression inventory: A self-rated scale for school-aged youngsters.* North Tonawanda, NY: Multi-Health Systems.

Kratochwill, T. R., & Morris, R. J. (Eds.). (1993). *Handbook of psychotherapy with children and adolescents.* Needham Heights, MA: Allyn & Bacon.

Kratochwill, T. R., & Shapiro, E. S. (2000). Conceptual foundations of behavioral assessment in the schools. In E. S. Shapiro & T. Kratochwill (Eds.), *Behavioral assessment in schools: Theory, research, and clinical foundations* (2nd ed., pp. 3–15). New York: Guilford Press.

Lahey, B., Applegate, B., Barkley, R., Garfinkel, B., McBurnett, K., Kerdyk, L., et al. (1994). DSM-IV field trials for oppositional defiant disorder and conduct disorder in children and adolescents. *American Journal of Psychiatry, 151,* 1163–1171.

Laurent, J., & Potter, K. I. (1998). Anxiety-related difficulties. In T. S. Watson and F. M. Gresham (Eds.), *Handbook of child behavior therapy* (pp. 371–392). New York: Plenum.

Lewinsohn, P. M. (1974). A behavioral approach to depression. In R. J. Friedman & M. M. Katz (Eds.), *The psychology of depression: Contemporary theory and research* (pp. 157–184). New York: Wiley.

Luiselli, J. (1978). Treatment of an autistic child's fear of riding a school bus through exposure and reinforcement. *Journal of Behavior Therapy and Experimental Psychiatry, 9,* 169–172.

MacDonald, M. L. (1975). Multiple impact behavior therapy in a child's dog phobia. *Journal of Behavior Therapy and Experimental Psychiatry, 6,* 317–322.

March, J. S., & Mulle, K. (1995). Manualized cognitive-behavioral psychotherapy for obsessive–compulsive disorder in childhood: A preliminary single case study. *Journal of Anxiety Disorders, 9,* 175–184.

Matson, J. L. (1989). *Treating depression in children and adolescents.* New York: Pergamon.

McConaughy, S., & Ritter, D. (2002). Best practices in multidimensional assessment of emotional or behavioral disorders. In A. Thomas & J. Grimes (Eds.), *Best practices in school psychology* (4th ed., pp. 1303–1320). Bethesda, MD: National Association of School Psychologists.

Merrell, K. W. (1999). *Behavioral, social, and emotional assessment of children and adolescents.* Mahwah, NJ: Erlbaum.

Merrell, K. W., & Walters, A. (1998). *Internalizing symptoms scale for children.* Austin, TX: Pro-Ed.

Miller, D. N., & Cole, C. L. (1998). Effects of social skills training on an adolescent with comorbid conduct disorder and depression. *Child and Family Behavior Therapy, 20,* 35–53.

Morris, R. J., & Kratochwill, T. R. (1998). Fears and phobias. In R. J. Morris & T. R. Kratochwill (Eds.), *The practice of child therapy* (3rd ed., pp. 91–131). Needham Heights, MA: Allyn & Bacon.

Morris, R. J., Shah, K., & Morris, Y. P. (2002). Internalizing behavior disorders. In K. L. Lane, F. M. Gresham, & T. E. O'Shaughnessy (Eds.), *Interventions for children with or at-risk for emotional and behavioral disorders* (pp. 223–241). Boston: Allyn & Bacon.

Poland, S., & Lieberman, R. (2002). Best practices in suicide intervention. In A. Thomas & J. Grimes (Eds.), *Best practices in school psychology* (4th ed., pp. 1151–1165). Bethesda, MD: National Association of School Psychologists.

Reynolds, C. R., & Kamphaus, R. (1992). *Behavioral Assessment System for Children.* Circle Pines, MN: American Guidance Service.

Reynolds, C. R., & Richmond, B. (1985). *Revised Children's Manifest Anxiety Scale.* Los Angeles: Western Psychological Services.

Reynolds, W. (1989). *Reynolds Child Depression Scale.* Odessa, FL: Psychological Assessment Resources.

Scotti, J., Morris, T. R., McNeil, C., & Hawkins, R. (1996). DSM-IV and disorders of childhood and adolescence: Can structural criteria be functional? *Journal of Consulting and Clinical Psychology, 64,* 1177–1191.

Severson, H. H., & Walker, H. M. (2002). Proactive approaches for identifying children at-risk for sociobehavioral problems. In K. L. Lane, F. M. Gresham, & T. E. O'Shaughnessy (Eds.), *Interventions for children with or at risk for emotional and behavioral disorders* (pp. 33–54). Boston: Allyn & Bacon.

Shapiro, E. S., & Kratochwill, T. R. (Eds.). (2000). *Behavioral assessment in schools: Theory, research, and clinical foundations* (2nd ed.). New York: Guilford Press.

Skiba, R., & Grizzle, K. (1992). Qualifications vs. logic and data: Excluding conduct disorders from the SED definition. *School Psychology Review, 21,* 23–28.

Skinner, B. F. (1953). *Science and human behavior.* New York: Macmillan.

Spielberger, C. (1973). *State-trait Anxiety Inventory for Children.* Palo Alto, CA: Consulting Psychologists Press.

Sugai, G., Horner, R. H., & Gresham, F. M. (2002). Behaviorally effective school environments. In M. Shinn, H. M. Walker, & G. Stoner (Eds.), *Interventions for academic and behavior problems: Preventive and remedial approaches* (2nd ed.). Bethesda, MD: National Association of School Psychologists.

Taylor, D. W. (1972). Treatment of excessive frequency

of urination by desensitization. *Journal of Behavior Therapy and Experimental Psychiatry, 3,* 311–313.

U.S. Department of Health and Human Services (1999). *Mental health: A report of the Surgeon General—executive summary.* Rockville, MD: U.S. Department of Health and Human Services, Substance Abuse and Mental Health Services Administration, Center for Mental Health Services, National Institutes of Health, National Institute of Mental Health.

Walker, H. M., Ramsey, E., & Gresham, F. M. (2004). *Antisocial behavior in schools: Evidence-based practices* (2nd ed.). Pacific Grove, CA: Thompson Wadsworth.

Walker, H. M., Reavis, K., Rhode, G., & Jenson, W. (1985). A conceptual model for delivery of behavioral services to behavior disordered children in education settings. In P. Bornstein & A. E. Kazdin (Eds.), *Handbook of clinical behavior therapy with children* (pp. 700–741). Homewood, IL: Dorsey.

Walker, H. M., & Severson, H. H. (1992). *Systematic Screening for Behavioral Disorders.* Longmont, CO: Sopris West.

Walker, H. M., Severson, H. H., & Feil, E. G. (1995). *Early screening project: A proven child-find process.* Longmont, CO: Sopris West.

Walker, H. M., & Shinn, M. R. (2002). Structuring school-based interventions to achieve integrated primary, secondary, and tertiary prevention goals for safe and effective schools. In M. R. Shinn, H. M.Walker, & G. Stoner (Eds.), *Interventions for academic and behavior problems II: Preventive and remedial approaches* (pp. 1–25). Bethesda, MD: National Association of School Psychologists.

Watson, T. S., & Kramer, J. J. (1992). Multimethod behavioral treatment of long-term selective mutism. *Psychology in the Schools, 29,* 359–366.

Watson, T. S., & Robinson, S. (1998). A behavior analytic approach for treatment depression. In T. S. Watson & F. M. Gresham (Eds.), *Handbook of child behavior therapy* (pp. 393–412). New York: Plenum.

Werry, J., Methuen, J., Fitzpatrick, J., & Dixon, H. (1983). Interrater reliability in DSM-III in children. *Journal of Abnormal Child Psychology, 11,* 341–354.

Wolpe, J. (1958). *Psychotherapy by reciprocal inhibition.* Stanford, CA: Stanford University Press.

15

Youth Delinquency

Prevention and Intervention

C. MICHAEL NELSON, PETER E. LEONE,
and ROBERT B. RUTHERFORD JR.

According to the first Office of Juvenile Justice and Delinquency Prevention (OJJDP) Juvenile Residential Facility Census in October 2000, 110,284 offenders younger than 21 were incarcerated in 3,061 juvenile facilities (Sickmund, 2002). Snyder (2001) reported that the number of child delinquents (juveniles between the ages of 7 and 12) handled in America's juvenile courts has increased 33% over the past decade. Recent changes in social policy and public attitudes concerning youths who engage in antisocial behavior have resulted in increasingly harsh penalties. Such policies as zero tolerance for misbehavior in school and the transfer out of youthful offenders to adult courts are symptomatic of a shift in focus from efforts to provide treatment to youths who display antisocial behavior to a focus on punishment, including incarceration. At the same time, research is demonstrating that youths with disabilities, mental health needs, and those from ethnic minority groups are significantly overrepresented in school suspension, expulsion, and dropout data, as well as in the juvenile delinquency system itself. This chapter reviews the literature that seeks to explain what factors place these youths at risk for involvement with the system, as well as their status in the system and the outcomes they experience upon returning to their communities. The research on interventions that attempt to (1) prevent youths from engaging in delinquent behavior or those who have offended from entering the system, (2) address their needs through educational services within the system, and (3) improve outcomes during transition and aftercare also is examined. Finally, questions and issues for future research involving youths who are involved, or are at risk of involvement, in the juvenile delinquency system are raised.

CHARACTERISTICS AND NEEDS OF YOUTHS INVOLVED IN THE JUVENILE DELINQUENCY SYSTEM

A consistent set of findings over several decades of research into the characteristics of incarcerated juveniles is that this population includes disproportionate numbers of youths who are ethnic minorities (especially African Americans and Hispanics); have experienced school failure, including illiteracy, suspension, expulsion, and dropping out; have disabilities recognized under the Individuals with Disabilities Education Act (IDEA); and have mental health diagnoses. For example, Galagher (1999) reported that 58.5% of the approximately 105,000 youths in private ju-

venile detention, correctional, and shelter facilities in 1997 were from ethnic minority
backgrounds (40% were African American
and 18.5% Hispanic). Foley (2001) conducted an extensive review of the research
concerning the academic characteristics of
incarcerated youths and found that, in general: (1) their assessed intellectual functioning has been at the low-average to average
range; (2) their academic achievement levels
range from fifth to ninth grade; (3) relative
to nonincarcerated students, they have
significant deficits in reading, math, and
written and oral language; (4) those who
recidivate have significantly lower levels of
intellectual and academic functioning than
those who do not; and (5) school failure is a
common experience among incarcerated
youth. A recent survey of state departments
of juvenile justice reported that, on average,
34.4% of youths in juvenile corrections
were served in special education programs
(Quinn, Rutherford, Leone, Osher, & Poirier,
in press), compared with a prevalence of approximately 10% in the public schools. The
existence of high rates of mental and emotional disorders among incarcerated youth
has been known for some time (Moffitt,
1990). Otto, Greenstein, Johnson, and Friedman (1992) reviewed epidemiological studies of juvenile offender populations, and
reported estimates of youth with psychiatric
disorders (including conduct disorders) as
high as 90%. More recently, Teplin, Abram,
McClellan, Dulcan, and Mericle (2002), in a
6-month prevalence study of detainees at the
Cook County (IL) Juvenile Temporary Detention Center, found nearly two-thirds of
boys and three-quarters of girls met criteria
for one or more psychiatric disorders. Based
on the prevalence of such disorders among
the incarcerated juvenile population, the juvenile delinquency system may be characterized as a "default system," because it is
where many youths who can't read, write,
or relate tend to end up when they drop out
or are forced out of school (Nelson, 2000;
Wollard, Gross, Mulvey, & Reppucci, 1992).

RISK AND RESILIENCE

The evidence just cited raises several questions about the possibility of a causal relationship between personal characteristics

and risk for involvement in delinquent
behavior. The first is whether the presence of
a condition, such as a disability, is itself a
risk factor. The answer to this question fundamentally is "no." Multiple factors are associated with antisocial behavior, and there
is no simple way to gauge their impact
(Christle, Nelson, & Jolivette, 2002). Moreover, risk factors that exist in young persons'
lives must be balanced against the influence
of factors that contribute to the development of resilience. Investigators probing the
backgrounds of youths involved with the
juvenile delinquency system have found basically the same features that appear in the
lives of youths who experience poor educational and life outcomes in general (e.g.,
dropping out of school, unemployment,
poor marital adjustment, substance abuse).
Moreover, these risk factors extend across a
variety of demographic, psychological, educational, and psychiatric attributes (e.g., ethnic minority status, economic disadvantage,
educational disability, psychiatric disorder).
Therefore, the following discussion focuses
on risk and resilience with regard to deviant
behavior in general, irrespective of a particular condition or diagnosis. Fortunately, there
is a sizable body of research to inform a discussion of risk and resilience.

Risk

Risk factors are conditions or situations that
are empirically related to particular outcomes. Welch and Sheridan (1995) define an
"at-risk" child as "any child or youth who,
due to disabling, cultural, economic, or
medical conditions, is (a) denied or has minimum equal opportunities and resources in a
variety of settings and (b) is in jeopardy of
failing to become a successful and meaningful member of his or her community (i.e.,
home, school, and business)" (p. 31). Risk
factors often occur in combination, and the
complex relationship among risks at particular developmental stages can increase the
chances for deviant behavior (Furlong &
Morrison, 2000; Garfinkel, 1997; Hawkins
et al., 2000).

Risk factors are both internal (i.e., physical and psychological characteristics of the
individual), and external (i.e., factors present in the environment, such as family functioning, school experiences, and peer associ-

ations). Years of epidemiological research have shown that psychological characteristics, such as cognitive deficits, hyperactivity, concentration problems, restlessness, risk taking, aggressiveness, early involvement in antisocial behavior, and beliefs and attitudes favoring deviancy, have a strong and consistent relationship to violent behaviors in boys (Christle et al., 2002). Limited intelligence has been associated with poor problem-solving skills, poor social skills, and risk for aggression and violence (Calhoun, Glaser, & Bartolomucci, 2001). Delinquent youths consistently score approximately eight points lower on tests of general intelligence than the general population of youths, regardless of race, family size, or economic status (Flannery, 1997).

The overrepresentation of ethnic minority youths in juvenile justice population statistics raises the question of whether race is a risk factor for delinquency. As Leone, Mayer, Malmgren, and Meisel (2000) observe, such a conclusion greatly oversimplifies the relationship between ethnicity and risk. Throughout their school experience, students of color remain at a disadvantage. Minority students, especially African Americans, are more likely to be identified as having mental retardation and emotional disturbance and less likely to be identified for programs for the gifted and talented (National Research Council, 2002). African American students are two to three times as likely to be suspended or expelled as other students (Skiba, Michael, Nardo, & Peterson, 2000). As these disadvantages pile up, it is not surprising that students of color are more likely to drop out of school (Gregory, 1996) and eventually become part of the overrepresentation of individuals of color in the correctional system. However, Pope and Snyder (2003) recently analyzed juvenile arrest data reported in the Federal Bureau of Investigation's National Incident-Based Reporting System for evidence of racial bias in juvenile arrests for violent crimes. They found no direct evidence of such bias; in fact, 1997 and 1998 arrest data suggested that "once a violent crime is reported to or witnessed by police, the likelihood of arrest is greater for white juvenile offenders than for non-white juvenile offenders" (p. 6). Arguably, poverty is the single most common risk factor among youths who experi-

ence poor educational and life outcomes, including academic failure, dropping out of school, unemployment, marital instability, substance abuse, homelessness, and criminal behavior (Christle et al., 2002; Scott, Nelson, & Liaupsin, 2001). For example, studies of factors associated with school dropout suggest that students who are likely to leave school without graduating could be identified at the time of birth, based on social class and family characteristics (Patterson, Reid, & Dishion, 1992). A connection has been established between poverty and school dropout for both general (Rumberger, 1987) and special education students (Rylance, 1997). Students who drop out of school tend to have backgrounds that include poverty, parents who are less well educated, homes in which academic skills such as reading are neither valued nor modeled, and the presence of multiple family stressors (e.g., drugs and alcohol, divorce, abuse) (Druian & Butler, 2001; Patterson et al., 1992).

Among the many external risk factors, conditions in the home have been studied extensively. Parent criminality, harsh and ineffective parental discipline, lack of parental involvement, family conflict, child abuse and/or neglect, and rejection by parents have been found to predict early onset and chronic patterns of antisocial behavior in children and youths (McEvoy & Welker, 2000; Patterson, Forgatch, & Stoolmiller, 1998). Other familial risk factors include parental attitudes favorable to violence, poor family management practices, and high residential mobility (Hawkins et al., 2000). The family's influence on a child's behavior is powerful and stable as well as generational in scope.

The risk factors described above are nested. For example, variables associated with the construct of poverty (e.g., family stability and interactions, verbal modeling, failure of educators to understand the characteristics and needs of students from poverty) interact to affect children's behavior in school and their academic performance. More youths who are poor ethnic minorities, have a disability or mental health problem, and come from homes that are disrupted or destabilized are found in the juvenile delinquency system than their prevalence in the general population would predict. Yet, it would be inaccurate to claim that any of these factors is a direct cause of delinquency. The vast majority of youths with these psychological or demographic characteristics do not engage in delinquent behavior, nor do they enter the juvenile delinquency system. Other risk factors, appearing later in the developmental process, increase the vulnerability of these youths to antisocial behavior.

For example, the effects of early risk factors are likely to be compounded when children enter school. Children whose family demographics and dynamics place them at risk are more likely to begin school less ready than their more typical peers to meet the academic and social demands placed on them. In school, teachers typically serving these children are from middle- or upper-income backgrounds and use a vocabulary and assume a level of familiarity with print materials above that of many children from low-income homes (Scott et al., 2001). Furthermore, if students exhibit aggressive and noncompliant behavior patterns learned at home, the stage is set for aversive interactions between the school and parents. In general, parents of high-risk children have been found to be less involved in their child's education, to have lower expectations for achievement outcomes, and to have poor relationships with teachers (Wehby, Harnish, Valente, Dodge, & Conduct Problems Research Group, 2002). Because of their histories of aversive interactions with the school, parents of at-risk students may avoid involvement with school personnel on behalf of their children.

While the educational system would seem to be an antidote for poor or unstable home environments, unfortunately this often appears not to be the case. Researchers have identified a number of factors in the school that may contribute to antisocial behavior. Flannery (1997) cited a number of school risk factors, including high student–teacher ratios, insufficient curricular and course relevance, overcrowded classrooms, poor building design, portable classrooms, and weak or inconsistent adult leadership. An overreliance on physical security measures, such as metal detectors, locker searches, and surveillance cameras, actually appears to increase the risk of school disorder (Johnson, Boyden, & Pittz, 2001).

School disciplinary practices, especially those that remove students from the instructional setting (i.e., in- or out-of-school suspension and expulsion) may alienate students and contribute to their academic failure. For example, students who experience high rates of suspension miss substantial amounts of academic instruction (Scott et al., 2001). Again, certain minority groups and students with disabilities are overrepresented in statistics on exclusionary school disciplinary practices. Recent investigations have found consistent evidence of significant ethnic minority overrepresentation in statistics on office referrals (Nelson, Gonzalez, Epstein, & Benner, 2003), suspension (Costenbader & Markson, 1998), expulsion (Skiba et al., 2000), and corporal punishment (Gregory, 1996; Shaw & Braden, 1990). Based on data summarized from a number of states, Leone et al. (2000) reported that special education students typically represent a disproportionate percentage of those suspended from school. McFadden, Marsh, Price, and Hwang (1992) found that black male students with disabilities were punished more severely than others for commission of the same offense.

Factors outside the school that put youths at risk for antisocial behavior include high levels of neighborhood disorganization (crime, drug selling, gangs, and poor housing) (Calhoun et al., 2001). Communities with high resident turnover, a large proportion of disrupted or single-parent families, and few adults to supervise or monitor children also create conditions that foster the development of youth antisocial behavior (Flannery, 1997; Hawkins et al., 2000). Limited opportunities for recreation or employment, the availability of firearms, and violence in the neighborhood are other risk factors that have been identified in communities (Dobbin & Gatowski, 1996; Loeber & Farrington, 2000).

Early involvement in antisocial or violent activity is a stable and strong predictor of later violent behavior (Hawkins et al., 2000; Laub & Lauristen, 1998). Involvement with peers who exhibit high-risk and deviant behavior has proven to be one of the best predictors of delinquency (Farmer & Cadwallader, 2000). Adolescents who are unpopular with conventional peers, and thus rejected by them, may find acceptance only in antisocial or delinquent peer groups.

Children who associate with deviant peer groups appear to go through a process of deviancy training, in which their peers teach them deviant norms and values. Over time, these relationships become stronger and more reinforcing, and the antisocial patterns and beliefs become more resistant to change.

Thus, the risk factors associated with antisocial behavior are multifaceted, interrelated, and change over time. There is a constant and progressive interplay between internal and external risks (Hanson & Carta, 1995). The larger the number of risk factors to which a child is exposed, the greater is the likelihood that he or she will engage in antisocial behavior (Hawkins et al., 2000). However, the impact of risk factors changes depending on when they occur in a youth's development, in what context, and under what circumstances. Moreover, approximately two-thirds of youths who are exposed to multiple risk factors across life domains do not engage in antisocial behavior (Bernard, 1997). The variable that appears to account for this phenomenon is the existence of certain "protective factors." Protective factors buffer or modify the effects of risk factors in a positive direction, contributing to the development of personal resiliency (Luthar & Cicchetti, 2000).

Resilience

Resilience is a characteristic that allows a person to make appropriate behavioral choices in the presence of multiple risk factors. Resilience may explain why persons are able to resist substance abuse, mental health problems, and criminal behavior even though they may be exposed to significant stress and adversity (Spekman, 1993). Resilience develops through the influence of protective factors, which serve to counteract the influence of risk factors. As with risk factors, protective factors can be classified as internal (individual) or external (family, school, community, and peer relations).

Internal protective factors are personal attributes that help individuals overcome risks, and consist of physical and psychological characteristics. Physical characteristics include good health and personal hygiene. Psychological protective factors include a range of skills and abilities, such as accommodating to changes in school or work schedules, having effective and efficient communication skills, and a wide range of social skills (Dobbin & Gatowski, 1996).

Cognitive skills, particularly those involving written and oral language expression and comprehension, are powerful protective factors in a society that relies heavily on the transmission and processing of information (Davis, 1999). In a meta-analysis of studies, Maguin and Loeber (1996) found that increases in academic performance were associated with decreases in rates of delinquency. Other cognitive factors that appear to be strong protective factors against antisocial behavior involve emotional and moral development. Emotional skills that foster resilience include being in control of one's actions and reactions, delaying gratification, being proactive, setting goals, making decisions about what to do rather than just letting things happen, taking responsibility for one's decisions, and engaging others when needed (Davis, 1999; Spekman, 1993). Researchers have found that when children were taught such moral concepts as empathy, impulse control, and anger management, concomitant reductions were observed in aggressive behaviors (McMahon, Washburn, Felix, Yakin, & Childrey, 2000). In addition, children who were involved in service learning projects and activities that contributed to the well-being of others displayed fewer problematic behaviors than those who were not involved in such activities (Davis, 1999).

External protective factors may be found in the home, school, and community. Researchers have identified three themes involving external protective factors that are common to each of these domains: (1) caring relationships, (2) positive and high expectations, and (3) opportunities for meaningful participation (Davis, 1999). In the home, many protective factors can promote resilience. An attachment to at least one family member who engages in proactive, healthy interactions with the child constitutes an important caring relationship. Caregivers also contribute to the development of a child's resilience by setting rules in the home, showing respect for the child's individuality, and being responsive and accepting of the child's behavior (Hanson & Carta, 1995).

In the schools, educators can help students develop resilience by providing positive and safe learning environments, setting high, yet achievable, academic and social expectations, and facilitating academic and social success (Furlong & Morrison, 2000). Youths who belong to a positive school social group (e.g., academic club or social organization) also are less likely to demonstrate antisocial behavior (Catalano, Loeber, & McKinney, 1999). Teachers are the most frequently encountered positive role models outside the family, and a caring relationship between student and teacher may be a strong protective factor. Teachers who offer trustworthiness, sincere interest, individual attention, and who use rituals and traditions in the classroom often are the determining factor in opening a child's mind to learning (Bernard, 1997; Davis, 1999; Garmezy, 1993).

A report from the Center on Crime, Communities, and Culture (1997) indicated that quality educational interventions may constitute the most effective and economical protective factors against delinquency. Alternative educational programs that include individualized instruction, rewards for positive behavior, goal-oriented work, and small class sizes have been effective in reducing dropout rates in many communities (Tobin & Sprague, 2000).

At the community level, neighborhoods can provide a context where youths are exposed to positive influences (Wandersman & Nation, 1998). Communities offer a network of social structures and organizations that potentially can deter youths from engaging in antisocial behavior. For example, mentors can teach youths strategies for avoiding trouble and interacting positively with others (Van Acker & Wehby, 2000). Because youths who are employed are less likely to be arrested, career counseling and job training can promote resilience (Calhoun et al., 2001). Recreational opportunities, volunteer activities, and well-organized after-school programs are other initiatives that foster and support resilience. Youths are more likely to commit crimes during after-school hours than at any other time of day; thus, after-school programs can be an effective crime prevention strategy (National Research Council, 2000). It has been demonstrated that after-school programs reduce juvenile crime and drug use (Terzian, 1994).

EDUCATIONAL PROGRAMMING FOR YOUTHS IN THE JUVENILE DELINQUENCY SYSTEM

The primary focus of educators and other professionals engaged in promoting positive academic and social outcomes for children and youths should be on keeping them out of juvenile and criminal courts and correctional facilities. However, for a myriad of reasons, including the presence of risk factors discussed in the preceding section, some children and youths are placed in correctional facilities prior to or following a hearing or trial. For example, a recent report to Congress by the U.S. General Accounting Office (2003) indicated that child welfare directors in 19 states and juvenile justice officials in 30 counties estimated that in fiscal year 2001 parents placed over 12,700 children into these systems so that their children could receive mental health services. Incarcerated youths, like their peers who are not incarcerated, have the same needs and, with few exceptions, rights to education and other programs that are designed to promote their development (Leone & Meisel, 1997).

Until relatively recently, programs in many correctional facilities represented some of the most chaotic and troublesome settings in which education services are offered (Leone, 1994). Class-action litigation in a number of states highlighted inadequate services and supports for incarcerated youths, particularly those with disabilities (Leone & Meisel, 1997). The increased visibility of the Correctional Education Association (CEA), the development of new organizations such as the Council of Educators of At-Risk and Delinquent Youth (CEARDY), the joint funding by the U.S. Departments of Education and Justice of the National Center for Education, Disability, and Juvenile Justice (EDJJ), and a number of new federal initiatives designed to support evidence-based instruction and appropriate transition services for incarcerated youths suggest that the status of educational services in juvenile corrections is beginning to change.

As we noted at the beginning of this chapter, the majority of detained and committed youths have moderate to severe skill deficits and prior school experiences marked by failure, truancy, and exclusion (Foley, 2001). A few students—more often girls than boys—perform at or above grade level. Therefore, academic programs for incarcerated youths need to accommodate a wide range of abilities and provide them with the opportunity to earn credits that will transfer to other schools after leaving juvenile corrections. Programs also need to provide differentiated instruction for students in short- and long-term facilities, meet the special education needs of students with disabling conditions, and provide prevocational or vocational training. Finally, as part of transition support, programs need to prepare students for engagement in continuing education and the world of work (Todis, Bullis, Waintrup, Schultz, & D'Ambrosio, 2001).

While the average length of stay in juvenile correctional facilities is 8 months (Snyder & Sickmund, 1999), the range for individual youths is wide. Many youths are confined in jails, detention centers, and other short-term facilities, where lengths of stay may range from several days to several months. Effective education programs in short-term facilities should focus on literacy, life skills training, and initial assessment of the educational and vocational aptitudes and aspirations of youth. Because the range in academic proficiency of incarcerated students is quite broad, educators in detention centers and jails need to use a variety of materials and strategies to ensure that all youths have successful experiences in the classroom. Similarly, life skills training centered on topics such as alcohol and other drug use, sexually transmitted diseases, legal rights and responsibilities, and career exploration can provide content for stimulating presentations and discussions in a detention center classroom.

In contrast to programs in short-term facilities, education programs in training schools or long-term facilities need to offer a range of programs and options for youths that include basic literacy instruction, academic course offerings associated with earning Carnegie Units or comparable units of instruction, GED preparation and testing, and prevocational and vocational coursework (National Center on Education, Disability, and Juvenile Justice, 2003; Leone, Meisel, & Drakeford, 2002). For students with significant cognitive, behavioral, or learning problems, literacy and functional skills instruction may be the most appropriate focus of an individualized education program (IEP).

There is a dearth of research information on educational interventions for incarcerated youths (Coffey & Gemignani, 1994; Rutherford, Griller-Clark, & Anderson, 2001; Rutherford, Quinn, Leone, Garfinkel, & Nelson, 2002). Much of the literature that does exist is descriptive and documents academic performance or social skills of youths. The paucity of research information may be associated with the difficulty in conducting controlled studies in jails, detention centers, and other correctional settings. The mobility of youth and the differing mandates of security and program staff create conditions that are not conducive to empirical investigations. In their review of the literature on academic practices in correctional education programs, Coffey and Gemignani (1994) reported that instructional practices "have all too long reflected the 'old' model, with heavy emphasis on remediation, drill and practice in the basics, and individualized student workbook exercises. . . . Generally, teachers and other staff seem to have rather low expectations of these students" (p. 81).

One of the more comprehensive studies of correctional education programming was an evaluation of the Chapter 1 (now Title 1) Neglected or Delinquent (N & D) Program (LeBlanc & Ratnofsky, 1991; Tashjian, LeBlanc, & Pfannensteil, 1991). A descriptive study of the programs indicated that education was a more integral part of the operation of youth facilities than of adult facilities. Further, programming in juvenile facilities was geared more toward preparing youths to return to public schools, whereas adult facilities' programs were designed to prepare youths for employment. A 10-month longitudinal study that was part of the N & D Program Evaluation included interviews with youths and documented their enrollment in academic and vocational classes. The investigators found that, while more than 75% of youths indicated they planned to return to school following their release, only half of all youths actually returned to school. Not surprisingly, youths who were enrolled in school at the time of their incarceration were more likely to return to school and remain in school after their return to the community (LeBlanc & Ratnofsky, 1991). The researchers found that students enrolled in N & D programs while incarcerated dropped out of school following release at the same rate as those not receiving services.

The National Juvenile Detention Association, in conjunction with the Center for Research and Professional Development, studied current practices in education in detention centers across the United States (Brooks & Histed, 2002). Thirty-six percent of the 350 directors or supervisors of education in detention facilities responded to a request for information about their programs. The descriptive data show a wide range of administrative arrangements, course offerings, supports, and instructional practices in detention center education programs. The low response rate makes it difficult to offer definitive statements about the status of services.

Several investigations have examined the effect of structured instructional activities on the reading performance of youth. Drakeford (2001) studied the effects of an intensive program on the oral reading fluency and reading placement scores of a group of incarcerated youths with a history of special education services. All youths were 17 years old and were performing at or below the 25th percentile for their age on standardized reading assessments. Using single-subject methodology, Drakeford found that 6 weeks of one-on-one tutorial sessions using direct instruction produced marked increases in oral reading rates from baseline to intervention phase. Additionally, all students' Corrective Reading Placement Test scores increased from pre- to postassessment, and students expressed positive changes in their attitudes toward reading and literacy on the Rhody-Secondary Reading Attitude Assessment.

In a similar investigation, Malmgren and Leone (2000) examined the impact of an intensive 6-week program of direct instruction and oral reading activities on the reading performance of 45 incarcerated youths. They found that students demonstrated significant gains on three of four subtests of the Gray Oral Reading Test (GORT-3) from pre- to posttesting. Student gains on the Comprehension subtest of the GORT were in the expected direction but were not statistically significant.

The Center on Crime, Communities, and Culture (1997) reviewed studies and reports of the effects of education programs in juvenile and adult corrections on recidivism and re-arrest rates. While this study provides little detail about the components and structure of correctional education programs reviewed, lower rates of recidivism and arrest consistently were associated with higher levels of literacy, completion of formal programs of study, and attainment of certificates and diplomas.

Drakeford (2001) reviewed unpublished reports describing evaluation of education programs in correctional facilities. As was true with the review conducted by the Center on Crime, Communities, and Culture (1997), he found that attainment of milestones such as GED certificates, high school diplomas, and completion of vocational programs was associated with lower rates of recidivism.

The limited evidence that does exist suggests that educational gains for incarcerated youths are associated with structured and intensive learning activities. Enrollment in an education program, *ipso facto*, has not been shown to produce educational gains, although achieving specific milestones, such as diplomas and certificates of completion, has been associated with lower rates of offending and re-arrest (Center on Crime, Communities, and Culture, 1997).

Effective education programs for students with disabilities have been developed in juvenile corrections. The most significant barriers to appropriate services often are conceptual. When educators, parents, or advocates experience difficulty in providing or obtaining appropriate services for incarcerated youth, it frequently is because staff or administrators believe it cannot be done in a correctional setting. Youths with disabilities who do not receive appropriate special education and related services may be more vulnerable to disciplinary sanctions in correctional settings (Leone, 1994). If education programs in juvenile corrections fail to adequately educate youths with disabilities and fail to implement appropriate instructional strategies, the likelihood is greater that youths will continue to experience trouble in the community after release.

Some juvenile correctional facilities have limited capacity to support appropriate educational services. Limited capacity can include inadequate classroom space, either because facilities were originally built without classrooms or because of overcrowding. When students are forced to attend academic classes in dayrooms, dining halls, or visiting areas, the number of distractions and the lack of support for instruction seriously compromise the quality of the services provided. Other impediments to operation of correctional education programs are institutional emphasis on security and control over education and treatment, inadequate funding, lack of administrative support, isolation of correctional school programs, poorly developed links between institutional programs and public schools, and lack of transition and aftercare services. Quality education programs also require collaboration among school, security, and treatment programs within juvenile correctional facilities.

OUTCOMES FOR YOUTHS AFTER RETURNING TO THEIR COMMUNITIES

As youths leave short-term detention centers and jails or long-term juvenile and adult correctional facilities, they need support to make the transition to school, work, and community and to keep from reoffending and being reincarcerated. This need is particularly critical for youths with disabilities. However, transition services and supports generally are the most neglected component of correctional education programming (Stephens & Arnette, 2000). Most juveniles released from secure care facilities are placed on probation or parole, where the agencies responsible for this function provide supervision and monitoring of youths to prevent their reoffending and reincarceration. Probation and parole officers generally have large caseloads and limited resources to support effective transition. These limitations, as well as the fact that these young people return to environments where the same external risk factors (e.g., family functioning, school experiences, and peer associations) that preceded their incarceration are found, likely account for the high recidivism rates for youth in the juvenile delinquency system. Positive transition outcomes for youth with disabilities who have been in the adult system are even less frequent.

Recidivism

Recidivism or offender re-arrest, reconviction, resentencing, and return to corrections, is a common phenomenon among juveniles and adults in this country (Cottle, Lee, & Heilbrun, 2001). Langan and Levin (2002) reported that 67.5% of the prisoners released in the United States in 1994 were re-arrested and that 51.8% were back in prison, serving time for a new sentence or for a technical violation of their parole. Juvenile recidivism data are equally alarming. Johnston (2003) reported that 24% of youths released from the Arizona Department of Juvenile Corrections had returned to custody within 1 year of their release. The rate rose to 37% within 2 years and 43.1% within 3 years of their release. For purposes of his study, recidivism was defined as recommitment to the juvenile corrections system for a new crime, revocation of parole and recommitment to juvenile corrections, or commitment to the adult corrections system. These recidivism estimates were considered to be low because they did not account for youths who may have been incarcerated in other states or in county jails and detention centers following their release from juvenile corrections. Bullis and his colleagues (Bullis & Yovanoff, 2002, 2003; Bullis, Yovanoff, Mueller, & Havel, 2002; Todis et al., 2001) conducted a 5-year longitudinal study of resilience among 531 adolescents transitioning from youth correctional facilities back into their communities. They found that approximately 60% of their sample returned to the juvenile correctional system or entered the adult correctional system during the time of the study.

Recidivism data for youths with disabilities are even more disturbing. In a retrospective analysis of the success rates or failures of youths with disabilities who were released from the Arizona Department of Juvenile Corrections, Johnston (2003) found that 69% had reoffended or violated their parole and were reincarcerated within one year of their release. Bullis et al. (2002) reported that, compared to nondisabled youths, youths with a disability were 2.8 times more likely to return to juvenile corrections at 6 months postrelease and 1.8 times more likely to return at 1 year following their release.

The relatively poor postrelease outcomes for youths with disabilities in the justice system are compounded by the fact that a significant proportion of the incarcerated juvenile population has been identified as disabled. As noted at the beginning of this chapter, Quinn et al. (in press) reported that 34.4% of the youths in juvenile detention and state departments of corrections facilities were identified as having a disability. This figure reflects only those youth who have been identified as having educational disabilities and are receiving special education services. In correctional education programs, a sizable number of other students have disabilities that have not been identified or have disabilities that are not included under IDEA. Therefore, it is likely that 50% or more of youths leaving correctional programs in fact have disabilities that affect their transition back to their home communities. Because youths with special education needs have such poor transition outcomes following incarceration, a number of attempts have been made to analyze both the risk factors that lead to further involvement in the justice system (Cottle et al., 2001) and the resiliency factors that lead to postincarceration success (Johnston, 2003; Yellin, 1996).

Transition and Aftercare

Transition for youths with disabilities in the justice system refers to a coordinated set of activities that are designed to promote movement from school to postschool activities and success as an adult. The term also refers to the passage of a student from the community (i.e., home, school, or work) to a correctional setting and back to the community again. In addition, it can refer to the passage of a student from one correctional setting to another (Griller-Clark, Rutherford, & Quinn, 2004).

Todis et al. (2001) have proposed the construct of *engagement* to analyze the outcomes of youths with disabilities leaving correctional facilities. They defined "engagement" according to the following criteria: (1) engaged in school and/or work; (2) not detained or committed since release; and (3) not institutionalized for substance abuse or emotional problems since release. Bullis and Yovanoff (2002) focused their analysis on the engagement status of formerly incarcerated youths who did not reenter the juvenile or adult correctional systems. These researchers compared students with and without disabilities on a number of selected variables and found that youths with disabilities were more likely to have failed a grade while in school, to have been committed for a person-related crime, and to have been last adjudicated for a felony in an urban setting. They suggest, however, that these students are more alike than different. Both students with and without disabilities had relatively low rates of engagement in school and/or work activities upon return to the community (Bullis & Yovanoff, 2002, 2003). These findings indicate that services focusing on educational placement and securing appropriate competitive work should be provided to incarcerated youths immediately after their return to the community.

In his analysis of the engagement status of youths with disabilities, Johnston (2003) found that immediate engagement upon release increases the likelihood that youths with disabilities will not recidivate within the first year of their release. Again, while only 31.9% of the participants in his study were successfully engaged at the end of the 1-year study, practices that assured immediate engagement upon release were responsible for students' sustained engagement.

INTERVENTION RESEARCH
A Note on Effective Practice

Both reactive and proactive approaches have been used to address youths who exhibit antisocial and delinquent behavior. Reactive approaches consist of interventions that involve treatment of existing problems after the fact, while proactive strategies take into account potential risks and attempt to prevent problems from becoming manifest. A critical variable in evaluating approaches used to address youths' antisocial behavior is the presence or absence of empirical support.

Traditional strategies used to address antisocial and delinquent behavior have focused on treatment of existing problems and rehabilitation of the offending youth (Winett, 1998). In general, these strategies have been implemented after the fact and involve aversive sanctions (e.g., corporal punishment, suspension, expulsion, and incarceration). The results of these approaches have not been positive (Leone et al., 2000). In fact, based on recidivism rates for juvenile offenders, incarceration is spectacularly ineffective. For example, the Annie E. Casey Foundation recently reported that 54 and 73% of youths released from confinement in Minnesota and Washington, respectively, were convicted of a new offense within 3 years of their release (ADVOCASEY, 2003). Morris (1987) suggested that corrections can be viewed as the "A" phase in a B–A–B experimental design to demonstrate how well the natural environment establishes and maintains social deviance. Why this may be the case was demonstrated in a classic study by Buehler, Patterson, and Furniss (1966), who studied the contingencies of reinforcement in three institutional programs for delinquent girls. They found that the behaviors of the staff members and the incarcerated youths fostered and sustained antisocial patterns of behavior. On the one hand, the staff inconsistently punished antisocial behavior while consistently ignoring instances of desired (prosocial) behavior exhibited by the girls. Moreover, staff members tended to remain on the periphery of the group, which reduced their ability to supervise and respond appropriately to the girls' behavior. On the other hand, the peer group consistently punished prosocial behaviors and reinforced antisocial behaviors with equal regularity. The models of antisocial behavior provided by peers were made all the more potent by the lack of reliable staff intervention.

Of course, rehabilitation and treatment is only one goal of incarcerating juveniles (and, compared with punishment, retribution, and protection of society, it perhaps is a minor goal for many correctional programs and the public). Unfortunately, the prevalence of incarcerated youths with serious mental health problems indicates a substantial need for treatment services, which often are inadequate in such settings (U.S. General Accounting Office, 2003; Otto et al., 1992). Moreover, when youths are incarcerated in adult correctional programs, they are unlikely to be provided with *any* mental health services. Despite their popularity, "tough on crime" policies, such as making it easier to try juveniles as adults (enacted in 49 states and the District of Columbia), have had very disappointing results. Transferring youths to adult jails to protect the public may sound tough and righteous; yet, studies have shown that youth who spend time in adult jails are more likely to be re-arrested for increasingly serious crimes compared to youth in juvenile facilities (Mendel, 2000). Even in communities, most of the resources committed to addressing antisocial and delinquent behavior continue to be invested in untested programs (Flannery, 1997) that lack accountability for the expenditures of public funds (Kramer, 2000; Mendel, 2000; see also Quinn and Poirier, Chapter 5, this volume).

Much attention recently has been directed at the need for both preventative and treatment interventions that have been established as effective by empirical research. Variously termed as "evidence-based," "research-based," or "scientifically based" practices, the presumption is that prevention and intervention strategies and programs are supported by research that demonstrates their efficacy. The specific criteria used to define these terms so that programs can be held accountable are somewhat elusive. For example, the Federal No Child Left Behind (NCLB) Act contains liberal references to "scientifically based practices." However, nowhere does this legislation define what constitutes such practice or how to determine whether a practice qualifies.

In contrast, several agencies such as the Center for the Study and Prevention of Violence (CSPV; 2000), the American Federation of Teachers (AFT; 2000), the Office of the Surgeon General (Satcher, 2001), and the Safe, Disciplined, and Drug-Free Expert Panel (Weinheimer, 2001) have outlined strict scientific evaluation criteria for identifying programs and practices that effectively prevent the development of violent behavior and substance abuse among children and youth. Although the specific criteria employed by each of the agencies differ, they contain several common elements. These are (1) the use of a sound experimental or evaluation design and appropriate analytical procedures, (2) empirical validation of effects, (3) clear implementation procedures, (4) replication of outcomes across implementation sites, and (5) evidence of sustainability.

These agencies have identified effective violence prevention programs that meet their criteria. Christle et al. (2002) reviewed the programs that have been identified and found that eight met criteria for at least two of these agencies. These include Functional Family Therapy (FFT), Multidimensional Treatment Foster Care, Multisystemic Therapy (MST), Prenatal Home Visitation by Nurses, Life Skills Training (LST), the Midwestern Prevention Project (MPP), the Bullying Prevention Program, and the Promoting Alternative Thinking Strategies (PATHS) program.

We would like to observe that policymakers, program developers, and the public unanimously insist that only programs and practices having demonstrated effectiveness, such as those cited above, be eligible for federal, state, and local governmental support. Regrettably, many current strategies lack evaluation research, and some strategies continue to be used even though they have proven to be ineffective (Nelson, 1997). Without empirical evidence, it is impossible to determine which programs have had significant positive effects. This lack of accountability, along with practitioners' failure to conduct systematic evaluations or to attend to empirical results, often have led policymakers to advocate for practices that are fashionable even when research studies offer evidence that they are ineffective. For example, juvenile correctional boot camps, based on the popular notion that delinquent youths need a strong dose of discipline, continue to operate in several states despite studies showing that graduates' recidivism rates are as high or higher than for youths placed in other correctional programs (Office of Juvenile Justice and Delinquency Prevention, 1996; Satcher, 2001). Prison-based education and literacy programs have been shown to be more effective than boot camps in reducing the recidivism rate of incarcerated youths (Center on Crime, Communities, and Culture, 1997).

In the following sections, we offer a tentative list of "best" or "promising" practices, based on direct research with at-risk or delinquent youths, empirical evidence from research with similar populations (e.g., students with emotional and behavioral disabilities), or a consensus of opinion by experts in the field. Due to the lack of suffi-

cient replicated studies in some areas with incarcerated juvenile populations (e.g., correctional programming, transition and aftercare), it sometimes is necessary to extrapolate from research findings with more heavily studied populations (e.g., youth with disabilities leaving public secondary education programs).

Recommended Prevention Practices

The CSPV, AFT, Office of the Surgeon General, and the Safe, Disciplined, and Drug-Free Expert Panel each have identified approaches that meet their criteria as effective practices. Although the focus of these initiatives has not been on delinquency prevention, it is reasonable to assume that efforts to prevent violence and substance abuse are close parallels. For example, while the CSPV focuses on the prevention of violence, several of the 11 programs that met their standards for a "blueprint" (e.g., Multisystemic Therapy, Functional Family Therapy, Life Skills Training, Big Brothers Big Sisters of America, and Promoting Alternative Thinking Strategies) are used with youths identified as delinquent or at risk for delinquency. In addition to the programs just cited, the 11 programs identified by CSVP as Blueprints include Multidimensional Treatment Foster Care, Prenatal Home Visitation by Nurses, the Midwestern Prevention Project (MPP), the Bullying Prevention Program, the Quantum Opportunities Program (QOP), and The Incredible Years Series.

Sherman (2003) conducted a comprehensive review of family-based crime prevention programs. He identified long-term frequent home visitation combined with preschool and family therapy by clinical staff as effective strategies for preventing delinquency. One of the best-known studies documenting the effects of early intervention on later criminal behavior is the longitudinal study comparing outcomes of at-risk children who participated in the Perry Preschool Program with those who did not (Berreauta-Clement, Schweinhart, Barnett, Epstein, & Weikart, 1985). The program included daily participation in a structured preschool curriculum with weekly home visits by teachers for a period of 30 weeks per year over a 2- to 3-year period. At age 19, youths who had participated in the experimental group had experienced a significantly lower arrest rate (7%) than those who were in the control group (31%). Lally, Mangione, and Honig (1988) conducted a longitudinal evaluation of the effects of weekly home visits over a 5-year period by teachers to high-risk preschool children and their mothers and reported similar findings: by the time the children reached the age of 15, 6% of youths in the experimental group had been arrested versus 22% of those in the control group.

Based on the combination of "bad demographics" associated with later undesirable outcomes for youths (e.g., families in poverty, single-parent homes, lack of exposure to good behavioral and educational models, high-crime neighborhoods, unavailability of community health and human services), children who are at risk for developing patterns of antisocial and delinquent behavior can be identified at a very young age—probably even before they are born. Furthermore, interventions that address the deleterious effects of these factors, especially when applied early, help children develop resilience. Long-term studies of the effects of early intervention programs, such as those just cited, are costly and therefore not common. However, it is clear from available research that efforts to improve parental skills and children's educational performance are effective deterrents to delinquency.

Recommended Practices in Juvenile Corrections Programs

Incarcerated youths need the stimulation and intellectual challenges that a well-developed education program can offer. Juveniles in correctional settings are entitled to educational services similar in quantity and quality to those available in communities (Rutherford et al., 2002). Students with disabilities are entitled to a free appropriate public education, including special education and related services. Irrespective of their classification or where they are housed within the detention or correctional setting, students who have not graduated from high school or who have not obtained a GED certificate are entitled to services that satisfy state requirements for completion of middle school or high school.

The research that does exist on academic programming in institutional settings suggests that intensive, highly structured instruction, particularly in reading, can promote dramatic gains in academic performance in a relatively short period of time. However, ensuring that students receive appropriate services requires that adequate administrative supports and procedures be in place. Records from previous schools or detention centers should be obtained within 2 weeks of students' admission to the facility. Upon release, students' records should be transferred within 2 weeks from the time they leave the correctional education program to the first public or private school or training program in which they enroll.

Appropriate programming requires sufficient numbers of qualified personnel to provide education and related services to all students. Those students in need of special education and related services should be identified, located, and evaluated within timelines prescribed by law and regulations. For students who previously have not been identified for special or compensatory education services but who struggle in the classroom, careful observation and implementation of academic supports and strategies are essential. As appropriate, staff people trained in screening, referral, and identification of students with disabilities are essential.

Students identified as being potentially disabled should receive a full and complete assessment by an appropriate evaluation team that includes specialists in the areas of the student's suspected disabilities. Procedures and a timeline for implementing IEPs are critical, especially given the difficulty of ensuring parental participation in the process. A proposed assessment plan should be forwarded to the student's parent, guardian, or surrogate parent within 15 days of referral to special education; IEP meetings should be held within 30 days of entry to the correctional education program; and IEPs should be developed or amended for students with previously identified disabilities in the correctional education program. Students with disabilities must be provided with classroom instruction in the amount and type specified in their IEPs. Sufficient and appropriate educational resources should be available to deliver special education services to accomplish each student's IEP goals. Goals and short-term objectives must be reviewed regularly by school staff to determine whether they are being met, whether specified services are being provided, and whether modifications are necessary. For all students who do not have a parent, surrogate parents (who are not employees of the correctional facility or of any agency providing services to the student) should be recruited, trained, and appointed to represent them at IEP meetings or to assist them in educational planning.

Recommended Transition Practices

Rutherford et al. (2002) have proposed transition practices for both short-term detention and long-term correctional programs. Transition experiences and outcomes for youths with disabilities often are disheartening. Obstacles that interfere with the provision of effective transition services in the juvenile delinquency system include lack of transition planning before release, inadequate professional development and specialized transition training for service providers, a significant lack of communication, coordination, and commitment among agencies that serve at-risk and delinquent youths, delays in transition planning in short-term and long-term correctional facilities due to difficulty in obtaining previous educational records, and lack of family involvement—one of the greatest challenges to the success of transition.

On the other hand, a number of practices have been proposed for overcoming barriers to effective transition from both short- and long-term correctional facilities (Coffey & Gemignani, 1994; Griller-Clark, Rutherford, Mathur, & McGlynn, 2001; Rutherford et al., 2002). Among the most important of these practices (especially for students with disabilities) are the immediate transfer of the youth's educational records from community schools to jails and detention centers to long-term correctional facilities and back to community schools, and a process for the immediate identification, evaluation, and placement of youths with disabilities. In addition, existing IEPs that include an individualized transition plan should be modified and implemented. Individualized preplacement transition planning and coordination with probation and parole officers to ensure

a continuum of services, care, and monitoring in the community also are essential steps for overcoming transition barriers and the dismal outcomes reported in the literature. Finally, a community-based transition system for maintaining youth placement and support after release from corrections can assist youths leaving secure facilities. Although research documenting effective transition practices for incarcerated youths is sparse, studies of variables associated with successful postschool outcomes of youths with disabilities from public education programs indicate that students who matriculate from an educational program, who participated in structured vocational and educational programs while in school, who left school with better academic skills, who gained work experience while in school, who have the social and employment skills needed to be successful in the workplace, and whose IEPs contained explicit transition plans experienced better outcomes (Carter & Wehby, 2003; deFur, 2003; Eisenman, 2003; Rylance, 1997). Furthermore, careful assessment of both youths' skills and the requirements of transition settings to establish an effective match consistently have been identified as best practices in transition programming (Neubert, 2003). These practices should be replicated in returning youths to communities from detention or corrections programs.

Youths in the juvenile delinquency system making the transition back to school and community often still are affected by the social and personal influences that contributed to the conduct that placed them in the justice system in the first place. Stephens and Arnette (2000) point out that many risk factors, such as "delinquent peer groups, poor academic performance, high crime neighborhoods, weak family attachments, lack of consistent discipline, and physical or sexual abuse" (p. 2), continue to exist following incarceration. In addition, these youths often return to school and the community with a variety of special service needs, including individual counseling, drug rehabilitation, and family counseling. Thus, structured supports, such as vocational training, adult mentor programs, and access to educational, health, and mental health services are critical to their successful adjustment.

As is true of prevention and services within correctional programs, the most effective transition or aftercare services for youths returning from secure care involve fostering resilience through developing and reinforcing internal and external protective factors, which serve to counteract the influence of risk factors (Armstrong, Dedrick, & Greenbaum, 2003). As noted earlier in this chapter, youths in correctional facilities and in transition must be exposed to such external protective factors as (1) caring and supportive adult relationships, (2) positive and high expectations for social, academic, and vocational behavior, and (3) opportunities for meaningful engagement in school, work, and the community (Davis, 1999).

CONCLUSIONS

As we hope this review has demonstrated, a great deal is known about delinquents and delinquency: their characteristics, demographics, risk factors, and which approaches to prevention and intervention seem to work better than others. Unfortunately, it appears that little of this knowledge has come to the attention of policymakers, or, if it has, it has failed to make a sufficient impression to influence public policy. Schiraldi (2000) pointed out that the makers of such policy get their information from the news media, not from the research literature. Perhaps the research community should examine its traditional dissemination practices (exclusive reliance on professional conferences and journals) and also consider an aggressive social marketing campaign that informs lawmakers and the public of certain realities, to wit:

• The present focus on "corrections" is misplaced. More often than not, it doesn't correct criminal behavior, and it is horribly expensive. In addition to the staggering expense of incarceration, taxpayers must shoulder the financial burden incurred by an underclass of citizens who lack the skills needed to be contributing members of society. While society needs protection from some offenders (e.g., those who are a danger to others, those who persistently engage in crimes against persons and property), scores of incarcerated persons (especially juveniles)

are not appropriately placed in correctional settings (see below).

• Many incarcerated youths have serious and complex problems (histories of physical abuse and neglect, homelessness, disabilities, mental health needs). The juvenile delinquency system is not equipped to address these needs. Again, when these youths return to their communities following incarceration, they overwhelm local human service resources.

• Programs and services should be proactive and forward-looking. Professionals and policymakers should work together to build networks of effective community services that include families, schools, afterschool programs, and vocational training, in addition to programs that address mental health, substance abuse, health, and welfare needs. Community services should focus on both prevention and aftercare, and funds currently being used to build more prisons should be diverted to support these efforts. Given the serious academic and social deficits displayed by youths in correctional settings, the term "rehabilitation," used to characterize programming, should be replaced with the term "habilitation," as the former implies restoration to a previously intact state, whereas habilitation more aptly suggests a focus on skills not yet mastered.

The research community can support this campaign by building the base of understanding regarding effective prevention, treatment, and aftercare practices. One place to focus these efforts is on conducting better assessments of the natural environments of antisocial and at-risk youths to improve prevention and intervention (including transition and aftercare) at the community level. The behavioral analyses of high-crime communities conducted by Stumphauser and his colleagues in the 1970s (Aiken, Stumphauzer, & Veloz, 1977; Stumphauser, Aiken, & Veloz, 1977) is a research model worth repeating. They demonstrated that the natural environment, including law enforcement practices, community attitudes and behaviors, and the absence of meaningful recreational and vocational opportunities broadly supported delinquent behavior. The explication of differential reinforcement contingencies that support antisocial behavior, in conjunction with Buehler et al.'s

(1966) documentation of reinforcement contingencies in juvenile correctional settings, strongly indicate that what has been done is ineffective and counterproductive. Contemporary researchers should replicate these studies. If similar results are obtained, program managers and policymakers must seriously consider better ways of doing business. Examination of the communities in which at-risk and delinquent youth are found, and to which incarcerated youths will return, could lead to more effective community programming to support the prevention of delinquency, as well as better programming inside the fence. Transition should drive programming at all three levels, and should begin with the question, What will youth need (in terms of skills and resources) to be productive or crime-free?

• The evidence supporting the importance of education in crime prevention needs to be highlighted and expanded. The Office of Special Education Program's funding of reading and behavior centers underscores policymakers' understanding that academic proficiency and behavioral performance are linked. The No Child Left Behind Act (2002) is a bold declaration of intention to increase the literacy of America's children. Professionals must work to ensure that the educational system doesn't leave any child behind because his or her behavior is challenging or disagreeable. The special education community can contribute to the improvement of NCLB by demonstrating the benefits of shifting emphasis from high-stakes accountability to individualized instruction.

Fortunately, efforts are under way in the federal government to identify effective practices and to disseminate information about these to professionals and parents. The U.S. Department of Education's Institute of Education Sciences has established the What Works Clearinghouse (*www.w-wc.org*). This clearinghouse is responsible for developing and updating Evidence Reports on topics nominated from the field. To be listed within a topic area, an intervention must be a replicable documented practice, product, or policy that is intended to have a beneficial impact on important student outcomes. Seven topics have been identified for year 1 (2003–2004): Interventions for Beginning Reading; Curriculum-Based Interventions for Increasing K–12 Math Achievement; Programs for Preventing High School Dropout; Programs for Increasing Adult Literacy; Peer-Assisted Learning in Elementary Schools: Reading, Mathematics, and Science Gains; Interventions for Elementary School English Language Learners: Increasing English Language Acquisition and Academic Achievement; and Interventions to Reduce Delinquent, Disorderly, and Violent Behavior in Middle and High Schools (Birman, 2003). In addition to a focus on literacy from the early school years into adulthood, the inclusion of the last topic, as well as preventing high school dropout rates, reflects the government's interest in addressing issues involving antisocial and delinquent behavior.

• Finally, researchers and policymakers should be cautious about which outcomes to use in evaluating the effectiveness of interventions for delinquency. Rates of reported juvenile crime, arrest, adjudication, and recidivism are convenient metrics; however, each has its weaknesses. The first two have been shown to significantly underestimate the actual rates of offending (Gehring, 2000). Similarly, adjudication is a measure of decisions made by juvenile courts, not of the behavior of juveniles. And, as Gehring (2000) points out, although recidivism is widely used as a gauge of the success of juvenile justice programs, it has numerous flaws, including lack of agreement on the definition, forcing data into a yes/no dichotomy, and the fact that it also reflects a set of decisions made by adults rather than being a clear measure of correctional success. Gehring concludes that "Until the 'get tough on crime' sentiment evolves into a 'get smart on crime' agenda, decision makers should be cautious about recidivism as a measure of . . . program success" (p. 204). Hopefully, future research on delinquency will contribute to the emergence of this agenda.

ACKNOWLEDGMENTS

Christine A. Christle and Kristine Jolivette, colleges of C. Michael Nelson at the University of Kentucky, contributed substantially to portions of this chapter.

REFERENCES

Aiken, T. W., Stumphauzer, J. S., & Veloz, E. V. (1977). Behavioral analysis of nondelinquent brothers in a high juvenile crime community. *Behavioral Disorders, 2,* 212–222.

ADVOCASEY Briefing. (2003, Spring). A matter: Forks in the road for juvenile justice. *ADVOCASEY, 5*(1). Retrieved May 20, 2003, from *http://www.aecf.org/publications/advocasey/spring2003/.*

American Federation of Teachers. (2000). *Building on the best, learning from what works: Five promising discipline and violence prevention programs.* Washington, DC: Author.

Armstrong, K. H., Dedrick, R. F., & Greenbaum, P. E. (2003). Factors associated with community adjustment of young adult with serious emotional disturbance: A longitudinal analysis. *Journal of Emotional and Behavioral Disorders, 11,* 66–76, 91.

Bernard, B. (1997). *Turning it around for all youth: From risk to resilience* (ERIC Document Reproduction Service No. ED 412 309).

Berreauta-Clement, J. R., Schweinhart, L. J., Barnett, W. S., Epstein, A. S., & Weikart, D. P. (1985). *Changed lives: The effects of the Perry Preschool Program on youths through age 19.* Ypsilanti, MI: High Scope Press.

Birman, B. (2003, July). *What works?* Plenary session, 2003. Office of Special Education Programs Research Project Directors' Conference, Washington, DC.

Brooks, C. C., & Histed, A.T. (2002). *The status of detention education programs.* East Lansing, MI: Center for Research and Professional Development, School of Criminal Justice, Michigan State University.

Buehler, R. E., Patterson, G. R., & Furniss, J. M. (1966). The reinforcement of behavior in institutional settings. *Behavior Research and Therapy, 4,* 157–167.

Bullis, M., & Yovanoff, P. (2002). Those who do not return: Correlates of the work and school engagement of formerly incarcerated youth who remain in the community. *Journal of Emotional and Behavioral Disorders, 10,* 68–78.

Bullis, M., & Yovanoff, P. (2003). Who are those guys? Examination of the demographic characteristics of incarcerated adolescents with and without disabilities. Eugene, OR: University of Oregon, Institute on Violence and Destructive Behavior.

Bullis, M., Yovanoff, P., Mueller, G., & Havel, E. (2002). Life on the "outs"—examination of the facility-to-community transition of incarcerated youth. *Exceptional Children, 69,* 7–22.

Calhoun, G. B., Glaser, B. A., & Bartolomucci, C. L. (2001). The juvenile counseling and assessment model and program: A conceptualization and intervention for juvenile delinquency. *Journal of Counseling and Development, 79,* 131–141.

Carter, E. W., & Wehby, J. H. (2003). Job performance of transition-age youth with emotional and behavioral disorders. *Exceptional Children, 69,* 449–465.

Catalano, R. F., Loeber, R., & McKinney, K. C. (1999). School and community interventions to prevent serious and violent offending. *Juvenile Justice Bulletin,* 1–12.

Center on Crime, Communities, and Culture. (1997). Education as crime prevention: Providing education to prisoners. *Research Brief* (Occasional Paper Series, No. 2). New York: Author.

Center for the Study and Prevention of Violence. (2000). Blueprints for violence prevention. Retrieved October 28, 2001, from University of Colorado at Boulder, Institute of Behavioral Science website: *http://www.colorado.EDU/cspv/.*

Christle, C. A., Nelson, C. M., & Jolivette, K. (2002). *Prevention of antisocial and violent behavior in youth: A review of the literature.* Retrieved July 15, 2002, from *http://www.edjj.org.*

Coffey, O. D., & Gemignani, R. M. (1994). *Effective practices in juvenile correctional education: A study of the literature and research 1980–1992.* Washington, DC: National Office for Social Responsibility.

Costenbader, V., & Markson, S. (1998). School suspension: A study with secondary school students. *Journal of School Psychology, 36,* 59–82.

Cottle, C. C., Lee, R. J., & Heilbrun, K. (2001). The prediction of criminal recidivism in juveniles: A meta-analysis. *Criminal Justice and Behavior, 28,* 367–394.

Davis, N. J. (1999). *Resilience: Status of the research and research-based programs.* Retrieved July 21, 2001, from *http://www.mentalhealth.org/school violence/5-28resilience.asp.*

deFur, S. H. (2003). IEP transition planning—from compliance to quality. *Exceptionality, 11,* 115–128.

Dobbin, S. A., & Gatowski, S. I. (1996). *Juvenile violence: A guide to research.* Reno, NV: National Council of Juvenile and Family Court Judges.

Drakeford, W. (2001). *The impact of an intensive program to increase the literacy skills of youth confined in juvenile corrections.* Unpublished doctoral dissertation, University of Maryland, College Park.

Druian, G., & Butler, J. A. (2001, June). Topical synthesis #1: Effective schooling practices and at-risk youth: What the research shows. Northwest Regional Educational Laboratory. Retrieved July 5, 2003, from *http://www.nwrel.org/scpd/sirs/1/topsyn1.html.*

Eisenman, L. T. (2003). Theories in practice: School-to-work transitions for youth with mild disabilities. *Exceptionality, 11,* 89–102.

Farmer, T. W., & Cadwallader, T. W. (2000). Social interactions and peer support for problem behavior. *Preventing School Failure, 44,* 105–109.

Flannery, D. J. (1997). *School violence: Risk, prevention, intervention, and policy* (Report No. RR93002016). Retrieved September 27, 2002, from *http://eric-web.tc.columbia.edu/monographs/uds109.*

Foley, R. M. (2001). Academic characteristics of incarcerated youth and correctional educational programs: A literature review. *Journal of Emotional and Behavioral Disorders, 9*, 248–259.

Furlong, M. J., & Morrison, G. M. (2000). The school in school violence. *Journal of Emotional and Behavioral Disorders, 8*, 71–82.

Galagher, C. A. (1999, March). Juvenile offenders in residential placement, 1997. *OJJDP Fact Sheet.* (Available from the U.S. Department of Justice, Office of Juvenile Justice and Delinquency Prevention, Washington, DC 20531).

Garfinkel, L. (1997). Youth with disabilities in the justice system: Integrating disability specific approaches. *Focal Point, 11*(1), 21–23.

Garmezy, N. (1993). Children in poverty: Resilience despite risk. *Psychiatry, 56*, 127–136.

Gerhing, T. (2000). Recidivism as a measure of correctional education program success. *Journal of Correctional Education, 51*, 197–205.

Gregory, J. F. (1996). The crime of punishment: Racial and gender disparities in the use of corporal punishment in the U.S. public schools. *Journal of Negro Education, 64*, 454–462.

Griller-Clark, H., Rutherford, R. B., Mathur, S. R., & McGlynn, M. (2001). Transition strategies for preventing recidivism of youth in the juvenile justice system. 56th Annual Correctional Education Association Conference, Scottsdale, Arizona.

Griller-Clark, H., Rutherford, R. B., & Quinn, M. M. (2004). Practices in transition for youth in the juvenile justice system. In D. Cheney (Ed.), *Transition of students with emotional or behavioral disabilities from school to community: Current approaches for positive outcomes,* (pp. 247–262). Arlington, VA: Division for Career Development and Transition/ Council for Children with Behavioral Disorders.

Hanson, M. J., & Carta, J. J. (1995). Addressing the challenges of families with multiple risks. *Exceptional Children, 62*, 201–212.

Hawkins, J. D., Herrenkohl, T. I., Farrington, D. P., Brewer, D., Catalano, R. F., Harachi, T. W., & Cothern, L. (2000). *Predictors of youth violence* (pp. 1–11). Washington, DC: Juvenile Justice Bulletin, Office of Juvenile Justice and Delinquency Prevention.

Johnson, T., Boyden, J. E., & Pittz, W. J. (Eds.). (2001). *Racial profiling and punishment in U.S. public schools: How zero tolerance policies and high stakes testing subvert academic excellence and racial equity.* Oakland, CA: Applied Research Center.

Johnston, J. W. (2003). *In the arena: Youth in transition from juvenile corrections to the community.* Unpublished doctoral dissertation. Arizona State University.

Kramer, R. C. (2000). Poverty, inequality, and youth violence. *Annals of the American Academy of Political and Social Science, 567*, 123–140.

Lally, J. R., Mangione, P. L., & Honig, A. S. (1988). The Syracuse Family Development Research Project: Long-range impact of an early intervention with low-income children and their families. In D. R. Powell (Ed.), *Annual advances in applied developmental psychology*: Vol. 3. *Parent education as early childhood intervention: Emerging directions in theory, research, and practice.* Norwood, NJ: Ablex. Retrieved June 2, 2003 from *http://www.ncjrs.org/works/.*

Langan, P. A., & Levin, D. J. (2002). *Recidivism of prisoners released in 1994.* Washington DC: Bureau of Justice Statistics, U.S. Department of Justice.

Laub, J. H., & Lauristen, J. L. (1998). The interdependence of school violence with neighborhood and family conditions. In D. S. Elliot, B. Hamburg, & K. R. Williams (Eds.), *Violence in American schools: A new perspective* (pp. 127–155). New York: Cambridge University Press.

LeBlanc, L.A., & Ratnofsky, A. (1991). Longitudinal study findings: National study of the ECIA Chapter 1 Neglected or Delinquent Program. *Unlocking learning: Chapter 1 in correctional facilities* (Contract No. 300-87-0124). Rockville, MD: Westat.

Leone, P. E. (1994). Education services for youth with disabilities in a state-operated juvenile correctional system: Case study and analysis. *Journal of Special Education, 28*, 43–58.

Leone, P. E., Mayer, M. J., Malmgren, K., & Meisel, S. M. (2000). School violence and disruption: Rhetoric, reality, and reasonable balance. *Focus on Exceptional Children, 33*(1), 1–20.

Leone, P. E., & Meisel, S. M. (1997). Improving education services for students in detention and confinement facilities. *Children's Legal Rights Journal, 17*, 1–12.

Leone, P. E., Meisel, S. M., & Drakeford, W. (2002). Special education programs for youth with disabilities in juvenile corrections. *The Journal of Correctional Education, 53*(2), 46–50.

Loeber, R., & Farrington, D. P. (2000). Young children who commit crime: Epidemiology, developmental origins, risk factors, early interventions, and policy implications. *Development and Psychopathology, 12*, 737–762.

Luthar, S. S., & Cicchetti, D. (2000). The construct of resilience: Implications for interventions and social policies. *Development and Psychopathology, 12*, 857–885.

Maguin, E., & Loeber, R. (1996). Academic performance and delinquency. In M. Tonry (Ed.), *Crime and justice: A review of research* (pp. 145–264). Chicago: University of Chicago Press.

Malmgren, K., & Leone, P. E. (2000) Effects of a short-term auxiliary reading program on the reading skills of incarcerated youth. *Education and Treatment of Children, 23*, 239–247.

McEvoy, A., & Welker, R. (2000). Antisocial behavior, academic failure, and school climate: A critical review. *Journal of Emotional and Behavioral Disorders, 8*, 130–140.

McFadden, A. C., Marsh, G. E., Price, B. J., & Hwang,

Y. (1992). A study of race and gender bias in the punishment of handicapped school children. *Urban Review, 24,* 239–251.

McMahon, M., Washburn, J., Felix, E. D., Yakin, J., & Childrey, G. (2000). Violence prevention: Program effects on urban preschool and kindergarten children. *Applied and Preventive Psychology, 9,* 271–281.

Mendel, R. A. (2000). *Less hype, more help: Reducing juvenile crime, what works—and what doesn't.* Washington, DC: American Youth Policy Forum.

Moffitt, T. E. (1990). Juvenile delinquency and attention deficit disorder: Boys' developmental trajectories from age 3 to age 15. *Child Development, 61,* 893–910.

Morris, E. K. (1987). Introductory comments: Applied behavior analysis in crime and delinquency: Focus on prevention. *The Behavior Analyst, 10*(1), 67–68.

National Center on Education, Disability, and Juvenile Justice. (2003). Unpublished class action litigation data involving youth with disabilities in juvenile and adult corrections. Available from *www.edjj.org.*

National Research Council. (2000). After-school programs to promote child and adolescent development: Summary of a workshop. In J. A. Gootman (Ed.), *Board on Children, Youth, and Families, Commission on Behavioral and Social Sciences and Education.* Washington, DC: National Academy Press.

National Research Council. (2002). Minority students in special and gifted education. In M. S. Donovan & C. T. Cross (Eds.), *Committee on Minority Representation in Special Education.* Washington, DC: National Academy Press.

Nelson, C. M. (1997). Aggressive and violent behavior: A personal perspective. *Education and Treatment of Children, 20,* 250–262.

Nelson, C. M. (2000). Educating students with emotional and behavioral disorders in the 21st century: Looking through windows, opening doors. *Education and Treatment of Children, 23,* 204–222.

Nelson, J. R., Gonzalez, J. E., Epstein, M. H., & Benner, G. J. (2003). Administrative discipline contacts: A review of the literature. *Behavioral Disorders, 28,* 249–281.

Neubert, D. A. (2003). The role of assessment in the transition to adult life process for students with disabilities. *Exceptionality, 11,* 63–75.

No Child Left Behind Act. (2002). Introduction: No Child Left Behind Act. Retrieved May 10, 2003, from *http://www.nochildleftbehind.gov/next/over view/index/html.*

Office of Juvenile Justice and Delinquency Prevention. (1996). *Juvenile boot camps: Lesson learned: Fact Sheet No. 36.* Washington, DC: U.S. Department of Justice.

Otto, R. K., Greenstein, J. J., Johnson, M. K., & Friedman, R. M. (1992). Prevalence of mental disorders among youth in the juvenile justice system. In J. J. Ccocozza (Ed.), *Responding to the mental health needs of youth in the juvenile justice system* (pp. 7–

48). Seattle, WA: National Coalition for the Mentally Ill in the Criminal Justice System.

Patterson, G. R., Forgatch, K. L., & Stoolmiller, M. (1998). Variables that initiate and maintain an early-onset trajectory for juvenile offending. *Development and Psychopathology, 10,* 531–547.

Patterson, G. R., Reid, J. B., & Dishion, T. J. (1992). *Antisocial boys:* Vol. 4. *A social interactional approach.* Eugene, OR: Castalia.

Pope, C. E., & Snyder, H. N. (2003, April). Race as a factor in juvenile arrests. *Juvenile Justice Bulletin.* Retrieved July 5, 2003, from *http://ojjdp.ncjrs.org.*

Quinn, M. M., Rutherford, R. B., Leone, P. E., Osher, D., & Poirier, J. M. (in press). Students with disabilities in detention and correctional settings. *Exceptional Children.*

Rumberger, R. W. (1987). High school dropouts: A review of issues and evidence. *Review of Educational Research, 57,* 101–121.

Rutherford, R. B., Griller-Clark, H., & Anderson, C. W. (2001). Treating offenders with educational disabilities. In J. B. Ashford, B. D. Sales, & W. H. Reid (Eds.), *Treating adult and juvenile offenders with special needs* (pp. 221–245). Washington, DC: American Psychological Association.

Rutherford, R. B., Quinn, M. M., Leone, P. E., Garfinkel, L., & Nelson, C. M. (2002). *Education, disability, and juvenile justice: Recommended practices.* Arlington, VA: Council for Children with Behavioral Disorders.

Rylance, B. J. (1997). Predictors of high school graduation or dropping out for youths with severe emotional disturbances. *Behavioral Disorders, 23,* 5–17.

Satcher, D. (2001). *Youth violence: A report of the Surgeon General.* Department of Health and Human Services. Retrieved October 3, 2001, from *http://surgeongeneral.gov/library/youthviolence/report.html.*

Schiraldi, V. (2000). *How distorted coverage of juvenile crime affects public policy* [Keynote address]. National Center for Education, Disability, and Juvenile Justice Loren M. Warboys Regional Forum. Retrieved February 15, 2001, from *http://www.edjj.org/schirladikeynote.html.*

Scott, T. M., Nelson, C. M., & Liaupsin, C. J. (2001). Effective instruction: The forgotten component in preventing school violence. *Education and Treatment of Children, 24,* 309–322.

Shaw, S. R., & Braden, J. P. (1990). Race and gender bias in the administration of corporal punishment. *School Psychology Review, 19,* 378–383.

Sherman, L. W. (2003). Family-based crime prevention. In L. W. Sherman, D. Goddfredson, D. MacKenzie, J. Eck, P. Reuter, & S. Bushway (Eds.), *Preventing crime: What works, what doesn't, what's promising.* A report to the United States Congress, prepared for the National Institute of Justice. College Park, MD: University of Maryland. Retrieved June 3, 2003, from *http://www.ncjrs.org/works/.*

Sickmund, M. (2002). Juvenile residential facility census, 2000: Selected findings. *Juvenile offenders and victims: National report series bulletin.* Retrieved July 5, 2003, from *http://ojjdp.ncjrs.org.*

Skiba, R. J., Michael, R. S., Nardo, A. C., & Peterson, R. (2000, June). The color of discipline: Sources of racial and gender disproportionality in school punishment. *Urban Review.* Retrieved March 26, 2003, from *http://www.indiana.edu/~safeschl/cod.pdf.*

Snyder, H. N. (2001). Epidemiology of official offending. In R. Loeber & D. P. Farrington (Eds.), *Child delinquents: Development, intervention, and service needs* (pp. 25–46). Thousand Oaks, CA: Sage.

Snyder, H. N., & Sickmund, M. (1999). *Juvenile offenders and victims: 1999 National report.* Washington, DC: National Center for Juvenile Justice, Office of Juvenile Justice and Delinquency Prevention.

Spekman, N. J. (1993). An exploration of risk and resilience in the lives of individuals with learning disabilities. *Learning Disabilities Research and Practice, 8,* 11–18.

Stephens, R. D., & Arnette, J. L. (2000). *From the courthouse to the schoolhouse: Making successful transitions.* Washington, DC: Juvenile Justice Bulletin, Office of Juvenile Justice and Delinquency Prevention, U.S. Department of Justice.

Stumphauser, J. S, Aiken, T. W., & Veloz, E. V. (1977). East side story: Behavioral analysis of a high juvenile crime community. *Behavioral Disorders, 2,* 76–84.

Tashjian, M. D., LeBlanc, L. A., & Pfannenstiel, J. C. (1991). Descriptive study findings: National study of the Chapter 1 Neglected or Delinquent Program. *Unlocking learning: Chapter 1 in correctional facilities* (Contract No. 300-87-0124). Rockville, MD: Westat.

Teplin, L. A., Abram, K. M., McClelland, G. M., Dulcan, M. K., & Mericle, A. A. (2002). Psychiatric disorders in youth in juvenile detention. *Archives of General Psychiatry, 59,* 1133–1143.

Terzian, R. R. (1994). The juvenile crime challenge: Making prevention a priority. Retrieved January 21, 2001, from *http://www.bsa.ca.gov/lhcdir/127rp.html.*

Tobin, T., & Sprague, J. R. (2000). Alternative education strategies: Reducing violence in school and the community. *Journal of Emotional and Behavioral Disorders, 8,* 177–186.

Todis, B., Bullis, M., Waintrup, M., Schultz, R., & D'Ambrosio (2001). Overcoming the odds: Qualitative examination of resilience among formerly incarcerated adolescents. *Exceptional Children, 68,* 119–139.

U.S. General Accounting Office (2003). *Child welfare and juvenile justice: Federal agencies could play a stronger role in helping states reduce the number of children placed solely to obtain mental health services* (GAO-03-397). Washington, DC: Author.

Van Acker, R., & Wehby, J. H. (2000). Exploring the social contexts influencing student success or failure: Introduction. *Preventing School Failure, 44(3),* 93–96.

Wandersman, A., & Nation, M. (1998). Urban neighborhoods and mental health: Psychological contributions to understanding toxicity, resilience, and interventions. *American Psychologist, 43,* 647–656.

Wehby, J. H., Harnish, J. D., Valente, E., Dodge, K. A., & Conduct Problems Research Group. (2002). *Parent involvement as a partial mediator of the role of socioeconomic status in child academic performance.* Nashville, TN: Vanderbilt University, Peabody College.

Weinheimer, A. (2001). Safe, disciplined, and drug-free schools expert panel: Exemplary programs. Washington, DC: U.S. Department of Education. Retrieved October 20, 2001, from *http://www.ed.gov/offices/OERI/ORAD/KAD/expert_panel/drug-free.html.*

Welch, M., & Sheridan, S. M. (1995). *Educational partnerships: Serving students at risk.* Fort Worth, TX: Harcourt Brace Jovanovich.

Winett, L. B. (1998). Constructing violence as a public health problem. *Public Health Reports.* Retrieved June 11, 2001, from *http://search.britannica.com:80/magazine/article?email=1&contentid=263941.*

Wollard, J. L., Gross, S. L., Mulvey, E. P., & Reppucci, N. D. (1992). Legal issues affecting mentally disordered youth in the juvenile justice system. In J. J. Cocozza (Ed.), *Responding to the mental health needs of youth in the juvenile justice system* (pp. 91–106). Seattle, WA: National Coalition for the Mentally Ill in the Criminal Justice System.

Yellin, E. M. (1996). *Resilience: A model of success for adjudicated youth.* Unpublished doctoral dissertation, Arizona State University, Tempe.

16

Research Issues in Autism Spectrum Disorders

DWIGHT P. SWEENEY *and* CHARLES D. HOFFMAN

The documented incidence of autistic spectrum disorder (ASD) is increasing at alarming rates, thereby creating a myriad of problems for schools and social service agencies seeking to serve this population. This chapter reviews limitations of past autism research, presents National Research Council (NRC, 2001) best-practice recommendations for research design and methodology, and describes recent American Psychological Association (2002) guidelines for the determination of treatment efficacy. Building on these recommendations and guidelines, an ecological/family context model for program evaluation and research is offered.

BACKGROUND

The dramatic increase in the number of children with autistic spectrum disorder (Gillberg, 1991; Wing, 1991) has brought with it the need to design and conduct sophisticated research on the efficacy of the large number of treatment options available for children with ASD. ASD is the currently preferred descriptor for a class of neurodevelopmental disorders that includes all of the disorders listed as pervasive developmental disorders (PDD) in the fourth edition of the *Diagnostic and Statistical Manual of Mental Disorders* (DSM-IV; American Psychiatric Associ-

ation, 1994). Specifically, ASD includes autistic disorder, Asperger's disorder, Rett's disorder, childhood disintegrative disorder (CDD), and pervasive developmental disorder not otherwise specified (PDD-NOS). Common clinical features of ASD include delays in communication or language, impaired social interactions, sensory processing problems, and the presence of "odd" or atypical behaviors. ASD may also coexist with mental retardation, cerebral palsy, epilepsy, attention-deficit/hyperactivity disorder (ADHD), obsessive–compulsive disorder (OCD), oppositional defiant disorder (ODD), or depression. Other characteristics typically found in children with autism may include aggressive and self-injurious behaviors (SIB), perseveration on interests and activities, dependence on routine, uneven developmental profiles, difficulties in sleeping, toileting, and eating, autoimmune irregularities, nutritional deficiencies, or gastrointestinal problems. Levels of functioning for children diagnosed with ASD range from mild to severe across multiple domains including intelligence, academic achievement, communication, social interaction, adaptive behavior, sensory-motor integration, sensory processing, and behavior (Schriebman, Heyser, & Stahmer, 1999; Schroeder, Reese, Hellings, Loupe, & Tessel, 1999). Despite increasing evidence that autism has a genetic or biological base and originates in the early stages of embryonic development, there are no current medical tests to diagnose the condition (Bailey, Phillips, & Rutter, 1996). Therefore, all diagnoses of ASD are based on observations of behavioral indicators such as atypical developmental profiles across the communication, social, and sensory domains. When other conditions are also present, it becomes extremely difficult to accurately diagnose the presence of ASD (Siegel, Pliner, Eschler, & Elliot, 1988). Usually a diagnosis of autism is not made before age 2. In many cases, the diagnosis of autism is not made until 3 years of age when the criteria necessary to meet the DSM-IV definition of autistic disorder are more readily apparent (Klin & Volkmar, 1999; Gillham, Carter, Volkmar, & Sparrow, 2000).

Instruments commonly used to screen for or diagnose ASD include the Childhood Autism Rating Scale (CARS; Schopler, Reichler, & Renner, 1988), the Gilliam Autism Rating Scale—Revised (GARS-R; Gilliam, 2002), The Autism Diagnostic Observation Schedule (ADOS; Lord, Rutter, DiLavore, & Risi, 2000), The Pervasive Developmental Disorders Screening Test–II (PDDST-II; Siegel, 2000), the Screening Test for Autism in Two-Year-Olds (Stone, Coonod, & Onsley, 2000), the Modified Checklist for Autism in Toddlers (M-CHAT; Robins, 2001), and the Australian Scale for Asperger's Syndrome (Garnett & Attwood, 1998), the Asperger Syndrome Diagnostic Scale (ASDS; Myles, Bock, & Simpson, 2000), and the Gilliam Asperger Disorder Scale (GADS; Gilliam, 2001).

Each of these instruments is targeted for different age ranges and has different psychometric properties. Further, some are intended to be completed by clinicians; others are to be completed by parents, teachers, or individuals familiar with the child. Therefore, researchers are encouraged to select the instruments with the best psychometric characteristics and those that are appropriate for the age range of children to be studied. As with all psychometric instruments, standard scores, developmental levels, indices, and other data obtained from these instruments need to be interpreted and reported within the limits of available normative data (Klin, Carter, & Sparrow, 1997).

For the past several years there has been increasing concern over the almost epidemic increase in the number of children being diagnosed with ASD. Within California, the Department of Developmental Services (CDDS) cited a 273% increase in the number of reported cases of ASD between 1987 and 1998 (California Department of Developmental Services; CDDS, 1999; Croen, Grether, Hoogstrate, & Selvin, 2002; see also Baker, 2002). Given concerns over this increase, the Medical Investigation of Neurodevelopmental Disorders (MIND) Institute completed a follow-up study that confirmed the increase in the incidence of ASD in California and that the increase is not due to changes in the diagnostic criteria or to underidentification in the past combined with overidentification in the present (Medical Investigation of Neurodevelopmental Disorders Institute; MIND, 2002). This trend has continued, as the CDDS has published an updated report indicating that between 1998 and 2002 the population of persons with autism served by the Developmental Services System in California increased by 97%. By including these new data, the overall number of identified persons with autism in California, not including those with Asperger's, Rett's, CDD, or PDD-NOS, has increased by 634% between 1987 and 2002 (CDDS, 2003). These statistics may actually underestimate the increase in incidence of ASD in California, as it has been estimated that only 75% to 80% of persons with ASD are registered with the Developmental Services System (CDDS, 2003). Thus, in California, autism is now more prevalent than childhood cancer, diabetes, or Down syndrome. Similar increases in the incidence of autism or ASD also have been reported in other regions of the United States (Yeargin-Allsopp et al., 2003). This dramatic rise in what used to be considered a low-incidence disorder has created unprecedented demands on health and social services agencies and schools to provide the full continuum of services for children with ASD and their families.

While no systematic epidemiological studies have been completed to determine the current incidence and prevalence rates for ASD, the epidemic-like increase cited in the available studies highlights the need for rigorous investigations to determine which treatment options have efficacy for children functioning across the spectrum. Such studies are needed to help determine which family supports and child interventions are most effective in reducing problematic behaviors across multiple settings and domains, thereby improving outcomes for children with ASD and their families. Given the wide range of functioning observed among children with ASD, these interventions will need to be examined by child functioning level across multiple domains, independent from diagnostic categories of disability (see Kasari, 2002; NRC 2001).

To date, most large-scale research on ASD has been confined to medical researchers seeking to determine the etiology of ASD. Little attention has been paid to the impact of a child with ASD on family integrity and sibling adjustment (Prizant & Rubin, 1999). Like prior research on the treatment efficacy of individual interventions, past studies examining family integrity and sibling adjustment have been limited by small sample size and have controlled for child diagnosis without examining the potential impact of functioning level or comorbidity with other conditions, independent of diagnosis, on the dependent measures (e.g., NRC, 2001). Only recently have researchers in the health and human services fields focused their research on treatment and interventions to reduce the impact of ASD on children and their families (see Kasari, 2002). Future research to identify behavioral interventions that consider the strengths, limitations, and competing demands on the child, his or her family, and his or her current educational placement will increase the likelihood of decreasing undesirable behaviors that reduce opportunities for normalization and negatively impact learning (Rudolph & Epstein, 2000).

It is essential that all future efficacy studies utilize functional analysis to identify positive replacement behaviors that will help to improve the learning outcomes and independence of each child (Durand, 1990, 1993; Gable, 1996; Lewis & Sugai, 1994). Such positive outcomes are essential since schools are increasingly finding themselves caught between the recent federal guidelines that "No child is left behind," ever increasing state and federal mandates for outcomes assessment, and the inclusion of all children in state or nationwide assessment programs. Finally, identifying effective behavioral management programs to be used by parents and nondisabled siblings (see Dyson, 1999) when working with their sister or brother with ASD will help maintain the integrity of the child's family unit and thereby likely reduce the need for more costly and restrictive out-of-home placements.

GUIDELINES FOR FUTURE RESEARCH

Given the concern about the rapid increase in the number of children with ASD and the resulting need to identify efficacious treatment options, the U.S. Department of Education's Office of Special Education Programs requested that the National Research Council (NRC) form a Committee on Educational Interventions for Children with Autism. One charge of this committee was to "create a framework for evaluating the scientific evidence concerning the effects and features of educational interventions for young children with autism" (NRC, 2001, p. 13). To carry out this component of their charge, the committee developed a set of guidelines for use in evaluating research studies to address areas of strength, limitations, and the overall quality of the evidence presented in these studies. The committee felt such guidelines were needed because

within the field of autism, there are many approaches to intervention that are widely disseminated but little researched. Some approaches have been greeted with great enthusiasm initially, but have relatively quickly faded out of general use, in part because of their failure to demonstrate worthwhile effects. Other approaches have withstood the test of time across sites and the children and families they serve, though they continue to be largely supported by clinical descriptions of effectiveness, rather than by formal evaluations. Yet wide use and respect cannot be interpreted as clear evidence of effectiveness; therefore, the committee elected to consider information about these approaches in light of more empirically oriented studies. (NRC, 2001, p. 14)

The guidelines developed by the committee were based on approaches identified by scientific societies, including the American Academy of Neurology (Filipek et al., 2000), the American Psychological Association (American Psychological Association, 2000), and the Society for Clinical Child Psychology (Lonigan, Elbert, & Johnson, 1998). Guidelines were provided for rating Internal Validity, External Validity/Selection Biases, and Generalization. Criteria for four levels were established within each of these areas with Level I being considered the most rigorous and Level IV the least rigorous. For example, to meet the Level I standard for Internal Validity, prospective studies must meet all of the criteria for Levels II–IV, and compare the intervention being studied to an alternative intervention or placebo in which evaluators of outcomes are blind to treatment status. Likewise, studies meeting the criteria for Level I in External Validity/Selection Biases would need to demonstrate random assignment of well-defined cohorts and adequate sample size for comparisons. Studies meeting the Level I standard for Generalization would need to show documented changes in at least one natural setting outside of the treatment environment and include social validity measures (NRC, 2001). Using these guidelines, the committee reviewed published research studies in the areas of social skills, communication, problem behavior, intervention methods, and sensory-motor integration.

The committee also noted that standards for conducting behavioral research have changed over time. Today's behavioral research is expected to use rigorously standardized measures, verify diagnoses, maintain independence between intervention and assessment, control for the effects of development, monitor treatment fidelity, match participants by intellectual and language levels, address generalization or maintenance of effects, and justify measures by their clinical value. Thus, the committee reported that, of the nine problem behavior studies reviewed, none reached the Level II criteria for Internal or External Validity. Approximately 55% met the Level II criteria for Generalization. Only 5% of the thirteen Intervention Methods studies reviewed met the Level I criteria for Internal and External Validity; none reached the Level I criteria for Generalization. These findings suggest an urgent need to increase the quantity and improve the quality of research to determine the efficacy of the multiple treatment options currently available.

To this end, the American Psychological Association has published *Criteria for Eval-*uating Treatment Guidelines* (American Psychological Association, 2002). The standards for determining treatment efficacy and clinical utility advocated by the American Psychological Association go beyond those called for by the NRC. Treatment efficacy is defined as "a valid ascertainment of the effects of a given intervention as compared with an alternative intervention or with no treatment, in a controlled clinical context. The fundamental question in evaluating efficacy is whether a beneficial effect of treatment can be demonstrated scientifically" (American Psychological Association, 2002, p. 1053). Clinical utility is defined as "(a) the ability of health care professionals to use and of patients to accept the treatment under consideration and (b) the range of applicability of that treatment" (American Psychological Association, p. 1056). Five criteria, some with subparts, are provided for determining treatment efficacy. The five primary criteria are:

1.0 Guidelines should be based on broad and careful consideration of the relevant empirical literature.
2.0 Recommendations on specific interventions should take into consideration the level of methodological rigor and clinical sophistication of the research supporting the intervention.
3.0 Recommendations on specific interventions should take into consideration the treatment conditions to which the intervention has been compared.
4.0 Guidelines should consider available evidence regarding patient–treatment matching.
5.0 Guidelines should specify the outcomes the intervention is intended to produce, and evidence should be provided for each outcome (American Psychological Association, 2002, pp. 1054–1055)

The American Psychological Association also provided four criteria, some with subparts, to assist in determining clinical utility. The four primary criteria are:

6.0 Guidelines should reflect the breadth of patient variables that may influence the clinical utility of the intervention.
7.0 It is recommended that guidelines take into account data on how differences between individual health care professionals may effect the efficacy of the treatment.

8.0 It is recommended that guidelines take into account information pertaining to the setting in which the treatment is offered.

9.0 Guidelines should take into account data on treatment robustness (American Psychological Association, 2002, pp. 1056–1057)

Further, 12 additional criteria are provided related to feasibility, cost considerations, and the guideline development process. Taken together, the NRC guidelines and the American Psychological Association criteria should be the benchmarks guiding all future research studies seeking to determine the efficacy, clinical utility, and probable generalization of any intervention or treatment program.

INTERVENTIONS NEEDING STUDY

As pointed out by the NRC, there has been a proliferation of intervention programs for children with ASD. While many of these interventions (e.g., applied behavioral analysis [ABA], Treatment and Education of Autistic and Related Communications Handicapped Children [TEAACH], Picture Exchange Communication System [PECS], etc.) are widely used and have obtained excellent results for some children with ASD, none of these interventions have been examined using designs that meet the standards for rigor, efficacy, and generalization called for by the NRC report or American Psychological Association criteria. Therefore, the following list of currently available treatments is provided for individuals seeking to validate the efficacy and clinical utility of these interventions. The list is not all-inclusive. It is simply representative, and no relative merit for any intervention is implied. However, it does demonstrate the wide variety of interventions available to parents, schools, or social service agencies.

1. Educational interventions
   a. Applied behavioral analysis (ABA)
   b. Treatment and Education of Autistic and Related Communications Handicapped Children (TEACCH)
   c. Daily life therapy (Higashi School)
   d. Lindamood–bell (Sensory Cognitive)
2. Nutritional supplements
   a. Vitamin therapy (B_6, C, and DMG)
   b. Cod liver oil (vitamin A)
3. Pharmacology
   a. Antipsychotics
   b. Anticonvulsants
   c. Antianxiety
   d. Antidepressants
   e. Beta blockers
   f. Opiate blockers
   g. Sedatives
   h. Stimulants
4. Speech and language therapy
   a. Picture Exchange Communication System (PECS)
   b. Communication books
   c. Augmentative communication devices
5. Computer programs
   a. Fast ForWord (Scientific Learning Corporation)
   b. Earobics (Cognitive Concepts)
   c. Train Time (Locu Tour)
6. Dietary interventions
   a. Casein/gluten-free diet
   b. Feingold program
   c. Allergy treatments
   d. Melatonin
7. Secretin
8. Anti-yeast therapy
9. Auditory integration training
10. Music therapy
11. Sensory integration therapy
12. Vision training
13. The Squeeze Machine
14. The Sun-Rise Program (Option Institute)
15. Facilitated communication
16. Floor-Time (Child-Centered Play Therapy)
17. Social Stories

PROPOSED MODEL FOR FUTURE RESEARCH

The authors have designed a model for future research that addresses many of the limitations of past research indicated in the NRC report. It will also serve to enable research in the area to better meet the American Psychological Association criteria for determining efficacy, clinical utility, and improve the potential for generalization. Importantly, the model also provides a conceptual base that relies on comprehensive assessment of the child with ASD and the salient characteristics of his or her ecological and familial context. In this regard, this approach addresses the need for multiple measures of child, sibling, and family functioning, and the accompanying need for comprehensive diagnostic data to control for differential child functioning levels across multiple domains. It also suggests the need for extensive demographic data to allow for specificity in the descriptions of the children and families being studied. The model outlined calls for large sample sizes, the availability of a matched control group, and merges past research from related disciplines (e.g., special education, child development, family process, etc.). Finally, it recommends the use of measures obtained from external sources to help establish the external validity of treatment effects. Recognizing the complexity of such a design, the following assumptions are offered as prerequisites for researchers wishing to use this model.

Assumptions of the Model

1. Access to a large sample (N = 100 or more) of willing participants who meet the criteria identified for study.
2. Availability of an equally large control group who meet the same criteria and are willing to participate to enable assessment of the effects of "doing nothing."
3. Use of random assignment to treatment and control groups.
4. Ability to collect multiple measures across multiple domains at multiple data points over a minimum 2-year period.
5. Ability to conduct long-term follow-up to assess stability of effects.
6. Partnership with agencies external to the treatment setting that can provide independent measures of effects needed to establish external validity (e.g., individualized education programs).
7. Ability to monitor treatment fidelity across multiple settings through direct observation, examination of treatment charts and notes, or through random videotape reviews.
8. Ability to provide treatment to non-treatment control groups during or immediately following the investigation.
9. Ability to examine data from children that do not complete the treatment program to determine if they differ from completers in any significant ways.
10. Ability to control for participants language, culture, and reading level when completing all research protocols and when interpreting treatment outcomes.

The following model is offered for consideration.

An Ecological/Family Context Model for Program Evaluation and Research

The conceptual and methodological model offered is derived from an ecologically based approach, which conceptualizes child development contextually (Bronfrenbrenner, 1992; Lerner, 1996) and acknowledges the family system as the primary crucible for developmental interactive processes and change (Minuchin, 1988). While the need for a family-centered approach to the study of childhood disability was indicated in the early 1990s (e.g., Sontag, 1996), efforts to this end have been impeded by a "lack of theory driven research, limited assessment tools, and research designs that are inadequate for capturing the complexities of the family process" (Quittner & DiGirolamo, 1998, p. 71). A contextual, ecological/family system's theoretical orientation provides the necessary contemporary conceptual frame for a program of evaluation and research to study children and adolescents with ASD and their families (Lerner, 1996; Prizant & Rubin, 1999; Schreibman, 2000). The associated methodology and research design necessarily include comprehensive assessment of the interrelated and interacting contextual influences that represent the full complexity of family processes and child development within an ecological framework.

Building on recent calls for the exploration of family variables in the assessment of intervention efficacy (CDDS, 2002; NRC, 2001; Prizant & Rubin, 1999; Quittner & DiGirolamo, 1998; Schreibman, 2000), the suggested model considers proximal family interaction patterns as central to the development of children with autism (Guralnick, 1997; Hauser-Cram, Warfield, Shonkoff, & Krauss, 2001). The comprehensive evaluation of children with ASD, and assessment of the interrelated domains of family functioning (e.g., Seligman, 1999) over time, will

enable the creation of a more complete picture of children and adolescents with ASD
and their families than has been available to
now. The methodology and related design
characteristics of the model are consistent
with improvements indicated as required to
advance research in the field (American Psychological Association, 2002; NRC, 2001)
and will permit the application of sophisticated statistical analyses, such as hierarchical linear regression modeling and structural
equation modeling (SEM), to the analyses of
intervention outcomes.

The overarching structure suggested is designed to move beyond the limitations of
unidirectional, unilevel approaches in prior
research (Hauser-Cram et al., 2001; Lerner,
1996; Sontag, 1996). Single-variable explanations in the literature have failed to account for the complexity and diversity of
causal pathways, interactive relationships,
and related outcomes that exist in the lives
of children with ASD and their families. As
Lerner indicates, the study of the processes
of child development using a child-in-con-
text approach, as in the one suggested here,
is at the cutting edge of contemporary developmental theory. Lerner states that this is
"the predominant conceptual frame for research in the study of human development"
(p. 781) and "the 'design criteria' imposed
on research, method and application pertinent to the study of any content area or dimension of the developing person" (p. 782).
Relying on the conceptualization of an integrated complex of causal factors within
which individual, familial, and social structural factors, as well as treatments, interact
and exert interrelated and variable influences (see Quittner & DiGirolamo, 1998)
requires a comprehensive, systematic approach, as in the one outlined.

In this model children are viewed as
nested within multilevel, hierarchical, environmental systems of influence: contexts that
comprise the interacting systems of their ecological reality (Bronfenbrenner, 1979, 1986,
1992; Lerner, 1991, 1996; Minuchin, 1988;
Overton, 1998; Thalen & Smith, 1998).
These reciprocally related contexts, and the
family members who populate the child's
developmental milieu, are considered as
components of a system made up of subsystems (or domains) that influence one another and the system as a whole synergisti-
cally, through the relationships among these

essential elements of the family constellation
(Sontag, 1996). As indicated, examination
of development as a joint function of child
characteristics and environmental characteristics (Bronfenbrenner, 1992) requires thorough appraisal of children and adolescents
with ASD, the key domains that constitute
the family and interfamilial relationships, as
well as the extrafamilial supports of the environment, longitudinally (Sontag, 1996).
Including intervention programs in this ecological vision of the child's world contributes enormously to the possibility for
successful program evaluation. Thorough
assessment of each child and the core elements of the system within which he or she
resides is required as the effectiveness or in-
effectiveness of a specific ingredient of an intervention may influence, and/or be influenced by, the related interacting domains.
Joining the evaluation of intervention programs with a basic research agenda will enable researchers to contribute substantively
to the understanding of how child characteristics and family dynamics interact with
interventions employed as well as to the understanding of related developmental dynamics and related adaptations of families.

Children and adolescents with ASD stand,
necessarily, at the center of this ecologically
based approach. The systematic assessment
of these children and their unique developmentally instigative characteristics is required, as they function as agents who
construct their development as well as respondents influenced by the multiple systems of ecological influence within which
they live (see Brandtstädter, 1998). The personal stimulus qualities and developmentally
structuring attributes (Bronfenbrenner, 1992;
Sontag, 1996) associated with ASD are viewed
as contributing to individually unique patterns of interactions within the family environment, as well as to differential responsiveness to intervention approaches, and
they have not been previously investigated in
conjunction with evaluation of the essential
domains of the child's environment. As suggested by NRC (2001), this suggests obtaining a level of detailed information regarding
the specific characteristics of each child's
disorder and coexisting conditions that goes
well beyond standard descriptive information routinely provided in intervention
research. Such comprehensive child assessment would permit much-needed precision

with regard to overall level of autistic involvement as well as child functioning within specific diagnostic domains. The impact of coexisting disabilities that influence child functioning might further explain differential treatment responses and, in turn, contribute to the necessary treatments by participant characteristics analyses that are of growing importance to this literature (CDDS, 2002; MIND, 2002). Examination of the level of child functioning as a continuous variable, both within and across domains, also supports the use of sophisticated statistical techniques, as in regression analyses, to create conceptual models designed to examine severity of impairment in relation to family and extrafamilial variables as well as treatment outcome in relation to both child and contextual variables.

A child's disabling condition is understood to interact with the contextual variables of his or her ecological reality, including treatment approaches, in complex and nonlinear ways that contribute to child and family adjustment (Seligman, 1999). Methodological limitations have led to there being insufficient attention paid to interactions between child factors, such as severity of autistic involvement and specific diagnosis on the spectrum of autism and/or coexisting conditions, and family variables such as parental stress (e.g., NRC, 2001) or sibling adjustment. The multifaceted interactional framework suggested and the evaluation of related systemic processes also require assessment of the essential domains of family functioning and of other core domains of potential influence. Family systems theory provides a structure composed of four subsystems requiring evaluation (Seligman): marital, parent–child, sibling, and extrafamilial. Relying on a set of carefully selected instruments, assessment of domains within each of these subsystems, as well as of individual parental functioning (e.g., Quittner & DiGirolamo, 1998) and other key family processes and resources, is considered an essential component of this contextual model.

Some Specific Methodological Suggestions

Centrally important components of the methodological approach suggested include the participation and assessment of a large number of children with ASD and their families who would participate on a long-term basis (i.e., a longitudinal design); the collection of extensive descriptive demographic information and comprehensive assessment of salient researcher identified ecological, familial, and related contextual domains; and, when possible, the random assignment of participants to an intervention and comparison groups methodology, to provide for the valid ascertainment of treatment efficacy (e.g., American Psychological Association, 2002).

Participants and Design

Given the heterogeneity that is a defining characteristic of ASD, and the requirements associated with the design and anticipated statistical analyses to be employed, it is suggested that 100 children with ASD and their families (parents or other primary care providers and siblings) represents the minimum number required to implement the model of evaluation and research outlined above effectively. A large number of participant children would support examination of the unique characteristics of children, including core coexisting conditions, in relation to treatment outcome measures (e.g., Kasari, 2002) and to indicated contextual indices and family features (NRC, 2001). A sufficiently large number of participants is required for the use of random assignment procedures, which, as indicated, are preferred to support the valid assessment of treatment effects (American Psychological Association, 2002; NRC, 2001).

If possible, it is best if children and families remain in the program a minimum of 2 years. This would allow longitudinal reexamination of intervention effectiveness by the testing of all children, parents, and siblings at entry into the program, and after specified periods of time (e.g., after 1 year and, then, at 2 years) or at the time of exiting the program. It is further recommended that some form of long-term follow-up (3–5 years) be used to verify the stability of treatment effects over time and across settings (generalization) (NRC, 2001; American Psychological Association, 2002).

Control Groups

Quasi-experimental designs relying on nonrandomized contrast groups may be used as the basis for evaluating treatment effectiveness (NRC, 2001, p. 200; Campbell & Stanley, 1963). When sufficient participant measures are available, each participant can be used as his or her own control over the course of the study (similar to the multiple baseline approach used in single-subject designs). Also, if available, a wait-list group could serve as a comparison, or "no-treatment," control group. All of these approaches support the determination of treatment efficacy in a manner consistent with the guidelines suggested by the American Psychological Association and the NRC.

Obtaining extensive demographic and other treatment history information for children and families entering an intervention program and those on a wait list may indicate that these groups are similar across these core indices at the same point in time. To further support the utility of this methodology, it may be possible to implement appropriate statistical controls for any a priori differences that may emerge between these respective groups. Use of a wait-list control would permit the possibility of matching groups with respect to obtained demographic or family domain indices, as well as for particular levels or component characteristics of a child's ASD. This approach would allow for the added power advantages associated with matched groups' statistical analyses to compare treatment efficacy for these respective groups or critical subgroups. Thus, despite limitations inherent in this methodological approach, comparing a treatment to a nontreatment wait-list control can support the determination of whether an intervention is efficacious and whether or not it has any adverse effects, compared to "doing nothing" (American Psychological Association, 2002). The same considerations would apply where there are alternative treatment sites associated with a particular program and, for example, specific treatments are implemented at one location but not at the other, and comparisons of effectiveness are made over time.

Given problems related to the comparability of groups, and consistent with the literature regarding treatment efficacy, or the valid ascertainment of the effects of an intervention compared with an alternative approach (e.g., American Psychological Association, 2002, p. 1053), the establishment of further methods of control using a random assignment approach is preferred (Kasari, 2002; NRC, 2001). Importantly, a large number of participants would permit the use of random assignment to compare treatment groups to no-treatment control groups and/or other treatments levels, as is required for rigorously designed intervention efficacy research (American Psychological Association, 2002; Kasari, 2002; NRC, 2001), and it is the approach recommended here. Further, consistent with applicable ethical concerns for the implementation of empirically valid treatment approaches for control groups (see NRC, 2001, p. 200), participants randomly assigned to any control groups or levels would begin treatment once the effectiveness of an intervention has been established. In this case, salient findings derived from the analyses of differences obtained for prior treatment groups could be examined for replication purposes, providing further evidence of efficacy and supporting the generalization of any findings.

Demographic Measures

As indicated, the collection of demographic information for participants needs to be extensive to ascertain the possible influence of these factors on child or family functioning or the interactive effect of such factors on treatment efficacy. Reports of the structural characteristics of the family (e.g., number and ages of children) and other extensive demographic information regarding participants and families (e.g., socioeconomic status) are essential components of the approach suggested. While not meant to be either complete or prescriptive, the following represents some key information for inclusion in the accumulation of relevant demographics.

Of course, the most important and therefore most extensive information garnered would be about the child with ASD. Researchers should obtain at least the following: age, gender, height, weight, and race, diagnosis information, current and past educational experiences, and medical and developmental status. Educational information, by way of further illustration, would include current classroom placement, grade level, cognitive level, total years in school, and length of the child's school day. Collection of information regarding whether the child met identified developmental milestones (e.g., as rolling over, sitting alone, and toilet training) on time and regarding the child's current level of communication (e.g., verbal) is also suggested. A full range of health and other related medical information would be collected, including a birth history (including any pregnancy difficulties) as well as any current or past major illnesses, hospitalizations, psychiatric concerns, injuries, allergies, special diets, seizure disorders, medications (including dosage and frequency of use), an immunization history and whether the child currently has a primary care physician. It is suggested that information be collected regarding the child's ongoing and historical experiences with related treatment services, such as adaptive physical education, speech therapy, in-home behavior therapy, physical therapy, psychotherapy, occupational therapy, neurological treatment, and so on.

Demographics collected for the parents would include their age, gender, ethnicity, occupation, household income, and educational level. Current and past marital history, other indicators of parental and family structure, as well as relevant health histories for the parents or other care providers should be ascertained. Additionally, demographics should be collected for any siblings who will be included in the research program, including their age, gender, educational level, classroom placement status, known disability, health problems, or developmental delays. It is important to note that all health data should be gathered and stored in a manner consistent with Health Insurance Portability and Accountability Act (HIPAA) and Family Educational Rights and Privacy Act (FERPA) guidelines (Turner & Foong, 2003; U.S. Department of Education, 2003).

Treatment Fidelity

To allow for replication and the determination treatment fidelity, all aspects of the intervention being studied need to be described in sufficient detail. For example, the criteria and process for selecting and grouping participants, along with descriptions of any specialized training or equipment required when implementing the intervention, will need to be sufficiently described so that all aspects of the study can be replicated by other researchers (NRC, 2001, pp. 227–228).

Domains Assessed

The following represent some suggestions of core child and contextual domains identified for evaluation. These evaluations should rely, wherever possible, on carefully selected and widely used published and, where required, literature-derived instruments. Longitudinal assessment, the inclusion of instruments recommended for the screening and diagnosis of autism, and using measures derived from multiple relevant sources are central to this approach (e.g., Filipek et al., 2000; Quittner & DiGirolamo, 1998).

Consistent with the purpose and effective implementation of the model, the assessments for the child with ASD include standardized measures of cognitive functioning (e.g., Wechsler Intelligence Scales; Wechsler, 1991), adaptive behavior (e.g., Vineland Adaptive Behavior Scales; Sparrow, Bala, & Cicchetti, 1984), as well as level of functioning and performance on standardized rating scales should be employed (e.g., the Gilliam Autism Rating Scale; Gilliam, 2002; and the Childhood Autism Rating Scale; Schopler et al., 1988).

In addition to obtaining the demographics outlined above, evaluations for each of the four subsystems based on the family systems theory, as well as of individual parental functioning and other key family processes and resources are essential for the contextual model. It is recommended that parent information should consist of measures assessing parental stress (e.g., Parenting Stress Index [PSI]; Abidin, 1995) and family functioning (e.g., Family Environment Scale [FES]; Moos & Moos, 1986). Parents' coping strategies and psychiatric symptomology, as well as their perception of available resources, self-esteem, and marital relationships (e.g., Dyadic Adjustment Scale [DAS]; Spanier, 1976), are also suggested. Parents can provide evaluations of siblings' overall social adjustment (e.g., Child Behavior Checklist; Achenbach, 1991), complete program evaluation instruments, and report on their perceptions of the program and its impact on their family. Sibling self-assessments may examine their self-concept (e.g., Piers-Harris, 1999) and depression (Kovacs, 1999), as well as their perceptions of their sibling's disability. Siblings who are old enough (11 years old and over on the FES) can complete a measure assessing their views of family functioning in addition to the assessments provided by their parents.

Importantly, scales identified for assessment purposes for many of the indicated domains also consist of relevant and useful subscales to test potentially impactful relationships within components of the overarching domains mentioned. In fact, given the empirical questions that may be addressed by the investigators, the availability of specific subscales on an evaluation instrument should be an important feature considered in an investigator's decision regarding the use of a specific instrument. For example, as parenting stressors could arise from either parent or child factors, the Parenting Stress Index provides separate parent (e.g., Competence, Isolation, and Attachment) and child (e.g., Demandingness, Mood, and Acceptability) domain scores (Rodrigues & Murphy, 1997).

Anticipated Statistical Analyses and Hypotheses

The ecologically based family systems model provides the conceptual underpinning for the comprehensive assessment and related procedures suggested. The methodological approach outlined provides for the specificity and concomitant sensitivity required for researchers to evaluate program effectiveness as well as to contribute substantively to the related literature. The research design (including the longitudinal component and the random assignment of participants suggested), the extensive demographic information obtained, and the detailed descriptions of the intervention programs are each seen as significant in this regard. The suggested array of measurement instruments, the relatively large number of children with ASD and family participants suggested, and the assessment of the level of child functioning as a continuous variable across and within diagnostic domains are also noteworthy. These latter components of the model, in particular, support the application of a range of sophisticated statistical analyses to address the complexity of family processes and treatment effects, including growth curve analysis (Burchinal & Applebaum, 1991),

hierarchical linear regression, and structural equation modeling directed to the analysis of the data (see NRC, 2001).

The sophisticated model outlined here would allow researchers to gauge intervention effectiveness within and across domains of the family system for specified assessment periods, and assess the interplay of factors that contribute to and/or are most affected by treatments employed. Change over time in the program could be examined for key domains for children, parents, the family system, and siblings on each of the multifarious associated measures selected by researchers using this model.

Treatment evaluations might begin with a repeated measures approach in which each child participant, parent, and family would be extensively assessed in relation to their own baseline level of performance obtained as they began an intervention. There is obvious merit in this part of the approach, particularly for tracking changes associated with unique characteristics of a parent, family or, in particular, a child with ASD. Thus, assessed changes on subscales of the full range of instruments employed would support the evaluation of specific treatment goals for the children with autism who participate (see Bailey et al., 1998; NRC, 2001).

As indicated, the methodology outlined relies, as well, on the ability to examine obtained changes in relation to a wait-list control or, preferably, to a control group formed using a random assignment procedure. This latter design approach—randomly assigning participant children and their families to levels of treatment—would provide for the most rigorous test of key hypotheses related to intervention efficacy. Based on random assignment and associated comparability of groups prior to the implementation of an intervention, this approach would provide the scientific basis for the testing of hypothesized improvements in child, parent, family, and sibling functioning for participants in different levels of treatment on the full range of assessment instruments employed (American Psychological Association, 2002). By proceeding in this way, significant improvements in functioning obtained for children with ASD or their parents randomly assigned to a treatment group, compared to a no-treatment group, would be readily attributable to the intervention rather than to unknown and/or uncontrolled variables associated with one group or the other. Comparisons using multivariate analyses of variance with treatment effects appraised for specified assessment periods on dependent measures within selected domains are useful statistical approaches, and these analyses are supported by the design outlined. Further, as indicated above, control group participants in the next stage of the design suggested would begin treatment. In this case, salient findings derived from analyses of differences obtained for initial treatment groups or levels could be examined and related hypotheses derived from these prior groups could be tested.

The comprehensive evaluation of children and their families supports exploration of the reciprocal and interactive relationship between level of child functioning and the wide range of family domains assessed. These analyses will enable contributions to the literature on processes and adaptations for families with a child with ASD (e.g., NRC, 2001: Schreibman, 2000). By way of example, regression analyses can be used to determine whether the level of child functioning predicts parental self-reports of their own functioning (e.g., stress) or accounts for significant levels of variance in the prediction of family or sibling functioning. Relationships between the range of measures selected to assess child functioning and dimensions of parental and family functioning can be examined at baseline, as families enter the program, as well as over the course of their participation. The examination of these relationships can be carried out as participant families begin the program, and then comparisons of the course of any indicated relationships can be compared for treatment and control conditions.

Similarly, and again consistent with the conceptual model, it is expected that improvements evidenced within key domains of the family will be associated with measurable positive changes in other domains. More specifically, with regard to participation in an intervention over time, the posited reciprocal nature of the variables assessed suggests examination of the relationship between anticipated improvements on indices of parent and family functioning as they, in turn, are associated with, or predictive of, positive changes in child functioning. For example, improvements in parents' views of their child's behavior or of their own parent-

ing role may each be related to improved child functioning. Hierarchical regression models can be developed to test these and other hypothesized relationships, based on the pertinent literature and on preliminary analyses of the data collected, to examine the relative contributions of the variables indicated. These models can also be used to explore the contributions of key contextual parent or family domain variables, socioeconomic factors, or other theoretically interesting contributors to positive changes in child functioning (overall, within specific diagnostic criteria, and over time). Importantly, where possible, measures of parent or family functioning found to be predictive of treatment effectiveness can then be used to inform the development of empirically based intervention strategies for parents and families.

Examination of the complexity of the impact of a child or adolescent with ASD within a family environment and the exploration of the potential influence of an intervention on this system will require more sophisticated statistical approaches than those described thus far. That these analyses, and the understanding that they will provide, would be available as tools of exploration and discovery further evidences the advantages of the approach outlined. The measures selected for inclusion would permit the application of multiple regression or structural equation modeling (SEM) to test for mediated or moderated effects (Holmbeck, 1997). For example, based on related literature, the mediating influence of a family variable assessed (e.g., cohesion) could be examined to determine if it serves to reduce any possible direct effect of level of child functioning on parental stress (see Quittner & DiGirolamo, 1998). If assessed, parental self-efficacy, shown to be an important factor in related parenting literatures (e.g., Coleman & Karraker, 2000; Hastings & Brown, 2002), may be found to mediate a negative relationship between level of child impairment and sibling adjustment. Hypothesized relationships cited earlier between parental and/or familial gains and indices of child improvement may be mediated by other assessed factors. For example, assessed levels of parent functioning (e.g., their anxiety or depression) may be found to reduce any positive influence of family factors examined on improvements in child functioning evidenced over time.

Quantitative or qualitative factors (e.g., gender, ethnicity, etc.) that can be anticipated to affect the direction or strength of the relationship between a predictor variable, as in the level of parental functioning, and a criterion measure, such as the level of child functioning, could be examined statistically as moderators of this relationship (Baron & Kenny, 1986; Holmbeck, 1997). The moderating, or interactive, effect of treatment condition as it influences the relationship between level of child functioning as a predictor variable and indices of family or parental functioning criterion factors also could be examined using this approach. By way of further example, the impact of severity of child functioning on a criterion measure of sibling adjustment could be examined to determine if the nature of any effect varies with treatment. Models developed to examine posited mediating or moderating effects of a range of assessed variables on key relationships between predictor and criterion factors should, again, rely on suggestions derived from the related literature and preliminary data analyses. Further, whether regression or SEM approaches are used, the mediating or moderating effects of variables should be examined and determined statistically.

In response to the universe of potential questions derived from this conceptual and methodological approach and the related literature, preliminary analyses can be carried out in order to contribute to the development of more comprehensive models for future confirmation. Figure 16.1 provides an example of a conceptual framework that might be tested by using SEM. Here, we have illustrated a complex model of hypothesized relationships that includes the prediction of parent and family functioning and sibling adjustment factors by a child functioning factor, as well as a hypothesized relationship between these latter factors. This model further suggests that parent and family functioning mediates the relationship between the other two factors, that this factor is moderated by SES, and that treatment influences consumer functioning.

The model depicted is, of course, preliminary and would probably be modified by the

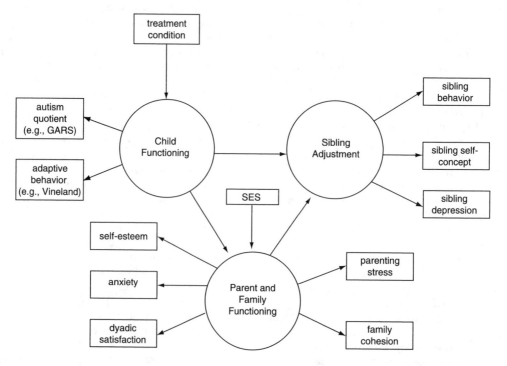

FIGURE 16.1. SEM (path) diagram for an example of a structural model suggesting relationships between the consumer, parent and family functioning, and sibling adjustment factors.

testing of simpler models, using multiple regression as well as SEM. For example, a model examining hypothesized relationships between the child functioning and sibling adjustment factors could be tested and examined for the potential moderating influence of treatment condition. Other indicators of these or other factors selected by researchers employing the methodological approach suggested would certainly be possible. Thus, in the latter regard, models that treat the parent and family functioning factor as separate factors could be tested.

SUMMARY

The dramatic increase in the occurrence of ASD in recent years indicates a compelling need for more rigorously designed and executed research in the area, particularly with regard to the identification of efficacious treatment options. To this end, the guidelines developed by NRC for the evaluation of existing intervention research (i.e., for rating a study's internal validity, external validity/selection biases, and generalization) were outlined. Using this framework to review the scientific quality of research studies on treatment effectiveness, the NRC concluded that there is an urgent need to increase the quantity and improve the quality of research to determine the efficacy of currently available treatment options for children with ASD and their families. The American Psychological Association's new *Criteria for Treatment Guidelines*, which provides standards for the scientific demonstration of any beneficial effects of a given treatment, were also summarized. The application of these more sophisticated approaches to validate the efficacy and clinical utility of a list of currently available treatments was suggested. Finally, an ecological/family conceptual model for program evaluation and research, designed to address many of the indicated limitations of past research, was presented. The assumptions of this approach were outlined, specific methodological details were provided, and related statistical benefits were discussed in relation to the NRC and American Psychological Association guidelines.

The increase in the prevalence of ASD has placed unprecedented demands on schools and social service agencies to provide appropriate services for this population. Therefore, it is imperative that researchers determine the efficacy and clinical validity of the myriad of treatment options available. Such findings will help ensure that schools and social service agencies have adequate research-based information to help choose the most cost-efficient and efficacious treatment options, thereby maximizing the potential benefit for each consumer served. The authors believe that efficacy studies based on the model described here will help provide the data needed for schools and social service agencies to make informed choices, thereby improving outcomes for children and adolescents with ASD.

REFERENCES

Abidin, R. R. (1995). *Parenting Stress Index* (3rd ed.) Odessa, FL: Psychological Assessment Resources.

Achenbach, T. M. (1991). *Child Behavior Checklist for Ages 4–18*. Burlington: University of Vermont.

American Psychiatric Association (1994). *Diagnostic and Statistical Manual of Mental Disorders* (4th ed.). Washington, DC: Author.

American Psychological Association. (2000). *Criteria for treatment guidelines*. Washington, DC: American Psychological Association.

American Psychological Association. (2002, December). Criteria for evaluation of treatment guidelines. *American Psychologist, 57*, 1052–1059.

Bailey, A., Phillips, W., & Rutter, M. (1996). Autism: Towards an integration of clinical, genetic, and neurological perspectives. *Journal of Child Psychology and Psychiatry, 37*, 89–126.

Bailey, D. B., Jr., McWilliam, R. A., Darkes, L. A., Hebbeler, K., Simeonsson, R. J., Spiker, D., & Wagner, M. (1998). Family outcomes in early intervention: A framework for program evaluation and efficacy research. *Exceptional Children, 64*, 313–328.

Baker, H. C. (2002). A comparison study of Autism Spectrum Disorder referrals 1997 and 1989. *Journal of Autism and Developmental Disorders, 32*, 121–125.

Baron, R. M., & Kenny, D. A. (1986). The moderator–mediator variable distinction in social psychological research: Conceptual, strategic, and statistical consideration. *Journal of Personality and Social Psychology, 51*, 1173–1182.

Brandtstädter, J. (1998). Action perspectives on human development. In W. Damon (Series Ed.) & R. M. Lerner (Vol. Ed.), *Handbook of child psychology: Vol. 1. Theoretical models of human development* (5th ed., pp. 807–864). New York: Wiley.

Bronfenbrenner, U. (1979). *The ecology of human de-*

velopment. Cambridge, MA: Harvard University Press.

Bronfenbrenner, U. (1986). Ecology of the family as a context for human development: Research Perspectives. *Developmental Psychology, 22,* 723–742.

Bronfenbrenner, U. (1992). Ecology systems theory. In R. Vasta (Ed.), *Annals of child development: Six theories of child development revised formulations and current issues.* (pp. 187–249). London: Jessica Kingsley.

Burchinal, M.R., & Applebaum, M. I. (1991). Estimating individual developmental functions: Methods and their assumptions. *Child Development, 62,* 23–43.

California Department of Developmental Services. (CDDS). (1999). Changes in the population of persons with autism and pervasive developmental disorders in California's Developmental Services system: 1987–1998. Sacramento, CA: Author.

California Department of Developmental Services. (CDDS). (2002). *Autism spectrum disorders: Best practice guidelines for screening, diagnosis and assessment.* Sacramento, CA: Author.

California Department of Developmental Services. (CDDS). (2003). *Autistic Spectrum Disorders: Changes in the California caseload: An update—1999 through 2002.* Sacramento, CA: Author.

Campbell, D. T., & Stanley, J. C. (1963). *Experimental and quasi-experimental designs for research.* Chicago: Rand McNally.

Coleman, P. K., & Karraker, K. H. (2000). Parenting self-efficacy among mothers of school-age children: Conceptualization, measurement, and correlates. *Family Relations, 49,* 13–24.

Croen, L. A., Grether, J. K., Hoogstrate, J., & Selvin, S. (2002). The changing prevalence of autism in California. *Journal of Autism and Developmental Disorders, 32,* 207–215.

Durand, V. M. (1990). *Severe behavior problems: A functional communication training approach.* New York: Guilford Press.

Durand, V. M. (1993). Functional assessment and functional analysis. In M. D. Smith (Ed.), *Behavior modification for exceptional children and youth.* Boston: Andover Medical.

Dyson, L. L. (1999). The Psychosocial functioning of school-age children who have siblings with developmental disabilities: Change and stability over time. *Journal of Applied Developmental Psychology, 20,* 253–271.

Filipek, P. A., Accardo, P. J., Ashwal, S., Baranek, G. T., Cook Jr., E. H., Dawson, G., et al. (2000). Practice parameters: Screening and diagnosis of autism. *American Academy of Neurology, 55,* 468–479.

Gable, R. A. (1996). A critical analysis of functional assessment: Issues for researchers and practitioners. *Behavioral Disorders, 22,* 36–40.

Garnett, M. S., & Attwood, A. J. (1998). The Australian Scale for Asperger's Syndrome. In A. J. Attwood (Ed.), *Asperger's syndrome: A guide for parents and professionals.* London: Jessica Kingsley.

Gillberg, C. (1991). Outcome in autism and autistic-like conditions. *Journal of Child and Adolescent Psychiatry, 30,* 375–382.

Gillham, J. E., Carter, A. S., Volkmar, F. R., & Sparrow, S. S. (2000). Toward a developmental operational definition of autism. *Journal of Autism and Developmental Disorders, 30,* 269–278.

Gilliam, J. E. (2001). *Gilliam Asperger Disorder Scale.* Austin, TX: Pro-Ed.

Gilliam, J. E. (2002). *Gilliam Autism Rating Scale-R.* Austin, TX: Pro-Ed.

Guralnick, M.J. (1997). Second-generation research in the field of early intervention. In M. J. Guralnick (Ed.), *The effectiveness of early intervention.* Baltimore, MD: Brookes.

Hastings, R. P., & Brown, T. (2002). Behavior problems of children with autism, parental self-efficacy, and mental health. *American Journal on Mental Retardation, 107,* 222–232.

Hauser-Cram, P., Warfield, M. E., Shonkoff, J. P., & Krauss, M. W. (2001). Children with disabilities: A longitudinal study of child development and parent well-being. *Monograph of the Society for Research in Child Development, 66,* 1–129.

Holmbeck, G. N. (1997). Toward terminological, conceptual, and statistical clarity in the study of mediators and moderators: Examples from the child-clinical and pediatric literature. *Journal of Consulting and Clinical Psychology, 65,* 599–610.

Kasari, C. (2002). Assessing change in early intervention programs for children with autism. *Journal of Autism and Developmental Disorders, 32,* 447–461.

Klin, A., Carter, A., & Sparrow, S. S. (1997). Psychological assessment. In D. J. Cohen & F. R. Volkmar (Eds.), *Handbook of autism and pervasive developmental disorders* (2nd ed.). New York: Wiley.

Klin, A., & Volkmar, F. R. (1999). Autism and other pervasive developmental disorders. In S. Goldstein & C. R. Reynolds (Eds.), *Handbook of neurodevelopmental and genetic disorders in children* (pp. 247–274). New York: Guilford Press.

Kovacs, M. (1999). *The Children's Depression Inventory (CDI).* North Tonawanda, NY: Multi-Health Systems.

Lerner, R. M. (1991). Changing organism—context relations as the basic process of development: A developmental contextual perspective. *Developmental Psychology, 27,* 27–32.

Lerner, R. M. (1996). Relative plasticity, integrity, temporality and diversity in human development: A developmental, contextual perspective about theory, process and method. *Developmental Psychology, 32,* 781–786.

Lewis, T. J., & Sugai, G. M. (1994). Functional assessment of problem behavior: A pilot investigation of the comparative and interactive effects of teacher and peer social attention on students in general education settings. *School Psychology Quarterly, 11,* 1–19.

Lonigan, C. J., Elbert, J. C., & Johnson, S. B. (1998). Empirically supported psychosocial interventions for children. *Journal of Clinical Child Psychology, 27,* 138–145.

Lord, C., Rutter, M., DiLavore, P. C., & Risi, S. (2000). *Autism Diagnostic Observation Schedule*. Los Angeles, CA: Western Psychological Services.

Medical Investigation of Neurodevelopmental Disorders Institute. (MIND). (2002). *The epidemiology of autism in California*. Davis, CA: Author.

Minuchin, P. P. (1988). Relationships within the family: A systems perspective on development. In R. A. Hinde & J. Stevenson-Hinde (Eds.), *Relationships within families: Mutual influences*. New York: Oxford University Press.

Moos, P. H., & Moos B. S. (1986). *Family Environment Scale manual*. Palo Alto, CA: Consulting Psychologists.

Myles, B., Bock, S., & Simpson, R. (1999). *Asperger Syndrome Diagnostic Scale*. Austin, TX: Pro-Ed.

National Research Council. (NRC). (2001). *Educating children with autism*. Washington, DC: National Academic Press.

Overton, W. F. (1998). Developmental psychology: Philosophy, concepts, and methodology. In W. Damon (Series Ed.) & R. M. Lerner (Vol. Ed.), *Handbook of child psychology: Vol. 1. Theoretical models of human development* (5th ed.). New York: Wiley.

Piers, E. V., & Harris, D. B. (1999). *The Piers-Harris Children's Self-Concept Scale*. Los Angeles, CA: Western Publishing Service.

Prizant, B. M., & Rubin, E. (1999). Contemporary issues in interventions for autism spectrum disorders: A Commentary. *Journal for the Association for Persons with Severe Handicaps*, 24, 199–208.

Quittner, A. L., & DiGirolamo, A. M. (1998). Family adaptation to childhood disability and illness. *Handbook of Pediatric Psychology and Psychiatry*, 2, 70–102.

Robins, D. L. (2001). The Modified Checklist for Autism in Toddlers: An initial study investigating the early detection of autism and pervasive developmental disorders. *Journal of Autism and Developmental Disorders*, 31, 131–144.

Rodriguez, C. M., & Murphy, L. E. (1997). Parenting stress and abuse potential in mothers of children with developmental disabilities. *Child Maltreatment*, 2, 245–252.

Rudolph, S., & Epstein, M. H. (2000). Empowering children and families through strength-based assessment. *Reclaiming Children and Youth*, 8, 207–209.

Schopler, E., Reichler, M. D., & Renner, B. (1988). *The Childhood Autism Rating Scale*. Los Angeles: Western Psychological Services.

Schreibman, L. (2000). Intensive behavioral and psychoeducational treatments for autism: Research needs and future directions. *Journal of Autism and Developmental Disorders*, 30, 373–378.

Schreibman, L., Heyser, L., & Stahmer, A. (1999). Autistic disorder: Characteristics and behavioral treatment. In N. A. Wieseler, R. H. Hanson, & G. Siperstein (Eds.), *Challenging behavior or persons with mental health disorders and severe developmental disabilities* (pp. 39–64). Reston, VA: American Association on Mental Retardation.

Schroeder, S. R., Reese, M., Hellings, J., Loupe, P., & Tessel, R. E. (1999). The causes of self-injurious behavior and their clinical implications. In N. A. Wieseler, R. H. Hanson, & G. Siperstein (Eds.), *Challenging behavior or persons with mental health disorders and severe developmental disabilities* (pp. 65–88). Reston, VA: American Association on Mental Retardation.

Seligman, M. (1999). Childhood disability and the family. In M. Seligman (Ed.), *Handbook of psychosocial characteristics of exceptional children* (pp. 111–131). New York: Kluwer Academic/Plenum.

Siegel, B. (2000). *The Pervasive Developmental Disorders Screening Test–II*. San Francisco, CA: Langley Porter Psychiatric Institute.

Siegel, B., Pliner, C., Eschler, J., & Elliot, G. R. (1988). How children with autism are diagnosed: Difficulties in identification of children with multiple developmental delays. *Journal of Developmental Behavioral Pediatrics*, 9, 199–204.

Sontag, J. C. (1996). Toward a comprehensive theoretical framework for disability research: Bronfenbrenner revisited. *Journal of Special Education*, 30, 319–344.

Spanier, G. B. (1976). Measuring dyadic adjustments: New scales for assessing the quality of marriage and similar dyads. *Journal of Marriage and the Family*, 38, 15–28.

Sparrow, S. S., Bala, D. A., & Cicchetti, D. V. (1984). *Vineland Adaptive Behavior Scale: Interview Edition*. Circle Pines, MN: American Guidance Service.

Stone, W. L., Coonrod, E. E., & Ousley, O. Y. (2000). Brief report: Screening Tool for Autism in Two-year-olds (STAT): Development and preliminary data. *Journal of Autism and Developmental Disorders*, 30, 607–612.

Thalen, E., & Smith, L. B. (1998). Dynamic systems theories. In W. Damon (Series Ed.) & R.M. Lerner (Vol. Ed.), *Handbook of child psychology: Vol. 1. Theoretical models of human development* (5th ed., pp. 563–634). New York: Wiley.

Turner, S., & Foong, S. (2003). Navigating the road to implementation of the Health Insurance Portability and Accountability Act. *American Journal of Public Health*, 93, 1806–1808.

U.S. Department of Education (2003). *Family Educational Rights and Privacy Act (FERPA)*. Retrieved October 3, 2003, from http:/www.ed.gov/policy/gen/guid/fpco/ferpa/index.html.

Wechsler, D. (1991). Wechsler Intelligence Scale for Children—III. San Antonio, TX: Psychological Corporation.

Wing, L. (1991). The relationship between Asperger's syndrome and Kanner's autism. In U. Frith (Ed.), *Autism and Asperger's Syndrome* (pp. 93–121). Cambridge, UK: Cambridge University Press.

Yeargin-Allsopp, M., Rice, C., Karapurkar, T., Doemberg, N., Boyle, C., & Murphy, C. (2003). Prevalence of autism in a U.S. metropolitan area. *Journal of the American Medical Association*, 289, 49–55.

PART IV

INTERVENTION AND TREATMENT RESEARCH

Introduction

C. Michael Nelson

What can be said about intervention and treatment research in the field of special education for students with emotional and behavioral disorders (EBD)? Alas, the first thing is, there hasn't been nearly enough of it. This is not to diminish the work of the many researchers who have labored throughout their careers to inform us about what works, for whom, and under what circumstances. Rather, this observation is based simply on the fact that our field has not been around for very many years. As Kauffman, Brigham, and Mock point out in Chapter 2 of this volume, experimentally verifiable interventions were not introduced until the middle of the 20th century. Prior to that time, attempts to improve the education of students with EBD were based largely on clinical intuition and psychoanalytic theory; treatment outcomes were presented as descriptive case studies (e.g., Berkowitz & Rothman, 1960; Bettelheim, 1950, 1967; Redl & Wineman, 1951). Moreover, as Steve Forness (personal communication, October 3, 2003) has observed, most of the research published in our journals focuses on diagnostic issues and characteristics of children with EBD. Intervention research requires more effort, in terms of ethical and experimental control, and more time to produce valid findings; therefore, it is less prevalent in the literature.

Fortunately, as the following chapters document, in the past 50 years much has been learned from treatment and intervention research with students who exhibit or who are at risk for EBD. Kauffman et al. (Chapter 2, this volume) acknowledge the contributions of behavioral psychology and applied behavior analysis to our knowledge of environmental variables that have functional influence on maladaptive child behavior, as well as exploring how to manipulate such factors as social attention, aversive stimuli, and instruction to achieve better educational and behavioral outcomes for our students. This is not to say that the current state of intervention science is without controversy, however. While agreement is widespread regarding desired outcomes for all students in American educational programs (i.e., literacy, productive citizenship, personal and vocational success), considerable disagreement exists with regard to specific outcomes for children and youths with EBD as a result of education and treatment programs. In the closing decades of the 20th century, educational programs were criticized as deemphasizing academic achievement while promoting behavioral control (Knitzer, 1982; Knitzer, Steinberg, & Flesch, 1990; Winett & Winkler, 1972). Although intervention research based on applied behavior analysis has been heralded for its ability to tease out functional relationships between student behavior and environmental stimuli, it also has been criticized for focusing on relatively microscopic outcomes (i.e., changes in rate and topography of specific targeted behaviors) as opposed to more "clinically significant" gains (e.g., improved adjustment, social acceptance, better quality of life, changes in clinical diagnosis, and reduced restrictiveness of educational and residential placement (Duchnowski, Kutash, & Friedman, 2002).

Much of this debate has centered on the way that student outcomes are measured. Behaviorists focus on specific target behaviors that are documented precisely; psychoeducational and medical practitioners gauge progress based on how well the student is functioning in more global terms that are measured by changes in self-concept and the perceptions of others on surveys, questionnaires, and rating scales; governments (state and federal) insist that outcomes be expressed in terms of standardized scores on norm-referenced instruments. Contributing to disagreements regarding outcomes and the measurement of outcomes is the postmodern idea that all knowledge is relative and that what can be known only amounts to personal narratives that are influenced by one's economic, racial, and other experiences (Danforth & Rhodes, 1997). Needless to say, the white noise created by these diverse perspectives makes it somewhat difficult to find a clear path through the claims and counterclaims regarding what works and what doesn't for students with EBD. A fortunate consequence of federal (No Child Left Behind Act [NCLB]) and state education improvement legislation is the creation of an expectation that practices should be supported by standards derived from scientific evidence of their effectiveness. However, most of the current standards apply to *all* students and are based on norm-referenced assessments of academic performance. As we practitioners in special education are well aware, norm-referenced standards don't match the characteristics, needs, and educational results of many children and youths with EBD. However, the field of special education has responded to the federal call for establishing standards for evidence-based practices. Groups of professionals currently are working to develop standards for validating contemporary single-subject, quantitative, and qualitative research methodologies (Odom, Gersten, Horner, Thompson, & Brantlinger, 2003).

Actually, efforts to establish standards for evidence-based practice and to identify strategies and programs that meet these standards have been in development for some time. A number of professional groups (e.g., American Federation of Teachers; Center for the Study and Prevention of Violence; Council for Exceptional Children; Division 12 Task Force of the American Psychological Association; Office of the Surgeon General; Safe, Disciplined, and Drug-Free Expert Panel; Task Force on Evidence-Based Interventions in School Psychology; U.S. Department of Education Institute of Education Sciences) have been engaged in sorting the knowledge base of practices into categories variously labeled "best practice," "promising practice," "blueprint programs," "promising programs," "empirically supported," and "well established and probably efficacious." While the criteria used to identify and classify practices vary among these initiatives, they contain several common elements: (1) the use of a sound experimental or evaluation design and appropriate analytical procedures, (2) empirical validation of effects, (3) clear implementation procedures, (4) replication of outcomes across implementation sites, and (5) evidence of sustainability. Over the years, a number of interventions used in the nation's schools, including those employed with students with EBD, have been shown to meet these criteria— among them, contingent praise, precorrection, precision requests, self-monitoring, direct instruction, curriculum-based measurement, classwide peer tutoring, group contingencies, response cost, token economies, time out, overcorrection, and some psychopharmacological interventions. Much of the research documenting the effectiveness of these interventions is reviewed in the following chapters.

These positive findings aside, a point made by Tankersley, Landrum, and Cook in Chapter 6 of this volume deserves emphasis. At the beginning of their chapter, they observe that "The base of rigorous, scientifically determined research that provides the foundation for special education is a significant achievement and signifies one of the things that is most right about the field" (p. 98). Later, they add an important caveat by Cook and Schirmer (2003) that the identification of effective practices is only meaningful to the extent that these practices are, in fact, applied (and applied with fidelity) to children and youths with disabilities. As Shakespeare would say, therein lies the rub. Tankersley and her colleagues document that we have good knowledge about what works; but, for a variety of reasons, we either fail to apply these interventions *at all*, or fail to apply them *as they were designed*. One critical issue is that practitioners are not aware of which practices are evidence-based and which are not. Tankersley et al. properly attribute this failing to teacher education and to a reliance on advertising and word-of-mouth for obtaining information rather than the research literature. Another issue is the often bemoaned tendency of interventionists not to implement behavioral interventions as they were planned and written. In my opinion, one reason that meta-analyses of psychopharmacological and behavioral interventions for attention-deficit/hyperactive disorder (ADHD) have found the former to have superior effect sizes (Forness, Kavale, & Davanzo, 2002) is that administration of a pill is regularly done with greater fidelity than implementation of a behavioral contingency.

Finally, it must be noted that there are no pat solutions—that is, interventions must be designed to fit characteristics of individual children, the settings in which interventions are applied, and the skill, willingness, and perseverance of interventionists. Given these parameters, it is unlikely that a uniformly applied, uniformly effective "packaged" intervention will ever be discovered. Consequently, despite a lack of consistently supportive evidence in the current school-based implementation literature (Sasso, Conroy, Peck Stichter, & Fox, 2001), the best advice is to develop individualized intervention plans around thorough ongoing assessments of student behavior in its relevant environmental contexts.

The chapters that follow aptly convey the diversity and range of research on interventions for students with EBD. In Chapter 17 Kimberly T. Kendziora summarizes the research documenting the deleterious effects of early-onset patterns of maladaptive and antisocial behavior in terms of their consequences for short- and long-term academic and social outcomes for children. Kendzoria also documents the negative effects of seri-

ous problem behavior on the providers of early childhood educational services, and the evidence she presents makes a strong case for improved training in behavior management procedures for all educators. She reports the findings of several meta-analyses of early childhood intervention programs specifically addressing behavior problems and points out a number of critical issues for researchers in this field. Kendziora makes the point that, especially with populations of young children, the distinction between early intervention and prevention is blurred, in that children with the most serious behavior problems tend to experience greater benefit from any kind of intervention than do children with milder forms of disordered behavior.

Dean E. Konopasek and Steven R. Forness's review of psychopharmacological treatment for children with EBD and related disorders (Chapter 18 of this volume) is important for two reasons. First, it documents the huge increase over the past decade and a half in the use of psychopharmacology in treating the broad range of children's emotional and behavioral disorders. The authors describe the emerging field of psychopharmacoepidemology, or the study of the prevalence and patterns in using psychoactive medications with children. Second, they review the various categories of medications, their indicators, effects, and side effects, as well as research documenting the outcomes of prescription drugs across many trials. Konopasek and Forness also provide a review of the Multimodal Treatment of ADHD (MTA) Study, which demonstrated that the administration of stimulant medication was significantly more effective than behavioral treatment and community care (a control group) and as effective as a combination of behavioral treatment and medication. Although such a large-scale study has yet to be conducted with other classes of psychoactive medications, the findings of the MTA study argue persuasively for greater partnerships between educational and medical interventionists.

In Chapter 19 Douglas Cheney and Michael Bullis review the research on school-to-community transition for adolescents with EBD, as well as the important issues that are raised by the postschool adjustment findings for these youths. At the beginning of their chapter, Cheney and Bullis discuss the unfortunate fact that *by law* transition services are restricted to youths who have been identified as having disabilities. They regard this as discriminating against the many youths without a disability label who nevertheless are in desperate need of assistance in making the transition from school (or incarceration) to adult life. Next, the authors summarize the historical and legal context that created a national focus on transition, and present reviews of transition research studies, including the National Longitudinal Research Study and studies conducted in several states. Anyone concerned with better outcomes for students with EBD who is not familiar with the postsecondary status of youths with emotional and behavioral challenges should read this summary carefully— but be forewarned: the findings are depressing. Fortunately, Cheney and Bullis follow this with comprehensive reviews of the research literature identifying factors that predict better outcomes and studies that document effective transition practices and programs. Their chapter concludes with a discussion of research issues and needs in the area of transition.

Chapter 20, by Nancy B. Meadows and Kay B. Stevens, offers a comprehensive review of research that focuses on teaching alternative or replacement behaviors as a strategy for intervening with individuals exhibiting a wide range of challenging behavior. Their review also provides an interesting historical account of the emergence of a focus on strengthening replacement behaviors, as opposed to simply reducing maladaptive behaviors. Meadows and Stevens's review is noteworthy too in that it documents intervention strategies based on differential reinforcement and explores the evolution of functional behavioral assessment from research involving individuals with developmental disabilities to the incorporation of functional assessment of behavior into behavior intervention planning for *all* students with disabilities, as required by the Individuals with Disabilities Act of 1997.

In Chapter 21, Lewis Polsgrove and Stephen W. Smith offer a thorough and insightful review of the research on teaching self-control to students with EBD. They provide an interesting background on the concept of self-control and the behavioral self-control processes of self-monitoring, goal setting, strategy selection and implementation, and self-evaluation and self-reinforcement. This is followed by a comprehensive review of the behavioral self-control and cognitive self-control literatures. The integration of these two lines of research in one review paper makes this a unique and engaging chapter.

Joseph C. Witt, Amanda M. VanDer Heyden, and Donna Gilbertson follow in Chapter 22 with an equally engaging analysis of the research literature on instruction and classroom management. In contrast to Lane's chapter on academic interventions (Chapter 24, this volume), Witt, VanDerHeyden, and Gilbertson focus on the research concerning *how* instruction is delivered, expectations are taught, and undesired classroom behavior is managed. These authors explicate a pyramidal model that demonstrates a hierarchical approach to addressing student behavior, from broad-based interventions that involve effective methods of delivering instruction, to teaching and reinforcing behavioral expectations and effective responses to inappropriate student behavior, and finally, to designing small-group and individual interventions based on functional behavioral assessments. This approach represents both a logical summary of the literature on these topics and a practical guide for making intervention decisions.

Chapter 23, by Kenneth A. Kavale, Sarup R. Mathur, and Mark P. Mostert, presents a review of the research on social skills training and teaching social behavior. The authors begin with a discussion of the parameters of social skills training, followed by a review of the best-researched social skills training programs, an explication of the nature of social skills deficits, and a summary of the research on teaching specific social skills. The chapter concludes with a summary of recent meta-analyses of social skills training research and a candid discussion of the experimental and social validity of the effects of such training.

Kathleen Lynne Lane's chapter on academic instruction and tutoring interventions (Chapter 24, this volume) is a thorough analysis of the recent literature covering a range of issues, including the academic characteristics of, and outcomes for, students with EBD. Lane's clear documentation that, as a group, these students present the greatest academic deficits, which are associated with the most dismal adult outcomes of any population of students with disabilities, provides a succinct justification for the current emphasis on addressing the academic needs of our student constituency. Her subsequent review of intervention research in the areas of reading, writing, and mathematics is systematic, thorough, and informative. Equally importantly, it documents the huge amount of research that remains to be done.

In Chapter 25, Carl J. Liaupsin, Kristine Jolivette, and Terrance M. Scott describe the research validating the effects of schoolwide behavior support on student behavior and school climate. The authors begin their review with a summary of evidence that the absence of proactive strategies for supporting desired behavior and responding to initial instances of disruptive behavior—and responding instead to maladaptive student behavior with harsh and inconsistent punishment—does not have a deterrent effect. Moreover, it destabilizes school climate. While the focus of this chapter is not on students with EBD specifically, Liaupsin et al. make a strong case for the logic of schoolwide prevention through universal interventions.

In the final chapter of this part, Chapter 26, Lucille Eber and Sandra Keenan shift the focus to students who present the most serious and complex intervention challenges faced by schools and other service providers—students who require highly coordinated multiagency services that address multiple life domains. Drawing upon the system of care and wraparound literature, Eber and Keenan show how the fragmented service delivery has neither served children and their families effectively in the past nor made good use of limited human and fiscal resources. They review the evolution of the system-of-care concept and how wraparound planning can be a useful tool for implementing coordinated services in school and community settings, especially when done in conjunction with the individualized education program process. Evaluation studies of system-of-care and wraparound planning are summarized, and the authors candidly describe research issues.

The recency of our field notwithstanding, the chapters in Part IV document the amazing amount and sophistication of research on treatment and interventions for students with EBD. And, while one may argue that some areas of intervention research do not receive sufficient emphasis, I believe they are an excellent sample of what we know regarding the interventions that work with our students. Moreover, these chapters (and those contained in Part V of this volume) offer much insight into the issues facing researchers, the gaps in our knowledge base, and directions for future research. In closing, it should be stressed that these chapters show not only how much has been done but also how relevant the research in any one area is to that being done in any other. Researchers and practitioners in the social sciences and helping professions have been accused of working in silos, in terms of the insularity that has typified such fields as mental health, juvenile justice, education, and medicine. Advocates for a system of care remind us of the need to remove barriers to transdisciplinary collaboration and to focus on child and family needs irrespective of the artificial boundaries established by our individual disciplines. This admonition is equally relevant to professionals working within a single discipline. Whether our focus is on academic achievement, social skills development, management of group and individual behavior, or self-mediated interventions, outcomes in any one area affect the total child. I trust that future generations of research will demonstrate that we have not overlooked this point.

REFERENCES

Berkowitz, P. H., & Rothman, E. P. (1960). *The disturbed child: Recognition and psychoeducational therapy in the classroom.* New York: New York University Press.

Bettelheim, B. (1950). *Love is not enough.* New York: Macmillan.

Bettelheim, B. (1967). *The empty fortress.* New York: Free Press.

Cook, B. G., & Schirmer, B. R. (2003). What is special about special education?: Introduction to the special series. *Journal of Special Education, 37,* 139.

Duchnowski, A. J., Kutash, K., & Friedman, R. M. (2002). Community-based interventions in a systems of care and outcomes framework. In B. Burns & K. Hoagwood (Eds.), *Community-based treatment for youth: Evidence-based interventions for severe emotional and behavioral disorders.* New York: Oxford University Press.

Forness, S. R., Kavale, K. A., & Davanzo, P. A. (2002). The new medical model: Interdisciplinary treatment and the limits of behaviorism. *Behavioral Disorders, 27,* 168–178.

Knitzer, J. (1982). *Unclaimed children: The failure of public responsibility to children and adolescents in need of mental health services.* Washington, DC: Children's Defense Fund.

Knitzer, J., Steinberg, Z., & Flesch, B. (1990). *At the school house door: An examination of programs and policies for children with behavioral and emotional problems.* New York: Bank Street College of Education.

Odom, S., Gersten, R., Horner, R., Thompson, B., & Brantlinger, E. (2003, July). *Validating evidence-based practices in special education: Multiple methodologies.* Presentation at the 2003 OSEP Research Project Directors' Conference, Washington, DC.

Redl, F., & Wineman, D. (1951). *Children who hate.* New York: Free Press.

Sasso, G. M., Conroy, M. A., Peck Stichter, J., & Fox, J. J. (2001). Slowing down the bandwagon: The misapplication of functional assessment for students with emotional or behavioral disorders. *Behavioral Disorders, 26,* 282–296.

Winett, R. A., & Winkler, R. C. (1972). Current behavior modification in the classroom: Be still, be quiet, be docile. *Journal of Applied Behavior Analysis, 5,* 499–504.

17

Early Intervention for Emotional and Behavioral Disorders

KIMBERLY T. KENDZIORA

Broadly speaking, research on early intervention is at a mature stage. We know that early intervention for children at risk due to poverty (e.g., Ramey, Campbell, & Ramey, 1999; Reynolds, Temple, Robertson, & Mann, 2001; Weikart & Schweinhart, 1992) and to low birth weight (e.g., Brooks-Gunn, Klebanov, Liaw, & Spiker, 1993) can produce lasting positive effects on cognitive development. Similarly, early intervention for young children with a range of disabilities is both well researched and widely implemented (Guralnick, 1991; Hauser-Cram, Warfield, Shonkoff, & Krauss, 2001; Shonkoff & Phillips, 2000). A current focus in early intervention research is not to determine *whether* programs work, but rather to identify *how* different types of intervention affect *specific outcomes* for children and families with varied vulnerabilities and opportunities (Guralnick, 1997; Shonkoff & Phillips, 2000).

One specific research emphasis that is receiving increasing attention in the early intervention arena is emotional or behavioral disturbance. Until relatively recently, behavior problems in early childhood such as marked noncompliance, temper tantrums, aggression, high activity level, and poor impulse control were considered to be typical of this developmental period, with few long-term implications for later adjustment. In-

deed, behavioral challenges are very common, affecting about 80% of all young children, peaking at about age 2 and declining thereafter (Tremblay et al., 1999). Pediatricians and other professionals often suggested to parents who expressed concern about these behaviors that their children would outgrow them. We now know that for some children this is not true. Without intervention, there are adverse short- and long-term outcomes of early severe emotional and behavioral problems (Campbell, 2002; Caspi, Elder, & Bem, 1987; Moffitt, 1993; Robins, 1978).

Part of the attention to early intervention for young children's behavior problems reflects the recognition of the importance that behavior plays in the education of children with or at risk of disabilities. Children's disruptive, noncompliant behavior can interfere with their learning and the learning of others. The challenges associated with educating students with severe problem behavior are substantial (Biglan, 1995; Kauffman, 1997; Sprague, Sugai, & Walker, 1998; Sugai & Horner, 1994; Walker, Colvin, & Ramsey, 1995). Although students with emotional or behavioral disturbances represent only 1–5% of a school's enrollment, they can account for more than 50% of the behavioral incidents handled by school personnel and consume significant amounts of educator and administrator time (Sugai, Sprague, Horner, & Walker, 2000; Taylor-Greene et al., 1997). The U.S. Department of Education has increasingly turned its attention to finding effective, practical strategies for addressing the urgent issue of supporting children with challenging behavior (e.g., allocating $8.7 million in 2001 to fund nine centers to study reading and behavior). One strategy for addressing challenging behavior is to provide services to children with emerging behavior problems *before school entry.*

Researchers and practitioners agree that early childhood is the best time to intervene when behavior problems are evident (Reid, 1993; Smith, 1988; Webster-Stratton & Taylor, 2001). In a meta-analysis of 80 studies of early intervention programs, Kim, Innocenti, and Kim (1997) computed and categorized 659 individual effect sizes,[1] most of which focused on cognitive benefits of early intervention. A graph of their data is presented in Figure 17.1. Essentially, Kim et al. found that, across studies, early intervention was consistently effective and produced positive effect sizes. For children with disabilities, the most powerful effects occurred when intervention began between 1½ and 3 years of age. Children with disabilities receiving intervention before 18 months of age tended to have the most severe disabilities and the worst prognoses. For children experiencing economic disadvantage, the largest effects were apparent at the earliest point of intervention. Although the authors noted

that children can benefit from intervention at any age, in general their analyses support the notion that "earlier is better." To date, very little research indicates an optimal time at intervention onset specifically for children with severely challenging behavior. Perhaps the only data come from the long-term outcome study of children from the Regional Intervention Program, in which Strain and his colleagues (Strain, Steele, Ellis, & Timm, 1982; Strain & Timm, 2001) observed that children who started the program earlier had better long-term behavioral outcomes.

The effectiveness of early intervention, taken together with the risk of poor outcomes, has made the implementation of early intervention programs for children at risk a clear national priority. In recognition of this priority, Congress mandated the Preschool Grants Program for Children with Disabilities in 1986, requiring states to make free and appropriate public education available to all children ages 3–5 with disabilities by the 1991–1992 school year. Congress also established the Early Intervention Program for Infants and Toddlers with Disabilities under Part C of the Individuals with Disabilities Education Act of 1997 (IDEA). In the 2000–2001 school year, almost 600,000 3- to 5-year-olds with disabilities were served in preschool programs (5% of the total population), and 230,853 children ages birth through 2, along with their families, were served under Part C (U.S. Department of Education, 2002). Despite the high

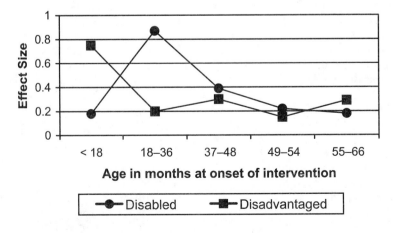

FIGURE 17.1. Early intervention effects by age of entry.

prevalence of severe behavioral challenges during this developmental period, only 1.4% of all preschoolers served under IDEA were categorized as having an emotional disturbance (U.S. Department of Education, 2002). It is very likely, however, that many of the preschoolers with speech or language impairments (55.2%) or developmental delays (24.9%) also had a variety of challenging behaviors that must be addressed for intervention to be successful (Kaiser, Cai, Hancock, Foster, & Hester, 2000).

The goal of this chapter is to provide a review of research in the field of early intervention for behavior disorders. I begin by considering the close connection between prevention and early intervention, and consider them together through the remainder of the chapter. I offer a rationale for intervening early in the development of behavior disorders and then review what effective early interventions look like and the probable pathways through which they achieve their benefits. I then identify and discuss four major areas that have been relatively underdeveloped in this research area: (1) early intervention for internalizing problems, (2) gender differences in early intervention, (3) how to disseminate effective early interventions, and (4) economic analysis of early interventions. Finally, I offer suggestions for future directions in early intervention research.

THE BLURRY LINE BETWEEN PREVENTION AND EARLY INTERVENTION

As research in early intervention has advanced, so too has prevention science. Within an educational context, prevention is generally regarded as the application of an intervention to the whole population of students rather than to specific children with problem behaviors (Colvin, Kame'enui, & Sugai, 1993). Schoolwide supports are thought to bolster the functioning of most students, with additional intervention needed for children at risk and those who are exhibiting some problems. A "triangle" diagram (depicted in Figure 17.2) that illustrates multiple levels of intervention has been widely disseminated and has been used to organize planning in many schools (Dwyer & Osher, 2000; Walker & Sprague, 1999).

Recent research on who benefits from preventive interventions blurs the lines in this diagram. Although prevention is directed nominally at those students with low risk, in multiple prevention studies, data have shown that it was the children at *highest* risk who benefited the most (Brown, 2003; Robertson, Greenberg, Kam, & Kusche, 2003). In examining the impact of a multicomponent preventive intervention for children in first and fifth grades, Stoolmiller, Eddy, and Reid (2000) found that the more aggres-

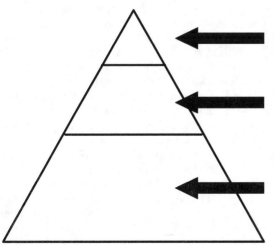

Provide Intensive Interventions
Provide coordinated, comprehensive, intensive, sustained, culturally appropriate child- and family-focused services and supports.

Intervene Early
Create services and supports that address risk factors and build upon protective factors for students at risk for severe academic or behavioral difficulties.

Build a Schoolwide Foundation
Support positive discipline, academic success, and mental and emotional wellness through a caring school environment teaching appropriate behaviors and problem-solving skills, positive behavioral support, and appropriate academic instruction.

FIGURE 17.2. A three-level approach to preventing school violence. Adapted from Dwyer and Osher (2000).

sive a child was initially, the greater the reduction in aggressive behavior at follow-up. Effect sizes ranged from essentially zero for children who were initially close to the mean to large for children who were initially highly aggressive. Similarly, Kellam and his colleagues followed students who were involved in a randomized trial of a classroom behavior management intervention implemented in first and second grades. They found that the most highly aggressive boys showed the largest improvements in off-task and disruptive behavior (Dolan et al., 1993; Kellam, Ling, Merisca, Brown, & Ialongo, 1998). At ages 19–21, the most aggressive 15% of boys who had been in the intervention condition had less substance use, antisocial personality disorder, and special education service use than controls, with no benefit either for low-risk boys or for any girls (Poduska, Kellam, Brown, Wang, & Ialongo, 2003; Schaeffer, Petras, Ialongo, Poduska, & Kellam, 2003).

Differential prevention effects have been observed in interventions outside of schools as well. In research on a home visitation program for expectant and new mothers to promote maternal and child health and prevent child abuse, benefits were most pronounced among unmarried, poor mothers (Olds, 2002; Olds et al., 1997). Center-based community preventive or early interventions also do little for low-risk children: surveys of families involved in Head Start have shown that program benefits differentially accrue to those with the most family risk factors (Zill et al., 2003).

The findings about prevention differentially benefiting high-risk children have two implications. First, it could be argued that early intervention is merely the selective application of prevention. The two types of intervention should certainly be considered together, because both benefit the same segment of the population. Second, the expectation that prevention provides some benefit to all children must be reconsidered. It may be that children at low risk simply have such low rates of the outcomes that are being prevented (e.g., aggression, low achievement) that "floor effects" make it impossible to demonstrate any intervention impact. If prevention does not affect these children, will efforts at "promotion" (e.g., of mental health or school bonding) have any impact?

One ripe area for future investigation will be what educators and social service providers can or should do to help children at low risk—those 80% at the bottom of the triangle—reach their full potential.

WHY INTERVENE EARLY?

Over the last decade, there has been an explosion in knowledge about how behavior disorders develop. The confluence of accumulating data from longitudinal studies and new methods for data analysis has enabled researchers to test specific theories of how behavior disorders emerge and change over time (Pettit & Dodge, 2003). These studies have provided an enormously compelling rationale for early intervention for behavior disorders. Seriously disruptive behavior is common enough to present challenges in every preschool or kindergarten classroom. Challenging behavior disrupts young children's school readiness, stresses teachers, and—without intervention—can become a lifelong concern.

Disruptive Behavior Is a Problem for About 10% of Young Children

Within the area of mental health concerns for preschool children, disruptive behaviors such as noncompliance, tantrums, aggression, high activity level, and poor impulse control represent the most commonly reported issues and represent the most frequent reason for referral to services (Arcelus, Gale, & Vostanis, 2001; Campbell, 2002; Costello & Janiszewski, 1990; Hoare, Norton, Chisholm, & Parry-Jones, 1996). Preschool teachers report that aggression and other disruptive behaviors are their biggest challenge in the classroom (Carpenter & Nangle, 2002; Gould, 2002). For example, Gould reported that for one Head Start grantee 60% of all disability and mental health referrals were for disruptive behavior.

In the Early Childhood Longitudinal Survey (ECLS), a nationally representative study of more than 22,000 kindergarten children, about 10% of children had challenging behavior (Raver & Knitzer, 2002; West, Denton, & Reaney, 2001; Zill & West, 2001). Teachers reported that 10% "often" or "very often" engaged in fights or easily lost their temper; according to parent reports, the rates for those items were between 15% and 33%. Parents reported that 18% of children showed signs of hyperactivity, and 13% had significant problems paying attention for sustained periods (Zill & West, 2001).

The ECLS also measured four family risk factors that are especially common among families targeted by early intervention efforts (such as Head Start): single parenthood, receipt of welfare or food stamps, mother has less than a high school education, and parent's primary language is other than English. About three-quarters of black or Latino families had one or more risk factors, compared with just over one-quarter of white families. Children from at-risk families were much more likely to be aggressive and have poor social skills.

With older children (ages 9 and up), it is possible to administer structured psychiatric interviews. Rigorous, nationally representative studies using this method have found that 10.3% of children have a disruptive behavior disorder (Shaffer et al., 1996). It is likely that the most challenging preschoolers are the same children who later meet diagnostic criteria for mental disorders. Behavior that is severe, that occurs at both home and at school, and that takes on different forms (hitting, screaming, running away) is most likely to persist (Loeber, 1990; Moffitt, 1993).

Kupersmidt and her colleagues presented these rates in a way that is especially meaningful for early childhood educators. In any classroom of about 20 children, at least two and as many as five children are likely to display noticeably and disturbingly high rates of aggressive, disruptive behavior (Kupersmidt, Bryant, & Willoughby, 2000). The challenge this represents to the teacher and to the other children can be overwhelming. Especially with an at-risk group of young children, it often takes only one child having a "wild" day to set off a chain of reactive behavior among other young children. Some teachers have good management skills and can address this—others do not. In a Baltimore study that randomly assigned children to first-grade classrooms (making the classrooms equivalent for child behavior), after 10 weeks with no intervention, about half the classrooms were fairly well managed and

half were chaotic (Kellam et al., 1998). There was little middle ground. For unprepared teachers, challenging behavior tended to overwhelm the classroom.

Challenging Behavior Impairs Children's School Readiness

Although leaders in the field of early intervention have long recognized the value of promoting early cognitive ability, recent research has highlighted the importance of also promoting early social and emotional competence for later school success (Raver & Knitzer, 2002; Shonkoff & Phillips, 2000). These findings are especially important, considering the increased emphasis on academic skills in kindergarten (Bracey, 2000). Even in early childhood settings, teachers need effective behavior management skills in order to prepare students for learning. Children who begin school with a repertoire of behaviors that are appropriate to the classroom are more ready to succeed in school.

Jimerson, Egeland, Sroufe, and Carlson (2000) showed that social and emotional factors measured during the preschool period are more powerful predictors of school dropout than later intelligence or achievement test scores. In the Head Start Family and Child Experiences Survey (FACES; Zill et al., 2003), ratings of children's behavior at the end of Head Start by parents and teachers predicted not only adjustment in kindergarten but also reading skills and general knowledge. Other studies have found strong associations from social and emotional measures beginning in the early primary grades. For example, Horn and Packard (1985) showed that poor impulse control and emotional problems in kindergarten or first grade were as good at predicting later achievement as intellectual ability and language. Griffin (1997) demonstrated that classroom behavior in kindergarten was significantly associated with reading at the end of first grade even after statistically removing the effects of IQ, mother's education, home literacy environment, entrance age, preschool experience, race, and gender. In general, research seems to show that poor socioemotional adjustment and conduct problems are associated with past, present, and future academic achievement problems

(Egeland, Kalkoske, Gottesman, & Erickson, 1990; Hinshaw, 1992; Loeber, 1990; Richman, Stevenson, & Graham, 1982).

The relation between academic achievement and challenging behavior is complex. The two tend to co-occur, even before school entry. Kaiser and her colleagues (2000) found that among 259 Head Start children those who had behavioral problems were more likely to have lower language scores than their peers without problems. Behavior problems may come first, getting in the way of learning language skills. Alternatively, poor communication skills may come first, producing behavior problems born of frustration and misunderstanding. It may be that both issues arise from common causes, such as prenatal exposure to drugs or alcohol or problematic parent–child interaction. Regardless of etiology, the co-occurrence of language delays and behavioral issues underscores the need for all educators to have a strong foundation in effective behavior management.

Another way that behavior problems impair school readiness is by interfering with the development of positive, productive peer relationships. Among preschool peers, aggressive behavior is very much noticed (Ladd & Mars, 1986) and, especially among boys, relatively stable (Ladd & Price, 1987). Aggressive behavior predicts peer rejection during both preschool (Ladd, Price, & Hart, 1988) and grade school (Coie & Kupersmidt, 1983; Dodge, 1983), which in turn is associated with a wide range of later difficulties, such as delinquency and academic failure (Campbell, 2002; Coie & Dodge, 1998; Rubin, Bukowski, & Parker, 1998). Children who are rejected by their achieving, socially skilled peers tend to flock together. These socially marginal groups become training grounds for ever more deviant behaviors (Dishion, 2000; Dishion & Andrews, 1995; Dishion, Capaldi, & Yoerger, 1999; Jessor & Jessor, 1977; La Greca, Prinstein, & Fetter, 2001; White, Pandina, & LaGrange, 1987).

Simply put, challenging behaviors get in the way of a child's ability to learn. Over time, children with socioemotional and problem behaviors at school fall further and further behind their peers. These children do not develop the motivation, concentration, and social skills necessary to be successful in school (Jimerson, Egeland, & Teo, 1999).

Challenging Behavior Wears out Teachers

The impact of challenging behavior on early childhood and primary grade staff can be profound. When staff members are continually exposed to extremely challenging behavior, the results can be early burnout, frustration, feelings of inadequacy, exhaustion, stress, anger, embarrassment, and disappointment (Strain, 2000). According to the most recent nationally representative data, among public school teachers who left the profession because of dissatisfaction with teaching as a career, student discipline problems were the number-one reason for leaving, followed by poor student motivation to learn and inadequate support from administration (National Center for Education Statistics, 1997).

When confronted with challenging behavior, teachers can find high-quality support hard to obtain. Because of the ongoing popularity of the topic of challenging behavior, the magazine of the National Association for the Education of Young Children (*Young Children*), the most widely read publication for early childhood teachers, has published many articles on how to address challenging behavior in the classroom (e.g., Bakley, 2001; Gartrell, 2001, 2002; Heath, 1994; Honig & Wittmer, 1996; Marshall, 1995; Ratcliff, 2001; Reinsberg, 1999; Schreiber, 1999; Watson, 2003). However, much of this advice reflects at best an incomplete understanding of the evidence base for best practices in behavior management. Perhaps because of the prevalence of unsupported advice or perhaps because of no advice at all, some teachers respond in ways that make matters worse. Teachers often reject children who behave in antisocial ways (Kupersmidt & Coie, 1990; Ladd, Birch, & Buhs, 1999; Shores & Wehby, 1999). In chaotic classrooms, researchers have observed low rates of teacher praise and little emphasis on individual responsibility and social competence, with the most challenging students receiving less support, nurturing, positive feedback, and instruction, as well as more criticism (Arnold et al., 1999; Brophy,

1996; McEvoy & Welker, 2000; Raver & Knitzer, 2002; Walker et al., 1995).

One outcome of teacher fatigue with challenging behavior is that aggressive children frequently are expelled from classrooms. In one Seattle clinic serving families of children ages 3–7 with conduct problems, more than 50% of the children had been asked to leave three or more schools by second grade (Webster-Stratton & Reid, 2002). The lack of teacher support and exclusion from the classroom lead to social and academic difficulties and contribute to the likelihood of future school dropout.

Without Intervention, Challenging Behavior Can Become a Lifelong Problem

The most compelling reason to intervene with early disruptive behavior is that, for some children, challenging behavior will become chronic, leading to poor academic, social, and personal outcomes. In one study, more than half of children ages 2–3 with a mental health disorder continued to have a disorder at ages 4–5, and two-thirds of 4- to 5-year-olds with disorders had similar diagnoses later on (Lavigne et al., 1998). Shaw and his colleagues (Shaw, Gilliom, Ingoldsby, & Nagin, 2003) have documented the continuity of behavior problems among very young boys. These researchers followed a sample of low-income mothers and their infant boys from ages 1½ to 8. Of 284 boys, 16 (5.6%) displayed chronically high levels of conduct problems over five waves of assessment. In comparison, 81% of boys had moderate or high levels of disruptive behavior at ages 2–3½ that declined markedly by age 8. Fourteen percent of boys had low levels of conduct problems in toddlerhood that virtually disappeared by age 8. In addition to identifying developmental trajectories of aggression from toddlerhood to middle childhood, Shaw et al. examined variables that predicted early and persistent aggression. After statistically controlling for variance associated with children's preschool verbal IQ, maternal age, and maternal education, boys' high levels of behavior problems at age 2 were predicted by their fearlessness as observed in a laboratory task and by mothers' depressive symptoms during

their sons' toddlerhood. The *persistence* of high levels of conduct problems from ages 1½ to 8 was predicted by fearlessness and observed maternal rejecting parenting. Thus, both individual and relationship variables may be important in identifying young children who will have ongoing problems with behavior.

The pattern of *ongoing* physical aggression observed by Shaw et al. (2003) is especially predictive of later social and personal problems. Recently, researchers from the United States, Canada, and New Zealand combined data from six longitudinal studies. Each study contained data on disruptive behavior problems beginning in early childhood and continuing at least until adolescence (Broidy et al., 2003). Chronic physical aggression during the elementary school years specifically increased the risk for both violent and nonviolent delinquency. Physical aggression retained its significant and independent influence on violent and nonviolent offending even when the potentially confounding influence of other disruptive behaviors was statistically controlled. In each of the six data sets, statistical modeling showed that a small group of boys—ranging from 4% to 10% of the samples—engaged in consistently high levels of physical aggression. Every study site also had a relatively large group of boys (the size varied from 15% to 60%) who engaged in almost no physical aggression, ever.

In the long term, then, young children whose disruptive behavior is severe and persistent are especially likely to have ongoing problems. More than half (53%) of children rated as having troublesome disruptive behavior by their kindergarten through third-grade teachers met psychiatric criteria for a disruptive behavior disorder at age 17½ (Egeland, Pianta, & Ogawa, 1996). In another study, children with very difficult temperaments at age 3 (10% of all children in a study of 1,037 children representative of the population) were interviewed at age 21 (Newman, Caspi, Moffitt, & Silva, 1997). The adults who had been difficult preschoolers reported higher levels of interpersonal conflict at home and in their romantic relationships. They were more likely to have been fired from a job, were more likely to have been victims of crime, and had the highest levels of adult antisocial behavior. Peers described them as unreliable and corroborated this profile of conflicted interpersonal adjustment across social contexts.

EFFECTIVE EARLY INTERVENTIONS FOR BEHAVIOR DISORDERS

Given the long-term significance of early challenging behavior, the importance of identifying effective interventions becomes paramount. Very few intervention studies have focused on preschoolers with challenging behavior who were otherwise typically developing, and published studies have generally shown modest results, even for lengthy interventions (Bryant, Vizzard, Willoughby, & Kupersmidt, 1999; Campbell, 2002). Well-developed, well-studied interventions have traditionally focused on the family and home setting for treating aggressive behavior in preschool-age children (e.g., Brestan & Eyberg, 1998; Patterson, Reid, & Dishion, 1992; Webster-Stratton, Hollinsworth, & Kolpacoff, 1989), whereas center-based intervention programs have more often focused on cognitive goals (e.g., Campbell & Ramey, 1995; Weikart, & Schweinhart, 1992). Ironically, cognitive-driven interventions that have also included social and emotional components (such as the Perry Preschool) have achieved some of their largest effects in the domain of social and behavioral adjustment, including reduced criminal behavior (Shonkoff & Phillips, 2000; Weikart, 1998).

Specific early intervention programs for behavior disorders that have been shown to be effective are reviewed in some detail in Conroy, Hendrickson, and Hester (Chapter 11, this volume). These include the *Regional Intervention Program* (Strain et al., 1982; Strain & Timm, 2001), *Incredible Years* (Webster-Stratton et al., 1989; Webster-Stratton, Reid, & Hammond, 2001), *First Steps to Success* (Golly, Sprague, Walker, Beard, & Gorham, 2000; Walker et al., 1998), and the *Fast Track Project* (Conduct Problems Prevention Research Group, 2000, 2002a). A comprehensive description of 32 effective prevention programs for school-age children may be found in Greenberg, Domitrovich, and Bumbarger (2000). Carey (1997) succinctly described the specific elements of effective behavioral interventions for preschool children, such as differential reinforcement, modeling, planned ignoring, reprimands, and time out.

In this section, rather than discussing individual early intervention programs, I will focus on what has been learned from meta-analyses and research syntheses of the early intervention literature. Specifically, what characteristics of early intervention programs are associated with effectiveness? And by what mechanisms do programs achieve their effects?

Characteristics of Effective Early Intervention

Although meta-analysis is often used to address the question of whether some intervention "works" in the global sense, when large numbers of studies are included, the relation between individual characteristics of those studies and observed effect sizes can be discerned. A pair of large meta-analyses published by Durlak and Wells (1997, 1998) provided exactly this kind of detail about qualities of preventive and early interventions for behavior disorders. Durlak and Wells (1997) coded 177 published prevention studies with respect to how the target population was selected (universal/all children, selective/at-risk children, or those about to experience some transition or milestone), whether the goal was change within individuals or change in an environment, and whether outcomes involved decreased problems or increased competencies. They found that most prevention programs both reduced children's problems and improved their competencies, with the average program participant surpassing the performance of 59–82% of those in control conditions. The effect sizes were comparable to those attained in well-established social and medical interventions. Prevention efforts aimed at teaching children ages 2–7 about feelings and behavior achieved an effect size of .70, and those teaching problem solving to children at these ages had an effect of .93—both very large effects. Prevention aimed at changing classrooms or schools had a mean effect size of .35, and interventions preparing children for school entry had an effect of .39. Overall, preventive interventions adopting a behavioral approach were more effective than were those adopting nonbehavioral methods (.49 vs. .25).

Durlak and Wells also examined results across 130 studies intervening with children who, based on some screening measure, showed some early signs of problems ("indicated prevention" in public health terms [Mrazek & Haggerty, 1994] also known as "secondary prevention"; Durlak & Wells, 1998). These interventions include the Primary Mental Health Project (Cowen et al., 1996), which began in 1957 and is currently implemented in over 300 schools across four states. This intervention involves systematic, brief screening of all primary school children and the subsequent provision of both direct and consultative services by trained nonprofessional "child associates." Other programs have targeted students' depression (Reynolds & Coats, 1986), aggression (Lochman, Burch, Curry, & Lampron, 1984), or social isolation (Gresham & Nagle, 1980). In their meta-analysis of these interventions, Durlak and Wells (1998) found very positive effects of such interventions overall, with particularly strong effect sizes for behavioral and cognitive-behavioral interventions (mean effect sizes of .51 and .53, vs. .27 for nonbehavioral interventions) and for interventions directed at disruptive or externalizing behavior problems (.72) compared to emotional or internalizing problems (.49), poor peer relations (.30), or low academic achievement (.26). Interventions targeting children under age 7 were the most powerful (.63, vs. .28 for children ages 7–11 and .43 for children over age 11).

Narrative syntheses of early intervention research have also illuminated program characteristics that are associated with effectiveness. Ramey and Ramey (1998), for example, enumerated six principles for maximizing the effectiveness of early intervention.

• *Principle 1: developmental timing.* Interventions that begin earlier in development and continue longer produce the greatest benefits.
• *Principle 2: program intensity.* Programs that involve greater contact time (more home visits per week, center hours per day, days per week, and weeks per year) produce larger positive effects than do less intensive interventions. In addition, the participants receiving the highest "dosage" of the intervention (those who attend regularly and participate actively) show the greatest developmental progress.
• *Principle 3: direct (vs. intermediary) provision of learning experiences.* For early intervention programs aimed at producing cognitive gains, providing direct educational experiences yields larger and longer-lasting benefits than does providing parent training to indirectly improve children's competence.
• *Principle 4: program breadth and flexibility.* Interventions that provide more comprehensive services (education, health, and social services) and use multiple routes to enhance children's development (working with both children and parents) generally have larger effects than do interventions that are narrower in focus.
• *Principle 5: individual differences in program benefits.* Children benefit from early intervention in a curvilinear fashion with respect to initial risk. Children with high biological risk or more severe disabilities do not benefit very much. As noted earlier, children at low risk also show little benefits. Children at high but not extreme risk seem to show the greatest benefit from early intervention or prevention.
• *Principle 6: environmental maintenance of development.* Program benefits diminish over time in the absence of environmental supports.

The more of these principles embodied by a given early intervention program, the more likely it is that the program will be effective.

Mechanisms of Early Intervention

In his comprehensive review of early family support and education interventions to prevent behavior disorders and delinquency, Yoshikawa (1994) identified two pathways through which early intervention programs are presumed to achieve their effects. One is the cognitive/school pathway, and another is the parenting/family pathway. The two pathways correspond roughly to two models of early intervention, with center-based early childhood education affecting cognitive development and school achievement, whereas home-based early family support affects parenting, child maltreatment, parental educational level, and attachment.

The cognitive/school pathway supposes that early interventions improve school readiness, which produces a positive reaction on the part of kindergarten teachers, followed by stronger bonding to school and better academic performance (Berrueta-Clement, Schweinhart, Barnett, & Weikart, 1987). Ramey and Ramey (1998) noted that early intervention that provides an educational foundation can increase children's intellectual skills so that they gain more from their experiences, as well as motivate children to seek out learning experiences. These variables are important for ongoing behavioral disorders. The theory underlying the Seattle Social Development project posits that promoting academic success in vulnerable children reduces the likelihood of delinquency, substance abuse, teen sexual activity, and violence (Hawkins, 1997). In the Chicago Longitudinal Study, children who completed preschool and kindergarten in Child–Parent Centers (and were provided with additional services in grades 1–3) had a significantly lower rate of juvenile arrests and significantly lower rates of grade retention and special education placement (Reynolds et al., 2001). In a separate longitudinal study that did not provide intervention, low IQ and need for remedial education at age 10 were shown to be powerful predictors of delinquency and adult criminal behavior (Werner & Smith, 1992).

The parenting/family pathway presumes that through family support and/or parent training, parents become better at socializing their children throughout childhood. When center-based programs such as High/Scope or Head Start promote active parental involvement, parents gain experience building proactive relationships with teachers that can support later academic performance (Zigler, Taussig, & Black, 1992). Parents' participation in intervention may help them adopt and support the kinds of behavioral expectations that will reduce the risk of later antisocial behavior. Parents may also have greater awareness of, and more actively promote, environmental opportunities for positive development (e.g., enrichment programs at school, positive peer groups) (Ramey & Ramey, 1998).

A third pathway through which early intervention may achieve improvements in young children's development is by directly affecting children's social and emotional functioning (Denham & Weissberg, in press). Children who become more aware of themselves, able to express emotions appropriately, and more aware of social conventions are likely to have more positive relationships with adults and peers, and will be more ready to participate productively in school. Adults can promote these qualities by responding sensitively to children, offering positive guidance with clear rules and limits, explicit teaching about emotions and behavior, modeling appropriate behaviors, and contingently responding to children's behavior (Denham & Weissberg, in press). Early intervention of this type may make children more willing and capable of meeting the behavioral standards set by parents, teachers, and other adults (Zigler et al., 1992). When children are given opportunities for successful involvement in social activities at a time in their lives when they are forming their identities, this could trigger a cycle of positive social exchange. With better socioemotional skills, children can access more facilitative teachers, parents, and peers (Ramey & Ramey, 1998).

ISSUES IN EARLY INTERVENTION RESEARCH

Despite the relatively advanced stage of early intervention research in general, several gaps in understanding remain. These include early intervention for internalizing problems, gender issues in early intervention, how to effectively disseminate and "scale up" effective early interventions, and economic analysis in early intervention research. The research that has been conducted in these areas has raised significant issues. I address each of these issues in turn.

Early Intervention for Internalizing Problems

To date, much more research attention has been devoted to understanding, treating, and preventing externalizing problems (disruptive behavior) than emotional problems such as anxiety, depression, and social withdrawal (National Advisory Mental Health Council Workgroup on Mental Disorders

Prevention Research, 1998). There have been both social and scientific reasons for this gap. First, studying anxiety and depression has not generally been a research priority because internalizing disorders tend not to be distressing to others—they're easier to ignore. Further, internalizing symptoms are differentially associated with personal qualities that tend to be valued by academic researchers, such as a scholastic orientation and meticulousness. For example, Weir and Gjerde (2002) asked nursery school teachers to classify children's preschool personalities using a Q-sort technique. Ten years later, the "overcontrolled" preschoolers were shy and restrained but also conscientious and intelligent. Prinstein and La Greca (2002) assessed 246 children in grades 4–6 and again 6 years later. Those children who identified with the peer group known as the "Brains" exhibited *increases* in internalizing distress between childhood and adolescence, whereas "Populars/Jocks" experienced significant *decreases* in internalizing distress across development.

A second social reason for the relative paucity of research on early interventions for internalizing disorders may be that they are more prevalent among girls than boys (e.g., Keiley, Lofthouse, Bates, Dodge, & Pettit, 2003), while research positions remain differentially populated by males (Task Force on Women in Academe, 2000). Gender bias has been implicated in the underrepresentation of women in heart disease research—a problem so serious that Congress enacted legislation in 1993 explicitly requiring the inclusion of women in clinical trials. It may also be that gender bias has contributed to the relative underdevelopment of research on internalizing problems.

There is also some scientific rationale for the lack of research on early interventions for internalizing behavior disorders. First, prevention or early intervention for internalizing problems may not be regarded as a high priority because some emotional disorders are regarded as very easy to treat when they emerge, responding to most active interventions (especially depression and simple phobias; Compton, Burns, Egger, & Robertson, 2002). Internalizing disorders may be harder to detect in early stages, as they are more weakly predicted from risk factors than are externalizing disorders (Ihle, Esser,

Schmidt, & Blanz, 2002). Even well-established constructs such as behavioral inhibition (e.g., Kagan, 1989) do not always predict later disorder (Kerr, Tremblay, Pagani, & Vitaro, 1997).

Whatever the reasons for the lack of research to date on early intervention for internalizing problems, the need for such work is clear. Anxiety disorders are the most prevalent mental disorders in childhood and adolescence, affecting about 13% of children (Costello et al., 1996). Further, between 10% and 15% of children and adolescents have some symptoms of depression (Smucker, Craighead, Craighead, & Green, 1986), and 5% have full-fledged major depression (Shaffer et al., 1996). Effective early interventions for internalizing problems could benefit very needy populations. Internalizing problems have been associated with a history of having a lower-quality physical home environment, maternal emotional unresponsiveness, and fewer stimulating experiences (Eamon, 2000). Bolger and Patterson (2001) showed, using a prospective longitudinal design, that parental neglect led to greater internalizing problems in primary school-age children. Fox and Calkins (1993; also Calkins & Fox, 2002) have shown in their research that socially withdrawn children not only were fearful of novelty as infants but also tended to have social histories including rejection and an ambivalent relationship with an insensitive parent. Thus, children with internalizing behavior disorders may benefit from early intervention efforts that include both individual and family components.

To date, there have been two studies examining preventive or early interventions for internalizing disorders among preschoolers and six investigating school-age children. First, LaFreniere and Capuano (1997) randomly assigned 42 anxious/withdrawn preschoolers either to an intervention targeting parent–child attachment or to a control group. Mothers in the intervention group showed more appropriate levels of control and less parental stress, and intervention children showed increased cooperation and enthusiasm, during mother–child interaction. Preschool teacher ratings showed significant improvement in children's social competence but not in their anxious and withdrawn behavior, although the latter did improve somewhat. Rapee and Jacobs (2002) pilot-tested a prevention program aimed at training parents of seven temperamentally anxious boys to reduce their young children's withdrawn and inhibited behaviors. The six-session cognitive-behavioral program addressed parental overinvolvement, modeling of anxiety, parent anxiety reduction, and exposure. Results showed marked changes in mothers' perceptions of withdrawn temperament and anxious symptoms that continued over the following 6 months. These data encourage a larger-scale investigation of parent education for the reduction of inhibited temperament in preschool children.

Among school-age children, six larger studies have been conducted. The only one to attempt to prevent an internalizing disorder (in this case, depression) among a whole school population was not successful (Clarke, Hawkins, Murphy, & Sheeber, 1993; they tried brief educational and behavioral skills curricula). Interventions applied to children who were selected through some screening procedure have been effective for both anxiety and depressive disorders. Of the remaining studies, three have been aimed at anxiety and two at depression.

To prevent anxiety, the Queensland Early Intervention and Prevention of Anxiety Project screened 1,786 7- to 14-year-old children and then assigned 128 of them to a 10-week combined child and parent cognitive-behavioral intervention or to a monitoring group (Dadds, Holland, Laurens, Mullins, Barrett, & Spence, 1999). Although both groups showed improvement at posttreatment, the group receiving the intervention was doing significantly better at 6-month and 2-year follow-ups. Another controlled trial (Roberts, Kane, Thomson, Bishop, & Hart, 2003) evaluated a preventive health curriculum aimed at reducing depressive and anxious symptoms in rural seventh graders. No intervention effects were found for depression, but children in the intervention group reported less anxiety than the control group after the program and at 6-month follow-up. Finally, among 489 sixth graders, Barrett and Turner (2001) also found that a 12-session cognitive-behavioral intervention reduced symptoms of anxiety at postintervention compared to controls.

Prevention of depressive symptoms among at-risk children has also proven successful. The Penn Depression Prevention Program targeted cognitive distortions among fifth- and sixth-grade students reporting either elevated depressive symptoms or high levels of parental marital conflict and low family cohesion. Initial results showed fewer self-reported depressive symptoms among intervention children (Jaycox, Reivich, Gillham, & Seligman, 1994). Continued follow-up across 2 years showed that, although depressive symptoms increased significantly over time for both the intervention and comparison groups, the children who received the intervention continued to have fewer symptoms than those who did not (Gillham, Reivich, Jaycox, & Seligman, 1995). In another intervention study, Clarke et al. (1995) implemented an early intervention with a sample of 9th- and 10th-grade suburban students with elevated depressive symptoms (but not disorder). They offered a 15-session cognitive-behavioral program. Although there were no significant differences at the end of the intervention, survival analyses that included assessments through 12 months postintervention indicated that there were significantly fewer youths with psychiatric diagnoses of major depressive disorder or dysthymia in the experimental condition compared to the controls.

A relatively more mature research area related to early intervention with internalizing disorders is suicide prevention. Recent summary reports of suicide prevention and intervention have arisen from such august institutions as the Institute of Medicine (Goldsmith, Pellmar, Kleinman, & Bunney, 2002), the U.S. Surgeon General (U.S. Public Health Service, 1999), and the government of British Columbia (White & Jodion, 1998). A collaborative of five U.S. government agencies has produced a *National Strategy for Suicide Prevention*, with its own website (*http://www.Mentalhealth.samhsa.gov/suicideprevention/*) and attendant resource center (*http://www.sprc.org/*). Despite this abundance of information and guidance, programs such as school-based suicide education programs and telephone hotlines that have little evidence supporting their efficacy are still relatively common (Burns & Patton, 2000). Even in more fully developed areas of research such as this, more work remains to be done.

Gender Differences in Early Intervention

Another gap in our understanding of early intervention has to do with differential effects of interventions on girls versus boys. Some preventive or early interventions have found effects for boys but not girls (e.g., Kellam et al., 1998); others have found equivalent effects for both boys and girls (e.g., Webster-Stratton et al., 2001); still others have excluded girls entirely because girls have fewer conduct problems to prevent (e.g., Tremblay, Masse, Pagani, & Vitaro, 1996). We know that gender differences in the prevalence of behavior disorders are robust, particularly for aggressive and depressive disorders (Crick & Zahn-Waxler, 2003; Eagly, 1987; Eagly & Steffen, 1986; Hyde, 1984; Kendziora et al., 2003; Maccoby & Jacklin, 1974, 1980). Why these differences exist and what implications this has for intervention have yet to be untangled.

For externalizing behavior, gender differences seem to be more closely tied to level or prevalence than to type or course of behavior. For example, Kendziora et al. (2003) examined the structure and development of teacher-rated aggression from first grade to middle school. The factor structure and developmental patterns were the same for boys and girls, but more boys than girls were aggressive, and when a child was aggressive, boys were more aggressive than girls were: the median level of boys' aggression was the same as the top quartile for girls'. Moffitt and Caspi (2001) found a similar result examining the development of antisocial behavior from ages 3 to 21 in a large community sample. They identified two pathways. *Life-course-persistent* antisocial behavior is associated with a high-risk early childhood, including poor parenting, neurocognitive problems, poor temperament, and behavior problems. In contrast, *adolescence-limited* antisocial behavior is associated with normal early childhood adaptation followed by association with delinquent peers in adolescence. Moffitt and Caspi showed that boys and girls showed the same patterns of risk and behavior but in very different numbers. Boys in the life-course-persistent pattern outnumbered girls by 10 to 1, with only 6 girls in the sample of 1,037 fitting this developmental pattern. The authors observed that little girls were less likely than were little boys to experience the early risks characteristic of the life-course-persistent pattern. In contrast, the male-to-female ratio for the adolescence-limited pattern was only 1.5 to 1, showing that adolescence is an especially sensitive period for the manifestation of externalizing problems in girls.

With respect to the development of internalizing disorders, Nolen-Hoeksema and Girgus (1994) reviewed the literature on the development of depression and concluded that the higher prevalence of depression among females beginning in adolescence occurs because girls are more likely than boys to carry risk factors for depression in earlier childhood. The risk factors cited included being unassertive, having a coping style that involves focusing on distress and passively ruminating about it rather than taking action, and focusing more on reciprocity than dominance in interpersonal interactions. Crick and Zahn-Waxler (2003) summarized a line of research showing that anxiety in childhood, which is also more common among girls (Zahn-Waxler, Klimes-Dougan, & Slattery, 2000), is a precursor to the development of problems with depression in adolescence and is another clear risk factor. They also argued that more research is needed to fully understand how girls' strong relational orientation can both exacerbate and protect them from the development of different kinds of disorders.

Dissemination and Going to Scale

Although early intervention is a mature field, the gap between research and practice is as much in evidence in this area as it is for other areas of behavior disorders. Researchers have tended to produce books, articles, and conference presentations that never leave the ivory tower. The audience for their work has often been limited to other researchers, scientific grant-giving agencies, tenure review boards, and graduate students. Practitioners who are absorbed in the daily demands of service provision (and perhaps under pressure to bill as many hours as possible) often have not found the time to read the journals that could support their work. When they do turn to the literature, they too often find it impenetrable or irrelevant.

Over the last decade or so, this situation has begun to change. In part, this change is in response to the unpleasant discovery that many interventions for a variety of mental and behavioral disorders work better in research-based settings than in community clinic settings (Henggeler, Melton, Brondino, Scherer, & Hanley, 1997; Weisz, Weiss, & Donenberg, 1992), and improving access to community interventions does not lead to improvement in children's behavior (Bickman, Guthrie, & Foster, 1995). Also contributing to this change is the rise of family advocacy within mental health, which results in demands for increased accountability on the part of community service providers (Hernandez & Hodges, 2001; Hoagwood, Jensen, Petti, & Burns, 1996; Stroul & Friedman, 1994).

The demand for accountability has led to the creation of numerous lists of "effective" or "evidence-based" interventions aimed at a variety of behavior disorders, but especially delinquency, violence, and/or drug use. The tremendous overlap in risk and protective factors for these problems means that the same interventions can address multiple concerns (Catalano, Berglund, Ryan, Lonczak, & Hawkins, 2002; Egeland et al., 1996). Because these concerns cross disciplinary and federal agency boundaries, multiple lists from multiple sources have included the same intervention programs, sometimes with different ratings (e.g., "promising" in one place but "model" in another). A very useful compilation of such lists may be found on the website of the Center for the Study and Prevention of Violence, at *http://www.colorado.edu/cspv/blueprints/matrix/matrix.pdf*. A major new effort to sort through the clutter in understanding what works is the U.S. Department of Education's new What Works Clearinghouse (*www.w-w-c.org*), which will apply uniform scientific standards to a wide range of educational interventions. Among the interventions reviewed during their first year (2003) are interventions to reduce delinquent, disorderly, and violent behavior.

Now that more is known about effective preventive and early interventions, the pressing challenge is to disseminate these interventions more widely. Schools and other community institutions have faced many challenges in maintaining "best practices" (Elias & Clabby, 1992; Gottfredson, 2001; Meyer, Miller, & Herman, 1993). For example, fewer than half of the schools involved in the Child Development Project achieved widespread changes in program practices by the end of 3 years of intervention (Battistich, Schaps, Watson, Solomon, & Lewis, 2000).

In a review of factors explaining why school-based prevention efforts do not work as well as they should, Gottfredson (2001) identified factors of the programs themselves, of schools, and of external pressures that affect implementation and maintenance. For example, school staff members must themselves perceive a real *need* for the program before they will implement it, especially if the program is complex or time-consuming. Too often, programs are handed down from administrators who do not take the time to listen to teachers and principals, understand their concerns and priorities, and ensure their buy-in. Effective dissemination requires that interventions be shaped from the very beginning by the end users (Jensen, 2003; Schoenwald & Hoagwood, 2001). Accordingly, some researchers have begun do devote specific attention to the development of community and institutional partnerships to support the successful implementation of preventive or early interventions (Conduct Problems Prevention Research Group, 2002b; Kellam, 2000).

In a provocative article, Rotheram-Borus and Duan (2003) identified four barriers to broad dissemination of effective interventions. These included (1) a researcher-driven system that relies on highly persistent individuals who devote their careers to the replication of their programs; (2) theoretical models that identify how targeted outcomes develop but not how they can change or be treated once developed; (3) lack of detail on how change is maintained over time; and (4) emphasis on "replication with fidelity" that does not allow local adaptation. Rotheram-Borus and Duan cited alternative models of successful intervention dissemination that involve either specified delivery models (e.g., D.A.R.E., Bureau of Justice Assistance, 1995, a generally ineffective program, is delivered by police departments and reaches 26 million children in the United States and 10 million internationally *per year*) or private enterprise (e.g., self-help books or groups such as Weight Watchers®).

Another model for the dissemination of effective services is through policy. Hawaii is currently engaged in a statewide effort to improve mental health practice for children by identifying evidence-based practices and launching a large-scale systematic training effort to support their use (Chorpita et al., 2002; Hawaii Department of Health, 2003). Through collaboration among the state's Department of Health, a university, and a family advocacy organization, research on effective psychosocial and pharmacological interventions for behavior disorders is continually reviewed and lists of effective treatments continually updated. Evaluation of this project's impact is still required (Jensen, 2002).

Economic Research in Early Intervention

If policymakers are to support the implementation of evidence-based preventive or early interventions for behavior disorders, research in this area must be more relevant to their needs. One way to bridge the research–policy gap is to include economic evaluation in research on early intervention. Economic evaluation asks, "Is a preventive or early intervention program 'worth it'?" (See also Quinn & Poirier, Chapter 5, this volume.) Statistically significant effects on targeted outcomes alone do not allow policymakers to judge whether the intervention is a good use of society's limited resources. Some prevention programs may take a broad approach and extend intervention to many individuals who would not develop problems even in the absence of the intervention. Interventions that require parents to leave work in order to participate in sessions may be costly due to lost wages. Moreover, some early intervention efforts are extravagantly expensive: the cost of implementing the Fast Track prevention program is about $40,000 for each high-risk child (Foster, Dodge, & Jones, 2003). Clearly, policymakers need guidance beyond effect sizes in order to make decisions about allocating resources.

Three early childhood programs have produced sound economic evaluations. Karoly and his colleagues (1998) summarized the economic research for two of these: the Perry Preschool program and the Elmira

Prenatal/Early Infancy project. The former was a center-based program for preschool children plus home visits for families aimed at promoting school achievement. The latter was a nurse home-visiting program to promote better health and parenting among poor, single mothers. Karoly et al. were interested in determining whether public funding of early intervention was warranted, and identified four types of savings to the government:

1. Increased tax revenues, resulting from increased employment by children and parents who had formerly been served by the program.
2. Decreased welfare outlays to participants plus reduced administrative costs.
3. Reduced expenditures for education, health, and other services (e.g., special education, emergency room visits, and stays in homeless shelters).
4. Lower criminal justice system costs (arrest, adjudication, and incarceration expenses).

Many program outcomes, such as personal well-being and higher IQs, produce savings that cannot be easily quantified. In addition, economic analyses are limited to the measured follow-up period.

Barnett (1993) conducted an economic analysis of the Perry Preschool program based on 25-year follow-up data. Karoly et al. (1998) adjusted the figures to 1996 dollars for their analysis, and showed that the savings to the government were $25,437 and the cost was $12,148, yielding a net savings of $13,289; a 2:1 ratio. Savings are due to benefits that occur as program children move from adolescence to adulthood: 40% of government savings was due to reduction in criminal justice cost, 26% to taxes on increased income, 25% to reduction in education services, and 9% due to reduction in welfare cost. There were no measurements of benefits to mothers, which could have dramatically increased the savings estimate.

For the Elmira program, data collected at an age 15 follow-up (Olds et al., 1997) allowed Karoly et al. to calculate that for high-risk families total savings for both child and mother were $24,694, compared to total cost of $6,083, yielding savings of $18,611 per family. This is a savings ratio of

4:1. More than 80% of the savings were due to behavior of the mother during the first 15 years of the child's life (mothers receiving the intervention were employed more and on welfare less). Most of the child savings were due to less crime over the child's lifetime. For lower-risk families involved in the project, there were no net savings.

A third early childhood intervention with a sound economic analysis is the Chicago Parent–Child Centers program (Reynolds et al., 2001). This school-based preschool plus follow-on program has operated continuously since 1967 in disadvantaged neighborhoods. In 1998 dollars (earlier figures were 1996 dollars), the program cost $9,931 per child and yielded $19,970 in government savings (reduction in use of educational services and criminal justice, plus taxes from increased employment)—a 2:1 ratio (Reynolds, 2000).

To date, there have been no economic analyses of programs targeting children with emerging behavior disorders, but at least two such efforts are under way. Foster (2002) is currently working on an economic evaluation of a preschool intervention with parent, teacher, and child components aimed at preventing conduct problems (the Incredible Years; Webster-Stratton et al., 2001). This analysis will include a fairly broad range of outcomes collected through grades 2–4 (including child behavior and health; educational, mental health, and social service use; parental employment; and caregiver strain). Kendziora (Bowdish, Albright, Bush, Kelly, & Kendziora, 2003) will conduct a limited economic evaluation of an intensive preschool intervention program for children with challenging behavior. She will include only educational outcomes (special education service use, disciplinary referrals, grades, test scores, graduation) but will have data at least through middle school on most students.

Across the few rigorous economic evaluations done to date, the conclusion that government savings ultimately exceed costs for early intervention programs means that public investment in these programs can be justified. There are additional monetary benefits to society for early interventions, as well as intangible benefits (i.e., well-being) that improve the value of such investments (Karoly et al., 1998). There are some areas of early

intervention programming that require further research in order to best inform policy. These include how to decide which services should be provided and at what developmental stage, and how best to target interventions to those who will benefit most.

FUTURE DIRECTIONS

Because of the relatively advanced stage of research in this area, I am relieved of the usual task of concluding with the blanket statement "more research needs to be done." More work *is* needed, but it needs to reflect the way this field has evolved and the new priorities of connecting research to practice and policy. Too much work has focused on developing new programs at the expense of disseminating effective interventions. Based on a scan of 1,034 federal initiatives related to prevention or early intervention across mental health, education, justice, and child welfare, Kendziora and Osher (1999) concluded, "Given the great overlap across agencies in the development of interventions, it may perhaps be time to slow down the development of new interventions, and proceed with the dissemination and much needed training in existing interventions that are known to work" (p. 10).

Practice in early intervention is also very well developed in the United States. Because of funding through the Individuals with Disabilities Education Act, Part C (for infants and toddlers with disabilities) and Part B (which includes preschoolers with disabilities), there is already an extensive network of providers and funding infrastructure supporting early intervention practice. Additionally, Early Head Start, Head Start, and many state prekindergarten programs provide a variety of early intervention services for young children who are at risk of poor school performance but who do not have identified disabilities. The federal government alone spent over $8.2 billion on early childhood education in the 2002 fiscal year (this does not include funding for child care or health services; White House, 2003).

Because of this established early intervention system, one avenue for productive future work is "practice-to-research." There are numerous programs successfully delivering early intervention for young children with emerging behavior disorders, and some even collect some data, but these "pockets of excellence" are unstudied. Jane Knitzer has done considerable work in the area of visiting and writing about particularly excellent early childhood intervention programs (e.g., Knitzer, 2000). It is up to researchers to pick up the gauntlet and build partnerships with these programs to systematically identify pathways of and models for success. One example of this kind of systematic evaluation of long-existing programs is Kendziora and Osher's evaluation of the almost 30 year-old Positive Education Program's Early Intervention Centers (EICs; see Bowdish et al., 2003). For this study, the researchers are using a matched-child design to compare academic outcomes of EIC children to children in district-based preschool programs, children not receiving special education until first grade, and typically developing peers. Results should be available in 2005.

Beyond the issues identified above as needing further attention, two final points must be made. Research in early intervention needs to be both more culturally competent and more inclusive of families. First, as the U.S. population becomes more diverse and as community-based early intervention programs adapt to their consumers' needs (Conway Madding, 2000), research needs to keep pace with this shift. Much more needs to be known about how to change the well-documented racial disparities in both access to services and attainment of positive outcomes once intervention is obtained (see the *Surgeon General's Report on Mental Health: Culture, Race and Ethnicity*; U.S. Department of Health and Human Services, 2001).

Finally, the consumers of preventive and early interventions—families themselves—must be more closely involved in all phases of the research process: identifying research questions, collecting data, interpreting results, and disseminating findings. Parental involvement has been a hallmark of early intervention practice (e.g., Goldberg, 1997), because in many ways parents are the engines of change in early intervention programs (Brooks-Gunn, Berlin, & Fuligni, 2000). However, families have typically been strangers to the research process. Early efforts to engage families in research usually defined the caregiver's role as an "advisor"

to the "professionals," who retained decision-making authority. Carpenter (1997) argued that adding parents' voices to the research process enhances the relevance of research to the day-to-day experience of caregiving. Turnbull, Friesen, and Ramirez (1998) outlined a participatory action research model with levels of family participation in research that can lead families from being research participants or reviewers of research to being co-researchers or research leaders, with professionals as advisors. When families are more involved in research, not only does the research itself benefit but also families become better informed and more able to make decisions about their children's care. Such "collective empowerment" (Turnbull, Turbiville, & Turnbull, 2000) can lead the next decade of research on early intervention for behavior disorders to a new level of usefulness.

NOTE

1. An effect size is a standardized statistic that is calculated to compare results across different studies. For intervention studies, effect size is often computed using d (Cohen, 1988), which is the combination of the mean of the intervention group minus the mean of the control group, divided by the pooled standard deviation. Effects are generally regarded as small at $d \approx .2$, medium when $d \approx .5$, large when $d \approx .8$.

REFERENCES

Arcelus, J., Gale, F., & Vostanis, P. (2001). Characteristics of children and parents attending a British Primary Mental Health Service. *European Child and Adolescent Psychiatry, 10,* 91–95.

Arnold, D. H., Ortiz, C., Curry, J. C., Stowe, R. M., Goldstein, N. E., Fisher, P. H., Zeljoja, A., & Yershova, K. (1999). Promoting academic success and preventing disruptive behavior disorders through community partnership. *Journal of Community Psychology, 27,* 589–598.

Bakley, S. (2001). Through the lens of sensory integration: A different way of analyzing challenging behavior. *Young Children, 56,* 70–76.

Barnett, W. S. (1993). Benefit–cost analysis of preschool education: Finding from a 25-year follow-up. *American Journal of Orthopsychiatry, 63,* 500–508.

Barrett, P., & Turner, C. (2001). Prevention of anxiety symptoms in primary school children: Preliminary results from a universal school-based trial. *British Journal of Clinical Psychology, 40,* 399–410.

Battistich, V., Schaps, E., Watson, M., Solomon, D., & Lewis, C. (2000). Effects of the Child Development Project on students' drug use and other problem behaviors. *Journal of Primary Prevention, 21,* 75–99.

Berrueta-Clement, J. R., Schweinhart, L. J., Barnett, W. S., & Weikart, D. P. (1987). The effects of early educational intervention on crime and delinquency in early adolescence and adulthood. In J. D. Burchard & S. N. Burchard (Eds.), *Primary prevention of psychopathology: Vol. 10. Prevention of delinquent behavior* (pp. 220–240). Newbury Park, CA: Sage.

Bickman, L., Guthrie, P. R., & Foster, E. M. (1995). *Evaluating managed mental health care: The Fort Bragg experiment.* New York: Plenum.

Biglan, A. (1995). Translating what we know about the context of antisocial behavior into a lower prevalence of such behavior. *Journal of Applied Behavior Analysis, 28,* 479–492.

Bolger, K. E., & Patterson, C. J. (2001). Pathways from child maltreatment to internalizing problems: Perceptions of control as mediators and moderators. *Development and Psychopathology, 13,* 913–940.

Bowdish, A., Albright, L., Bush, S., Kelly, D., & Kendziora, K. (2003, June). *Family centered early intervention: Practice and research.* Symposium presented at the 2003 Building on Family Strengths Conference, Portland, OR.

Bracey, G. W. (2000). A children's garden no more. *Phi Delta Kappan, 81,* 712–713.

Brestan, E. V., & Eyberg, S. M. (1998). Effective psychosocial treatments of conduct-disordered children and adolescents: 29 years, 82 studies, and 5,272 kids. *Journal of Clinical Child Psychology, 27,* 180–189.

Broidy, L. M., Nagin, D. S., Tremblay, R. E., Bates, J. E., Brame, B., Dodge, K. A., Fergusson, D., Horwood, J. L., Loeber, R., Laird, R., Lynam, D. R., Moffitt, T. E., Pettit, G. S., & Vitaro, F. (2003). Developmental trajectories of childhood disruptive behavior disorders and adolescent delinquency: A six-site, cross-national study. *Developmental Psychology, 39,* 222–245.

Brooks-Gunn, J., Berlin, L. J., & Fuligni, A. S. (2000). Early childhood intervention programs: What about the family? In J. P. Shonkoff & S. J. Meisels, (Eds.), *Handbook of early childhood intervention* (2nd ed., pp. 549–588). New York: Cambridge University Press.

Brooks-Gunn, J., Klebanov, P. K., Liaw, F., & Spiker, D. (1993). Enhancing the development of low-birthweight, premature infants: Changes in cognition and behavior over the first three years. *Child Development, 64,* 736–753.

Brophy, J. (1996). *Teaching problem students.* New York: Guilford Press.

Brown, C. H. (2003, June). *Methodologic issues in variation in impact among universal prevention programs.* Paper presented at the 11th annual meeting of the Society for Prevention Research, Washington, DC.

Bryant, D., Vizzard, L. H., Willoughby, M., & Kupersmidt, J. (1999). A review of interventions for preschoolers with aggressive and disruptive behavior. *Early Education and Development, 10,* 47–68.

Bureau of Justice Assistance (1995). *Drug Abuse Resistance Education (D.A.R.E.) Fact Sheet.* Document #FS000039. Retrieved from *http://www.ncjrs.org/pdffiles/darefs.pdf.*

Burns, J. M., & Patton, G. C. (2000). Preventive interventions for youth suicide: A risk factor-based approach. *Australian and New Zealand Journal of Psychiatry, 34,* 388–407.

Calkins, S. D., & Fox, N. A. (2002). Self-regulatory processes in early personality development: A multilevel approach to the study of childhood social withdrawal and aggression. *Development and Psychopathology, 14,* 477–498.

Campbell, F. A., & Ramey, C. T. (1995). Cognitive and school outcomes for high-risk African American students in middle adolescence: Positive effects of early intervention. *American Educational Research Journal, 32,* 743–772.

Campbell, S. B. (2002). *Behavior problems in preschool children: Clinical and developmental issues* (2nd ed.). New York: Guilford Press.

Carey, K. T. (1997). Preschool interventions. In A. P. Goldstein & J. C. Conoley (Eds.), *School violence intervention: A practical handbook* (pp. 93–106). New York: Guilford Press.

Carpenter, B. (1997). Empowering parents: The use of the parent as researcher paradigm in early intervention. *Journal of Child and Family Studies, 6,* 391–398.

Carpenter, E. M., & Nangle, D. W. (2002). The Compass program: Addressing aggression in the classroom. *Head Start Bulletin,* Issue No. 73, 27–28.

Caspi, A., Elder, G. H., & Bem, D. J. (1987). Moving against the world: Life course patterns of explosive children. *Developmental Psychology, 23,* 308–313.

Catalano, R. F., Berglund, M. L., Ryan, J. A. M., Lonczak, H. S., & Hawkins, J. D. (2002). Positive youth development in the United States: Research findings on evaluations of positive youth development programs. *Prevention and Treatment, 5,* Article 15. Article retrieved from *http://journals.apa.org/prevention/.*

Chorpita, B. F., Yim, L. M., Donkervoet, J. C., Arensdorf, A., Amundsen, M. J., McGee, C., Serrano, A., Yates, A., Burns, J. A., & Morelli, P. (2002). Toward large-scale implementation of empirically supported treatments for children: A review and observations by the Hawaii Empirical Basis to Services Task Force. *Clinical Psychology: Science and Practice, 9,* 165–190.

Clarke, G. N., Hawkins, W., Murphy, M., & Sheeber, L. (1993). School-based primary prevention of depressive symptomatology in adolescents: Findings from two studies. *Journal of Adolescent Research, 8,* 183–204.

Clarke, G. N., Hawkins, W., Murphy, M, Sheeber, L. B., Lewinsohn, P. M., & Seeley, J. R. (1995). Targeted prevention of unipolar depressive disorder in an at-risk sample of high school adolescents: A randomized trial of a group cognitive intervention. *Journal of the American Academy of Child and Adolescent Psychiatry, 34,* 312–321.

Cohen, J. (1988). *Statistical power analysis for the behavioral sciences* (2nd ed.). Hillsdale, NJ: Erlbaum.

Coie, J. D., & Dodge, K. A. (1998). Aggression and antisocial behavior. In W. Damon (Series Ed.) and N. Eisenberg (Vol. Ed.), *Handbook of child psychology: Vol. 3. Social, emotional, and personality development* (5th ed., pp. 779–862). New York: Wiley.

Coie, J. D., & Kupersmidt, J. B. (1983). A behavioral analysis of emerging social status in boys' groups. *Child Development, 54,* 1400–1416.

Colvin, G., Kame'enui, E.J., & Sugai, G. (1993). School-wide and classroom management: Re-conceptualizing the integration and management of students with behavior problems in general education. *Education and Treatment of Children, 16,* 361–381.

Compton, S, N., Burns, B. J., Egger, H. L., & Robertson, E. (2002). Review of the evidence base for treatment of childhood psychopathology: Internalizing disorders. *Journal of Consulting and Clinical Psychology, 70,* 1240–1266.

Conduct Problems Prevention Research Group. (2000). Merging universal and indicated prevention programs: The fast track model. *Addictive Behaviors, 25,* 913–927.

Conduct Problems Prevention Research Group. (2002a). Evaluation of the first 3 years of the fast track prevention trial with children at high risk for adolescent conduct problems. *Journal of Abnormal Child Psychology, 30,* 19–36.

Conduct Problems Prevention Research Group. (2002b). The implementation of the Fast Track Program: An example of a large-scale prevention science efficacy trial. *Journal of Abnormal Child Psychology, 30,* 1–17.

Conway Madding, C. (2000). Maintaining focus on cultural competence in early intervention services to linguistically and culturally diverse families. *Infant-Toddler Intervention, 10,* 9–18.

Costello, E. J., Angold, A., Burns, B. J., Stangl, D. K., Tweed, D. L., Erkanli, A., & Worthman, C. M. (1996). The Great Smoky Mountains Study of Youth. Goals, design, methods, and the prevalence of DSM-III-R disorders. *Archives of General Psychiatry, 53,* 1129–1136.

Costello, E. J., & Janiszewski, S. (1990). Who gets treated? Factors associated with referral in children with psychiatric disorders. *Acta Psychiatrica Scandinavica, 81,* 523–529.

Cowen, E. L., Hightower, A. D., Pedro-Carroll, J. L., Work, W. C., Wyman, P. A., & Haffey, W. G. (1996). *School-based prevention for children at risk: The Primary Mental Health Project.* Washington, DC: American Psychological Association.

Crick, N. R., & Zahn-Waxler, C. (2003). The development of psychopathology in females and males: Current progress and future challenges. *Development and Psychopathology, 15,* 719–742.

Dadds, M. R., Holland, D. E., Laurens, K. R., Mullins, M., Barrett, P. M., & Spence, S. H. (1999). Early intervention and prevention of anxiety disorders in children: Results at 2-year follow-up. *Journal of Consulting and Clinical Psychology, 67,* 145–150.

Denham, S., & Weissberg, R. P. (in press). Social-emotional learning in early childhood: What we know and where to go from here. In E. Chesebrough, P. King, M. Bloom, & T. P. Gulotta (Eds.), *A blueprint for the promotion of pro-social behavior in early childhood.* New York: Kluwer Academic/Plenum.

Dishion, T. J. (2000). Cross-setting consistency in early adolescent psychopathology: Deviant friendships and problem behavior sequelae. *Journal of Personality, 68,* 1109–1126.

Dishion, T. J., & Andrews, D. W. (1995). Preventing escalation in problem behaviors with high-risk young adolescents: Immediate and 1-year outcomes. *Journal of Consulting and Clinical Psychology, 63,* 538–548.

Dishion, T. J., Capaldi, D. M., & Yoerger, K. (1999). Middle childhood antecedents to progressions in male adolescent substance use: An ecological analysis of risk and protection. *Journal of Adolescent Research, 14,* 175–205.

Dodge, K. A. (1983). Behavioral antecedents of peer social status. *Child Development, 54,* 1386–1399.

Dolan, L. J., Kellam, S. G., Brown, C. H., Werthamer-Larsson, L., Rebok, G. W., Mayer, L., Laudolff, J., Turkkan, J., Ford, C., & Wheeler, L. (1993). The short-term impact of two classroom-based preventive interventions on aggressive and shy behaviors and poor achievement. *Journal of Applied Developmental Psychology, 14,* 317–345.

Durlak, J. A., & Wells, A. M. (1997). Primary prevention mental health programs for children and adolescents: A meta-analytic review. *American Journal of Community Psychology, 25,* 115–152.

Durlak, J. A., & Wells, A. M. (1998). Evaluation of indicated preventive intervention (secondary prevention) mental health programs for children and adolescents. *American Journal of Community Psychology, 26,* 775–802.

Dwyer, K., & Osher, D. (2000). *Safeguarding our children: An action guide.* Washington, DC: U.S. Departments of Education and Justice, American Institutes for Research.

Eagly, A. H. (1987). *Sex differences in social behavior: A social role interpretation.* Hillsdale, NJ: Erlbaum.

Eagly, A. H., & Steffen, V. J. (1986). Gender and aggressive behavior: A meta-analytic review of the social psychological literature. *Psychological Bulletin, 100,* 309–330.

Eamon, M. K. (2000). Structural model of the effects of poverty on externalizing and internalizing behaviors of four- to five-year-old children. *Social Work Research, 24,* 143–154.

Egeland, B., Kalkoske, M., Gottesman, N., & Erickson, M. F. (1990). Preschool behavior problems: Stability and factors accounting for change. *Journal of Child Psychology and Psychiatry, 31*, 891–910.

Egeland, B., Pianta, R., & Ogawa, J. (1996). Early behavior problems: Pathways to mental disorders in adolescence. *Development and Psychopathology, 8*, 735–749.

Elias, M. J., & Clabby, J. F. (1992). *Building Social Problem Solving Skills: Guidelines from a School-Based Program.* San Francisco: Jossey-Bass.

Foster, E. M. (2002, July). *Success and CBAS: An Economic Evaluation of the Incredible Years.* Paper presented at the Oregon Social Learning Center. Retrieved from *http://www.personal.psu.edu/faculty/e/m/emf10/papers/CBASOverview.ppt.*

Foster, E. M., Dodge, K. A., & Jones, D. (2003). Issues in the economic evaluation of prevention programs. *Applied Developmental Science, 7*, 76–86.

Fox, N. A., & Calkins, S. D. (1993). Pathways to aggression and social withdrawal: Interactions among temperament, attachment, and regulation. In K. H. Rubin & J. B. Asendorpf (Eds.), *Social withdrawal, inhibition, and shyness in childhood* (pp. 81–100). Hillsdale, NJ: Erlbaum.

Gartrell, D. (2001). Replacing time-out: Part one— Using guidance to build an encouraging classroom. *Young Children, 56*, 8–16.

Gartrell, D. (2002). Replacing time-out: Part two— Using guidance to maintain an encouraging classroom. *Young Children, 57*, 36–43.

Gillham, J. E., Reivich, K. J., Jaycox, L. H., & Seligman, M. E. P. (1995). Prevention of depressive symptoms in schoolchildren: Two-year follow-up. *Psychological Science, 6*, 343–351.

Goldberg, S. (1997). *Parent involvement begins at birth: Collaboration between parents and teachers of children in the early years.* Needham Heights, MA: Allyn & Bacon.

Goldsmith, S. K., Pellmar, T. C., Kleinman, A. K., & Bunney, W. E. (Eds.). (2002). *Reducing suicide: A national imperative.* Washington, DC: National Academies Press.

Golly, A., Sprague, J., Walker, H. M., Beard, K., & Gorham, G. (2000). The First Step to Success Program: An analysis of outcomes with identical twins across multiple baselines. *Behavioral Disorders, 25*, 170–182.

Gottfredson, D. C. (2001). *Schools and delinquency.* New York: Cambridge University Press.

Gould, B. (2002). Early childhood behavior specialist: *Head Start Bulletin,* Issue No. 73, 37–38.

Greenberg, M. T., Domitrovich, C., & Bumbarger, B. (2000). *Preventing mental disorders in school-age children: A review of the effectiveness of prevention programs.* State College, PA: Penn State University. Retrieved from *http://www.prevention.psu.edu/cmhs.pdf.*

Gresham, F. M., & Nagle, R. J. (1980). Social skills training with children: Responsiveness to modeling and coaching as a function of peer orientation. *Journal of Consulting and Clinical Psychology, 48*, 718–729.

Griffin, E. A. (1997, April). *The role of children's social skills in achievement at kindergarten entry and beyond.* Paper presented at the 62nd Biennial Meeting of the Society for Research in Child Development, Washington, DC.

Guralnick, M. J. (1991). The next decade of research on the effectiveness of early intervention. *Exceptional Children, 58*, 174–183.

Guralnick, M. J. (1997). Second-generation research in the field of early intervention. In M. J. Guralnick (Ed.), *The effectiveness of early intervention: Second generation research* (pp. 3–20). Baltimore: Brookes.

Hauser-Cram, P., Warfield, M. E., Shonkoff, J. P., & Krauss, M. W. (2001). Children with disabilities: A longitudinal study of child development and parent well-being. *Monographs of the Society for Research in Child Development, 66*, 3, Serial No. 266.

Hawaii Department of Health. (2003). *Child and adolescent mental health services strategic plan 2003–2006.* Retrieved from *http://www.hawaii.gov/health/camhd/reports/camhd_plan.pdf.*

Hawkins, J. D. (1997). Academic performance and school success: Sources and consequences. In R. P. Weissberg, T. P. Gullotta, R. L. Hampton, R. A. Ryan, & G. R. Adams (Eds.), *Healthy children 2010: Vol. 8. Enhancing children's wellness. Issues in children's and families' lives* (pp. 278–305). Thousand Oaks, CA: Sage.

Heath, H. E. (1994). Dealing with difficult behaviors— Teachers plan with parents. *Young Children, 49*, 20–24.

Henggeler, S. W., Melton, G. B., Brondino, M. J., Scherer, D. G., & Hanley, J. H. (1997). Multisystemic therapy with violent and chronic juvenile offenders and their families: The role of treatment fidelity in successful dissemination. *Journal of Consulting and Clinical Psychology, 65*, 821–833.

Hernandez, M., & Hodges, S. (Eds.). (2001). *Developing outcome strategies in children's mental health.* Baltimore: Brookes.

Hinshaw, S. P. (1992). Academic underachievement, attention deficits, and aggression: Comorbidity and implications for intervention. *Journal of Consulting and Clinical Psychology, 60*, 893–903.

Hoagwood, K., Jensen, P. S., Petti, T., & Burns, B. J. (1996). Outcomes of mental health care for children and adolescents: I. A comprehensive conceptual model. *Journal of the American Academy of Child and Adolescent Psychiatry, 35*, 1055–1063.

Hoare, P., Norton, B., Chisholm, D., & Parry-Jones, W. (1996). An audit of 7000 successive child and adolescent psychiatry referrals in Scotland. *Clinical Child Psychology and Psychiatry, 1*, 229–249.

Honig, A. S., & Wittmer, D. S. (1996). Helping children become more prosocial: Ideas for classrooms, families, schools, and communities. *Young Children, 51*, 62–70.

Horn, W., & Packard, T. (1985). Early identification of learning problems: A meta-analysis. *Journal of Educational Psychology, 77,* 597–607.

Hyde, J. S. (1984). How large are gender differences in aggression? A developmental meta-analysis. *Developmental Psychology, 20,* 722–736.

Ihle, W., Esser, G., Schmidt, M. H., & Blanz, B. (2002). Childhood and adolescent predictors of mental disorders from childhood to early adulthood. *Kindheit und Entwicklung, 11,* 201–211. Abstract retrieved from Psych Info Accession Number 2002-06907-001.

Jaycox, L. H, Reivich, K. J., Gillham, J., & Seligman, M. (1994). Prevention of depressive symptoms in school children. *Behaviour Research and Therapy, 32,* 801–816.

Jensen, P. S. (2002). Putting science to work: A statewide attempt to identify and implement effective interventions. *Clinical Psychology: Science and Practice, 9,* 223–224.

Jensen, P. S. (2003). Commentary: The next generation is overdue. *Journal of the American Academy of Child and Adolescent Psychiatry, 42,* 527–530.

Jessor, R., & Jessor, S. L. (1977). *Problem behavior and psychosocial development.* New York: Academic Press.

Jimerson, S. R., Egeland, B., Sroufe, L. A., & Carlson, B. (2000). A prospective longitudinal study of high school dropouts: Examining multiple predictors across development. *Journal of School Psychology, 38,* 525–549.

Jimerson, S. R., Egeland, B., & Teo, A. (1999). A longitudinal study of achievement trajectories: Factors associated with change. *Journal of Educational Psychology, 91,* 116–126.

Kagan, J. (1989). Temperamental contributions to social behavior. *American Psychologist, 44,* 668–674.

Kaiser, A. P., Cai, X., Hancock, T. B., Foster, E. M., & Hester, P. P. (2000). Parent-reported behavior problems and language delays in boys and girls enrolled in Head Start. *Behavioral Disorders, 26,* 26–41.

Karoly, L. A., Greenwood, P. W., Everingham, S. S., Hoube, J,. Kilburn, M. R., Rydell, C. P., Sanders, M., & Chiesa, J. (1998). *Investing in our children: What we know and don't know about the costs and benefits of early childhood interventions.* Santa Monica, CA: Rand.

Kauffman, J. M. (1997). *Characteristics of emotional and behavior disorders of children and youth* (6th ed.). Columbus, OH: Merrill.

Keiley, M. K., Lofthouse, N., Bates, J. E., Dodge, K. A., & Pettit, G. S. (2003). Differential risks of covarying and pure components in mother and teacher reports of externalizing and internalizing behavior across ages 5 to 14. *Journal of Abnormal Child Psychology, 31,* 264–283.

Kellam, S. G. (2000). Community and institutional partnerships for school violence prevention. *Preventing School Violence: Plenary Papers of the 1999 Conference on Criminal Justice Research and Evaluation—Enhancing Policy and Practice Through Research, Volume 2.* NCJ 180972 (pp. 1–21). Washington, DC: National Institute of Justice.

Kellam, S. G., Ling, X., Merisca, R., Brown, C. H., & Ialongo, N. (1998). The effect of the level of aggression in the first grade classroom on the course and malleability of aggressive behavior into middle school. *Development and Psychopathology, 10,* 165–185.

Kendziora, K. T., Greenbaum, P. E., Kellam, S. G., Brown, C. H., Vanfossen, B. E., Poduska, J. M., & Ialongo, N. (2003, June). *Gender and age differences in teacher-rated aggression: A longitudinal analysis from first grade to middle school.* Paper presented at the 11th annual meeting of the Society for Prevention Research, Washington, DC.

Kendziora, K. T., & Osher, D. (1999). *Federal Agency prevention initiatives.* Unpublished document. Washington, DC: Center for Effective Collaboration and Practice, American Institutes for Research.

Kerr, M. M., Tremblay, R. E., Pagani, L., & Vitaro, F. (1997). Boys' behavioral inhibition and the risk of later delinquency. *Archives of General Psychiatry, 54,* 809–816.

Kim, Y., Innocenti, M., & Kim, J. (1997). *When should we begin? A comprehensive review of age at start in early intervention.* Paper presented at the Annual World Congress of the International Association for the Scientific Study of Intellectual Disabilities, Helsinki, Finland. ERIC No. ED403725.

Knitzer, J. (2000). Early childhood mental health services: A policy and systems development perspective. In J. P. Shonkoff & S. J. Meisels (Eds.), *Handbook of early intervention* (pp. 416–438). New York: Cambridge University Press.

Kupersmidt, J. B., Bryant, D., & Willoughby, M. T. (2000). Prevalence of aggressive behaviors among preschoolers in Head Start and community child care programs. *Behavioral Disorders, 26,* 42–52.

Kupersmidt, J. B., & Coie, J. D. (1990). Preadolescent peer status, aggression, and school adjustment as predictors of externalizing problems in adolescence. *Child Development, 61,* 1350–1362.

Ladd, G. W., Birch, S. H., & Buhs, E. S. (1999). Children's social and scholastic lives in kindergarten: Related spheres of influence? *Child Development, 70,* 1373–1400.

Ladd, G. W., & Mars, K. T. (1986). Reliability and validity of preschoolers' perceptions of peer behavior. *Journal of Clinical Child Psychology, 15,* 16–25.

Ladd, G. W., & Price, J. M. (1987). Predicting children's social and school adjustment following the transition from preschool to kindergarten. *Child Development, 58,* 1168–1189.

Ladd, G. W., Price, J. M., & Hart, C. H. (1988). Predicting preschoolers' peer status from their playground behaviors. *Child Development, 59,* 986–992.

LaFreniere, P. J., & Capuano, F. (1997). Preventive intervention as means of clarifying direction of effects in socialization: Anxious-withdrawn preschoolers case. *Development and Psychopathology, 9,* 551–564.

La Greca, A. M., Prinstein, M. J., & Fetter, M. D. (2001). Adolescent peer crowd affiliation: Linkages with health-risk behaviors and close friendships. *Journal of Pediatric Psychology, 26,* 131–143.

Lavigne, J. V., Arend, R., Rosenbaum, D. Binns, H. J., Christoffel, K. K., & Gibbons, R. D. (1998). Psychiatric disorders with onset in the preschool years: I. Stability of diagnoses. *Journal of the American Academy of Child and Adolescent Psychiatry, 37,* 1246–1254.

Lochman, J. E., Burch, P. R., Curry, J. F., & Lampron, L. B. (1984). Treatment and generalization effects of cognitive-behavioral and goal-setting interventions with aggressive boys. *Journal of Consulting and Clinical Psychology, 52,* 915–916.

Loeber, R. (1990). Development and risk factors of juvenile antisocial behavior and delinquency. *Clinical Psychology Review, 10,* 1–41.

Maccoby, E. E., & Jacklin, C. N. (1974). *The psychology of sex differences.* Stanford, CA: Stanford University Press.

Maccoby, E. E., & Jacklin, C. N. (1980). Sex differences in aggression: A rejoinder and reprise. *Child Development, 51,* 964–980.

Marshall, H. H. (1995). Beyond "I like the way . . . " *Young Children, 50,* 26–28.

McEvoy, A., & Welker, R. (2000). Antisocial behavior, academic failure, and school climate: A critical review. *Journal of Emotional and Behavioral Disorders, 8,* 130–140.

Meyer, A., Miller, S., & Herman, M. (1993). Balancing the priorities of evaluation with the priorities of the setting: A focus on positive youth development programs in school settings. *Journal of Primary Prevention, 14,* 95–113.

Moffitt, T. E. (1993). Adolescence—limited and life-course-persistent antisocial behavior: A developmental taxonomy. *Psychological Review, 100,* 674–701.

Moffitt, T. E., & Caspi, A. (2001). Childhood predictors differentiate life-course persistent and adolescence-limited antisocial pathways among males and females. *Development and Psychopathology, 13,* 355–375.

Mrazek, P. J., & Haggerty, R. J. (Eds.). (1994). *Reducing risks for mental disorders: Frontiers for preventive intervention research.* Washington, DC: National Academy Press.

National Advisory Mental Health Council Workgroup on Mental Disorders Prevention Research. (1998). *Priorities for Prevention Research at NIMH.* Bethesda, MD: National Institutes of Health/National Institute of Mental Health. NIH Publication No. 98-4321.

National Center for Education Statistics (1997). *Schools and Staffing Survey. Characteristics of Stayers, Movers, and Leavers: Results from the Teacher Follow-up Survey: 1994–95.* Washington, DC: U.S. Department of Education, Office of Educational Research and Improvement. Document # NCES 97-450. ·Retrieved from *http://nces.ed.gov/pubs97/97450.pdf.*

Newman, D. L., Caspi, A., Moffitt, T. E., & Silva, P. A. (1997). Antecedents of adult interpersonal functioning: Effects of individual differences in age three temperament. *Developmental Psychology, 33,* 206–217.

Nolen-Hoeksema, S., & Girgus, J. S. (1994). The emergence of gender differences in depression during adolescence. *Psychological Bulletin, 115,* 424–443.

Olds, D. L. (2002). Prenatal and infancy home visiting by nurses: From randomized trials to community replication. *Prevention Science, 3,* 153–172.

Olds, D. L., Eckenrode, J., Henderson, C. R., Kitzman, H., Powers, J., Cole, R., Sidora, K., Morris, P., Pettit, L. M., & Luckey, D. (1997). Long-term effects of home visitation on maternal life course and child abuse and neglect: 15-year follow-up of a randomized trial. *Journal of the American Medical Association, 278,* 637–643.

Patterson, G. R., Reid, J. B., & Dishion, T. J. (1992). *Antisocial boys.* Eugene, OR: Castalia.

Pettit, G. S., & Dodge, K. A. (2003). Violent children: Bridging development, intervention, and public policy. *Developmental Psychology, 39,* 187–188.

Poduska, J. M., Kellam, S. G., Brown, C. H., Wang, C. P., & Ialongo, N. (2003, June). *Effects of a classroom behavior intervention in 1st and 2nd grades on cumulative use of services for problems with behavior, feelings, drugs, or alcohol by young adulthood.* Paper presented at the 11th annual meeting of the Society for Prevention Research, Washington, DC.

Prinstein, M., & La Greca, A. M. (2002). Peer crowd affiliation and internalizing distress in childhood and adolescence: A longitudinal follow-back study. *Journal of Research on Adolescence, 12,* 325–351.

Ramey, C. T., Campbell, F. A., & Ramey, S. L. (1999). Early intervention: Successful pathways to improving intellectual development. *Developmental Neuropsychology, 16,* 385–392.

Ramey, C. T., & Ramey, S. L. (1998). Early intervention and early experience. *American Psychologist, 53,* 109–120.

Rapee, R. M., & Jacobs, D. (2002). The reduction of temperamental risk for anxiety in withdrawn preschoolers: A pilot study. *Behavioural and Cognitive Psychotherapy, 30,* 211–216.

Ratcliff, N. (2001). Use the environment to prevent discipline problems and support learning. *Young Children, 56,* 84–88.

Raver, C. C., & Knitzer, J. (2002). *Ready to enter: What research tells policymakers about strategies to promote social and emotional school readiness among three- and four-year-olds.* New York: National Center on Children in Poverty.

Reid, J. B. (1993). Prevention of conduct disorder before and after school entry: Relating interventions to developmental findings. *Development and Psychopathology, 5,* 243–262.

Reinsberg, J. (1999). Understanding young children's behavior. *Young Children, 54,* 54–57.

Reynolds, A. J. (2000). *Success in early intervention: The Chicago Child–Parent Centers.* Lincoln, NE: University of Nebraska Press.

Reynolds, A. J., Temple, J. A., Robertson, D. L., & Mann, E. A. (2001). Long-term effects of an early childhood intervention on educational achievement and juvenile arrest: A 15-year follow-up of low-income children in public schools. *Journal of the American Medical Association, 285,* 2339–2346.

Reynolds, W. M., & Coats, K. I. (1986). A comparison of cognitive behavioral therapy and relaxation training for the treatment of depression in adolescents. *Journal of Consulting and Clinical Psychology, 54,* 653–660.

Richman, N., Stevenson, J., & Graham, P. J. (1982). *Pre-school to school: A behavioural study.* San Diego, CA: Elsevier/Academic Press.

Roberts, C., Kane, R., Thomson, H., Bishop, B., & Hart, B. (2003). The prevention of depressive symptoms in rural school children: A randomized controlled trial. *Journal of Consulting and Clinical Psychology, 71,* 622–628.

Robertson, E., Greenberg, M., Kam, C. M., & Kusche, C. (2003, June). *Who is likely to be impacted by universal intervention: Findings from the PATHS curriculum.* Paper presented at the 11th annual meeting of the Society for Prevention Research, Washington, DC.

Robins, L. N. (1978). Sturdy childhood predictors of adult antisocial behavior: Replications from longitudinal studies. *Psychological Medicine, 8,* 611–622.

Rotheram-Borus, M. J., & Duan, N. (2003). Next generation of preventive interventions. *Journal of the American Academy of Child and Adolescent Psychiatry, 42,* 518–526.

Rubin, K. H., Bukowski, W., & Parker, J. G. (1998). Peer interactions, relationships, and groups. In W. Damon (Series Ed.) and N. Eisenberg (Volume Ed.), *Handbook of child psychology: Vol. 3. Social, emotional, and personality development* (5th ed., pp. 619–700). New York: Wiley.

Schaeffer, C. M., Petras, H., Ialongo, N., Poduska, J., & Kellam, S. (2003). Modeling growth in boys' aggressive behavior across elementary school: Links to later criminal involvement, conduct disorder, and antisocial personality disorder. *Developmental Psychology, 39,* 1020–1035.

Schoenwald, S. K., & Hoagwood, K. (2001). Effectiveness, transportability, and dissemination of interventions: What matters when? *Psychiatric Services, 52,* 1190–1197.

Schreiber, M. E. (1999). Time-outs for toddlers: Is our goal punishment or education? *Young Children, 54,* 22–25.

Shaffer, D., Fisher, P., Dulcan, M. K., Davies, M., Piacentini, J., Schwab-Stone, M. E., Lahey, B. B., Bourdon, K., Jensen, P. S., Bird, H. R., Canino, G., & Regier, D. A. (1996). The NIMH Diagnostic Interview Schedule for Children Version 2.3 (DISC-2.3): Description, acceptability, prevalence rates, and performance in the MECA Study. Methods for the Epidemiology of Child and Adolescent Mental Disorders Study. *Journal of the American Academy of Child and Adolescent Psychiatry, 35,* 865–877.

Shaw, D. S., Gilliom, M., Ingoldsby, E. M., & Nagin, D. S. (2003). Trajectories leading to school-age conduct problems. *Developmental Psychology, 39,* 189–200.

Shonkoff, J. P., & Phillips, D. A. (Eds.). (2000). *From neurons to neighborhoods: The science of early childhood development.* Washington, DC: National Academies Press.

Shores, R. E., & Wehby, J. H. (1999). Analyzing the classroom social behavior of students with EBD. *Journal of Emotional and Behavioral Disorders, 7,* 194–199.

Smith, B. J. (1988). *Does early intervention help? ERIC Digest #455.* ERIC No. ED295399.

Smucker, M. R., Craighead, W. E., Craighead, L. W., & Green, B. J. (1986). Normative and reliability data for the Children's Depression Inventory. *Journal of Abnormal Child Psychology, 14,* 25–39.

Sprague, J., Sugai, G. H., & Walker, H. M. (1998). Antisocial behavior in schools. In S. Watson & F. M. Gresham (Eds.), *Child behavior therapy: Ecological considerations in assessment, treatment, and evaluation* (pp. 451–474). New York: Plenum.

Stoolmiller, M., Eddy, J. M., & Reid, J. B. (2000). Detecting and describing preventive intervention effects in a universal school-based randomized trial targeting delinquent and violent behavior. *Journal of Consulting and Clinical Psychology, 68,* 296–306.

Strain, P. (2000, December). *Establishing environments in which children can succeed and develop positive behaviors.* Presentation at the National Head Start Child Development Institute, Washington, DC.

Strain, P. S., Steele, P., Ellis, T., & Timm, M. A. (1982). Long-term effects of oppositional child treatment with mothers as therapists and therapist trainers. *Journal of Applied Behavior Analysis, 15,* 163–169.

Strain, P. S., & Timm, M. A. (2001). Remediation and prevention of aggression: An evaluation of the Regional Intervention Program over a quarter century. *Behavioral Disorders, 26,* 297–313.

Stroul, B. A., & Friedman, R. M. (1994). *A system of care for children and youth with severe emotional disturbances.* Washington, DC: Georgetown University, CASSP Technical Assistance Center.

Sugai, G., & Horner, R. (1994). Including students with severe behavior problems in general education settings: Assumptions, challenges, and solutions. In J. Marr, G. Sugai, & G. Tindal (Eds.), *The Oregon conference monograph* (Vol. 6, pp. 102–120). Eugene, OR: University of Oregon.

Sugai, G., Sprague, J. R., Horner, R. H., & Walker, H. M. (2000). Preventing school violence: The use of office discipline referrals to assess and monitor schoolwide discipline interventions. *Journal of Emotional and Behavioral Disorders, 8,* 94–101.

Task Force on Women in Academe. (2000). *Women in*

academe: Two steps forward, one step back. Washington, DC: American Psychological Association.

Taylor-Greene, S., Brown, D., Nelson, L., Longton, J., Gassman, T., Cohen, J., Swartz, J., Horner, R., Sugai, G., & Hall, S. (1997). Schoolwide behavioral support: Starting the year off right. *Journal of Behavioral Education, 7,* 99–112.

Tremblay, R. E., Japel, C., Perusse, D., Boivin, M., Zoccolillo, M., Montplaisir, J., & McDuff, P. (1999). The search for the age of "onset" of physical aggression: Rousseau and Bandura revisited. *Criminal Behavior and Mental Health, 9,* 8–23.

Tremblay, R. E., Masse, L. C., Pagani, L., & Vitaro, F. (1996). From childhood physical aggression to adolescent maladjustment: The Montreal prevention experiment. In R. DeV. Peters & R. J. McMahon (Eds.), *Preventing childhood disorders, substance abuse, and delinquency* (pp. 268–298). Thousand Oaks, CA: Sage.

Turnbull, A. P., Friesen, B. J., Ramirez, C. (1998). Participatory action research as a model for conducting family research. *Journal of the Association for Persons with Severe Handicaps, 23,* 178–188.

Turnbull, A. P., Turbiville, V., & Turnbull, H. R. (2000). Evolution of family–professional partnerships: Collective empowerment as the model for the early twenty-first century. In J. P. Shonkoff & S. J. Meisels (Eds.), *Handbook of early childhood intervention* (2nd ed., pp. 630–650). New York: Cambridge University Press.

U.S. Department of Education. (2002). *Twenty-fourth annual report to Congress on the implementation of the Individuals with Disabilities Education Act.* Washington, DC: U.S. Government Printing Office.

U.S. Department of Health and Human Services. (2001). *Mental health: culture, race, ethnicity: A supplement to mental health: A report of the Surgeon General..* Rockville, MD: U.S. Department of Health and Human Services, Public Health Service, Office of the Surgeon General.

U.S. Public Health Service. (1999). *The Surgeon General's Call to Action to Prevent Suicide 1999.* Washington, DC: Author.

Walker, H. M., Colvin, G., & Ramsey, E. (1995). *Antisocial behavior in school: Strategies and best practices.* Pacific Grove, CA: Brooks/Cole.

Walker, H. M., Kavanagh, K., Stiller, B., Golly, A., Severson, H. H., & Feil, E. G. (1998). First Step to Success: An early intervention approach for preventing school antisocial behavior. *Journal of Emotional and Behavioral Disorders, 6,* 66–80.

Walker, H. M., & Sprague, J. R. (1999). The path to school failure, delinquency, and violence: Causal factors and some potential solutions. *Intervention in School and Clinic, 35,* 67–73.

Watson, M. (2003). Attachment theory and challenging behaviors: Reconstructing the nature of relationships. *Young Children, 58,* 12–20.

Webster-Stratton, C., Hollinsworth, T., & Kolpacoff, M. (1989). The long-term effectiveness and clinical significance of three cost-effective training programs for families with conduct-problem children. *Journal of Consulting and Clinical Psychology, 57,* 550–553.

Webster-Stratton, C., & Reid, M. J. (2002). *The incredible years classroom management teacher training program: Content, methods, and process.* Unpublished manuscript. University of Washington, Seattle, WA.

Webster-Stratton, C., Reid, M. J., & Hammond, M. (2001). Preventing conduct problems, promoting social competence: A parent and teacher training partnership in Head Start. *Journal of Clinical Child Psychology, 30,* 238–302.

Webster-Stratton, C., & Taylor, T. (2001). Nipping early risk factors in the bud: Preventing substance abuse, delinquency, and violence in adolescence through interventions targeted at young children (0–8 years). *Prevention Science, 2,* 165–192.

Weikart, D. P. (1998). Changing early childhood development through educational intervention. *Preventive Medicine: An International Journal Devoted to Practice and Theory, 27,* 233–237.

Weikart, D. P., & Schweinhart, L. J. (1992). High/Scope preschool program outcomes. In J. McCord & R. E. Tremblay (Eds.), *Preventing antisocial behavior: Interventions from birth through adolescence* (pp. 67–86). New York: Guilford Press.

Weir, R. C., & Gjerde, P. F. (2002). Preschool personality prototypes: Internal coherence, cross-study replicability, and developmental outcomes in adolescence. *Personality and Social Psychology Bulletin, 28,* 1229–1241.

Weisz, J. R., Weiss, B., & Donenberg, G. R. (1992). The lab versus the clinic: Effects of child and adolescent psychotherapy. *American Psychologist, 47,* 1578–1585.

Werner, E., & Smith, R. S. (1992). *Overcoming the odds: High risk children from birth to adulthood.* Ithaca, NY: Cornell University Press.

West, J., Denton, K., & Reaney, L. M. (2001). *The kindergarten year: Findings from the Early Childhood Longitudinal Study, kindergarten class of 1998–1999.* Washington, DC: National Center for Education Statistics.

White, H. R., Pandina, R. J., & LaGrange, R. (1987). Longitudinal predictors of serious substance use and delinquency. *Criminology, 3,* 715–740.

White, J., & Jodion, N. (1998). *"Before-the-fact" interventions: A manual of best practices in youth suicide prevention.* Vancouver, BC: University of British Columbia.

White House. (2003). *Funding for early childhood care and education.* Washington DC: Author. Document retrieved from *http://www.whitehouse.gov/infocus/earlychildhood/sect3.pdf.*

Yoshikawa, H. (1994). Prevention as cumulative protection: Effects of early family support and education on chronic delinquency and its risks. *Psychological Bulletin, 115,* 28–54.

Zahn-Waxler, C., Klimes-Dougan, B., & Slattery, M. J. (2000). Internalizing problems of childhood and adolescence: Prospects, pitfalls, and progress in understanding the development of anxiety and depression. *Development and Psychopathology, 12*, 443–466.

Zigler, E. F., Taussig, C., & Black, K. (1992). Early childhood intervention: A promising preventative for juvenile delinquency. *American Psychologist, 47*, 997–1006.

Zill, N., Resnick, G., Kim, K., O'Donnell, K., Sorongon, A., McKey, R. H., Pai-Samant, S., Clark, C., O'Brien, R., & D'Elio, M. A. (2003, May). *Head Start FACES 2000: A whole-child perspective on program performance.* Washington, DC: Administration for Children and Families.

Zill, N., & West, J. (2001). *Entering kindergarten: A portrait of American children when they begin school: Findings from the Condition of Education 2000.* Washington, DC: National Center for Education Statistics.

18

Psychopharmacology in the Treatment of Emotional and Behavioral Disorders

DEAN E. KONOPASEK *and* STEVEN R. FORNESS

Research over the past 15 years has demonstrated a steady, if not dramatic, increase in the use of psychopharmacology to treat children and adolescents with emotional or behavioral disorders (EBD; Connor, 2002; Emslie, Walkup, Pliszka, & Ernst, 1999; Rowland et al., 2002; Zima & Bussing, 2004). Major advances in the field of psychopharmacology have led to a significant, albeit sometimes criticized, shift in our view of the role medication has played in the treatment of child and adolescent mental health disorders. This chapter reviews current literature regarding the epidemiology and pharmacological treatment of children with EBD, considerations surrounding the medical model as it relates to special education decision making, and issues of collaboration and cooperation between special education, the family, and the medical community.

BEHAVIORAL VERSUS PSYCHOPHARMACOLOGICAL TREATMENT

Within special education, the behavioral model has long been the "gold standard" of treatment for children with EBD (Kauffman,

2001), with medical intervention (i.e., psychotropic medication) offered as an adjunct therapy, at best. Under this view of the medical model it was assumed that factors such as underlying psychodynamic conflicts or minimal brain dysfunction were the etiologies of disordered school behavior or learning. It was further assumed that these factors required diagnoses and treatment before practical school intervention could be effectively begun. This was our common interpretation of the medical model from within the field of special education, a view that has now been out of favor for so long that most special education professionals today do not remember its ever having been acceptable. As Forness and Kavale (2001) noted, "Such an interpretation of the medical model, at least at that moment in our understanding, probably deserved to be vilified" (p. 269).

More recently, major advances have been made in child and adolescent psychopharmacology, advances which suggest that psychopharmacologic treatment may even exceed the effectiveness of psychosocial intervention (MTA Cooperative Group, 1999a, 1999b; Zima & Bussing, 2004). Additionally, improvements in diagnoses, brain imaging, medical treatment of child psychiatric disorders, and the emerging field of pediatric psychopharmacoepidemiology have served to help shape a "new" medical model of special education. This new model suggests that screening for psychiatric diagnoses and possible referral for psychopharmacologic intervention need to be *added* to existing behavioral or psychosocial treatment for many children with EBD rather than viewed as a distinct, separate alternative (Forness, Kavale, & Davanzo, 2002). This new conception suggests that, for a significant number of children with EBD, diagnoses that lead to possible psychopharmacologic therapy are critical to successful intervention. The odds in favor of the relevance of this model to effective treatment of classroom behavior problems are too great to ignore (Forness & Kavale, 2001).

PSYCHOPHARMACOEPIDEMIOLOGY

Pediatric psychopharmacoepidemiology is a relatively new field, focusing on studying the prevalence and patterns of the use of psychiatric medications with children (Forness, Kavale, Sweeney, & Crenshaw, 1999). Data over the past decade point to the increasingly widespread use of psychopharmacologic medications, with as many as 2–4% of children in general education, 15–20% of children in special education, and 40–60% of children in residential facilities receiving medication treatment (Gadow, 1997; Olfson, Marcus, Weissman, & Jensen, 2002; Vitiello & Hoagwood, 1997). Zima and Bussing (2004) note that, during the 10-year period between 1987 and 1996, the use of psychotropic medications overall, as prescribed to children and adolescents, increased nearly three times, with increases for stimulants and antidepressants being particularly high. They go on to caution, however, that these increasing trends should not be interpreted as representing overprescribing or inappropriate use of medications for children. In fact, most evidence over the past several years suggests that stimulant medication may actually be significantly *underprescribed* (Riddle, Labellarte, & Walkup, 1998; Walkup, 2003). Data suggest that prescription rates for stimulants and related medications are well below conservative prevalence estimates for attention-deficit/

hyperactivity disorder (ADHD; Forness & Kavale, 2001; Gadow, 1997; Jensen, 2002; Jensen et al., 1999; Pappadopulos & Jensen, 2001).

In addition to increases in psychopharmacologic interventions for school-age children, studies have also found increases in the application of many of these medications for preschoolers, particularly the stimulants (Connor, 2002; Greenhill et al., 2003). With the development of newer and safer medications to treat depression (e.g., selective serotonin reuptake inhibitors [SSRIs], "novel" antidepressants), their use has correspondingly increased significantly (Emslie et al., 1999). Coincidentally, use of tricyclic antidepressants (TCAs) has decreased, owing to safety concerns, sedating qualities, and monitoring difficulties (Geller, Reising, Leonard, Riddle, & Walsh, 1999). The use of neuroleptics has also steadily increased, associated in part with the development of atypical antipsychotic drugs that appear to be more effective and safer, with fewer untoward side effects (Findling, Gilmore, & McNamara, 2001; Patel, Sanchez, Johnsrud, & Crismon, 2002).

STIMULANTS AND RELATED MEDICATIONS FOR ADHD

ADHD is one of the most common disorders of childhood and adolescence, conservatively affecting 3–5% of all school-age children in the United States (American Psychiatric Association, 1994; Barkley, 1998). Developmentally inappropriate levels of inattention, hyperactivity, and impulsivity diagnostically characterize ADHD. At least some of these symptoms must have appeared prior to 7 years of age and must persist to a degree that significantly impairs the child's functioning in more than one setting (e.g., home and school). It is considered a neurobiological disorder with considerable evidence supporting a genetic basis (Sunohara et al., 2000; Thapar, Harrington, Ross, & McGuffin, 2000; Weiss, Hechtman, & Weiss, 2000). Treatment options for ADHD have typically focused on pharmacology, behavioral/psychosocial interventions, or a combination of both (Fine et al., 2003; Purdie, Hattie, & Carroll, 2002). The following sections will focus on pharmacological treatment, describing three main classes of medications used in the treatment of ADHD; stimulants, antidepressants, and other agents.

Stimulants

Over 60 years ago it was observed that stimulants appeared to reduce disruptive behaviors now associated with ADHD (Bradley, 1937). Today, stimulants are the mainstay of pharmacologic treatments for ADHD. They include methylphenidate, dextroamphetamine, magnesium pemoline, and amphetamine/dextroamphetamine. Variations of methylphenidate have also been marketed under other trade names, including Concerta, Focalin, Metadate, and Methylin (see Table 18.1). Methylphenidate accounts for about 90% of prescribed medication for ADHD (Julien, 2001). One other stimulant, methamphetamine, is used very infrequently to treat ADHD. Adderall and Concerta have been found to be as effective as methylphenidate (Findling, Short, & Manos, 2001; Grcevich, Rowane, Marcellino, & Sullivan-Hurst, 2001; Newcorn, 2001; Rapport, Gerber, & Lau, 2002). Stimulants are rapidly absorbed in the bloodstream after ingestion, resulting in a relatively quick onset of action, then are rapidly metabolized by the liver. Consequently, multiple doses are generally required to sustain the desired effect over time.

The procedure used to determine the type and dosage of medication to use is called an algorithm. The algorithm for psychopharmacologic treatment of ADHD is relatively straightforward since much is known about the disorder and stimulants have been well studied (Pliszka et al., 2003). This algorithm begins with a low dose of methylphenidate, increasing the dosage until therapeutic effects are reached or until side effects preclude further use of the drug. If methylphenidate is not satisfactory, the next step is to try dextroamphetamine or Adderall. Pemoline is not recommended as an initial treatment choice due to a risk of potentially fatal liver failure (American Academy of Pediatrics, 2001). If desired treatment results are still not obtained, the next step is generally a nonstimulant medication, such as one of the tricyclic antidepressants or an atypical antidepressant (bupropion or venlafaxine). Antihypertensive medications, such as clonidine, may also be prescribed (American Academy of Child and Adolescent Psychiatry, 2002).

It may appear paradoxical to treat a seemingly overactive child with a stimulant medication. Biologically, attention difficulties related to ADHD seem to be attributed to dysfunction in the region of the brain associated with cognitive/attention processing, manifested by reduced neurotransmitter availability (Bush et al., 1999). Stimulants increase concentrations of the neurotransmitters dopamine and, to a lesser extent, norepinephrine and serotonin. This increase in neurotransmitter availability results in improved cognition, memory, and attention.

The side effects of stimulants are typically mild and tend to diminish over time. As noted in Table 18.1, the most common side effects are decreased appetite, stomachache, headache, insomnia, and irritability (American Academy of Pediatrics, 2001). Some concern has been raised regarding growth delay associated with stimulants. Although some studies have found little or no decrease in either height or weight in later life, other studies have reached conflicting conclusions, indicating the need for additional research into stimulants' long-term effects (Rapport & Moffitt, 2002; Vitiello, 2001). All stimulants are controlled substances, administered through the U.S. Drug Enforcement Administration (DEA). Although concern has frequently been raised regarding the potential for treatment with stimulants to lead to either dependence or an increased risk of illicit drug use later on, research has not borne this out (Barkley, Fischer, Smallish, & Fletcher, 2003; Chilcoat & Breslau, 1999; Wilens, Faraone, Biederman, & Gunawardene, 2003).

Evidence supporting the effectiveness of stimulants in the treatment of ADHD is unequivocal (American Academy of Child and Adolescent Psychiatry Official Action, 2002; Forness & Kavale, 2001; Greenhill et al., 2001). The most comprehensive empirical multimodal study ever undertaken to address the treatment of young children with ADHD was initiated by the National Institute of Mental Health (NIMH) in 1995 (MTA Cooperative Group, 1999a, 1999b). Referred to as the Multimodal Treatment of ADHD (MTA), six sites around the United States and a site in Canada participated in

TABLE 18.1. Stimulant and Nonstimulant Medications for ADHD

Generic name	Trade name	Forms	Dosages	Duration	Side effects
			Stimulants		
Methylphenidate	Concerta	Extended release	18 mg 27 mg 36 mg 54 mg	8–12 hours	Loss of appetite, insomnia, stomachache, headache, irritability, and anxiety
	Focalin	Immediate action	2.5 mg 5.0 mg 10 mg	4–5 hours	
	Metadate	Extended release	10 mg 20 mg	6–8 hours	
	Methylin	Immediate action	5.0 mg 10 mg 20 mg	3–4 hours	
		Extended release	10 mg 20 mg	6–8 hours	
	Ritalin	Immediate action	5.0 mg 10 mg 20 mg	3–4 hours	
		Sustained release	20 mg	6–8 hours	
Dextroamphetamine	Dexedrine	Immediate action	5 mg 10 mg	4–6 hours	
		Sustained release	5 mg 10 mg 15 mg	6–10 hours	
Pemoline	Cylert	Immediate action	18.75 mg 37.5 mg 75 mg	6–8 hours	Pemoline is usually not a first-line treatment due to increased risk of liver failure
Amphetamine/ dextroamphetamine	Adderall	Immediate action	5 mg 7.5 mg 10 mg 12.5 mg 15 mg 20 mg 30 mg	4–6 hours	
		Extended release	5 mg 10 mg 15 mg 20 mg 25 mg 30 mg	8–10 hours	
			Nonstimulants		
Atomoxetine	Strattera	Immediate action	10 mg 18 mg 25 mg 40 mg 60 mg	5–8+ hours	Upset stomach, loss of appetite, dizziness, fatigue, mood swings
Modafinil	Provigil	Immediate action	100 mg 200 mg	6–8 hours	Headache, nausea, anxiety, insomnia, dry mouth

the 14-month study, which involved 579 children between 7 and 10 years of age, all diagnosed with the combined type of ADHD (inattention *and* hyperactivity). Participants were randomized to one of four possible treatment groups. One group served as a community control (CC). Subjects in this group were not given any specific treatment, but two-thirds of the parents sought out stimulant treatment through community physicians on their own over the course of the study. A second group received medication alone (MED). Children in this group received methylphenidate unless the response was inadequate, in which case they were administered another second-line medication according to the algorithm as indicated above. The third group received intensive psychosocial treatment (BEH), based largely on behavioral principles. This included parent training classes (both individual and group), child-focused behavioral therapy, an intensive summer treatment program, and school-based interventions. School-based training involved comprehensive teacher training and consultation, a "shadow" aide for the child, and a daily report card linked to home consequences. A fourth group (COMB) received a combination of the BEH and MED treatment regimes. Regarding the efficacy of medication in the treatment of ADHD, the results of the study were clear. Despite the intensive treatment regimen of the BEH group, stimulant medication (MED) was not only significantly more effective than behavioral treatment or community care alone, but on the vast majority of different outcome measures was as effective as behavioral and medication treatments combined (MTA Cooperative Group, 1999a, 1999b). Interestingly, combined treatment also tended to improve scores on reading tests and on ratings of social skills on long-term follow-up if children remained on medication (Arnold et al., 2000).

More recently, Swanson et al. (2001) reported normalization findings (no ADHD symptomology) at the end of the 14-month MTA study. On a 4-point scale on which a score of 0 meant "no ADHD symptoms," 1 meant "some," 2 meant "pretty much," and 3 meant "very much," all groups scored above 2 prior to treatment, with no differences among groups. After treatment, 25% of the CC group had normalized—that is, scored at an average of below 1 on the 4-point scale, compared to 34% of the BEH group. For the MED group, 56% had normalized after 14 months, and in the COMB group the normalization rate was 68%. In other words, behavioral intervention alone led to a complete reduction in ADHD in only about one-third of the children, compared to nearly a two-thirds reduction in the combined group. On follow-up, 10 months after completion of the study, these four groups held their respective positions on this variable, with the CC group at 27% normalized, BEH at 32%, MED at 38%, and the COMB group at 48%. Although children in the MED and COMB groups lost some ground relative to children in the other groups, the combined behavioral and medication treatment was still 1.5 times better than the behavioral treatment on follow-up (Arnold et al., 2000). Collectively, these findings clearly demonstrate the effectiveness of stimulant medication as a treatment for ADHD symptomology but, more importantly, indicate that best practice is usually a combination of medication and behavioral therapy.

Antidepressants Used to Treat ADHD

Although antidepressants will be described in greater detail in a following section of this chapter, they are also used in the treatment of ADHD (refer to Table 18.2 in the next section). Tricyclic antidepressants (TCAs) have been used for this purpose since the 1960s (Geller et al., 1999; Kollins, Barkley, & DuPaul, 2001). Today, their use is generally limited to cases where ADHD symptoms have been either unresponsive to or adversely affected by stimulants (American Academy of Child and Adolescent Psychiatry, 2002). A second class of antidepressants, represented by the selective serotonin reuptake inhibitors (SSRIs), is also occasionally used, but there is some debate over the efficacy of SSRIs as a treatment for ADHD (Emslie et al., 1999). The "atypical" or "novel" antidepressants have also been studied as second-line treatments for ADHD and seem to be quite promising (Conners et al., 1996; Hudziak et al., 2000; Kotler et al., 2000; Newcorn, 2001).

Other Medications for ADHD

Atomoxetine represents the first nonstimulant medication specifically approved for ADHD by the U.S. Food and Drug Administration (FDA). Recent studies, along with earlier clinical trials, show therapeutic results that rival those of methylphenidate without the abuse potential associated with stimulants (Heiligenstein et al., 2000; Kratochvil et al., 2002). Another medication, modafinil, appears promising but is more expensive and is recommended only as a second- or third-line drug for ADHD (Rugino, 2002). Clonidine and guanfacine, both antihypertensive medications, have been used to treat ADHD, although generally in combination with methylphenidate (Hazell & Stuart, 2003; Julien, 2001).

MEDICATIONS FOR DEPRESSION AND DISORDERS OF MOOD

Although childhood onset of depressive or other mood disorders does not occur as often as ADHD, it is not uncommon and may conservatively affect over 2% of children and at least twice that number of adolescents (Birmaher & Brent, 1998). There are essentially three major types of mood disorders described in the fourth edition of the *Diagnostic and Statistical Manual of Mental Disorders* (DSM-IV): depression, dysthymia, and bipolar disorder (American Psychiatric Association, 1994). Bipolar disorders in children are relatively rare and difficult to diagnose, due to less distinct patterns of cycling than occur in adults, but become more common during adolescence and early adulthood. Antidepressants or mood stabilizers are the second most often prescribed medication for children and adolescents, with some evidence to suggest that they may now have surpassed stimulants in frequency of use (Safer, 1997; Sweeney, Forness, Kavale, & Levitt, 1997). Emslie et al. (1999) reviewed the extant literature regarding the safety and efficacy of nontricyclic medications in the treatment of depressive and anxiety disorders in children and adolescents. They addressed two major questions in conducting their research: (1) Comparing adults and children, are there differences in the pharmacokinetics, safety, and efficacy of the antidepressants under study? and (2) Are depressive and anxiety disorders in children and adults similar? Regarding the first question, although drug therapy for childhood depressive disorders is generally similar to that employed for adults, they were quick to point out that only basic pharmacologic data are available for children and adolescents. Therefore, they strongly recommended that ongoing efficacy studies involving children and adolescents be conducted. Regarding the second question they found that, in general, there are more similarities than dissimilarities in adult and childhood depressive disorders and anxiety.

Five different types of antidepressants and mood stabilizers will be discussed in this section: TCAs, SSRIs, "novel" or "atypical" antidepressants, monoamine oxidase inhibitors (MAOIs), and lithium.

TCAs

The TCAs (see Table 18.2) are classified by their unique three-ring chemical structure. They have been used to treat depressive disorders, anxiety disorders, and panic disorders in adults for many years. The TCAs have also been used in children for the same disorders, although recent research has generally not supported their efficacy as a treatment of pediatric depressive disorders (Geller et al., 1999; Wagner & Ambrosini, 2001). Also, much concern has been raised as to their safety in this population (Braconnier, Le Coent, & Cohen, 2003). Geller et al. (1999) concluded that continued use of TCAs for children and adolescents needs to be carefully weighed against serious risks of lethal overdose and reports of sudden unexplained death. The availability of safer and easier to monitor medications now make the TCAs less attractive as treatment for pediatric psychiatric disorders. Consequently, TCAs are typically no longer used as a drug of first choice in the treatment of depressive disorders or anxiety (Walsh, 1998).

SSRIs

A relatively new class of antidepressant medications, the SSRIs, has become widely

TABLE 18.2. Antidepressants

Class	Generic name	Trade name	Side effects
TCAs	Amitriptyline Desipramine Doxepin Imipramine Nortriptyline Protriptyline Trimipramine	Elavil Norpramin Sinequan Tofranil Pamelor Vivactil Surmontil	Sedation, fatigue, nervousness, dry mouth, tremors, blurred vision
SSRIs	Citalopram Escitalopram Fluoxetine Fluvoxamine Paroxetine Sertraline	Celexa Lexapro Prozac Luvox Paxil Zoloft	Stomach upset, insomnia, dizziness, headache, blurred vision, dry mouth
"Novel" or "atypical" Antidepressants	Bupropion Mirtazapine Venlafaxine Trazodone Nefazodone	Wellbutrin Remeron Effexor Desyrel Serzone	Tremor, insomnia, headache/dizziness, nausea, dry mouth
MAOIs	Phenylzine Selegiline Tranylcypromine	Nardil Eldepryl Parnate	Drowsiness, dizziness, abdominal pain, hypertensive crisis[a]
Lithium	Lithium carbonate	Eskalith Lithobid Lithonate Lithotabs	Nausea/vomiting, headache, tremor, weight gain

[a]Hypertensive crisis can be fatal. Use of MAO inhibitors requires strict dietary vigilance.

used to treat depressive disorders and anxiety (see Table 18.2). The first of these drugs, fluoxetine, was approved by the FDA in 1988 and is currently the only SSRI specifically approved by the FDA for use with children and adolescents 7–17 years of age for depression and obsessive–compulsive disorder (OCD; U.S. Food and Drug Administration, 2003). Since then, several other SSRIs have been introduced (Table 18.2). Ongoing research continues to support the relative safety and efficacy of the SSRIs in pediatric populations (Bostic, Prince, Brown, & Place, 2001; Emslie et al., 2002; Nixon, Milin, Simeon, Cloutier, & Spenst, 2001; Pine, 2002). Two recent studies (Rosack, 2002; Simon, Cunningham, & Davis, 2002) found no effect for maternal use of SSRIs on either congenital malformations or developmental delay. They did note a slightly decreased birth weight and earlier delivery associated with maternal SSRI exposure.

An NIMH study currently under way, the Treatment for Adolescents with Depression Study (TADS), is viewed as an important "next step" in depression research. The TADS is designed to directly compare the effectiveness of four treatment conditions on major depressive disorder in adolescents, specifically, (1) cognitive behavioral therapy alone, (2) clinical trial of medication (fluoxetine) alone, (3) a combination of both, and (4) placebo only. Preliminary data from the second and third phases of the trial are under review with findings released sometime in 2004 (Emslie et al., 2002; Treatment for Adolescents with Depression Study Team, 2003).

"Novel" or "Atypical" Antidepressants

These medications are chemically unrelated to either the TCAs or SSRIs. In general, most have fewer side effects than TCAs and are more selective in their chemical action (Forness et al., 1999). Both venlafaxine and bupropion are occasionally used to treat ADHD (Garland, 2003). Treatment of depression with mirtazapine has been associated with agranulocytosis, a rare but serious and potentially fatal blood disorder.

MAOIs

The MAOIs represent an effective alternative class of medications used to treat major depressive disorder. The MAOIs act by blocking the action of enzymes that metabolize specific neurotransmitters, primarily serotonin and norepinephrine. Phenylzine and tranylcypromine are MAOIs that have been used for many years to treat depression. Selegiline, the newest of the MAOIs, is used primarily as a treatment for Parkinson's disease but has been studied as a treatment for major depression (Bodkin & Amsterdam, 2002). The MAOIs are seldom, if ever, used as a first-line treatment for major depressive disorder due to the risk of potentially life-threatening hypertensive crisis if foods containing tyramine are consumed (Emslie et al., 1999). These foods include aged cheeses, certain alcoholic beverages, canned or dried meats, certain fruits and vegetables (e. g., avocados, bananas, fava beans), caffeine, colas, and chocolate. *Note that this list in by no means exhaustive and includes only a few representative food types.*

The treatment algorithm for depressive disorders typically begins with the SSRIs, followed by the "novel" or "atypical" agents, after which the TCAs or MAOIs may be considered. Compared to the stimulants, antidepressants take substantially longer to elicit the desired therapeutic steady-state response, often measured in weeks rather than hours.

Lithium

Lithium has been used for over half a century as the primary treatment choice for bipolar disorder. It is currently the only medication approved as maintenance therapy for bipolar disorder in individuals 12 years of age and older (Young & Scahill, 2002). It has also been used in combination with other mood stabilizers for depression that seems resistant to standard medical treatment, as well as a treatment for aggression and certain behavioral disorders in children with developmental disorders (Forness et al., 1999). Pharmacologically, lithium promotes balance of multiple neurotransmitter systems. It has a fairly narrow therapeutic range, requiring regular blood-level monitoring to avoid overdosage. Lithium toxicity is a medical emergency and may require inpatient hospital treatment. Side effects include headache, tremor, and weight gain (see Table 18.2). Carbamazepine is also used as a treatment for bipolar disorder. It has a wider therapeutic range than lithium and fewer negative side effects, but both are often used in combination (Carlson et al., 2003).

MEDICATIONS FOR ANXIETY DISORDERS

The term "childhood anxiety disorder" refers to a constellation of psychiatric diagnoses, including separation anxiety disorder, generalized anxiety disorder (GAD), specific phobias, social phobias, obsessive–compulsive disorder, selective mutism, and posttraumatic stress disorder (PTSD) (Nemeroff, 2001). Together, these disorders affect as many as 13% of children and youth, more than any other childhood psychiatric disorder. Treatment options for anxiety disorders typically include either psychosocial therapy (often cognitive-behavioral therapy) or medication. This section will focus on three classes of medications used to treat anxiety disorders: anxiolytic (antianxiety) medications, adrenergic agents, and antidepressants.

Anxiolytics

The anxiolytics are nearly synonymous with benzodiazepines, since they have been the drug of choice for decades for the short-term treatment of anxiety and insomnia. The first benzodiazepine, chlordiazepoxide, was introduced in the 1960s as a treatment for anxiety. Since then, 14 additional benzodiazepines have been developed as anxiolytic agents (see Table 18.3). The benzodiazepines are easy to use, have relatively low toxicity, and are tremendously effective in relieving anxiety (Julien, 2001). However, they are controlled substances under DEA Schedule IV (abuse may lead to limited physical or psychological dependence) and are generally used for acute rather than chronic anxiety due to the risk of producing dependency.

Adrenergic Medications

Adrenergic agents influence the secretion or absorption of adrenaline and noradrenalin, both neurotransmitters involved in blood pressure regulation, cardiac output, and arousal. Clonidine is an antihypertensive medication which, in addition to its antianxiety effects, has also been used to treat Tourette's syndrome and ADHD (Sweeney et al., 1997). Another antihypertensive medication, guanfacine, has also been used to treat anxiety in children. Finally, buspirone is a newer antianxiety medication that shows much promise in the treatment of anxiety disorders.

Propranolol belongs to a group of adrenergic medications called "beta-blockers." These drugs are primarily used in the management of cardiovascular disorders, exerting their effect by lowering blood pressure and heart rate and stabilizing cardiac functioning. Although not approved by the FDA for psychiatric disorders, propranolol has been used to treat PTSD, anxiety, and panic disorders, as well as behavior disorders in children with mental retardation. Riddle et al. (1999) reviewed the extant literature regarding the efficacy and safety of anxiolytic medications, adrenergic agents, and the opiate antagonist naltrexone in the treatment of various psychiatric disorders in children and adolescents. They found that there were virtually no controlled studies to support use of these drugs for treatment of psychiatric disorders, pointing to the need for significant double-blind placebo studies of these drugs with this population.

Antidepressants

The SSRIs have become widely used in the treatment of various types of anxiety disorders. The SSRIs have high tolerance levels, relatively few negative side effects, and lack the need for blood-level monitoring. A significant number of studies have been conducted investigating their effectiveness in treating a variety of specific anxiety disorders.

The National Institute of Mental Health has supported the development of research units in pediatric psychopharmacology (RUPPs). The purpose of the RUPPs has focused on short-term efficacy and safety studies of psychotropic medications commonly used in children and adolescents with mental disorders. Several RUPP studies are currently under way. One study focused on fluvoxamine as a

TABLE 18.3. Benzodiazepines

Generic name	Trade name	Side effects[a]
Long-acting agents		
Diazepam	Valium	
Chlordiazepoxide	Librium	
Flurazepam	Dalmane	
Halazepam	Paxipam	
Prazepam	Centrax	
Chlorazepate	Tranxene	
		Sedation, drowsiness, ataxia, lethargy, mental confusion, motor and cognitive impairments, disorientation
Intermediate-acting agents		
Lorazepam	Ativan	
Clonazepam	Klonopin	
Quazepam	Dormalin	
Estazolam	ProSom	
Short-acting agents		
Midazolam	Versed	
Oxazepam	Serax	
Temazepam	Restoril	
Triazolam	Halcion	
Alprazolam	Xanax	

[a] Side effects of the benzodiazepines are generally dose-related extensions of the intended or main effects.

treatment for anxiety disorders (Research Unit in Pediatric Psychopharmacology, 2001). The group studied 238 children ages 6–17 who met the criteria for social phobia, separation anxiety disorder, or GAD, and who had received psychological treatment for at least 3 weeks without improvement. Children were randomly assigned to either a control or experimental (fluvoxamine) group. Results indicated a 76% response from the fluvoxamine group, compared to a 29% response from the control group, based on the Clinical Global Impressions–Improvement scale. In a follow-up study (Research Units in Pediatric Psychopharmacology, 2002), participants in the first RUPP investigation entered a 6-month treatment phase to examine (1) long-term maintenance of response in fluvoxamine responders, (2) acute response to fluoxetine in fluvoxamine nonresponders, and (3) acute response to fluvoxamine in placebo nonresponders. Results indicated that anxiety symptoms remained low in 94% of subjects who initially responded to fluvoxamine. Among fluvoxamine nonresponders who were switched to fluoxetine, 71% improved. Among 48 placebo nonresponders placed on fluvoxamine, 56% showed clinically significant improvement.

A significant number of other research studies point to the effectiveness of SSRIs in the treatment of various types of anxiety disorders. Consequently, the SSRIs are now

TABLE 18.4. Pharmacological Treatments by Specific Anxiety Disorder

Specific anxiety disorder	Medication	Class
Separation anxiety	Fluvoxamine	SSRI
Generalized anxiety disorder	Venlafaxine	Atypical antidepressant
	Buspirone	Azapirone
	Fluvoxamine	SSRI
Specific phobias	Paroxetine	SSRI
Social phobia	Clonidine	Adrenergic agent
	Alprazolam	Benzodiazepine
	Clonazepam	Benzodiazepine
	Phenylzine	MAOI
	Citalopram	SSRI
	Fluoxetine	SSRI
	Fluvoxamine	SSRI
	Paroxetine	SSRI
Obsessive–compulsive disorder	Citalopram	SSRI
	Fluoxetine	SSRI
	Paroxetine	SSRI
	Sertraline	SSRI
	Clomipramine	TCA
Selective mutism	Fluoxetine	SSRI
Posttraumatic stress disorder	Fluvoxamine	SSRI
	Paroxetine	SSRI
Panic disorder	Clonidine	Adrenergic agent
	Guanfacine	Adrenergic agent
	Alprazolam	Benzodiazepine
	Citalopram	SSRI
	Fluvoxamine	SSRI
	Paroxetine	SSRI

Note. This list is not exhaustive, but reflects use of these medications for specific anxiety disorders reflected in the research reviewed.

becoming a first-line treatment for such disorders (American Academy of Child & Adolescent Psychiatry, 2002; Cook et al., 2001; Davidson, 1998; Masi et al., 2001; Riddle et al., 2001; Thompson, Ebbesen, & Persson, 2001). Table 18.4 (on p. 361) presents a summary of various medications used in the treatment of anxiety disorders.

MEDICATIONS FOR SCHIZOPHRENIA AND PSYCHOTIC DISORDERS

Schizophrenia and related psychotic conditions are rare in children, although somewhat more common in teenagers (Findling et al., 2001). Approximately one-third of people with schizophrenia develop symptoms during their teenage years. Since adolescent-onset schizophrenia is typically associated with a poor outcome, early effective pharmacological treatment is critical (Sporn & Rapoport, 2001). Some 70% of patients treated with antipsychotic medications show significant improvement in psychotic symptoms (Hoff & Kremen, 2003).

Classical Antipsychotics

Prior to the 1950s the only available pharmacological treatment for schizophrenic disorders was sedation. Although sedatives exerted a significant calming effect, they did nothing to treat the hallucinations and delusions symptomatic of schizophrenia. In the early 1950s chlorpromazine, a drug typically used as a calming agent prior to surgery, was found to have the additional effect of reducing the positive symptoms associated with schizophrenia (Julien, 2001). These symptoms included delusions, hallucinations, disorganized speech, and/or grossly disorganized or catatonic behavior (American Psychiatric Association, 1994). Other drugs belonging to the same class (phenothiazines) exerted similar effects. These drugs, among other neuroleptic medications developed in the late 1950s and 1960s, became known as "typical" or "classical" antipsychotics (Table 18.5) and were the mainstay of pharmacologic treatment for the next two decades.

Atypical Antipsychotics

In the early 1990s, a new group of medications was developed to treat schizophrenia (Table 18.5). Collectively known as "atypical" or "novel" antipsychotic agents, these drugs have the advantage over the classical medications in that they are effective not only for positive symptoms of schizophrenia but negative symptoms as well. Negative symptoms of schizophrenia include flattened affect, restrictions in thought and speech production, and reduced goal-directed behavior (American Psychiatric Association,

TABLE 18.5. Antipsychotic Medications

Class	Generic name	Trade name	Side effects
Typical or "classical" antipsychotics	Chlorpromazine Haloperidol Thiothixene Thioridazine Fluphenazine Trifluoperazine Perphenazine Mesoridazine Prochlorperazine Loxapine Pimozide	Thorazine Haldol Navane Mellaril Prolixin Stelazine Trilafon Serentil Compazine Loxitane Orap	Sedation/fatigue, agitation/ restlessness, dizziness, anticholinergic effects, extrapyramidal side effects, tardive dyskinesia, neurolpetic malignant syndrome
Atypical or "novel" antipsychotics	Quetiapine Risperidone Clozapine Olanzapine Ziprasidone Aripiprazole	Seroquel Risperdal Clozaril Zyprexa Geodon Abilify	Dizziness, headache, drowsiness, anticholinergic effects, weight gain, tardive dyskinesia, neuroleptic malignant syndrome

1994). These medications also tend to be less sedating and have reduced extrapyramidal side effects (EPS). As a result, the atypical antipsychotics are generally used as the "first-line" treatment for schizophrenia and other psychotic disorders (Findling et al., 2001). Clozapine was the first atypical antipsychotic released in the United States. Due to the risk of potentially fatal agranulocytosis, however, it is now used only for treatment-resistant schizophrenia. Other atypical antipsychotics, including risperidone, olanzapine, quetiapine, and ziprasidone, have been studied extensively as effective first-line treatments for schizophrenia and other psychotic disorders (Findling et al., 2003; Stigler, Posey, & McDougle, 2003).

Although the side effect profile for the typical and atypical antipsychotics is similar, there are differences, primarily in degree. Common side effects associated with all antipsychotics fall into three general categories: EPS, anticholinergic effects, and sedation. Tremors, nervousness, pacing, hand wringing, and similar features are symptomatic of EPS. These symptoms are also collectively referred to as "Parkinsonian features." Anticholinergic effects include dry mouth, blurred vision, constipation/diarrhea, sweating, and nausea, among others. Side effects associated with atypical antipsychotic medications include sedation and EPS, although generally to a lesser extent than observed with the classical antipsychotics. Weight gain is perhaps the most significant negative side effect associated with the atypical antipsychotics, especially olanzapine and risperidone (Bryden, Carrey, & Kutcher, 2001; Campbell, Rapoport, & Simpson, 1999; Martin et al., 2000; Ratzoni et al., 2002). Aripiprazole, the newest of the atypical antipsychotics, however, appears to produce very little associated weight gain. Both the classical and atypical antipsychotics can still produce dyskinesias, either tardive dyskinesia or withdrawal dyskinesia, from long-term use. Campbell et al. (1997) studied 118 children with autism who were treated with haloperidal between 1979 and 1994. Nearly 34% of the children in this study developed dyskinesias (primarily withdrawal). The prevalence was somewhat higher in girls.

Both the typical and atypical antipsychotics are used to treat psychiatric conditions other than schizophrenia. Conduct disorder has long been treated with antipsychotic medication. Among the atypical drugs, risperidone has been studied, with promising results (Findling et al., 2000). A study group sponsored by the Center for the Advancement of Children's Mental Health at Columbia University examined the use of antipsychotics for aggressive youths and concluded that antipsychotic medications, both typical and atypical, may be effective in the treatment of aggression. They recommended that, if antipsychotic medications are indicated, a trial of an atypical antipsychotic should be used first (Pappadopulos et al., 2003; Schur et al., 2003). They also recognized the need for more research regarding the efficacy of these medications in pediatric populations.

Antipsychotic medications are also used to treat autism. Haloperidol, thiothixene, molindone, pimozide, risperidone, and olanzapine have all been studied, either clinically or anecdotally. Arnold et al. (2003) found that risperidone was superior to placebo in reducing symptoms of irritability in children with autism, an area of major concern for parents. Malone, Cater, Sheikh, Choudhury, and Delaney (2001) conducted a pilot study comparing olanzapine and haloperidol in children with autistic disorder. Their findings suggest olanzapine may be an effective treatment for children with autism, although they caution that more long-term placebo-controlled studies are needed. Motor and vocal tics associated with Tourette's syndrome have also been responsive to treatment with antipsychotic medications. Haloperidal has long been used and, more recently, risperidone and ziprasidone have shown promise as effective treatments (Campbell et al., 1999; Sallee et al., 2000).

ISSUES OF COLLABORATION

At the outset of this chapter we attempted to reinforce the notion that psychopharmacologic intervention needs to be added to the list of traditional behavioral or psychosocial treatments for many children with EBD rather than considered as a separate, discreet option. The extensive and growing body of research documenting the effectiveness of medication in the treatment of emotional and behavioral disorders in children and adolescents is unequivocal. The question remains: How can the educational system, the family, and the medical community join together to provide the optimal diagnostic, prescriptive, and evaluative service to children with EBD? Effective collaboration is the key.

Forness and Kavale (2001) have outlined a series of steps that should be added to the diagnostic/prescriptive process for children with E/BD. *Step 1* involves screening for a psychiatric diagnosis when emotional or behavioral problems seem resistant to standard behavioral procedures and/or when attentional or disruptive behaviors suggest possible underlying psychiatric disorders. *Step 2* involves screening for any secondary diagnoses that might also be present. As an example, a primary diagnosis of ADHD with no apparent secondary diagnosis may suggest that referral to a pediatrician might be sufficient. If a secondary diagnosis is identified, a psychiatric referral may be indicated since comorbidity may complicate pharmacological treatment.

The remaining steps involve collaboration with prescribing physicians. *Step 3* involves providing feedback to parents regarding the possibility that a treatable psychiatric disorder may be present and that a referral to a physician may be warranted. *Step 4* entails assisting the physician with any further diagnostic information needed through the school. This may include copies of assessment reports, checklists, or other information for the parents to take to their child's physician. *Step 5* involves providing classroom baseline and treatment effectiveness data to the physician, which can assist in tracking the efficacy of pharmacological intervention, should it be indicated. *Step 6* is ongoing and involves providing extended support and monitoring once the appropriate type and dose of medication is determined. Systematic and frequent monitoring is critical during the titration phase of psychopharmacological intervention. Parents and teachers are in a key position to observe the emergence of main (intended) effects as well as side effects and share this information with the physician. School professionals also need to be prepared to provide assistance to parents and physicians over the long term.

Teachers and other "nonmedical" professionals need to be better informed about the medications used to treat psychiatric disorders, as well as the risks and benefits of placing children and adolescents on psychoactive medications (Forness, Walker, & Kavale, 2003). Konopasek (2004) has prepared a series of "medication fact sheets" designed to provide basic information about psychiatric medications to address this issue.

Collaboration is a complex and critically important process. Kollins et al. (2001) and Wilens (2001) offer excellent discussions of the school's role in this process. Adding this new medical model to special education, as described in the opening of this chapter, requires careful consideration as to how school professionals will operationalize their collaborative efforts. Active and cooperative collaboration between the school, the family, and the physician will help maximize both the immediate and long term effects of psychopharmacological intervention.

REFERENCES

American Academy of Child and Adolescent Psychiatry. (2002, October). *New research spotlights promising treatments for GAD, OCD, and ADHD.* Poster session presented at the American Academy of Child and Adolescent Psychiatry, San Francisco, CA.

American Academy of Child and Adolescent Psychiatry Official Action. (2002). Practice parameters for the use of stimulant medications in the treatment of children, adolescents, and adults. *Journal of the Academy of Child and Adolescent Psychiatry, 41,* 26S–49S.

American Academy of Pediatrics. (2001). Clinical practice guideline: Treatment of the school-aged child with attention-deficit/hyperactivity disorder. *Pediatrics, 108,* 1033–1044.

American Psychiatric Association. (1994). *Diagnostic and statistical manual of mental disorders* (4th ed.). Washington, DC: Author.

Arnold, L. E., Jensen, P. S., Hechtman, L., Hoagwood, K., Greenhill, L., & MTA Cooperative Group (2000, October). *Do MTA treatment effects persist? New follow-up at 2 years.* Paper presented at the annual meeting of the American Academy of Child and Adolescent Psychiatry, New York.

Arnold, L. E., Vitiello, B., McDougal, C., Scahill, L., Shaw, B., Gonzalez, N. M., Chuang, S., Davies, M., Hollway, J., Aman, M. G., Cronin, P., Koenig, K., Kohn, A., McMahon, D. J., & Tierney, E. (2003). Parent-defined target symptoms respond to risperidone in RUPP autism study: Customer approach to clinical trials. *Journal of the American Academy of Child and Adolescent Psychiatry, 42,* 1443–1450.

Barkley, R. A. (1998). *Attention-deficit hyperactivity disorder: A handbook for diagnosis and treatment* (2nd ed.). New York: Guilford Press.

Barkley, R. A., Fischer, M., Smallish, L., & Fletcher, K. (2003). Does the treatment of attention-deficit/hyperactivity disorder with stimulants contribute to drug use/abuse? A 13-year prospective study. *Pediatrics, 111,* 97–109.

Birmaher, B., & Brent, D. (1998). Practice parameters for the assessment and treatment of children and adolescents with depressive disorders. *Journal of the American Academy of Child and Adolescent Psychiatry, 37*(10, supplement), 63–83.

Bodkin J. A., & Amsterdam J. D. (2002. Transdermal selegiline in major depression: A double-blind, placebo-controlled, parallel-group study in outpatients. *American Journal of Psychiatry, 159,* 1869–1875.

Bostic, J. Q., Prince, J., Brown, K., & Place, S. (2001). A retrospective study of citalopram in adolescents with depression. *Journal of Child and Adolescent Psychopharmacology, 11,* 159–166.

Braconnier, A., Le Coent, R., & Cohen, D. (2003). Paroxetine versus clomipramine in adolescents with severe major depression: A double-blind, randomized, multicenter trial. *Journal of the American Academy of Child and Adolescent Psychiatry, 42,* 22–29.

Bradley, C. (1937). The behavior of children receiving benzedrine. *American Journal of Psychiatry, 94,* 577–585.

Bryden, K. E., Carrey, N. J., & Kutcher, S. P. (2001). Update and recommendations for the use of antipsychotics in early-onset psychoses. *Journal of Child and Adolescent Psychopharmacology, 11,* 113–130.

Bush, G., Frazier, J. A., Rauch, S. L., Seidman, L. J., Whalen, P. J., Jenike, M. A., Rosen, B. R., & Beiderman, J. (1999). Anterior cingulate cortex dysfunction in attention-deficit hyperactivity disorder revealed by MRI and the counting stroop. *Biological Psychiatry, 45,* 1542–1552.

Campbell, M., Armenteros, J. L., Malone, R. P., Adams, P. B., Eisenberg, Z. W., & Overall, J. E. (1997). Neuroleptic-related dyskinesias in autistic children: A prospective, longitudinal study. *Journal of the American Academy of Child and Adolescent Psychiatry, 36,* 835–843.

Campbell, M., Rapoport, J. L., & Simpson, G. M. (1999). Antipsychotics in children and adolescents. *Journal of the American Academy of Child and Adolescent Psychiatry, 38,* 537–545.

Carlson, G. A., Jensen, P. S., Findling, R. L., Meyer, R. E., Palabrese, J., DelBello, M. P., Emslie, G., Flynn, L., Goodwin, F., Hellander, M., Kowatch, R., Kusumakar, V., Laughren, T., Leibenluft, E., McCracken, J., Nottelmann, E., Pine, D., Sachs, G., Schaffer, D., Simar, R., Strober, M., Weller, E. D., Wozniak, J., & Youngstrom, E. A., (2003). Methodological issues and controversies in clinical trials with child and ad-

olescent patients with bipolar disorder: Report of a consensus conference. *Journal of Child and Adolescent Psychiatry, 13,* 13–27.

Chilcoat, H., & Breslau, N. (1999). Pathways from ADHD to early drug use. *Journal of the American Academy of Child and Adolescent Psychiatry, 38,* 1347–1354.

Conners, C, K., Casat, C. D., Gualtieri, C. T., Weller, E., Reader, M., Reiss, A., Weller, R. A., Khayrallah, M., & Ascher, J. (1996). Bupropion hydrochloride in attention deficit disorder with hyperactivity. *Journal of the American Academy of Child and Adolescent Psychiatry, 35,* 1314–1321.

Connor, D. F. (2002). Preschool attention deficit hyperactivity disorder: A review of prevalence, diagnosis, neurobiology, and stimulant treatment. *Developmental and Behavioral Pediatrics, 23,* S1–S9.

Cook, E. H., Wagner, K. D., March, J. S., Biederman, J., Landau, P., Wolkow, R., & Messig, M. (2001). Long-term sertraline treatment of children and adolescents with obsessive–compulsive disorder. *Journal of the American Academy of Child and Adolescent Psychiatry, 40,* 1175–1181.

Davidson, J. R. T. (1998). Pharmacotherapy of social anxiety disorder. *Journal of Clinical Psychiatry, 59,* 47–51.

Emslie, G. J., Heiligenstein, F. H., Wagner, K. D., Hoog, S. L., Ernest, D. E., Brown, E., Nilsson, M., & Jacobson, J. G. (2002). Fluoxetine for acute treatment of depression in children and adolescents: A placebo-controlled, randomized clinical trial. *Journal of the American Academy of Child and Adolescent Psychiatry, 41,* 1205–1215.

Emslie, G. J., Walkup, J. T., Pliszka, S. R., & Ernst, M. (1999). Nontricyclic antidepressants: Current trends in children and adolescents. *Journal of the American Academy of Child and Adolescent Psychiatry, 38,* 517–528.

Findling, R. L., Gilmore, H. M., & McNamara, N. K. (2001). The pharmacotherapy of child and adolescent psychotic disorders. *Child and Adolescent Psychopharmacology News, 6*(1), 1–4.

Findling, R. L., McNamara, N. K., Branicky, L. A., Schluchter, M. D., Lemon, E., & Blumer, J. L. (2000). A double-blind pilot study of risperidone in the treatment of conduct disorder. *Journal of the American Academy of Child and Adolescent Psychiatry, 39,* 509–516.

Findling, R. L., McNamara, N. K., Youngstrom, E. A., Branicky, L. A., Demeter, C. A., & Schulz, S. C. (2003). A prospective, open-label trial of olanzapine in adolescents with schizophrenia. *Journal of the American Academy of Child and Adolescent Psychiatry, 42,* 170–175.

Findling, R. L., Short, E. J., & Manos, M. J. (2001). Developmental aspects of psychostimulant treatment in children and adolescents with attention-deficit/hyperactivity disorder. *Journal of the American Academy of Child and Adolescent Psychiatry, 40,* 1441–1447.

Fine, A. H., Kotkin, R. A., Fowler, M., Forness, S. R., Jensen, P. S., Kapz, M., Lerner, M., Posner, M. I., Swanson, J. M., & McKandliss, B. D. (2003). Future directions in the holistic treatment of children with learning and attention disorders: Concerns and guidelines. In A. H. Fine and R. A. Kotkin (Eds). *Therapist's guide to learning and attention disorders* (pp. 443–476). New York: Academic Press.

Forness, S. R., & Kavale, K. A. (2001). Ignoring the odds: Hazards of not adding the new medical model to special education decisions. *Behavioral Disorders*, 26, 269–281.

Forness, S. R., Kavale, K. A., & Davanzo, P. A. (2002). The new medical model: Interdisciplinary treatment and the limits of behaviorism. *Behavioral Disorders*, 27, 168–178.

Forness, S. R., Kavale, K. A., Sweeney, D. P., & Crenshaw, T. M. (1999). The future of research and practice in behavioral disorders: Psychopharmacology and its school implications. *Behavioral Disorders*, 24, 305–318.

Forness, S. R., Walker, H. M., & Kavale, K. A. (2003). Psychiatric disorders and their treatment: A primer for teachers. *Teaching Exceptional Children*, 36(2), 42–49.

Gadow, K. D. (1997). An overview of three decades of research in pediatric psychopharmacoepidemiology. *Journal of Child and Adolescent Psychopharmacology*, 7, 219–236.

Garland, J. E. (2003). Use of venlafaxine in child and adolescent psychiatry. *Child and Adolescent Psychopharmacology News*, 8(5), 1–4.

Geller, B., Reising, D., Leonard, H. L., Riddle, M. A., & Walsh, B. T. (1999). Critical review of tricyclic antidepressant use in children and adolescents. *Journal of the American Academy of Child and Adolescent Psychiatry*, 38, 513–516.

Grcevich, S., Rowane, W. A., Marcellino, B., & Sullivan-Hurst, S. (2001). Retrospective comparison of Adderall and methylphenidate in the treatment of attention deficit hyperactivity disorder. *Journal of Child and Adolescent Psychopharmacology*, 11, 35–41.

Greenhill, L. L., Jensen, P. S., Abikoff, H., Blumer, J. L., DeVeaugh-Geiss, J., Fisher, C., Hoagwood, K., Kratchovil, C. J., Lahey, B. B., Laughren, T., Leckman, J., Petti, T., Pope, K., Shaffer, D., Vitiello, B., & Zenah, C. (2003). Developing strategies for psychopharmacological studies in preschool children. *Journal of the American Academy of Child and Adolescent Psychiatry*, 42, 406–414.

Greenhill, L. L., Swanson, J. M., Vitiello, B., Davies, M., Clevenger, W., Wu, M., Arnold, L. E., Abikoff, H. B., Bukstein, O. G., Conners, C. K., Elliott, G. R., Hechtman, L., Hinshaw, S. P., Hoza, B., Jensen, P. S., Kraemer, H. C., March, J. S., Newcorn, J. H., Severe, J. B., Wells, K., & Wigal, T. (2001). Impairment in deportment responses to different methylphenidate doses in children with ADHD: The MTA titration trial. *Journal of the American Academy of Child and Adolescent Psychiatry*, 40, 180–187.

Hazell, P. L., & Stuart, J. E. (2003). A randomized controlled trial of clonidine added to psychostimulant medication for hyperactive and aggressive children. *Journal of the American Academy of Child and Adolescent Psychiatry*, 42, 886–894.

Heiligenstein, J. J., Spenser, T. J., Faries, D. E., Biederman, J., Kratochvil, C., & Conners, C. K. (2000, October). *Efficacy of tomoxetine vs. placebo in pediatric outpatients with ADHD*. Paper presented at the annual meeting of the American Academy of Child and Adolescent Psychiatry, New York.

Hoff, A. L., & Kremen, W. S. (2003). Neuropsychology in schizophrenia: An update. *Current Opinion in Psychiatry*, 16, 149–155.

Hudziak, J., Brigidi, B., Marte, B., Stranger, C., Bergersen, T., & Rudiger, L. (2000, October). *Bupropion SR in the treatment of stimulant-responsive ADHD adolescents*. Paper presented at the annual meeting of the American Academy of Child and Adolescent Psychiatry, New York.

Jensen, P. S. (2002, Fall). Is ADHD overdiagnosed and overtreated? A review of the epidemiologic evidence. *Emotional and Behavioral Disorders in Youth*, 95–97.

Jensen, P. S., Kettle, L., Roper, M. S., Sloan, M. T., Dulcan, M. K., Hoven, C., Bird, H. R., Bauermeister, J. J., & Payne, J. D. (1999). Are stimulants over-prescribed? Treatment of ADHD in four communities. *Journal of the American Academy of Child and Adolescent Psychiatry*, 38, 797–804.

Julien, R. M. (2001). *A primer of drug action*. New York: Worth.

Kauffman, J. M. (2001). *Characteristics of emotional and behavioral disorders of children and youth* (7th ed.). Upper Saddle River, NJ: Merrill/Prentice Hall.

Kollins, S. H., Barkley, R. A., & DuPaul, G. J. (2001). Use and management of medications for children diagnosed with attention deficit hyperactivity disorder (ADHD). *Focus on Exceptional Children*, 33(5), 1–24.

Konopasek, D. E. (2004). *Medication fact sheets*. Longmont, CO: Sopris West.

Kotler, L., Findling, R., Fried, J., Shuang, S., Lemon, E., Branicky, L., Tosyali, C., & Greenhill, L. (2000, October). *An open label study of venlafaxine in children and adolescents with ADHD*. Paper presented at the annual meeting of the American Academy of Child and Adolescent Psychiatry, New York.

Kratochvil, C. J., Heiligenstein, J. H., Dittmann, R., Spencer, T. J., Biederman, J., Wenicke, J., Newcorn, J. H., Casat, C., Milton, D., & Michelson, D. (2002). Atomoxetine and methylphenidate treatment in children with ADHD: A prospective, randomized, open-label trial. *Journal of the American Academy of Child and Adolescent Psychiatry*, 41, 776–784.

Malone, R. P., Cater, J., Sheikh, R. M., Choudhury, M. S., & Delaney, M. A. (2001). Olanzapine versus haloperidol in children with autistic disorder: An open pilot study. *Journal of the American Academy of Child and Adolescent Psychiatry*, 40, 887–894.

Martin, A., Landau, J., Leebens, P., Ulizio, K., Cicchetti, D., Scahill, L., & Leckman, J. F. (2000). Risperidone-associated weight gain in children and adolescents: A retrospective chart review. *Journal of Child and Adolescent Psychopharmacology, 10,* 259–268.

Masi, G., Toni, C., Mucci, M., Millepiedi, S, Mata, B., & Perugi, G. (2001). Paroxetine in child and adolescent outpatients with panic disorder. *Journal of Child and Adolescent Psychopharmacology, 11,* 151–157.

MTA Cooperative Group. (1999a). A 14-month randomized clinical trial of treatment strategies for attention-deficit/hyperactivity disorder. *Archives of General Psychiatry, 56,* 1073–1086.

MTA Cooperative Group. (1999b). Moderators and mediators of treatment response for children with attention-deficit/hyperactivity disorder. *Archives of General Psychiatry, 56,* 1088–1096.

Nemeroff, R. (2001, Summer). Update on evidence-based treatments for childhood anxiety disorders. *Emotional and Behavioral Disorders, 1*(3), 62–64.

Newcorn, J. H. (2001, Summer). New medication treatment for ADHD. *Emotional and Behavioral Disorders in Youth, 1*(3), 59–61.

Nixon, M. K., Milin, R., Simeon, J. G., Cloutier, P., & Spenst, W. (2001). Sertraline effects in adolescent major depression and dysthymia: A six-month open trial. *Journal of Child and Adolescent Psychopharmacology, 11,* 131–142.

Olfson, M., Marcus, S. C., Weissman, M. M., & Jensen, P. S. (2002). National trends in the use of psychotropic medications in children. *Journal of the American Academy of Child and Adolescent Psychiatry, 41,* 514–521.

Pappadopulos, E., & Jensen, P. S. (2001, Spring). What school professionals, counselors, and parents need to know about medication for emotional and behavioral disorders in kids. *Emotional and Behavioral Disorders in Youth, 1*(2), 35–37.

Pappadopulos, E., MacIntyre, J. C., Crismon, M. L., Findling, R. L., Malone, R. P., Derivan, A., Schooler, N., Sikich, L., Greenhill, L., Schur, S. B., Felton, C. J., Kranzler, H., Rube, D. M., Sverd, J., Finnerty, M. Ketner, S., Siennick, S. E., & Jensen, P. S. (2003). Treatment recommendations for use of antipsychotics for aggressive youth (TRAAY). Part II. *Journal of the American Academy of Child and Adolescent Psychiatry, 42,* 145–161.

Patel, N. C., Sanchez, R. J., Johnsrud, M. T., & Crismon, M. L. (2002). Trends in antipsychotic use in a Texas Medicaid population of children and adolescents: 1996–2000. *Journal of Child and Adolescent Psychopharmacology, 12,* 221–229.

Pine, D. S. (2002). Treating children and adolescents with selective serotonin reuptake inhibitors: How long is appropriate? *Journal of Child and Adolescent Psychopharmacology, 12,* 189–203.

Pliszka, S. R., Lopez, M., Crimson, M. L., Toprac, M. G., Hughes, C. W., Emslie, G. J., & Boemer, C. (2003). A feasibility study of the children's' medication algorithm project (CMAP) for the treatment of ADHD. *Journal of the American Academy of Child and Adolescent Psychiatry, 42,* 279–287.

Purdie, N., Hattie, J., & Carroll, A. (2002). A review of the research on interventions for attention deficit hyperactivity disorder: What works best? *Review of Educational Research, 72,* 61–99.

Rapport, M. D., Gerber, T. N., & Lau, C. (2002). Methylphenidate and Adderall treatment for children with ADHD: Has therapeutic equivalence been demonstrated? *Child and Adolescent Psychopharmacology News, 7*(2), 4–10.

Rapport, M. D., & Moffitt, C. (2002). Attention deficit hyperactivity disorder and methylphenidate: A review of the height/weight, cardiovascular, and somatic complaint side effects. *Clinical Psychology Review, 22,* 1107–1131.

Ratzoni, G., Gothelf, D., Brand-Gothelf, A., Reidman, J., Kikinzon, L., Gal, G., Phillip, M., Apter, A., & Weizman, R. (2002). Weight gain associated with olanzapine and risperidone in adolescent patients: A comparative prospective study. *Journal of the American Academy of Child and Adolescent Psychiatry, 41,* 337–343.

Research Unit in Pediatric Psychopharmacology. (2001). Fluvoxamine for the treatment of anxiety disorders in children and adolescents. *New England Journal of Medicine, 344,* 1279–1285.

Research Unit in Pediatric Psychopharmacology. (2002). Treatment of pediatric anxiety disorders: An open-label extension of the research units on pediatric psychopharmacology anxiety study. *Journal of Child and Adolescent Psychopharmacology, 12,* 175–188.

Riddle, M. A., Bernstein, G. A., Cook, E. H., Leonard, H. L., March, J. S., & Swanson, J. M. (1999). Anxiolytics, adrenergic agents, and naltrexone. *Journal of the American Academy of Child and Adolescent Psychiatry, 38,* 546–556.

Riddle, M. A., Labellarte, M. J., & Walkup, J. T. (1998). Pediatric psychopharmacology: Problems and prospects. *Journal of Child and Adolescent Psychopharmacology, 8,* 87–97.

Riddle, M. A., Reeve, E. A., Yaryura-Tobias, J. A., Yang, H. M., Claghorn, J. L., Gaffney, G., Greist, J. H., Holland, D., McConville, B. J., Pigott, T., & Walkup, J. T. (2001). Fluvoxamine for children and adolescents with obsessive–compulsive disorder: A randomized, controlled, multicenter trial. *Journal of the Academy of Child and Adolescent Psychiatry, 40,* 222–229.

Rosack, J. (2002). Study finds no link between antidepressants, birth defects. *Psychiatric News, 37*(18), 1–2.

Rowland, A. S., Umbach, D. M., Stallone, L., Naftel, A. J., Bohlig, E. M., & Sandler, D. P. (2002). Prevalence of medication treatment for attention deficit-hyperactivity disorder among elementary school children in Johnston County, North Carolina. *American Journal of Public Health, 92,* 231–234.

Rugino, T. A. (2002). Modafinil: A treatment alternative for children with ADHD. *Child and Adolescent Psychopharmacology News, 7*(6), 5–7.

Safer, D. J. (1997). Changing patterns of psychotropic medications prescribed by child psychiatrists in the 1990s. *Journal of Child and Adolescent Psychopharmacology, 7,* 267–274.

Sallee, F. R., Kurlan, R., Goetz, C. G., Singer, H., Scahill, L., Law, G., Dittman, V. M., & Chappell, P. B. (2000). Ziprasidone treatment of children and adolescents with Tourette's syndrome: A pilot study. *Journal of the American Academy of Child and Adolescent Psychiatry, 39,* 292–299.

Schur, S. B., Sikich, L., Findling, R. L., Malone, R. P., Crismon, M. L., Derivan, A., MacIntyre, J. C., Pappadopulos, E., Greenhill, L., Schooler, N., Van Orden, K., & Jensen, P. S. (2003). Treatment recommendations for the use of antipsychotics for aggressive youth (TRAAY). Part I: A review. *Journal of the American Academy of Child and Adolescent Psychiatry, 42,* 132–144.

Simon, G. E., Cunningham, M. L., & Davis, R. L. (2002). Outcomes of prenatal antidepressant exposure. *American Journal of Psychiatry, 159,* 2055–2061.

Sporn, A., & Rapoport, J. L. (2001). Childhood onset schizophrenia. *Child and Adolescent Psychopharmacology News, 6*(2), 1–4.

Stigler, K. A., Posey, D. J., & McDougle, C. J. (2003). Atypical antipsychotic: Efficacy and tolerability in well-designed trials. *Child and Adolescent Psychopharmacology News, 8*(1), 8–11.

Sunohara, G. A., Roberts, W., Malone, M., Schachar, R. J., Tannock, R., Basile, V. S., Wigal, T., Wigal, S. B., Schuck, S., Moriarty, J., Swanson, J. M., Kennedy, J. L., & Barr, C. L. (2000). Linkage of the dopamine D4 receptor gene and attention-deficit/hyperactivity disorder. *Journal of the American Academy of Child and Adolescent Psychiatry, 39,* 1537–1542.

Swanson, J. M., Kraemer, H. C., Hinshaw, S. P., Arnold, L. E., Conners, C. K., Abikoff, H. B., Clevenger, W., Davies, M., Elliot, G. R., Greenhill, L. L., Hechtman, L., Hoza, B., Jensen, P. S., March, J. S., Newcorn, J. H., Owns, E. B., Pelham, W., Schiller, E., Severe, J. B., Simpson, S., Vitiello, B., Wells, K., Wigal, T., & Wu, M. (2001). Clinical relevance of the primary findings of the MTA: Success rates based on severity of ADHD and ODD symptoms at the end of treatment. *Journal of the American Academy of Child and Adolescent Psychiatry, 40,* 168–179.

Sweeney, D. P., Forness, S, R., Kavale, K. A., & Levitt, J. G. (1997). An update on psychopharmacologic medication: What teachers, clinicians, and parents need to know. *Intervention in School and Clinic, 33,* 4–21.

Thapar, A., Harrington, R., Ross, K., & McGuffin, P. (2000). Does the definition of ADHD affect heritability? *Journal of the American Academy of Child and Adolescent Psychiatry, 39,* 1528–1536.

Thompson, P. H., Ebbesen, C., & Persson, C. (2001). Long-term experience with citalopram in the treatment of adolescent OCD. *Journal of the American Academy of Child and Adolescent Psychiatry, 40,* 895–902.

Treatment for Adolescents with Depression Study Team (2003). Treatment for adolescents with depression study (TADS): Rationale, design, and methods. *Journal of Child and Adolescent Psychiatry, 42,* 531–542.

U.S. Food and Drug Administration. (2003). Food and Drug Administration approvals. *Medscape Pharmacists, 4,* 1–14.

Vitiello, B. (2001). Long-term effects of stimulant medications on the brain: Possible relevance to the treatment of attention deficit hyperactivity disorder. *Journal of Child and Adolescent Psychopharmacology, 11,* 25–34.

Vitiello, B., & Hoagwood, K. (1997). Pediatric psychopharmacoepidemiology: Clinical applications and research priorities in children's mental health. *Journal of Child and Adolescent Psychopharmacology, 7,* 287–290.

Wagner, K. D., & Ambrosini, P. J. (2001). Childhood depression: Pharmacological therapy/treatment (Pharmacotherapy of childhood depression). *Journal of Clinical Child Psychology, 30,* 88–97.

Walkup, J. T. (2003). Increasing use of psychotropic medications in children and adolescents: What does it mean? *Journal of Child and Adolescent Psychopharmacology, 13,* 1–3.

Walsh, B. T. (Ed.). (1998). *Child psychopharmacology.* Washington, DC: American Psychiatric Press.

Weiss, M., Hechtman, L., & Weiss, G. (2000). ADHD in parents. *Journal of the American Academy of Child and Adolescent Psychiatry, 39,* 1059–1061.

Wilens, T. E. (2001). *Straight talk about psychiatric medications for kids.* New York: Guilford Press.

Wilens, T. E., Faraone, S. V., Biederman, J., & Gunawardene, S. (2003). Does stimulant therapy of attention deficit hyperactivity disorder beget later substance abuse? Meta-analytic review of the literature. *Pediatrics, 111,* 179–185.

Young, C. M., & Scahill, L. (2002). Lithium in children and adolescents. *Child and Adolescent Psychopharmacology News, 7*(4), 10–12.

Zima, B. T., & Bussing, R. (2004). Child mental health services. In H. I. Kaplan & B. J. Sadock (Eds.), *Comprehensive textbook of psychiatry* (8th ed., pp. 482–500). Philadelphia: Lippincott.

19

The School-to-Community Transition of Adolescents with Emotional and Behavioral Disorders

DOUGLAS CHENEY *and* MICHAEL BULLIS

The transition of students with disabilities from high school to community and young adulthood does not come easily for most of the members of this diverse population. Research findings paint a dismal picture for many adolescents with emotional and behavioral disorders (EBD) upon leaving public school, a process that is unsuccessful for most. Once in the community as adults, a large portion will experience grave challenges in becoming employed, securing assistance from community-based social service agencies, enrolling in any type of postsecondary education, and establishing enduring supportive relationships. Yet, an emerging body of work suggests that there are interventions that can foster a successful transition for many.

Before beginning this review, it necessary to address an important issue that has been discussed elsewhere in this volume but deserves special mention here—at least as it relates to transition. An unfortunate truism of the educational and social service systems in our country is that access to these services is predicated in large part on an adolescent having a disability. Much has been written about the vagaries of diagnosing EBD in the fields of education (e.g., Forness & Knitzer,

1992) and psychology (Achenbach, 1985; Achenbach & Edelbrock, 1978). Suffice it to say that the identification process for EBD is far from perfect and probably underidentifies a large number of adolescents who could and should be so identified and who could and should receive educational and social services as a result of this condition. In line with this fact, we use the EBD term broadly to include both adolescents who have been formally identified with an educational disability or psychiatric label and also those adolescents who do not have a diagnostic label but who exhibit extreme behavioral disorders and who are sufficiently deviant from the norm to mandate some type of specialized transition assistance (e.g., adolescents who are incarcerated for criminal behavior).

This chapter includes five sections. We first provide a brief historical and legal foundation for the transition initiative and its associated mandates and services. Following this, we summarize selected follow-up studies on the transition experiences of adolescents with EBD and provide a section on factors associated with transition success for this population. The fourth section addresses transition-related assessment procedures and interventions. The chapter ends with a discussion of the implications of this review for future research and practice.

HISTORICAL AND LEGAL FOUNDATIONS

Transition became a key issue in special education in 1984 when Madeline Will, then Assistant Secretary of Education, proclaimed that improving the postschool work outcomes of students with disabilities needed to become a national priority (Will, 1984). Since then, federally funded programs and mandates have clarified the importance of transition services and numerous studies have addressed outcomes of students with disabilities. The 1990 Amendments to the Individuals with Disabilities Education Act provided the first defined transition services in federal law as follows:

> A coordinated set of activities for a student, designed within an outcome-oriented process that promotes movement from school to post-school activities, including post-secondary education, vocational training, integrated employment (including supported employment), continuing and adult education, adult services, independent living, or community participation. The coordinated set of activities must be based on the individual student's needs, taking into account the student's preferences and interests, and must include instruction, community experiences, the development of employment and other post-school adult living objectives, and, if appropriate, acquisition of daily living skills and functional vocational evaluation. (Individuals with Disabilities Act of 1990)

The 1997 Amendments to IDEA expanded on previous transition mandates by requiring that the individualized education program (IEP) include a statement of transition services, updated annually, for all students beginning at age 14 (or younger, if determined by the IEP team). Transition services must consider the student's course of study and components of the student's IEP must refer to these courses of study, whether they are academic or vocational. Once the student reaches the age of 16, the transition plan also is required to include, if appropriate, a statement of interagency responsibilities or needed linkages. All statements in the transition plan are intended to provide the necessary instruction, related services, and community experiences to enhance the post-school outcomes of the student. A student with a disability must be invited to participate in this planning process so that his or her interests in school, work, and community will be taken into consideration in developing the transition plan. Finally, adult service providers or other community agency representatives that might provide the student services are to be invited to the transition planning meetings held by the school team (U.S. Department of Education, 1999).

Clearly, the law has been developed so that a process, a product, and outcomes are delineated to enhance the postschool outcomes for all students with disabilities. Although some data suggest these outcomes are improving for many youths with disabilities, youths with EBD are still struggling to successfully earn credits in high school and complete their diplomas (U.S. Department of Education, 2000). The next section presents findings from studies that suggest that students with EBD have yet to achieve the desired results in school and the community that other youths with or without disabilities achieve.

LONGITUDINAL TRANSITION STUDIES

The focus on outcomes articulated in Will's (1984) original paper on transition and the legal mandates on transition through federal legislation focused initially and in large part on describing the school-to-community transition process and outcomes for adolescents with disabilities. This section summarizes the transition results for a national sample of adolescents with EBD and other disabilities recognized under the umbrella of special education, as well as several state-level studies.

The National Longitudinal Transition Study

As a result of the national focus on transition (Edgar, 1987, 1988; Hasazi, Gordon, & Roe, 1985; Will, 1984), the U.S. Office of Special Education and Rehabilitative Services funded the National Longitudinal

Transition Study (NLTS) in 1987. This study began as a 5-year study conducted by SRI International with a national sample of 8,000 youths ranging in ages from 13 to 21 who had received special education and related services between 1985 and 1986. An initial sample of 450 school districts serving students in special education was randomly selected from 14,000 school districts nationally, and approximately 300 school districts and 25 special schools agreed to participate in the study. Data on study participants were collected from phone interviews with their parents, from a survey of educators in their schools, and from the students' school records (Marder, 1992).

Of the students with EBD, 1,321 contacts were attempted, and 41% of them were unsuccessful. Of the remaining 59%, 584 interviews were completed, and data on an additional 89 students were obtained through the surveys and record reviews. Although numerous analyses have been conducted on the NLTS data, we report the major findings regarding employment, education, social experiences, and affiliation with community-based agencies. Two years after leaving school, 59.3% of students with EBD were employed; 3–5 years after leaving school this dropped to 52.6%. A total of 19% had lost a job between these two data points, and 23.7% had been employed during this time period. Of those employed 3–5 years after high school, their median hourly wage was $3.35 (D'Amico & Blackorby, 1992). By comparison, for the total sample of students with disabilities, 40.8% were unemployed 3–5 years after high school, and for the students without disabilities only 31% were unemployed 3–5 years after high school.

In regard to education, only 57.8% of students with EBD were enrolled in some form of vocational education, compared with 64.8% of all students with disabilities (Valdes, Williamson, & Wagner, 1990; Wagner, 1991). Further, 58.6% of the students with EBD dropped out of school, as compared to 37.1% of all students with disabilities (Wagner, Blackorby, Cameto, & Newman, 1993). These dropout data are significant due to their high association with poor employment and community adjustment. Postsecondary enrollment fared no better for young adults with EBD. In the 2 years after leaving

high school, only 17% of participants with EBD were enrolled in postsecondary education programs. In the 3–5 years after leaving high school, this index rose to 25.6% and was comparable to students with learning disabilities entering postsecondary programs. In comparison, 53.1% of students in general population were enrolled in postsecondary education 2 years after high school, rising to 68.6% 3 years after high school (Wagner et al., 1993).

Most students with EBD have a difficult time achieving independent living status in the first 5 years after high school. During this time period, 40.2% of the participants with EBD were living independently, compared to 37.4% of all participants with disabilities (Newman, 1992). Additionally, 25.6% of youths with EBD became parents, and almost 50% were arrested while in high school (Wagner & Shaver, 1989), and 58% were arrested within the 3- to 5-year period after leaving high school (Wagner, 1991).

Finally, only 5.7% of participants with EBD received services from vocational rehabilitation, compared to 12.7% with other disabilities (Marder, Wechsler, & Valdes, 1993). According to parent reports regarding their son or daughter with EBD, 43.9% of participants with EBD had a need for personal counseling, but only 27.1% received such services (Marder et al., 1993).

More recently, the Office of Special Education Programs of the U.S. Department of Education commissioned the National Longitudinal Transition Study-2 (NLTS2). In this study, a second cohort of students was added for comparative purposes. In contrast to the 1987 study, this study included students who were between 15 and 17 years old and who were enrolled in special education in 2001. To make the distribution of students in the two samples equivalent, a subset of youths were selected from each cohort to make valid comparisons. Two major findings stand out at this time for students with EBD. First, half of all students with disabilities in the 2001 cohort were receiving related or support services, as opposed to one-third of the sample in 1987. This was most significant in the area of EBD, where a 20 percentage point increase was noted for mental health services. Secondly, and less positive, was the finding that the overall dropout rate for students with disabilities had been cut in half, but youths with EBD had the highest dropout rate in 1987 and had no decrease over time (Wagner, Cameto, & Newman, 2003).

Selected State Studies

Seminal studies in the 1980s brought attention to the problematic outcomes of students with EBD: (1) Hasazi, Gordon, and Roe (1985) in Vermont; (2) Edgar and colleagues' studies in the state of Washington (Edgar & Levine, 1987; Neel, Meadows, Levine, & Edgar, 1988); (3) Mithaug, Horiuchi, and Fanning (1985) study in Colorado; and (4) the Frank, Sitlington, and Carson (1991) study in Iowa. In these studies, students with special education disabilities (including EBD and other disabilities, such as specific learning disabilities) who had graduated from or left school within the states were interviewed regarding their transition adjustment in the community. Hasazi et al. (1985), Edgar (1988), and Mithaug et al. (1985) conducted these interviews by telephone and relied upon the former student or a family member as the primary informants. Frank, Sitlington, and Carson (1991) conducted their interviews through a mixture of in-person and phone interviews, speaking with the young adults as their primary respondents, with parents serving as a secondary source. Mithaug et al. (1985) contacted the young adults. Edgar (1988) collected data from both former students and parents, while Neel et al. (1988) relied upon parents as the source of information. Brief summaries of the results of these studies follow. In the Hasazi et al. (1985) and Mithaug et al. (1985) studies, the total samples were composed of young people with disabilities other than EBD; thus, their results—while having potential implications for adolescents with EBD—should be viewed with a degree of caution.

Hasazi et al. (1985) studied the postschool employment experiences of a sample of 459 former students with disabilities from nine school districts in Vermont who left school between 1979 and 1983. A total of 130 (28%) had dropped out of high school before earning a completion document, 296 (66%) had last been placed in high school in a resource room, and 129 (29%) had been in a special class; the majority (N = 292,

65%) were male. No data were gathered on the respondents' special education labels, but some portion of the sample did include persons who had been labeled as EBD during high school. Of the total sample, 301 (66%) were interviewed regarding their employment achievements. The majority of the respondents (N = 166, 55%) were competitively employed, typically in a full-time job (N = 111, 37%). The authors found that the following variables were associated with employment status at the time of the interview: sex (males were more likely to be employed), last high school program (respondents from resource rooms were more likely to be employed than students from a special class), manner of exit from high school (graduates were more likely to be employed), and part-time work during high school and summer work experience (persons who were involved in either type of placement were more likely to be employed).

Mithaug et al.'s (1985) target sample was 234 special education students who had graduated from 45 school districts in Colorado between 1978 and 1979. These students were identified as having mental retardation, perceptual/communication disabilities, emotional or behavioral disorders, and physical disabilities. Unfortunately, the results were not disaggregated by disability group. The authors expected to identify about 16% of the population as EBD but actually identified as such and interviewed only 12% of the population, or 37 students. Nearly two-thirds of the graduates lived at home, with little indication of financial independence, but with most (82%) having held at least one job. At the time of the interview, 69% of respondents were working. Most respondents (64%) also felt satisfied with their lives.

Neel et al. (1988) identified a subsample of students with EBD who had been part of Edgar and Levine's (1987) statewide study of students with disabilities who had graduated or aged out of high school in 21 school districts in the state of Washington between 1978 and 1986. Of the 4,157 students identified in the 21 districts, 2,077 were successfully contacted, and 160 were classified as "severely behaviorally disabled," Washington State's term for EBD. The school districts were determined to be representative of the urban, suburban, and rural locations, as well as the ethnic distribution, in the state of Washington. In addition, a cohort of students without disabilities was identified for comparison purposes. Neel et al. (1988) found that 17% of their sample was in postsecondary education programs, as opposed to 47% of the cohorts without disabilities. At the time of interview, 60% of the students with EBD were employed, as contrasted with 73% of the nondisabled respondents, with most finding the jobs through family or friends. Although most of the youths exceeded minimum-wage levels, they were still earning relatively low wages on their jobs. School and employment status also were tabulated as a measure of student engagement in structured activities. The proportion with unengaged time, defined as neither working nor in school, at 31% was higher for students with EBD, as compared to only 8% of the students without disabilities. More than two-thirds (72%) of parents reported their sons/daughters did not use other community agencies or services, and more than half of youths with EBD (58%) and nondisabled youths (66%) were still living with their parents at the time of data collection.

Frank et al.'s (1991) study identified a sample of students with disabilities from the graduating classes of 1985 and 1986 in 15 area education agencies in Iowa. Of the total sample of 2,476 students who were formerly enrolled in special education, 293 had been identified as behaviorally disordered, and 200 were interviewed and included in the data analyses. Frank et al. (1991) found that the majority of students (graduates and dropouts) were living with their parents, yet a greater percentage of dropouts (26%, compared to 15%) were living independently. Almost twice as many graduates as dropouts were employed (58%, compared to 30%), and about the same percentage of graduates and dropouts reported they had attended some sort of postsecondary education (40%). Postsecondary experiences differed for each group, however, with graduates reporting community college as the most frequent experience (20%) and dropouts reporting military service (25%) as most frequent and attendance at community college (10%) as less frequent. Of those who were employed, most were either laborers or service workers, dropouts were earning more than graduates, and most jobs were found through family or friend networks.

A final group of studies with relevance to this chapter and population were conducted by Bullis and his colleagues on the facility-to-community transition of adolescents who were incarcerated in Oregon (Bullis, 1994; Bullis, Yovanoff, Havel, & Mueller, 2001). They examined the facility-to-community transition experiences of a random sample of 531 youths with and without disabilities who were incarcerated in the Oregon Youth Authority (OYA), the state's juvenile correctional system. Data were gathered on the students' educational, personal, and criminal histories and on the services they received while in the juvenile correctional system. After leaving OYA or being placed on parole, youths were interviewed, and, if possible, a family member was included at 6-month intervals to profile each youth's community adjustment experiences. The participants' continuing associations with OYA and the adult correctional systems was examined by accessing extant state databases from those two agencies regarding their respective populations.

Analysis of the demographic characteristics of the sample (Bullis & Yovanoff, in press-a) indicated that the majority (58%) had special education disabilities, which were split roughly evenly between specific learning disabilities and emotional disorders. Comparison between those with and without disabilities revealed that participants with disabilities were more likely to have been retained a grade while in school, committed to the juvenile correctional system for a person-related crime, and last adjudicated for a felony in an urban setting.

A recent article profiling the facility-to-community transition experiences of the 531 formerly adjudicated youths on parole focused on predicting "engagement" (a combination of work, education, and remaining *in* the community and *out* of the juvenile or adult correctional systems) (Bullis, Yovanoff, Mueller, & Havel, 2002). The authors employed a simple predictive model composed of sex, ethnicity, disability status, and type of crime for which the participant was committed to OYA, with engagement at two points in time after release from OYA: 6 months and 12 months postexit after leaving the juvenile correctional system. In this and a second study (Bullis & Yovanoff, 1997), 12 months postexit was the point in time after which virtually all "age-eligible" youths (i.e., youths who turn 18 years of age generally do not to return to the juvenile correctional system because they "age out" of that system) did *not* to return to the juvenile correctional system. Stated differently, if a formerly incarcerated youths did not return to the juvenile correctional system during the 12 months following release, it was extremely unlikely that he or she would return after that point in time.

Participants who *were* engaged at time 1, compared to participants who were *not* engaged at time 1, were 2.38 times *less likely* to return to OYA at time 2 and 3.22 times *more likely* to be engaged at time 2. Disability also was associated with community adjustment, but in a negative manner. Participants with a disability, compared to participants without a disability, were 2.80 times *more likely* to return to OYA at time 1, 1.83 *times more likely* to return to OYA at time 2, and 2.22 times *less likely* to be engaged at time 2. Gender displayed a varied association with community adjustment. Females, compared to males, were 3.85 times *less likely* to be engaged at time 1 but 2.63 times *less likely* to return to OYA at time 2. Neither cultural/ethnic minority status nor type of crime committed by participants of OYA (person-related vs. property) displayed statistically significant associations with engagement at time 1 or time 2.

In a further analysis of the dataset (Bullis & Yovanoff, in press-b), the impact of community-based social services on the engagement of the participants with disabilities was studied. At time 1, only 28% of the sample received services from mental health. Those who did receive such services were *2.25* times *more likely* to be engaged at time 1 as compared to participants who did not receive such services. Somewhat surprisingly, few participants received services from any other agencies, so the researchers aggregated social services into an omnibus variable including all other *community-based agencies*; participants who received services from community-based agencies other than mental health were *1.96* times *more likely* to be engaged at time 1 as compared to participants who did not receive such services. Given the clear association of engagement

status at time 1 with engagement status at time 2 and remaining in the community, these results carry critical implications for the transition process.

Summary of Findings

Generally, longitudinal studies on the community transition of adolescents with EBD have found that they have a high dropout rate when compared to both typically developing peers and to peers with other disabilities. When both graduates and nongraduates with EBD are considered together, they both have limited levels of success in their transition to adulthood (Wood & Cronin, 1999). Adolescents with EBD, both upon their return to the community and later as young adults, have a lower employment rate, typically earn low wages in the labor or service sectors, have difficulties with interpersonal skills, have mental health issues, and have higher arrest rates than their peers (Bullis & Cheney, 1999). Finally, few of these young adults enter postsecondary education programs, thus further limiting their career paths and ultimate success in employment and quality of life as adults (U.S. Department of Education, 1994, 2000).

PREDICTIVE FACTORS

There is an emerging literature regarding predictive factors that influence school, work, and community success. Rylance (1998) used the NLTS database to explore four primary predictors—family characteristics (parents' education, household income, and 1 vs. 2 parents at home), personal characteristics (gender; age; ethnicity; ability to tell time, count, read, and use a telephone; and self-care), receipt of counseling, and receipt of vocational training while in school—with postschool employment for 412 students with EBD. A regression analysis was conducted using these variables from wave 1 data of the NLTS (students who exited school before 1990) as the predictors for the dependent variable (employment status), for student data from wave 2 in 1990–1991. The predictor variables accounted for only 13% of the variance of employment status after 1 year, with the personal and family variables explaining 11% of the variance and school variables accounting for 2% of the variance. The author concluded that, while showing a low level of variance, the school related-variables exerted "sufficient strength" to significantly predict postschool employment. These findings are consistent with those of the National Longitudinal Transition Study research (D'Amico, 1991; D'Amico & Blackorby, 1992; Heal & Rusch, 1995).

Benz, Lindstrom, and Yovanoff (2000) conducted two studies to examine the transition outcomes in education and employment for students with disabilities. In the first study, they examined student and program factors that predicted receipt of a high school diploma and placement in employment or continuing education at program exit. In the first study, 10% of the total sample of 709 students had EBD in this first study. The authors used eight variables in their predictive model that are associated with transition failure, and which also are frequently associated with EBD: absenteeism, suspension, high school dropout, unstable living situation, prior arrest, substance use or abuse, and pregnancy. Students with one or more risk factors were less likely to graduate unless they had completed four or more of the transition goals included on their IEP. Two program-related variables—holding two or more jobs while in the transition program and completing four or more transition goals—predicted student engagement in productive work or continuing education after exiting the program. The authors also computed the cumulative effects of these variables and found that staying in the transition program for a year or more, holding two or more jobs while in the program, and completing four or more transition goals resulted in a fourfold increase in the probability of graduation for students with risk factors and a twofold increase for those without such factors.

In the second study, the authors used focus groups to examine the program participants' perceptions of the most meaningful and important help they received to achieve their education and transition goals. A total of 45 participants in six communities who had completed 4 years in the transition program attended the focus group interviews. Themes from these interviews suggested that students found the transition program much more meaningful than regular high school participation. Further, the respondents believed that the transition program offered more individualized services, consistent support from staff members, and the persistent reminders and efforts to help them succeed. Finally, the youths suggested that the transition program provided additional opportunities to explore career options and learn skills to help them succeed at work and in their school and personal lives. The findings across both studies highlight providing students individualized attention to meet the educational requirements of graduation and the vocational preparation and exploration to succeed in work. Some suggestions to meet this individualized programming are to work with the students to develop self-determined curricula and to enhance collaboration across agencies so that integrated work and academic programs are available for students to apply learning and earn credits in community settings.

Scanlon and Mellard (2002) examined the school experiences of 172 students with disabilities through interviews in person or on the phone. Participants were either presently in high school or had dropped out to pursue the General Education Development (GED) diploma as an optional degree. Most students (114, 66%) had learning disabilities, while 18 (10%) had EBD. The rest of the sample had multiple, physical, or communication disabilities. The authors were interested in these students' perceptions of the impact of their disability on their school experiences and daily living. The authors were also interested in gaining an understanding as to how the experiences of students with learning disabilities (LD) and EBD intersect around the issue of dropping out of school. Across all disabilities, students reported attendance problems and lack of interest in the curriculum as the key factors leading to leaving school. Also, across all groups, students who stayed in school until at least the 11th grade were more likely to obtain a GED. Since most students in the LD/EBD categories reported they had average to very good reading abilities, the authors suggested that some of the students with LD were misidentified and probably displaying behaviors more consistent with those of students with EBD. Students with EBD were more likely to achieve in adult education programs, which may provide a context where the individuals have greater academic success. The authors concluded that students with EBD are likely to find adult education programs less antagonizing and more accepting of their emotional or behavioral issues. The authors suggest these issues need to be addressed to improve programs for these students and to keep them in school to completion of the diploma.

Corbett and Clark (2002) studied the influence of the types and amounts of vocational programming on the postschool outcomes of youths and young adults with EBD. They completed a retrospective analysis of school records for 305 students with EBD who exited secondary education programs between 1990 and 1997 in a large school district in Florida. They found a significant negative correlation between vocational education and dropout, suggesting that greater participation in vocational education was associated with lower rates of dropping out. Vocational education and on-the-job training were also significantly correlated with earnings, with greater amounts of generic vocational education and on-the-job training being related to higher earnings after high school.

Todis, Bullis, D'Ambrosio, Schultz, and Waintrup (2001) used an ethnographic approach to study the factors associated with young adults recently released from corrections facilities who were successful in their current work and living situations. Most of the 15 respondents in the study came from unstable homes and had issues with drug use and financial problems, but a few were from middle- or upper-middle-class backgrounds without financial issues. The respondents noted their parents were unprepared to deal with the challenges they presented when they began middle school. During their time in corrections facilities, these youths described how the structure of the facility helped them to quit using drugs, develop a regular daily schedule, and benefit from improved sleep and health. The point-and-level systems the facilities placed them on clarified daily expectations to be successful. Many received their GED or high school diploma while incarcerated through small classes and individualized programs, and reported making personal connections with at least one adult staff member at the facilities. Youths reported having reflective time during their sentence, and this helped them plan and prepare for their future. Upon return to their communities, they were placed back with families who provided a cheap place to live, but peers and family conflicts led to incidents of drug use and illegal activities. Most females became pregnant soon after their release, although parenting seemingly had a stable effect on their lives. Three groups emerged after leaving correctional facilities: those who never reoffended and did well, those who were less successful and just getting by, and those who reoffended and struggled with ongoing substance abuse and mental health issues. The authors suggest that transition supports be greatly expanded for this group of youths to include employment and housing support, in addition to counseling services, drug treatment, and close mentoring by an adult, along with school support and parent support.

ASSESSMENT PROCEDURES AND INTERVENTIONS

Bullis and Cheney (1999) reviewed two demonstration projects to identify promising practices for the transition of youths and young adults with EBD. They concluded that several program elements impacted student outcomes, based on results from the projects. These included: (1) placing transition programs for students with EBD off-campus from public high schools; (2) having low staff-to-student ratios (1:12–15); (3) having transition and career education specialists as staff members; (4) having these staff members organize and coordinate community-based social services as appropriate for each individual's needs; and (5) using a zero-rejection policy with unconditional care for the students. They also recommended that such programs should include the following program elements: (1) intake and functional assessment, (2) personal futures planning for the youth, (3) a community-based wraparound process for service delivery, (4) competitive employment, (5) flexible educational experiences, (6) social skills programs, and (7) long-term coordinated support and follow-up services.

These recommendations are similar to those offered by others. Edgar's (1987) earliest proposals asserted that programs for these youths should focus on functional vocational programs. Indeed, Edgar (1988) believed that work was the mainstay of these youths' community success. More recently, Harvey (2001) reiterated the importance of making vocational education and career awareness the primary goals of students with EBD secondary education experience. Maag and Katsiyannis (1998) emphasized the significance of social skills training, and Frank and Sitlington (1997) added as especially important both employment and postsecondary enrollment in college for this group, along with social skills training. Kohler (1993), Corbett and Clark (2002), and Walker and Bunsen (1995) emphasized the relationship between vocational experience in school with future ability to obtain and maintain competitive employment, as well as the need to coordinate services across agencies in the community. In considering these findings for youths with EBD, Wood and Cronin (1999) concluded that secondary programs for youths with EBD must focus on increasing high school graduation, increasing vocational training and employment as curriculum components, and improving the transition planning process by having a transition specialist coordinate services across multiple agencies.

There are two clear areas of research relating to the foregoing points. The first relates to the development of functional assessments of transition skills. The second describes and evaluates model demonstration transition programs specifically for adolescents with EBD.

Assessment Studies

In the early 1990s, Bullis and his colleagues began a series of studies based on the premise that youths with EBD needed greater specificity in assessment approaches relating to social and vocational functioning. Bullis and Davis (1999) argued that traditional assessments such as intelligence and personality tests were not as relevant to the transition or rehabilitation field as were "functional assessments" of individual's actual employability, education, and community living skills. In line with Cohen and Anthony's (1984) conclusion that psychiatric symptoms and diagnoses did not predict vocational outcomes, while measures of vocational skills did, Bullis and Davis (1999) contended that functional assessments of the youths' skills and targeted interventions would lead to more effective transition programming and, ultimately, better transition outcomes.

Bullis and colleagues focused on the development of functional assessments for social skills of youths with EBD in vocational and community settings. Bullis, Nishioka-Evans, Fredericks, and Davis (1993) identified job-related behaviors of youths with EBD, using the behavior analytic model (Goldfried & D'Zurilla, 1969). This content-analytic approach identified relevant social interactions for this population and provided a range of response alternatives to each situation typical of the target population. Bullis and Davis (1996) subsequently conducted factor analyses of the field-test data from this initial project to establish two measures with adequate psychometric characteristics: one focusing on job-related knowledge and the other on ratings of social skills in the workplace. In a complementary project, Bullis, Bull, Johnson, and Johnson (1994) identified community-based social behaviors for persons with EBD and factor analyzed the field test data to establish knowledge measures of social skills relevant to community living and the rating scales of these skills (Bullis & Davis, 1997).

The development of these measures is a helpful step forward for assisting educators and transition specialists in their work with youths with EBD. They have utility in identifying the strengths and weaknesses of social behavior in work and the community. The assessments can be used to develop goals and objectives in the youth's transition plans. The tests are also useful in preparing intervention strategies since they identify whether the youth's problems are due to knowledge deficits, skill deficits, or a combination of both. The authors concede that further large-scale use of the measures is needed to provide further information on their reliability and validity. Further, they suggest that the tests will have utility when directly linked to social skills curricula to potentially affect positive social outcomes for youths with EBD in the school and community.

In another approach to assessing student factors influencing success in high school, Kortering, Brazeil, and Tompkins (2002) completed interviews with 33 students with EBD who were in ninth (76%), tenth (18%), or eleventh (6%) grades. Interview questions addressed how students' perceived the best and worst parts of high school, the advantages or disadvantages of staying in school, supports to help them stay in school, recommendations to help youths stay in school, how they had been helped by teachers, and their views of a high school diploma. Students' best classes allow them to socialize, provide for some physical outlet, and emphasized science. Worst classes were those that were boring and had negative teacher interactions. Staying in school and receiving a diploma were viewed as important. Supports for staying in school were highly variable, from policy changes to family support to textbooks and scheduling. The IEP was recommended by the authors as a means of dealing with the variability of these requests for support. Curriculum changes, such as better textbooks, flexible scheduling, and methods to help them deal effectively with peers, were recommended by the students. The authors suggested that these changes could be integrated into students' IEPs. Finally, several of the students indicated that teachers who provided individual help, were amiable, offered encouragement, and made learning an enjoyable experience were most appreciated and effective with them.

Transition Programs

Throughout the 1990s, the federal government made a concerted effort to expand its funded-research projects from those focusing on follow-up outcomes of youths with EBD to studies of interventions assessing improved service delivery components and models. These intervention projects had as their dependent variables improvements in outcomes in education, employment, and community living for students with EBD. Along with research on interventions to impact outcomes, a growing literature has begun on program evaluation of secondary programs for students with EBD.

RENEW (Rehabilitation, Empowerment, Natural Supports, Education, and Work)

The RENEW program was initially funded in 1995 by a grant from the Rehabilitation Services Administration. It was designed to improve the transition outcomes of youths and young adults with EBD and implemented in Manchester, New Hampshire. In its first three years, RENEW served over 25 youths, and results on the first cohort of 18 young adults found that 17 of the 18 completed high school or its equivalent and half (9) entered postsecondary education. The cohort averaged 28 hours per week of work and its members' wages significantly exceeded the minimum wage ($6.18 versus $4.25). These youths also reported after 2 years in the project that they were much more satisfied with their work, schooling, progress toward goals, and handling of life problems (Cheney, Hagner, Malloy, Cormier, & Bernstein, 1998; Hagner, Cheney, & Malloy, 1999; Malloy, Cheney, Hagner, Cormier, & Bernstein, 1998).

Job Designs

Job Designs was located at a mental health treatment center outside a small town in Oregon and funded through a series of federal, state, and local grants or contracts from 1989 to 2000 (Bullis & Fredericks, 2002; Bullis, Fredericks, et al., 1994). Between 1992 and 1995, 79 youths with EBD were accepted into Job Designs, who were referred from the mental health facility (i.e., youths who were exiting the facility to live in the community) or from community-based agencies serving youths in the immediate locale. A total of 71% of those in the program were placed in one or more competitive jobs, worked more than 20 hours per week, and were paid above the minimum wage. Of the 53 who left the program, 21% dropped out of school, 30% completed high school, and 49% maintained enrollment in some type of educational program. Overall, project participants were satisfied with their involvement in the Job Designs and reported that the staff were helpful and helped them gain important skills in the program.

Job Designs and RENEW shared some common features (Bullis & Cheney, 1999).

Neither was located on a high school campus, as their participants had not been successful in the high school setting and were not interested in participating in the high school curriculum. The programs had low staff-to-participant ratios (i.e., 1 staff person for every 12–15 adolescents) in order to meet each person's individualized and intensive needs. Each program had a case manager who focused on career and educational aspects of transition for these youths and young adults. This relationship between youths and the transition specialist was considered critical to the programs' success. The programs practiced zero-reject or unconditional care, providing services to the clients during some difficult times. Even when youths exhibited risky, dangerous, or illegal behavior, they were continued in the programs.

TIP (Transition to Independence Process)

The TIP system frames the strategies that guide practices with young people with EBD and the community collaborations that facilitate successful movement into the domains of employment, educational opportunities, living situations, and community life (Clark, Pschorr, Well, Curtis, & Tighe, 2004). The application of the TIP system has been evaluated through its implementation in the Jump on Board for Success (JOBS) Transition program in several communities in Vermont. Youths who participate in the JOBS Transition program meet Vermont's ACT 264 criteria for severe emotional disturbance and are 14–20 years of age at the time of admission. The JOBS Transition program focuses on person-centered planning and tailoring supports and services to the young person's needs and interests in employment, education, living situation, and community life adjustment. The goals of this program are to secure paid employment for these youths, increase community integration, acquire appropriate living/job skills, decrease dependence on assistance programs (e.g., welfare, social security insurance), and improve the self-confidence of participants.

From 1994 to 2001, 80 individuals with EBD were graduated from the JOBS Transition programs across three Vermont communities. The pre- and postcomparison findings for these 80 graduates showed that changes in a positive direction on the following outcome indicators included (1) graduating from high school or earning a GED (from 53% to 83%); (2) having high school dropouts earn a GED (from 48% to 60%); (3) involvement in the corrections system (from 43% to 13%); (4) living in an independent residential placement (from 25% to 5%); (5) reducing services from community mental health agencies (from 80% to 7%); and (6) receiving social security or welfare benefits (from 51% to 15%). From entry into the program to discharge, changes occurred in the anticipated direction across *each* of these indicators.

ARIES (Achieving Rehabilitation, Individualized Education, and Employment Success)

The ARIES project for adolescents with EBD (Bullis, Moran, Todis, Benz, & Johnson, 2002) was funded for 3 years by the federal Rehabilitation Services Administration. Unlike the projects described above, however, it was operated jointly by staff from the University of Oregon and the Springfield, Oregon, School District, and located within the public school system. A total of 85 participants were referred to ARIES through the schools, vocational rehabilitation, and other community agencies (e.g., corrections, mental health). Each participant was assigned a district-employed transition specialist who worked in conjunction with that individual and, when appropriate, his/her family to develop a service delivery plan and to then access and secure necessary services. Competitive vocational placements were secured for participants, and support was provided for their educational placements. Self-determination was emphasized through each participant's central role in choosing and developing his or her service plan in conjunction with the transition specialist. ARIES participants achieved a relatively high degree of educational achievement. Of the 59 participants who formally exited the program, 36 (61%) completed an educational program, but 31(53%) indicated they did not want to pursue any educational goals (e.g., postsecondary education, specialized technical training) in the future. Conversely, of the 23 participants who had not received one of the above-mentioned school completion documents, 20 (87%) indicated that they wanted to achieve some sort of educational training after leaving the program. Qualitative evaluation of the project indicated that participants, educators, and social service staff viewed the ARIES model as effective in meeting the needs of the adolescents with EBD and provided a critical place within the continuum of services offered through the schools.

FUTURE RESEARCH IN TRANSITION OF YOUTHS WITH EBD

Current results focusing on the transition of youths with EBD are in their infancy. The NLTS and NLTS2 studies have provided the field with evidence of the most problematic outcomes for these youths, but we have yet to complete intervention studies with enough scientific rigor to reach clear conclusions on evidence-based practices for youths with EBD. This section addresses what we believe to be the major research areas in this field in the next decade.

Assessment

Research in the area of assessing the transition skills of youths with EBD is in need of large-scale use of the measures to provide further information on their reliability and validity. If these large-scale studies establish such validity, then the functional measures proposed by Bullis and Davis (1996, 1997) could serve as an evidence-based assessment approach to developing goals and objectives in youths' transition plans. The tests also could be a valid approach to identifying a youth's knowledge or skill deficits. These findings would be particularly valuable for special education teachers and transition specialists as they develop and revise IEPs and transition plans.

Further research also is needed on how best to use student input in the transition process. Kortering et al.'s (2002) findings suggest that we need to use qualitative measures to analyze student input in their transition plans and the subsequent success or failure of these plans. It would appear from the early findings of Kortering et al. that students view school as a social setting more than an academic setting and that these vari-

ables need to be considered for the staying power of school to lead students with EBD toward school completion.

Intervention Research

Of the four intervention programs reviewed in this chapter, none of them has included over 100 students during the reported intervention time. Because only those youths who described their outcomes, which also were analyzed by the researchers, were included, all would be considered a sample of convenience and a sample of voluntary participants. Random assignment was not used, nor was it necessarily considered as a positive approach to identifying students for these studies. Sampling issues present a rather large challenge to our efforts in studying evidence-based practices for students with EBD.

One sampling issue is how to use randomization in such studies. Considering that transition programs are developed at high schools as the site, the unit of evaluation would typically be the school. A district and research team could develop different transition programs based on recommendations of the projects reviewed, randomly assign students with EBD to each high school, and compare intervention effects. This probably would not be a popular approach based on family or student desires in light of Kortering et al.'s suggestions, and would likely receive resistance in the community.

Additionally, the intervention components and intensity levels are difficult to control when two schools are compared. It is difficult to assess variables such as the nature of the relationship between the student and the transition specialist, although the projects reviewed emphasize the importance of this relationship and the necessity of keeping the student/specialist ratio low. This brings to mind the research of Patterson (1982) and the type of parenting style that is most effective with youths. When permissive, authoritative, and authoritarian styles were considered, the authoritative parent—one who is caring and warm but who sets clear limits— often is most effective. Further analyses of personal characteristics of transition specialists and secondary special educators may be warranted to determine the impact of the provider's interpersonal style on the youth's transition outcomes and the best way to "pair" transition specialists with these youths (e.g., are there certain types of staff members and students who work best with one another?).

Level or dosage effects of interventions may also be important to assess. The projects reviewed suggested that a package of intervention elements is required to improve the transition outcomes of these youths. This package includes flexible education programs, vocational awareness and placements, low specialist-to-student ratios, coordinated care in the community, and social skills training. What is not known is the influence of each of these variables on the ultimate community adjustment of these youths. This influence would be best assessed by a large-scale study of at least 100 youths and the foregoing variables analyzed in a regression analysis to determine the amount of variance each contributes to community adjustment. Conducting such a large "N" study while controlling for fidelity of implementation of the independent variables also presents a challenge to this type of research.

Perhaps a more pragmatic model for analysis is required in this research on transitions that is more closely aligned with programmatic evaluation than with experimental investigations. In this line of research, stable and consistently employed intervention approaches would be investigated over a number of years in a transition program. Student outcomes would then be assessed and, given that positive outcomes would be obtained, the program could be disseminated and replicated at other sites. This approach is more likely to be useful in high school and community approaches addressing the needs of youths with EBD.

One challenge in program evaluation is to coordinate the efforts and procedures of the research and practice teams. That is, high school programs often are not able to collect and analyze complete data from community agencies for each student; thus, collaboration between research teams, community agencies, and school districts—much as has occurred in the programs described above—is necessary. Further, the research team needs to identify replication sites to expand the models developed to other communities and

regions with different demographics such as socioeconomics, urban/suburban/rural populations, and ethnic differences. Our recommendations for transition programs may vary based on findings from urban centers as opposed to rural settings.

Finally, virtually all of the research studies conducted on adolescents with EBD are constrained by time and funding limits. Most adolescents, both typically developing and those with disabilities including EBD, display numerous educational, vocational, and living changes between the ages of 16 and 25. Longitudinal studies are essential to follow students with EBD who successfully complete educational and vocational programs into their early adulthood, which requires long-term contact and interviewing procedures of these young adults at ages through their 20s. This long-term follow-up would allow for adult experiences to be identified that could serve as the ultimate standards of adjustment for persons with EBD as young adults in our society.

We conclude this chapter with a final thought. Adolescence and young adulthood is a strange and difficult time period for all us—and especially for young people with EBD. This is the time of life when bodily changes slow and a great "evening" of peoples occurs coincident with entry into the work world and adult roles. Work, daily schedules, bills, wages—issues that may have seemed foreign to a high school student—assume more importance and relevance as a person leaves public school and force a youth into life patterns and responsibilities like those of the very adults that students couldn't understand months earlier. Because of the relevance of the content addressed in transition programs, we strongly believe that effective interventions can make both immediate and long-term differences in the lives of youths with EBD.

It would be naive, however, to believe that such programs will be effective with all youths with EBD. There may be times when the changes in a youth may not be seen for some years, until he or she is ready to use the skills that have been learned. The challenge is to try to serve these youths in the best way possible and to continue those efforts as needed for these youths as they climb the slippery slope to adulthood.

REFERENCES

Achenbach, T. (1985). *Assessment and taxonomy of child and adolescent psychopathology.* Beverly Hills, CA: Sage.

Achenbach, T., & Edelbrock, C. (1978). The classification of child psychopathology. A review and analysis of empirical efforts. *Psychological Bulletin, 85,* 1275–1301.

Benz, M. R., Lindstrom L., & Yovanoff, P. (2000). Improving graduation and employment outcomes of students with disabilities: Predictive factors and student perspectives. *Exceptional Children, 66,* 509–529.

Bullis, M. (1994). *Investigation of the institution-to-community transition of adolescents with emotional and behavioral disorders.* Funded grant proposal, Office of Special Education Programs, Field Initiated Research Studies.

Bullis, M., Bull, B., Johnson, P., & Johnson, B. (1994). Identifying and assessing the community-based social behaviors of adolescents and young adults with emotional and behavioral disorders. *Journal of Emotional and Behavioral Disorders, 2,* 173–189.

Bullis, M., & Cheney, D. (1999). Vocational and transition intervention for adolescents and young adults with emotional or behavioral disorders. *Focus on Exceptional Children, 31*(7), 1–24.

Bullis, M., & Davis, C. (1996). Further examination of job-related social skills measures for adolescents and young adults with emotional and behavioral disorders. *Behavioral Disorders, 21,* 161–172.

Bullis, M., & Davis, C. (1997). Further examination of community-based social skills measures for adolescents and young adults with emotional and behavioral disorders. *Behavioral Disorders, 23,* 29–39.

Bullis, M., & Davis, C. (Eds.). (1999). *Functional assessment procedures in transition and rehabilitation for adolescents and adults with learning disorders.* Austin, TX: Pro-Ed.

Bullis, M., & Fredericks, H. D. (Eds.). (2002). *Vocational and transition services for adolescents with emotional and behavioral disorders: Strategies and best practices.* Champaign, IL: Research Press.

Bullis, M., Fredericks, H. D., Lehman, C., Paris, C., Corbitt, J., & Johnson, B. (1994). Description and evaluation of the Job Design project for adolescents and young adults with emotional or behavioral disorders. *Behavioral Disorders, 19,* 254–258.

Bullis, M., Moran, T., Todis, B., Benz, M., & Johnson, M. (2002). Description and evaluation of the ARIES project: Achieving rehabilitation, individualized education, and employment success for adolescents with emotional disturbance. *Career Development for Exceptional Individuals, 25,* 41–58.

Bullis, M., Nishioka-Evans, V., Fredericks, H. D., & Davis, C. (1993). Identifying and assessing the job-related social skills of adolescents and young adults with emotional and behavioral disorders. *Journal of Emotional and Behavioral Disorders, 1,* 236–250.

Bullis, M., & Yovanoff, P. (1997). *Return to close custody: Analysis of the Oregon Youth Authority's data set.* Eugene, OR: Institute on Violence and Destructive Behavior, University of Oregon.

Bullis, M., & Yovanoff, P. (in press-a). More alike than different? Comparison of formerly incarcerated adolescents with and without disabilities. *Journal of Child and Family Studies.*

Bullis, M., & Yovanoff, P. (in press-b). The importance of getting started right: Further analysis of the facility-to-community transition of formerly incarcerated adolescents. *Journal of Special Education.*

Bullis, M., Yovanoff, P., Havel, M. E., & Mueller, G. (2001). *Transition research on adjudicated adolescents in community settings: Final report on the TRACS project.* Eugene, OR: Institute on Violence and Destructive Behavior, University of Oregon.

Bullis, M., Yovanoff, P, Mueller, G., & Havel, E. (2002). Life on the "outs"—Examination of the facility-to-community transition of incarcerated adolescents. *Exceptional Children, 69,* 7–22.

Cheney, D., Hagner, D., Malloy, J., Cormier, G., & Bernstein, S. (1998). Transition services for youth and young adults with emotional disturbance: Description and initial results of project RENEW. *Career Development for Exceptional Individual, 21,* 17–32.

Clark, R., Pschorr, O., Well, P., Curtis, P., & Tighe, T. (2004). Transition into community roles for young people with emotional/behavioral difficulties: Collaborative systems and program outcomes. In D. Cheney (Ed.), *Transition of students with emotional/behavioral disabilities* (pp. 201–226). Arlington, VA: Council for Children with Behavioral Disabilities and Division for Career Development and Transition, The Council for Exceptional Children.

Cohen, B., & Anthony, W. (1984). Functional assessment in psychiatric rehabilitation. In A. Halpern & Fuhrer (Eds.), *Functional assessment in rehabilitation* (pp. 79–100). Baltimore: Brookes.

Corbett, W. P., & Clark, H. B. (2002). Employment and social outcomes associated with vocational programming for youths with emotional or behavioral disorders. *Behavioral Disorders, 27,* 358–370.

D'Amico, R. (1991). The world of work awaits: Employment experiences during and shortly after secondary school. In M. Wagner, L. Newman, R. D'Amico, E. D. Jay, P. Butler-Nalin, C. Marder, & R. Cox. (Eds.), *Youth with disabilities: How are they doing? The first comprehensive report from the National Longitudinal Transition Study of Special Education Students* (pp. 8-1–8-55). Menlo Park, CA: SRI International.

D'Amico, R., & Blackorby, J. (1992). Trend in employment among out-of school youth with disabilities. In M. Wagner, R. D'Amico, L. Marder, L. Newman, & J. Blackorby (Eds.), *What happens next? Trends in postschool outcomes of youths with disabilities* (pp. 4-1–4-47). Menlo Park, CA: SRI International.

Edgar, E. B. (1987). Secondary programs in special education. Are many of them justifiable? *Exceptional Children, 53,* 555–561.

Edgar, E. B. (1988). Employment as an outcome for mildly handicapped students. *Focus on Exceptional Children, 21,* 1–8.

Edgar, E. B., & Levine, P. (1987). *Special education students in transition: Washington state data, 1976–1986.* Seattle: University of Washington, Experimental Education Unit.

Forness, S. R., & Knitzer, J. (1992). A new proposed definition and terminology to replace "serious emotional disturbance" in the Individuals with Disabilities Education Act. *School Psychology Review, 21,* 12–20.

Frank, A. R., & Sitlington, P. L. (1997). Young adults with behavioral disorders before and after IDEA. *Behavioral Disorders, 23,* 40–56.

Frank, A. R., Sitlington, P. L., & Carson, R. (1991). Transition of adolescents with behavioral disorders—Is it successful? *Behavioral Disorders, 16,* 180–191.

Goldfried, M., & D'Zurilla, T. (1969). A behavioral-analytic model for assessing competence. In C. D. Spielberger (Ed.), *Current topics in clinical and community psychology* (Vol. 1, pp. 151–195). New York: Academic Press.

Hagner, D., Cheney, D., & Malloy, J. (1999). Career-related outcomes of a model transition demonstration for young adults with emotional disturbance. *Rehabilitation Counseling Bulletin, 42,* 228–242.

Harvey, M. (2001). Vocational–technical education: A logical approach to dropout prevention secondary special education. *Preventing School Failure, 45*(3), 108–113.

Hasazi, S. B., Gordon, L. R., & Roe, C. A. (1985). Factors associated with the employment status of handicapped youth exiting high school from 1979 to 1983. *Exceptional Children, 51,* 445–469

Heal, L., & Rusch, F. (1995). Predicting employment for students who leave special education high school programs. *Exceptional Children, 61,* 472–487.

Individuals with Disabilities Education Act of 1990, 20 U.S.C. #1400 seq.

Kohler, P. D. (1993). Best practices in transition: Substantiated or implied? *Career Development for Exceptional Individuals, 16,* 107–121.

Kortering, L., Braziel, P., & Tompkins, J. (2002). The challenge of school completion among youths with behavioral disorders: Another side of the story. *Behavioral Disorders, 27,* 142–154.

Maag, J., & Katsiyannis, A. (1998). Challenges facing successful transition for youth with E/BD. *Behavioral Disorders, 23,* 209–221.

Malloy, J., Cheney, D., Hagner, D., Cormier, G., & Bernstein, S. (1998). Personal futures planning for youth and young adults with emotional and behavioral disorders. *Reaching Today's Youth, 2,* 22–30.

Marder, C. (1992). Secondary students classified as seriously emotionally disturbed: How are they being served: Menlo Park, CA: SRI International.

Marder, C., Wechsler, M., & Valdes, K. (1993). *Services for youth with disabilities after secondary school.* Menlo Park, CA: SRI International.

Mithaug, D., Horiuchi, C., & Fanning, P. (1985). A report on the Colorado statewide follow-up of special education students. *Exceptional Children, 51,* 397–404.

Neel, R. S., Meadows, N. B., Levine, P., & Edger, E. B. (1988). What happened after special education: A statewide follow-up study of secondary students who have behavior disorders. *Behavioral Disorders, 13,* 209–216.

Newman, L. (1992). A place to call home: Residential arrangements of out-of-school youth with disabilities. In M. Wagner, R. D'Amico, C. Marder, L. Newman, & J. Blackorby (Eds.), *What happens next?: Trends in postschool outcomes of youth with disabilities* (pp. 5-1–5-35). Menlo Park, CA: SRI International.

Patterson, G. (1982). *Coercive family processes.* Eugene, OR: Castalia.

Rylance, B. J. (1998). Predictors of post-high school employment for youth identifies as severely emotionally disturbed. *The Journal of Special Education, 32,* 184–192.

Scanlon, D., & Mellard, D. (2002). Academic and participation profiles of school-age dropouts with and without disabilities. *Exceptional Children, 68,* 239–258.

Todis, B., Bullis, M., D'Ambrosio, R., Schultz, R., & Waintrup, M. (2001). Overcoming the odds: Qualitative examination of resilience among adolescents with antisocial behaviors. *Exceptional Children, 68,* 119–139.

U.S. Department of Education. (1994). *The sixteenth annual report to Congress on the implementation of the Individuals with Disabilities Education Act.* Washington, DC: Author.

U.S. Department of Education. (1999). *The twenty-first annual report to Congress on the implementation of the Individuals with Disabilities Education Act.* Washington, DC: Author.

U.S. Department of Education. (2000). *The twenty-second annual report to Congress on the implementation of the Individuals with Disabilities Eduation Act.* Washington, DC: Author.

Valdes, K., Williamson, C., & Wagner, M. (1990). *The national longitudinal transition study of special education students: Vol 3. Youth categorized as emotionally disturbed.* Palo Alto, CA: SRI International.

Wagner, M. (1991). *The benefits associated with vocational education for young people with disabilities.* Menlo Park, CA: SRI International.

Wagner, M., Blackorby, J., Cameto, R., & Newman, L. (1993). *What makes a difference: Influences on postschool outcomes of youth with disabilities.* Menlo Park: SRI International.

Wagner, M., Cameto, R., & Newman, L. (2003). *Youth with disabilities: A changing population. A report of findings from the National Longitudinal Transition*

Study (NLTS) and the National Longitudinal Transition Study-2 (NLTS2). Menlo Park, CA: SRI International.

Wagner, M., & Shaver, D. (1989). *Educational programs and achievements of secondary special education students: Findings from the National Longitudinal Transition Study.* Menlo Park, CA: SRI International.

Walker, R., & Bunsen, T. D. (1995). After high school: The status of youth with emotional behavioral disorders. *Career Development for Exceptional Individuals, 18,* 97–107.

Will, M. (1984). *OSERS program for the transition of youth with disabilities: Bridges from school to working life.* Washington, DC: Office of Special Education and Rehabilitation.

Wood, H. J., & Cronin, M. E. (1999). Students with emotional/behavioral disorders and transition planning: What the follow-up studies tell us. *Psychology in the School, 36,* 327–345.

20

Teaching Alternative Behaviors to Students with Emotional and Behavioral Disorders

NANCY B. MEADOWS *and* KAY B. STEVENS

The purpose of this chapter is to examine the history and current trends related to teaching alternative behaviors to students with emotional and behavioral disorders. "Alternative behavior" is defined, followed by a brief review of research tracing the history of teaching alternative behaviors, including definitions, descriptions, and research related to differential reinforcement. The issues of generalization and social validity as they relate to teaching appropriate social skills are addressed. Finally, the identification of appropriate alternative social behaviors based on outcome analysis and functional behavioral assessment is reviewed.

Teaching alternative behavior involves teaching and reinforcing behaviors to replace challenging or maladaptive behaviors. The purpose of teaching alternative behaviors is to assist individuals who habitually exhibit maladaptive behaviors to learn more socially acceptable ways to behave. Children and youths with emotional and behavioral disorders (EBD) consistently exhibit bizarre, inappropriate, unacceptable, and/or maladaptive behaviors; thus, they experience minimal tolerance from others and often fail in school, work, and personal relationships.

Professional terminology related to the process of teaching alternative behaviors changes from time to time, but the objective

of identifying socially appropriate behaviors and attempting to embed them in the repertoires of students with maladaptive behaviors remains constant. On the surface, the process appears simple: (1) target challenging/maladaptive behaviors that are not socially acceptable, (2) target alternative behaviors that are recognized as socially acceptable, and (3) implement an intervention to teach and/or reinforce the acceptable behavior. However, while researchers have studied the process for decades, their results clearly have illustrated that the process is anything but simple.

Research related to teaching alternative behaviors has a relatively long tradition, (Deitz & Repp, 1973), although the practice is often omitted in traditional teacher education curricula. The 1997 reauthorization of the Individuals with Disabilities Education Act mandates that functional behavioral assessments (FBA; see Fox & Gable, Chapter 8, this volume) be conducted to identify specific problems and replacement behaviors, as well as the historical and environmental factors that maintain problem behaviors. This mandate was the result of special educators' efforts to bring a systematic approach to the analysis and treatment of problem behaviors. The idea of the federal government's mandating procedures in special education is not new (e.g., individualized education programs, least restrictive environment, due process, etc.). While mandates often are based on logical and well-meaning ideas or theories, they usually precede the knowledge and capability of the field to respond effectively. As a result, the federal law requires that an FBA be conducted for students with disabilities who exhibit specific types of challenging behaviors. The law also states that interventions be designed based on the FBA. The interventions must include positive behavioral supports that respond to the individual needs of the student. "Best practice" suggests that continuous assessment of the learner's progress and the effectiveness of the interventions be conducted and interventions adjusted until positive results are attained. This has renewed efforts in the area of assessing students' problem behaviors and teaching alternative behaviors.

The terms "alternative" and "replacement" behaviors can be synonymous, but they also can differ somewhat in meaning depending on the researchers' operational definition and purpose. *Alternative behavior* is seen throughout the literature, while *replacement behavior* is a more contemporary term, which is used by some researchers to describe the process of identifying the function of maladaptive behavior and establishing a curriculum to teach/facilitate specific replacement behaviors based on the function of the maladaptive behaviors. (This process will be addressed later in the chapter.) While processes for developing assessment and interventions to teach or increase alternative behaviors have varied somewhat, the variance appears to be more in the sophistication of the process and less in the actual interventions.

HISTORICAL PERSPECTIVE REGARDING TEACHING ALTERNATIVE BEHAVIORS

We begin our look at teaching alternative behaviors with work from the 1960s. Populations of students with severe, pervasive behavioral disorders resulting from a variety of etiologies typically served as subjects for this research. The idea of teaching alternative behaviors evolved out of a body of work with children with autism and developmental delays. One of the prominent features of

autism is the general inability to use expressive language with clear communicative intent (Kanner, 1943). Similar communication deficits also are found in children with pervasive disorders, such as mental retardation (Talkington, Hall, & Altman, 1971) or schizophrenia (Shodell & Reiter, 1968).

For many years, the primary work with children exhibiting such language deficits was to attempt to teach spoken language (Reichle & Keogh 1986). In the late 1960s and early 1970s, researchers began to investigate behavioral differences between verbal and nonverbal children with mental disorders. For example, Shodell and Reiter (1968) studied the prevalence and frequency of self-mutilative behaviors in verbal and nonverbal children with schizophrenia. The results of their study indicated that nonverbal children were significantly more likely to self-mutilate and did so more frequently than verbal children.

In 1971 Talkington, Hall, and Altman hypothesized that individuals with mental retardation for whom communication was impossible, even for expressing basic needs, had higher levels of frustration. Drawing on the "frustration–aggression hypothesis" (Dollard, Doob, Miller, Moyer, & Sears, 1939), Talkington et al. (1971) predicted that higher levels of frustration would manifest in higher levels of aggressive behaviors in nonverbal children. Talkington and his colleagues tested this theory with individuals with mental retardation who were matched across numerous variables. Two groups were created: noncommunicating and communicating. All participants were rated across nine categories of aggressive behaviors. Results indicated that the noncommunicating group exhibited significantly more aggressive behaviors than the group that could communicate. However, none of the aggressive categories involved harm to self or others. Talkington and his colleagues' interpretation was that the behavior was triggered by frustration and that the aggressive behavior served a function, in that it earned the individual desired attention (function).

As this new paradigm took shape, educational programs for children with disabilities that previously had been confined to speech-based language programs began to develop methods for reaching nonverbal children (Reichle & Keogh, 1986). Educators of children with autism began to consider that the complex nature of interactive language rather than the inability to develop speech skills was the key factor that limited communicative exchanges (LaVigna, 1978). Therefore, alternative nonverbal modes of communication were sought as a substitute for vocal speech. These new modes of communication represented some of the first uses of alternative behaviors in the treatment of individuals with severe disabilities. Among the early techniques that enjoyed moderate success when used as alternative communication were sign language (Fulwiler & Fouts, 1976), "total communication" (Creedon, 1973), visual symbols (Premack & Premack, 1974), symbolic gestures (Sage, 1978), and word cards (LaVigna, 1978). The hope was that teaching students alternative ways to communicate would decrease their frustration and aggressive behaviors.

In early attempts to suppress problem behaviors, interventionists employed predominantly aversive strategies, which included contingent electric shock (Lovaas & Simmons, 1969), time out (Zeilberger, Sampen, & Sloane, 1968), response cost (Iwata & Bailey, 1974), contingent restraint (Gaylord-Ross, Weeks, Lipner, & Gaylord-Ross, 1983), and extinction (Lovaas, Freitag, Gold, & Kassorla, 1965). In all of these techniques, response-contingent administration of punishment or withholding of reinforcement was directly linked to the learner's performance of an undesired behavior.

The success of these aversive strategies demonstrated that individuals diagnosed with autism or other pervasive developmental delays could indeed learn and benefit from the presentation of aversive stimuli (Meyer & Evans, 1986). However, while the strategies decreased inappropriate behaviors, no appropriate behaviors were being taught to take the place of the maladaptive behaviors; therefore, the learner often continued to use the intolerable/inappropriate form of behaviors when the threat of punishment was not present. In other words, behaviors that decreased in the treatment setting did not necessarily generalize to settings where treatment was not conducted. In addition, during the late 1970s and early 1980s, educators began to express ethical and legal concerns about the use of aversive

methods. Deleterious side effects of punishment procedures were noted, such as recurring and increased aggressive responses from the learner and implementation difficulties in community and home settings (Donnellan, LaVigna, Negri-Shoultz, & Fassbender, 1988). These issues prompted researchers and educators to search for less punitive methods of reducing problem behaviors. At the same time, these methods also were being applied to individuals with less severe disabilities who exhibited challenging behavior (e.g., students with emotional and behavioral disorders), and caregivers and practitioners were voicing similar ethical and procedural concerns.

Differential Reinforcement

One trend researchers began to investigate was based on the principles of reinforcement and its potential as a behavior reduction procedure. In general, learning theory dictates that reinforcement of desired behaviors will increase the likelihood and frequency of such behaviors. These reinforcement-based techniques are antithetical to punishment procedures, as they call for differential reinforcement of desired behaviors while limiting or providing no attention or reinforcement to undesired behaviors.

Four commonly used differential reinforcement procedures are (1) differential reinforcement of low rates of responding (DRL; Deitz & Repp, 1983); (2) differential reinforcement of other behaviors (or the omission of target behavior) (DRO; Deitz & Repp, 1983); (3) differential reinforcement of incompatible behavior (DRI; Deitz & Repp, 1983); and (4) differential reinforcement of alternative behaviors (DRA; Ayllon, Layman, & Burk, 1972; Deitz & Repp, 1983; O'Brien & Repp, 1990). Descriptions of each of the differential reinforcement procedures are included in texts that focus on treatment of students with discipline problems and emotional/behavioral disorders and date back to the 1970s (e.g., Deitz & Hummell, 1978; Sulzer-Azaroff & Mayer, 1977). An overview of the four procedures identified above demonstrates a portion of the historical evolution of these procedures.

Differential reinforcement of low rates of responding, or DRL, refers to assisting a learner to decrease behaviors that are inappropriate only because they occur too frequently (Webber & Scheuermann, 1991). For example, asking for a hall pass to use the restroom is not in itself an inappropriate behavior; however, doing so three or four times during an hour-long class period (a medical problem not withstanding) is inappropriate and disruptive. Many behaviors are problems only because of their frequency of occurrence. In our example, the teacher's goal may be for the students to leave the room to go to the restroom only once during a 1-hour period. Therefore, the teacher provides reinforcement for gradual or complete reduction of the target behavior. The DRL procedure has been demonstrated to decrease talking-out behavior (Deitz & Repp. 1973), inappropriate social behaviors and vocalizations (Dampf, 1977), and stereotypical behavior in learners with profound retardation (Singh, Dawson, & Manning, 1981).

Differential reinforcement of other behaviors, or DRO, is much like DRL except it refers to reinforcing a student for not exhibiting a target behavior at all for a designated period of time. Some authors identify this technique as "differential reinforcement of behavior omission" (Deitz & Repp, 1983). Others refer to it as "differential reinforcement of zero rates of behavior" (Webber & Scheuermann, 1991). The only real difference between DRL and DRO is that in the latter case only zero occurrence of the target behavior will be reinforced. A DRO procedure is used with behaviors that cannot be tolerated such as fighting, destruction of property, and threatening to injure oneself or others. Early research examples include eliminating self-injurious behaviors (Repp, Deitz, & Speir, 1974) and exhibitionism (Lutzker, 1974).

Differential reinforcement of incompatible behaviors, or DRI, (also called *differential reinforcement of competing behaviors*), requires reinforcement of behaviors that are structurally incompatible with the undesired target behavior (Deitz & Repp, 1983). For example, a child who is truant to school would be reinforced for coming to school, as it is physically impossible for the child to be absent and present at the same time. Differential reinforcement of incompatible behavior does not require that the learner perform a particular behavior determined by the teacher—only that the behavior performed is topographically incompatible with the target behavior (Deitz & Repp, 1983). It is the practice of "catch 'em being good." An early research example is using DRI to decrease disruptive and talking-out behaviors of students with mild retardation (Hall et al., 1971).

Finally, *differential reinforcement of alternative behaviors,* or DRA, is similar to DRI because both methods specifically foster the performance of behaviors other than the target behavior. However, the key difference between DRA and the other differential reinforcement procedures is the identification of a specific target behavior or behaviors that offer productive alternatives to the target behavior (Deitz & Repp, 1983). Unlike DRO, reinforcement in DRA strategies is limited to the selected alternative behavior(s). As described in Alberto and Troutman (2003), the alternative behaviors are not required to be physically incompatible with the target behavior, as in DRI strategies. The alternative behavior must help the learner function in more appropriate ways, and it must result in reinforcement that is as easily and quickly obtained as the reinforcement gained in response to the inappropriate behaviors. If the function or outcome of the learner's behavior is not met, maintenance and generalization of the alternative behavior(s) will suffer and competing behaviors that historically have been reinforced will resume. Programming for maintenance and generalization by way of selecting specific alternative behaviors that are functional for the learner is critical.

While all the differential reinforcement procedures are designed to decrease inappropriate behavior, DRA specifically requires corresponding reinforcement of adaptive behaviors in an attempt to enhance the learner's repertoire of appropriate responses. Thus, DRA actually sets out to target and teach new alternative behaviors. Since this chapter focuses on teaching alternative behaviors, guidelines and recommendations for implementing DRI and DRA are addressed.

Two general approaches are recommended for DRA interventions (Mace & Roberts, 1993). The first requires that a general type or types of desired behavior (e.g., nonaggressive behavior toward peers) are identified and defined as the alternative response(s) to be reinforced on a variable reinforcement schedule. Second, the educator or therapist may identify one particular alternative response (e.g., sharing toys) to be used in place of the target behavior. Ideally, this alternative response will effectively replace the undesired behavior and serve the same function.

However, many variables must be considered when implementing the DRA procedure. Donnellan and her colleagues (1988) identified seven essential variables that educators must consider when devising DRA protocols.

1. *Absence of motor behavior as the alternative response.* Users of DRA may experience limited success if the identified alternative behavior involves lack of movement or the absence of behavior (e.g., sitting quietly) rather than doing something that enhances the child's functional behavior (e.g., coloring).

2. *Topographically similar versus dissimilar.* Alternative responses that are topographically dissimilar to the target behavior are recommended. Alternative responses should require movement that is physically or structurally different from the target behavior.

3. *Topographically compatible versus incompatible.* Defined alternative responses will be more successful if they are structurally incompatible with the target behavior. If spitting were identified as the target behavior, singing would be a topographically incompatible alternative response as it is very difficult to sing and spit at the same time.

4. *The 100% rule.* Theoretically, the 100% rule states that the target behavior and the alternative response or responses defined should represent 100% of the universe of possibilities for behavior in the identified situation. Therefore, the learner is either performing the target behavior or one of the alternative responses—no other options exist. Donnellan et al. (1988) provided the example of a child whose target is "out-of-seat" behavior. An alternative response that would satisfy the 100% rule would be in seat and engaged in academic behaviors.

5. *The schedule of reinforcement and intervention.* Reasonable parameters must be set when employing a DRA intervention.

The interventionist must decide the schedule of reinforcement (e.g., continuous or intermittent) that can be delivered easily and as planned. In addition to the schedule of reinforcement, the educator or therapist must also determine the length, duration, and location of the intervention.

6. *The status of the alternative response prior to intervention.* Educators must determine the presence and frequency of the alternative response during baseline procedures. The response must already exist in the child's behavioral repertoire in order to be reinforced. If the child lacks the defined alternative response, additional procedures (e.g., prompting, direct teaching) must be implemented to ensure acquisition of the desired behavior.

7. *Identification and specification of reinforcement.* When implementing DRA, the educator or therapist must clearly explain to the learner the desired alternative response and the specific reinforcers that will be available contingent on exhibiting that response, as well as the target behavior that will no longer be reinforced. Clarity and consistency are key elements in DRA.

Deitz and Repp (1983) offered additional recommendations for successful implementation of DRA. First, alternative behaviors should be selected based on their ability to benefit the learner by increasing their appropriate behavioral repertoire, thus improving social skills. Second, an educator may reinforce appropriate alternative responses in the learner's peers, as well as the learner, giving the opportunity for students to learn via imitating appropriate models of the desired behavior.

Despite the potential of DRA, several drawbacks exist related to its implementation. Typically, corrective or aversive consequences are not used when implementing DRA, which can lead to increased intervention time. In addition, problem behaviors that continue to receive reinforcement in other settings may not generalize (Bregman & Gerdtz, 1997; Polsgrove & Reith, 1983), and minimal empirical evidence exists regarding the isolated use of DRA (Bregman & Gerdtz, 1997). In fact, in 1990 O'Brien and Repp conducted a 20-year review of reinforcement-based reduction techniques used to decrease maladaptive behavior in populations with severe or profound retardation. Only three studies were identified where participants received isolated DRA interventions; therefore, no analysis or interpretation of DRA data were included in the review.

Treatment Packages Including DRA

Several researchers (Deitz & Repp, 1983; Luiselli, 1984) have suggested the use of DRA procedures in combination with techniques that respond to the problem behaviors when they occur. Combined treatment packages that include DRA have been used with success for reducing various maladaptive behaviors. One such combination technique is the use of positive practice overcorrection, which requires students to repeat an alternative, appropriate behavior multiple times contingent on exhibiting an inappropriate behavior. One purpose of positive practice overcorrection is to teach the learner, through repeated practice, an alternative behavior that represents a more appropriate response to the situation. Preator and Jenson (1984) tested a positive practice overcorrection model to decrease inappropriate touching of objects by a 6-year-old child with autism. Initially, an overcorrection procedure was implemented that consisted of the boy raising and lowering his arms for approximately 3 minutes immediately following an episode of inappropriate hand usage. After a period of 15 weeks, inappropriate hand usage had decreased but continued to be a problem. At this point, a DRA training phase was added that required the boy to ask for permission to touch objects. The results indicated that overcorrection alone was moderately effective in reducing inappropriate touching behavior. However, when DRA was added to overcorrection, an immediate and lasting decrease was noted in the target behavior.

Mulick, Schroeder, and Rojahn (1980) conducted research that included a package of four treatments: (1) extinction, (2) DRO, (3) DRI, and (4) extinction with DRA to decrease vomiting behavior in a 15 year-old boy with profound retardation. Vomiting behavior was most reduced in the DRI condition, followed by the extinction-DRA intervention. However, the extinction-DRA

condition evidenced the highest mean rate of positive behavior acquisition (playing with toys), rendering this condition the most successful in teaching alternative behaviors.

Estevis and Koenig (1994) conducted research on stereotypic rocking, using a cognitive behavioral approach that incorporated the reinforcement of alternative responses. The study participant was an 8-year-old boy with average intelligence who was congenitally blind. The intervention, designed to reduce his rocking behavior, included both cognitive and DRA components. The alternative response was defined as clasping his hands together and was reinforced when he performed this behavior in lieu of rocking. Simultaneously, the child engaged in self-talk or whispered a predetermined self-monitoring script that discouraged rocking behavior. The results indicated that the child's rocking behavior was reduced significantly by using this treatment package approach.

THE FORM AND FUNCTION OF BEHAVIOR

Prior to the mid-1980s, the majority of research efforts using DRA were focused on suppression of inappropriate behaviors, such as those described above, even though interventions also taught and reinforced alternative behaviors. However, as early as 1978, scholars were beginning to revive a principle originally presented by Premack (1959) almost two decades earlier. This principle held that behaviors are maintained through the pairing of contingent and instrumental responses. A contingent response is regarded as any activity or response that serves as reinforcement for another activity, known as the instrumental response (Bernstein & Ebbesen, 1978). This theoretical pairing posits that, for example, acting-out behavior (the instrumental response or form of the behavior), followed consistently by teacher attention (the contingent response or function of the behavior), will be maintained despite the intention of the teacher's attentive response (i.e., punishment or reprimand). Reinforcement researchers began to differentiate between the form (e.g., using profanity) of the target behavior and its intended function (e.g., getting attention). Differential reinforcement of alternative behaviors provided the perfect opportunity to bridge the gap between theory and practice when considering form and function. The primary motivation behind defining alternative responses is to enhance the child's universe of adaptive and desirable behavior (Mace & Roberts, 1993). Alternative responses can be specifically designed to teach a new, acceptable behavior that will replace the previous form while still achieving the same function. In 1980 Stainback and Stainback wrote, "It can be expected that in the future educators will spend more time on curricular activities that will involve how to build appropriate behavior rather than focusing undue amounts of time on how to eliminate or reduce maladaptive behavior" (1980, p. 270).

Functional Communication Training

From the form and function theory, as it relates to behavior problems, came a technique called "functional communication training" (FCT; Carr & Durand, 1985). FCT is used when an individual's inappropriate behavior is exhibited in order to earn some external reinforcement. The inappropriate behavior has communicative intent; it occurs to bring about a specific outcome or set of outcomes. FCT teaches individuals alternative appropriate responses that bring about the same outcome as their inappropriate behavior. An assumption that underlies the theory is that individuals who demonstrate bizarre, maladaptive behaviors often are doing so in an effort to communicate. The form of their behaviors, although atypical, likely has a clear communicative intent or function (however, the individual's "intent" to use the behavior may not be deliberate).

Functional communication training is a type of DRA (Fisher, Kuhn, & Thompson, 1998). When comparing DRA and FCT, Fisher and his colleagues stated that "FCT is somewhat unique in that, by design, the alternative response (a) specifies its reinforcer . . . , (b) requires minimal response effort . . . , (c) is reinforced on a dense schedule . . . , and (d) can be used to obtain reinforcement across environmental contexts" (p. 1).

Using procedures similar to those used in FCT, educational researchers are investigating school interventions to teach a variety of appropriate social skills to students with EBD who exhibit troublesome behaviors that may result in rejection, involvement in disciplinary actions, and/or removal from naturalistic settings (Sugai & Lewis, 1998, Walker, Schwartz, Nippold, Irvin, & Noell, 1994; Zaragoza, Vaughn, & McIntosh, 1991). FCT, typically conducted in clinical or institutional settings, has helped lead us to functional social skills training implemented in school settings. However, teaching social skills in schools is somewhat new and requires that researchers and practitioners consider a variety of related issues such as skill maintenance and generalization, the social validity of alternative social skills, and procedures for identifying alternative social behaviors.

MAINTENANCE AND GENERALIZATION OF ALTERNATIVE BEHAVIORS

Systematically teaching and reinforcing functional alternative behaviors in no way ensures that the learner will use these alternative behaviors in settings and contexts that historically have not supported such behaviors. In many instances, educators teach alternative behaviors based on a mainstream value system not shared by the learner. For example, teaching a student to ignore another student's provocations may clash with everything the learner has observed, understood, and performed in other settings within similar contexts. Students with challenging behaviors have used those behaviors habitually in an effort to function in their worlds. To them, their behaviors define who they are; therefore, new alternative behaviors must also work for the learner. Educators must assist the learner in selecting alternative behaviors, teaching him or her when and how to use the behaviors, and practicing change.

In a classic and often cited work by Stokes and Baer (1977), a series of programming considerations are provided to educators and therapists to understand the role and function of behavior maintenance and generalization. While many of the considerations seem common sense, the actual implementation of maintenance and generalization procedures frequently is overlooked, resulting in learner failure as he or she falls back on the more natural and comfortable competing behaviors to the ones being taught.

Stokes and Baer's (1977) recommendations for facilitating maintenance and generalization include (1) assessing the learner's use of new behaviors across settings and contexts and supplying support when the learner's efforts to engage in such behaviors are absent or limited; (2) teaching alternative behaviors in the natural environments where they will be needed rather than in contrived settings (e.g., counseling sessions, special education classrooms, institutions); (3) practicing through role play or actual events to help the learner experience reinforcement for engaging in the alternative behavior(s); and (4) working with the learner's significant others (i.e., parents, teachers, school staff, extended family members, peers) to ensure that all understand and can provide consistency with regard to expectations and interventions. Planning and implementing programs for maintenance and generalization often is more difficult than teaching alternative behaviors. As with any intervention, one of the major challenges is the degree to which treatment gains extend beyond the parameters of the treatment condition (Kerr & Nelson, 2002).

SOCIAL VALIDITY OF ALTERNATIVE BEHAVIORS

According to Wolf (1978), social validity refers to the feasibility, desirability, and effectiveness of an intervention in teaching alternative behaviors. Kerr and Nelson (2002) define social validation as the "degree to which significant others agree that a behavior should be changed, approve of a particular behavioral intervention, or concur that intervention has been effective" (p. 461). Social validity is of great importance when identifying specific alternative behaviors for intervention. When planning to teach students with challenging behaviors, we must assess the social validity of interventions as well as the potential outcomes of the intervention being used. We must ask the questions Wolf proposed:

- Can we actually conduct the intervention—is it a feasible undertaking?
- Do we find the intervention and all its ramifications worthwhile—is it a desirable undertaking?
- Will the intervention enhance the learner's accessibility to an improved life—does it have potential effectiveness?

These questions are answered subjectively by the learner and significant others in the learner's life. As Wolf suggests, subjectivity has its place when making decisions about our abilities to facilitate life changes. The questions of social validity must be considered with care and clear understanding as we attempt to teach alternative behaviors to students who can not make or are not making good decisions regarding their own behaviors.

Valid Social Skills

The concept of social validity provides a basis for identifying alternative social behaviors that are relevant to students with EBD (Maag, 1999). Walker emphasized the importance of social validity in his set of "Cardinal Rules for Conducting Social Skills Training" (Walker, Todis, Holmes, & Horton, 1988; Walker et al., 1994). Walker considers the critical first step in both the selection and training of social skills to be the validation of the new skills by the targeted consumer groups—parents, teachers, the students themselves. In addition, the overall efficacy of social skills training depends on the integration of newly taught skills into a student's behavioral repertoire and their use in natural settings.

Identifying and teaching alternative social behaviors that students also consider socially valid has been a primary concern of Gresham and his colleagues throughout their research. According to Gresham (1986), a "social validity definition" of social competence involves socially significant behaviors that others consider socially acceptable and that predict important social outcomes (Gresham, Sugai, & Horner, 2001). Instruction focuses on identifying and teaching "valid" social skills—those that predict important outcomes such as "peer acceptance, significant others' judgments of social skill, academic achievement, positive feelings of self-worth, and positive adaptation to school, home and community environments" (Gresham & Elliott, 1993, p. 139).

Valid Social Skill Interventions

Interventions developed to teach alternative social behaviors are based on the underlying premise that new behaviors can be taught. Although many factors influence and often serve as barriers to the acquisition of alternative social behaviors, it is assumed that social skills are learned responses that are acquired in much the same way as other skills. The learning may be planned (e.g., as in direct instruction of social skills), or unplanned (e.g., trial and error, observations) but the premise is that new social skills can be taught (Sugai & Lewis, 1998). Zaragoza et al. (1991), in a review of studies from 1980 through 1990, found that alternative social behaviors targeted for intervention typically fall into two categories: problem-solving skills or specific social behaviors. For example, Amish and colleagues developed an intervention program for students with EBD to teach specific problem-solving skills such as identifying the problem, developing alternative solutions, and evaluating consequences (Amish, Gesten, Smith, Clark, & Stark, 1988.) Gresham and Nagle (1980) used coaching and modeling techniques with third- and fourth-grade students to teach specific skills such as asking for and giving information. In other studies, researchers have used a combination of approaches to teach both specific social skills and problem-solving skills. For example, Rutherford and colleagues (Rutherford, Anderson, DiGangi, & Chipman, 1992) developed social skills curricula for students that are based on the identification of specific social skills and that incorporate direct instruction and problem-solving strategies.

There is a general consensus, however, that even though students have learned alternative behaviors through social skills instruction, there has been very little success in increasing overall social competence of children with behavior problems (Gresham et al., 2001). "Modest" and "less than dramatic" effects have been reported in several meta-analyses of social skills interventions (Forness & Kavale, 1996; Kavale & Forness, 1995; Kavale, Mathur, Forness, Rutherford, & Quinn, 1997; Mathur, Kavale, Quinn, Forness, & Rutherford, 1998). One explanation offered is that the social skills targeted for instruction were not socially valid for students. That is, they may be important social skills for the adults who wrote the curriculum, but the students do not perceive the skills as producing socially valid outcomes. As a result, students who are considered socially incompetent may not increase their levels of social acceptance even if specific skills are mastered (Gresham, 1986; Mathur & Rutherford, 1996; Winnett, Moore, & Anderson, 1991). Gresham et al. (2001) have offered another explanation: social skills training interventions fail to match the types of social skills deficits that students exhibit. Most social skills curricula are written with the assumption that students have an "acquisition deficit." Alternative behaviors are taught because it is assumed that students have not learned or are missing an important step in performing the social skills targeted for instruction (Gresham, 1986; Gresham et al., 2001). However, some students may have a performance deficit, and, even though they have "mastered" a social skill, they may not "perform" the skill at appropriate times (Gresham, 1986). Interventions differ depending on the type of skill deficit a student has. Rather than focusing on just learning alternative behaviors, students may need to learn when and under what conditions to perform the behavior.

It may be that students do not use a particular social skill because a competing behavior is more efficient and reliable in getting their needs met (Gresham et al., 2001). Horner and Billingsly (1988) looked at the effects of competing behavior on the generalization and maintenance of adaptive behaviors and found that competing behaviors often are more reliable and more efficient in producing desired outcomes for the student than socially appropriate behaviors. The student also has had more practice using the competing behavior, which increases the likelihood of it being used. Typically, the competing antisocial or maladaptive behavior is immediately reinforced, requires less effort to perform, and produces more consistent results.

IDENTIFYING ALTERNATIVE BEHAVIORS

In the 1980s, many studies focused on identifying socially competent and incompetent children, primarily on the basis of adult and peer judgments (Asher & Hymel, 1981; Dodge, 1985; Dodge, McClaskey, & Feldman, 1985; Gresham, 1986). Numerous assessment devices such as peer sociometric interviews, nomination and rating scales, teacher-rating instruments, and parent rating scales were developed. Putallaz and Gottman (1981) labeled such judgments "indicator variables" because they indicate the existence of a problem but do not explain its nature. Which behaviors or skills actually differentiate socially competent from incompetent children, or how those skills might be acquired, remained unclear (Putallaz, 1983; Walker, Shinn, O'Neill, & Ramsey, 1987). It has been argued that, in order to develop instruments that contribute to the planning of social skills interventions for each individual child, an assessment that links inappropriate behaviors to the function they serve for the child would be more effective (Lewis, Sugai, & Colvin, 1998).

Determining the Function of Behavior

Every chain of behaviors produces an effect that meets a need or function for an individual. In fact, it is the reinforcement received by reaching this social/behavioral goal that shapes the specific behaviors exhibited by the child (Neel & Cessna, 1993; Neel, Cheney, Meadows, & Gelhar, 1992). Determining the "function" of a behavior requires identification of the relationships that exist between the students' behaviors and their desired outcomes. To be most effective, interventions should include alternative behaviors that the student can substitute for problem behaviors and still reliably achieve his or her desired social goal or outcome. As we discussed earlier in the chapter, these are often referred to as replacement behaviors because they meet the student's needs and produce socially valid outcomes.

Outcome Analysis

Outcome analysis is based on two important concepts: the outcome that occurs as a result of the behavior and replacement behaviors (Neel & Cessna, 1993). Behavioral outcomes refer to the functional relationship between the behaviors we observe and the outcome achieved by the child. When a child acts, even with behaviors that we view as disordered, his behavior produces a result. This result or outcome can be viewed as the function (purpose) *of* the behavior The functions of students' behaviors are not always easy to determine and may require multiple observations and anecdotal records in order to generate a correct hypothesis. Behavioral functions common to most children include accessing a reinforcer (e.g., social attention, tangible object) or escape or avoidance of an aversive stimulus (e.g., undesired activity, person, or context). It is important to correctly identify the function of a student's behavior in order to teach appropriate replacement behaviors that will generalize across times, settings, and individuals. For example, if the teacher has determined that the function of a child's disruptive behavior is to "escape" a math activity because it is the only way he or she knows how to deal with frustration, targeted replacement behaviors would focus on teaching new skills for escaping a frustrating activity (e.g., asking for help, taking a short break from the activity). The teacher does not try to change the behavioral function but rather offers instruction in replacement behaviors that achieve the desired behavioral function.

Functional Behavioral Assessment

Lewis et al. (1998), in a schoolwide study involving 110 students in first through fifth grades, found that social skills instruction, when paired with group contingencies, produced only moderate reductions in the overall level of problem behavior observed during lunch, recess, and transition. Their results pointed to the need for further individualized assessment and intervention in order to identify social behaviors that students perceive as socially valid. Lewis et al. recommended the use of functional assessment to identify replacement social skills that meet the individual student's needs.

Naturalistic functional assessment (NFA) uses direct observation and focuses on identifying naturally occurring environmental factors that may predict or maintain problematic behaviors (Repp & Horner, 1999;

Sugai & Lewis, 1998). According to Repp and Horner (1999), functional assessment identifies the function of problem behavior from baseline data without any artificial manipulations in the classroom. NFA assumes there are relationships between problematic social behaviors and environmental factors and, most importantly, gives indications of the conditions under which behaviors will reoccur and/or be sustained. When the information collected during the functional assessment is accurate and the hypothesis reliably describes the social interaction, "valid" and "contextually relevant" alternative social skills are targeted as replacement behaviors, thereby increasing the likelihood that students will engage in these behaviors. According to Sugai and Lewis (1998), "Because of its practical utility and technical adequacy, the functional assessment technology has been identified as a preferred practice when assessing social behaviors" (p. 147).

According to Quinn, Gable, Rutherford, Howell, and Hoffmann (1999), changing focus from the student's behaviors alone to the functions of those behaviors is at the core of functional assessment. It is also possible that the student may find that engaging in a behavior to achieve one need might lead to another function being fulfilled (Quinn et al., 1999). For example, a student who swears at a teacher in order to escape an activity might find that such behavior also gains positive attention from peers.

Behavior Improvement Plans

The purpose of functional behavioral assessment is to identify replacement behaviors that are taught and reinforced through a behavior improvement plan (BIP). Behavior improvement plans include strategies for teaching "functionally equivalent replacement behaviors (i.e., behavior that serves the same purpose but is more acceptable)" (Quinn et al., 1999). Quinn and her colleagues have developed guidelines for selecting interventions that match the functions identified during the functional assessment process. They recommend choosing the least intrusive and the least complex intervention that is also closely aligned with the function of the behavior and will be the most likely to

positively change student behavior quickly and easily. Viable interventions have system-wide support, have shown prior evidence of effectiveness with the targeted behavior, and are likely to promote a replacement behavior that will occur and be reinforced in the natural environment (Quinn et al., 1999).

CONCLUSION

As we have discussed in this chapter, research related to teaching alternative behaviors has a relatively long tradition. Through research and practice, we have grown more sophisticated in our knowledge of how best to assist individuals who habitually exhibit maladaptive behaviors in learning more socially acceptable ways to behave. Professional terminology related to the process of teaching alternative behaviors has changed over time, but the objective of identifying socially appropriate behaviors and attempting to embed them in the repertoires of students with maladaptive behaviors remain constant. On the surface, teaching alternative behaviors seems to be a simple process: (1) target challenging/ maladaptive behavior that are not socially acceptable, (2) target alternative behaviors that are recognized as socially acceptable, and (3) implement an intervention to teach and/or reinforce the acceptable behavior. However, as noted earlier, the research results discussed in this chapter have clearly illustrated that the process is anything but simple.

REFERENCES

Alberto, P. A., & Troutman, A. C. (2003). *Applied behavior analysis for teachers* (6th ed.). Upper Saddle River, NJ: Merrill/Prentice Hall.

Amish, P. L., Gesten, E. L., Smith, J. K., Clark, H. B., & Stark, C. (1988). Social problem-solving training for severely emotionally and behaviorally disturbed children. *Behavioral Disorders, 13*, 175–186.

Asher, S. R., & Hymel, S. (1981). Children's social competence in peer relations: Sociometric and behavioral assessment. In K. A. Dodge (Ed.), *Social competence in children* (pp. 125–157). Chicago: University of Chicago Press.

Ayllon, T., Layman, D., & Burk, S. (1972). Disruptive behavior and reinforcement of academic performance. *Psychological Record, 22*, 315–323.

Bernstein, D. J., & Ebbesen, E. B. (1978). Reinforcement and substitution in humans: A multiple-response analysis. *Journal of Experimental Analysis of Behavior, 30,* 243–253.

Bregman, J. D., & Gerdtz, J. (1997). Behavioral interventions. In D. J. Cohen & F. R. Volkmar (Eds.), *Handbook of autism and pervasive developmental disorders* (2nd ed., pp. 606–630). New York: Wiley.

Carr, E. G., & Durand, V. M. (1985). Reducing behavior problems through functional communication training. *Journal of Applied Behavior Analysis, 18,* 111–126.

Creedon, M. (1973). *Language development in nonverbal autistic children using a simultaneous communication system.* Paper presented at the annual meeting of the Society for Research in Child Development, Philadelphia, PA.

Dampf, P. M. (1977). The elimination of an inappropriate response to adult direction. *Education and Treatment of Children, 1,* 19–22.

Deitz, S. M., & Hummel, J. H. (1978). *Discipline in the schools: A guide to reducing misbehavior.* Englewood Cliffs, NJ: Educational Technology.

Deitz, S. M., & Repp, A. C. (1973). Decreasing classroom misbehavior through the use of DRL schedules of reinforcement. *Journal of Applied Behavior Analysis, 6,* 457–463.

Deitz, D. E., & Repp, A. C. (1983). Reducing behavior through reinforcement. *Exceptional Education Quarterly, 3,* 34–46.

Dodge, K. A. (1985). Facets of social interaction and the assessment of social competence in children. In B. H. Schneider, K. H. Rubin, & J. E. Ledingham (Eds.), *Children's peer relations: Issues in assessment and intervention* (pp. 3–22). New York: Springer-Verlag.

Dodge, K. A., McClaskey, C. L., & Feldman, E. (1985). Situational approach to the assessment of social competence in children. *Journal of Consulting and Clinical Psychology, 53,* 344–453.

Dollard, J., Doob, L. W., Miller, N. E., Moyer, D. P., & Sears, R. R. (1939). *Frustration and aggression.* New Haven, CT: Yale University Press.

Donnellan, A. M., LaVigna, G. W., Negri-Shoultz, N., & Fassbender, L. L. (1988). *Progress without punishment: Effective approaches for learners with behavior problems.* New York: Teachers College Press.

Estevis, A. H., & Koenig, A. J. (1994). A cognitive approach to reducing stereotypic body rocking. *Re:View, 26,* 119–126.

Fisher, W. W., Kuhn, D. E., & Thompson, R. H. (1998). Establishing discriminative control of responding using functional and alternative reinforcers during functional communication training. *Journal of Applied Behavior Analysis, 31,* 543–560.

Forness, S. R., & Kavale, K. A. (1996). Training social skill deficits in children with learning disabilities: A meta-analysis of the research. *Learning Disability Quarterly, 19,* 2–13.

Fulwiler, R. L., & Fouts, R. S. (1976). Acquisition of American sign language by a noncompliant autistic child. *Journal of Autism and Childhood Schizophrenia, 6,* 43–51.

Gaylord-Ross, R. J., Weeks, M., Lipner, C., & Gaylord-Ross, C. (1983). The differential effectiveness of four treatment procedures in suppressing self-injurious behavior among severely handicapped students. *Education and Training of the Mentally Retarded, 18,* 38–44.

Gresham, F. M. (1986). Conceptual issues in the assessment of social competence in children. In P. S. Strain, M. J. Guralnick, & H. M. Walker (Eds.), *Children's social behavior: Development, assessment and modification* (pp. 143–179). New York: Academic.

Gresham, F. M., & Elliott, S. N. (1993). Social skills intervention guide: Systematic approaches to social skills training. In J. E. Zins & M. J. Elias (Eds.), *Promoting student success through group interventions* (pp. 137–158). New York: Hawthorne.

Gresham, F. M., & Nagle, R. J. (1980). Social skills training with children: Responsiveness to modeling and coaching as a function of peer orientation. *Journal of Consulting and Clinical Psychology, 48,* 718–729.

Gresham, F. M., Sugai, G., & Horner, R. H. (2001). Interpreting outcomes of social skills training for students with high-incidence disabilities. *Exceptional Children, 67,* 331–344.

Hall, R. V., Willard, D. Goldsmith, S., Emerson, M., Owen, M., Davis, F., & Porcia, E. (1971). The teacher as observer and experimenter in the modification of disrupting and talking out behaviors. *Journal of Applied Behavioral Analysis, 4,* 141–149.

Horner, R. H., & Billingsly, F. (1988). The effects of competing behavior on the generalization and maintenance of adaptive behavior in applied settings. In R. H. Horner, G. Dunlap, & R. Koegel (Eds.), *Generalization and maintenance: Lifestyle changes in applied settings* (pp. 197–220). Baltimore: Brookes.

Iwata, B. A., & Bailey, J. S. (1974). Reward versus cost token systems: An analysis of the effects on students and teacher. *Journal of Applied Behavior Analysis, 7,* 567–576.

Kanner, L. (1943). Autistic disturbances of affective contact. *Nervous Child, 2,* 217–250.

Kavale, K. A., & Forness, S. R. (1995). Social skills deficits and training: A meta-analysis of the research in learning disabilities. In T. E. Scruggs & M. A. Mastropieri (Eds.), *Advances in learning and behavioral disabilities* (Vol. 9, pp. 119–160). Greenwich, CT: JAI Press.

Kavale, K. A., Mathur, S. R., Forness, S. R., Rutherford, R. B., & Quinn, M. M. (1997). Effectiveness of social skills training for students with behavior disorders: A meta-analysis. In T. E. Scruggs & M. A. Mastropieri (Eds.), *Advances in learning and behavioral disabilities* (Vol. 11, pp. 1–26). Greenwich, CT: JAI Press.

Kerr, M. M., & Nelson, C. M. (2002). *Strategies for addressing behavior problems in the classroom* (4th ed.). Upper Saddle River, NJ: Merrill/Prentice Hall.

LaVigna, G. W. (1978). Communication training in mute autistic adolescents using the written word. In *Readings in autism* (pp. 154–163). Guilford, CT: Special Learning.

Lewis, T. J., Sugai, G. M., & Colvin, G. (1998). Reducing problem behavior through a school-wide system of effective behavioral support: Investigation of a school-wide social skills training program and contextual interventions. *The School Psychology Review*, 27, 446–459.

Lovaas, O. I., Freitag, G., Gold, V. J., & Kassorla, I. C. (1965). Experimental studies in childhood schizophrenia: Analysis of self-destructive behaviors. *Journal of Experimental Child Psychology*, 2, 67–84.

Lovaas, O. I., & Simmons, J. Q. (1969). Manipulation of self-destruction in three retarded children. *Journal of Applied Behavior Analysis*, 2, 143–157.

Luiselli, J. K. (1984). Effects of brief overcorrection on stereotypic behavior of mentally retarded students. *Education and Treatment of Children*, 7, 125–138.

Lutzker, J. R. (1974). Social reinforcement control of exhibitionism in a profoundly retarded adult. *Mental Retardation*, 12, 46–47.

Maag, J. W. (1999). *Behavior management*. San Diego: Singular.

Mace, F. C., & Roberts, M. L. (1993). Factors affecting selection of behavioral interventions. In J. Reichle & D. P. Wacker (Eds.), *Communicative alternatives to challenging behavior: Integrating functional assessment and intervention strategies* (pp. 113–133). Baltimore: Brookes.

Mathur, S. R., Kavale, K. A., Quinn, M. M., Forness, S. R., & Rutherford, R. B. (1998). Social skills interventions with students with emotional and behavioral problems: A quantitative synthesis of single-subject research. *Behavioral Disorders*, 23, 193–201.

Mathur, S. R., & Rutherford, R. B. (1996). Is social skills training effective for students with emotional or behavioral disorders? Research issues and needs. *Behavioral Disorders*, 22, 21–28.

Meyer, L. H., & Evans, I. M. (1986). Modification of excess behavior: An adaptive and functional approach for educational and community contexts. In R. H. Horner, L. H. Meyer, & H. D. B. Fredericks (Eds.), *Education of learners with severe handicaps: Exemplary service strategies* (pp. 315–350). Baltimore: Brookes.

Mulick, J. A., Schroeder, S. R., & Rojahn, J. (1980). Chronic ruminative vomiting: A comparison of four treatment procedures. *Journal of Autism and Developmental Disorders*, 10, 203–213.

Neel, R. S., & Cessna, K. K. (1993). Behavioral intent: Instructional content for students with behavior disorders. In K. K. Cessna (Ed.), *Instructionally differentiated programming* (pp. 31–40). Denver: Colorado Department of Education.

Neel, R. S., Cheney, D., Meadows, N. B., & Gelhar, S. (1992). Interviewing middle school students to determine problematic social tasks in school settings. In R. B. Rutherford & S. R. Mathur (Eds.), *Severe behavior disorders of children and youth* (Vol. 15, pp. 57–67). Reston, VA: Council for Children with Behavioral Disorders.

O'Brien, S., & Repp, A. C. (1990). Reinforcement-based reductive procedures: A review of 200 years of their use with persons with severe or profound retardation. *Journal of the Association for Persons with Severe Handicaps*, 15, 148–159.

Polsgrove, L., & Reith, H. J. (1983). Procedures for reducing children's inappropriate behavior in special education settings. *Exceptional Education Quarterly*, 3, 20–33.

Preator, K. K., & Jenson, W. R. (1984). Overcorrection and alternative response training in the reduction of an autistic child's inappropriate touching. *School Psychology Review*, 13, 107–110.

Premack, D. (1959). Toward empirical behavioral laws: Positive reinforcement. *Psychological Review*, 66, 219–233.

Premack, D., & Premack, A. J. (1974). Teaching visual language to apes and language-deficient persona. In R. L. Schiefelbusch & L. L. Lloyd (Eds.), *Language perspectives: Acquisition, retardation, and intervention*. Baltimore: University Park Press.

Putallaz, M. (1983). Predicting children's sociometric status from their behavior. *Child Development*, 54, 1417–1426.

Putallaz, M., & Gottman, J. (1981). Social skills and group acceptance. In S. Asher & J. Gottman (Eds.), *The development of friendship: Description and intervention* (pp. 116–149). New York: Cambridge University Press.

Quinn, M. M., Gable, R. A., Rutherford, R. B., Howell, K. W., & Hoffmann, C. C. (1999). *Addressing student problem behavior—Part III: Creating positive behavioral intervention plans and supports*. Washington, DC: Center for Effective Collaboration and Practice.

Reichle, J., & Keogh, W. J. (1986). Communication instruction for learners with severe handicaps: Some unresolved issues. In R. H. Horner, L. H. Meyer, & H. D. B. Fredericks (Eds.), *Education of learners with severe handicaps: Exemplary service strategies* (pp. 189–219). Baltimore: Brookes.

Repp, A. C., Deitz, S. M., & Speir, N. C. (1974). Reducing stereotypic responding of retarded persons by the differential reinforcement of other behavior. *American Journal of Mental Deficiency*, 79, 279–284.

Repp, A. C., & Horner, R. H. (1999). *Functional analysis of problem behavior: From effective assessment to effective support*. Belmont, CA: Wadsworth.

Rutherford, R. B., Anderson, K. A., DiGangi, S. A., & Chipman, J. L. (1992). *Teaching social skills: A practical instructional approach*. Ann Arbor, MI: Exceptional Innovations.

Sage, W. (1978). Classrooms for the autistic child. In *Readings in autism* (pp. 99–105). Guilford, CT: Special Learning Corporation.

Shodell, M. J., & Reiter, H. H. (1968). Self-mutilative

behavior in verbal and nonverbal schizophrenic children. *Archives of General Psychiatry, 19,* 453–455.

Singh, N., Dawson, M. J., & Manning, P. (1981). Effects of spaced responding DRL on the stereotyped behavior of profoundly retarded persons. *Journal of Applied Behavior Analysis, 14,* 521–526.

Stainback, S., & Stainback, W. (1980). *Educating children with severe maladaptive behaviors.* New York: Grune and Stratton.

Stokes, T. F., & Baer, D. M. (1977). An implicit technology of generalization. *Journal of Applied Behavior Analysis, 10,* 349–367.

Sugai, G., & Lewis, T. J. (1998). Preferred and promising practices for social skills instruction. In E. L. Meyen, G. A. Vergason, & R. J. Whelan, (Eds.) *Educating students with mild disabilities* (pp. 137–162). Denver: Love.

Sulzer-Azaroff, B., & Mayer, G. R. (1977). *Applying behavior analysis procedures with children and youth.* New York: Holt.

Talkington, L. W., Hall, S., & Altman, R. (1971). Communication deficits and aggression in the mentally retarded. *American Journal of Mental Deficiency, 76,* 235–237.

Walker, H. M., Schwartz, I. E., Nippold, M. A., Irvin, L. K., & Noell, J. W. (1994). Social skills in school-age children and youth: Issues and best practices in assessment and intervention. *Topics in Language Disorders, 14*(3), 70–82.

Walker, H. M., Shinn, M. R., O'Neill, R. E., & Ramsey, E. (1987). A longitudinal assessment of the development of antisocial behavior in boys: Rationale, methodology, and first year results. *Remedial and Special Education, 8,* 7–16.

Walker, H. M., Todis, B., Holmes, D., & Horton, G. (1988). *The ACCESS Program.* Austin, TX: Pro-Ed.

Webber, J., & Scheuermann, B. (1991). Accentuate the positive: Eliminate the negative! *Teaching Exceptional Children, 24*(1), 13–19.

Winnett, R. A., Moore, J. F., & Anderson, E. S. (1991). Extending the concept of social validity: Behavior analysis for disease prevention and health promotion. *Journal of Applied Behavior Analysis, 24,* 215–230.

Wolf, M. M. (1978). Social validity: The case for subjective measurement, or how applied behavior analysis is finding its heart. *Journal of Applied Behavior Analysis, 11,* 203–214.

Zaragoza, N., Vaughn, S., & McIntosh, R. (1991). Social skills interventions and children with behavior problems: A review. *Behavioral Disorders, 16,* 260–275.

Zeilberger, J., Sampen, S. E., & Sloane, H. N. (1968). Modification of a child's behavior problems in the home with the mother as therapist. *Journal of Applied Behavior Analysis, 1,* 47–53.

21

Informed Practice in Teaching Self-Control to Children with Emotional and Behavioral Disorders

LEWIS POLSGROVE *and* STEPHEN W. SMITH

Without appropriate intervention, children who display high and consistent levels of emotional and behavioral disorders (EBD) are at significant risk of enduring a lifetime of difficulties, including school failure, social rejection, low self-esteem, depression, antisocial behavior, delinquency, substance abuse, adult adjustment problems, unemployment, and possible institutionalization (Kauffman, 2001; Walker, Colvin, & Ramsey, 1995; Wolf, Braukmann, & Ramp, 1987). Fortunately, over the past four decades research has advanced our understanding of the etiology of children's EBD and its treatment. A large body of evidence from applied studies has clearly documented that early, intense, multimodal, culturally sensitive, behaviorally based, and ecologically anchored interventions offer an effective strategy for ameliorating EBD of children and adolescents. These components, when properly implemented, have been shown to produce significant and long-lasting changes in reducing socially inappropriate, oppositional, and antisocial behavior (Borduin et al., 1995; Nelson, Scott, & Polsgrove, 1999; Strain & Timm, 2001; Walker, Sprague, Close, & Starlin, 2000).

As school years represent a critical period in the psychosocial development of children and adolescents, recent research on school-wide (contextual) interventions has concentrated on reducing the probability of behavioral and discipline issues through appropriate instruction, increasing awareness of socially appropriate behavior, and teaching students social skills. This approach has shown encouraging results (Sugai & Horner, 2002; Lewis & Sugai, 1999). However, most evidence-based interventions in natural settings for children and adolescents have relied extensively on adult-centered or external methods of controlling inappropriate behavior primarily through applied behavior analysis (ABA) techniques: stimulus control, contingent reinforcement, and various behavior reduction procedures (Alberto & Troutman, 2001; Polsgrove, 1991; Wolery, Bailey, & Sugai, 1988).

Numerous studies have shown that ABA strategies can produce powerful outcomes in a variety of settings. However, they have important limitations. First, they may be used to advance the values and goals of institutional programs over those of individuals (Kazdin, 1980). Second, it has long been recognized that children with EBD often have limited behavioral repertoires and are largely guided by what Mussen, Conger, and Kagan (1969) identified as "external considerations of probable reward or punishment" (p. 514) rather than internal standards and mechanisms of behavioral guidance. Thus, exclusive use of external behavioral control may foster dependence that may affect students' capacity to resist negative external influences (Goldstein, 1988). Third, natural environments are notorious for lacking the quality of guidance or consistency of reinforcement necessary for children to acquire and maintain appropriate behavior. In school settings, for example, most teachers have little training in dealing with problems posed by students with EBD (Schumm & Vaughn, 1992), and their rejection of students who show problematic behavior is well documented (e.g., Curci & Gottlieb, 1990). Fourth, most behaviors are situation-specific, that is, those learned in one situation do not automatically generalize to new settings, nor are they maintained over time (Stokes & Baer, 1977). Finally, students with EBD often have faulty perceptions of social situations and lack the requisite skills for establishing effective social interactions, maintaining motivation, or effectively controlling their emotional reactions to stressful situations (Freedman, Rosenthal, Donahoe, Schlundt, & McFall, 1978; Lochman & Dodge, 1994). Thus, these students require considerable training in these areas plus additional support for attempts at improving their performance. These elements are frequently unavailable in standard school programs.

Behavioral control is surely an important issue in interventions for students with EBD (Nelson et al., 1999). Perhaps the most important ultimate goal for this population, however, concerns teaching skills to regulate their behavior. Thus armed, students with EBD would be better able to control their emotional reactions, adjust to complex social situations, deal with challenging academic and social difficulties, manage anxiety, and achieve personal goals. More importantly, in learning to better manage their behavior, students with EBD could reduce their dependence on external sources of control and thereby increase their freedom of choice, self-determination, and self-esteem (Wehmeyer, Agran, & Hughes, 2000; Worell & Nelson, 1974).

The importance of teaching students behavioral self-control often is overlooked in behavioral intervention programs for controlling the behavior of students with EBD. However, there exists a considerable theoretical framework and research literature on behavioral self-regulation from which practitioners can draw to guide training efforts in this area. In this chapter, we will provide an overview of the theoretical underpinnings of self-regulation, review applied studies, and offer recommendations for training and research in this area.

PERSPECTIVE ON SELF-CONTROL
Issues of "Freedom" and Responsibiilty

The issue of whether an individual has free choice over his or her actions or whether these are controlled by environmental variables has a long and important history in the psychology literature. This debate often lies at the crux of acrimonious exchanges in the literature on special education concerning the human dignity of individuals with disabilities and their rights to self-determination. A major influence on American psychology during the 20th century, Skinner (1953) viewed human behavior as determined and controlled, if not immediately then ultimately, by environmental variables. This approach has drawn considerable criticism from those embracing a "humanistic" philosophy, which emphasizes the role of human dignity and an intrinsic locus of control over behavior (Rogers & Skinner, (1956). While offering entertainment value for philosophers in the social sciences, this debate, like the nature–nurture controversy, has remained unresolved as an "either–or" hypothesis. That is, humans are not simply automatons who act solely at the behest of the environment (Thoreson & Mahoney, 1974).

Perhaps the most viable resolution of the issue of behavioral locus of control resides in recognizing reciprocity between environmental variables and individual behavior. That is, while the environment clearly shapes behavior, an individual has considerable capacity for altering the environment (Bandura, 1986, Patterson, Dishion, & Chamberlain, 1993). A major advance in this area occurred with the recognition that, although not observable directly, internal stimuli, or "private events," nevertheless play a crucial role in determining behavior. Skinner (1953) recognized this early on, but because these are scientifically inaccessible he concentrated his research on environmental causation. Acceptance of the idea that behavioral determinants are not exclusively external requires an explanation of other mechanisms of control. Thus, in the mid-1960s hybrid behavioral and cognitive explanations of these began appearing in the literature. Homme (1965) posited that individuals can have the capacity to recognize and manipulate cognitive stimuli ("coverants") to control their behavior. Bandura's (1969) seminal analysis argued that environmental stimuli provide information to the behaver, who then makes decisions to respond to these based upon the probability of one response producing a desired outcome over another. The response selection and form of the behavior are guided by internal antecedents such as previous memories and imaginal and verbal stimuli. External feedback related to an overt response shapes the probability of future responses. From this perspective human behavior can be best explained in terms of a complex interaction of cognitive and environmental stimuli. The source or "locus" of control, however, has considerable situational dependence and may vary along a continuum from primarily external (e.g., when in confinement) to primarily self-directed control (e.g., when engaged in creative activity) (Thoreson & Mahoney, 1974),

It has been well documented that children and youths with EBD have difficulty controlling their emotions, interpreting social situations, and adjusting to external demands. Due to their limited behavioral repertoires, many react to external stimuli in stereotypical patterns: labile, aggressive, impulsive, inadequate, and/or inappropriate behaviors that carry with them considerable "response cost." These reactions put them at risk for academic failure or social rejection and may result in restriction of opportunities and even loss of freedom (Bierman, Greenberg, & Conduct Problems Prevention Research Group, 1996; Dodge & Frame, 1982; Lochman, Dunn, & Klimes-Dougan, 1993; Walker et al., 1995). While the traditional role of teachers of these students clearly requires use of strategies for controlling their problematic behaviors, teaching

them alternative responses is equally important as a means of maximizing their emotional, social, and behavioral development and freedom. Such instruction thus prepares students to responsibly exercise "free will." Worell and Nelson (1974) defined social freedom in terms of "the number and range of acceptable response alternatives" the individual has available in a given situation (p. 5). They view the teacher's role as providing both structure (external control) and freedom of choice that will "facilitate and enhance the competence, self-regulation and self-actualization of each individual student" (p. 4).

Fortunately, teachers of today have at their disposal an array of evidence-based strategies they can employ in tandem with standard behavior management strategies to teach children behavioral self-control (SC). Individual studies and research syntheses consistently have shown these to produce significant effects in natural settings (Kazdin, 1978; Kazdin & Weisz, 2003; Nelson, Smith, Young, & Dodd, 1991; Polsgrove, 1979; Robinson, Smith, Miller, & Brownell, 1999). However encouraging these results, available evidence suggests that training students with EBD in behavioral SC is not standard practice in classrooms across the country. One of the main conclusions Knitzer, Steinberg, and Fleisch (1990) drew in their national study of school programs for these students was that, in most programs they observed, "obedience predominates over responsibility, punishment over logical consequences, [and] systematic, coherent attempts to help them gain control over their problems is the exception, not the rule" (p. 64). One reason educators appear to adhere to this status quo concerns a limited awareness by practitioners of SC theory and research on effective methods for teaching students behavioral self-regulatory strategies. In the following section we provide an overview of the related theory and research.

Definition of Self-Control

A familiarity with key ideas is required to fully appreciate research and training issues related to behavioral self-control. One continuing area of misunderstanding seems to lie with the definition itself. A major advance in understanding how individuals control their behavior began with Skinner's (1953) observation that the process involved both response(s) to be controlled and a repertoire of controlling behaviors. Later researchers recognized that the term "self-control" best described the *end result* of a succession of self-regulatory measures used by an individual to control his or her behavior (Kanfer & Karoly, 1972; Thoresen & Mahoney, 1974). These allow the individual to forgo immediately reinforcing events in order to gain access to more desirable delayed consequences or outcomes (Goldfried & Merbaum, 1973). Thus, in exercising behavioral self-regulation an individual acts independently of what one would predict based upon the immediately available external consequences and is more reliant (presumably) on internal controlling responses. Moreover, theorists generally assume that effective SC is not necessarily due to an inherent character trait, but learned from either trial and error or social learning experiences (Goldfried & Merbaum, 1973; Thoresen & Mahoney, 1974).

Process of Self-Control

The SC process is complex and, as it involves considerable cognitive behavior, difficult to document objectively. Observers on the topic generally recognize that situational variables, internal states, and cognitive and behavioral abilities are critical in determining the effectiveness of self-regulation. Such abilities involve a capacity to: (1) accurately observe one's own behavior, (2) recognize current behavior as inadequate or inappropriate, (3) identify the behavior(s) that is problematic, (4) recognize behavior required in a given situation, (5) select and implement a set of strategies to effectively regulate behavior, and (6) objectively evaluate performance and alter it accordingly. However, the self-regulatory process is considerably more involved. To provide a perspective on this complex process we turn now to presenta-

tion of a self-regulation model originally developed by Kanfer and Karoly (1972) and modified for our discussion.

Kanfer and Gaelick (1986) observed that much of our interaction with the environment consists of smooth behavioral sequences or chains that operate in an automatic mode. However, when unexpected environmental demands disrupt these patterns, new responses are required and self-regulation processes, if these are available to the individual, are then initiated. These may be categorized in four stages.

Self-Monitoring

The first stage of the SC process, self-monitoring, is initiated when a negative or potentially negative consequence occurs that prompts an individual to observe his or her overt behavior and identify problematic behaviors, perhaps even counting instances of these (see Figure 21.1). As a function of these observations, the person may compare his or her current performance with pervious performances and/or that of others in the same situation. This exercise may result in recognition of a discrepancy between external criteria and the person's performance and may lead to an important crossroad—that of commitment to change. This component is critical to self-regulation, as it represents an acceptance by the individual of responsibility for behavioral change (Kanfer & Gaelick, 1986). Commitment to change may consist of a simple verbalized intention statement or a written contract (Rutherford & Polsgrove, 1981).

Goal Setting

The second stage of the process involves goal setting. Based upon information from the self-monitoring activity, the individual may set behavioral objectives specifying the target behavior(s), degree of change desired, and perhaps a time frame. Goals may be

Stage One		Stage Two	Stage Three	Stage Four
Self-Monitoring →	Discrepancy Detection →	Commitment to Change →	Goal Setting →	Strategy Selection & Implementation →	Self-Evaluation/ Self-Reinforcement

FIGURE 21.1. Behavioral self-regulation model.

adopted from external performance standards or acquired as a function of the social learning process.

Strategy Selection and Implementation

Once goals are established, an individual selects an approach to use in changing his or her behavior in the strategy selection and implementation phase. This may involve review and implementation of a variety of behavioral or cognitive strategies intended to produce positive long-range outcomes.

Self-Evaluation/Self-Reinforcement

In the self-evaluation stage of the self-regulation process, an individual compares his or her performance with previously established goals as well as the adequacy of the behavior change strategy for meeting these goals. Failure to meet previously established standards (presumably) occasions a negative evaluation and a change in strategies, lowering of goals, or reappraisal of the situation. Self-evaluation also leads to the final phase of the process, the contingent administration (or withholding) of self-reinforcement.

Based on results of the self-evaluation of performance, an individual determines the appropriateness of allowing him- or herself access to reinforcing events. Behavior that has failed to meet goal-related criteria (presumably) would go unrewarded, while that which has met or exceeded criteria would signal the appropriateness of allowing oneself to engage in some form of reinforcing event. Although theorists generally consider self-reinforcement essential to maintaining the SC process in the absence of external controls, they generally agree that initiating and maintaining self-regulatory strategies depend on the anticipation and availability of external reinforcement (Bandura & Perloff, 1967; Kanfer & Karoly, 1972; Thoresen & Mahoney, 1974). Individuals may spend countless hours and exert considerable self-denial, for example, in earning a college degree with the ultimate goal of being employed in a rewarding and more lucrative profession. Moreover, an essential factor for training individuals in self-control involves services of a competent instructor/therapist. This mentor should be knowledgeable regarding SC theory and capable of

teaching and shaping self-regulatory skills through the use of modeling, prompting and cuing (stimulus control), and reinforcement procedures (Goldstein, 1988; Kanfer & Gaelick, 1986). There exists a robust literature in successfully training children with EBD to use self-regulation skills in natural environments. The following section will describe typical applications and provide examples of these.

BEHAVIORAL SELF-CONTROL INTERVENTIONS

The behavioral approach to SC grew out of laboratory studies in which animals were taught over a series of trials to forego immediate reinforcement in order to earn a larger reward (more food) at some point in the future (e.g., Jackson & Hackenberg, 1996). Such studies raised the question as to whether the "self" in humans exerted control over behavior or whether this was simply the effect of undetected environmental contingencies operating (Skinner, 1953). Unlike animals, however, humans have a capacity to delay immediate gratification through the use of "verbal mediators" between external contingencies operating in a situation and natural or learned impulses (Hughes & Lloyd, 1993). An individual's ability to control his or her behavior requires a number of teachable skills involving recognition of a need for behavioral self-control, identification of the special behaviors that need to be controlled, and application of self-regulatory strategies. One approach to teaching individuals behavioral "self-regulation" involves providing them with instruction in manipulating *external* variables to decrease impulsive behavior or delaying immediate reinforcement as a means of avoiding punishment and gaining access to more highly rewarding long-range consequences. Key to this instructional process is the availability of external support in the form of direct instruction of the skills and reinforcement of successive approximations at applying these. External support is then faded as the individual acquires independent ability to regulate his or her own behavior. In some cases this training may involve manipulating environmental variables to increase a student's commitment to change in the form of his or her selecting a behavior of lower probability—one that is in one's long-range best interest—over one that is immediately reinforcing. A variety of behavioral approaches have been evaluated in natural settings. These include, but are not limited to, self-monitoring, goal setting, environmental planning, behavioral rehearsal and precorrection, self-evaluation, and self-reinforcement. While internalization of self-regulatory strategies may occur in these applications, they do not utilize the teaching students to manipulate verbal, emotional, or imaginal stimuli (cognitions), as do primarily cognitive approaches to teaching self-regulation.

Studies on Self-Monitoring

In the literature on SC, "self-monitoring" (SM) takes on a variety of meanings. Thus, the term may refer to the simple noninstrumental observation of one's ongoing overt behavior, observation plus judgment of its adequacy in meeting ongoing interoceptive, proprioceptive, or exteroceptive social and environmental contingencies), or observation and recording of overt or covert behavior (Gottman & McFall, 1972; Kanfer & Gaelick, 1986; Thoresen & Mahoney, 1974). Although the SM construct often is discussed separately from other components of the SC process, it functions in concert with these in applications.

Self-monitoring has been found useful in academic and social interventions involving children with EBD. This population is prone to automatically respond to "provocative" stimuli impulsively and inappropriately, often with little awareness or concern for the long-term consequences of their behavior. Typically, the immediate "payoffs" for such reactions are gaining social attention and escaping task demands. The teacher may withdraw the assignment to avoid the student's escalating his or her behavior and possibly requiring physical intervention—a classroom version of the negative reinforcement trap (Patterson, 1982). Patterson and his colleagues, among others, have documented that children's coercive and aggressive behavioral repertoires develop from extensive observational and direct instruction in antisocial behavior (Patterson, 1982; Patterson, Dishion, & Chamberlain, 1993). After exposure to thousands of learning "trials" these behaviors become learned to an automatic level and emitted even under the most innocuous circumstances. Teachers who are responsible for working with such children thus face two important training goals: "deautomatizing" inappropriate patterns of behavior and teaching more acceptable "replacement" alternatives. A starting place for the SC process would involve teaching students to observe their problem behavior(s) in addition to situational variables that may occasion the behavior and its resulting consequences.

In search of alternatives to external control methods and interventions for generalizing and maintaining treatment gains, a spate of studies has investigated the role of SM in teaching school children to regulate their behavior. Early school-based studies on SM focused on establishing its reactive properties as an intervention option and investigated its power to produce positive behavioral outcomes with external cues and reinforcement. In one of the first studies, Broden, Hall, and Mitts (1971) compared the effects of SM, SM plus teacher praise, and praise-only strategies. One student in this study recorded her "study" behavior whenever she chose to do so during class periods. Although a brief baseline and prior student commitment may have skewed results, self-monitoring appeared to effect an increase in task attention; a result that was enhanced with the addition of a teacher praise component. In a replication study, having a second student record instances of his talking out without permission produced initial suppression, but, following a second baseline, his disruptive behavior increased.

In a similar study by Gottman and McFall (1972) one-half of a class of high school students from low-income backgrounds were asked to tally instances when they spoke out in class discussions; the other half were instructed to record times they felt like speaking out in class discussions but did not. In a crossover design, after a week of SM the instructions were reversed for each of the groups. Multiple-time series analysis revealed significantly higher class oral participation rates and improvement in daily class grades during periods when students recorded positive contributions than when they recorded their refraining from participation.

Another school study of the effects of SM with early elementary students (Glynn, Thomas, & Shee, 1973) clearly demonstrated that SM could maintain effects of high rates of on-task behavior. In a sequel Glynn and Thomas (1974) reported that self-recording introduced as an initial intervention produced positive but unstable changes in children's on-task behavior, but this practice plus providing opportunity for students to exchange their records for free-time activities resulted in stable and clinically significant increases in task attention. These studies suggested that SM may be an effective behavior change strategy under certain conditions. Later studies on SM have replicated and extended previous results to different populations, target behaviors, and broader issues, employing more sophisticated methodology than earlier studies.

Of primary interest in this chapter are the effects of SM with children and adolescents with EBD. Levendoski and Cartledge (2000) found cuing children with EBD to record their on-task behavior at 10-minute intervals resulted in significant increases in both their task attention as well as their academic productivity. In an interesting twist to immediate self-recording the teacher in Carr and Punzo's (1993) study first explained the importance of academic achievement and then taught three secondary students with behavioral disorders to record, post hoc, the results of their academic accuracy and productivity on independent task assignments. Using a multiple-baseline design, introduction of the SM phase was staggered for each student across reading, math, and spelling. Prior to the intervention, accuracy on assignments and productivity was low and erratic. Training in SM resulted in considerable improvements and stability in these academic behaviors for each student. In addition, on-task behavior improved noticeably with introduction of the SM phase, and the students were reported to "spontaneously engage in goal-setting" (p. 249).

In addition to academic applications, studies on SM have shown it to be effective for maintaining social skills training objectives. A multiple-baseline study by Kiburz, Miller, and Morrow (1984) taught the social skills of greeting and thanking others and initiating conversations to an adolescent with EBD enrolled in a residential center. Following this training, the youngster was taught to monitor these skills in three different settings and reported the results to his supervisor. Data collected by an independent observer showed that SM maintained and, in some cases, even accelerated the use of these skills. Moore, Cartledge, and Heckaman (1995) reported SM to be effective in facilitating the generalization and maintenance of game-related social skills taught to three secondary students in an EBD class from the training situation to an applied setting.

Ironically, only a few studies have also investigated the effects of SM in increasing attention to task and reducing disruptive behaviors. For example, Dunlap et al. (1995) investigated the effects of a SM training program on the task-engagement and disruptive behaviors of two children with EBD. Self-recording in this study required the students to evaluate, cued by a tone tape at 1-minute intervals, whether they were on-task, quiet, in seat, asked for appropriate assistance, asked for permission to speak, and responded appropriately. A classroom consultant also independently kept records of the students' behavior at each cued interval, and the student received praise and bonus points for backup reinforcers for accurately matching the consultant's records. Results for each student were carefully monitored. The data clearly indicated that the introduction of SM procedures increased and stabilized task attention and decreased rather high rates of disruptive behavior for both students under a variety of experimental conditions. Dunlap et al. interpreted these results as providing further evidence of the reactivity of SM and its capacity to improve student performance in conjunction with other classroom management procedures.

Several studies on SM have involved the use of videotape feedback. For example, Shear and Shapiro (1993) investigated the effects of training students to observe video recordings of their classroom behavior. Participants were enrolled in an elementary school classroom for children with EBD. Three students in an "observation-only" group were required to watch an unedited videotape of their behavior; the other three students watched a videotape of themselves with their disruptive behavior edited out (for an undisclosed reason) and recorded instances of their on- and off-task behaviors. Observations of the student's disruptive classroom behavior were conducted immediately following their video-observation sessions. Self-recording, as defined by the procedures in this study, had little effect on reducing disruptive behavior for any of the students.

In contrast to the Shear and Shapiro study in which the students viewed and evaluated their behavior independently, Lonnecker, Brady, McPherson, and Hawkins (1994) incorporated video self-observation into a SC training package, which included self-modeling, discrimination training, and behavioral rehearsal. In this study the classroom behavior of two second graders, who were identified as the most disruptive and uncooperative members of a special education class of children with EBD, were videotaped. In individual training sessions, the students were shown footage of two vignettes in which they were behaving appropriately and one vignette of behaving inappropriately (self-modeling). A behavior coach pointed out the "trouble spots" on the tape and queried the student as to the antecedents of his or her behavior and replacement alternatives (discrimination training). Next, the students and trainer rehearsed alternative cooperative behaviors with the trainer playing the role of teacher or classmate and providing positive feedback and encouragement for using these in the live classroom situation. Daily home-to-school behavioral report cards and social approval for improving behavior from teachers and administrators completed the intervention package.

Lonnecker et al. employed a multiple-baseline design across subjects and two other classes comparing baseline, video training, and fading phases in which training sessions were gradually withdrawn. Cooperative behaviors of both students showed considerable improvement over the course of the study such that attending to task and speaking in moderated voices were observed at a stable 100% incidence in all three classes by the end of the study. Similarly, inappropriate behavior gradually declined and stabilized at zero in all three classes. These investigators concluded that the use of videotaped classroom behavior combined with incident-specific training offered an economical, effective, generalizable, and durable intervention package.

The studies reviewed on SM indicate that this strategy can be employed in a variety of ways and offers an effective and economic alternative to traditional external management procedures for students with EBD. Self-monitoring has potential for increasing student attention to task, academic productivity, and reducing their inappropriate behavior. In addition, some evidence suggests that, if used in tandem with external contingencies and discrimination training, SM may provide a mechanism for generalizing improvements in academic and behavioral performance over settings and across time. Despite the potential for SM to produce positive outcomes with children with EBD, we find research on this strategy limited, for the most part, to compressed time frames and single settings. Nevertheless, it appears to be a very useful and effective strategy for practitioners to use in teaching children to regulate their behavior, especially when combined with appropriate training and external reinforcement.

Studies on Goal Setting

The setting of performance standards is an integral component in the SC process. As with any environmentally adaptive behavior, however, considerable variability has been noted in the ability to set goals and persist in efforts to accomplish these (Zimmerman, 1996). Bandura (1977) proposed the construct "effectance motivation" to describe the degree to which an individual displays approach, exploratory, and problem-solving behaviors. Those who are highly motivated in this regard are considered to be internally motivated. They perceive themselves as able to effectuate positive outcomes and set performance standards and "persist in their efforts until their performances match self-prescribed standards" (Bandura, 1977, p. 193).

While foundational studies comparing self-regulation skills and perceived self-efficacy of students with EBD are not available, clinical reports and strong circumstantial evidence suggest that these are major deficits for this population. Among their other difficulties, most students with EBD express symptoms of inattention, impulsiveness, learned helplessness, task avoidance, factors that undoubtedly contribute to high rates of academic underachievement and school failure (Kauffman, 2001). Zimmerman (1996) reported considerable evidence that underachievers typically are low in essential academic learning skills, self-control, and self-efficacy. Thus, it would be within reason to conclude that many students in the "underachiever" ranks are those with EBD. As school failure is a strong predictor of later adjustment problems, a major objective of teachers who have students with EBD or are at risk for this condition should involve training them to set, and strive to achieve, academic and personal goals.

From a theoretical perspective training in goal setting (GS) may have several positive outcomes, including more accurate self-monitoring, enhanced awareness of external social and academic standards, recognition of standards versus performance discrepancies, increased likelihood of commitment to behavioral change, and acquisition of a more reality-based and accurate self-evaluation system (Kanfer & Gaelick, 1986). Goal setting also may be immediately motivating. Kelley and Stokes (1984) observed that the act of identifying contingencies for reinforcement could "serve as a discriminative stimulus for goal achievement" (p. 224). In their summary of GS research, Locke and Latham (2002) identified four advantages to training involving GS. First, it focuses attention on task-relevant activities and away from irrelevant activities. Second, setting goals is motivating, especially when challenging tasks are provided along with feedback on effort and performance. Third, goals encourage persistence at a task, which is an important skill for many students to learn. Fourth, GS activates the use of planning skills and problem-solving strategies and increases the likelihood that students will use problem-solving strategies to enhance their performances in other settings.

Despite the central importance of goal setting to the SR process, scant attention has been given to this strategy as a reactive component in effecting positive changes in behavior (cf. Nelson et al., 1991). Most studies on this issue have addressed the effectiveness of GS on academic performances involving nondisabled students and those with academic deficits and cognitive processing disorders. These nevertheless offer information on the effectiveness of goal setting that can be applied in teaching children with EBD. For example, in an early study comparing both external and student-set contingencies, versus no reinforcement conditions, Felixbrod and O'Leary (1973) found no differences in academic performances between the two experimental groups. However, students in the first two groups demonstrated significantly higher performance on math problems solved correctly than students assigned to the no-reinforcement condition. They concluded that setting performance standards was effective in increasing student productivity, but self-imposed standards were as effective as externally assigned standards under certain conditions.

One of the first studies investigating the effects of GS with students displaying academic difficulties (Lovitt & Curtiss, 1969) showed that allowing students to set their own criteria for reinforcement increased academic productivity compared with teacher-determined contingencies. Goal setting has also been broadly effective in other studies with children with learning disabilities and mental retardation in improving motivation, persistence at tasks, and productivity (Copeland & Hughes, 2002).

In a foundational study on the effects of GS, Kelley and Stokes (1984) employed a systematic multiple-baseline design comparing the effects of external versus self-set goals involving eight students at risk for EBD. Although student-determined goals were not as effective as externally set contingencies, they were effective in maintaining moderate levels of student productivity. The investigators concluded that, with appropriate training in contingency setting, students are likely to learn to set "reasonable" standards for their behavior. Other studies have shown GS to be an effective complementary strategy in completing homework assignments (Miller & Kelley, 1994), helping to control anger (Lochman, Burch, Curry, & Lampron, 1984), and planning and recruiting social support for transition from residential institutions (Balcazar, Keys, & Garate-Serafini, 1995).

In general, teaching students GS skills appears to exert a positive motivating influence on their behavior and perhaps eventually leads to a greater sense of accomplishment and self-efficacy (Zimmerman, 1996). While the current literature offers considerable promise, research has yet to clarify several issues: the extent to which GS alone contributes to increased improvements in academic and social functioning, the relative effectiveness of external versus self-determined goals, the conditions necessary for the optimal use of GS, or its effectiveness in teaching students to control unacceptable risk taking and aggressive and antisocial behaviors.

Studies on Self-Evaluation and Self-Reinforcement

Another component in the SC process involves an individual's evaluation of the adequacy of a recent performance vis-à-vis previous personal performances or those of a social model, externally set standards, or requirements of the physical environment (Kanfer & Gaelick, 1986; Thoresen & Mahoney, 1974). The concepts of self-monitoring and self-evaluation are intertwined in the literature, often making it difficult to discern what SC procedure is under scrutiny in a particular study. Perhaps the simplest way to differentiate between these activities would be to restrict the term "self-monitoring" to those operations in which the individual observes and records his or her behavior in some fashion but covertly judges the adequacy of the performance in some undetected way. Thus differentiated, self-evaluation (SE), from a behavioral self-control perspective, can be defined as the operations of observing one's behavior and making some overt comparison of current performance with publicly defined goals. Another close association in the literature exists between SE and self-reinforcement (SR). The latter may be defined as the contingent access to reinforcing events that an individual may allow or deny him- or herself as a presumed function of performance evaluations. As studies investigating the effects of SE typically involve an SR component, in the following discussion we will consider these in tandem.

A series of ground-breaking studies on SE/SR laid the foundation for those to follow. In one of the earliest of these, Bolstad and Johnson (1972) demonstrated that, following exposure to a token reinforcement system, highly disruptive primary school students could maintain treatment gains when taught to accurately evaluate and contingently reinforce themselves. The performance of two SE + SR groups in this study were significantly superior to those of a group who received external reinforcement and two control groups.

Kaufman and O'Leary (1972) were among the first to investigate the effects of SE on secondary students with EBD. Following a token reinforcement program, adolescents assigned to an after-school class in a psychiatric facility were asked to evaluate their performance and to award themselves tokens (SR) based on maintaining low levels of inappropriate academic and social behaviors. The students maintained behavioral improvements for 7 days in the absence of the teacher-directed token system. In a follow-up study, Santogrossi, O'Leary, Romanczyk, and Kaufman (1973) compared the effectiveness of SE on several disruptive behaviors of a similar group of students enrolled in an after-school remedial reading program. A component analysis involved rules + social reinforcement + occasional reprimands, SE, token economy + SE, and SE + SR. The results demonstrated that SE alone was ineffective in improving behavior over baseline levels. Installment of the token system reduced disruptive behaviors to nil. Introduction of the SE + SR condition initially maintained low levels of inappropriate behavior established in the token phase, but these ultimately returned to baseline levels. In the SE + SR condition students began lying about their performances and continued to be unruly even when a token phase was installed. These results introduced a caveat regarding the use of SE and SR, suggesting that these techniques are probably most judiciously used as maintenance strategies following full exposure to a systematic token reinforcement program.

Related studies probed the latter hypothesis. Drabman, Spitalnik, and O'Leary (1973) studied the effects of teaching SE and SR to eight elementary school students from "adjustment" classes who displayed an average 86% disruptive behavior during baseline. Following baseline the teacher introduced a token system in which she awarded students five points at 15-minute intervals for being in seat, on-task, nondisruptive, sitting appropriately, nonaggressive, and completing assignments and praised them for "appropriate behavior." This program reduced to 28% the targeted behaviors. In a "matching" phase students awarded themselves one to five points every 15 minutes based upon their performance while the teacher continued to rate them. If their ratings matched hers within 1 point, they received the same number of points they awarded themselves; if they matched the teacher's points exactly, they received a bonus point; if they were two or more points away from the teacher's rating, they received no points.

In four phases the opportunity to earn bonus points was slowly faded until the SE phase of the study. Then, students continued to award themselves points but were allowed to exchange for backup reinforcers (SR) the exact number of points they gave themselves in each of the SE periods. The teacher continued to rate and praise the students for appropriate behavior and exact matching, but she never overrode the students' ratings in the SE phase. During the SE+SR phase, students maintained the low levels of inappropriate behavior established in the token phase. Unlike the situation in earlier studies these low rates generalized to "control" periods when the opportunity to earn points was unavailable. Moreover, the students did not attempt to fudge on their SE or maximize reinforcement. Three "serendipitous" effects reported were that peer pressure appeared to minimize inflated ratings, peer reinforcement may have acted in support of appropriate behavior, and students gained over 7 months' performance in their reading vocabulary during the 2-month training period.

In a replication and extension of the previous study, conducted over 4½ months, Turkewitz, O'Leary, and Ironsmith (1975) employed 12 phases to investigate a SC training program: baseline, GS alone, GS + SE, token reinforcement, matching points + fading (3 phases), no matching, fading backup reinforcers (3 phases), and no backups. Results indicated that externally assigned goals had some initial effect on reducing disruptive behavior, while SE alone was ineffective. As in the Drabman et al. (1973) study, the token system produced dramatic reductions in targeted behaviors. These improvements

both generalized to nonreinforcement control periods and were largely sustained when the opportunity to earn reinforcement was withdrawn. However, advancement in reading skill was not witnessed in the latter studies.

A second generation of SE + SR studies has focused on using these strategies to promote generalization and maintenance of treatment gains made by students with EBD. Rhode, Morgan, and Young (1983) provided perhaps the most convincing case that a carefully planned and executed SE + SR training program can be quite powerful in shaping appropriate classroom behaviors and facilitating their transfer to regular class settings. Using Turkewitz et al.'s (1975) procedures, these investigators taught eight students in a special education resource room to control their behavior through SE + SR.

Observations of the students' ongoing performance were collected both in the special and regular education classes. The data show that SE + SR training enabled students to achieve high (90–100%) and stable rates of appropriate behavior in the resource room. These gains did not automatically transfer to the regular class setting, however, until the same procedures were introduced there. When SE + SR procedures were introduced into the regular class setting, appropriate classroom behavior for six of the students reached levels equivalent to that of regular classroom peers, and the other two students significantly improved their appropriate behavior over baseline. These results offer clear evidence that SC training can produce powerful generalization effects. A replication of this study with three children identified as seriously emotionally disturbed using simplified matching and fading procedures demonstrated similar results for two of the students. Although the third student was able to achieve high and stable appropriate behaviors in the resource room using SE + SR procedures, these improvements did not transfer to the regular classroom.

Two recent studies demonstrated that guided SE + SR procedures have potential for generalizing appropriate peer interactions from training situations to unstructured activity settings. Kern-Dunlap et al. (1992) videotaped the peer interactions of five middle school students enrolled in a special class for children with EBD during the activity period. Following a baseline period, students were taken to a training room and watched (SM) 10 minutes of videotaped footage of their interacting with peers in the activity period from the previous day. The tape was stopped at 30-second intervals, and a behavioral coach asked them to identify appropriate and inappropriate behaviors. Appropriate behaviors were praising, encouraging, or helpful statements to a peer while playing a game; inappropriate behaviors were commands, insulting remarks, or disruptive noises or gestures. Students marked "yes' on a recording sheet if they showed appropriate behavior (SE), "no" if they thought their behavior was inappropriate.

A behavioral "coach" also rated students' behavior. When they marked "no," the coach reviewed with them how they could have behaved more appropriately. Students gave themselves one point for each of their "yes" ratings (SR) and received a bonus point if their rating matched that of the coach. Points were exchangeable for small backup reinforcers after each session. In a multiple-baseline design across students, four of the five showed significant increases in the number of desirable social interactions they displayed toward peers, and all five of the students showed clear reductions in socially undesirable interactions. Investigators explained these results as due to the training in alternative behavior, reinforcement for exhibiting appropriate social interactions, and training sessions providing discriminative stimuli for the students to develop rule-governed behavior.

In a component analysis and partial replication of the earlier study, Kern et al. (1995) compared the effects on the behavior of three elementary school students with EBD of (1) reinforcing students for meeting externally set goal reductions in appropriate behavior the preceding day, versus (2) reinforcement + discussion of appropriate and inappropriate behavior of their classroom interactions, versus (3) videotaped feedback + SE + SR, as per the earlier study. The rewards/goal condition had little effect on improving appropriate behavior for the students, while the rewards + discussion condition appeared to have a minimal effect on two of the students. Introduction of the videotaped feedback + SE + SR condition

produced clear improvements in appropriate behavior and reductions in inappropriate behavior in all three students. A companion study, which explored a more economical application of earlier studies, was conducted with eight students with EBD in a psychiatric day-school class. The students were shown a videotape of the entire class and asked to individually rate their behavior (SE). If these ratings matched those of the teacher or facilitator, these were added to those of other students for a classwide delayed reinforcement. All eight students clearly improved their incidence of appropriate behavior and reduced their inappropriate behavior.

In summary, a review of major studies involving the teaching of behavioral SC strategies to children with EBD indicates that these offer a means of transferring to them skills for developing self-determination. In our view, the literature, albeit thin in some areas, nevertheless provides convincing evidence that SM, GS, and SE/SR used judiciously with a combination of external guidance and support can be quite effective in improving academic responses and social behaviors.

Taken together, these studies demonstrate that simply having students set goals or imposing them and evaluating their behavior may be most effective when prior training is provided. Under certain conditions SE + SR can result in the generalization of appropriate behavior across class periods and distinctly different settings plus maintain positive treatment outcomes over time. Perhaps the primary guidance these studies offer teachers for instructing students in behavioral SC would involve *first* establishing control over critical inappropriate behaviors using a structured environment (e.g., token system); *second*, embedding in this system the training of students in SM, GS, and SE/SR procedures; and *third*, gradually fading external support while shaping appropriate use of these strategies by the student.

Cross-setting generalization can be accomplished by using specific instruction and rehearsal of appropriate behavior, congruous training methods applied by adults in the transfer setting, and the gradual fading of external supports to minimal levels. Even after students demonstrate they are able to set realistic goals, accurately observe and evaluate their behavior, and contingently reinforce themselves for meeting performance standards, however, continual external reinforcement and even periodic "booster" training sessions appear important for maintaining newly acquired self-regulatory skills.

COGNITIVE SELF-CONTROL INTERVENTIONS

In conjunction with behavioral SC strategies, practitioners may select from a host of cognitive-behavioral approaches to teach students with EBD to regulate their behavior. In the self-regulation model discussed previously (Figure 21.1.), cognitive-behavioral approaches reside in the "strategy selection and implementation" component. The term "cognitive-behavior modification" (CBM) has been used widely in the literature on SC and refers to the manipulation of internal stimuli such as thoughts to control internal and external behavior. Within this framework cognitive stimuli are viewed as internal behaviors analogous to external behaviors. As these "private events" are unobservable, however, there is no way to verify that changes in behavior are the result of an individual's manipulation of cognitive stimuli or simply his or her learning to respond more discriminately to external contingencies. Thus, introduction of the notion of CBM has generated considerable debate in the psychological literature (cf. Bandura, 1969; Skinner, 1953). Although it is improbable this issue will be resolved, a succession of controlled studies, critical research reviews, and meta-analyses have shown that teaching cognitive behavioral skills to children and youth with EBD produces significant positive changes in their behavior (Dush, Hirt, & Schroeder, 1989; Robinson et al., 1999; Whalen et al., 1985).

Cognitive-behavioral strategies offer a dimension of self-control not covered by strictly behavioral approaches. Following appropriate training, these are generated and applied by the individual. Theoretically, at least, they offer a portable mechanism to guide behavior in various settings. Instruction in CBM has been used successfully to address various emotional and behavioral difficulties of children and youths including anxiety, phobias, hyperactivity, impulsivity, disruptiveness, and aggression. This typically involves teaching students to identify internal and external "triggers" that cue the behavior and use internal stimuli such as self-statements, logical problem solving, visualization, and physiological feedback as tools to control their behavior. The typical approach to training involves modeling of the self-controlling responses by the instructor and imitation and rehearsal of the strategy by the student, with corrective feedback and reinforcement for performing the desirable behavioral alternative. CBM training has been used extensively and successfully to teach students to manage their social and situational problems (e.g. Goldstein, 1988). Although classroom applications of the use of visualization have been rare, modern athletes often manipulate images to enhance their performance through envisioning themselves succeeding in competition (e.g., Reed, 2002). Some studies have used relaxation training to teach children to control physiological functions (e.g., anxiety) that impede performance (Luiselli, Steinman, Marholm, & Steinman, 1981; Mullins & Christian, 2001).

Development of Cognitive-Behavioral Interventions

Cognitive SC has its roots in behavior therapy, in which therapists use modeling, feedback, and reinforcement to change behavior. This approach heavily employs the use of self-instructions that are covert statements that guide decisions and actions needed to successfully complete a task, meet social interactions, or modulate emotional reactions. The underlying assumption of self-instruction is that a person's thoughts, perceptions, and other cognitive events mediate or affect behavior. This notion, however, is not without the understanding that behavior has multiple determinants. Within the broad cognitive-behavioral view that incorporates cognitive self-control, there are interpersonal, cognitive, and social factors that interact to cause emotional or behavioral disorders (Reinecke, Datillio, & Freeman, 1996). Of importance is that the cognitive-behavioral approach has as its foundation the empirical tradition of the early behavioral movement.

Early in the 1960s, researchers were expanding their research into cognitive processes by looking at attention, memory, problem solving, self-referent speech, and attributions, so much so that Dember (1974) proclaimed that psychology had gone "cognitive" (Hughes, 1988). Cognitive-semantic therapists such as Ellis (1962) and Beck (1976) were among the first to demonstrate empirically that verbal behavior could alter nonverbal behavior effectively, contributing to the "cognitive revolution" in mainstream psychology (see Meichenbaum, 1993). Similarly, Mahoney (1974) and Meichenbaum (1977) expanded traditional conditioning paradigms to develop a multidimensional approach that included covert processes (i.e., cognition). They argued that strict reliance on operant and classical conditioning failed to predict or explain complex patterns of human behavior accurately, such as impulsivity or aggression. Moreover, ignoring the vital role of cognition resulted in techniques that temporarily altered behavior but did not teach useful strategies or effect lasting change (Hughes, 1993). Since theorists considered the internalization of self-statements fundamental to developing self-control, deficient or maladaptive self-statements were seen to contribute significantly to a spectrum of childhood behavior problems including anxiety, impulsivity, hyperactivity, and aggression (Mahoney, 1974; Meichenbaum, 1977).

Foundational investigations explored the capacity of self-instructions for changing behavior. For example, Meichenbaum and Goodman's (1971) seminal study compared the effects of modeling alone with modeling and self-instructional training on decreasing impulsive behavior. The results supported the superiority of a combined approach. Such basic research established the reactivity of major components of the CBM process. Kendall & Braswell (1982) later noted that cognitive-behavioral techniques for the remediation of social deficits can incorporate cognitive, behavioral, emotive, and developmental strategies, using rewards, modeling, role plays, and self-evaluation. Eventually, what was known about the effects of behavior therapy was combined with an emerging set of data in cognitive psychology to build what can be called a new "coping template" (Kendall, 1993). It was Bandura (1986), however, whose social

cognitive theory helped cognitive-behavioral interventions gain prominence.

After significant work in the 1960s, Bandura rejected the unidirectional explanation of behavior. Bandura believed that behavior is not exclusively controlled by the environment and argued instead that human behavior can be explained through a triadic reciprocal model wherein behavior, personal factors and cognition, and the environment operate interactively. This reciprocal model explains the role of symbolic or cognitive learning processes, a person's self-regulation of behavior, and the interdependence of personal and environmental influences. Thus, Bandura was able to bridge the gap between behavioral theorists and cognitive psychologists while, at the same time, influencing the practice of behavior therapy by applying social or cognitive learning theory to clinical problems. As such, Bandura's social-cognitive theory has important implications for working with students who exhibit emotional or behavioral disorders.

Extending the cognitive framework, Dodge and his colleagues (see Dodge, 1980; Dodge & Frame, 1982; Dodge & Newman, 1982; Dodge & Somberg, 1987; Dodge & Tomlin, 1987) demonstrated that aggressive children tend to misinterpret social cues, often attributing hostile intent to others even when given evidence to the contrary. Further, aggressive children display other cognitive deficits when compared to normal peers, including *limited problem-solving ability*, impulsive social decision making, inattention to social cues, poor social reasoning, lack of empathy, and poor perspective taking. Dodge accounts for social competence levels as well as the likelihood of inappropriate aggression on the basis of a social information processing model involving five steps: (1) receiving and perceiving social input, (2) interpretation, (3) response search, (4) response decision, and (5) response enactment that determine how environmental events are internalized and responses selected. Presumably, children who behave unacceptably lack skills required to understand others' intentions (step 2) and/or to generate and select appropriate responses in social situations (steps 3 and 4).

Spivack and Shure (Spivack, 1973; Spivak, Platt, & Shure, 1976; Spivak & Shure, 1974) also found a relation between aggressive behavior and deficits in social information processing. Similarly, D'Zurilla and his colleagues (D'Zurilla & Goldfried, 1971; D'Zurilla & Nezu, 1980) defined effective problem solving as a cognitive-behavioral process that (1) generates a variety of alternative responses to a problem and (2) facilitates evaluation of consequences to implement the most appropriate choice. They cited studies (e.g., Allen, Chinsky, Larcen, Lochman, & Selinger, 1976) verifying that use of a problem-solving procedure improved how elementary students coped with anger. More recent studies of the characteristics of aggressive children and the effects of CBIs (see Conduct Problems Prevention Research Group [CPPRG], 1999a; CPPRG, 1999b; Daunic, Smith, & Miller, 2004; Robinson, Smith, & Miller, 2002) indicate that teaching students cognitive strategies can decrease hyperactivity/impulsivity and disruption/aggression and strengthen prosocial behavior.

Applications of Cognitive-Behavioral Interventions

Cognitive-behavioral interventions (CBIs) offer teachers strategies for replacing problem behaviors with more appropriate ones. Through CBI, students can be equipped with procedures to modify their thoughts and beliefs, thereby promoting self-regulation (Robinson et al., 1999). The CBI approach provides self-instructional strategies (i.e., using inner speech or self-talks) for individuals to modify their underlying cognition to produce therapeutic change. The CBI model engages and supports the reciprocal nature of internal cognitive events and overt behavior change through teaching strategies that guide a person's performance to reduce inappropriate behaviors.

These strategies have been used in various combinations in classroom training situations. As with behavioral SC applications, appropriate instruction is critical to a student's acquisition of cognitive-behavioral skills. Observational learning plays a central role in the cognitive-behavioral training process, and it is thus important for teachers to model the cognitive skills they want their students to acquire. For example, teachers can "think out loud" as they talk about how they might handle their own problems, eval-uate the outcome, and learn from experience. Their explanations of the cognitive strategies they used and their metacognitive awareness of those strategies (i.e., thinking about their thinking) serve as a powerful model for students to emulate.

Through the use of CBIs, teachers and other professionals can also target cognitive distortions that cause some children and adolescents to exhibit inappropriate behavioral responses in social situations. The CBI approach can include strategic instruction in useful communication skills and cognitive problem solving to interact with others effectively and appropriately. There is emerging evidence that CBM is an effective and economical approach to altering behavior of children and youth (Robinson et al., 1999); yet, closer scrutiny of the efficacy and efficiency of CBM is warranted, especially in school settings (Smith, 2002). Meta-analyses conducted by Dush et al. (1989) and Robinson et al. (1999) offer insight into the effects of CBI used with children and youth.

Dush and his colleagues analyzed 48 studies to measure the observed effects of self-statement modification (SSM), a specific form of cognitive therapy, on childhood behavior disorders. Participants in these studies exhibited a variety of significant problem behaviors: social anxieties, phobias, disruptiveness, hyperactivity, impulsivity, antisocial behavior, aggression, and delinquency. The participants were in school settings, hospitals, residential treatment facilities, and outpatient clinics. Dush et al. found that children and youths exposed to SSM experienced half of a standard deviation greater gain, on the average, than the control groups; yet, the commingled diagnostic categories demonstrated the need for a more refined selection of studies specific to interventions conducted only in school settings. As a result, Robinson et al. (1999) found 23 studies that targeted the reduction of hyperactivity/impulsivity and/or aggression in school settings using CBI. With this meta-analysis, the mean effect size across all the studies was 0.74, and 89% of the studies had treatment participants who experienced greater gains on both posttest and maintenance measures when exposed to a treatment with a cognitive component. Additionally, they noted that their meta-analytic findings indicated that CBI implemented in school settings resulted in treatment effects that were maintained following intervention.

Strategy Training

There are a variety of approaches for remediating significant behavioral problems based on the cognitive-behavioral approach. Problem solving, self-instructional training (SIT), attribution training, cognitive restructuring, relaxation training, and verbal mediation have all been found to be effective for improving behavior (cf. Hughes, 1988; Kaplan, 1995). In this section, however, we will focus on problem solving and SIT as examples of strategy training using a cognitive-behavioral approach. Problem solving is valuable for academic survival as well as social adjustment (Kendall & Braswell, 1982); it is a lifetime skill, and students who learn to generate their own solutions to problems are less likely to resist behavior change than when instructed by adults (Spivack & Shure, 1974). We will also examine SIT because it is a teaching strategy used to teach academic and behavioral skills involving cognitive modeling as an essential component.

Problem Solving

Early in the 1970s, Spivack, Shure, and colleagues investigated the effects of strategic instruction in social problem solving, with generally positive results. Successful social problem solving requires the individual to assess relevant cognitive processes, accurately interpret social cues, generate and evaluate potential subsequent social responses, implement a selected response, and monitor overt performance. This complex set of cognitive and overt behaviors can lead to social success for individuals (i.e., social competence) or create situations where others react negatively to their social interactions.

When children and youths with EBD become proficient at applying problem-solving strategies in social or personal situations that may cause them anxiety, frustration, or anger, they can improve their chances of meeting social adjustment demands, accomplishing a variety of social challenges successfully, and becoming proficient at self-control rather than continually relying on adults to help them. As with most cognitive-

behavioral interventions, problem solving is based on a series of sequential steps, with the ultimate goal of self-control. Problem solving incorporates a "how-to-think" framework for students to use when modifying their behavior rather than receiving explicit "what-to-think" instructions from a teacher. Most importantly, problem solving becomes a student-operated system, thus allowing students to generalize their newly learned behavior much more than teacher-operated systems that rely on external reward and punishment procedures (Harris & Pressley, 1991). Although listed somewhat differently in different contexts or curricula, the problem-solving steps generally include:

1. Recognizing that a problem exists.
2. Defining the problem in terms of the goal(s).
3. Generating alternative solutions.
4. Evaluating the solutions.
5. Designing a plan and carrying it out.
6. Determining how well the plan worked.

These steps can be demonstrated when a competent student attempts to solve a math word problem. First, the student approaches the problem systematically (recognizing that a problem exists), or he is likely to "guess" incorrectly if the solution that came to mind first is attempted as the answer. Second, the student has to figure out what the problem was asking for (defining the problem) and what information is needed to solve it. The student then moves on to attempt several possible solutions (generating solutions) before deciding on one (evaluating the solution). The next step is to attempt to answer the problem with the selected solution (designing a plan and carrying it out). When the plan is completed, the student evaluates how useful the strategy was (i.e., correct or wrong answer) when the answer was eventually revealed (determining how well the plan worked).

These steps are essentially the same, whether they are used to solve a math problem or a personal/social problem. Teachers can help their students learn to apply the steps to anger-provoking situations, social conflicts, or personal dilemmas. A variety of teaching techniques are used to help students learn and conduct the skill, including modeling, instruction in divergent thinking, brainstorming solutions, and behavioral rehearsal through contrived and original role plays. Teachers can use this approach with their class as they collaboratively plan classroom rules and procedures. The skills students develop in learning to solve social problems should help them cope with everyday challenges, reduce disruptive or aggressive behavior, and contribute to a positive climate and a more smoothly managed classroom.

Self-Instructional Training

Self-instructional training (SIT) is a strategy for teaching any sequential thinking skill such as problem solving, handling frustration, managing anger, or resisting peer pressure. Through a teacher's instruction, students learn to think through the step-by-step components of the required behavior. Just as with problem solving, SIT can be applied to skill instruction in a variety of learning situations.

The theoretical framework underlying SIT is based on the collective work of Luria (1961) and Vygotsky (1962), who argued that individuals learn to regulate their own behavior by progressing through several developmental stages. Initially, children learn what is expected through the speech of others, such as parents or teachers, who tell them what to do and what not to do. For example, a parent might say to a toddler, "Don't touch the stove, Jamie, because it is hot and could hurt you." At the early toddler stage, Jamie's behavior is being regulated through her mother's speech. As Jamie develops, she learns to tell (or remind) herself what to do in certain situations, recalling that her mother has told her in the past "No, don't touch. It's hot!"—and then looks at her parents to see their reaction. At this stage, Jamie is learning to regulate her behavior through her own overt speech. Next, Jamie would internalize the speech, as she begins simply to think "Don't touch, it could be hot," rather than having to say it aloud. Finally, Jamie no longer has to tell herself not to touch the stove, because she has repeated these instructions to herself, first overtly and then covertly, until the behavior has become automatic—meaning she knows how to judge a stove's condition.

This developmental model applies to any type of learning that involves cognitive processing. The following five practice steps, first developed by Meichenbaum, are involved in teaching students to use self-instructions (Hinshaw & Erhardt, 1991):

1. Cognitive modeling: adult (teacher) talks aloud while performing task.
2. Overt external guidance: adult instructs (aloud) while student performs task.
3. Overt self-guidance: student instructs self aloud while performing task.
4. Faded overt self-guidance: student instructs self in a whisper while performing task.
5. Covert self-instruction: student uses inner speech to instruct self while performing task.

The shorthand version of these steps is: teacher says, teacher does; teacher says, student does; student says, student does; student whispers, student does; student thinks, student does (Kaplan, 1995).

Cognitive Modeling

Cognitive modeling allows students access to the thinking processes of experts who possess the skill being taught. It is most often the case that individuals see the end result of a solution that a person has arrived at but not the cognitive process and step-by-step approach taken. Bandura (1986) showed that successful models are those who have status, skill competence, and power or authority. Teachers, hopefully, would be appropriate models for most students, and through overt verbalizing of their thought strategies they can reveal how they arrived at an acceptable solution. For example, a teacher who is using SIT to teach the steps of anger management to her students may start the teaching sequence by cognitively modeling how she successfully handled an anger-provoking situation. Cognitive modeling would be the first step (i.e., teacher says, teacher does) of the multistep process. Similar to problem solving, SIT can be a useful teaching tool for teachers who would use, in addition to modeling, verbal rehearsal, behavioral rehearsal through contrived and original role plays to practice the skill, and possibly a mnemonic for remembering the thinking steps. Smith, Siegel,

O'Connor, and Thomas (1994) used the ZIPPER mnemonic (Zip your mouth, Identify the problem, Pause, Put yourself in charge, Explore choices, Reset) to teach elementary special education students to reduce anger and aggression. Smith et al. first used cognitive modeling to teach the ZIPPER strategy that consisted of 20 verbal and physical self cues (e.g., using zipper motion across mouth, taking deep breaths, pointing to head and saying "What can I do?") that were gradually faded out over six sessions of instruction. Results indicated that students learned the mnemonic and were able to reduce their unwanted behavior, maintaining their decreased levels of anger and aggression over time.

Kaplan (1995) recommends that we keep the following helpful hints in mind when using SIT with students:

1. Use peer teaching whenever possible so that students get to practice performing the steps for another student.
2. Help students remember the steps by starting with only a few, and/or by using visual prompts such as a card on their desk with the steps listed as they are beginning the skill.
3. Have students put the steps in their own words to facilitate ownership and remembering.
4. Use SIT first with motor or academic skills (teaching first graders how to write a capital G, teaching fourth graders how to find the topic sentence in a paragraph, or teaching high school students how to find the hypotenuse of a triangle) that are unemotional and nonthreatening before moving to social situations that may provoke anger or frustration.
5. Review/rehearse self-statements frequently.
6. Encourage students to use self-talk in situations other than the classroom and report back to the class about their experiences.

Teaching students how to think rather than telling them what to think (and what to do) is a powerful strategy and one that pays lifelong dividends. As students go through critical transitions associated with progressing through school, they must learn to become more independent from adult guidance and develop self-reliance to meet the challenges of a complex and constantly changing world successfully. Through teaching problem solving and using self-instructional training, teachers can foster the skills that will help students develop independence and self-control.

CBI Packages

Etscheidt (1991) employed a three-group comparison study to investigate the effects of a CBI to decrease the aggressive behaviors of students with EBD. The first group received the CBI, the second group received the CBI and a positive consequence (e.g., listening to music at the end of class), and the third group (control) received neither the CBI nor the positive consequence.

Etscheidt's CBI was adapted from the *Anger Coping Program* (Larsen & Lochman, 2002), which provides instruction for students to change aggressive responses by modifying their thinking processes about the circumstances surrounding situations. The instruction also included strategies to help students in developing, evaluating, and selecting appropriate alternative responses. Etscheidt's goals included increasing self-awareness, identifying a student's reaction to peer influences, providing avenues to identify problem situations, and using problem-solving techniques. The problem-solving component increased a student's ability to identify, evaluate, and select alternative solutions for a specific social situation.

In Etscheidt's program, students used a five-step strategy to effectively approach a problem situation:

1. *Stop and think before acting.* Students are taught to restrain aggressive responses through the use of covert speech.
2. *Identify the problem.* Students are required to distinguish the specific aspects of a problematic situation that may elicit an aggressive response.
3. *Develop alternative solutions.* Students generate at least two alternative solutions to a problematic situation:
   a. Thinking about something else until able to relax
   b. Moving to another location in the room to avoid further provocation.
4. *Evaluate the consequences of possible so-*

lutions. Students assessed the benefits of each possible solution.

5. *Select and implement a solution.* The students carried out the selected alternative.

Etscheidt indicated that the two groups who received the CBI demonstrated more SC than the control group students. In fact, the students in the control group exhibited significantly more aggressive behaviors than those who received the training. Finally, Etscheidt found that the addition of a positive consequence did not significantly increase the effectiveness of the CBI.

Smith and Daunic (2003) are studying the effects of a CBI, the *Tools for Getting Along: Teaching Students to Problem-Solve* curriculum, on fourth- and fifth-grade students who exhibit behavioral problems. Preliminary results indicate that the curriculum can help students reduce their aggression and classroom disruption, and the effects can be maintained. The curriculum is designed to help students develop positive solutions to social problems. The curriculum has a problem-solving framework that uses understanding and dealing with frustration and anger as a vehicle for instruction. Anger management was chosen as the instructional focus since anger is a frequent correlate of disruptive and aggressive behavior and can be preceded by frustration. The lessons include anger management and problem-solving concepts similar to Etscheidt's program, employing a sequential strategy for students to use when approaching a problem situation. *Tools for Getting Along* also uses direct instruction, modeling, guided practice, and independent practice for skill development, along with opportunities for skill generalization.

Teachers who use *Tools for Getting Along* help students develop self-management of behavior through the purposeful manipulation of overt speech and, eventually, the use of covert verbalizations. Teachers are encouraged to use paired or small-group learning and enhance generalization by having students solve real-life problems. For example, a "Tool Kit" provides students with cumulative review, practice, and periodic opportunities to relate learned concepts to their experiences at home or school. A self-monitored point system is used throughout the instruction to reward participation. Teachers instruct students to self-assign points for completing the Tool Kit and participating appropriately in class.

The *Anger Coping Program* (Larson & Lochman, (2002) was designed to remediate aggressive and defiant behaviors of elementary students. Weekly lessons are built around five main concepts: goal setting, self-talk, anger concepts, alternatives to anger, and social perspective taking. Goal setting is the basis for homework that is reviewed at the beginning of each lesson. This is the component that uses a student's real-life experiences to increase generalization of the learned skills. For example, a student's goal may be "I will not act on my anger if someone calls me a name when we are playing in the neighborhood." Self-talk is taught using modeling and practicing during role plays to control anger and stay calm. Anger concepts include an exploration of the emotions, thoughts, and physiological responses when angry. Alternatives to anger are explored and evaluation of each alternative is taught to help students arrive at a feasible, effective, and ultimately successful resolution. The intent of social perspective taking is to help students understand that there are different outcomes from assuming different perspectives in a variety of situations. Social perspective taking can reduce misinterpretations of events, misperceptions, and social cue distortions that can lead to aggression. *Anger Coping* allows students to take turns to provide a variety of perspectives of hypothetical and real-life situations.

SUMMARY AND RECOMMENDATIONS

Perhaps the most important measure of the effectiveness of treatment programs and special education classes for children and youth with EBD is their successful transition and adaptation to natural settings. As school districts move increasingly toward inclusion, teaching these students skills that enhance their chances of academic survival and social acceptance in regular education classrooms takes on increasing importance. Their acquisition of such competencies is essential to maximizing their self-determination and freedom of choice, an outcome many special educators accept as the ultimate aim of educating children with disabilities (Wehmeyer et al., 2000). Unfortunately, what little information we have on the effectiveness of educational programs for students with EBD suggests these are largely inadequate in providing the type of natural experiences and transitional competencies they require for assuming managerial responsibilities for themselves (Grosenick, George, George, & Lewis, 1991; Knitzer et al., 1990).

While recent studies have shown that restructuring educational settings through positive behavior support and wraparound programs can improve services for these students (e.g., Eber, Sugai, Smith, & Scott, 2002); Lewis & Sugai, 1999), the transfer and continuation of academic progress and improvements in social behavior of students with EBD made in clinical programs and special education classes may be further enhanced through teaching them self-regulation skills. This solution requires both sound research and well-trained personnel. Here we summarize our findings on issues related to research on teaching children behavioral and cognitive SC and offer recommendations on improving practice.

Research Issues

In this chapter we presented considerable evidence from controlled studies that teaching behavioral and cognitive self-regulation strategies to children and adolescents with learning and behavior problems produces positive and generalizable outcomes. Issues related to teaching students behavioral and cognitive SC remains an active topic of concern for researchers and evidence in this area continues to mount. However, as others before us, we found the research base limited in some areas and murky as to what variables were responsible for observed results (Hughes & Lloyd, 1993; Hughes, Ruhl, & Misra, 1989).

Although a number of studies have shown that children and youths with EBD can learn to use behavioral and cognitive self-regulation strategies, we are virtually unknowledgeable about how their self-monitoring, goal-setting, self-evaluation, and self-reinforcement practices and cognitive strategies compare with those of peers. Equally, little information is available on variables that affect commitment to behavioral change of students with EBD. What is more, little is

known about which CBI components facilitate behavior change and the possible interaction effect with individual (i.e., teacher and student) attributes. Being better informed on these issues would allow us to tailor training programs in behavioral and cognitive SC for this population. Some answers would be helpful to such basic questions as: What behavioral and cognitive strategies are most effective in securing a commitment to behavioral change from students with EBD? How do the goal-setting, self-evaluation, and self-reinforcement practices and cognitive frameworks of this population differ from those of students without EBD? How do commitment and self-regulatory practices and the cognitive processes of these students change in relation to failure and success, and in academic and social situations? How do we assess self-regulatory skills?

Despite the potential benefits of training students with EBD in behavioral and cognitive self-regulation, studies that have addressed cross-setting generalization and long-term maintenance of treatment gains remain sparse. Some studies have indicated that generalization can occur with appropriate training and careful programming of cross-setting generalization (e.g., Rhode et al., 1983), but, as yet, we have virtually no sense of the long-term effects of this training (Hughes & Lloyd, 1993). In addition to more research on self-control, more *refined* research is needed. An important variable looming in the background of SC studies of all types concerns the unmonitored effects of a major rival hypothesis: adventitious external reinforcement. In classroom studies, for example, the effects of one or more self-regulatory strategies may be more parsimoniously explained by changes in teachers' expectancies/instructions (i.e., demand characteristics) or their frequency of social attention or other forms of reinforcement.

A frequent problem in studies involving the training of SC concerns the participation of the teacher or investigator in collecting data. It is essential for observers and other data collectors to be both naive to the purpose of the study and independent of the classroom environment. How, for example, can one conclude that a student's behavioral or cognitive *self*-regulation produces observed effects when the investigator actively participates in cuing and reinforcing appropriate behaviors or collecting data? Other possible contaminating variables that are left unaccounted for in SC studies include alterations of the classroom ecology, simultaneous operation of other behavioral control or social learning programs, and variations in the training procedures.

CBIs and behavioral SC interventions are typically delivered as treatment packages consisting of repeated cognitive and behavioral practice. What is not known at this time is an acceptable or sufficient level of exposure to treatment that can bring about adequate behavior change that is long-lasting. CBI researchers (e.g., Heinicke, 1989; Lochman, 1992; Whalen, Henker, & Hinshaw, 1985) have investigated treatment exposure and duration and found, understandably, that increased exposure (i.e., total time) resulted in greater gains and that a minimum of 10–12 sessions was necessary. Lochman (1985) manipulated total exposure and duration of treatment using the Anger Coping Program and found that students who received 18 weeks (one lesson per week) achieved greater gains than those who received 12, and that booster sessions (i.e., lessons after completion of the curriculum that provide review and practice) improved long-term effects on classroom behavior (Lochman, 1992). Beyond these few preliminary studies, little is known about the amount of treatment needed to bring about significant and long-term behavior change that makes a difference in social competence.

In summary, although some particularly well-controlled studies have provided encouraging results, we join earlier reviewers of the literature in adopting an optimistic but skeptical position on the effectiveness of behavioral and cognitive SC training (Hughes & Lloyd, 1993; Hughes, Ruhl, & Misra, 1989). Hughes and Lloyd (1993) put it most succinctly: "*We think the question of why self-management techniques work remains unanswered*" (p. 421; emphasis added).

Personnel Training Issues

Regardless of the robustness of a particular research literature on academic or social interventions with children, practitioners must be appropriately trained in their application and, as importantly, be convinced that these will lead to positive outcomes. Research limitations aside, the consistently positive results associated with behavioral and cognitive SC training merit their widespread adoption in intervention programs for students with EBD. As we observed earlier, the application of these practices in educational settings appears largely underutilized.

Wehmeyer et al.'s (2000) national survey of over 1,200 special educators revealed that, although a majority of special education teachers have taught students self-management strategies, only a small percentage reported they incorporated SC instruction into the daily curriculum. Several explanations were given for this discrepancy in results. First, teacher preparation in this area appears to be inadequate. Only one-quarter of respondents reported receiving graduate training in teaching children SC strategies, and only 12% were exposed to this information in their undergraduate programs. Nearly 70% of the teachers said they received their information on SC through journal articles, conferences, and workshops. Second, as curricula and materials are often set by state standards, teachers responding to the survey reported they lacked the authority to depart from standard practices. Third, the major barrier to implementing SC procedures concerned the teacher's belief that the students would not benefit from instruction in self-determination.

As the tide of program accountability steadily rises, positive educational outcomes become increasingly important. Perhaps the most effective intervention with students with EBD involves the use of "tried-and-true" traditional interventions such as differential reinforcement, token economies, and behavior reduction procedures (Alberto & Troutman, 2001). It is possible then that special educators weigh the cost–benefit ratio of acquiring additional training in SC strategies and incorporating these approaches and decide that the research results are not convincing enough to justify the effort. However, considering that schools are moving increasingly to inclusive classrooms and the potential long-term benefits that instruction in SC can provide, it seems most critical that, in addition to training in applied behavior analysis and cognitive instruction, teachers of these children have training in SC strategies. The anticipation of positive outcomes related to an intervention and being skilled in implementing it are not the only considerations that determine its adoption and use, however.

The social validity of any classroom intervention (i.e., judgments of students, teachers, and parents about whether an intervention is fair, reasonable, and appropriate) can influence how often it is used, independent of its efficacy (Wolf, 1978). Thus, understanding how socially valid an intervention is in specific contexts often determines its viability (Bierman et al., 1996; Coie, Underwood, & Lochman, 1991; Hope & Bierman, 1998) and its likelihood of implementation and dissemination (Smith & Farrell, 1993). To enlist teachers in acquiring the complex skills for teaching behavioral and cognitive SC to children with EBD, it is essential to develop positive beliefs and attitudes toward the importance, feasibility, and relevance of these approaches (Kazdin, 1980; Kazdin & Cole, 1981).

Regardless of the setting, classroom teachers need behavior change strategies that are efficient and can be implemented into their daily instructional routines to lessen the negative effects of aberrant classroom behavior. The model frequently used in the reduction of behavior problems is to pull students from their regular education classrooms or to place students in special programs to provide skill remediation in small-group settings. Once targeted, students are likely to be further identified by peers as deviant because they were identified in need of extra out-of-class programming or through their special program placement. Thus, experts recommend that educators teach typically functioning peers alongside students with behavior problems to (1) diminish hostile exchanges among students and biased responding, (2) minimize stigmatization of students with or at risk for EBD, (3) increase all children's skills, (4) facilitate skill reinforcement throughout the school day, and (5) maximize generalization (see Lochman et al., 1993; Walker et al., 1995). In addition to other benefits, it is more cost-efficient for classroom teachers to deliver self-control strategies within the regular classroom than to assign additional staff to teach target students in separate settings. Despite the compelling reasoning of providing universal treatment to a wide range of students, little

is known about how educators can arrange effective, universal self-control programming. Obviously, this is an area of SC research that will require significant attention.

Understanding how teacher variables (e.g., attitudes about classroom management/discipline style, use of supportive classroom practices, openness to innovative practices) relate to treatment outcomes becomes critical for effective and efficient delivery of SC in classrooms. Coie et al. (1991) point out that teachers are often overworked or unwilling to consider programs that are unrelated to academics. Teachers who are particularly stressed because of the necessity to meet state-mandated performance standards may see curricula not directly related to academics as "nonessential," and their attitude may affect students' response to the intervention. CPPRG (1999b) examined the impact of teacher/classroom variables in their study of a CBI for elementary students and found that (1) the level of a teacher's conceptual understanding, (2) how well teachers helped students generalize learned skills outside of designated curriculum time, and (3) the effectiveness of teachers' classroom management were significantly related to teacher ratings of student behavior following treatment. This research suggests that it is the teacher's acceptance and skill at using a classroom model that most affects student outcomes.

Similarly, Hirschstein, Van Shoiack, and Beretvas (2000) found that teacher behavior not formally part of the program may affect student outcomes. The amount of democratic practices or support of emotion regulation in the classroom significantly contributed to the variance observed in students' social competence scores. Democratic practices involved students in generating or evaluating solutions to a social problem, discussing opportunities for problem solving, having students work cooperatively, and asking students to help make a decision affecting the class. Support of emotion regulation consisted of discussions about using anger management and problem-solving strategies, cognitive modeling of their perspectives (i.e., thinking aloud), and prompting students in conflict to use their learned cognitive strategies. Hirschstein et al. further concluded that teacher support for emotion regulation and perspective taking improved ratings of students' antisocial behavior. Supportive practices, then, is an area of needed concentration in future research on the effectiveness of CBIs in the classroom because of the influence that teachers can have on student outcomes. Beyond that, future research should address the conditions that contribute to the development of supportive practices.

Assisting students with EBD who display significant social and behavior problems to achieve acceptable levels of self-control remains a complicated and often an elusive goal. We believe the SC approach to affect behavior change holds much promise. There is a continuing need for evidence-based, reliable, and context-relevant methods to teach children to control their behavior and thereby reduce their dependence on external methods of control. The research community in our field has achieved significant knowledge gains toward this end. Appropriately implemented, current behavioral and cognitive self-control strategies offer effective methods for assisting students to become more successful in academic and social settings. Yet, we do not have a complete picture of the multiplicity of self-control components and approaches and how these interrelate. As with many educational interventions, additional research is needed to provide teachers and other educational professionals with more powerful interventions they need to impact positively the lives of students who exhibit emotional and behavioral disorders.

REFERENCES

Alberto, P., & Troutman, A. (2001). *Applied behavior analysis for teachers* (6th ed.). Columbus, OH: Merrill.

Allen, G. J., Chinsky, J. M., Larcen, S. W., Lochman, J. E., & Selinger, H. V. (1976). *Community psychology and the schools: A behaviorally oriented multilevel preventive approach*. Hillsdale, NJ: Erlbaum.

Balcazar, F. E., Keys, C. B., & Garate-Serafini, J. (1995). Learning to recruit assistance to attain transition goals. *Remedial and Special Education, 16*, 237–246.

Bandura, A. (1969). *Principles of behavior modification*. New York: Holt, Rinehart, & Winston.

Bandura, A. (1977). Self-efficacy: Toward a unifying theory of behavioral change. *Psychological Review, 34*, 191–215.

Bandura, A. (1986). *Social foundations of thought and action: A social cognitive theory*. Englewood Cliffs, NJ: Prentice-Hall.

Bandura, A., & Perloff, B. (1967). The relative efficacy of self-monitored and externally imposed reinforcement systems. *Journal of Personality and Social Psychology, 7*, 111–116.

Beck, A. T. (1976). *Cognitive therapy and the emotional disorders*. New York: International Universities Press.

Bierman, K. L., Greenberg, M. T., & Conduct Problems Prevention Research Group. (1996). Social skills training in the Fast Track Program. In R. D. Peters & R. J. McMahon (Eds.), *Preventing childhood disorders, substance abuse, and delinquency* (pp. 65–89). Thousand Oaks, CA: Sage.

Bolstad, O. D., & Johnson, S. M. (1972). Self-regulation in the modification of disruptive classroom behavior. *Journal of Applied Behavior Analysis, 5*, 443–454.

Borduin, C. M., Mann, B. J., Cone, L. T., Henggeler, S. W., Fucci, B. R., Blaske, D. M., & Williams, R. A. (1995). Multisystemic treatment of serious juvenile offenders: Long-term prevention of criminality and violence. *Journal of Consulting and Clinical Psychology, 63*, 569–557.

Broden, M., Hall, R. V., & Mitts, B. (1971). The effect of self-recording on the classroom behavior of two eighth-grade students. *Journal of Applied Behavior Analysis, 4*, 191–199.

Carr, S. C., & Punzo, R. P. (1993). The effects of self-monitoring of academic accuracy and productivity on the performance of students with behavioral disorders. *Behavioral Disorders, 18*, 241–250.

Coie, J. D., Underwood, M., & Lochman, J. E. (1991). Programmatic intervention with aggressive children in the school setting. In D. J. Pepler & K. H. Rubin (Eds.), *The development and treatment of childhood aggression* (pp. 389–410). Hillsdale, NJ: Erlbaum.

Conduct Problems Prevention Research Group (CPPRG). (1999a). Initial impact of the Fast Track prevention trial for conduct problems: I. The high-risk sample. *Journal of Consulting and Clinical Psychology, 67*, 631–647.

Conduct Problems Prevention Research Group (CPPRG). (1999b). Initial impact of the Fast Track prevention trial for conduct problems: II. Classroom effects. *Journal of Consulting and Clinical Psychology, 67*, 648–657.

Copeland, S. R., & Hughes, C. (2002). Effects of goal setting on task performance of persons with mental retardation. *Education and Training in Mental Retardation and Developmental Disabilities, 37*, 40–57.

Curci, R. A., & Gottlieb, J. (1990). Teachers' instruction of non-categorically grouped handicapped children. *Exceptionality, 1*, 239–248.

Daunic, A. P., Smith, S. W., & Miller, M. D. (2004). *Preventing aggression among elementary students in high-risk schools: Preliminary trial of a universal cognitive-behavioral intervention*. Manuscript submitted for publication.

Dember, W. N. (1974). Motivation and the cognitive revolution. *American Psychologist, 29,* 161–168.

Dodge, K. A. (1980). Social cognition and children's aggressive behavior. *Child Development, 51,* 162–170.

Dodge, K. A., & Frame, C. (1982). Social cognitive biases and deficits in aggressive boys. *Child Development, 53,* 620–635.

Dodge, K. A., & Newman, J. (1982). Biased decision-making processes in aggressive boys. *Journal of Abnormal Psychology, 90,* 375–379.

Dodge, K. A., & Somberg, D. (1987). Hostile attributional biases among aggressive boys as exacerbated under conditions of threat to self. *Child Development, 58,* 213–224.

Dodge, K. A., & Tomlin, A. (1987). Utilization of self-schema as a mechanism of interpersonal bias in aggressive children. *Social Cognition, 5,* 280–300.

Drabman, R. S., Spitalnik, R., & O'Leary, K. D. (1973). Teaching self-control to disruptive children, *Journal of Abnormal Psychology, 82,* 10–16.

Dunlap, G., Clarke, S., Jackson, M., Wright, S., Ramos, E., & Brinson, J. (1995). Self-monitoring of classroom behaviors with students exhibiting emotional and behavioral challenges. *School Psychology Quarterly, 10,* 165–177.

Dush, D. M., Hirt, M. L., & Schroeder, H. E. (1989). Self-statement modification in the treatment of child behavior disorders: A meta-analysis. *Psychological Bulletin, 106,* 97–106.

D'Zurilla, T. J., & Goldfried, M. R. (1971). Problem solving and behavior modification. *Journal of Abnormal Psychology, 78,* 107–126.

D'Zurilla, T. J., & Nezu, A. M. (1980). A study of the generation-of-alternative process in social problem solving. *Cognitive Therapy and Research, 4,* 67–72.

Eber, L., Sugai, G., Smith, C. R., & Scott, T. M. (2002). Wraparound and positive behavioral interventions and supports in the schools. *Journal of Emotional and Behavioral Disorders, 10,* 171–180.

Ellis, A. (1962). *Reason and emotion in psychotherapy.* New York: Lyle Stuart.

Etscheidt, S. (1991). Reducing aggressive behavior and increasing self-control: A cognitive-behavioral training program for behaviorally disordered adolescents. *Behavioral Disorders, 16,* 107–115.

Felixbrod, J. L., & O'Leary, K. D. (1973). Effects of reinforcement on children's academic behavior as a function of self-determined and externally imposed contingencies. *Journal of Applied Behavior Analysis, 6,* 241–250.

Freedman, B. J., Rosenthal, L., Donahoe, C. P., Jr., Schlundt, D. G., & McFall, R. M. (1978). A social-behavioral analysis of skill deficits in delinquent and nondelinquent adolescent boys. *Journal of Consulting and Clinical Psychology, 46,* 1448–1462.

Glynn, E. L., & Thomas, J. D. (1974). Effect of cueing on self-control of classroom behavior. *Journal of Applied Behavior Analysis, 7,* 299–306.

Glynn, E. L., Thomas, J. D., & Shee, S. M. (1973). Behavioral self-control of on-task behavior in an elementary classroom. *Journal of Applied Behavior Analysis, 6,* 105–113.

Goldfried, M. R., & Merbaum, M. (1973). *Behavior change through self-control.* New York: Holt.

Goldstein, A. P. (1988). *The prepare curriculum.* Champaign, IL: Research Press.

Gottman, J., & McFall, R. (1972). Self-monitoring effects in a program for potential high school dropouts. *Journal of Consulting and Clinical Psychology, 39,* 273–281.

Grosenick, J. K., George, M., George, N., & Lewis, T. J. (1991). Public school services for behaviorally disordered students: Program practices in the 1980s. *Behavioral Disorders, 16,* 87–96.

Harris, K. R., & Pressley, M. (1991). The nature of cognitive strategy instruction: Interactive strategy construction. *Exceptional Children, 57,* 392–404.

Heinicke, C. M. (1989). Psychodynamic psychotherapy with children: Current status and guidelines for future research. In B. B. Lahey & A. E. Kazdin (Eds.), *Advances in clinical child psychology* (Vol. 12, pp. 1–26). New York: Plenum Press.

Hinshaw, S. P., & Erhardt, D. (1991). Attention-deficit hyperactivity disorder. In P. C. Kendall (Ed.), *Child and adolescent therapy: Cognitive behavioral procedures* (pp. 98–128). New York: Guilford Press.

Hirschstein, M., Van Schoiack, L., & Beretvas, S. N. (2000, April). *Effects of a social-emotional learning program on student behavior: A multilevel analysis.* American Educational Research Association, New Orleans.

Homme, L. E. (1965). Perspectives in psychology: XXIV. Control of coverants, the operants of the mind. *Psychological Record, 15,* 501–511.

Hope, T. L., & Bierman, K. L. (1998). Patterns of home and school behavior problems in rural and urban settings. *Journal of School Psychology, 36,* 45–58.

Hughes, C. A., & Lloyd, J. W. (1993). An analysis of self-management. *Journal of Behavioral Education, 3,* 401–425.

Hughes, C. A., Ruhl, K. L., & Misra, A. (1989). Self-management with behaviorally disorder students in school settings: A promise unfulfilled? *Behavioral Disorders, 4,* 250–262.

Hughes, J. H. (1988). *Cognitive behavior therapy with children in schools.* New York: Pergamon.

Hughes, J. H. (1993). Behavior therapy. In T. R. Kratochwill & R. J. Morris (Eds.), *Handbook of psychotherapy with children and adolescents* (pp. 185–220). Boston: Allyn & Bacon.

Jackson, K., & Hackenberg, T. D. (1996). Token reinforcement and self-control in pigeons. *Journal of the Experimental Analysis of Behavior, 66,* 29–49.

Kanfer, F. H., & Gaelick, L. (1986). *Self-management methods.* In F. H. Kanfer & A. P. Goldstein (Eds.). *Helping people change* (pp. 283–345). New York: Pergamon.

Kanfer, F. H., & Karoly, P. (1972). Self-control: A

behavioristic excursion into the lion's den. *Behavior Therapy, 3,* 398–416.

Kaplan, J. S. (1995). *Beyond behavior modification.* Austin, TX: Pro-Ed.

Kauffman, J. M. (2001). *Characteristics of emotional and behavioral disorders of children* (7th. ed.). Columbus, OH: Merrill/Prentice Hall.

Kaufman, K. F., & O'Leary, K. D. (1972). Reward, cost and self-evaluation procedures for disruptive adolescents in a psychiatric hospital school. *Journal of Applied Behavior Analysis, 5,* 293–309.

Kazdin, A. E. (1978). *History of behavior modification.* Baltimore: University Park Press.

Kazdin, A. E. (1980). Acceptability of alternative treatments for deviant child behavior. *Behavior Therapy, 13,* 259–273.

Kazdin, A. E., & Cole, P. M. (1981). Attitudes and labeling biases toward behavior modification: The effects of labels, content, and jargon. *Behavior Therapy, 12,* 56–58.

Kazdin, A. E., & Weisz, J. R. (Eds.). (2003). *Evidence-based psychotherapies for children and adolescents.* New York: Guilford Press.

Kelley, M., & Stokes, T. (1984). Student–teacher contracting with goal-setting for maintenance. *Behavior Modification, 8,* 223–244.

Kendall, P. C. (1993). Cognitive-behavioral therapies with youth: Guiding theory, current status, and emerging developments. *Journal of Consulting and Clinical Psychology, 61,* 235–247.

Kendall, P. C, & Braswell, L. (1982). Cognitive-behavioral self control therapy for children: A component analysis. *Journal of Consulting and Clinical Psychology, 50,* 672–689.

Kern, L., Wacker, D. P., Mace, F. C., Falk, G. D., Dunlap, G., & Kromrey, J. D. (1995). Improving the peer interactions of students with emotional and behavioral disorders through self-evaluation procedures: A component analysis and group application. *Journal of Applied Behavior Analysis, 28,* 47–59.

Kern-Dunlap, L., Dunlap, G., Clarke, S., Childs, K. E., White, R. L., & Steward, M. P. (1992). Effects of a videotape feedback package on the peer interactions of children with serious behavioral and emotional challenges. *Journal of Applied Behavior Analysis, 25,* 355–364.

Kiburz, C. S., Miller, S. R., & Morrow, L. W. (1984). Structured learning using self-monitoring to promote maintenance and generalization of social skills across settings for a behaviorally disordered adolescent. *Behavioral Disorders, 19,* 47–55.

Knitzer, J., Steinberg, Z., & Fleisch, B. (1990). *At the schoolhouse door.* New York: Bank Street College of Education.

Larson, J., & Lochman, J. E. (2002). *Helping schoolchildren cope with anger: A cognitive-behavioral intervention.* New York: Guilford Press.

Levendoski, L. S., & Cartledge, G. (2000). Self-monitoring for elementary school children with serious emotional disturbances: Classroom applications for

increased academic responding. *Behavioral Disorders, 25,* 211–234.

Lewis, T. J., & Sugai, G. (1999). Effective behavior support: A systems approach to proactive schoolwide management. *Focus on Exceptional Children, 31*(6), 1–24.

Lochman, J. E. (1985). Effects of different treatment lengths in cognitive behavioral interventions with aggressive boys. *Child Psychiatry and Human Development, 16,* 45–56.

Lochman, J. E. (1992). Cognitive-behavioral intervention with aggressive boys: Three-year follow-up and preventive effects. *Journal of Consulting and Clinical Psychology, 60,* 426–432.

Lochman, J. E., Burch, P. R., Curry, J. F., & Lampron, L. B. (1984). Treatment and generalization effects of cognitive-behavioral and goal-setting interventions with aggressive boys. *Journal of Consulting and Clinical Psychology, 52,* 915–916.

Lochman, J. E., & Dodge, K. A. (1994). Social-cognitive processes of severely violent, moderately aggressive, and nonaggressive boys. *Journal of Consulting and Clinical Psychology, 62,* 366–374.

Lochman, J. E., Dunn, S. E., & Klimes-Dougan, B. (1993). An intervention and consultation model from a social cognitive perspective: A description of the Anger Coping Program. *School Psychology Review, 22,* 458–471.

Locke, E. A., & Latham, G. P. (2002). Building a practically useful theory of goal setting and task motivation: A 35-year odyssey. *American Psychologist, 57,* 705–717.

Lonnecker, C., Brady, M. P., McPherson, R., & Hawkins, J. (1994). Video self-modeling and cooperative classroom behavior in children with learning and behavior problems: Training and generalization effects. *Behavioral Disorders, 20,* 24–34.

Lovitt, T. C., & Curtiss, K. A. (1969). Academic response rate as a function of teacher and self-imposed contingencies. *Journal of Applied Behavior Analysis, 2,* 49–53.

Luiselli, J. K., Steinman, D. L., Marholm, D., & Steinman, W. M. (1981). Evaluation of progressive muscle relaxation with conduct-problem, learning disabled children. *Child Behavior Therapy, 3,* 41–55.

Luria, A. R. (1961). *The role of speech in the regulation of normal and abnormal behaviors.* New York: Liveright.

Mahoney, M. J. (1974). *Cognition and behavior modification* Cambridge, MA: Ballinger.

Meichenbaum, D. H. (1977). *Cognitive-behavior modification: An integrative approach.* New York: Plenum.

Meichenbaum, D. H. (1993). Changing conceptions of cognitive behavior modification: Retrospect and prospect. *Journal of Consulting and Clinical Psychology, 61,* 202–204.

Meichenbaum, D. H., & Goodman, J. (1971). Training impulsive children to talk to themselves: A means of developing self-control. *Journal of Abnormal Psychology, 77,* 115–126.

Miller, D. L., & Kelley, M. L. (1994). The use of goal-setting and contingency contracting for improving children's homework performance. *Journal of Applied Behavior Analysis, 27,* 73–84.

Moore, R., Cartledge, G., & Heckaman, K. (1995). The effects of social skill instruction and self-monitoring on anger-control, reactions-to-losing and reactions-to-winning behaviors of ninth-grade students with emotional and behavioral disorders. *Behavioral Disorders, 20,* 253–266.

Mullins, J. L., & Christian, L. (2001). *Research in Developmental Disabilities, 22,* 449–462.

Mussen, P. H., Conger, J. J., & Kagan, J. (1969). *Child development and personality.* New York: Harper & Row.

Nelson, C. M., Scott, T. M., & Polsgrove, L. (1999). *A Revisitation of the Behavioral Perspective on Emotional/Behavioral Disorders: Assumptions and their Implications for Education and Treatment.* CEC Monograph Series. Reston, VA: Council for Exceptional Children.

Nelson, J. R., Smith, D. J., Young, R. K., & Dodd, J. M. (1991). A review of self-management outcome research conducted with students who exhibit behavioral disorders. *Behavioral Disorders, 16,* 169–179.

Patterson, G. R. (1982). *Coercive family process.* Eugene, OR: Castalia.

Patterson, G. R., Dishion, T. J., & Chamberlain, P. (1993). Outcomes and methodological issues relating to treatment of antisocial children. In T. R. Giles (Ed.), *Handbook of effective psychotherapy.* New York: Plenum.

Polsgrove, L. (1979). Self-control: Methods for child training. *Behavioral Disorders, 4,* 116–130.

Polsgrove, L. (Ed.). (1991). *Reducing undesirable behaviors. CEC Mini-Library Series.* Reston, VA: Council for Exceptional Children.

Reed, C. L. (2002). Chronometric comparisons of imagery to action: Visualizing versus physically performing springboard dives. *Memory and Cognition, 30,* 1169–1178.

Reinecke, M. A., Datillio, F. M., & Freeman, A. (1996). General issues. In M. A. Reinecke, F. M. Datillio, & A. Freeman (Eds.). *Cognitive therapy with children and adolescents: A case book for clinic practice.* New York: Guilford Press.

Rhode, G., Morgan, D. P., & Young, R. (1983). Generalization and maintenance of treatment gains of behaviorally handicapped students from resource rooms to regular classrooms using self-evaluation procedures. *Journal of Applied Behavior Analysis, 16,* 171–188.

Robinson, T. R., Smith, S. W., & Miller, M. D. (2002). Effect of a cognitive-behavioral intervention on responses to anger by middle school students with chronic behavior problems. *Behavioral Disorders, 27,* 256–271.

Robinson, T. R., Smith, S. W., Miller, M. D., & Brownell, M. T. (1999). Cognitive behavior modification of hyperactivity-impulsivity and aggression: A meta-analysis of school-based studies. *Journal of Educational Psychology, 91,* 195–203.

Rogers, C. R., & Skinner, B. F. (1956). Some issues concerning the control of human behavior: A symposium. *Science, 124,* 1057–1066.

Rutherford, R. B., & Polsgrove, L. (1981). Behavioral contracting with behaviorally disordered children and youth: An analysis of the clinical and experimental literature. *Monograph in Behavioral Disorders,* Arizona State University, 49–69.

Santogossi, D. A., O'Leary, K. D., Romanczyk, R. G., & Kaufman, K. F. (1973). Self-evaluation by adolescents in a psychiatric hospital school token program. *Journal of Applied Behavior Analysis, 6,* 227–287.

Schumm, J. S., & Vaughn, S. (1992). Planning for mainstreamed special education students: Perceptions of general classroom teachers. *Exceptionality, 3,* 81–98.

Shear, S. M., & Shapiro, E. (1993). Effects of using self-recording and self-observations in reducing disruptive behavior. *Journal of School Psychology, 31,* 519–534.

Skinner, B. F. (1953). *Science and human behavior.* New York: Free Press.

Smith, S. W. (2002, August). *Applying cognitive-behavioral techniques to social skills instruction* (ERIC Digest no. E630). Arlington, VA: ERIC Clearinghouse on Disabilities and Gifted Education.

Smith, S. W., & Daunic, A. P. (2003). *Technical Report #9: Tools for getting along: Teaching students to problem-solve.* Gainesville, FL: Department of Special Education, University of Florida.

Smith, S. W., & Farrell, D., T. (1993). Level system use in special education: Classroom intervention with prima facie appeal. *Behavioral Disorders, 18,* 251–264.

Smith, S. W., Siegel, E. M., O'Connor, A. M., & Thomas, S. B. (1994). Effects of cognitive-behavioral training on angry behavior and aggression of three elementary-aged students. *Behavioral Disorders, 19,* 126–135.

Spivack, G. (1973). A conception of healthy human functioning. *Research and evaluation report #15.* Philadelphia: Hahnemann Medical College and Hospital.

Spivack, G., Platt, J., & Shure, M. B. (1976). *The problem-solving approach to adjustment.* San Francisco: Jossey-Bass.

Spivack, G., & Shure, M. B. (1974). *Social adjustment of young children: A cognitive approach to solving real-life problems.* San Francisco: Jossey-Bass.

Stokes, T. F., & Baer, D. M. (1977). An implicit technology of generalization. *Journal of Applied Behavior Analysis, 10,* 349–367.

Strain, P. S., & Timm, M. (2001). Remediation and prevention of aggression: An evaluation of the regional intervention program over a quarter century. *Behavioral Disorders, 26,* 297–313.

Sugai, G., & Horner, R. H. (2002). Introduction to the special series on positive behavior support in schools. *Journal of Emotional and Behavioral Disorders, 10,* 130–135.

Thoreson, C. E., & Mahoney, M. J. (1974). *Behavioral self-control.* New York: Holt.

Turkewitz, H., O'Leary, K. D., & Ironsmith, M. (1975). Generalization and maintenance of appropriate behavior through self-control. *Journal of Consulting and Clinical Psychology, 43,* 577–583.

Vygotsky, L. (1962). *Thought and language.* Cambridge, MA: MIT Press.

Walker, H. M., Colvin, G., & Ramsey, E. (1995). *Antisocial behavior in school: Strategies and best practices.* Pacific Grove, CA: Brooks/Cole.

Walker, H. M., Sprague, J. R. Close, D. W., & Starlin, C. M. (2000). What is right with behavior disorders: Seminal achievements and contributions of the behavior disorders field. *Exceptionality, 8*(1), 13–28.

Wehmeyer, M. L., Agran, M., & Hughes, C. (2000). A national survey of teachers' promotion of self-determination and student-directed learning. *Journal of Special Education, 34,* 58–68.

Whalen, C. K., Henker, B., & Hinshaw, S. P. (1985). Cognitive-behavioral therapies for hyperactive children: Premises, problems, and prospects. *Journal of Abnormal Child Psychology, 13,* 391–410.

Wolery, M. R., Bailey, D. P., & Sugai, G. (1988). *Effective teaching: Principles and procedures of applied behavior analysis with exceptional students.* Boston: Allyn & Bacon.

Wolf, M. M. (1978). Social validity: The case for subjective measurement or how applied behavior analysis is finding its heart. *Journal of Applied Behavior Analysis, 11,* 203–214.

Wolf, M. M., Braukmann, C. J., & Ramp, K. A. (1987). Serious delinquent behavior as part of a significantly handicapping condition: Cures and supportive environments. *Journal of Applied Behavior Analysis, 20,* 347–359.

Worell, J., & Nelson, C. M. (1974). *Managing instructional problems.* New York: McGraw-Hill.

Zimmerman, B. J. (1996). Enhancing student academic and health functioning: A self-regulatory perspective. *School Psychology Quarterly, 11,* 47–66.

22

Instruction and Classroom Management

Prevention and Intervention Research

Joseph C. Witt, Amanda M. VanDerHeyden,
and Donna Gilbertson

There are few goals that are as important to teachers and schools as having safe, well-managed schools and classrooms. "Discipline" and safety are routinely at the top of national surveys about topics that teachers consider important or in need of improvement. It is therefore surprising that research that systematically focuses on classroom management has remained relatively stagnant over the past several years. The classic work of researchers in the 1980s (Brophy, 1983; Emmer, Evertson, & Anderson, 1980) continues to be widely cited in contemporary treatises on classroom management. Hence, current best practice for teachers continues to be a mix of proactive strategies (e.g., teaching rules, routines, and procedures) and reactive strategies for responding to problems once they do occur (e.g., behavior plans). That the research in support of these ideas, ancient by most standards, continues to be widely cited as "best practice" is an anomaly, given that many other topics pertaining to learning (e.g., phonemic awareness) and behavior (e.g., functional analysis) have generated numerous published reports.

Like many other domains of knowledge, research pertinent to classroom management has become more specialized as the field has matured. It is not that research has not been conducted that is new, useful, and important; instead, the new research is both broader and deeper. The research has broadened in the sense that the importance of other areas of teaching and learning (e.g., the fundamentals of curriculum and instruction) to child behavior in the classroom has been explored further. At the same time, research has increased our depth of understanding about many subareas of classroom management. For example, research on functional assessment has helped us to understand how better to prevent and respond to serious behavior problems.

The purpose of this chapter is to review some important recent developments that are pertinent to the body of knowledge about classroom management. Although we will briefly review foundational research, more thoroughgoing treatments of that literature are available elsewhere (Doyle, 1986). More specifically, the purpose of this effort is to provide a review of the literature with an eye toward the implications for practices that may derive from the research. To maintain some focus on practice and to provide an organization for the chapter, we will structure what follows around a simple pyramid model.

A PYRAMID MODEL OF CLASSROOM MANAGEMENT

A persistent belief among some school-based professionals is that behavior problems, once observed and properly understood, can be corrected, usually through the application of a negative consequence. For example, when a teacher observes a student swearing in class, the "problem-solving" machinery of the school goes into action, and it is decided that the child will be sent to the office every time he swears. Alternatively, the child might get a reward for "not swearing." Case closed. Problem solved. Next day, the same child begins to do a perfect voice imitation of the teacher that is even more annoying. That behavior is added to the list of violations. And so it goes. A closer analysis, of course, might reveal a lack of attention to some basic issues. For example, the child might routinely be asked to do academic work for which he lacks prerequisite skills. Alternatively, the teacher may have planning gaps creating several 5- to 10-minute blocks of time each day when the students are supposed to sit quietly and do nothing while the teacher prepares for the next lesson.

Experienced teachers, behavior specialists, and others recognize that it is virtually impossible to manage problem behaviors once they occur if certain prerequisites are not in place. First, the teacher must be competent to teach the academic subjects, the curriculum must be appropriate for the students, and instruction must provide opportunities to learn, practice, and receive feedback. If children cannot perform expected work, if there is a lack of consequences for doing or not doing the academic work, and/or if the teacher is not competent to teach the subject matter, then there is no behavior management program in existence that can produce enduring behavior change in such a classroom.

Second, children in a classroom must know what is expected of them behaviorally.

There are two basic reasons children do not behave appropriately in the classroom: either they *can't* do it or they *won't* do it (Bandura, 1969). The first step is to ensure that each student knows what and how to do what is expected. Students must be taught rules, procedures, and teacher expectations. For example, teaching positive behaviors, reminding students to use the behaviors during times when behavior problems are likely, and then closely monitoring student behavior produces marked reductions in behavior problems (Colvin, Sugai, Good, & Lee, 1997). Using this approach, however, is based upon the questionable assumption that teachers can articulate appropriate expectations, which they then systematically teach and consequence.

Finally, *if* there is a solid academic program and *if* positive behavioral expectations have been taught by teachers, *then* strategies for responding to behavior problems can be successful. There are two reasons for this assertion. First, there will be fewer behavior problems to which the teacher must respond. Second, because the classroom context supports and encourages appropriate behavior, consequential procedures are more likely to be effective, and "doing the right thing" is more likely to be reinforcing.

We propose a problem-solving model of assessment for classroom behavior. Problem-solving models of assessment have been written about most frequently with respect to academic performance problems (Good & Kaminski, 1996; Shinn, 1995). The first stage of a problem-solving model involves measuring the degree to which fundamental features of the environment are operating as they should be (i.e., adequacy of the instructional environment). An indicator of whether or not preventative measures are adequate is the behavior performance of most of the other children in the class. If the majority of the class is performing well, then it is likely that adequate prevention methods are being implemented consistently in the classroom. On the other hand, if many children in the class exhibit off-task behavior during instruction or do not consistently comply with classroom rules and routines or teacher commands, then adequacy of classroom management becomes suspect. When many children in a class exhibit behaviors that interfere with effective instruction, classwide intervention is indicated. Once a classwide problem has been ruled out or resolved through intervention, then individual child problems can be considered. For individual child problems, a behavioral intervention might be attempted prior to launching a full functional analysis, which often is expensive and beyond the skills of many school-based teams. A powerful intervention that attempts to control for several of the most common causes or functions of problem behavior is ideal. In planning this "broad-band" type of intervention, the interventionist should think in terms of maximizing the probability of desired behaviors (academic productivity) and minimizing the probability of behaviors that interfere with academic productivity (Mace & Roberts, 1986). Hence, reinforcing academic productivity and blocking reinforcement for lack of academic productivity may be sufficient to correct behavior problems for most children. Progressing through an intervention sequence of whole class to individual child has been shown to have a positive effect on reducing overidentification of children for special education by improving accurate identification (Gresham, 2002). These effects have been observed because poor performance due to lack of motivation and/or inadequate instruction and practice are ruled out prior to individual assessment. Hence, more restrictive treatments are avoided by applying the problem-solving model. With disruptive behavior, the same sequence can be applied. Logically, similar benefits could be attained: reducing overidentification (because behavior problems are successfully treated prior to identification) and avoiding more restrictive treatments or placements (e.g., special education referral or a succession of ineffective and increasingly restrictive treatments). These benefits derive as a result of moving from an exclusive focus on the child to a focus on children as they interact with the environment.

This chapter will be organized around these three integrated strands necessary for classroom management:

- Are academic skills taught appropriately?
- Are positive behavioral expectations taught appropriately?
- Are teacher responses to inappropriate behavior consistent and accurate?

These three areas are depicted in Figure 22.1. The pyramid structure implies that each layer is foundational for the next layer. Conceptually, this is true. In practice, teachers will put all three *in place more or less concurrently during the first few weeks of school. In the sections that follow, we will review literature pertinent to each of these major rubrics.*

ARE ACADEMIC SKILLS TAUGHT APPROPRIATELY?

The first level of the pyramid model of classroom management presented in Figure 22.1 focuses on appropriate instructional activities. There are a number of important advantages of focusing on instruction when evaluating the effectiveness of classroom management. First, classroom management occurs during instructional activities. Second, recent studies have identified many curricular (what is taught) and instructional (how curriculum is taught) variables that are frequently linked with challenging behavior (Kern, Choutka, & Sokol, 2002). Modifications of these variables not only have reduced problem behaviors but also have enhanced academic productivity. Thus, a clear relationship exists between the learning environment and undesirable behavior. This relationship indicates strategies that a teacher can employ to remediate problems. Third, utilization of variables that fit naturally within the context of classroom instructional activities may reduce or eliminate the need for additional resources or intrusive behavior intervention plans. Finally, an initial targeting on severe behavior with intensive interventions may exceed the teacher's skill level, particularly if current strategies are unable to successfully reduce minor problems. Managing behavior problems first by simply changing instructional methods allows the teacher to alter less complicated but critically relevant factors that are necessary to enhance all students' academic performance.

Focusing on instruction first changes the goal of classroom management in an important way. Rather than focusing only on changing problem behavior, classroom management is directed at modifying the daily instructional variables that directly influence

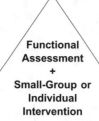

Functional
Assessment
+
Small-Group or
Individual
Intervention

Level 3:
Are Teacher Responses to
Inappropriate Behavior
Consistent and Accurate?
Assess next level if class observation indicates that
an effective consequential plan for rule compliance
and infractions is consistently used—and yet
behavior problems persist for a few students.

Level 2: Are Positive Behavioral Expectations
Taught and Managed Appropriately?
Assess next level if classwide assessment indicates that the majority of
students are following rules and the majority of class time is spent on
academic activities—and yet behavior problems persist.

Level 1: Are Academic Skills Taught Appropriately?
Assess next level if classwide assessment indicates that the majority of students
are adequately performing on grade-level skills—and yet behavior problems persist.

FIGURE 22.1. The pyramid model of classroom management.

academic productivity. Importantly, this approach upholds educators' primary role of providing a supportive environment that promotes academic gains and enables the child to participate to the greatest degree possible in the general education curriculum. In order to increase participation in activities that meet the environmental demands, the functional goal becomes teaching students how to perform critical skills such as reading and writing. This goal is important given that children with challenging behaviors frequently perform at lower academic levels than their peers and make slower progress in special education programs than students with only learning disabilities (Anderson, Kutash, & Duchnowski, 2001).

Fortunately, recent research has increasingly demonstrated a number of ways teachers can manage teaching and curriculum variables to facilitate learning while promoting positive classroom behavior and reducing behavior problems including aggression and self-injury (Dunlap, Kern, & Worcester,

2001). Given the relationship between instruction and behavior problems, the goal of this section is to answer the following question: How can teachers manage their classroom teaching in such a way that students are both learning more and behaving in a manner that interrupts learning less? Based on empirical findings from this literature, two key academic areas should be evaluated to determine their effects on student behaviors: instructional tasks and management of instruction.

Instructional Tasks

A recent emphasis on nonaversive approaches has spurred the development of proactive procedures that focus on the identification of events or conditions that occur *prior* to problem behaviors. The intent of this assessment is to implement interventions that alter, eliminate, or replace instructional variables in a manner that reduces the likelihood of problem behavior occurring. A majority of studies investigating the relationship between instructional variables and problem behavior have concentrated on task difficulty based on the assumption that problem behavior will occur if disruptive behaviors successfully lead to escape or avoidance of an aversive academic task (e.g., Center, Deitz, & Kaufman, 1982; Weeks & Gaylord-Ross, 1981). In general, these studies have found that difficult tasks are associated with increased levels of problem behaviors. For example, DePaepe, Shores, Jack, and Denny (1996) found that students completed more work and exhibited more on-task behavior when completing work with 90% or more accuracy as compared to 75% or less accuracy. Gilbertson, Witt, Dufrene, and Duhon (in press) further demonstrated that greater percentages of on-task behavior were obtained when students with behavior problems were given work they were able to complete both accurately and fluently. However, students generally maintained higher levels of on-task performance at lower fluency levels if they were concurrently receiving instructional intervention to *increase academic performance to mastery levels*. The Gilbertson et al. study was interesting in that it showed concomitant improvements in behavior as a function of an *instructional* intervention incorporating practice, feedback, and incentives. This latter finding represents an important practical implication for teachers who need interventions that will provide for adequate skill acquisition and proficiency with an increase in appropriate classroom behaviors since teachers are not typically teaching "easy" material that students have already mastered. Thus, these results suggest that students' disruptive behaviors may decrease if children are given simple, effective instruction at a level where academic gains or adequate change in slope of performance can be obtained.

Researchers have demonstrated that functional assessment can be used to differentiate between academic tasks that are associated with the occurrence of problem behaviors from those that are associated with acceptable behaviors (Dunlap et al., 2001). The tasks that are found to be associated with high occurrence of problem behaviors can then be modified to reduce problem behaviors in a manner similar to antecedents that occasion acceptable behaviors. Using this approach, problem behaviors that occurred with task difficulty or demand have been reduced in two ways. First, decreasing the amount of effort needed to perform the task has modified tasks by altering task requirements, changing ways to complete the task, providing frequent breaks, and programming shorter task time periods (Kern et al., 2002). Second, tasks have been modified to make the task less aversive or have enhanced the task with more reinforcing components. For example, giving students a choice of task (Dunlap et al., 1994), embedding high probability completed tasks with low-probability tasks (Horner, Day, Sprague, O'Brien, & Heathfield, 1991), and modifying task preference (Blair, Umbreit, & Bos, 1999) reduced classroom problem behaviors. Many of these curriculum adjustments may be feasible approaches that potentially enhance all students' on-task performance as opposed to just benefiting one student. However, it is important to note that modifications of instructional tasks are most likely effective due to changes in contingencies that follow academic performance (Smith & Iwata, 1997). For example, a decrease in task difficulty may lead to fewer errors, which in turn leads to more praise or diminishes the reinforcing effects of escape, or shorter task durations decrease the delay between starting work and teacher attention or escape.

To date, few studies have included an empirical evaluation of the effects of curricular modifications on academic performance, on-task performance, and disruptive behaviors. For example, Penner, Frank, and Wacker (2000) developed instructional modifications based on functional assessment results that identified classroom variables that were highly associated with problem behaviors for three students exhibiting classroom disruptive behaviors. Individual interventions were then designed to increase academic performance although disruptive behavior was also evaluated. Two instructional modifications purposely designed to ease task effort and increase peer attention effectively enhanced academic performance and decreased problem behavior. Specifically, a combination of completing assignments on computer with peer tutoring was effective for one student, while a combination of shortened assignment and peer tutoring was effective for a second student. Miller, Gunter, Venn, Hummel, & Wiley (2003) also found that both academic and on-task measures improved when extensive work examples were paired with either a shortened math assignment or functional writing activity. Results from a study conducted by Skinner, Hurst, Teeple, and Meadow (2002) demonstrated that on-task behavior and work completion during seat work increased in students with emotional disturbance when math problems were interspersed with a small percentage of easier problems.

Realistically, it is futile to try to manage behavior when students are working at a frustrational level that hinders skill acquisition (Gickling & Armstrong, 1978). Thus, task difficulty is a highly relevant variable that should be initially considered when problem behaviors are encountered in a classroom. A simple assessment of a student's performance in grade-level materials quickly indicates whose performance falls sharply below peers or critical benchmarks. One well-researched screening tool, curriculum-based assessment (CBA), has been utilized to determine instructional placement and evaluate effectiveness of instructional programming (Shinn, 1998). Briefly, CBA involves the administration of brief probes composed of a subset of critical curriculum skills that the student is expected to know over a certain period of time. One advantage of CBA is that administration is simple and time-efficient since the administration of each probe requires only 1–5 minutes. More importantly, child performance functions as an indicator of whether or not there are problems with the basic characteristics of instruction in the classroom. For example, if many students exhibit poor academic performance and/or on-task behavior in a class, then instructional adequacy is suspect. If students fail to increase performance when instructional level or task difficulty is adjusted, there may be a deficit in teaching methods serious enough or consistent enough to affect the critical behavior of interest in schools, that is, academic performance.

Thus, instructional level is one parameter that has a strong impact on academic and classroom social behavior that can easily be assessed and set at an appropriate level before a more complicated assessment, training, and intervention plan is considered. We recommend that this be the first assessment step conducted and reviewed when problem behaviors occur. When students are performing below an instructional level, effective instruction can be given at an appropriate level to determine if learning occurs at an adequate rate with a concurrent decrease in problem behaviors. The results of a classwide assessment presented in Figure 22.2 provide an illustration of a classwide screening using a 2-minute math worksheet consisting of grade-level math skills. Figure 22.2 displays the math scores from a classwide screening that was administered in a fourth-grade classroom in March. To facilitate decision making, the students' scores are displayed from the lowest to highest math scores. A math benchmark is shown on the graph to indicate the instructional level for math skills for fourth grade (Shapiro, 1996). Additionally, as can be seen in Figure 22.3, the students in March were on-task 58% of the time while completing a math worksheet. According to findings by Shinn, Walker, Stieber, and Ramsey (1987), the average on-task performance observed for students during a number of school activities was approximately 70%. As in this case, a high percentage of student disruptive and off-task behavior is often associated with low academic performance. The intervention, which was to provide guided practice using materials that were at the student's instructional level, resulted in improvements in both behavior and academic performance in April, once students were able to successfully complete their work (see Figure 22.3). More involved intervention strategies are attempted only if students fail to respond to this level of intervention performed with documented integrity in the classroom.

Management of Instruction

There are two common functions of problem behaviors that are linked to poor academic performance and that impact instructional strategies. Some students may choose to engage in inappropriate behaviors because academic tasks are too difficult and disruption allows them to escape the task. Other students possess the necessary skills to perform the tasks expected in class, but for some reason they choose to engage in problem behavior instead of correct work com-

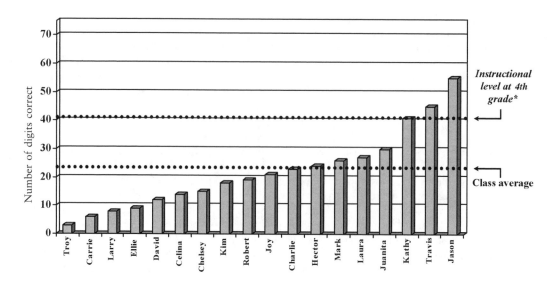

FIGURE 22.2. Performance of each child in a fourth-grade class during a classwide screening. Each bar represents the number of digits correct in 2 minutes for each child in the class on a math worksheet sampling a fourth-grade math skill. The dotted lines indicate performance at or above a national norm and the average score of all students.

*National norm for fourth grade.

pletion. A skill-deficit problem suggests that professional attention be focused on instructional strategies and work level, whereas a performance deficit requires that attention be directed at antecedents and consequences of behaviors related to what the student is supposed to be doing and not supposed to be doing. Duhon et al. (in press), for example, identified students with either skill or performance deficits after conducting a brief

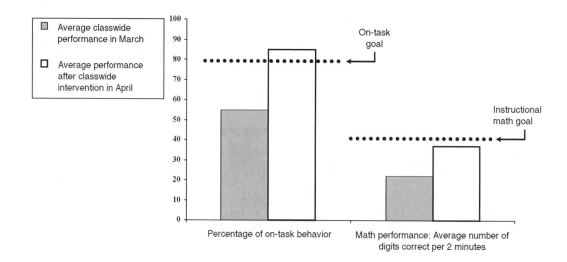

FIGURE 22.3. Pre-and postevaluation of classroom behavior and academic performance following intervention.

condition that provided students with the opportunity to earn an incentive if they performed within an instructional level on an academic task similar to a poorly performed class assignment. If a student demonstrated an appropriate skill level with incentives, then this result suggested that the child exhibited a performance deficit and would most likely benefit from a contingency-based intervention. Conversely, when a student was not able to perform within an instructional level, then the child exhibited a skill deficit and would benefit from an instructional intervention.

Although students exhibiting skill deficits require instructional changes, all students are more likely to do the work if positive contingencies are present for work productivity. In the classroom, students have many concurrent response choices that compete with work completion (Mace & Roberts, 1986). According to the *matching law* (Herrnstein, 1970, 1972; McDowell, 1982), given concurrent operants, individuals are more likely to perform the response at a rate roughly equivalent to the amount of reinforcement associated with that response. Relative rate of reinforcement (frequency), quality, immediacy (delay to reinforcement), and response cost (effort) influence the choice such that the individual will perform the easiest response that results in the fastest, highest-quality, and densest schedule of reinforcement. Individuals will sample both reinforcement schedules at roughly the rate of reinforcement, all other variables being equal, meaning individuals will continue to exhibit both responses (i.e., inappropriate and appropriate behavior) to earn available reinforcement. An understanding of this formula is necessary to maximize at all times the probability of correct or desired responding while minimizing the probability of undesired responding. Further, at least a rudimentary understanding of the effect of reinforcer satiation is needed for behavior management to be successful. If the critical goal is academic growth, then it is important that behaviors that result directly in academic productivity be reinforced. One classic study by Ayllon and Roberts (1974), for example, demonstrated that a token reinforcement system, which was solely contingent upon increases in academic performance, resulted in increased academic

performance with a corresponding decrease in rates of disruptive behaviors. Hence, applying the contingency to work completion rather than on-task behavior positively influenced behavior and increased academic growth. Additionally, these results were obtained without further modifications during instruction and practice.

Consequences for academic performance can be relatively simple. For example, frequent feedback delivered promptly after academic work completion appears to be more effective than frequent praise for most students (Waxman & Walberg, 1991). For example, corrective feedback given promptly after academic work completion is a critical factor that enhances academic performance and on-task behavior (Waxman & Walberg, 1991). Moreover, feedback is equally effective if provided from peers, teachers, public posting, and computers (Graham, 1999). Praise also has a positive effect on on-task behavior and academic performance (Sutherland & Welby, 2001; Waxman & Walberg, 1991). Despite these simple strategies, observational studies investigating student–teacher interactions (Shores & Wehby, 1999) have generally found that students diagnosed with emotional and behavioral disorders receive teacher attention primarily for inappropriate behavior and receive low rates of positive interactions. Once students choose to attempt academic tasks, variables designed to support accurate skill acquisition must occur. Now, effective task presentation, modeling, and guided practice with immediate error correction matched to the level of acquisition (McKee & Witt, 1990) become critical teacher behaviors.

One consistent finding of effective teaching research is that active student responding is robustly related to academic achievement (Brophy, 1986; Gettinger & Stoiber, 1999; Greenwood, 1996). Students who frequently practice learned skills are able to integrate and organize information more quickly and accurately and apply these skills in the completion of higher-level objectives. Moreover, effective teachers with few disruptions and high achievement actively *do many things to optimize successful student responding*. For example, teachers who spend more time providing guided practice to supervise initial task performance have students who are more engaged during independent seatwork (McKee & Witt, 1990). During guided practice, increased pace, choral response, and response cards concurrently increase response opportunities and increase on-task behavior when students are first learning a skill (Munk & Repp, 1994). During independent seatwork, altering the response mode during practice (verbal or written) or providing instructional support results in increased opportunities to respond (Skinner, 1996). However, research suggests that few teachers of students with behavior problems consistently implement effective teaching strategies (Gunter & Denny, 1996). In fact, several studies further suggest that less instruction is provided to students who frequently exhibit problem behaviors than to appropriately behaved students (Carr, Taylor, & Robinson, 1991). Results from observational studies in the classroom suggest that academic responses are also dismally low for students with EBD (Sutherland & Wehby, 2001).

If effective instructional strategies are actively implemented, then most children will behave appropriately and *learn*. A simple outcome measure, such as correct responses per minute, dynamically indicates the degree to which instruction has had the desired effect. Whereas this type of assessment may also indicate an instructional programming or delivery problem, the results have limited treatment implications without further assessment. A number of systematic formal observation tools for evaluating instructional environments exist (e.g., the Instructional Environmental System; Ysseldyke & Christenson, 1993). Yet, these assessments may be complicated and time-consuming, and many items are not expressed in operational terms. To date, few studies have empirically validated the degree with which these assessments directly link to interventions that increase academic productivity and decrease problem behaviors.

An extensive list of effective variables such as those in Table 22.1 are primarily based on low to moderate correlations with few high correlations between teacher behavior and student achievement (Brophy, 1986). Thus, these behaviors are more of a guideline for effective strategies that may vary with changes in context or when used in conjunction with other procedures. Researchers warn against the danger of using these types of lists to evaluate teaching and basing decisions on the number of successful procedural compliances rather than adequate academic gains (Brophy, 1986; Ysseldyke & Elliot, 1999).

Ideally, positive student behavior change would result quickly with implementation of a few key teaching procedures; however, there is little empirical evidence thus far to specify such a reliable simple approach. To ensure effective results, a "train–test–train–test" cycle is the best approach to use until desired relevant student behavior change is obtained. Beginning with the simplest relevant variable and progressing to more complex analyses until the problem is resolved, obtaining frequent dynamic measures of academic performance upon which to judge the adequacy of the solution may be the best approach. For example, instructional level may first be assessed. Next, management of contingencies for work completion is a relatively simple procedure to observe and implement once instructional level is assessed and adjusted, if needed. If adequate progress still does not occur, practice may be assessed to determine whether a sufficient number of opportunities to respond occur. If a sufficient number of opportunities to respond were observed but high error rates also were observed, then additional acquisition-level instruction with immediate corrective feedback might be attempted (Haring, Lovitt, Eaton, & Hansen, 1978), and so on.

ARE POSITIVE BEHAVIORAL EXPECTATIONS TAUGHT AND MANAGED APPROPRIATELY?

If the academic program is fundamentally sound, the next level in the pyramid (Figure 22.1) is that expected behaviors must be taught and consistently managed by teachers. Effective instruction depends upon time being disproportionately allocated to instruction or academic management, as opposed to being allocated to organization of students and responding to misconduct. Managing positive behavioral expectations in the classroom decreases problem behaviors and increases academically engaged time. Rules, rules management, and classroom routines provide a structure within which positive behavioral expectations are

TABLE 22.1. Effective Instructional and Environmental Variables

Daily review and checking of previous work

Pretests

Presenting information and materials

Background knowledge
Clarity of goals/objectives
States main ideas during and after lesson
Advanced organizers such as outlines
Brief presentations with explicit teaching
Step-by-step presentations that are well sequenced using a learning hierarchy approach
Modeling examples
Specific and concrete procedures
Prompts signals between transitions between content steps/materials
Checking for student understanding
Questions with 3-second wait time
Preparing students for practice

Providing practice

Guided student practice
    Opportunity to respond (e.g., response cards, choral practice, oral questions, written)
    Pace
    Errorless learning strategies
    Monitoring
    Questioning

Independent practice
    Frequent student responses
    Type of task
    Pace
    Short duration
    High success rate in work accuracy
    Monitoring
    Procedures to get help
    Procedures when work is completed
    Peer tutoring

Providing feedback regarding academic performance

Goal setting
Specific
Corrective
Promptly
Praise
Graded work and homework

Note. Data from Brophy (1996); McKee and Witt (1990); Waxman and Walberg (1991); and Ysseldyke and Elliot (1999).

built. Lack of rule clarity, absence of consistent consequences for rule violations, and ineffective instruction practices in schools are related to aggressive and noncompliant child behaviors (Mayer, 1995; Walker, Colvin, & Ramsey, 1995).

Rules are a set of positive behavior expectations designed to promote an organized, productive, and cooperative environment. Studies have indicated that effective teachers post rules in the classroom and that student behavior is directly influenced by how rules are taught and managed (Emmer, 2001). To evaluate rule compliance, a simple tally of rule violations during a classroom observation can be used to estimate rate of rule compliance. A high number of rule violations during an observation suggests that students do not know how to perform the expected rule behavior, rules are unclear, rules are not consistently managed, and/or compliance with rules is neither monitored nor consequenced. In the case of high rates of rule violations, rules may need to be re-identified and operationalized in coordination with the teacher, taught or retaught to the students, and implemented with a system for delivering positive and aversive consequences, depending on compliance. A number of management systems have effectively increased student compliance with rules. From least intrusive to most intrusive, these strategies range from praise, precorrection (Colvin et al., 1997), precision commands (Rhode, Jenson, & Reavis, 1998), indiscriminable contingencies (Rhode et al., 1998), group contingencies (Gresham & Gresham, 1982), overcorrection (Carey & Bucher, 1983), response cost (Kelley & McCain, 1995; Proctor & Morgan, 1991; Witt & Elliot, 1982), and token economies (Musser, Bray, Kehle, & Jenson, 2001). Regardless of the strategy that the teacher prefers to use, the key factors that influence compliance are intensive student training on rules and rule consequences followed by teacher monitoring, immediate and consistent response to rule infractions, and frequent acknowledgement of rule compliance. Without a plan for managing rule compliance, teachers may react in a manner that may trigger more intense reactions from students. For example, an upset teacher may argue, yell, or invade a student's space publicly in front of his or her peers. This type of teacher reaction often leads to students responding in the same manner. Few studies have directly compared the effects of various rule types and management on academic performance and/or problem behaviors. However, in most rule compliance studies, rules have targeted behaviors that decreased disruptions (e.g., staying seated, raising hands, keeping quiet, and hands and feet to oneself), whereas one or two rules may have targeted academic tasks (e.g., work completion and following directions) (Malone & Tietjens, 2000). Most teachers use between five and six rules on average that target how to speak, interact, move, handle supplies, and complete assignments (Howard & Norris, 1994).

In addition to rules, effective teachers use classroom routines to increase academic time. By definition, classroom routines are specific procedures for accomplishing daily activities in the shortest possible period of time. For example, students can be responsible for certain jobs such as handing out papers, grading papers, moving into and out of small groups, lining up, and turning in work with little disruption. When routines consistently are being used, students appear to know what to do with few prompts, and they move quickly (i.e., within 1–2 minutes) from one activity to another. In contrast, an ineffective teacher may take 15 minutes to organize students and materials between two activities. Given that there are typically at least 15 transitions per day, these teachers lose a considerable amount of teaching time to managing student behavior (LaFleur, Witt, Naquin, Harwell, & Gilbertson, 1998). Further, longer transition times have been linked to increased disruptive behavior (Emmer, 2001). LaFluer et al. (1998) demonstrated that teachers who consistently used more than 2 minutes to transition from one activity to another were able to decrease transitions after teaching students a simple transition routine. Briefly, students learned to quietly respond to a teacher signal, listen to directions, and follow those directions within a given time limit. Effective teachers spend a great deal of time planning routines and then actively teaching students how to perform the behaviors expected during routine activities (Emmer, 2001), preserving instructional time and preventing behaviors that interfere with learning.

In summary, any strategy that positively influences *both* student achievement and classroom behaviors will ultimately produce increases in academic time and successful engagement at the appropriate task level. Once it is shown that academic skills and positive behavioral expectations are managed in a manner that enhances academic progress and on-task behavior for most students, then a small percentage of students will be revealed as clearly needing more intensive services (Sugai, Sprague, Horner, & Walker, 2000). For this small percentage of students who fail to respond to classwide academic and behavioral management systems, individual behavior support in the classroom is more likely needed to target individual learning characteristics and social needs.

ARE TEACHER RESPONSES TO INAPPROPRIATE BEHAVIOR CONSISTENT AND ACCURATE?

Thus far, level 1 of the pyramid depicted in Figure 22.1 focused on activities that can be categorized as *preventive*. We now begin to focus on classroom management activities that are *reactive*—those that would be used if all the proven prevention activities are implemented and are not effective. Even the best teachers will have a small percentage of children who do not respond to an array of best prevention practices. As already mentioned, research indicates that effective and ineffective teachers are no different in their response to inappropriate behavior in the classroom. Effective teachers are distinguished from ineffective teachers in how thoroughly they implement proven preventive strategies. In this section, we will discuss what teachers may do once the problem behavior has occurred.

The most commonly used "interventions" for problem behavior in the classroom are weak and nonspecific treatments, such as discussion, repeating, and removal. Most alarming, ineffective treatments are likely to be replaced with increasingly restrictive and ineffective treatments in an escalating cycle (Walker et al., 1995). For example, treatment frequently involves talking with the teacher outside of the classroom, but talking alone is generally a weak and ineffective method for producing actual behavior change. In as many as 75% of cases, children exhibiting antisocial behaviors are assigned to highly restrictive in-school and out-of-school placements. Children exhibiting disruptive behaviors are likely to be identified as experiencing school problems early in their schooling careers but are not likely to benefit from the services that are provided there and subsequently experience a more pronounced risk for school failure, placement in special education classrooms, and eventual dropout, as compared to same-age at-risk peers (Walker, Shinn, O'Neill, & Ramsey, 1987). It is important to note that demographic variables, referral source and reason, and IQ scores have not been found to differ between "behavior disordered" dropouts and "behavior disordered" graduates. However, the number of previous drop-outs, transfers to other schools, and changes in service placements (usually from less to more restrictive) are generally associated with higher rates of dropouts, compared to graduates. Traditionally, practitioners have focused on the assessment of child variables to the exclusion of environmental variables that may affect student performance in the classroom setting. Treatment has been guided by pragmatism, resource availability, or skill level of the treatment agent, as opposed to adjusting child–environment fit. The effects of increasingly restrictive and ineffective treatments are experienced, perhaps most acutely, by students exhibiting low-tolerance behaviors. Among the least-tolerated behaviors are noncompliance, disruption, and aggression (Nelson, Rutherford, Center, & Walker, 1991). The intervention most frequently attempted by many teachers to deal with child noncompliance and aggression is referral to special education, and the resulting placements are among the most restrictive for these students.

Methods that rely on early universal screening and implementation of prevention/intervention, beginning with the classroom basics (e.g., communicating classroom rules daily, teaching students the prosocial skills they are expected to perform, and increasing adult monitoring in problem areas during problem times) described in the previous section and progressing as merited to more involved assessment and intervention strategies, are likely to be the most efficient and the most effective. Most importantly, practitioners should use assessment strategies that link directly to effective intervention. Robust effects for decreased student disruptions, fewer discipline problems, decreased dropout and suspension rates, increased academic engagement, and increased positive feelings among students and staff have been obtained by implementing function-based interventions in the regular classroom setting (Mayer, 1995).

FUNCTIONAL ASSESSMENT

The pyramid depicted in Figure 22.1 makes use of *group* oriented strategies at level 3. Group strategies will be effective for most but not all students. At the top of the pyramid is Functional Assessment, leading to the design of intervention. This conceptualization is consistent with a multitiered invention approach where, based upon resistance to less intense interventions, children "graduate" to interventions that are more prescriptive, intensive, and individualized (Gresham, 2002). For behavior problems that have not responded to group-oriented best practices, the next tier will frequently involve a functional assessment of the behaviors exhibited by the child and, based upon the functional assessment, the design of an intervention.

When an individual child problem must be addressed, ideally because the child has not adequately responded to the lower-tier efforts at promoting positive classroom behavior, functional assessment is superior to topography-based treatments. Functional analysis data link directly to treatment by identifying potential predictor or maintaining variables that can be manipulated to alter the response–reinforcer relationship. Because no specific form of treatment has been shown to be sufficiently effective across behavioral topographies, contingencies, and situations, function-specific treatments are superior in reducing problematic behaviors and increasing appropriate behaviors (Iwata, Vollmer, Zarcone, & Rodgers, 1993). Indeed, functional analyses have yielded effective treatments for a wide variety of behavior problems including aggression (Vollmer, Ringdahl, Roane, & Marcus, 1997), disruption (Fisher, Lindauer, Alterson, & Thompson, 1998), pica (Piazza et al., 1998), tantrums (Vollmer, Northup, Ringdahl, LeBlanc, & Chauvin, 1996), and compliance with instruction (Noell, VanDerHeyden, Gatti, & Whitmarsh, 2001). Functional analysis involves exposing an individual to several conditions in which specific environmental variables are directly manipulated to determine their effect on the target behavior. An elevated rate of behavior in a given condition suggests that the target behavior is maintained by the contingencies in effect for that condition. The four conditions most commonly used are attention, escape, alone, and play (Derby et al., 1992; Iwata, Dorsey, Slifer, Bauman, Richman, 1982, 1994). In the attention condition, the therapist provides attention in the form of expressions of concern or disapproval (e.g., "Stop, you may hurt yourself") contingent on the occurrence of the target behavior. The attention condition is designed to evaluate the effect of positive reinforcement in the form of attention on the target behavior. In the escape condition, the therapist presents tasks using a graduated prompt procedure (verbal instruction, modeling, physical guidance) approximately every 30 seconds. The client is provided a brief escape from instructions contingent on occurrence of the target behavior. The escape condition is designed to evaluate the effect of negative reinforcement in the form of escape from instructions on the target behavior (Carr & Newsom, 1985). In the alone condition, the treatment room is relatively devoid of stimuli, no therapist is present, and there are no programmed contingencies in effect for the target behavior. This condition is designed to determine if responding persists in the absence of social stimulation (i.e., automatic reinforcement). In the play condition, the client is engaged with a preferred activity, no demands are presented, and a fixed schedule of attention is delivered. The play condition serves as a control condition for the assessment and is arranged to decrease the individual's motivation to engage in the aberrant behavior, simulating an enriched environment. Conditions are typically conducted in a multielement design, counterbalancing the order of conditions across days. The therapist determines by visual inspection the programmed contingency or contingencies that appear to be functionally related to the aberrant behavior.

Because of the promising effects of functional analysis procedures with persons with developmental disabilities, school-based researchers and practitioners have adopted and expanded the methods for use in classroom settings with typically developing children (Broussard & Northup, 1995; Sasso et al., 1992; Noell et al., 2001; Taylor & Romanczyk, 1994) and children with diagnoses such as attention-deficit/hyperactivity disorder (DuPaul, Eckert, & McGoey, 1997; Gulley & Northup, 1997).

The 1997 revisions to the Individuals with Disabilities Act (IDEA), requiring functional assessment of behavior problems, represented an appropriate response to the evidence indicating the effectiveness of function-based treatments in reducing problem behaviors and restrictive placements. Yet, the implementation of so-called functional behavior assessment in the schools has not followed the evidence. Perhaps because systems were ill equipped and unprepared in the basic skills necessary to perform accurate functional assessment, most systems have adopted rating scales or interviews to identify the function of disruptive behavior in the classroom. Because the individuals charged with administering and interpreting these scales are typically untrained in the basics of behavior analysis, they are not capable of accurately collecting the right information, identifying response–reinforcer relationships, and translating these findings into effective intervention. One unfortunate side effect of the primary focus on functional behavior assessment as a tool for managing disruptive behavior in classrooms is that all the nonspecific sources of variance (e.g., inadequate instruction, poor management of precorrection activities, absence of feedback, procedural integrity) have become lost. Stone (1994) has stated, "Instead of a stable consensus regarding best teaching practices, there seems only an unending succession of innovations." (p. 234). We would add that these innovations are rarely properly operationalized, implemented, and evaluated for effectiveness, which may explain why they are so quickly replaced.

There seems to be an evolving consensus in educational policy that practice be guided by data. That is, practitioners should seek to use strategies that are supported by the best evidence available. There is a wealth of information on effective instructional techniques (e.g., within-stimulus prompting, errorless learning, time-delay prompting, fading procedures, controlling establishing operations, establishing behavioral fluency), and yet many of these strategies, and more importantly the conceptual/mathematical paradigm upon which they are built, are unknown to those who work in classrooms. Procedures such as template matching, or identifying the reinforcement schedule that effectively maintains desired levels of appropriate behavior in one setting (i.e., treatment), and then systematically programming the same schedule in the goal setting (i.e., regular classroom) followed by systematic fading to approximate natural occurrence in

the classroom, represent powerful applications of functional assessment data (Ager & Shapiro, 1995; Hoier, McConnell, & Pallay, 1987). Instructional fading (fading in instructional demands during intervention), where disruptive behavior appears to be maintained by escape from instructional tasks, is a logical strategy to eliminate the escape contingency (Horner et al., 1991). However, teachers must ultimately increase task difficulty, and studies have found that escape extinction was necessary to maintain the effects initially achieved with reduction of task demands (Zarcone, Iwata, Mazaleski, & Lerman, 1994). Evidence exists to inform the use of function-based treatments (e.g., instructional fading with extinction) and non-function-based treatments (e.g., time out; Mace, Page, Ivancic, & O'Brien, 1986). However, with respect to instructional planning and implementation, this level of precision is not needed for most children. For most children, effective teaching will correctly establish new skills and result in less disruption. For example, a broad-band intervention that controls for many of the variables associated with effective instruction could be attempted.

So, a typical math intervention begins with an instructional-level task. The teacher (or peer tutor) helps the student to correctly complete the first two rows of the worksheet, followed by independently timed practice for a score. Contingent reward (choice from a treasure chest or activity menu) depends on the number of correct items in 2 minutes plus error reduction or below minimum number. Once errors are reduced, the intervention is changed slightly to promote fluency. Next, the child practices flashcards with the teacher or peer tutor for 3 minutes, followed by independently timed practice for a score and reward contingent upon beating the previous highest score. This type of broad-band intervention controls for many effective teaching variables such as sequencing, mass opportunities to respond, corrective feedback and timing of corrective feedback, maximizing motivation to respond, short time intervals, and rich attention schedule. A similar approach to behavior can be adopted.

From our view, the key lies in the precision with which research findings from well-controlled studies can be translated into real-world settings with children with less significant deficits, with a keen focus on collecting the most meaningful information in the briefest amount of time to get the best outcome (efficiency) in choosing an assessment tool and corresponding intervention. For children who do not respond to basic effective instruction in the classroom, other more complicated strategies should be applied. Most educational practice may be considered "sloppy" or imprecise, and yet it works for most students (Stone, 1994). Individuals who are trained to change one variable at a time based on the best evidence available and monitor the effectiveness of that change prior to making another may be rare. Also, effective strategies that superficially appear simple may be difficult for teachers to implement. For example, Wolery, Anthony, Snyder, Werts, and Katzenmeyer (1997) found that teachers required training to correctly implement a constant time-delay prompting procedure and that only after teachers correctly implemented the procedure was the desired change in child behavior observed. Management of behavior is more difficult than academic problems in that a child may present an infinite number of behaviors to a teacher at any time and the teacher *on the fly* must respond to the behavior in an effective way. Finally, in contrast with academic responding, for low-tolerated behaviors in the classroom, such as aggression, the treatment goal may be 100% during the first treatment session, whereas a more gradual trend of improvement may be tolerated for academic responses.

Studies have demonstrated that treatment integrity is a variable that may not be assumed and must be directly measured and ensured (Gresham, 1991; Wickstrom, Jones, LaFleur, & Witt, 1998). Currently no requirement exists to guarantee that students are actually provided with legally mandated interventions in the regular classroom setting, which is a critical loophole in the system. Teacher "reinforcement" for correctly implementing behavior plans may be increased problem behavior in the short term if extinction burst occurs. Hence, the treatment agent must plan not only for the contingencies that affect child behavior but also for the contingencies that affect whether or not the intervention is likely to be correctly implemented over time. Use of a problem-solving model (beginning with simple solutions and moving to more complicated solutions using dynamic academic indicators to track effectiveness at each step) will avoid treatment agents becoming "bogged down" in an extended interpretation of functional analysis, descriptive analysis, and interview data.

CONCLUSION AND SUGGESTIONS FOR RESEARCH

We began this chapter by suggesting that research activity pertaining to traditional classroom management topics (e.g., rules, routines, etc.) has been somewhat dormant over the past 10 years. Instead, this review focused on research relevant to instructional and other variables that have been linked to changes in student classroom behavior. This review might be considered a review of newer parts, pieces, and components that, if properly combined and used, lead to improvements in student behavior and *perhaps* academic achievements. For example, a teacher who pays careful attention to basic principles of instructional design (i.e., sequencing, pacing, feedback) is going to have more success on both the academic side and the behavior side of the equation than a teacher who is ignorant of instructional design.

At the level of practice, the pieces and parts reviewed here must be integrated in a manner that is practical and usable by schools. Numerous "packages" have been developed that assist teachers in putting forth an integrated classroom management plan. Strategies have ranged from school-wide token economies to more "student-centered" approaches. The most advanced and supported system to date appears to be positive behavior support (PBS). What, from our review, seems to be missing with most packages is a comprehensive evaluation of these more comprehensive and integrated systems. PBS appears to have the most research support and has documented that office referrals and other variables improve as a result of using PBS (Taylor-Greene et al., 1997).

Schools, now more than ever, are focused on improving academic outcomes for children and not merely having students be still, quiet, and docile. Hence, a comprehensive evaluation of "classroom management" would examine both academic and behavior outcomes. Such an evaluation might include important outcomes such as office referrals, but it also would include classroom compliance rates, academic engaged time, and other variables that relate to student achievement and school safety. This type of evaluation probably does not exist because it is a daunting task. Perhaps, however, it is time for classroom management researchers to "step up to the plate" and show how an integrated system of best practices leads to more effective schools.

At a minimum, this needed research would appear to have to address the following questions (see Figure 22.4 for a schematic view):

• What should be trained? Which specific classroom management practices should be included in a comprehensive model?
• How should training occur? How can teachers and other professionals be trained to use these practices with fidelity? How can we be sure they are fully trained?
• How can training outcomes be documented? Documentation of training outcomes must include some documentation that teachers know what to do, actually do it in a real setting, and do it consistently in the real setting with real students.
• How can the ongoing use of the management practices be documented? Once teachers are trained, then the *evaluation* of the model can *begin*. Once evaluation begins, there is a requirement that ongoing fidelity to the model be continually monitored. Degradations in the fidelity of the model are likely for some teachers. How much treatment strength is acceptable? What research designs will help us to learn the extent to which such degradations covary with decreased effects?
• What outcomes will be measured? In addition to behavior, it will be important to show that the model improves academic achievement. Ideally, the evaluation of academic performance will include ongoing continuous progress monitoring.

It is important that this type of comprehensive evaluation be conducted. Researchers, especially in the area of reading, have made

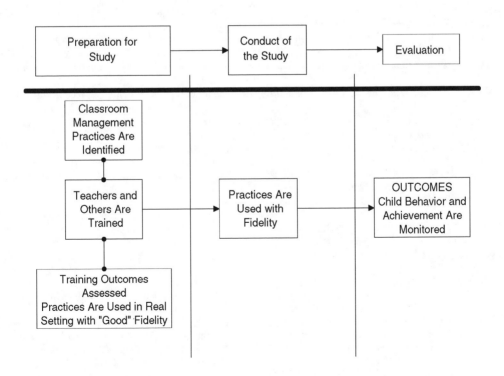

FIGURE 22.4. This figure illustrates the various components of a comprehensive evaluation of a classroom management package or system.

great strides over the past 10 years in conducting comprehensive longitudinal investigations that have identified the important curricular and instructional variables that lead to a reduction of children who are not successful in reading. Behavior is inherently more difficult to study than reading. However, behavior is critically important, and the comprehensive evaluation of a useful behavioral model is overdue.

Certainly previous research has contributed a great deal to our understanding of classroom management. However, it is time for a comprehensive evaluation focusing on: What is the most efficient and practical way to do business, how much does it cost to do it well, and what positive academic outcomes might we expect?

REFERENCES

Ager, C. L., & Shapiro, E. S. (1995). Template matching as a strategy for assessment of and intervention for preschool students with disabilities. *Topics in Early Childhood Special Education, 15*, 187–218.

Anderson, J. A., Kutash, K., & Duchnowski, A. J. (2001). A comparison of the academic progress of students with EBD and students with LD. *Journal of Emotional and Behavioral Disorders, 9*, 106–115.

Ayllon T., & Roberts, M. D. (1974). Eliminating discipline problems by strengthening academic performance. *Journal of Applied Behavior Analysis, 7*, 71–76.

Bandura, A. (1969). *Principles of behavior modification.* New York: Holt.

Blair, K., Umbreit, J., & Bos, C. (1999). Using functional assessment and children's preferences to improve the behavior of young children with behavioral disorders. *Behavioral Disorders, 24*, 151–166.

Brophy, J. E. (1983). Classroom organization and management. *Elementary School Journal, 83*, 265–285.

Brophy, J. (1986). Teacher influences on student achievement. *American Psychologist, 41*, 1069–1077.

Broussard, C. D., & Northup, J. (1995). An approach to functional assessment and analysis of disruptive behavior in regular education classrooms. *School Psychology Quarterly, 10*, 151–164.

Carey, R. G., & Bucher, B. (1983). Positive practice overcorrection: The effects of duration of positive practice on acquisition and response reduction. *Journal of Applied Behavior Analysis, 16*, 101–109.

Carr, E. G., & Newsom, C. (1985). Demand-related tantrums: Conceptualization and treatment. *Behavior Modification, 9*, 403–426.

Carr, E. G., Taylor, J. D., & Robinson, S. (1991). The effects of severe behavior problems in children on the teaching behavior of adults. *Journal of Behavior Analysis, 24*, 523–535.

Center, D. B., Dietz, S. M., & Kaufman, M. E. (1982). Student ability, task difficulty and inappropriate classroom behavior. *Behavior Modification, 6*, 355–374.

Colvin, G., Sugai, G., Good, R., & Lee, Y. (1997). Using active supervision and precorrection to improve transition behaviors in an elementary school. *School Psychology Quarterly, 12*, 344–363.

DePaepe, P. A., Shores, R. E., Jack, S. L., & Denny, R. K. (1996). Effects of task difficulty on the disruptive and on-task behavior of students with severe behavior disorders. *Behavioral Disorders, 21*, 216–225.

Derby, K. M., Wacker, D. P., Sasso, G., Steege, M., Northup, J., Cigrand, K., & Asmus, J. (1992). Brief functional assessment techniques to evaluate aberrant behavior in an outpatient setting: A summary of 79 cases. *Journal of Applied Behavior Analysis, 25*, 713–721.

Doyle, W. (1986). *Classroom organization and management.* In M. Wittrock (Ed.) The *handbook of research on teaching* (3rd ed., pp. 392–431). New York: Macmillan.

Duhon, G. J., George H., Noell, G. H, Witt, J. C., Freeland, J. T., Dufrene, B. A., et al. (in press). Identifying academic skill and performance deficits: An examination of brief and extended assessments. *School Psychology Review.*

Dunlap, G., dePerczel, M., Clarke, S., Wilson, D., Wright, S., & White, R. (1994). Choice making to promote adaptive behavior for students with emotional and behavioral challenges. *Journal of Applied Behavior Analysis, 27*, 505–518.

Dunlap, G., Kern, L., & Worcester, J. (2001). ABA and academic instruction. Focus on Autism and Other Developmental Disabilities. *School Psychology Review, 16*, 129.

DuPaul, G. J., Eckert, T. L., & McGoey, K. E. (1997). Interventions for students with attention-deficit/hyperactivity disorder: One size does not fit all. *School Psychology Review, 26*, 369–381.

Emmer, E. T. (2001). Classroom management: A critical part of educational psychology with implications for teacher education. *Educational Psychologist, 36*, 103–113.

Emmer, E. T., Evertson, C. M., & Anderson, L. M. (1980). Effective classroom management at the beginning of the school year. *Elementary School Journal, 80*, 219–231.

Fisher, W. W., Lindauer, S. E., Alterson, C. J., & Thompson, R. H. (1998). Assessment and treatment of destructive behavior maintained by stereotypic object manipulation. *Journal of Applied Behavior Analysis, 31*, 513–527.

Gettinger, M., & Stoiber, K. C. (1999). Excellence in teaching: Review of instructional and environmental variables. In C. R. Reynolds & T. Gutkin (Eds.). *The handbook of school psychology* (3rd ed., pp. 933–958). New York: Wiley.

Gickling, E. E., & Armstrong, D. L. (1978). Levels of

instructional difficulty as related to on-task behavior, task completion, and comprehension. *Journal of Learning Disability, 11,* 32–39.

Gilbertson, D., Witt, J. C., Dufrene, B., & Duhon, G. (in press). *The effect of various rates of academic response on on-task behavior.*

Good, R. H., & Kaminski, R. A. (1996). Assessment for instructional decisions: Toward a proactive/prevention model of decision-making for early literacy skills. *School Psychology Quarterly, 11,* 326–336.

Graham, S. (1999). Handwriting and spelling instruction for students with learning disabilities: A review. *Learning Disabilities Quarterly, 22,* 78–96.

Greenwood, C. R. (1996). The case for performance-based instructional models. *School Psychology Quarterly, 11,* 283–296.

Gresham, F. M. (1991). Assessment of treatment integrity in school consultation and prereferral intervention. *School Psychology Review, 18,* 37–50.

Gresham, F. M. (2002). Responsiveness to intervention: An alternative approach to the identification of learning disabilities. In R. Bradley, L. Danielson, & D. Hallahan (Eds.), *Identification of learning disabilities: Research to practice* (pp. 467–519). Mahwah, NJ: Erlbaum.

Gresham, F. M., & Gresham, G. N. (1982). Interdependent, dependent and independent group contingencies for controlling disruptive behavior. *Journal of Special Education, 16,* 101–110.

Gulley, V., & Northup, J. (1997). Comprehensive school-based behavioral assessment of the effects of methylphenidate. *Journal of Applied Behavior Analysis, 30,* 627–638.

Gunter, P. L., & Denny, R. K. (1996). Research issues and needs regarding teacher use of classroom management strategies. *Behavioral Disorders, 22,* 15–20.

Haring, N. G., Lovitt, T. C., Eaton, M. D., & Hansen, C. L. (1978). *The fourth R: Research in the classroom.* Columbus, OH: Merrill.

Herrnstein, R. J. (1970). On the law of effect. *Journal of the Experimental Analysis of Behavior, 13,* 243–266.

Herrnstein, R. J. (1972). Derivatives of matching. *Psychological Review, 86,* 486–495.

Hoier, T. S., McConnell, S., & Pallay, A. G. (1987). Observational assessment planning and evaluating educational transitions: An initial analysis of template matching. *Behavioral Assessment, 9,* 5–19.

Horner, R. H., Day, H. M., Sprague, J. R., O'Brien, M., & Heathfield, L. T. (1991). Interspersed requests: A nonaversive procedure for reducing aggression and self-injury during instruction. *Journal of Applied Behavior Analysis, 24,* 265–278.

Howard, N. A., & Norris, M. R. (1994). *Source, characteristics, and perceived effectiveness of classroom rules.* Paper presented at the Kentucky Grow Conference, Kentucky. (ERIC Document Reproduction Service ED 395 855).

Iwata, B. A., Dorsey, M. F., Slifer, K. J., Bauman, K. E., & Richman, G. S. (1982). Toward a functional analysis of self-injury. *Analysis and Intervention in Developmental Disabilities, 2,* 3–20.

Iwata, B. A., Dorsey, M. F., Slifer, K. J., Bauman, K. E., & Richman, G. S. (1994). Toward a functional analysis of self-injury. *Journal of Applied Behavior Analysis, 27,* 197–209.

Iwata, B. A., Vollmer, T. R., Zarcone, J. R., & Rodgers, T. A. (1993). Treatment classification and selection based on behavioral function. In R. Van Houten & S. Axelrod (Eds.), *Behavior analysis and treatment* (pp. 101–125). New York: Plenum.

Kelley, M. L., & McCain, A. P. (1995). Promoting academic performance in inattentive children: The relative efficacy of school-home notes with and without response cost. *Behavior Modification, 19,* 339–356.

Kern, L., Choutka, C. M., & Sokol, N. G. (2002). Assessment-based antecedent interventions used in natural settings to reduce challenging behavior: An analysis of the literature. *Education and Treatment of Children, 25,* 113–130.

LaFleur, L., Witt J. C., Naquin, G., Harwell, V., & Gilbertson D. M. (1998). Use of coaching to enhance classroom management by improvement of student transitioning between classroom activities. *Effective School Practices, 17,* 79–82.

Mace, F. C., Page, T. J., Ivancic, M. T., & O'Brien, S. (1986). Effectiveness of brief time-out with and without contingent delay: A comparative analysis. *Journal of Applied Behavior Analysis, 19,* 79–86.

Mace, F. C., & Roberts, M. L. (1986). Factors affecting selection of behavioral interventions. In J. Reichle & D. P. Wacker (Eds.), *Communication and language series: Vol. 3. Communicative alternatives to challenging behavior: Integrated functional assessment and intervention strategies* (pp. 113–133). Baltimore: Brookes.

Malone, B. G., & Tietjens, C. L. (2000). Re-examination of classroom rules: The need for clarity and specified behavior. *Special Services in the Schools, 16,* 159–170.

Mayer, G. R. (1995). Preventing antisocial behavior in the schools. *Journal of Applied Behavior Analysis, 28,* 467–478.

McDowell, J. J. (1982). The importance of Herrnstein's mathematical statement of the law of effect for behavior therapy. *American Psychologist, 37,* 771–779.

McKee, W. T., & Witt, J. C. (1990). Effective teaching: A review of instructional and environmental variables. In T. B. Gutkin & C. R. Reynolds (Eds.), *The handbook of school psychology* (pp. 823–847). New York: Wiley.

Miller, K. A., Gunter, P. L., Venn, M. L., Hummel, J., & Wiley, L. P. (2003). Effects of curricular and materials modifications on academic performance and task engagement of three students with emotional or behavioral disorders. *Behavioral Disorders, 28,* 130–149.

Munk, D., & Repp, A. (1994). The relationship between instructional variables and problem behavior: A review. *Exceptional Children, 60,* 390–401.

Musser, E. H., Bray, M. A., Kehle, T. J., & Jenson, W. R. (2001). Reducing disruptive behavior in students with serious emotional disturbance. *School Psychology Review, 30*, 294–304.

Nelson, C. M., Rutherford, R. B., Center, D. B., & Walker, H. M. (1991). Do public schools have an obligation to serve troubled children and youth? *Exceptional Children, 57*, 406–415.

Noell, G. H., VanDerHeyden, A. M., Gatti, S. L., & Whitmarsh, E. L. (2001). Functional assessment of the effects of escape and attention on students' compliance during instruction. *School Psychology Quarterly, 16*, 253–269.

Penner, D. A., Frank, A. R., & Wacker, D. P. (2000). Instructional accommodations for adolescent students with severe emotional or behavioral disorders. *Behavioral Disorders, 25*, 325–343.

Piazza, C. C, Fisher, W. W., Hanley, G. P., LeBlanc, L. A., Worsdell, A. S., Lindauer, S. E., et al. (1998). Treatment of pica through multiple analyses of its reinforcing functions. *Journal of Applied Behavior Analysis, 31*, 165–189.

Proctor, M., & Morgan, D. (1991). Effectiveness of a response cost raffle procedure on the disruptive classroom behavior of adolescents with behavior problems. *School Psychology Review, 20*, 97–109.

Rhode, G., Jenson, W. R., & Reavis, H. K. (1998). *The tough kid book: Practical classroom management strategies.* Longmont, CO: Sopris West.

Sasso, G. M., Reimers, T. M., Cooper, L. J., Wacker, D., Berg, W., Steege, M., et al. (1992). Use of descriptive and experimental analyses to identify the functional properties of aberrant behavior in school settings. *Journal of Applied Behavior Analysis, 25*, 809–821.

Shapiro, E. S. (1996). *Academic skills problems: Direct assessment and intervention* (2nd ed.). New York: Guilford Press.

Shinn, M. R. (1995). Best practices in curriculum-based measurement and its use in a problem-solving model. In A. Thomas & J. Grimes (Eds.), *Best practices in school psychology* (Vol. 3, pp. 547–567). Washington DC: National Association of School Psychologists.

Shinn, M. R. (1998). *Advanced applications of curriculum-based measurement.* New York: Guilford Press.

Shinn, M. R., Walker, H. M., Stieber, S., & Ramsey, E. (1987). Antisocial behaviors in school settings: Initial differences in an at-risk and normal population. *Journal of Special Education, 21*, 69–84.

Shores, R. E., & Wehby, J. H. (1999). Analyzing the classroom social behavior of students with EBD. *Journal of Emotional and Behavioral Disorders, 7*, 194–199.

Skinner, C. H. (1996). Increasing learning rates by increasing student response rates: A summary of research. *School Psychology Quarterly, 1*, 313–325.

Skinner, C. H., Hurst, K. L., Teeple, D. F. & Meadow, S. O. (2002). Increasing on-task behavior during mathematics independent seat-work in students with emotional disturbance by interspersing additional brief problems. *Psychology in the Schools, 39*, 647–659.

Smith, R. G., & Iwata, B. A. (1997). Antecedent influences on behavior disorders. *Journal of Applied Behavior Analysis, 30*, 343–375.

Stone, J. E. (1994). Developmentalism's impediments to school reform: Three recommendations for overcomng them. In R. Gardner III, D. M. Sainato, J. O. Cooper, T. E. Heron, W. L. Heward, J. W. Eshleman, & T. A. Grossi (Eds.), *Behavior analysis in education: Focus on measurably superior instruction* (pp. 233–253). Pacific Grove, CA: Brooks/Cole.

Sugai, G., Sprague, J. R., Horner, R. H., & Walker, H. M. (2000). Preventing school violence: The use of office discipline referrals to assess and monitor school-wide discipline interventions. *Journal of Emotional and Behavioral Disorders, 8*, 94–101.

Sutherland, K. E., & Wehby, J. H. (2001). Exploring the relationship between increased opportunities to respond to academic requests and the academic and behavioral outcome of students with EBD. *Remedial and Special Education, 22*, 13–121.

Taylor, J. C., & Romanczyk, R. G. (1994). Generating hypotheses about the function of student problem behavior by observing teacher behavior. *Journal of Applied Behavior Analysis, 27*, 251–265.

Taylor-Greene, S., Brown, D., Nelson, L., Longton, J., Gassman, T., Cohen, J., Swartz, J., Horner, R. H., Sugai, G., & Hall, S. (1997). School-wide behavioral support: Starting the year off right. *Journal of Behavioral Education, 7*, 99–112.

Vollmer, T. R., Northup, J., Ringdahl, J. E., LeBlanc, L. A., & Chauvin, T. M. (1996). Functional analysis of severe tantrums displayed by children with language delays: An outclinic assessment. *Behavior Modification, 20*, 97–115.

Vollmer, T. R., Ringdahl, J. E., Roane, H. S., & Marcus, B. A. (1997). Negative side effects of noncontingent reinforcement. *Journal of Applied Behavior Analysis, 30*, 161–164.

Walker, H. M., Colvin, G., Ramsey, E. (1995). *Antisocial behavior in schools: Strategies and best practices.* Pacific Grove, CA: Brooks/Cole.

Walker, H. M., Shinn, M. R., O'Neill, R. E., & Ramsey, E. (1987). A longitudinal assessment of the development of antisocial behavior in boys: Rationale, methodology, and first-year results. *Remedial and Special Education, 8*(4), 7–16.

Waxman, H. C., & Walberg, H. J. (1991). *Effective teaching: Current research.* Berkeley, CA: McCutchan.

Weeks, M., & Gaylord-Ross, R. (1981). Task difficulty and aberrant behavior in severely handicapped students. *Journal of Applied Behavior Analysis, 14*, 19–36.

Wickstrom, K. F., Jones, K. M., LaFleur, L. H., & Witt, J. C. (1998). An analysis of treatment integrity in school-based behavioral consultation. *School Psychology Quarterly, 13*, 141–154.

Witt, J. C., & Elliot, S. E. (1982). The response cost lottery: A time efficient and effective classroom intervention. *Journal of School Psychology, 20,* 155–161.

Wolery, M., Anthony, L., Snyder, E. D., Werts, M. G., & Katzenmeyer, J. (1997). Training elementary teachers to embed instruction during classroom activities. *Education and Treatment of Children, 20,* 40–58.

Ysseldyke, J. E., & Christenson, S. L. (1993). *The instructional environmental system—II.* Longmont, CO: Sopris West.

Ysseldyke, J. E., & Elliot, J. (1999). Effective instructional practices: Implications for assessing educational environments. In T. B. Gutkin & C. R. Reynolds (Eds.), *The handbook of school psychology* (pp. 497–512). New York: Wiley.

Zarcone, J. R., Iwata, B. A., Mazaleski, J. L., & Lerman, D. C. (1994). Reemergence and extinction of self-injurious behavior during stimulus (instructional) fading. *Journal of Applied Behavior Analysis, 27,* 307–316.

23

Social Skills Training and Teaching Social Behavior to Students with Emotional and Behavioral Disorders

KENNETH A. KAVALE, SARUP R. MATHUR,
and MARK P. MOSTERT

A lack of social competence plays a significant role in the social, educational, and psychological adjustment of students with emotional and behavioral disorders (EBD) (Gresham, 1998) and represents a defining characteristic for this group of children. Generally, splintered or inadequate social skills are often associated with negative social outcomes, including psychiatric and self-regulation problems, internalizing and externalizing behavior disorders (Merrell & Gimpel, 1998), as well as low self-concept, peer rejection, loneliness, and problems with social relationships with peers and authority figures (Asher & Hymel, 1981). Unsurprisingly, many students with EBD do not engage in enough positive social interactions to reinforce appropriate behavior for increased social acceptance. As a result, many students with EBD become trapped in ineffective and negative social interaction cycles that hinder social competence and acceptance. Further, a strong relationship between social skills deficits and externalizing disorders may result in referrals for mental health services and higher rates of delinquent behaviors. Positive experiences, therefore, are critical in promoting appropriate social responses among these students, given that interpersonal problems, social isolation, and poor social adjustment during childhood are reasonable predictors of psychiatric or mental health problems, possible institutionalization, and involvement with the legal and justice systems later in life.

Because many students with EBD are socially incompetent, researchers have assumed that that these students exhibit social skills deficits simply because they have not had the opportunity to learn and practice more desirable and appropriate behaviors. On this basis, researchers have recently attempted to provide a structured, explicit way of teaching the requisite skills for social success. While there are many versions of this approach, they are usually subsumed under the term "social skills training." The purpose of social skills training is to promote overall social effectiveness in students with EBD by teaching them acceptable social behaviors and skills. Such training generally includes (1) selecting social skills needing improvement, (2) demonstrating, explaining, or modeling these skills, (3) practicing these skills while being coached, (4) providing feedback and reinforcement during practice, and (5) identifying social situations where the skill might be usefully applied. As with any intervention, the efficacy of social skills training is an important question. One purpose of this chapter is to answer the question posed by Mathur and Rutherford (1996): Is social skills training effective with students with emotional or behavioral disorders? We summatively (1) address problems in the conceptual framework of social competence, social skills, and social skills training; (2) examine several findings related to the effectiveness of social skills training; and (3) provide some suggestions for improving social skills interventions.

CONCEPTUAL FRAMEWORK

Beginning with Moreno's (1934) work on peer popularity and social preferences, there has been interest in social skills and the possibility of teaching discrete behaviors. One enduring problem, however, has been how best to define social skills (Gresham, 1986). Walker, Colvin, and Ramsey (1995) defined social skills as a set of behaviors that (1) allows individuals to initiate and maintain positive social relationships, (2) contributes to peer acceptance and to a satisfactory school adjustment, and (3) allows an individual to cope effectively and adaptively with larger (and therefore more demanding) social environments. Ultimately, social skills are behaviors that are assumed to represent the theoretical construct of social competence (Dodge, Pettit, McClaskey, & Brown, 1986). For example, McFall (1982) distinguished between *social competence* as a summative judgment of an individual's behavior by significant social agents (parents, teachers, peers) and *social skills* as specific actions that individuals use in responding to everyday social tasks. For social competence, Vaughn and Hogan (1990) identified four components: (1) positive relations with others, (2) accurate and age-appropriate social cognition, (3) absence of maladaptive behaviors, and (4) effective social behaviors (social skills). The effectiveness of these skills in producing positive social outcomes is the basis for making judgments about social competence.

As a theoretical trait, social competence must demonstrate construct validity (Cronbach & Meehl, 1955) because it proposes a set of skills evolved from theories of social functioning, which may or may not be true and accurate depictions of what it means to be socially competent. Construct validity problems exist in many aspects of assessing cognitive and emotional function. For example, the concept of intelligence is a classic example of the need for construct validation. Early attempts to validate "intelligence" through specific psychomotor and psychophysical skills were abandoned when they did not correlate with other behavioral evidence of intelligence (e.g., school grades). That is, the expected and logical relationships between variables were not confirmed. Later, Binet constructed alternative tasks logically related to intelligence, and the tasks requiring complex cognitive abilities were found to be related to other variables in a manner expected of a measure of intelligence. Henceforth, intelligence was characterized by construct validity.

The construct of social competence has been integral to the definition of mental retardation (MR) and emotional disturbance (ED). The definition of MR includes two relevant and necessary conditions: low intellectual functioning and inadequate adaptive behavior. Adaptive behavior refers to the effectiveness and degree with which individuals meet the standard of self-sufficiency and social responsibility expected of their age and cultural group (Leland, Shellhaas, Nihira, & Foster, 1967). To assess adaptive behavior, a number of adaptive behavior scales were developed, but all possessed some technical problems (Clausen, 1972). Nevertheless, adaptive behavior scales were periodically revised to improve their psychometric characteristics. Part of the process included attempts to move away from an implied face validity to studies of construct validation. Meyers, Nihira, and Zetlin (1979) reviewed 26 adaptive behavior measures and found a number with adequate construct validity. Thus, some adaptive behavior scales reflect universal and enduring dimensions, which provide confidence in judgments about social competence. Similarly, the federal definition of ED includes "an inability to build or maintain satisfactory interpersonal relationship with peers and teachers" as one of the defining criteria of ED. To assess the interpersonal relationships of students with EBD, four assessment procedures are commonly used: (1) observation, (2) behavioral rating scales, (3) sociometric techniques, and (4) self-report. Although some of these procedures have a great deal of appeal to clinicians and researchers, these procedures are not totally reliable because of limited psychometric qualities, inaccuracy of behavioral data, and observer subjectivity. For example, single-subject studies have mostly used observation procedures to examine changes in social behaviors of students with EBD in naturalistic or contrived situations. These studies often report observer drift, limited interrater reliability, and few opportunities for valid social comparison across peer groups and settings.

In response to these criticisms, some researchers have argued for a multimethod approach that focuses on a comprehensive base of information to obtain an aggregated picture of social functioning (Walker et al, 1995). Group design studies have often employed standardized behavioral rating scales, such as the Behavioral Assessment System for Children (BASC; Reynolds & Kamphaus, 1992), a multimethod system that includes a teacher rating scale, a parent rating scale, a self-report scale, a direct observation form to be used in a classroom, and a questionnaire evaluating developmental history. Although BASC has high internal consistency and test–retest reliability, its interrater reliability is only within moderate ranges. None of these procedures assists in providing relevant information contributing to a better understanding of the construct of social competence. Some researchers in psychology and psychopathology argue that the use of aggregated multiple assessments actually increases error variance due to covariation between similar variables assessed by different procedures. Clearly, future research should provide empirical validation for these stances (Merrell & Gimpel, 1998).

As with other attempts to assess "process" variables, social skill assessments currently used for identifying students with EBD do not demonstrate an adequate level of construct validity. Although many social skill assessments are technically sound, information about construct validity is limited. Consequently, there are difficulties in measuring social skills and the effects of social skills training (Maag, 1989; Vaughn & Haager, 1994). At this time, therefore, problems with construct validity preclude researchers from being confident about what they are measuring. Without construct validation, it is possible that whatever is measured may be neither critical dimensions of social competence nor something defined in a manner that permits a logical undergirding to what is eventually defined and verified as social competence.

The question of construct validity assumes even more importance when a distinction is made between social skill deficits and performance deficits. A social skill deficit implies that a child does not actually possess the necessary skill levels to perform in a socially competent fashion. In contrast, a performance deficit suggests that the social skill is part of the child's repertoire but is not performed. For performance deficits, teaching is not required; rather, these children require an incentive-based management approach that prompts, cues, and reinforces existing social skills. Social skill deficits, on the other hand, require direct teaching. However, without higher levels of construct validation, questions arise about what exactly is being taught and whether or not the particular skill is an important contributor to social competence.

The issue of construct validity is also a factor affecting social validity. Essentially, social validity refers to the acceptance of an individual's behavior as it conforms to community and cultural standards of conduct. Gresham (1986) postulated three components for social validity. *Social significance* refers to perceptions about the goals and purposes of social skills intervention. Therefore there must be a clear rationale for why social skills are being taught, which social skills are being taught, and what outcomes are expected. With enhanced understanding of social competence and the nature of social skills, a stronger rationale is possible to establish behavioral efficacy levels for success in the home, school, and community.

The second component of social validity is *social importance*, which refers to the nature of the behavior change accrued from training and whether or not the change makes a difference for the student with EBD. These are important considerations when it has been shown that social skills training efforts too often focus on skills that have no demonstrated relationship to improved outcomes. Several training programs such as

ASSET (see Sheldon, Sherman, Schumaker, & Hazel, 1984) and ACCESS (see Williams, Walker, Holmes, Todis, & Fabre, 1989) have been very careful in the rationale and procedures used to select social skills for their curricula. These efforts, however, deal with content validity and, while there was general agreement about the importance of the skills included, significant variation existed among consumers about the relative importance attached to individual skills. These variations might be minimized with enhanced construct validation.

The final component of social validity is *social acceptability*. Are the training methods and techniques acceptable to all parties involved? Did students approve of these methods? Would these methods be used again? Again, although the answers to such questions are essentially subjective judgments, construct validation might provide a more empirical basis in making these judgments more objective.

Construct validity is also an important consideration when dealing with forms of "process" training. Social skills represent "processes" that, if deficient, are trained in an effort to enhance functioning. The enduring problem surrounding process training is that processes are unobservable and only outcomes can be observed. What can be concluded when the product (outcome) demonstrates only limited improvement? In actuality, little can be concluded because there is little insight into the process, that is, the actual internal human functioning that produced the social skill. Poor outcomes may, therefore, be due to these unseen factors or to more overt vaiables such as measurement problems or ineffective teaching strategies.

Issues related to social skills training for students with EBD parallel similar problems in other areas of special education. Specifically, special education has a long history of limited success with process training (see Kavale & Forness, 1999), reflecting poor construct validity underlying whatever "process" is being inculcated. A classic example is found in the area of visual perception and the Frostig program. The Frostig test was designed to assess five specific and separate visual-perceptual subareas that could then be inculcated as needed. However, construct validation efforts could not support these five areas as distinct and independent entities. Consequently, it was not at all clear exactly what was being taught except visual perception in some general sense. Not surprisingly, Frostig training showed limited effectiveness (Kavale, 1984). Until construct validation of social skills is advanced, the same problems experienced in other areas of special education in defining, measuring, and training process skills will tend to limit EBD research in enhancing social functioning.

The construct of s*ocial skills training* includes a set of instructional procedures that usually incorporate the components of modeling, practice, reinforcement, and programming for generalization (Mathur & Rutherford, 1989, 1994). Using these components, students are taught specific social skills such as complimenting others, initiating conversations, asking appropriate questions, or appropriately interacting with peers and authority figures.

It is clear that the effectiveness of social skills instruction needs to go beyond simple skills acquisition. Socially valid skills that are learned must then be generalized and maintained over time. While the need for social skills training for students with antisocial behavior and conduct problems is self-evident, the effectiveness of these interventions remains uncertain, especially in producing prolonged and socially valid treatment effects (Webster-Stratton, Reid, & Hammond, 2001). Thus, while initial social skills training might be necessary, it is not sufficient unless it can be transformed into appropriate behavior across settings and conditions. In this regard, Gresham (1998) noted that social skills training has not produced specifically large, socially valid, long-lasting, or generalizable changes for students with EBD. There is, therefore, a need to explore factors, barriers, and issues that influence the successful implementation of social skills training (Ang & Hughes, 2001; McConaughy, Kay, & Fitzgerald, 2001).

SOCIAL SKILL TRAINING PROGRAMS

In order to strengthen the social skill repertoires of students with EBD, training programs specifically designed to teach interpersonal skills have been developed (e.g.,

Goldstein, 1988; Rutherford, Chipman, DiGangi, & Anderson, 1992; Walker, McConnell, Holmes, Todis, Walker, & Golden, 1983). In the 1980s, Arnold Goldstein and his colleagues developed a structured learning approach to teaching social skills called Skillstreaming that involved four instructional components: modeling, role playing, performance feedback, and transfer of training. The purpose of modeling was to expose the learners to several examples of expert performance in various situations. After modeling the skills, learners were provided opportunities for rehearsal, using role play across a spectrum of social situations where the learned skills might be needed. The students were provided with constructive feedback on relevant aspects of their role-play performance and were asked to complete homework assignments in the hope that this would enhance application and transfer of the learned social skill to different settings. Using the components of direct instruction, the Skillstreaming programs were structured around three age levels: preschool, elementary, and adolescent. Manuals and scripted skill lessons were available for each level.

Another example, the ACCEPTS program (Walker et al., 1983) also uses a direct instruction approach, where skills are taught individually following the basic instructional sequence shown in Table 23.1. These programs presume that systematic and direct instruction of social skills can assist in developing the effective social response patterns necessary for establishing positive relationships, thereby serving the ultimate purpose of social skills instruction, which is to build a repertoire of efficient social behavioral patterns that not only replace undesirable or maladaptive behaviors but also contribute to the social competence of students with EBD (Mathur & Rutherford, 1996).

However, herein lies a major conceptual tension, because at the core of these endeavors are the terms "social competence" and "social skills." Although these two terms are often used interchangeably, they should not be considered equivalent. Social competence refers to an individual's overall interpersonal

---

TABLE 23.1. ACCEPTS Instructional Sequence

Step 1: Definition and guided discussion
      a. Teacher presents skill definition, followed by student oral response.
      b. Teacher leads students in a guided discussion of skill application and a range of examples.

Step 2: Positive example
      a. Teacher presents first video scene example showing appropriate skills application, *or*
      b. Teacher models an example of appropriate skill application.
      c. Debrief episode.

Step 3: Negative example
      a. Teacher presents second video scene (non-example) demonstrating failure to use skill or incorrect skill application, *or*
      b. Teacher models a non-example demonstrating failure to use skill or incorrect skill application.
      c. Debrief episode.

Step 4: Review and restate skill definition
      a. Teacher reviews skill definition.
      b. Student oral response.

Step 5: Positive example
      a. Teacher presents a third video scene of appropriate skill application, *or*
      b. Teacher models a second example of appropriate skill application.
      c. Debrief episode.

Step 6: Activities
      a. Teacher *models* a range of activities that exemplify or expand upon skill production.
      b. Teacher presents students with *practice* activities and role-play situations designed to build skill mastery.

functioning, but is viewed differently by different investigators. For example, Hops (1983) asserts that "competence is a summary term which reflects social judgment about the general quality of an individual's performance in a given situation" (p. 4). Another view of social competence combines social skills and adaptive behavior (Gresham, 1986), which together promote independent social functioning (Leland, 1978). A contrasting view emphasizes social interaction and reciprocity as the basis of social competence (McConnell, 1987). The concept of interaction includes two behaviors: initiation by the subject and response by peers or adults. When positive social interactions are naturally reinforced, social reciprocity is more likely to develop.

On the other hand, social skills are situation-specific behaviors that enhance effective participation in social situations. The concept of social skills from a behavioral perspective is based on the assumption that "specific identifiable skills form the basis for socially competent behavior" (Hops, 1983, p. 4). Gresham (1986) defined social skills along three dimensions: peer acceptance, behavioral skills, and social validity. For *peer acceptance*, the effectiveness of social skills training is evaluated in terms of how well peers accept the target student, as measured by sociometric assessment techniques. The higher the acceptance of the target student by his or her peers, the more successful the training is thought to be. In terms of an emphasis on behavioral skills, social skills are defined through specific, objective behavioral steps and strategies that maximize the opportunities for positive social reinforcement while simultaneously reducing the likelihood of punishment. Students learn social skills using a task-analytic approach that follows a stepwise progression from simple to complex behaviors. The *behavioral skills* approach emphasizes functional behavioral assessment of antecedents and consequences of specific behaviors in order to first define the behavioral skills in operational terms and then to provide closely targeted remedial programming. In terms of *a social validity* definition, the emphasis is on the social significance and meaningfulness of social skills. Here the goal of social skills intervention is to target specific social behaviors that predict important social outcomes.

Such outcomes are commonly measured by behavioral rating scales to evaluate judgments about student social performance.

Clearly, different definitions result in different emphases in how students with EBD are evaluated and taught. Although no universally agreed-upon definition of social skills exists, many common definitional components are identified and targeted in social skills training programs. According to Walker et al. (1995), social competence is demonstrated when students are capable of (1) maximizing their chances of reinforcement from support networks, (2) meeting task-related demands imposed by teachers and peers, and (3) demonstrating flexibility in their social functioning.

ETIOLOGY OF SOCIAL SKILLS DEFICITS

As Gresham (1998) noted, many social skills research studies have employed social skills interventions without regard to the etiology of the social skills deficits. Thus, another problem in operationalizing what is meant by social skills training is the tendency to treat the symptoms rather than the underlying cause and the assumption that different underlying causes dictate different training approaches. Therefore, a clear rationale for providing social skills interventions should rest on whether they are geared (1) toward students who have never learned the skills, or (2) toward those who possess the skills but need to shape, reform, enhance, or increase the frequency of these skills. However, students with EBD may well possess both acquisition and performance deficits. Acquisition deficits may be associated with developmental delays or limited social opportunities for social learning. Performance deficits may be associated with, for example, a lack of motivation, the dominance of other psychological factors, and a lack of opportunity to use the social skills they possess.

TEACHING SOCIAL SKILLS

The definition of EBD implicitly includes deficits in social functioning (Kavale, Forness, & Mostert, in press). Consequently, social skills training has become a primary intervention for students with EBD (Rutherford, Quinn, & Mathur, 1996). Like any intervention, social skills training needs to be evaluated: Is it possible to teach students to initiate and to maintain positive social relationships, to establish positive peer acceptance, to establish satisfactory school adjustment, and to gain the ability to cope effectively and adaptively with the larger social environment? The task of judging the efficacy of social skills training is difficult because the target social competencies cover a wide range of behaviors. Researchers tend to pay more attention to the definition of dependent variables in terms of prosocial behaviors and less attention to the components that are used in the social skills interventions to increase those behaviors. As we have noted already, this is of particular concern given that accurate conclusions about interventions cannot be determined if social skill components for implementation are not accurately reported. Although research reviews provide partial insight into the effectiveness of social skills interventions, they often fail to offer information on the specific instructional components and how these components contribute to the overall functioning of students with EBD. Consequently, research investigating effectiveness involves significant problems in definition, sampling, measurement, and design. These difficulties make any conclusions tentative in the light of suggestions showing only modest effects (e.g., Zaragoza, Vaughn, & McIntosh, 1991). Further, the complexities associated with social skills training make it difficult to interpret the real meaning of "modest effects," thereby constricting the scope of recommendations that can be offered.

META-ANALYSIS OF SOCIAL SKILLS TRAINING

Kavale, Mathur, Forness, Rutherford, and Quinn (1997; see also Quinn, Kavale, Mathur, Rutherford, & Forness, 1999) used the methods of meta-analysis to gain greater insights into the efficacy of social skills training. Meta-analysis produces a quantitative research synthesis that offers the possibility of a more precise determination of intervention efficacy (Lipsey & Wilson, 1993). The methods of meta-analysis are well known (e.g., Glass, McGaw, & Smith, 1981),

and a number of advances have served to enhance the objectivity and verifiability of the technique (e.g., Cooper & Hedges, 1994; Hedges & Olkin, 1985). Further, analytical guidelines are now available in special education (see Mostert, 1996, 2001, 2003; Mostert & Kavale, 2001).

The initial step in meta-analysis is to collect a representative and inclusive set of research studies investigating the efficacy of social skills training. A sampling framework was constructed that included (1) on-time databases using the descriptors EBD and social skills training, (2) reference lists from review articles, (3) bibliographies from individual research reports, and (4) a hand search of recent relevant journals. The search revealed that both group and single-subject designs were available in the EBD social skills training literature. Thus, a comprehensive evaluation requires the inclusion of group and single-subject designs.

The potential pool of studies was reduced because many did not meet the following inclusion criteria: (1) expository articles with no data, (2) studies without a clearly defined EBD population, (3) studies without an appropriate outcome assessment, or (4) studies with outcome data that did not permit the calculation of an appropriate meta-analytic metric. These exclusions left a pool of 35 studies to serve as the database.

For group design studies, the primary statistic in meta-analysis is the effect size (ES) that permits the quantification and standardization of individual study findings. Methods for calculating ES outcomes may take several forms (see Bangert-Drowns, 1986), but we chose the procedures suggested by Glass et al. (1981), where the ES for calculating the efficacy of social skills training was defined by

$$ES = \frac{M_T - M_C}{SD_C}$$

where M_T is the mean (average) score of the treatment (EBD) group on an outcome measure, M_C is the mean (average) score of the control (comparison) group on an outcome measure, and SD_C is the standard deviation of the control (comparison) group.

To enhance the ES estimates, procedures developed by Hedges and Olkin (1985) and

Hunter and Schmidt (1990) were applied, when appropriate, to correct for either small sample size, violation of parametric assumptions, or artifactual variance. The Glass procedures for meta-analysis calculate an individual ES for each comparison in a study and then aggregate them into discrete groupings to investigate dimensions of interest. Before synthesis begins, the appropriate unit of analysis must be determined. Because studies may yield more than one ES measurement, analysis can be based on either individual ES regardless of the number calculated for a study or on a single ES per study based on a weighted average. Three analyses were performed to determine which unit of analysis was appropriate. First, the correlation between ES and number of comparisons per study was calculated and was not significant ($r = .055$), indicating no pattern of statistical dependency. Second, the intrastudy correlation coefficient was calculated, and the obtained value ($p = .562$) indicated that the ES in the same study were more similar than the ES in another study. Finally, individual ES versus weighted average study ES aggregations were tested for homogeneity (see Hedges & Olkin, 1985), and the test statistic (Q) was not significant, indicating that pooling individual ES from different studies was appropriate. These analyses suggested that aggregation could proceed with individual ES.

Since the investigation did not sample from a single population, it was necessary to test whether the parameter variance was zero ($V^2 = 0$). The procedure suggested by Hedges and Olkin (1985), analogous to F tests in a random effects model, was used. The test statistic was not significant and suggests that the studies used shared a common ES parameter and could be combined into more discrete aggregations.

Finally, it was necessary to determine whether the obtained sample of studies was large enough to answer questions about the efficacy of social skills training for students with EBD. Rosenthal (1979) addressed the so-called file drawer problem, the potential bias caused by the greater likelihood of published research to show positive findings. Orwin (1983) developed a method, based on ES level, for calculating a fail-safe number (N_{fs}) of studies that would ensure an ES above the criterion level. The calculated N_{fs}

of 9 indicates that the obtained database ($N = 35$) was sufficient for ruling out the "file drawer" problem as a rival hypothesis.

In group-design studies, an ES may be interpreted like a z score and thus shows the level of improvement associated with social skills training. An ES of +1.00 indicates a one standard deviation superiority for the training group, which means that 84% of those receiving training were better off than a comparison group receiving no training. On average, training would move subjects to the 84th percentile, which would indicate a 34 percentile rank gain on an outcome measure compared to comparison subjects who remain at the 50th percentile.

THE EFFECTS OF SOCIAL SKILLS TRAINING

The 35 group-design studies included 1,123 subjects who were 67% male with an average age of 11.53 years and average IQ of 94. From the 35 studies, 328 ES measurements were calculated and produced the following: average ES = 0.199 ($SD = 0.541$), ES range = −1.321 to +2.136, ES median = 0.161; indicating a modest positive skew, 27% negative ES, suggesting that in at least one out of four cases better outcomes were found for students receiving *no* social skills training. The average ES of 0.199 indicated that the average student would advance from the 50th percentile to the 58th percentile as a result of social skills training and would be better off than 58% of students receiving no such training. These are very modest grains, and according to Cohen's (1988) classification of ES magnitude, would be deemed "small."

One major variable in assessing outcomes was represented by the different individuals who were asked to evaluate subjects' behavior. The findings for five different raters are shown in Table 23.2.

Teachers appeared to perceive the greatest benefit from social skills training (ES = 0.223). Only slightly lower were the perceptions of peers and students with EBD themselves. In all three cases, the evaluators were above the overall average (0.199), suggesting that social skills training may produce a more positive classroom environment.

Experimenters did not appear to view social skills training as effective as did teachers

TABLE 23.2. Effects of Social Skills Training Observed by Different Raters

Rater	Mean ES	Standard deviation of ES	Number of ES	Power rating
Teacher	0.223	0.425	73	Small
Self	0.217	0.592	83	Small
Peer	0.215	0.387	44	Small
Experimenter	0.188	0.611	60	Small
Parent	0.153	0.599	68	Small

(ES = 0.188). Apparently, a more positive classroom environment does not transfer to the home environment, where parents perceived training to be least effective (ES = 0.153). No differences, however, were found among raters, $F (5,323) = 1.79$, $p < .25$, and ES for all raters can be considered "small." Although some modest trends emerged in the rater analysis, the primary finding of limited efficacy for social skills training was supported.

The evaluation of social skills training includes a number of factors that range from general to specific indices. It is therefore instructive to aggregate ES data into groupings that include broad dimensions of prosocial behaviors, problem behavior, and finally specific behavior traits. The findings appear in Table 23.3.

These findings reflect several global results. First, prosocial behaviors demonstrated a better than "average" (i.e., ES = 0.199) response to training that would translate into a 10 percentile rank gain on outcome measures. Thus, training has a modest positive effect on the global construct of prosocial behavior. Second, and perhaps more significant, problem behaviors appeared to be more resistant to treatment. Unlike prosocial behaviors, all problem behaviors showed a *below*-average (i.e., ES = 0.199) response to training.

The findings for problem behavior also showed some contradictory results. For ex-

TABLE 23.3. Effects of Social Skill Training by Construct

Construct	Mean ES	Standard deviation of ES	Number of ES	Power rating
Prosocial behavior				
Social relations	0.267	0.667	13	Small
Social behavior	0.266	0.475	16	Small
Social problem solving	0.258	0.617	22	Small
Social ability	0.221	0.373	21	Small
Problem behavior				
Family relations	0.198	0.396	9	Small
School relations	0.177	0.440	21	Small
Social communication	0.176	0.736	28	Small
Disruptive	0.131	0.569	21	Small
Specific behaviors				
Anxiety	0.422	0.256	8	Medium
Adjustment	0.268	0.200	10	Small
Cooperation	0.256	0.513	12	Small
Interaction	0.241	0.371	34	Small
Self-concept/esteem	0.164	0.446	17	Small
Aggression	0.129	0.486	20	Small

ample, the greatest improvement was in the area of family relations even though parents appeared to observe the least improvement (ES = 0.153). Such findings suggest caution, but it remains important to note that the ESs involved are quite small. A very small effect was found for disruptive behavior, suggesting that it is likely resistant to change. The modest 5 percentile gain demonstrates the difficulties in treating conduct disorder (CD). Although school relations revealed some improvement, the level was below the more positive perceptions noted by teachers and peers. Thus, the notion of school relations needs greater specification, especially in the way it relates to teachers and peers.

Specific behavior traits demonstrated a variable response to training. The largest effect was for anxiety, usually defined as a persistent feeling of anxiousness unrelated to specific environmental events. This is a positive outcome that suggests it is possible to treat a trait symptomatic of EBD. Although the reduction in anxiety may permit a student to better cope with stressful situations, it is not known how the reduced anxiety level is related to learning new social skills. Consistent with findings about prosocial behavior, three traits (adjustment, cooperation, and interaction) exceeded the overall mean (0.199) and appear to reflect the more positive perceptions among teachers, peers, and students with EBD themselves. Although pooled self-ratings were slightly positive (ES = 0.217), the positive perceptions did not hold for the (well-below-average) ES for self-concept/esteem (0.164). With self-concept/esteem being among the better measured traits (e.g., Piers–Harris Self-Concept Scale, Coopersmith Self-Esteem Inventory), it appears that, while things may appear better, students with EBD do not yet feeling better about themselves. The smallest ES (0.129) was for aggression, suggesting it is also a trait resistant to change, much like disruptive behavior. It thus appears that the symptoms of CD are difficult to treat, and behaviors such as sustained levels of aggression against other people and property may be useful as part of a formal diagnosis for EBD (Rutherford & Nelson, 1995).

Social skills were assessed with a variety of measures, with the largest effects found when the assessments were based on perceptions about behavior change. The more formal and structured behavior ratings/checklists appeared less sensitive than sociometric procedures (ES = 0.157 vs. 0.234). The sociometric findings reflected the positive effects for cooperation and interaction, unsurprising considering that sociometric measures often rely on peer nominations and peer ratings. The ES for peers as raters was also better than average among the other four sets of participants (ES = 0.215). Further, any social skill enhancement appears to have limited effect on personality as evidenced by the small ES (0.122) found for formal personality assessments. Essentially no effect was found on tests of academic achievement, suggesting that social skill interventions do not influence academic performance.

JUDGING THE EFFECTIVENESS OF SOCIAL SKILLS TRAINING

When groups of students with EBD were provided with social skills interventions, only modest changes in behavior were produced. The overall ES of 0.199 would be deemed small, and only 58% of students with EBD would accrue benefits. Across a variety of variables, uniformly small effects were found. For example, duration of treatment had no influence on outcomes. The average training program lasted about 12 weeks, with students receiving about 2½ hours of training per week. When aggregated into two groupings representing "more" or "less" than the average 12 weeks of training, no differences were found. A similar analysis for age ("younger" vs. "older") revealed no differences. Additionally, for both length of training and age, there was no significant correlation with ES, suggesting that these variables had little association with outcomes.

Research quality did not influence findings. Using criteria provided by Campbell and Stanley (1966) and Lytton and Romney (1991), individual studies were rated with respect to research quality (high, medium, low). Most studies (65%) fell in the medium category and produced an ES that closely approximated the overall ES (0.174 vs. 0.199). No differences were found among ES associated with research quality, F $(z, 325) = 1.34$, $p < .25$. The research investigating social skills training for students with EBD is generally well designed and adequate for the purposes of assessing efficacy.

Although remaining in the "small" range, some variation in ES magnitude was found. For example, modest differences were found for different raters of program effectiveness. When evaluated in a school context, treatment effects were perceived to be slightly higher than when evaluated by parents at home. This finding may reflect either the lack of generalization from school to home or possible observer bias when raters are aware of being involved in a research investigation.

Little difference was found among specific constructs describing prosocial behavior, although all were at a level higher than the overall mean. In comparison, all assessments of problem behavior were below the overall mean level, with disruptive behavior being the poorest responder. These findings were affirmed when specific behavior traits were analyzed. For example, aggression appeared to be particularly resistant to intervention and accounts for the small ES associated with disruptive behavior. In summary, the findings seem to suggest that social skills training may be more effective in promoting prosocial behaviors rather than reducing disruptive behaviors, which may require alternative treatment (e.g., positive behavioral interventions and supports).

VALIDATING THE EFFECTS OF SOCIAL SKILLS TRAINING

In a meta-analysis investigating the effectiveness of social skills training for students with learning disability (LD), Kavale and Forness (1995; see also Forness & Kavale, 1996), found an overall ES of 0.211. A total of 53 studies were included that were comparable with respect to demographic variables. In general, ES estimates were quite comparable, and none was above the 0.300 level, indicating only modest changes in behavior. The ES would again be deemed "small" and, as for findings related to students with EBD, only 58% of students with LD would accrue benefits as a result of social skills training. The findings for students with LD would appear to confirm and validate the findings for students with EBD and

indicate that social skills training produced only minimal improvements for most students with high incidence, mild disabilities.

The EBD literature also included a large proportion of single-subject studies evaluating social skills training that provide further insight into the efficacy of social skill interventions. Because data between group and single-subject designs are not immediately comparable, questions arise about the appropriate methodology for their quantitative synthesis. In their meta-analysis, Mathur, Kavale, Quinn, Forness, and Rutherford (1998) chose the percentage of nonoverlapping data points (PND) described by Scruggs, Mastropieri, and Casto (1987a) as an equivalent ES statistic. The PND method requires the examination of graphed data from each study to determine the number of nonoverlapping data points between baseline and treatment phases of the study.

The synthesis of single-subject research is more controversial than the methods used for group designs. Historically, synthesis of single-subject research has been based on "visual inspection" methods (Parsonson & Baer, 1978), but such procedures using parametric (Gentile, Roden, & Klein, 1974) and nonparametric (Levin, Marascuilo, & Hubert, 1978) statistical tests all possessed problems limiting their usefulness.

Scruggs et al. (1987a) suggested that the PND index may eliminate statistical problems related to assumptions about independence, normality, and homogeneity when applying parametric techniques. While the PND procedure was challenged (Salzberg, Strain, & Baer, 1987) it was also defended as the most unencumbered technique for synthesizing single-subject research (Scruggs, Mastropieri, & Casto, 1987b). Although remaining entirely defensible (e.g., Scruggs & Mastropieri, 1998), Strain, Kohler, and Gresham (1998) objected to the logic and interpretation of the PND methodology, but Kavale, Mathur, Forness, Quinn, and Rutherford (2000) demonstrated how the PND method has provided an objective, replicable, and valid means of synthesizing single-subject research.

The PND may be interpreted in a straightforward manner: the larger, the better. If, for example, PND = 100%, then the treatment would be deemed highly effective, while PND = 0% represents no treatment effectiveness. Within the context of applied behavior analysis, a PND of 75% or better probably indicates a useful treatment because, in substantially more instances, behavior shows improvement over that demonstrated during baseline.

Mathur et al. (1998), across 64 single-subject research studies that produced 463 graphs from which a PND could be calculated, reported a mean PND of 62%, with 47 graphs showing 0% and 103 graphs showing 100% PND. There was thus a tendency toward more positive treatment, but the mean PND (62%) indicates only modest intervention efficacy by falling between the 50% (moderate) and 75% (good) figures. The correlation between PND and number of data points in the intervention phase was not significant ($r = .086$, $p < .10$), suggesting no relationship between outcome and length of training.

The single-subject research did not investigate as many skills as the group research, but several variables permitted aggregation. The findings are shown in Table 23.4. The largest PND (66%) was associated with interaction and, although below the benchmark 75% level, there appears to be some success in fostering more interaction. Social behavior encompassed a variety of skills such as, for example, interpersonal relations, conduct, and on-task performance. The PND for the aggregated social behavior was 63%, a level comparable to the overall PND. The large associated SD suggests caution in interpreting these effects. The smallest PND (59%) was found for communication, suggesting limited success in this area. There was a difference between the PND for interaction and communication ($t (330) = 2.06$, $p < .05$), suggesting greater benefit from training directed at increasing interaction. These findings are thus consistent with the Kavale et al. (1997) group design meta-

analysis and appear to further validate previous findings that social skills training produced limited changes in behavior.

QUESTIONING THE EFFECTIVENESS OF SOCIAL SKILLS TRAINING

Overall, then, small effects were associated with social skills training, a conclusion seemingly at variance with conventional wisdom attesting to its efficacy. Although other meta-analyses (e.g., Beelman, Pfingston, & Losel, 1994; Schneider & Byrne, 1985; Vaughn et al., 2003) found higher-average ES for social skills training efficacy, they focused on a broader spectrum of children receiving social skills interventions, not students with EBD exclusively. For example, Ang and Hughes (2001) found an ES of .62 favoring social skills training for students demonstrating externalizing behavior problems. Because the outcome assessments (behavior ratings and observations) focused on externalizing behaviors, the training effects appear to reduce primary symptomology, but whether or not the improvement can be generalized to social skills seems problematic.

These issues emphasize why the definition of social skills is critical. Does a child with conduct disorder (CD) or oppositional defiant disorder (ODD) whose social behavior improves (e.g., becomes less aggressive) also become more socially competent? In an evaluation of a social skills curriculum, Webster-Stratton et al. (2001) found greater success in reducing conduct problems than in improving social problem solving. Thus, social skills training may be useful in treating antisocial behavior, but whether there is generally improved social competence is not clear. For students with EBD whose symptom complex includes a lack of social competen-

TABLE 23.4. Effects of Training on Social Skills in Single-Subject Research

Variable	Number of data points	Mean PND	Standard deviation of PND	Power rating
Interpretation	213	66	34	Moderate
Social behavior	121	63	40	Moderate
Communication	119	59	27	Moderate

cies but no externalizing behavior, the findings reported by Kavale et al. (1997) and Mathur et al. (1998) may reflect the reality that social skills training for students with EBD has not produced particularly large or socially important behavior changes.

Although an ES of 0.199 is small in statistical terms, the question arises whether any numerically positive effect might be practically or clinically meaningful in the contexts where the treatment is applied (Sechrest & Yeaton, 1982). Rosenthal and Rubin (1982) provided an intuitively appealing way to index practical significance in the binomial effect size display (BESD), that is, the proportion of treatment versus control subjects above a common success threshold (defined arbitrarily as the median). For example, in an evaluation of the efficacy of 156 psychological, educational, and behavioral treatments, Lipsey and Wilson (1993) found a mean ES of 0.47 that, in BESD terms, means a 62% success rate for a treatment group versus a control group with a 38% success rate. Although an ES of 0.47 is termed "medium" in statistical terms, a 24-percentage-point spread between treatment and control success rates appears to possess practical significance. The ES of 0.199 in BESD terms translates into a 55% versus 45% success rate for treatment and control groups, respectively. The 10-percentage-point spread in success rates is fairly small and does not seem to possess practical significance. Thus, in terms of both statistical and practical considerations, social skills training cannot easily be endorsed as an effective way of teaching social skills to children with EBD.

Besides the theoretical and psychometric issues alluded to earlier, other factors may contribute to the modest effects found for social skills training. One problem surrounds subject sampling. Training effects appear larger for specific diagnoses like CD or ODD, but smaller effects seem associated with a more general EBD designation that may be related to the way subjects are selected. In the Kavale et al. (1997) meta-analysis, a majority of studies selected subjects on the basis of the presence or absence of specific social skills deficits, with a formal EBD label being a secondary consideration. Two difficulties are obvious in such a selection procedure: (1) the extent to which a subject is "truly" EBD is indeterminate and

(2) the identified social skill deficit may be more severe than anticipated, making it more resistant to treatment than a "milder" deficit associated with the constellation of behaviors defining EBD. Consequently, determining the effectiveness of social skills training for the "typical" EBD student is difficult.

The very nature of the social skills training programs may also contribute to the limited findings of effectiveness. A majority of the experimental studies developed training programs specifically designed for the study's research purposes. Such experimental programs represent an amalgam of techniques that may individually possess face validity, but the total program may not possess the requisite content validity. This caveat is particularly cogent since most studies did not include any pilot testing to evaluate how well the program met its intended purposes. Although the effectiveness of such programs was modest, the present findings left unanswered whether or not social skills training itself was effective. More positive outcomes may result from carefully constructed and tested training programs.

The nature of the social skills training programs may introduce additional difficulties as well. The training activities were usually group-administered, contrary to the notion of special education being specially designed individualized instruction. Thus, the intervention may not "fit" an individual student's needs. The structured design of training programs limits the flexibility of practitioners in choosing the social skills to be taught and does not easily allow for modifying training when interventions appear to be having little effect on social functioning. Consequently, group training programs may lack social validity, the pivotal notion that positive social skills are those deemed important by others in the same context (Mathur & Rutherford, 1996).

The length of training may also contribute to limited efficacy. The average social skills training program was for 2.5 hours per week for 12 weeks, for a total of 30 hours (see Kavale et al., 1997). With the average subject being 10 years old, the observed social skill deficits were relatively long-standing, and 30 hours may be insufficient to ameliorate such enduring deficits. For example, there would be little reason to expect significant changes in reading achievement after 30 hours of training for students with severe and persistent reading difficulties. Such temporal truncation may preclude the modification of basic elements of social competence. Similarly, while social skill deficits may require more training time; it is not clear whether more training consistently produces larger effects.

Social validity data need to be assessed at the onset of social skills intervention to provide important information about the significance of the goals, acceptability of social skills procedures, and importance of potential outcomes (Gresham, 1986). The best chance for successful fidelity and integrity of implementation of social skills interventions depends upon how well these interventions are defined and operationalized by researchers and practitioners. While this area of research is still some way from accomplishing this, when aspects of intervention and definition have become clearer, they must be implemented with integrity to produce the desired social outcomes of overall competent functioning of students with EBD.

CONCLUSION

Although a popular adjunct intervention, social skills training does not appear to significantly influence social functioning in students with EBD. Given the importance of developing social skills to deal effectively with social situations and the adverse consequences of not doing so (Elliott & Gresham, 1993), these findings were disappointing.

As a "special" intervention, social skills training must be placed in the context of other "special" process training practices like perceptual-motor training (ES = 0.39). Unlike "special" interventions, however, social skills training, as a relatively new and evolving methodology, cannot yet be dismissed. Although disappointing, the limited efficacy should not cause undue pessimism because social skills training must still be considered an *experimental* intervention that requires further specification to answer a number of theoretical, psychometric, and design questions. We agree with Gresham (1998), who suggested that social skills training should not be either razed or remodeled but rather rebuilt as part of a com-

prehensive treatment for students with EBD. Until that time, social skills training must be viewed as an intervention that has received limited empirical support but, nevertheless, should be viewed as one which "should be refined and customized—certainly not eliminated!" (Quinn et al., 1999, p. 62).

REFERENCES

Ang, R. P., & Hughes, J. N. (2001). Differential benefits of skills training with antisocial youth based on group composition: A meta-analytic investigation. *School Psychology Review, 31*, 164–185.

Asher, S. R., & Hymel, S. (1981). Children's social competence in peer relations: Sociometric and behavioral assessment. In J. D. Wine & M. D. Smye (Eds.), *Social competence* (pp. 125–151). New York: Guilford Press.

Bangert Drowns, R. L. (1986). Review of development in meta-analytic methods. *Psychological Bulletin, 99*, 388–399.

Beelmann, A., Pfingston, U., & Losel, F. (1994). Effects of training social competence in children: A meta-analysis of recent evaluation studies. *Journal of Clinical Child Psychology, 23*, 260–271.

Campbell, D. T., & Stanley, J. C. (1966). *Experimental and quasi-experimental designs for research.* Chicago, IL: Rand McNally.

Clausen, J. (1972). Quo vadis, AAMD? *Journal of Special Education, 6*, 51–60.

Cohen, J. (1988). *Statistical power analysis for the behavioral sciences* (2nd ed.). Hillsdale, NJ: Erlbaum.

Cooper, H., & Hedges, L. V. (Eds.). (1994). *Handbook of research synthesis.* New York: Sage.

Cronbach, L. J., & Meehl, P. E. (1955). Construct validity in psychological tests. *Psychological Bulletin, 52*, 281–302.

Dodge, K. A., Pettit, G. S., McClaskey, C. L., & Brown, M. (1986). A social information processing model of social competence in children. In M. Perlmutter (Ed.), *Cognitive perspectives on children's social and behavioral development* (pp. 77–125). Hillsdale, NJ: Erlbaum.

Elliott, S. N., & Gresham, F. M. (1993). Social skills interventions for children. *Behavior Modification, 17*, 287–313.

Forness, S. R., & Kavale, K. A. (1996). Treating social skill deficits in children with learning disabilities: A meta-analysis of the research. *Learning Disability Quarterly, 19*, 2–13.

Gentile, J. R., Roden, A. H., & Klein, R. D. (1974). An analysis of variance model for the intrasubject replication design. *Journal of Applied Behavior Analysis, 5*, 193–198.

Glass, G. V., McGaw, B., & Smith, M. L. (1981). *Meta-analysis in social research.* Beverly Hills, CA: Sage.

Goldstein, A. P. (1988). *The prepare curriculum: Teaching prosocial competencies.* Champaign, IL: Research Press.

Gresham, F. M. (1986). Conceptual and definitional issues in the assessment of social skills: Implications for classification and training. *Journal of Clinical Child Psychology, 15,* 16–25.

Gresham, F. M. (1998). Social skills training: Should we raze, remodel, or rebuild? *Behavioral Disorders, 24,* 19–25.

Hedges, L. V., & Olkin, I. (1985). *Statistical methods for meta-analysis.* New York: Academic Press.

Hops, H. (1983). Children's social competence and skills: Current research practices and future directions. *Behavior Therapy, 14,* 3–18.

Hunter, J. E., & Schmidt, F. L. (1990). *Methods of meta-analysis: Correcting error and bias in research findings.* Newbury Park, CA: Sage.

Kavale, K. A. (1984). A meta-analytic evaluation of the Frostig test and training program. *The Exceptional Child, 31,* 134–141.

Kavale, K. A., & Forness, S. R. (1995). Social skill deficits and training: A meta-analysis of the research in learning disabilities. In T. E. Scruggs & M. A. Mastropieri (Eds.), *Advances in learning and behavioral disabilities* (Vol. 9, pp. 119–160). Greenwich, CT: JAI Press.

Kavale, K. A., & Forness, S. R. (1999). *Efficacy of special education and related services.* Washington, DC: American Association on Mental Retardation.

Kavale, K. A., Forness, S. R., & Mostert, M. (in press). Defining emotional or behavioral disorders: The quest for affirmation. In P. Garner, F. Yuen, P. Clough, & T. Pardeck (Eds.), *Handbook of emotional and behavioral difficulties in education.* London: Chapman/Sage.

Kavale, K. A., Mathur, S. R., Forness, S. R., Quinn, M. M., & Rutherford, R. B. (2000). Right reason in the integration of group and single-subject research in behavioral disorders. *Behavioral Disorders, 25,* 142–157.

Kavale, K. A., Mathur, S. R., Forness, S. R., Rutherford, R. B., & Quinn, M. M. (1997). Effectiveness of social skills training for students with behavior disorders: A meta-analysis. In T. E. Scruggs & M. A. Mastropieri (Eds.), *Advances in learning and behavioral disabilities* (Vol. 11, pp. 1–26). Greenwich, CT: JAI Press.

Leland, H. (1978). Theoretical considerations of adaptive behavior. In A. Coulter & H. Morrow (Eds.), *Adaptive behavior: Concepts and measurements* (pp. 21–44). New York: Grune & Stratton.

Leland, H., Shellhaas, M., Nihira, K., & Foster, R. (1967). Adaptive behavior: A new dimension in the qualification of the mentally retarded. *Mental Retardation Abstracts, 4,* 359–387.

Levin, J. R., Marascuilo, L., & Hubert, L. J. (1978). *N* = 1 nonparametric randomization tests. In T. R. Kratchowill (Ed.), *Single-subject research: Strategies for evaluating change* (pp. 167–196). New York: Academic Press.

Lipsey, M. W., & Wilson, D. B. (1993). The efficacy of psychological, educational, and behavioral treatment: Confirmation from meta-analysis. *American Psychologist, 48,* 1181–1209.

Lytton, H., & Romney, D. (1991). Parent's differential socialization of boys and girls: A meta-analysis. *Psychological Bulletin, 190,* 267–296.

Maag, J. W. (1989). Assessment in social skills training: Methodological and conceptual issues for research and practice. *Remedial and Special Education, 53,* 519–529.

Mathur, S. R., Kavale, K. A., Quinn, M. M., Forness, S. R., & Rutherford, R. B. (1998). Social skills interventions with students with emotional and behavioral problems: A quantitative synthesis of single-subject research. *Behavioral Disorders, 23,* 193–201.

Mathur, S. R., & Rutherford, R. B. (1989). Analysis of literature on social competence of behaviorally disordered children and youth. In R. B. Rutherford & S. A. DiGangi (Eds.), *Monograph in severe behavior disorders of children and youth* (Vol. 12, pp. 72–86). Reston, VA: Council for Children with Behavioral Disorders.

Mathur, S. R., & Rutherford, R. B. (1994). Success of social skills training with delinquent youth: Some critical issues. In T. E. Scruggs & M. A. Mastropieri (Eds.), *Advances in learning and behavioral disabilities* (Vol. 8, pp. 147–160). Greenwich, CT: JAI Press.

Mathur, S. R., & Rutherford, R. B. (1996). Is social skills training effective with students with emotional or behavioral disorders? Research needs and issues. *Behavioral Disorders, 22,* 21–28.

McConaughy, S. H., Kay, P. J., & Fitzgerald, M. (2001). How long is long enough? Outcomes for a school-based prevention program. *Exceptional Children, 67,* 21–34.

McConnell, S. R. (1987). Entrapment effects and the generalization and maintenance of social skills training for elementary school students with behavioral disorders. *Behavioral Disorders, 12,* 252–263.

McFall, R. (1982). A review and reformulation of the concept of social skills. *Behavioral Assessment, 4,* 1–33.

Merrell, K. W., & Gimpel, G. A. (1998). *Social skills of children and adolescents: Conceptualization, assessment, and treatment.* London: Erlbaum.

Meyers, C. E., Nihira, K., & Zetlin, A. (1979). The measurement of adaptive behavior. In N. R. Ellis (Ed.), *Handbook of mental deficiency: Psychological theory and research* (2nd ed., pp. 431–481). Hillsdale, NJ: Erlbaum.

Moreno, J. (1934). *Who shall survive? A new approach to the problem of human interrelations.* Washington, DC: Nervous and Mental Disease.

Mostert, M. P. (1996). Reporting meta-analyses in learning disabilities. *Learning Disabilities Research and Practice, 11*(1), 2–14.

Mostert, M. P. (2001). Characteristics of meta-analyses reported in mental retardation, learning disabilities, and emotional and behavioral disorders. *Exceptionality, 9,* 199–225.

Mostert, M. P. (2003). Meta-Analyses in mental retardation. *Education and Training in Developmental Disabilities, 38,* 229–249.

Mostert, M. P., & Kavale, K. A. (2001). Evaluation of research for usable knowledge in behavioral disorders: Ignoring the irrelevant, considering the germane. *Behavioral Disorders, 27,* 51–67.

Orwin, R. G. (1983). A fail-safe N for effect in meta-analysis. *Journal of Educational Statistics, 8,* 157–159.

Parsonson, B. S., & Baer, D. M. (1978). The analysis and presentation of graphic data. In T. R. Kratchowill (Ed.), *Single subject research: Strategies for evaluating change* (pp. 101–166). New York: Academic Press.

Quinn, M. M., Kavale, K. A., Mathur, S. R., Rutherford, R. B., & Forness, S. R. (1999). A meta-analysis of social skills interventions for students with emotional and behavioral disorders. *Journal of Emotional and Behavioral Disorders, 7,* 54–64.

Reynolds, C. R., & Kamphaus, R. W. (1992). *The Behavioral Assessment System for Children.* Circle Pines, MN: American Guidance Services.

Rosenthal, R. (1979). The "file drawer problem" and tolerance for null results. *Psychological Bulletin, 86,* 638–641.

Rosenthal, R., & Rubin, D. B. (1982). A simple, general purpose display of magnitude of experimental effect. *Journal of Educational Psychology, 74,* 166–169.

Rutherford, R. B., Chipman, J., DiGangi, S. A., & Anderson, K. (1992). *Teaching social skills: A practical instructional approach.* Ann Arbor, MI: Exceptional Innovations.

Rutherford, R. B., & Nelson, C. M. (1995). Management of aggressive and violent behavior in the schools. *Focus on Exceptional Children, 27*(7), 1–13.

Rutherford, R. B., Quinn, M. M., & Mathur, S. R. (1996). *Effective strategies for teaching appropriate behaviors to children with emotional and behavioral disorders.* Reston, VA: Council for Children with Behavioral Disorders.

Salzberg, C. L., Strain, P. S., & Baer, D. M. (1987). Meta-analysis for single-subject research: When does it clarify, when does it obscure? *Remedial and Special Education, 8,* 43–48.

Schneider, B., & Bryne, B. M. (1985). Children's social skills training: A meta-analysis. In B. Schneider, K. Rubin, & J. Ledingham (Eds.), *Children's peer relations: Issues in assessment and intervention* (pp. 175–192). New York: Springer-Verlag.

Scruggs, T. E., & Mastropieri, M. A. (1998). Summarizing single-subject research. *Behavior Modification, 22,* 221–243.

Scruggs, T. E., Mastropieri, M. A., & Casto, G. (1987a). The quantitative synthesis of single-subject research: Methodology and validation. *Remedial and Special Education, 8,* 24–33.

Scruggs, T. E., Mastropieri, M. A., & Casto, G. (1987b). Response to Salzberg, Strain, and Baer. *Remedial and Special Education, 8,* 49–52.

Sechrest, L., & Yeaton, W. H. (1982). Magnitude of experimental effects in social science research. *Evaluation Review, 6,* 579–600.

Sheldon, J., Sherman, J., Schumaker, J., & Hazel, S. (1984). Developing a social skills curriculum for mildly handicapped adolescents and young adults: Some problems and approaches. In S. Braaten, R. B. Rutherford, & C. A. Kardash (Eds.), *Programming for adolescents with behavioral disorders* (Vol. 1, pp. 105–116). Reston, VA: Council for Children with Behavioral Disorders.

Strain, P. S., Kohler, F. W., & Gresham, F. M. (1998). Problems in logic and interpretation with quantitative syntheses of single-case research: Mathur and colleagues (1998) as a case in point. *Behavioral Disorders, 24,* 74–85.

Vaughn, S., & Haager, D. (1994). The measurement and assessment of social skills. In G. R. Lyon (Ed.), *Frames of reference for the assessment of learning disabilities* (pp. 555–570). Baltimore: Brookes.

Vaughn, S., & Hogan, A. (1990). Social competence and learning disabilities: A prospective study. In H. L. Swanson & B. K. Keogh (Eds.), *Learning disabilities: Theoretical and research issues* (pp. 175–191). Hillsdale, NJ: Erlbaum.

Vaughn, S., Kim, A., Morris Sloan, C. V., Hughes, M. T., Elbaum, B., & Sridhar, D. (2003). Social skills interventions for young children with disabilities: A synthesis of group design studies. *Remedial and Special Education, 24,* 2–15.

Walker, H. M., Colvin, G., & Ramsey, E. (1995). *Antisocial behavior in schools: Strategies and best practices.* Pacific Grove, CA: Brooks/Cole.

Walker, H. M.., McConnell, S., Holmes, D., Todis, B., Walker, J., & Golden, N. (1983). *The Walker Social Skills Curriculum: The ACCEPTS Program.* Austin, TX: Pro-Ed.

Webster-Stratton, C., Reid, J., & Hammond, M. (2001). Social skills and problem-solving training for children with early-onset conduct problems: Who benefits? *Journal of Child Psychology and Psychiatry, 42,* 943–952.

Williams, S. L., Walker, H. M., Holmes, D., Todis, B., & Fabre, T. (1989). Social validation of adolescent social skills by teachers and students. *Remedial and Special Education, 10,* 18–27, 37.

Zaragoza, N., Vaughn, S., & McIntosh, R. (1991). Social skills interventions and children with behavior problems: A review. *Behavioral Disorders, 16,* 260–275.

24

Academic Instruction and Tutoring Interventions for Students with Emotional and Behavioral Disorders

1990 to the Present

KATHLEEN LYNNE LANE

By definition, students with emotional disturbances (ED; Individuals with Disabilities Education Act [IDEA], 1997), are characterized by internalizing and externalizing behavior patterns (Achenbach, 1991) that impede academic, social, and behavioral progress. Behavioral and social deficits of these youngsters have been well documented over the past 25 years, as evidenced by numerous treatment outcome studies (e.g., Mathur, Kavale, Quinn, Forness, & Rutherford, 1998; Zaragoza, Vaughn, & McIntosh, 1991) and ample assessment tools such as the Systematic Screening for Behavior Disorders (SSBD; Walker & Severson, 1992), the Early Screening Project (ESP; Walker, Severson, & Feil, 1995), the Social Skills Rating System (Gresham & Elliott, 1990), the Walker–McConnell Scale of School Adjustment (Walker & McConnell, 1995), and the Child Behavior Checklist (CBCL; Achenbach, 1991).

However, until relatively recently, little attention has been devoted to academic is-

sues for students with emotional and behavioral disorders (EBD) (Lane, Gresham, & O'Shaughnessy, 2002; Lane & Wehby, 2002). The lack of attention to academic issues may stem, in part, from (1) the tendency of teacher preparation programs to focus predominantly on the social and behavioral characteristics and needs of this population (Lane, Gresham, et al., 2002); (2) negative teacher–student interactions documented in self-contained classrooms serving students with emotional and behavioral disorders (Shores, Jack, Gunter, Ellis, DeBriere, & Wehby, 1993); and (3) the misconception held by many educators that students must behave properly before academic learning is possible (O'Shaughnessy, Lane, Gresham, & Beebe-Frankenberger, 2003).

In addition, recent research exploring the relationship between academic underachievement—particularly in the area of reading—and externalizing behavior disorders suggests that, in some instances, students may act out to avoid aversive academic tasks. Tasks may be aversive because the instructional level does not coincide with the student's ability level either because the tasks are too difficult or too easy (Gickling & Armstrong, 1978; Gunter, Denny, Jack, Shores, & Nelson, 1993; Umbreit, Lane, & Dejud, 2004).

The nature of the relationship between academic underachievement and externalizing behaviors patterns continues to be a focal point in the EBD research and teaching communities (Hinshaw, 1992; Lane, Gresham, et al., 2002; Lane & Wehby, 2002). Yet, regardless of the causal relationships between these domains, it is clear that attention must be devoted to understanding how to better teach students with ED and, more broadly, students with or at risk for EBD. It is imperative that the research community identify effective, efficient strategies and procedures for building these students' academic skills to enable maximum participation in the general education curriculum. If we continue to identify these students, place them in restrictive environments, and address only their social and behavioral needs, we run the risk of further handicapping these students (Lane, 2003; Lane, Gresham, et al., 2002). Even if their socio-behavioral deficits and excesses (Gresham, 2002) were remediated in these environments and the students could return to the general education setting, they would likely have tremendous gaps in their academic content knowledge and skill levels making it difficult to succeed in the general education environment. Consequently, we must identify the most effective, efficient methods for instructing these students who clearly demonstrate academic deficits that adversely influence their educational performance (IDEA, 1997; Lee, Sugai, & Horner, 1999).

ACADEMIC CHARACTERISTICS

As compared to typically developing students in general education environments, students with EBD exhibit moderate to severe, broad academic deficits (e.g., Greenbaum et al., 1996; Mattison, Spitznagel, & Felix, 1998; Nelson, Benner, Lane, & Smith, in press; Scruggs & Mastorpieri, 1986; Wagner, 1995; Wilson, Cone, Bradley, & Reese, 1986). Not only do students with EBD per-

form below general education students, these discrepancies are evident in multiple areas (e.g., reading, math, written expression, science; Scruggs & Mastropieri, 1986). In addition to performing below typically developing students, evidence suggests that students with EBD may exhibit greater academic deficits relative to students with learning disabilities (LD) and mild mental retardation (MMR; Gajar, 1979). However, evidence is mixed (Gajar, 1979), with some studies indicating that students with EBD actually outperform students with LD (Epstein & Cullinan, 1983) and MMR (Wagner, 1995; Wilson et al., 1986).

The prevalence of academic deficits does not appear to improve over time. Some evidence suggests that deficits remain stable (Mattison, Hooper, & Glassberg, 2002) or even worsen (Greenbaum et al., 1996; Nelson et al., in press) as students progress through school. A recent cross-sectional study conducted by Nelson and colleagues of 155 kindergarten through 12th-grade students with EBD found prevalence rates of achievement deficits to be high and more pronounced with adolescents. Further, adolescents evidenced more comorbid academic deficits than did elementary-age students with EBD. This broadening scope of deficits appears to more be characteristic of the EBD population than the LD population. A longitudinal study by Anderson, Kutash, and Duchnowski (2001) revealed that, while students with LD made significant growth in reading over time, similar growth was not experienced by students with EBD. Although the degree of similarity between students with EBD and students with LD in academic achievement is not clearly established, what is clear is that students with EBD, as compared to students with LD, experience less positive outcomes (Anderson et al., 2001).

ACADEMIC AND ADULT OUTCOMES

Academic and adult outcomes for this population are poor at best. In terms of academic performance, students with ED earn lower grades and have a higher course failure rate than any other disability group (Lee et al., 1999; U.S. Department of Education, 1994). Sixteen percent of students with ED are required to repeat a given grade; this rate is more than double the retention rate for general education students (Wagner, 1995). Moreover, the school dropout rate for students receiving special education services exceeds 50% (Wagner, Blackorby, Cameto, & Newman, 1993). This is particularly alarming given that dropout status is highly correlated with postsecondary outcomes, including negative employment and poor community adjustment (Carson, Sitlington, & Frank, 1995). In brief, students with academic deficiencies and behavioral problems are highly likely to experience academic failure, school dropout, and propensities toward criminality, unemployment, substance abuse, and mental health services (Kauffman, 2001; Kazdin, 1993; Lee et al., 1999; Offord & Bennett, 1996; Walker, Colvin, & Ramsey, 1995).

Given the poor academic performance of students with EBD and the negative academic outcomes associated with poor performance, it is essential that the field of EBD identify evidence-based instructional strategies and curricular programs to better serve this population (Lee et al., 1999). This chapter reviews the literature pertaining to academic interventions in the areas of reading, written expression, and mathematical skills as conducted with students with EBD. Content includes the results of a systematic literature review, a discussion of limitations in each content area, and recommendations for future academic interventions for students with and at risk for EBD.

METHOD

A systematic review of the literature was conducted to identify studies published between 1990 and 2003 involving academic interventions for students with or at risk for emotional and behavioral disorders. Electronic searches of the psychology (Psych Info) and ERIC data bases were conducted, using all possible combinations of the following three sets of terms and their derivatives: (1) aggression, conduct disorder, defiant, disruptive, oppositional, antisocial, problem behavior, emotional or behavioral disorders, or emotionally disturbed, (2) treatment, intervention, studies, remediation, training, instruction, and (3) reading,

literacy, academic, mathematics, writing, or spelling. Next, hand searches of *Behavioral Disorders* and *Journal of Emotional and Behavioral Disorders*, two journals dedicated to students with EBD, were conducted.

Inclusion Criteria

Studies meeting the following criteria were included in this review: (1) examined school-based academic instructional intervention(s) directed by an interventionist, teacher, or peer, (2) involved school-age participants with or at risk for emotional and behavioral disorders, (3) published between 1990 and 2003, and (4) reported student outcomes on either academic performance or academic-related behaviors. "School-based" referred to studies conducted in a school setting in either a special or general education environment. Investigations conducted in clinical settings or in juvenile detention centers were excluded (Greene, 1996; Malmgren & Leone, 2000; Simpson, Swanson, & Kunkel, 1992).

"Academic instructional interventions" referred to reading, writing, and mathematical interventions conducted by an interventionist, teacher, or peer inclusive of tutoring interventions. Interventions focusing on curricular modification such as adjusting task difficulty (DePaepe, Shores, Jack, & Denny, 1996), task length (Miller, Gunter, Venn, Hummel, & Wiley, 2003), choice or level of interest (Clarke et al., 1995; Cole, Davenport, Bambara, & Ager, 1997; Kern, Bambara, & Fogt, 2002), medium preference (Kern, Delaney, Clarke, Dunlap, & Childs, 2001), environmental adjustments (Ervin et al., 2000), self-regulatory procedures (e.g., self-monitoring, Carr & Punzo, 1993; Glomb & West, 1990; Levendoski & Cartledge, 2000), or feedback modifications (e.g., McLaughlin, 1992) were excluded (Barton-Arwood, 2003). Also excluded were packaged interventions that included academic interventions implemented in conjunction with social or behavioral interventions if the design did not permit analysis of the isolated effects of the academic intervention component (e.g., Kamps, Kravits, Rauch, Kamps, & Chung, 2000; Kamps, Kravits, Stolze, & Swaggart, 1999). This resulted in excluding peer tutoring interventions that were combined with other modifications such as self-monitoring, shortened assignments, or computer usage (Penno, Frank, & Wacker, 2000). Interventions incorporating reinforcement procedures to motivate student performance (e.g., Cochran, Feng, Cartledge, & Hamilton, 1993; Cybriwsky & Schuster, 1990; Harper, Mallette, Maheady, Bentley, & Moore, 1995; Lane, 1999; Lane, O'Shaughnessy, Lambros, Gresham, & Beebe-Frankenberger, 2001; Locke & Fuchs, 1995; McCurdy, Cundari, & Lentz, 1990; Skinner, Smith, & McLean, 1994) were included, however.

Participants must have been kindergarten through 12th-grade students in one of the following categories based on categories specified in a review of functional assessment-based interventions for students with EBD (Lane, Umbreit, & Beebe-Frankenberger, 1999): (1) at risk for behavior problems; (2) emotionally disturbed (ED), a category specified in the Individuals with Disabilities Education Act (IDEA, 1997) requiring special services; (3) emotional and behavioral disorders (EBD), which includes more global behavioral problems; (4) oppositional defiant disorders (ODD) or conduct disorders (CD), psychiatric diagnoses delineated in the *Diagnostic and Statistical Manual of Mental Disorders* (DSM-IV; American Psychiatric Association, 1994); (5) EBD and either an educational label (learning disability, other health impairment, or speech and language) or psychiatric label (ODD, CD, depression); (6) attention-deficient/hyperactivity disorder (ADHD) and behavioral concern (ADHD + at risk or EBD), to include students with identified attention problems and behavior patterns (e.g., coercion, noncompliance) that place them at risk for behavior disorders; and (7) ADHD and diagnosed behavioral problem in either educational (ADHD + ED) or psychiatric (ADHD + ODD or CD) domains. Students with dual diagnoses of mental retardation and behavioral disorders were excluded, as these students, due to low cognitive abilities, traditionally participate in life skills curricula rather than the more traditional core academic curricula (Browder & Shear, 1996; Schloss, Alper, Arnold-Reid, Aylward, & Dudenhoeffer, 1995).

Studies published from 1990 to the present were included to identify recent investigations targeting academic instruction and to avoid unnecessary overlap with other review articles (e.g., Coleman & Vaughn, 2000; Ruhl & Berlinghoff, 1992). Dissertation articles and book chapters were excluded from this review to ensure that only referenced research studies were included.

Finally, studies must have reported student outcome data on either academic performance or academic-related behaviors (e.g., task engagement). Studies with a narrative report excluding actual data were excluded (Edwards & Chard, 2000), as were studies reporting only problem behaviors (e.g., disruption, Hogan & Prater, 1993).

If an article's abstract suggested a possible fit with the above inclusion criteria, the article was obtained and read to determine actual eligibility. Each study was read and coded for the following variables: participant characteristics (number, gender, age, grade level, and label), instructional setting, intervention focus and setting, research design and dependent variables, results, and components related to valid inference making (accuracy of the dependent variable, fidelity of the independent variable, generalization and maintenance, and social validity; Lane, Beebe-Frankenberger, Lambros, & Pierson, 2001).

RESULTS

A total of 25 articles with data on 199 participants met the criteria for inclusion: 14 articles targeting reading instruction, 1 on writing instruction, and 11 on mathematic instruction (see Table 24.1). This paper provides a review of participant characteristics, intervention focus and setting, research design and dependent variables, components related to valid inference making, and outcomes of each instructional area.

Reading

Participant Characteristics

Eight of the 14 articles were published after 1997, with the remaining 6 articles published between 1990 and 1997. A total of 128 students participated in these studies, with students ranging in age from 5 to 14 years of age. Three studies were conducted in middle schools (Locke & Fuchs, 1995;

TABLE 24.1. Academic Intervention Studies with Students with and at Risk for Emotional and Behavioral Disorders: 1990 to Present

Author (Journal, year)	Participant characteristics and instructional setting	Purpose	Intervention and intervention setting	Research design and dependent variables	Components related to valid inference making	Outcomes
Reading						
Babyak, Koorland, & Mathes (*BD*, 2000)	N = 4; males; ages 10–11; grades 4–5; S1 BD, SLD, ADHD; S2 BD, SL; S3 BD; S4 SLD; public summer school program for students with BD	To examine the effects of story mapping instruction on reading comprehension skills of students with BD who had reading deficits	Story mapping instruction (with reinforcement: behavioral system) Separate classroom with the last 6 sessions held at a summer camp (*n* = 1) or students' homes (*n* = 2)	Repeated measures multiple-baseline across subjects A–Baseline B–Story Mapping C–Guided Practice (GP) D–Independent Practice (IP) DV1: *story retell* DV2: *passage comprehension* story elements DV 3: *main idea probes* DV4: *social validity* (SV)	RDV: M, R TI: M, R SV: T (M), S (M, R), Consumers (M, R) G: not mentioned M: not mentioned	*Story retells*: Percentage of correct responses were higher during GP or IP relative to baseline. *Story elements*: Percentages of correct responses increased. *Main idea*: Little change for 3 students. *SV*: Students rated the intervention favorably. Volunteers correctly identify 85% retells.
Cochran, Feng, Cartledge, & Hamilton (*BD*, 1993)	N = 16; males; ages 7–11; grades 2 (*n* = 8) and 5 (*n* = 8); BD; self-contained elementary school for students with BD	To determine the effectiveness of African American males with BD as cross-age peer tutors	Peer tutoring: 4 fifth-grade students with BD tutored 4 second-grade students with BD; the remaining students served as comparison students; reinforcement component (praise, stickers) present Library or home economics room.	Group comparisons using descriptive procedures DV1: *sight words* DV2: *rating scales* Social Skills Rating System (SSRS), teacher, student DV3: *direct observation cooperative statements* DV4: *SV student interviews* DV5: *SV teacher questionnaire*	RDV: M, R TI: not mentioned SV: T (M, R), S (M, R), G: not mentioned M: M, R	*Sight words*: Increased for all. Few academic gains for tutors. *Rating scales*: Improved social skills and problem behavior scores for tutees and tutors. Only tutees made academic gains. *Cooperative statements*: Increases in academic cooperative statements and decreases in uncooperative statements. *SV*: Favorable remarks by students and teachers.
Dawson, Venn, & Gunter (*BD*, 2000)	N = 4; 3 males, 1 female; ages 7–8; grades 1 (*n* = 2) and 2 (*n* = 2); EBD; resource special education classroom	To determine the effects of teacher- and computer-provided modeling on the reading performance of students with EBD	Reading previews. conditions: no-reading model (NM); computer model (CM); teacher model (TM) Resource classroom	Alternating treatment design conditions: no model, computer model, and teacher model DV1: mean *number of correct* words read per minute DV2: mean *percentage* of words read *correctly*	DV: M, R TI: not mentioned SV: T (M, R), S (not mentioned) G: not mentioned M: not mentioned	*Number correct*. Students, cumulatively, read more words correctly under TM and CM conditions as compared to NM. *Percentage correct*. Students read greater percentages of words correctly in (1) CM as compared to NM; and (2) TM relative to CM and NM.
Falk & Wehby (*BD*, 2001)	N = 6; males; ages 5–6; grade K; S1–4 SL; S5 ED; S6 OHI–ADHD; self-contained room for students with EBD at an urban elementary school	To examine the effectiveness of the peer tutoring component of kindergarten PALS (K-PALS) in improving early reading skills of kindergarteners with EBD	K-PALS peer tutoring; point system for reinforcement Self-contained room for students with EBD	Multiple-baseline across tutoring pairs A–Prebaseline: B–Baseline: C–K-PALS DV1: *letter-naming* DV2: *letter-sound* DV3: *segmenting* DV4: *blending*	RDV: M, R TI: M, R SV: not mentioned G: not collected M: not collected	*Letter-naming* outcomes not reported. *Letter-sound* increases for 4 of the 6 students during the tutoring phase. *Segmenting* scores were inconsistent. *Blending* skills improved for 5 of the 6 students.

Lane (*JEBD*, 1999)	N = 39; 23 males, 16 females; ages 6–7; grade 1; at risk; general education classroom	To determine if an academic or social skills intervention is more effective in decreasing problem behavior and increasing academic skills of first-grade students at risk for antisocial behavior	Academic intervention (AI), Phonological Awareness Training for Reading (PATR), social skills intervention (SSI), or treatment contact control (TCC) group; reinforcement component Empty classroom, office, outside, and in a cafeteria	Mixed model, repeated measures, hierarchical analysis of variance Three time points: onset, end, 3-weeks later DV1: teacher ratings *SSRS* DV2: *Critical Events Index (CEI)* DV 3: *Word Attack* DV 4: *TOPA* DV 5: Social Validity *(SV)* Teacher: *IRP-15 and Interview* DV 6: Social Validity *(SV)* Student: *Children's Intervention Rating Profile and Interview*	RDV: M, R TI: M, R SV: T (M, R), S (M, R) G: not mentioned M: M, R	Social and academic skills of students in the AI group did not change over time at a different rate than the skills of the students in the SSI or TCC groups on any DVs. AI group showed significant increases in *TOPA* scores. Although the AI group made some gains in *word attack* and *SSRS social skills*, the gains were insignificant. *Maintenance.* No significant changes for the AI group between post and follow-up phases. *SV.* Favorable ratings.
Lane, O'Shaughnessy, Lambros, Gresham, & Beebe-Frankenberger (*JEBD*, 2001)	N = 7; 5 males, 2 females; ages 74–92 months; grade 1; at-risk; general education classroom	To examine the efficacy of phonological awareness training with first-grade students at risk for conduct, attention, and early reading problems	Intervention: Phonological Awareness Training for Reading (PATR); reinforcement of participation. Private rooms (conference room or empty classroom) at each elementary school	Multiple-baseline across groups A–Baseline B–Intervention, PATR C–Post D–Follow-up DV1: nonsense word fluency (*NWF*) DV2: correct words per minute (*CWPM*) DV3: total disruptive behavior (*TDB*) DV4: negative social interactions (*NSI*) DV 5: Social Validity (SV) Teacher DV 6: SV Student	RDV: M, R TI: M, R SV: T (M, R), S (M, R) G M: M, R	*NWF.* Substantial, lasting gains in word attack skills. *CWPM.* Improvements between baseline and intervention phases with 5 students improving into the postintervention phase. *TDB.* Decreases in TDB from baseline to intervention phases. *NSI.* All but 1 student showed decreases in NSI between baseline and interventions. Two improved into follow-up phases. *SV.* In general, favorable ratings.
Lane, Wehby, Menzies, Gregg, Doukas, & Munton (*ETC*, 2002)	N = 7; 4 males, 3 females; ages 6–8; grade 1; at risk; general education classroom	To examine the efficacy of a supplemental early literacy program for first-grade students at risk for antisocial behavior who were nonreponsive to a schoolwide literacy and behavioral intervention	John Shefelbine's *Phonics Chapter Books* General education class during the traditional school day	Multiple-baseline across groups A–Baseline B–Intervention, PATR C–Post D–Follow-up DV1: Nonsense word fluency (*NWF*) DV2: Oral reading fluency (*ORF*) DV3: Total disruptive behavior (*TDB*) DV4: Negative social interactions (*NSI*) DV5: Social Validity (SV) Teacher DV 6: SV Students	RDV: M, R TI: M, R SV: T (M, R), S (M, R) G: not mentioned M: M, R follow-up	*NWF.* Strong progress despite initial variability. *ORF.* Increased for all students who finished. *TDB.* Strong decreases between baseline and post phases for students who finished. Levels dropped to 0 in follow-up. *NSI.* All but 1 student showed decreases between baseline and post intervention phases. *SV.* Teacher ratings were mixed. Four students provided positive ratings.

(continued)

TABLE 24.1. (*continued*)

Author (Journal, year)	Participant characteristics and instructional setting	Purpose	Intervention and intervention setting	Research design and dependent variables	Components related to valid inference making	Outcomes
Locke & Fuchs (*JEBD*, 1995)	N = 3; male; age 11; grade 5; S1 SED; S1 SED; S1 SED; ADHD; ODD; self-contained classroom for children with BD in an urban general education middle school.	To examine the effects of peer-mediated instruction in the area of reading on task engagement and social interactions of students with BD educated in a self-contained classroom	Peer mediated instruction (PMI)— limited to partner reading; dyad points awarded for following procedures Self-contained class	ABAB withdrawal A–Baseline PMI–Training B–PMI-1 A–Withdrawal B–PMI DV1: *on-task* DV2: *positive interaction* (PI) DV3: *Social Validity* (SV)	RDV: M, R TI: informally SV: consumers (M, R) G: not mentioned M: not mentioned	*On-task*. On-task increased during treatment phases relative to baseline with high average percentage of nonoverlapping data points. *Positive interaction*. Mean PI levels were lower during withdrawal phases relative to treatment phases. *SV*. Significant differences for on-task and positive interactions.
McCurdy, Cundari, & Lentz (*ETC*, 1990)	N = 2; male; ages 8–9; grade NS; SED; private laboratory for children with behavior disorders	To examine the efficacy of two direct teaching strategies (time delay and trial-and-error) with opportunities to observe instruction	Trail-and-Error (TE) vs. Time Delay (TD); Direct Instruction (DI) vs. Observational Learning (OL); pennies for reinforcement Small office and two classrooms	Multiple-baseline design across paired word lists A–Baseline B–Instruction C–Maintenance DV1: *number of correct words read*	RDV: M, R TI: M, R SV: not mentioned G: not mentioned M: M, R	*Number of correct sight words read*. Few differences between strategies. Few differences in DI and OL phases, with DI yielding slightly better results. *Maintenance*. Maintained high levels of words read correctly for words learned in DI and OL phases.
Scott & Shearer-Lingo (*PSF*, 2002)	N = 3; male; age NS; grade 7; EBD class (label not assigned); self-contained middle school classroom.	To examine the effect of a repeated reading instruction strategy on the reading and task engagement of three middle school students with EBD.	Repeated readings using 2 programs: Teach Your Child to Read (TYC) and Great Leaps (GL); reinforcement provided to 1 student Classroom (n = 2) and library (n = 1)	Multiple-baseline across subjects A–Baseline B–TYC – 2 weeks C–GL DV1: *Oral reading fluency* DV2: *On-task*	RDV: M, R TI: M SV: not mentioned G: not mentioned M: not mentioned	*ORF*: Students showed the greatest gains during GL. *On-task*: Stable during baseline with slight improvement during TYC. Strong improvement (near 90%) during GL.
Skinner, Cooper, & Cole (*JABA*, 1997)[a]	N = 1; male; age 12; grade 5; BD; attending a school for students with behavior and learning disorders	To compare the effects of rapid and slow presentations on rates of accurate oral reading.	Listening preview presentation rates: rapid and slow oral presentation Small office at the school	Multielement design Baseline: silent previewing DV1: *Words correct per minute*	RDV: M, R TI: M, R SV: not mentioned G: not assessed M: not assessed	Listening previews result in greater increases in rates of accurate reading as compared to silent previewing, with the best results in the slow preview presentation.
Skinner, Johnson, Larkin, Lessley, & Glowacki (*JEBD*, 1995)	N = 3; 2 males, 1 female; ages 7–9; S1 (Charles) ADHD, ODD; S2 (Susan) ADHD, MMR; S3 nonspecific organic mental disorder with ADHD; residential school for children with EBD	To determine the effects of reading word lists with slow and fast presentation rates on reading accuracy and oral reading rates	Tape words; fast-taped words (FTW, 1 second); slow-taped words (STW, 5 seconds); assessment only (AO) S2 S3; intermittent assessment only (IAO) S1 Observation room adjacent to the classroom.	Adapted alternating = treatment design DV1: Number of *words read correctly* (WRC). DV2: number of *words read correctly per minute* (WRCPM) DV3: number of *seconds required to read word lists during assessments* (SRWL)	RDV: M, R TI: M, R SV: T (inferred) G: not mentioned M: M (S2 only)	FTW and STW yielded higher increases in accuracy and rates of accurate reading as compared to assessment conditions. STW produced greater increases DV1 & 2 reading compared to FTW for S1 and S3. S2 showed no difference in accuracy trends between FTW and STW. *Maintenance*: S2 Maintained increases across all word lists.

| Skinner, Smith, & McLean (*BD*, 1994). | *N* = 3, 2 males, 1 female; ages 9–11; grade NS; S1 EBD: ADHD, ODD, CD; S2 EBD, ADHD, ODD, CD; S3 EBD, CD + mild depressive disorders; private laboratory school for students with EBD | To compare the effects of immediate and 5-second intertrial intervals on sight-word mastery rates with three elementary students with BD and learning problems | Intertrail intervals (ITI) duration (immediate and 5-second delay); tangible reinforcers provided

Observation room adjacent to the students' classroom | Adapted alternating treatment design
A–Pretreatment
B–Intervention
C–Maintenance

DV1: number of *sight words* mastered | RDV: M, R
TI: M, R
SV: not mentioned
G: not mentioned
M: M, R | *Sight words.* Modeling treatments were more effective in increasing sight-word accuracy compared to the no treatment phase. There were no clear differences in sight-word acquisition rate in either ITI phase. *Maintenance.* Lasting increases in sight-word accuracy (12 weeks). |
| Spencer, Scruggs, & Mastropieri (*BD*, 2003) | *N* = 30; 70% male; ages, grade 7, male = 157.8 months; grade 8 males = 168.6 months; grades 7 (*n* = 12) and 8 (*n* = 18); ED, MH, or OHI; alternative middle school for students with EBD | To examine the effectiveness of an explicit strategy instruction (paragraph summary strategy) within a social studies class using peer tutoring with middle school students with EBD | Peer tutoring (social studies): Treatment 1: students served as peer tutors using a paragraph summary strategy Treatment 2: Traditional instruction

Classroom | Crossover design

DV1: *multiple-choice and open-ended chapter pre/posttests*
DV2: *weekly quizzes*
DV3: *summarization pre/posttests*
DV4: *time-on-task*
DV5: *student satisfaction* survey
DV6: *qualitative Measure* (teacher data) | RDV: M, R
TI: M
SV: T (M, R), S (M, R)
G: not mentioned
M: not mentioned | Resulted in improved achievement on *weekly quizzes* and *multiple-choice* tests and higher engaged *time-on-task*. Effects were not evident on *open-ended tests* or on *summary sentence or summary strategy.* *Survey and Qualitative Measures*: Most students and teachers rated peer tutoring favorably. |

Writing

| McLaughlin (*BD*, 1991) | *N* = 10; male; 10 years, 6 months, to 12 years, 8 months; elementary (grade level not specified); BD (by state and federal criteria); self-contained classroom. | To examine the effectiveness of personalized instruction (PSI) with and without same-day retakes in teaching spelling to students with BD | Personalized instruction with and without same-day retakes

Self-contained classroom | Single Case Design ABCABC
A–traditional,
B–PSI + no retakes,
C–PSI + retakes

DV1: *number of lessons passed* by entire class with 100%
DV2: *spelling* data for three student (high, middle, and lowest achieving)
DV3: *social validity* (SV) questionnaire | RDV: M, R
TI: M, R
SV: S (M, R)
G: not mentioned
M: not mentioned | PSI + no retakes resulted in the number of students *passing*. PSI + retakes resulted in further improvement (*M* = 6.2). Replication phases yielded similar results. Effects were true of· the high, medium, and low performing students. *SV*: students had strong preferences for PSI + retakes and rated their performance as best under the PSI + retakes. |

Mathematics

| Cade & Gunter (*BD*, 2002) | *N* = 3; male; ages 11–14; grade NS; SED; special day school for students with SED | To determine the effectiveness of a mnemonic to solve basic division calculations (divison-by-7 facts) with a student with EBD | Intervention: using a mnemonic to solve basic division fact calculations (seven songs and tapping drill)

Classroom at the special day school | Multiple-baseline across subjects using a multiple-probe technique.
A–Baseline
B–Mnemonic Training

DV1: *percentages* of response *correct* (PC) | RDV: M, R
TI: not assessed
SV: not mentioned
G: not mentioned
M: M, R (S1, S2 only) up to 6 days | Student's *PC* scores on division facts increased to 100% after two sessions. *Maintenance*: S1, S2 only. Skills maintained with respective PC scores of 100 and 96%. |

(continued)

TABLE 24.1. (*continued*)

Author (Journal, year)	Participant characteristics and instructional setting	Purpose	Intervention and intervention setting	Research design and dependent variables	Components related to valid inference making	Outcomes
Cybriwsky & Schuster (*RASE*, 1990)	N = 1; male; age 10; grade NS; BD; self-contained classroom for students with BD in an integrated public elementary school	To examine the effectiveness of time delay procedures in teaching 15 multiplication facts to a student with BD	Constant time-delay reinforcement system (bonus tickets) used during probe and training sessions. Sessions took place at a table in the front of the self-contained classroom	Multiple probe design across behaviors probe, training, maintenance DV1: *correct anticipation responses* DV2: *correct wait responses* DV3: *Percentage of Student Errors*	RDV: M, R TI: M, R SV: not mentioned G: M, R M: M, R	A 4-second constant time delay procedure resulted in increased correct responses and lower error rates (2.8%). *Maintenance*: Correct responding sustained 8 weeks and generalized to other settings, materials, and person.
Franca, Kerr, Reitz, & Lambert (*ETC*, 1990)	N = 8; male; ages 13–16; grade NS; middle school; ED/BD self-contained classroom in a private school for EBD students.	To examine the effectiveness of same-age peer tutoring (fractions) on the academic and social behavior of middle school students with BD.	Intervention: peer tutoring in fractions; social reinforcement Self-contained classroom	Multiple-baseline across 4 tutor–tutee dyads. DV1: *Correct rate (CR)* DV2: *Error rate (ER)*. DV3: *Sociometric status* DV4: *Self-concept* DV5: *Attitude toward math* (pre-post) DV6: *Social interaction* (positive, PSI, and negative, NSI, verbal interactions between tutor and tutee)	RDV: M, R TI: M, R (informally) SV: T (not mentioned) S (M, R) G: not mentioned M: M, R (social interactions of Dyads 1 and 2) Follow-up	Increased CR and decreased ER for tutors and tutees. Few changes in *sociometric status*. *Self-concept* results inconsistent. Small positive changes in some tutors' scores. Tutees and tutors showed improved *attitude toward math*. Significant increases in PSI and fewer NSI between tutors and tutees. *Maintenance.* Tutors held PSI and NSI levels. *Social Validity*: Favorable.
Harper, Mallette, Maheady, Bentley, & Moore (*JBE*, 1995)[b]	N = 1; age 9; grades 3–5; grade NS for ED; 1 with ED; self-contained classroom for children with mild disabilities.	To examine the effectiveness of classwide peer tutoring in increasing the rate and accuracy of acquiring 100 subtraction items with students with mild disabilities	Classwide peer tutoring; reinforced with daily point earning and public display Resource room	Alternating treatment design (variant) DV1: *accuracy of responding* weekly quiz DV2: *short-term maintenance* (1 week) DV3: *long-term maintenance* (17 days) DV4: *rate of accurate responding* DV5: *student satisfaction* (SV)	RDV: M, R TI: M, R (R - inferred) SV: T (not mentioned) S (M, R) G: not mentioned M: M, R	Subtraction accuracy was 47%. This student showed 99% at post test and 100% retention at both short- and long-term data collection points. *Accurate responding*: only class averages available—students showed improvements. *SV.* All students reported that CWPT was helpful socially and academically.
Jolivette, Wehby, & Hirsch (*BD*, 1999)	N = 3; male; ages 9–10; grade NS; S1 ADHD; S2 Autism; S3 EBD; self-contained summer school class for students receiving services for EBD	To examine the effects of an academic strategy identification procedure that addresses computation skills and strategy usage	Intervention: three instructional strategies directly linked to results of a structural analysis of the task-related skills were designed for each student; no reinforcement In class	Design: Strategy testing, replication, strategy implementation, probe DV1: *Accuracy of math responses* (percentage of correct responses) on math worksheets.	RDV: M, R TI: M, R SV: not mentioned G: not mentioned M: not mentioned	Each student's accuracy percentages increased with the introduction of the identified strategies.
Lee, Sugai, & Horner (*JPBI*, 1999)	N = 2; male; age 9; grade 3; S1 EBD + learning problems; S2 EBD + ADHD; S1 self-contained classroom; S2 resource room; special education classroom for special education	To determine the effects of using instruction in component skills designed to increase task accuracy on the occurrence of problem and off-task behaviors demonstrated by 2 students with EBD.	Intervention: individualized component skills instruction for the first and second set of difficult tasks; no reinforcement Special education classroom.	A-B-A within-subject reversal. Instructional Analysis: C1-A-C2-A-C3-A or C1-A-C2-A within-subject alternating treatment designs DV1: *Problem behavior* DV2: *Off-task behaviors* DV3: *Percentage of correct answers*	RDV: M, R TI: not mentioned SV: T (M, R), S (not mentioned) G: not mentioned M: not mentioned	When instruction in component skills was introduced on difficult tasks, increases in performance were observed along with reductions in escape-motivated, off-task, and problem behaviors.

Lee & Zentall (*BD*, 2002)	Study 1 N = 17; 16 male, 1 female; ages 8–14 years; grade NS; ADHD + ODD/CD Study 2 N = 17; 16 males, 1 female; ADHD + ODD/CD; two private urban schools for children with BD serving students ages 8 to 14	To examine the effects of within-task stimulation and competing visual stimulation on the mathematics performance and behavior of students with ADHD and behavioral concerns	Study 1: within-task stimulation; low within-task stimulation (LWS) and high within-task stimulation (HWS) (single-digit addition problems) Study 2: Competing visual stimulation; same as above plus low-competing stimulation (LCS) and high-competing stimulation (HCS) Office or conference room.	Study 1 Counterbalanced design (group) DV1: *number of problems attempted* DV2: *number of problems completed correctly* DV3: *Talking/noise making* DV4: *Visually off task* DV5: *Torso movement* DV6: *Limb movement* Study 2 Same as above, plus DV7: *Looks to competing stimulation monitor.*	Study 1 RDV: M, R TI: not mentioned SV: not mentioned G: not mentioned M: not mentioned Study 2 RDV: M, R TI: not mentioned SV: not mentioned G: not mentioned M: not mentioned	Study 1: Completed more problems and more problems correctly with HWS condition relative to LWS condition. DV3, DV4, and DV5 were higher in LWS than HWS. Order effects: more DV3, DV4, and DV5 when students received HWS prior to LWS. Study 2: Completed more problems and more problems correctly in the LCS than in the HCS conditions. DV7 higher in HCS than LCS conditions. Order effects: students with LCS condition on day 1 showed less DV5 than those with HCS first.
McWhirter & Bloom (*BD*, 1994)	N = 3; male; ages 11–15; grades 6-8, middle school; behaviorally and emotionally handicapped; self-contained intensive intervention public classroom.	To examine the effects of a student-operated business curriculum on on-task behavior of middle school students with BD	Intervention: business-related math intervention; ongoing classroom management program, which included a reinforcement component In the classroom	Single-subject ABAB design A–Baseline B–Business-related math intervention DV1: *On-task behavior* (+/-)	RDV: M, R TI: not mentioned SV: T (M, R), S (not mentioned) G: not mentioned M: not mentioned	On-task behavior increased for all students during the intervention phase. On-task behavior decreased in the return to baseline phase and substantially increased once the intervention was reintroduced.
Nelson, Johnson, & Marchand-Martella (*JEBD*, 1996)	N = 4; male; ages 8–9; grade 3; BD; enrolled in self-contained behavior intervention classroom under the school-related eligibility criteria for BD; mainstreamed for the entire school year	To compare the effectiveness of direct instruction, cooperative learning, and independent learning instructional practices on the on-task and disruptive behavior of elementary students with BD	Intervention: comparing direct instruction, cooperative learning, and independent learning in mathematics (content areas in math were also presented randomly) Experimental elementary classroom	Design: alternating treatments design in which conditions were presented in randomized order DV1: *On-task* DV2: *Disruptive behavior*	RDV: M, R TI: during training, not during intervention SV: not mentioned G: not mentioned M: not mentioned	Higher rates of on-task and lower rates of disruption during DI relative to CL and IL. Minimal overlap in data between DI and CL or IL conditions. Considerable overlap on both DVs between CL and IL.
Skinner, Ford, & Yunker (*BD*, 1991)	N = 2; male; ages 9–11; grade NS; BD; university-affiliated residential school for students with behavioral disorders	To explore the interaction between topography (written and verbal response) and the rates or numbers of responses occasioned by an academic intervention	Intervention: cover, copy, compare with verbal (VCCC) or written responses (WCCC) required (multiplication); reinforcement (stickers) for participation Testing room or empty classroom	Adapted alternating treatment design, baseline intervention; WCCC, VCCC, and NT were implemented in random order during each session DV1: *number of digits correct* per minute DV2: *Percentage of problems correct*	RDV: M, R TI: during training SV: not assessed G: not assessed M: not assessed	VCCC condition resulted in greater fluency and accuracy of multiplication facts than WCCC or NT across the last nine intervention sessions

Note. Only data for students with ED are reported.

Grade: NS, not specified. *Journal Titles: BD, Behavioral Disorders; ETC, Education and Treatment of Children; JABA, Journal of Applied Behavior Analysis; JBE, Journal of Behavioral Education; JEBD, Journal of Emotional and Behavioral Disorders; PSF, Preventing School Failure; JPBI, Journal of Positive Behavior Interventions; RASE, Remedial and Special Education; Labels: ADHD,* attention-deficit/hyperactivity disorder; *BD,* behavioral disorder; *CD,* conduct disorder; *EBD,* emotional and behavioral disorders; *ED,* emotional disorder; *MMR,* mild mental retardation; *ODD,* oppositional defiant disorder; *SED,* serious emotional disorder; *SL,* speech–language disorder; *SLD,* specific learning disability. OHI = other health impaired S1, subject 1 (etc.). DV, dependent variables. *Components: RDV,* reliability of the dependent variables; *TI,* treatment integrity; *SV,* social validity; *T,* teacher; *S,* student; *G,* generalization; *M,* maintenance. *Categories: M,* mentioned; *R,* reported.

[a] Only data for students with behavioral concerns are reported.

[b] Data only reported for ED; other 7 students' data not reported.

Scott & Shearer-Lingo, 2002; Spencer, Scruggs, & Mastropieri, 2003), 10 in elementary schools, and 1 was not specified (Skinner, Cooper, & Cole, 1997). Seventy-four percent of the students ($n = 91$) were male and 26% ($n = 33$) female. Fifty-three students (41%) were identified by their teachers as at risk for emotional and behavioral disorders; 5 (4%) had an emotional disturbance (formerly "seriously emotionally disturbed"), as specified in IDEA; 1 (%) had an emotional disturbance or psychiatric conduct problem (e.g., conduct disorder or oppositional defiant disorder) and ADHD; 25 (20%) had a label of emotional and behavioral disorder (or behavioral disorder); 14 (11%) had a label of EBD and an educational (e.g., learning disability or speech and language impairment) or psychiatric (e.g., conduct disorder or oppositional defiant disorder) problem; and 30 (23%) had the ED only or EBD + educational or psychiatric label (however, the exact numbers of students in each category were not specified; see Spencer et al., 2003). In some instances, the student's classification was inferred. For example, in Cochran et al. (1993), Scott and Shearer-Lingo (2002), Skinner et al. (1997), and Skinner et al.'s (1994) studies, the authors did not explicitly state that the students had behavioral disorders; however, they stated that students were receiving their education in a self-contained classroom for students with EBD.

Students were in a variety of education settings, ranging from general education classrooms (53 students; Lane, 1999; Lane, O'Shaughnessy, et al., 2001; Lane, Wehby, et al., 2002), resource rooms (4 students; Dawson, Venn, & Gunter, 2000), self-contained rooms in a general education school (9 students; Falk & Wehby, 2001; Locke & Fuchs, 1995), day schools serving EBD populations (56 students; Babyak, Koorland, & Mathes, 2000; Cochran et al., 1993; McCurdy et al., 1990; Skinner et al., 1997; Skinner et al., 1994; Spencer et al., 2003), and residential schools for students with behavioral disorders (3 students; Skinner, Johnson, Larkin, Lessley, & Glowacki, 1995). In one instance (Scott & Shearer-Lingo, 2002), it was not possible to determine if students were in a self-contained classroom at a general education school or in a self-contained classroom at a special education school.

Interventions: Focus and Settings

Four studies (Cochran et al., 1993; Falk & Wehby, 2001; Locke & Fuchs, 1995; Spencer et al., 2003) focused on peer-tutoring interventions, and four examined the utility of specific curricular programs such as Phonological Awareness Training for Reading (Lane, 1999; Lane, O'Shaughnessy, et al., 2001), John Shefelbine's *Phonics Chapter Books* (Lane, Wehby, et al., 2002), and Teach Your Child to Read in 100 Easy Lessons and Great Leaps (Scott & Shearer-Lingo, 2002). The remaining studies explored the effects of story mapping (Babyak et al., 2000), reading previews (Dawson et al., 2000), listening previews (Skinner et al., 1997), trial-and-error and time-delay procedures (McCurdy et al., 1990), taped words (Skinner et al., 1995), and intertrial intervals (Skinner et al., 1994).

Intervention intensity, or dosage, was explicitly stated in three studies (Lane, 1999; Lane, O'Shaughnessy, et al., 2001; Lane, Wehby, et al., 2002), inferred in three studies (Babyak et al., 2000; Cochran et al., 1993; Locke & Fuchs, 1995), and, in the remaining studies, could not be determined, given insufficient information regarding the number, length, or frequency of intervention sessions. From the information available, interventions ranged in length from less than 5 hours (Locke & Fuchs, 1995) to 15–17 hours in instructional time (Babyak et al., 2000; Cochran et al., 1993; Lane, O'Shaughnessy, et al., 2001; Lane, Wehby, et al., 2002).

The majority of the studies ($n = 8$) were conducted in settings other than the existing classroom, with sessions conducted in separate classrooms (Babyak et al., 2000), the library (Cochran et al., 1993), conference rooms or offices (Lane, O'Shaughnessy, et al., 2001; Skinner et al., 1997), and observation rooms (Skinner et al., 1995, Skinner et al., 1994). Five studies conducted the intervention in the student's classroom, and one study (Scott & Shearer-Lingo, 2002) conducted some sessions in the library and others in the classroom.

Research Design and Dependent Variables

As was the case in the Coleman and Vaughn (2000) review, the majority of the studies employed single-case methodologies ($n = 12$). Specific designs included multiple baseline (n = 6; Babyak et al., 2000; Falk & Wehby, 2001; Lane, O'Shaughnessy, et al., 2001; Lane, Wehby, et al., 2002; McCurdy et al., 1990; Scott & Shearer-Lingo, 2002), alternating treatments (n = 3; Dawson et al., 2000; Skinner et al., 1995; Skinner et al., 1994), withdrawal (n = 1; Locke & Fuchs, 1995), cross-over (n = 1; Spencer et al., 2003), and multielement (n = 1; Skinner et al., 1997) designs. Two studies used group methodologies ranging from descriptive (Cochran et al., 1993) to multivariate procedures (Lane, 1999) to examine group differences.

Outcome variables included academic, behavioral, and social domains, including reading probes (e.g., letter naming, sight words, story retells, passage comprehension, number of words read correctly), direct observations of student behavior (e.g., task engagement, disruptive behavior, and social interactions), rating scales (teacher and parent perspectives; Cochran et al., 1993), and standardized measures of reading performance (e.g., Test of Phonological Awareness; Lane, 1999; Lane, O'Shaughnessy, et al., 2001; Lane, 2003). Several studies addressed only academic measures such as percentage of sight words correct, comprehension passages, and oral reading fluency (Babyak et al., 2000; Dawson et al., 2000; Falk & Wehby, 2001; McCurdy et al., 1990; Skinner et al., 1997; Skinner et al., 1995; Skinner et al., 1994), whereas one study monitored only sociobehavioral measures such as on-task behavior, disruptive behavior, or social engagement (Locke & Fuchs, 1995). Some studies assessed a combination of variables such as (1) sight words, behavior ratings, and direct observation of cooperative statements (Cochran et al., 1993); (2) early literacy probes and direct observations of behavior (Lane, O'Shaughnessy, et al., 2001; Lane, Wehby, et al., 2002); (3) oral reading fluency and on-task behaviors (Scott & Shearer-Lingo, 2002); and (4) weekly quizzes, pre- and postmeasures, and on-task behavior (Spencer et al., 2003).

Components Related to Valid Inference Making

To draw valid inferences about intervention outcomes, it is essential that certain components be included in intervention design and implementation. These components include reliability of the dependent variables, integrity of the independent variables (Gresham, 1989), social validity, and generalization and maintenance (Lane & Beebe-Frankenberger, 2004). As expected, all 14 studies (100%) mentioned and reported the reliability of the dependent variables. However, only 12 studies (86%) mentioned treatment integrity, and only 10 studies (71%) actually reported levels of implementation (one of which reported informal observations; Locke & Fuchs, 1995).

All but five studies (Falk & Wehby, 2001; McCurdy et al., 1990; Scott & Shearer-Lingo, 2002; Skinner et al., 1997; Skinner et al., 1994) assessed social validity from teacher, student, or parent perspectives. Eight studies assessed social validity from the teacher perspective; however, only seven studies reported the outcomes. Of these eight studies, six also mentioned and reported social validity outcomes from the students' perspectives, and one also mentioned and reported social validity from consumer perspectives (Babyak et al., 2000). Locke and Fuchs (1995) also assessed and reported social validity from the consumer perspective.

Seven studies mentioned and reported maintenance data on one or more participants. None of the studies assessed generalization of responses, behaviors, or settings. Only four studies (Lane, 1999; Lane, O'Shaughnessy, et al., 2001; Lane, Wehby, et al., 2002; Skinner et al., 1995) included all components.

Outcomes

Despite the limited pool of reading interventions (n = 14), academic instruction in reading resulted in improved reading skills and, in several instances, improved behaviors. Although space does not permit a detailed synopsis of each study, a brief analysis of studies follows.

Results of the peer tutoring studies reviewed indicate that peer tutoring interventions involving cross-age (Cochran et al., 1993) and same-age (Falk & Wehby, 2001; Locke & Fuchs, 1995; Spencer et al., 2003) peers produced increases in sight words (Cochran et al., 1993), letter-sound naming (Falk & Wehby, 2001), blending (Falk & Wehby, 2001), and chapter quizzes before and after the intervention (Spencer et al.,

2003). In addition to improved academic skills, tutors and tutees also exhibited higher levels of task engagement (Locke & Fuchs, 1995; Spencer et al., 2003) and cooperative statements (Cochran et al., 1993). While peer tutoring did not always results in equal gains for tutors and tutees (Cochran et al., 1993), social validity outcomes suggest that peer tutoring is generally rated favorably by teachers, students (Cochran et al., 1993; Spencer et al., 2003), and consumers (Locke & Fuchs, 1995).

Three of the four studies examining the effectiveness of specific curricular programs resulted in improved early literacy skills (Lane, O'Shaughnessy, et al., 2001; Lane, Wehby, et al., 2002; Scott & Shearer-Lingo, 2002), lower levels of disruptive behavior in the classroom (Lane, O'Shaughnessy, et al., 2001; Lane, Wehby, et al., 2002), improved social interactions on the playground (Lane, O'Shaughnessy, et al., 2001; Lane, Wehby, et al., 2002); and higher levels of task engagement (Scott & Shearer-Lingo, 2002). All but one study (Lane, 1999) showed relatively strong effects.

Only one study (Babyak et al., 2000) explored the effects of story mapping on reading comprehension. The 17-hour intervention was effective in improving the reading skills of all 4 participants, as measured by story retells and passage comprehension measures. Although little movement was observed on the main idea probes, students rated the intervention favorably.

The remaining studies examined the effects of reading previews (Dawson et al., 2000), listening previews (Skinner et al., 1997), trial-and-error and time-delay procedures (McCurdy et al., 1990), taped words (Skinner et al., 1995), and intertrial intervals (Skinner et al., 1994) on improving reading fluency and accuracy. In brief, teacher models resulted in students reading more words correctly as compared to computer models and no model conditions. However, computer models resulted in a higher mean number of correct words read and percentage of words read correctly than the no-modeling condition (Dawson et al., 2000). Thus, this study speaks to the effectiveness of modeling, whether teacher- or computer-delivered, on reading performance of students with EBD. Listening previews produced higher rates of reading accuracy relative to silent previewing. Further, the mean number of

words correct was higher and the mean error rates were lower in the slow preview condition in comparison to the rapid oral presentation (Skinner et al., 1997). Listening to fast and slow taped words yielded higher improvements in accuracy and rates of accurate reading related to assessment-only conditions (Skinner et al., 1995), with two of the three subjects performing better in the slow taped word condition. Immediate and 5-second delay intertrial intervals (Skinner et al., 1994) were more successful in increasing sight words mastered, compared to the no-treatment condition. Both ITI conditions resulted in lasting (12-week) increases in sight word accuracy.

Collectively, these studies were largely effective in fulfilling the intended purposes, as evidenced by the desired changes in the academic variables selected to monitor student progress. In several studies, collateral effects on behavioral and social interaction measures were evident (Cochran et al., 1993; Lane, O'Shaughnessy, et al., 2001; Lane, Wehby, et al., 2002; Locke & Fuchs, 1995; Scott & Shearer-Lingo, 2002). However, this body of literature has limitations.

Limitations

As evidenced above, the research base of empirically validated methods of providing reading instruction to students with and at risk for EBD is sparse. This is particularly disturbing given that reading is a keystone skill that permits or restricts access to all other learning (Adams, 1990; O'Shaughnessy et al., 2003; Walker et al., 1995; Walker & Severson, 2002). The majority of the studies focus on intervening at the elementary level ($n = 10$), with little attention to middle school efforts ($n = 3$). Although the interventions produced favorable outcomes for the student participants, a number of limitations are evident. Specifically, these limitations include (1) a paucity of students with a total absence of reading treatment-outcome studies at the high school level; (2) limited research conducted in the existing classroom context; (3) narrow content scope, often of brief duration, with most investigations addressing phonetic skills and sight word acquisition and only one study focusing on comprehension skills (Babyak et al., 2000); (4) designs that lack the components necessary to draw accurate conclusions about intervention outcomes (Lane, Beebe-Franken-berger, et al., 2001); (5) outcome measures also of narrow scope; (6) reports that provide insufficient information to determine intervention intensity; and (7) limited replications. These limitations will be discussed in more detail, and recommendations to address these limitations will be provided in the final section of this chapter, "Recommendations."

Writing

Academic interventions targeting written expression of students with or at risk for EBD represent, by far, the least developed instructional area of the three examined in this chapter. Of the five articles identified for possible inclusion, only one article met all inclusion criteria (McLaughlin, 1992). Although Hogan and Prater (1993) examined the effects of peer tutoring on spelling and vocabulary, the intervention also included a self-management component, making it impossible to examine the isolated effects of peer tutoring on on-task, academic, and disruptive behavior. Glomb and West (1990) also examined the effects of a self-management procedure (WATCH) on the thoroughness, accuracy, and neatness of adolescent students' creative writing assignments. Edwards and Chard (2000) examined the effects of systematic instruction in story elements and narrative summary writing on the writing skills and academic engagement of 22 students with EBD ranging in age from 11 to 16 years. However, the study was excluded, as explicit student outcome data were not presented. Only a general narrative description of student outcomes was provided.

McLaughlin (1992) examined the effects of a personalized system of instruction (PSI) with and without a same-day retake component on the spelling performance of 10 elementary-age male students with behavioral disorders. The 45-minute instructional block took place in a self-contained classroom. Students worked at their own rate, receiving tutoring from a teacher or student who had mastered the material. Posttests were recorded on cassette tapes for use in the listening centers on Fridays. Single-case methodology, an A-B-C-A-B-C design, was used to evaluate student outcomes. Results indicated that more spelling tests were passed by the entire class with 100% accuracy when PSI was in place. The number of lessons passed by the entire class increased even further when retakes were permitted. These effects were true of high-, medium-, and low-performing students ($n = 3$). Social validity data, which were collected from the student perspective, indicated that students preferred PSI + retakes to PSI alone and baseline conditions. Further, they indicated that they performed best under the PSI + retakes condition. This study was limited by an absence of treatment integrity and generalization data.

Limitations

Writing has the potential to serve as an important expressive skill for students with or at risk for EBD (Tindal & Crawford, 2002). Specifically, writing could provide these youngsters with a socially appropriate method of obtaining recognition and expressing their thoughts, which, in turn, may serve as an appropriate replacement behavior to other less desirable methods of communication (e.g., verbal and physical aggression). Tindal and Crawford (2002) suggest that writing be viewed in a social context with attention to the purpose, audience, and type of discourse. As such, writing could be used as an important medium to teach students with or at risk for EBD. It is imperative that additional treatment outcome studies be conducted to explore the instructional and behavioral outcomes associated with improved written expression skills, ranging from basic production (e.g., spelling) to more sophisticated forms of writing (e.g., compositions). Further, future investigations need to include design features and components necessary to draw valid inferences about intervention outcomes.

Mathematics

Participant Characteristics

Half of the 10 articles predated the 1997 reauthorization of the IDEA, whereas the remaining articles were published between 1999 and 2000. The 10 articles contained 11 studies and included 61 participants ranging in age from 8 to 16 years old. Two studies were conducted in middle schools (Franca, Kerr, Reitz, & Lambert, 1990;

McWhirter & Bloom, 1994), six in elementary schools (Cade & Gunter, 2002; Cybriwsky & Schuster, 1990; Harper et al., 1995; Jolivette, Wehby, & Hirsch, 1999; Lee et al., 1999; Nelson, Johnson, & Marchand-Maretella, 1996), and three studies did not specify school level (Lee & Zentall, 2002; Skinner, Ford, & Yunker, 1991). Ninety-five percent of the students ($n = 58$) were male and 3% ($n = 2$) were female (note: In one study [Harper et al., 1995]), gender was not reported for the student with ED). None of the students was identified by his or her teachers as being at risk for emotional and behavioral disorders; 4 (7%) had an emotional disturbance (formerly "seriously emotionally disturbed") as specified in IDEA prior to the 1997 reauthorization; 34 (56%) had an emotional disturbance or psychiatric conduct problem (e.g., conduct disorder or oppositional defiant disorder) and ADHD; 19 (31%) had a label of emotional and behavioral disorder (or behavioral disorder); 3 (5%) had a label of EBD and an educational (e.g., learning disability or speech and language impairment) or psychiatric (e.g., conduct disorder or oppositional defiant disorder) problem; and 1 (2%) was in the behavioral concern with ADHD category. In some instances, the student's classification was inferred. For example, Cybriwsky and Schuster (1990) stated that the students were placed in a self-contained classroom for students with BD in an integrated public elementary school. Franca et al. (1990) stated that students were in a self-contained classroom in a private school for "emotionally disturbed/behavioral disordered students" (p. 111).

Students were in relatively restrictive settings as compared to those in the reading interventions. Ten studies were conducted in self-contained classrooms, half of which were in self-contained schools (Cade & Gunter, 2002; Franca et al., 1990; Jolivette et al., 1999; Lee & Zentall, 2002) and one in a residential school serving students with behavioral disorders (Skinner et al., 1991).

Interventions: Focus and Settings

Two studies (Franca et al., 1990; Harper et al., 1995) focused on peer-tutoring interventions, both of which involved same-age peers. Five studies examined the effectiveness of specific strategies, including (1) mnemonics to teach "sevens" division facts (Cade & Gunter, 2002); (2) structural analysis-derived strategies, Say It Before You Do It and Permanent Model, to teach computational skills (Jolivette et al., 1999); (3) cover, copy, and compare with verbal and written responses to teach multiplication facts (Skinner et al., 1991); (4) individualized component skills instruction to teach unknown skills in addition, subtraction, and multiplication operations (Lee et al., 1999); and (5) direct instruction, cooperative learning, and independent learning to teach multiplication, visual patterns, and numerical patterns (Nelson et al., 1996).

Two studies by Lee and Zentall (2002) examined the effects of low and high within-task stimulation (Study 1) as well as the additive effects of low and high competing stimuli (Study 2) in teaching single-digit addition problems. The remaining two studies explored the effects of constant time delay (zero versus 4-second delay) in teaching multiplication facts (Cybriwsky & Schuster, 1990) and the impact of a business-related math intervention on task engagement (McWhirter & Bloom, 1994).

Intervention intensity, or dosage, was explicitly stated in one study (Cybriwsky & Schuster, 1990). Six studies (Franca et al., 1990; Jolivette et al., 1999; Lee & Zentall, 2002; McWhirter & Bloom, 1994; Nelson et al., 1996; Skinner et al., 1991) provided enough information to compute the total duration of interventions. The remaining studies lacked the requisite information (e.g., number, length, or frequency of intervention treatment time) or included a range of information (e.g., intervention lasted 20–35 minutes) making it impossible to determine exact intervention intensity. From the information available, interventions ranged in length from less than 1 hour (Skinner et al., 1991) to approximately 9 hours (McWhirter & Bloom, 1994).

Four of the studies were conducted in settings other than the instructional setting with sessions conducted in a work area outside of the classroom (Cade & Gunter, 2002), office or conference room (Lee & Zentall, 2002), or a testing room or empty classroom (Skinner et al., 1991). The remaining studies were conducted in the actual classrooms.

Research Design and Dependent Variables

All but two studies (Lee & Zentall, 2002) employed single-case methodologies (n = 10). The most common methodologies were alternating treatment (n = 4; Harper et al., 1995; Lee et al., 1999; Nelson et al., 1996; Skinner et al., 1991) and multiple baseline (n = 2; Cade & Gunter, 2002; Franca et al., 1990) followed by withdrawal, rapid reversal, and multiple probe designs. The two group design studies used counterbalanced designs (Lee & Zentall, 2002).

Outcome variables included academic, behavioral, and social domains such as (1) Percentage of correct responses (Cade & Gunter, 2002; Cybriwsky & Schuster, 1990; Franca et al., 1990; Harper et al., 1995; Jolivette et al., 1999; Lee et al., 1999; Skinner et al., 1991); (2) Percentage of errors (Cybriwsky & Schuster, 1990; Franca et al., 1990); (3) Sociometric, self-concept, and attitudinal measures (Franca et al., 1990); (4) Body movement (Lee & Zentall, 2002); (5) Task engagement (Lee et al., 1999; McWhirter & Bloom, 1994; Nelson et al., 1996); and (6) Disruptive behavior (Nelson et al., 1996).

The majority of the studies assessed only academic behaviors. However, four studies addressed academic performance and sociobehavioral outcomes (e.g., Franca et al., 1990; Lee et al., 1999; Lee & Zentall, 2002). Two studies (McWhirter & Bloom, 1994; Nelson et al., 1996) did not monitor academic performance. Instead, they assessed task engagement, an academic-related behavior.

Components Related to Valid Inference Making

As with the reading and writing interventions, all studies (n = 11; 100%) mentioned and reported the reliability of the dependent variables. However, only four studies (36%) mentioned and reported treatment integrity, one of which did so informally (Franca et al., 1990). Cade and Gunter (2002) and Nelson and colleagues (1996) mentioned that the absence of treatment integrity during intervention implementation was a limitation of their investigations. Skinner et al. (1991) and Nelson et al. (1996) did assess procedural integrity during the training phase. Four studies assessed and reported social validity, with two studies assessing it from the teacher's perspective (Lee et al., 1999; McWhirter & Bloom, 1994) and two from the student's perspective (Franca et al., 1990; Harper et al., 1995). Four studies mentioned and reported maintenance data on one or more participants (Cade & Gunter, 2002; Cybriwsky & Schuster, 1990; Franca et al., 1990; Harper et al., 1995), one of which also included generalization data (Cybriwsky & Schuter, 1990). Only three studies included treatment integrity, social validity, and maintenance components (Cybriwsky & Schuster, 1990; Franca et al., 1990; Harper et al., 1995).

Outcomes

The scope of mathematical interventions, like reading interventions, was limited. However, the outcomes were favorable. Peer-tutoring studies resulted in academic gains, as evidenced by higher levels of correct responding (Franca et al., 1990; Harper et al., 1995). Franca and colleagues (1990) reported increased correct rates and decreased incorrect rates for both tutor's and tutee's fraction worksheets. However, changes in sociometric status were mixed with minimal changes observed. Data suggest that tutors, as compared to tutees, may have gained more prestige from classmates. Similar findings were observed on self-concept ratings. However, tutors and tutees showed improved attitude toward math from baseline to intervention phases. Social validity data indicated that students would have preferred to switch roles. Results of Harper and colleagues' (1995) study of classwide peer tutoring (CWPT) indicated that CWPT was effective in improving accuracy of responding on weekly subtraction quizzes. The one student with ED scored 99% accuracy during posttesting and 100% retention during short-term and long-term maintenance data collection phases. All students rated CWPT favorably.

Studies focusing on specific strategies also produced desired outcomes. Cade and Gunter's (2002) use of musical mnemonics to teach "sevens" division facts increased the percentage of correct division facts computed on independent work samples, with scores increasing to 100% after two sessions. Two studies for which maintenance data were collected experienced strong retention of skills, with percentage correct scores of 100% and 96%.

Jolivette and colleagues (1999) used structural analysis of task-related skills (e.g., direct observation, preference assessment, and error analysis) to identify strategies to teach computational skills. The identified strategies, Say It Before You Do It (*n* = 1) and Permanent Model (*n* = 2), resulted in improved accuracy of math responses on worksheets. However, the authors indicated that it was difficult to determine strategy usage in the absence of visible or verbal repeated cues.

Skinner et al. (1991) examined the relationship between topography and number of responses occasioned by a cover, copy, and compare (CCC) intervention. CCC with verbal responses (VCCC) resulted in higher fluency and accuracy of multiplication facts than CCC with a written response (WCCC) or the no-treatment condition over the last nine sessions. VCCC resulted in more than twice the number of correct responses relative to WCCC for two students.

Lee et al. (1999) employed individualized component skills instruction to teach unknown skills in addition, subtraction, and multiplication operations to three third-grade students. Instruction in component skills resulted in increased percentage of correct math problems as well as decreased percentage of intervals with problem and off-task behaviors.

Nelson et al. (1996) compared the effectiveness of direct instruction (DI), cooperative learning (CL), and independent learning (IL) in teaching multiplication, visual patterns, and numerical patterns on-task engagement and disruptive behavior of elementary-age students with BD. Results suggest clear behavioral differences between conditions with higher levels of task engagement and lower levels of disruption during DI as compared to CL and IL. One limitation of this study is the absence of data to determine academic performance levels.

The remaining studies focused on stimulation, timing, and curricular interventions. Lee and Zentall (2002) examined the effects

of low and high within task stimulation (study 1) as well as the additive effects of low and high competing stimuli (study 2) in teaching single-digit addition problems. Results of study 1 suggested that students completed more problems and more problems accurately in the high within-task stimulation (HWS) condition than in the low within-in-task stimulation (LWS). Movement, talking, and visual off-task behaviors were lower in the LWS than in the HWS condition. Order effects indicated that behavioral levels were higher when students received LWS after HWS. Results of study 2 revealed that students completed more problems and more problems correctly in the low competing visual stimulation (LCS) condition than in the high competing stimulus (HCS) condition. Students glanced at the competing stimulation monitor less frequently in the LCS than in the HCS. Order effects indicated less torso movement with students in the LCS phase than those students who were in the HCS on day 1.

Cybriwsky and Schuster (1990) examined the impact of time-delay procedures in teaching 15 multiplication facts to a 10-year-old student with BD. Results suggest that a 4-second constant time-delay procedure was effective in teaching unknown multiplication facts within approximately 1 hour of instruction. In addition, the intervention was associated with low error rates. Results were maintained over an 8-week period and generalized to other environments, materials, and persons.

McWhirter and Bloom (1994) evaluated the effects of a student-operated business curriculum on task engagement. Findings of a withdrawal design revealed higher levels of on-task behavior for all students during the intervention phases relative to baseline.

In general, these studies resulted in improved academic skills and in one instance (e.g., Franca et al., 1990) resulted in collateral effects in socio-behavioral measures. However, this body of work has several of the limitations noted in the reading instruction literature.

Limitations

As with the case of reading instruction, few treatment-outcome studies exploring mathematics instruction were identified. Again, the majority of the studies focused on elementary-age students ($n = 6$), with few studies of students at the middle school level ($n = 2$) and no investigations at the high school level. Participants were predominantly male, and the interventions demonstrated, for the most part, the desired changes in the dependent measures. Still, similar limitations persist, including (1) an absence of investigations with high school students, (2) strong focus on base skills (e.g., addition, subtraction, multiplication, and division facts), with no attention to applied problem solving skills, (3) designs that did not include components such as treatment integrity, social validity, and generalization and maintenance, (4) narrowly defined outcome measures, (5) lack of information regarding actual intervention duration, and (6) limited replications.

RECOMMENDATIONS

Students with and at risk for EBD, by definition, are characterized by maladaptive behavior patterns, limited social skills, and academic underachievement. To date, most treatment-outcome studies with this population have focused on the behavioral and social domains. This lack of attention to academic issues is alarming, considering that students with EBD show moderate to severe academic deficits relative to typically developing peers (Greenbaum et al., 1996; Mattison et al., 1998) and may have more academic deficits relative to students with other high-incidence disabilities (e.g., LD), although results of the latter point are inconclusive. Of further concern is the fact that academic deficits, like externalizing behavior patterns, do not appear to improve over time in the absence of intervention efforts (Greenbaum et al., 1996; Nelson et al., in press).

This chapter reviewed the literature pertaining to academic interventions in the areas of reading, written expression, and mathematical skills as conducted with students with EBD. Treatment-outcome studies of reading, writing, and mathematical instruction for students with and at risk for EBD conducted to date have provided a

solid foundation from which to launch additional inquiries. However, the following limitations were noted: population focus, breadth issues (population, replication, content scope), design features (components related to valid inference making, outcome measures), and reporting (dosage, implications for replication).

Population Focus

In the field of EBD we have a variety of terms representing psychiatric (ODD, CD), educational (ED), and research-related communities (BD, EBD, externalizing, and internalizing; Kauffman, 2001). This lack of continuity of terminology poses challenges in many areas, such as identification and service delivery, communication between educational and mental health professions, and investigations of these students (Lane, Gresham, et al., 2002). In addition, the range of terminology used to refer to these learners poses challenges when synthesizing the literature. For example, in several instances, students representing self-contained classes for students with EBD were included in these investigations. Yet, often these students did not have a formal diagnosis of ED as specified in IDEA. It is quite possible that students exhibited behavior patterns typical of students with the more global term of EBD. However, the following questions remain unanswered: Which students are we studying? Should we restrict our investigations to only those students with certified emotional disturbances? Or should we broaden the research focus, as many researchers have, to include students with high-incidence disabilities who demonstrate aberrant behaviors?

To interpret accurately the efficacy of various instructional programs and approaches, it is necessary to clearly define the population of interest. Research by Gresham, MacMillan, and Bocian (1998) suggests that multidisciplinary teams are less than accurate when determining special education eligibility and ineligibility. Results indicated that school teams show rather low rates of agreement with authoritative or research-based definitions of mild-disability groups. They conclude that school teams are making classification decisions based on perceived educational needs rather than strict adherence to specified cutoff scores and definitions. Given the lack of precision in determining eligibility as the tendency toward sympathy placements, it may be more sagacious to avoid relying exclusively on school-assigned labels (e.g., LD or ED). Instead, it may be better to focus our research efforts on a broader range of students (e.g., EBD) rather than restricting our work to a more narrowly defined group of learners. Further, this decision to "go wide" may also help to avoid false negatives (e.g., not providing intervention support to students with or at risk for behavioral problems who may or may not be receiving services under a different educational label, e.g., LD). The consequences of a false negative are particularly detrimental when one considers the negative outcomes associated with antisocial behavior patterns in general (Walker & Severson, 2002).

Breadth Issues

Another limitation of the current research base pertains to breadth issues. Specifically, there is (1) insufficient work across the age span, (2) a lack of systematic investigations across content area curricular scopes, and (3) limited replications.

Age Span

Reading and mathematical interventions have largely occurred at the elementary level with some investigations at the middle school level. Yet, none of the studies identified in this review was conducted at the high school level. One possible explanation for the lack of academic instruction investigations may stem from concerns on the part of the researchers regarding actually getting students to attend and participate in the intervention. The literature suggests that poor school attendance is typical of many students with and at risk for EBD at the high school level, in part because students have the desire and means (e.g., transportation) to participate in more reinforcing activities (e.g., socializing off-campus) than school participation. Although the task of intervening with high school students with EBD may appear to be a daunting task, this area of inquiry is sorely needed. To not provide academic instruction to students with and at

risk for EBD is irresponsible. Questions remain not only about how to teach these students but also about "what" to teach them as well. Perhaps the focus should shift to more of a functional skills curriculum to assist these students in transitioning from school to work, or more broadly, to life given that poor postsecondary outcomes often await students with ED (e.g., unemployment, impaired social relationships, and access to mental health services; Wagner, 1995; Walker et al., 1995; Walker & Severson, 2002).

Content Area Curricular Scopes

To become a proficient reader, writer, or mathematician, students must develop competence in a wide range of interrelated skills. For example, becoming a competent reader involves numerous skills (e.g., phonemic awareness, phonetic skills, sight-word vocabulary, fluency skills, and comprehension strategies). For readers to make transitions from learning to read to reading to learn (Fry & Lagomarsino, 1982) students must develop the above-mentioned skills. Reading instruction in early literacy skills is clearly a logical starting point, given that reading problems broaden over time, creating tremendous differences in the reading performance of "good" and "poor" readers (Juel, 1991; Stanovich, 1986). However, students must also develop additional skills (e.g., comprehension strategies) to be able to extract meaning from text. To date, limited investigations have been conducted to identify efficient, effective strategies for teaching higher-level skills (e.g., reading comprehension) to students with or at risk for EBD in reading (Babyak et al., 2000; Locke & Fuchs, 1995). Further, no studies have been conducted to explore higher-level skills in mathematics (e.g., applied problem solving) or written expression (e.g., composing text).

Replication

Many studies reviewed employed single-case methodologies. To establish external validity of the intervention procedures examined, replication is essential (Gay & Airasian, 2000; Johnston & Pennypacker, 1993). With the exception of studies examining the utility of Torgeson and Bryant's (1994) Phonological Awareness Training for Reading program with at-risk students (Lane, 1999; Lane, O'Shaughnessy, et al., 2001) and the effects of within-task and competing stimuli (Lee & Zentall, 2002) in math instruction, none of the studies reviewed included replications with students with and at risk for EBD. However, some studies did represent extensions of instructional programs or strategies conducted with other disability categories such as ITI (e.g., Skinner et al., 1994), peer-assisted learning strategies (Falk & Wehby, 2001; Locke & Fuchs, 1995), classwide peer tutoring (Harper et al., 1995), mnemonics (Cade & Gunter, 2002), and cover–copy–compare (Skinner et al., 1991).

Limitations in breadth call for a systematic investigation of instructional strategies and programs across the grade span (kindergarten through 12th grade) with instructional foci that cover the range of skills necessary to develop competence in the given content area. Single short-term studies are insufficient to generalize results to student with and at risk for EBD. Therefore, it is imperative that studies be replicated to promote external validity. Similarly, it is important that these systematic investigations of programs and strategies across the age span also investigate outcomes for identified (e.g., ED or, more broadly, EBD) and nonidentified learners (e.g., at risk for EBD) to determine if these groups of students are equally responsive to intervention efforts.

Design Features

The studies reviewed are also limited, in some cases, by a lack of attention to components necessary for drawing accurate conclusions about intervention outcomes. In brief, several studies did not include treatment integrity, social validity, and generalization and maintenance data. Further, several investigations included only a narrow scope of outcome measures.

Components Related to Valid Inference Making

Several reviewed studies lacked some of the components (e.g., treatment integrity, generalization and maintenance, and social validity) that were needed to draw valid in-

ferences about intervention outcomes. Although all studies assessed and reported interrater reliability of the dependent variables, several studies did not report the accuracy, or fidelity, of implementation of the independent variable—the intervention (Gresham, 1989). This is particularly troubling given that accurate conclusions about interventions cannot be determined if the degree of implementation is not reported. For example, if treatment integrity data are not collected and the intervention does not produce the desired results, it is not possible to determine whether the intervention failed due to poor implementation or a poorly designed intervention. This "curious double standard" of providing careful attention to the accuracy of dependent variables and less attention to the accuracy of independent variables has been noted in other bodies of literature as well (Gresham, MacMillan, Beebe-Frankenberger, & Bocian, 2000).

In addition, several studies also lacked data on the extent to which gains were sustained over time (maintenance) and generalization to nontraining conditions (e.g., across persons, settings, or behaviors; Dunlap, 1993; Lane & Beebe-Frankenberger, 2004). If the ultimate goal of academic instruction intervention efforts is to determine the extent to which specific programs or techniques produce lasting increases in students' academic skills that can be used beyond the training conditions, then generalization and maintenance must be assessed.

Social validity data are also lacking from many studies reviewed. Social validity, when assessed at the onset of intervention, provides important information about the parties' perceptions of the significance of the goals, acceptability of procedures, and importance of potential outcomes (Lane, Beebe-Frankenberger, et al., 2001; Wolf, 1978). Social validity ultimately has implications for intervention effectiveness. For example, if the intervention is viewed as socially valid, then the intervention is likely to be implemented as designed. If treatment integrity is high and the intervention sound, then the intervention is likely to produce the desired outcomes—lasting changes that sustain and generalize. If interventions are perceived as socially valid at the end of the intervention, it is also likely that the desired goals were significant, the procedures acceptable, and the outcomes important. This information collectively enlightens research and practice. As researchers we have the skills to design effective interventions—in theory. However, if the intervention is tedious and resource laden (e.g., insufficient time, materials, and effort), it is likely to be perceived as socially invalid, implemented with low integrity, and will ultimately fail to produce the desired outcomes. Collectively, these components provide the information necessary to accurately interpret intervention outcomes and inform future research and practice.

Outcome Measures

Several studies employed a narrow range of outcome measures that prohibit identification of collateral effects of improved academic skills on social and behavioral performances within and beyond the classroom setting, as well as perceptions of academic, social, and behavioral performance (e.g., teacher and parent rating scales). Researchers recommend assessment practices based on the principle of multioperationalism (Gresham, Lane, & Lambros, 2001). This involves assessing performance from multiple perspectives (e.g., parent, teacher, students, and record review) using a range of methodologies (e.g., direct observation, curriculum-based measurement, rating scales, interviews, and permanent products). Although single-case design does not support the use of some of these measures, future studies using group design methodologies would be wise to address the principle of multiple operationalism.

Future investigations could be enhanced by designing studies to include: (1) accuracy of intervention implementation, (2) social validity from consumers' perspectives prior to and at the conclusion of intervention implementation, (3) generalization, not only over time (maintenance) but also across settings, persons, and responses, and (4) a range of outcome measures to assist in assessing generalizing of effect.

Reporting

A final limitation of the studies reviewed concerns reporting procedures. Many studies provided only partial information about the intervention features and the intervention dosage. For example, rather than explicitly stating the number of hours of intervention, often only partial information was provided, making it difficult—or impossible—to determine exact intervention time. The absence of this information has implications for research and practice. If insufficient information on intervention features and implementation logistics are not presented, replication efforts become more challenging. In addition, educators have greater difficulty determining the feasibility of implementing the strategies or curriculum in their classrooms. Given that many studies occurred outside of the actual classroom environment (e.g., Babyak et al., 2000; Cade & Gunter, 2002; Cochran et al., 1993; Lee & Zental, 2002; Lane, 1999; Lane, O'Shaughnessy, et al., 2001; McCurdy et al., 1990; Skinner et al., 1991; Skinner et al., 1995; Skinner, 1994), it is essential that information on intervention duration and implementation procedures be provided so that researchers and educators can draw conclusions about how to bring these techniques into the classroom during the traditional school day.

SUMMARY

Providing effective, efficient instruction to students with and at risk for EBD is a pressing concern that has captured the attention of the research and teaching communities, given the challenges these students pose within and beyond the school setting. Recent events such as the No Child Left Behind Act (Frounier, 2002) and the President's Commission on Excellence in Special Education have served to further stimulate interest in how to better serve this group of youngsters (Barton-Arwood, 2003). Studies conducted to date have produced promising results, as evidenced by improved early-literacy skills, computational skills, and spelling. Some evidence also exists to suggest that improved academic competence is associated with improved social and behavioral performance as well (Cochran et al., 1993; Franca et al., 1990; Lane, O'Shaughnessy, et al., 2001; Lane, Wehby, et al., 2002; Lee et al., 1999; Lee & Zentall, 2002; Scott & Shearer-Lingo, 2002; Spencer et al., 2003).

However, this body of literature is characterized by key limitations including (1) an unclear population focus, (2) concerns regarding breadth of the students involved, the content scope explored, and the replication of studies, (3) the limited presence of design features needed to draw accurate conclusions about intervention outcomes, and (4) insufficient reporting procedures. Future investigations of academic instruction with this population can be enhanced by addressing these limitations while developing and systematically exploring instructional strategies and programs for students with and at risk for EBD across the K–12 grade span.

REFERENCES

Achenbach, T. M. (1991). *Manual for the child behavior checklist/4–18 and 1991 profile.* Burlington: University of Vermont, Department of Psychiatry.

Adams, M. J. (1990). *Beginning to reading: Thinking and learning about print.* Cambridge, MA: MIT Press.

American Psychiatric Association. (1994). *Diagnostic and statistical manual of mental disorders* (4th ed.). Washington, DC: Author.

Anderson, J. A., Kutash, K., & Duchnowski, A. J. (2001). A comparison of the academic progress of students with EBD and students with LD. *Journal of Emotional and Behavioral Disorders, 9,* 106–115.

Babyak, A. E., Koorland, M., & Mathes, P. G. (2000). The effects of story mapping instruction on the reading comprehension of students with behavioral disorders. *Behavioral Disorders, 25,* 239–258.

Barton-Arwood, S. (2003). *Comorbid reading and behavioral deficits among young students with emotional/behavioral disorders.* Unpublished doctoral dissertation. University of California, Riverside, Riverside, CA.

Browder, D., & Shear, S. (1996). Interspersal of known items in a treatment package to teach sight words to students with behavior disorders. *Journal of Special Education, 29,* 400–413.

Cade, T., & Gunter, P. L. (2002). Teaching students with severe emotional or behavioral disorders to use a musical mnemonic technique to solve basic division calculations. *Behavioral Disorders, 27,* 208–214.

Carr, S., & Punzo, R. (1993). The effects of self-monitoring of academic accuracy and productivity on the performance of students with behavioral disorders. *Behavioral Disorders, 18,* 241–250.

Carson, R. R., Sitlington, P. L., & Frank, A. R. (1995). Young adulthood for individuals with behavioral disorders: What does it hold? *Behavioral Disorders, 20,* 127–135.

Clarke, S., Dunlap, G., Foster-Johnson, L., Childs, K.

E., Wilson, D., White, R., & Vera, A. (1995). Improving the conduct of students with behavioral disorders by incorporating student interests into curricular activities. *Behavioral Disorders, 20,* 221–237.

Cochran, L., Feng, H., Cartledge, G., & Hamilton, S. (1993). The effects of cross-age tutoring on the academic achievement, social behaviors, and self-perceptions of low-achieving African-American males with behavioral disorders. *Behavioral Disorders, 18,* 292–302.

Cole, C. L., Davenport, T. A., Bambara, L. M., & Ager, C. L. (1997). Effects of choice and task preference on the work performance of students with behavior problems. *Behavioral Disorders, 22,* 65–74.

Coleman, M., & Vaughn, S. (2000). Reading interventions for students with emotional/ behavioral disorders. *Behavioral Disorders, 25,* 93–104.

Cybriwsky, C., & Schuster, J. (1990). Using constant time delay procedures to teach multiplication facts. *Remedial and Special Education, 11,* 54–59.

Dawson, L., Venn, M. L., & Gunter, P. L. (2000). The effects of teacher versus computer reading models. *Behavioral Disorders, 25,* 105–113.

DePaepe, P., A., Shores, R. E., Jack, S. L., & Denny, R. K. (1996). Effects of task difficulty on the disruptive and on-task behavior of students with severe behavior disorders. *Behavioral Disorders, 21,* 216–225.

Dunlap, G. (1993). Promoting generalization: Current status and functional considerations. In R. V. Houten & S. Axelrod (Eds.), *Behavior analysis and treatment* (pp. 269–296). New York: Plenum.

Edwards, L., & Chard, D. J. (2000). Curriculum reform in a residential treatment program: Establishing high academic expectation for students with emotional and behavioral disorders. *Behavioral Disorders, 25,* 259–263.

Epstein, M. H., & Cullinan, D. (1983). Academic performance of behaviorally disordered and learning-disabled pupils. *Journal of Special Education, 17,* 303–307.

Ervin, R. A., Kern, L., Clarke, S., DuPaul, G. J., Dunlap, G., & Friman, P. C. (2000). Evaluating assessment-based intervention strategies for students with ADHD and comorbid disorders within the natural classroom context. *Behavioral Disorders, 25,* 344–358.

Falk, K. B., & Wehby, J. H. (2001). The effects of peer-assisted learning strategies on the beginning reading skills of young children with emotional or behavioral disorders. *Behavioral Disorders, 26,* 344–359.

Fournier, R. (2002, January 9). Education overhaul signed. *The Associated Press syndicated article in the Riverside Press Enterprise,* pp. A1, A9.

Franca, V. M., Kerr, M. M., Reitz, A. L., & Lambert, D. (1990). Peer tutoring among behaviorally disordered students: Academic and social benefits to tutor and tutee. *Education and Treatment of Children, 3,* 109–128.

Fry, M. A., & Lagomarsino, L. (1982). Factors that influence reading: A developmental perspective. *School Psychology Review, 11*, 239–250.

Gajar, A. (1979). Educable mentally retarded, learning disabled, emotionally disturbed: Similarities and differences. *Exceptional Children, 45*, 470–472.

Gay, L. R., & Airasian, P. (2000). *Educational research: Competencies for analysis and application* (6th ed.). Columbus, OH: Merrill.

Gickling, E., & Armstrong, D. (1978). Levels of instructional difficulty as related to on-task behavior, task completion, and comprehension. *Journal of Learning Disabilities, 11*, 559–566.

Glomb, N., & West, R. P. (1990). Teaching behaviorally disordered adolescents to use self management skills for improving the completeness, accuracy, and neatness of creative writing homework assignments. *Behavioral Disorders, 15*, 233–242.

Greenbaum, P. E., Dedrick, R. F., Friedman, R. M., Kutash, K., Brown, E. C., Lardierh, S. P., & Pugh, A. M. (1996). National Adolescent and Child Treatment Study (NACTS): Outcomes for children with serious emotional and behavioral disturbance. *Journal of Emotional and Behavioral Disorders, 4*, 130–146.

Greene, J. F. (1996). Effects of an individualized structured language curriculum for middle and high school students. *Annals of Dyslexia, 46*, 97–121.

Gresham, F. M. (1989). Assessment of treatment integrity in school consultation and prereferral intervention. *School Psychology Review, 18*, 37–50.

Gresham, F. M. (2002). Social skills assessment and instruction for students with emotional and behavioral disorders. In K. L. Lane, F. M. Gresham, & T. E. O'Shaughnessy (Eds.), *Interventions for children with or at risk for Emotional and Behavioral Disorders* (pp. 242–258). Boston: Allyn & Bacon.

Gresham, F. M. & Elliott, S. N. (1990). *Social Skills Rating System (SSRS)*. Circle Pines, MN: American Guidance Service.

Gresham, F. M., Lane, K. L., & Lambros, K. (2000). Comorbidity of conduct and attention deficit hyperactivity problems: Issues of identification and intervention with "fledgling psychopaths." *Journal of Emotional and Behavioral Disorders, 8*, 83–93.

Gresham, F. M., MacMillan, D. L., Beebe-Frankenberger, M. E., & Bocian, K. M. (2000). Treatment integrity in learning disabilities intervention research: Do we really know how treatments are implemented? *Learning Disabilities Research and Practice, 15*, 198–205.

Gresham, F. M., MacMillian, D. L., & Bocian, K. M. (1998). Agreement between school study team decisions and authoritative definitions in classification of students at-risk for mild disabilities. *School Psychology Quarterly, 13*, 181–191.

Gunter, P., Denny, R. K., Jack, S., Shores, R. E., & Nelson, C. M. (1993). Aversive stimuli in academic interactions between students with serious emotional disturbance and their teachers. *Behavioral Disorders, 18*, 265–274.

Harper, G. F., Mallette, B., Maheady, L., Bentley, A. E., & Moore, J. (1995). Retention and treatment failure in classwide peer tutoring: Implications for further research. *Journal of Behavioral Education, 5*, 399–414.

Hinshaw, S. P. (1992). Externalizing behavior problems and academic underachievement in childhood and adolescence: Causal relationships and underlying mechanisms. *Psychological Bulletin, 111*, 127–155.

Hogan, S., & Prater, M. A. (1993). The effects of peer tutoring and self-management training on on-task, academic, and disruptive behaviors. *Behavioral Disorders, 18*, 118–128.

Individuals with Disabilities Education Act Amendments of 1997. Public Law No. 105-17, Section 20, 111 Stat. 37 (1997). Washington, DC: U.S. Government Printing Office.

Johnston, J. M., & Pennypacker, H. S. (1993). *Strategies and tactics of behavioral research* (2nd ed.). Hillsdale, NJ: Erlbaum.

Jolivette, K., Wehby, J. H., & Hirsch, L. (1999). Academic strategy identification for students exhibiting inappropriate classroom behaviors. *Behavioral Disorders, 24*, 210–221.

Juel, C. (1991). Beginning reading. In R. Barr, M. L. Kamil, P. B. Mosenthal, & P. D. Pearson, (Eds.). *Handbook of reading research* (Vol. 2, pp. 759–788). Mahwah, NJ: Erlbaum.

Kamps, D., Kravits, T., Rauch, J., Kamps, J. L., & Chung, N. (2000). A prevention program for students with or at risk for ED: Moderating effects of variation in treatment and classroom structure. *Journal of Emotional and Behavioral Disorders, 8*, 141–154.

Kamps, D., Kravits, T., Stolze, J., & Swaggart, B. (1999). Prevention strategies for at-risk students and students with EBD in urban elementary schools. *Journal of Emotional and Behavioral Disorders, 7*, 178–188.

Kauffman, J. M. (2001). *Characteristics of emotional and behavioral disorders of children and youth* (7th ed.). Columbus, OH: Merrill.

Kazdin, A. E. (1993). Treatment of conduct disorders: Progress and directions in psychotherapy research. *Development and Psychopathology, 5*, 277–310.

Kern, L., Bambara, L., & Fogt, J. (2002). Class-wide curricular modification to improve the behavior of students with emotional or behavioral disorders. *Behavioral Disorders, 27*, 317–326.

Kern, L., Delaney, B., Clarke, S., Dunlap, G., & Childs, K. (2001). Improving the classroom behavior of students with emotional and behavioral disorders using individualized curricular modifications. *Journal of Emotional and Behavioral Disorders, 9*, 239–247.

Lane, K. L. (1999). Young students at risk for antisocial behavior: The utility of academic and social skills interventions. *Journal of Emotional and Behavioral Disorders, 7*, 211–233.

Lane, K. L. (2003). Identifying young students at risk for antisocial behavior: The utility of "teachers as tests." *Behavioral Disorders, 28*, 360–389.

Lane, K. L., & Beebe-Frankenberger, M. E. (2004). *School-based interventions: The tools you need to succeed.* Boston: Allyn & Bacon

Lane, K. L., Beebe-Frankenberger, M. E., Lambros, K. M., & Pierson, M. E. (2001). Designing effective interventions for children at-risk for antisocial behavior: An integrated model of components necessary for making valid inferences. *Psychology in the Schools, 38,* 365–379.

Lane, K. L., Gresham, F. M., & O'Shaughnessy, T. E. (2002). Identifying, assessing, and intervening with children with or at risk for behavior disorders: A look to the future. In K. L. Lane, F. M. Gresham, & T. E. O'Shaughnessy (Eds.), *Interventions for children with or at risk for emotional and behavioral disorders* (pp. 317–326). Boston: Allyn & Bacon.

Lane, K. L., O'Shaughnessy, T. E., Lambros, K. M., Gresham, F. M., & Beebe-Frankenberger, M. E. (2001). The efficacy of phonological awareness training with first-grade students who have behavior problems and reading difficulties. *Journal of Emotional and Behavioral Disorders, 9,* 219–231.

Lane, K. L., Umbreit, J., & Beebe-Frankenberger, M. E. (1999). A review of functional assessment research with students with or at-risk for emotional and behavioral disorders. *Journal of Positive Behavioral Interventions, 1,* 101–111.

Lane, K. L., & Wehby, J. H. (2002). Addressing antisocial behavior in the schools: A call for action. *Academic Exchange Quarterly, 6,* 4–9.

Lane, K. L., Wehby, J. H., Menzies, H. M., Gregg, R. M, Doukas, G. L., & Munton, S. M. (2002). Early literacy instruction for first-grade students at-risk for antisocial behavior. *Education and Treatment of Children, 25,* 438–458.

Lee, Y. Y., Sugai, G., & Horner, R. H. (1999). Using an instructional intervention to reduce problem and off-task behaviors. *Journal of Positive Behavior Interventions, 1,* 195–204.

Lee, D. L., & Zentall, S. S. (2002). The effects of visual stimulation on the mathematics performance of children with Attention Deficit/Hyperactivity Disorder. *Behavioral Disorders, 27,* 272–288.

Levendoski, L. S., & Cartledge, G. (2000). Self-monitoring for elementary school children with serious emotional disturbances: Classroom applications for increased academic responding. *Behavioral Disorders, 25,* 211–224.

Locke, W. R., & Fuchs, L. S. (1995). Effects of peer-mediated reading instruction on the on-task behavior and social interaction of children with behavior disorders. *Journal of Emotional and Behavioral Disorders, 3,* 92–99.

Malmgren, K. W., & Leone, P. E. (2000). Effects of a short-term auxiliary reading program on the reading skills of incarcerated youth. *Education and Treatment of Children, 23,* 239–247.

Mathur, S. R., Kavale, K. A., Quinn, M. M., Forness, S. R., & Rutherford, R. B. (1998). Social skills interventions with students with emotional and behavioral problems: A quantitative synthesis of single-subject research. *Behavioral Disorders, 23,* 193–201.

Mattison, R. E., Hooper, S. R., & Glassberg, L. A. (2002). Three-year course of learning disorders in special education students classified as behavioral disorder. *Journal of the American Academy of Child and Adolescent Psychiatry, 41,* 1454–1461.

Mattison, R. E., Spitznagel, E. L., & Felix, B. C. (1998). Enrollment predictors of the special education outcome for students with SED. *Behavioral Disorders, 23,* 243–256.

McCurdy, B. L., Cundari, L., & Lentz, F. E. (1990). Enhancing instructional efficiency: An examination of time delay and the opportunity to observe instruction. *Education and Treatment of Children, 13,* 226–238.

McLaughlin, T. F. (1992). Effects of written feedback in reading on behaviorally disordered students. *Journal of Educational Research, 85,* 312–315.

McWhirter, C. C., & Bloom, L. A. (1994). The effects of a student-operated business curriculum on the on-task behavior of students with behavioral disorders. *Behavioral Disorders, 19,* 136–141.

Miller, K. A., Gunter, P. L., Venn, M. L., Hummel, J., & Wiley, L. P. (2003). Effects of curricular and materials modifications on academic performance and task engagement of three students with emotional or behavioral disorders. *Behavioral Disorders, 28,* 130–149.

Nelson, J. R., Benner, G. J., Lane, K. L., & Smith, B. W. (in press). An investigation of the academic achievement of K-12 students with emotional and behavioral disorders in public school settings. *Exceptional Children.*

Nelson, J. R., Johnson, A., & Marchand-Martella, N. (1996). Effects of direction instruction, cooperative learning, and independent learning practices on the classroom behavior of students with behavioral disorders: A comparative analysis. *Journal of Emotional and Behavioral Disorders, 4,* 53–62.

Offord, D. R., & Bennett, K. H. (1996). Conduct disorder. In L. T. Hechtman (Ed.), *Do they grow out of it? Long-term outcomes of childhood disorders* (pp. 77–99). Washington, DC: American Psychiatric Association.

O'Shaughnessy, T. E., Lane, K. L., Gresham, F. M, & Beebe-Frankenberger, M. E. (2003). Children placed at risk for learning and behavioral difficulties: Implementing a school-wide system of early identification and prevention. *Remedial and Special Education, 24,* 27–35.

Penno, D. A., Frank, A. R., & Wacker, D. P. (2000). Instructional accommodations for adolescent students with severe emotional or behavioral disorders. *Behavioral Disorders, 25,* 325–343.

Ruhl, K. L., & Berlinghoff, D. H. (1992). Research on improving behaviorally disordered students' academic performance: A review of the literature. *Behavioral Disorders, 17,* 178–190.

Schloss, P., Alper, S., Young, H., Arnold-Reid, G., Aylward, M., & Dudenhoeffer, S. (1995). Acquisition of functional sight words in community-based recreation settings. *Journal of Special Education, 29,* 84–96.

Scott, T. M., & Shearer-Lingo, A. (2002). The effects of reading fluency instruction on the academic and behavioral success of middle school students in a self-contained EBD classroom. *Preventing School Failure, 46,* 167–173.

Scruggs, T. E., & Mastropieri, M. A. (1986). Academic characteristics of behaviorally disordered and learning disabled students. *Behavioral Disorders, 11,* 184–190.

Shores, R. E., Jack, S. L., Gunter, P. L., Ellis, D., DeBriere, T. J., & Wehby, J. H. (1993). Classroom interactions of children with behavior disorders. *Journal of Emotional and Behavioral Disorders, 1,* 27–39.

Simpson, S., Swanson, J., & Kunkel, K. (1992). The impact of an intensive multisensory reading program on a population of learning-disabled delinquents. *Annals of Dyslexia, 42,* 54–66.

Skinner, C. H., Cooper, L., & Cole, C. L. (1997). The effects of oral presentation previewing rates on reading performance. *Journal of Applied Behavior Analysis, 30,* 331–333.

Skinner, C. H., Ford, J. M., & Yunker, B. D. (1991). A comparison of response requirements on the multiplication performance of behaviorally disordered students. *Behavioral Disorders, 17,* 56–65.

Skinner, C. H., Johnson, C. W., Larkin, M. J., Lessley, D. J., & Glowacki, M. L. (1995). The influence of rate of presentation during taped-words interventions on reading performance. *Journal of Emotional and Behavioral Disorders, 3,* 214–223.

Skinner, C. H., Smith, E. S., & McLean, J .E. (1994). The effects of intertribal interval duration on sight-word learning rates in children with behavioral disorders. *Behavioral Disorders, 19,* 98–107.

Spencer, V. G., Scruggs, T. E., & Mastropieri, M. A. (2003). Content area learning in middle school social studies classrooms and students with emotional or behavioral disorders: A comparison of strategies. *Behavioral Disorders, 28,* 77–93.

Stanovich, K. E. (1986). Matthew effects in reading: Some consequences of individual differences in the acquisition of literacy. *Reading Research Quarterly, 21,* 360–406.

Tindal, G., & Crawford, L. (2002). Teaching writing to students with behavior disorders: Metaphor and medium. In K. L. Lane, F. M. Gresham, & T. E. O'Shaughnessy (Eds.), *Interventions for children with or at risk for emotional and behavioral disorders* (pp. 3–17). Boston: Allyn & Bacon.

Torgesen, J. K., & Bryant, B. R. (1994). *Phonological awareness training for reading.* Austin, TX: Pro-Ed.

Umbreit, J., Lane, K. L., & Dejud, C. (2004). Improving classroom behavior by modifying task difficulty: The effects of increasing the difficulty of too-easy tasks. *Journal of Positive Behavior Interventions, 6,* 13–20.

U.S. Department of Education. (1994). *National agenda for achieving better results for children and youth with serious emotional disturbance.* Washington, DC: Office of Special Education Programs.

Wagner, M. M. (1995). Outcomes for youths with serious emotional disturbance in secondary school and early adulthood. *The Future of Children, 5*(2), 90–111.

Wagner, M. M., Blackorby, J., Cameto, R., & Newman, L. (1993). *What makes a difference? Influences on post-school outcomes of youth with disabilities.* Menlo Park, CA: SRI International.

Walker, H. M., Colvin, G., & Ramsey, E. (1995). *Antisocial behavior in school: Strategies and best practices.* Albany, NY: Brooks/Cole.

Walker, H. M., & McConnell, S. (1995). *The Walker-McConnell Scale of Social Competence and School Adjustment.* Austin, TX: Pro-Ed.

Walker, H. M., & Severson, H. H. (1992). *Systematic Screening for Behavior Disorders (SSBD): User's guide and technical manual.* Longmont, CO: Sopris West.

Walker, H. M., & Severson, H. H. (2002). Developmental prevention of at-risk outcomes for vulnerable antisocial children and youth. In K. L. Lane, F. M. Gresham, & T. E. O'Shaughnessy (Eds.), *Interventions for children with or at risk for emotional and behavioral disorders* (pp. 177–194). Boston: Allyn & Bacon.

Walker, H. M., Severson, H. H., & Feil, E. G. (1995). *Early screening project: A proven child find process.* Longmont, CO: Sopris West.

Wilson, L., Cone, T., Bradley, C., & Reese, J. (1986). The characteristics of learning disabled and other handicapped students referred for evaluation in the state of Iowa. *Journal of Learning Disabilities, 19,* 553–557.

Wolf, M. M. (1978). Social validity: The case for subjective measurement or how applied behavior analysis is finding its heart. *Journal of Applied Behavior Analysis, 11,* 203–214.

Zaragoza, N., Vaughn, S., & McIntosh, R. (1991). Social skill intervention and children with behavior problems: A review. *Behavioral Disorders, 16,* 260–275.

25

Schoolwide Systems of Behavior Support

Maximizing Student Success in Schools

CARL J. LIAUPSIN, KRISTINE JOLIVETTE,
and TERRANCE M. SCOTT

Every school has a student body representing a range of behaviors from pleasant to rude, compliant to defiant, and all the ground in between. Some of these students are obvious and memorable, while others find ways to blend into the background and avoid notice, even when their behaviors are often less than desirable. School personnel do not need complicated screening instruments or professional in-service training to find these most challenging students, because their behaviors make them obvious (Walker, Colvin, & Ramsey, 1995). As such, one might reasonably ask why, if these students are so obvious, we cannot simply round them up, intervene, and thereby create trouble-free school environments by dealing with the most problematic of students. However, there are two logical lines of reasoning and evidence suggesting why such simple solutions have not and will not be effective.

First, while it is true that the majority of disciplinary referrals generally can be accounted for by approximately 10% of the school population (Sugai, Sprague, Horner, & Walker, 2000), there is a second level of students whose behaviors are not as obvious but tend to escalate when not addressed early. Placing all of a school's resources into responding to students with the most challenging behaviors is a never-ending battle, as the next group is growing just below their radar. While not obvious to the discipline system, these behaviors are noticed by teachers who indicate that, on a daily basis, these less intense but more frequent problem behaviors (e.g., off-task, noncompliant, distractibility) are as challenging and disruptive of students' learning time as the dangerous or defiant behaviors associated with the most challenging students (Furlong, Morrison, & Dear, 1994; Petersen, Pietrzak, & Speaker, 1998; Stephenson, Linfoot, & Martin, 2000).

As further evidence that focusing solely on the most challenging students is an ineffective method of creating positive environments, attempts at profiling students to predict and prevent only the most dangerous or disruptive behaviors (e.g., assault, menacing, weapons) have been wholly unsuccessful (American Psychological Association, 1993). While we know those who are likely to have problems, we are unable to predict with complete accuracy the worst behaviors or their perpetrators. Effective intervention for challenging behaviors must focus on prevention and early intervention among all students in the school.

Second, intervention for students with challenging behavior has historically been reactive, exclusionary, and ineffective. A survey conducted during the 1996–1997 school year found that more than 75% of all schools reported having zero-tolerance policies for various student offenses and an increase in the presence of law enforcement officers and metal detectors (U.S. Departments of Education and Justice, 1999). However, evidence suggests that such measures have been ineffective, or even counterproductive, in preventing school violence (Hyman & Perone, 1998; Mayer & Leone, 1999). Evidence strongly suggests that once students exhibit challenging behaviors in the school, they are far less likely to receive the same levels and quality of academic instruction from that point forward (Carr, Taylor, & Robinson, 1991), thereby exacerbating the problem by creating an environment in which the predictors of problem behavior are more firmly in place.

In addition, students identified as exhibiting behavioral difficulties will be exposed to more negative interactions with adults in the school (Van Acker, Grant, & Henry, 1996; Wehby, Symons, & Shores, 1995). These students also face tougher disciplinary codes—often based purely upon negative perceptions and expectations (Skiba, Peterson, & Williams, 1997). When used as the chief strategy to reduce problem behavior, exclusion is both inequitable and ineffective. Still, schools continue to exclude students with challenging behaviors as a first-level response, and often without any more proactive instructional strategies for future problem prevention (Contenbader & Markson, 1994). As a result, males and those from disadvantaged backgrounds (i.e., minorities) are grossly overrepresented in removal from the school and eventual dropout (Panko-Stilmock, 1996; Rylance, 1997; Skiba et al., 1997). Again, it is clear that effective intervention for challenging behaviors must focus on prevention and early intervention among all students in the school.

The development of a response that is effective among all students in a school necessarily requires the combined implementation of several elements. First, responses should incorporate a systemic process to ensure that all of the school's stakeholders are involved in the effort and that the school develops policies and procedures that will sustain a schoolwide intervention effort. Second, schoolwide responses should take a proactive approach that prevents and reduces the occurrence of problem behaviors and saves scarce intervention resources for the most challenging of behavioral issues. Third, both the broad-based and student-specific decisions made by the administrators, staff, students, and parents/families should be informed through the collection and evaluation of relevant data. Finally, to ensure effective outcomes, schoolwide systems for managing challenging behavior should, to the greatest degree possible, implement research-based and research-validated practices.

The purpose of this chapter is to provide a brief background with regard to existing and emerging schoolwide systems of behavior support. Numerous systems change processes and programs effectively incorporate the characteristics of schoolwide systems of behavior support, including Peacebuilders (Embry, Flannery, Vazsonyi, Powell, & Atha, 1996), Project ACHIEVE (Knoff & Batsche, 1995), Effective Behavior Support (Lewis & Sugai, 1999), and Positive Behavior Support (Sugai, Horner, et al., 1999). Rather than focusing on specific programs, this chapter explores the theoretical and empirical research that is typical of such programs. More specifically, this chapter describes the characteristics of schoolwide systems of behavior support, issues surrounding the evaluation of the expected outcomes of such systems, current research on positive outcomes, and weaknesses in the literature that should drive future research.

CHARACTERISTICS OF EFFECTIVE SCHOOLWIDE SYSTEMS

The impetus of schoolwide systems of behavior support is a focus on an integrated approach to assess and intervene in the areas found to be problematic (Freeman, Smith, & Tieghi-Benet, 2003). These areas may include student behavior and achievement, staff roles and responsibilities, and academic and social programs. Sugai and Horner (2002) define schoolwide systems of behavior support as a process in which a school's staff "focuses on decreasing the number of new cases of a problem behavior or situations by ensuring and maintaining the use of the most effective practices for all students" (p. 131). There are four salient characteristics of effective schoolwide systems: shared vision, leadership, collaborative effort, and data-based evaluation. These four characteristics, when combined with evidence-based academic and social interventions, strategies, and instructional practices, increase the likelihood of schools providing appropriate learning environments that are proactive and preventative in nature for all students (Nelson, Martella, & Marchand-Martella, 2002).

Shared Vision

The first characteristic of effective schoolwide systems of behavior support is for the staff of the school to have a shared vision. This means that a majority of the staff agree that there are predictable barriers and roadblocks as well as predictable behavioral patterns within the school that hinder appropriate student academic and social growth (Scott & Hunter, 2001). Barriers, roadblocks, and predictable behavioral patterns can be identified when staff meet and brainstorm about where, when, and under what conditions students are most likely to engage in problematic behaviors or to fail academically or socially. This brainstorming includes staff sharing of experiences, looking at existing data (e.g., from office referrals), and discussing current school practices (e.g., What do we do when a student fails academically or socially?). Also, it is important that staff members come to a consensus on how to prevent and minimize the identified barriers and roadblocks so that seamless implementation and coordination of a set of evidence-based practices and preventative restructuring can occur (Warren et al., 2003). This consensus revolves around a set of objectives and goals to be achieved through implementation of a plan for schoolwide behavior support that matches school and student needs with evidence-based practices. A shared vision among staff includes a time commitment. The length of time is dependent on the nature of agreed-upon objectives and goals and students' abilities to meet them (e.g., some schoolwide behavior support plans call for 1–5 years' worth of staff

commitment) (Chapman & Hofweber, 2000; Warren et al., 2003).

Leadership

Another key characteristic of effective schoolwide systems is the support and commitment of the school administration. Once staff members identify the barriers and roadblocks to their students' success and agree upon a plan to prevent further student failure and to promote student academic and social success, leadership by administrators and staff needs to be encouraged. Administrative leadership can take on many forms but should be consistent and visible (Colvin & Fernandez, 2000). For example, the administration may provide financial support (i.e., money to support professional development activities on specific academic or social evidence-based practices) (Taylor-Greene & Kartub, 2000), staffing support (i.e., reallocation of staffing patterns and/or the number of staff members available; Kartub, Taylor-Greene, March, & Horner, 2000), and other required resources (i.e., purchase of a computerized data collection program that analyzes trends and patterns in referrals (Sadler, 2000). In addition, staff leadership is needed to provide the day-to-day implementation and monitoring of the schoolwide system of behavior support. For example, a schoolwide team can be convened that represents each "subgroup" within the school to monitor staff implementation of the schoolwide behavior support plan, to facilitate staff discussions of the effectiveness or noneffectiveness of the plan based on the collected data, and to be a liaison with school administration (Scott, 2001).

Collaborative Effort

Once a majority of staff members are committed, share a common vision, and are provided administrative leadership capabilities, schools are ready to collaborate on the schoolwide system of behavior support. This collaborative effort centers on a set of agreed-upon academic and social expectations that will be taught, modeled, and reinforced by all staff. In addition, the specific roles of staff need to be agreed upon, with the strengths of each person highlighted. For example, a staff member with training and experience with token systems may be in charge of designing a reinforcement system for all students and for training staff who will be implementing such a program. Another example would be a set of staff members who evaluate the pros and cons of the current reading programs the school is using, research alternative reading programs, and then provide training to new teachers or teachers who request retraining on how to implement the agreed-upon curricula. It is important to note that the overall effects, either positive or negative, of a schoolwide system of behavior support is influenced by staff effort, attitude, and motivation (Freeman et al., 2003). Therefore, any changes in school practices should include staff members as collaborators in all decisions, not just as implementers.

Data-Based Evaluation

Schoolwide systems of behavior support are based on the premise that staff use data to make informed decisions regarding the changes needed within the school to promote student success and to prevent further student failure. Making data-based decisions requires that schools establish open and ongoing communications among staff members and the administration, with open sharing of data collected. The overall effectiveness of a schoolwide system of behavior support is based on the data collected and their relationship to the objectives and goals of the plan. Schools should collect data from a variety of sources, using multiple measures and methods. Typical measures used include data on office referrals (Nakasato, 2000; Scott, 2001), student achievement (Colvin & Fernandez, 2000; Nelson, Benner, Reid, Epstein, & Currin, 2002), and suspensions (Scott, 2001). Once data are collected, schools may use a variety of data summary tools to analyze the data and make decisions regarding the efforts of staff in future applications of the plan for schoolwide behavior support. For example, some schools have used the School-Wide Evaluation Tool (SET) (Nersesian, Todd, Lehmann, & Watson, 2000; Sugai, Lewis-Palmer, Todd, & Horner, 1999). No matter how data are collected, staff should be provided with visual displays

of the data through graphs and/or tables so that future decisions can be made objectively while continuing to build consensus (Nakasato, 2000).

While developing the four characteristics of schoolwide behavior support will prepare a school to undertake systems change, it also is imperative that schools embed three foci into efforts to provide all students in the school with a supportive and appropriate learning environment. These foci include schoolwide ecological manipulations, academic and social expectations, and specific disciplinary policies and procedures (Nelson et al., 2002).

Ecological Manipulations

Schoolwide systems of behavior support focus on areas in and around the school where behavioral problems exist. These areas typically are identified through existing data and voiced by staff or students. Once these areas are confirmed to be contributing to student academic and/or social failure, decisions need to be made as to how to prevent future problems. Ecological manipulations can be time- and cost-efficient methods for preventing future failure and promoting success. Ecological manipulations are an important aspect of schoolwide systems of behavior support when predictable patterns of failure and success are known. These manipulations may revolve around changes in physical arrangements, policies, and routines. For example, if a barrier or roadblock to student success is found to be a physical feature of the school, such as placement of the lunchroom tables that create long lines or a building design problem that creates "blind spots" in the hallways, manipulations may include rearranging the lunchroom tables to allow for smoother student traffic patterns or installing mirrors in the "T" section of hallways to allow for 100% visibility of students. If a barrier or roadblock to student success is a policy issue, such as lack of student monitoring in the hallways during transitions, manipulations may include a change in staffing patterns and responsibilities so that during transitions staff members stand in their classroom doorways, with an additional staff person situated in the highest-traffic areas. Finally, if school routines, such as too many students in the hallways at once or insufficient time allocated for student transitions, are contributing to patterns of student failure, manipulations may include dismissing or transitioning students by area or grade level in a staggered fashion or increasing the amount of time students have to transition from class to class. Any ecological manipulations that are implemented should be made in response to collected data, agreed upon by staff, supported by the administration, and include training and practice for all staff responsible for implementing the changes.

Academic and Social Expectations

An agreed-upon set of academic and social expectations is a primary element of any schoolwide system of behavior support. The social expectations for all students typically center on five or fewer positively stated behaviors. These expectations are likely to differ across age groups. Settings for primary-aged students may have only three simple rules, such as "be respectful, be responsible, and be safe" (Horner, Sugai, Todd, and Lewis-Palmer, in press, p. 12), while secondary settings might include up to five rules, such as these that were developed for a middle school: "be respectful, be responsible, follow direction, keep hands and feet to self, be there—be ready" (Taylor-Greene & Kartub, 2000, p. 233).

The set of positively worded social expectations should then be operationally defined for each school environment. For instance, a school may determine that in the classroom "be respectful" means using appropriate language and taking turns. In the lunchroom, "be respectful" may be considered to include keeping the tables clean and using a soft voice. As schools develop expectations, they should endeavor to reflect the social values of stakeholders in the educational environment as well as the common language of the school and local community (Horner et al., in press).

The process for communicating the expectations to students should be explicit but can take various forms. For example, staff may teach, model, and reinforce social expectations through preplanned role plays or embed social expectation lessons into the ongoing activities and interactions between staff and students (Fox & Little, 2001). For some students, more detailed and individualized instruction in the social domain may be warranted. For these students, a functional behavioral assessment may help staff (1) determine the factors maintaining the problem behavior, (2) select appropriate alternate or replacement behaviors, and (3) develop a response that includes instruction in specific social skills.

Academic expectations for all students typically focus on improvement over past performance (e.g., using school test data or individual data). For example, staff may implement a "contest" for the grade levels that earn the most "A" and "B" grades for the semester or for the students who are most improved. For students with individualized education programs (IEPs), growth and achievement of academic expectations may be measured in terms of mastery of long- and short-term objectives. In addition, schoolwide supports are needed to promote student growth on the agreed-upon academic and social expectations. Specific supports are determined by staff, based on the needs of the students and the goals or objectives of the plan. Examples of supports may include predictable rules and expected behaviors during different periods of the school day (Nelson et al., 2002), social skills instruction (Fox, Dunlap, & Cushing, 2002), and group contingencies, or rewards (Scott, 2001). In all, students are far more likely to achieve the schoolwide academic and social expectations if reinforced and encouraged to do so.

Disciplinary Policies and Procedures

It is imperative that, to the greatest degree possible, agreed-upon disciplinary policies and procedures be fairly and equally applied by all staff, including the administration. Inconsistency on the part of adults in addressing problematic student behavior is known to decrease the effectiveness of a well-designed and well-intended program. Some schools may decide to implement an integrated approach to addressing disciplinary issues, such as using student assistance teams (Lohrmann-O'Rourke et al., 2000) and wraparound planning (Eber, Sugai,

Smith, & Scott, 2002). When predictable patterns for failure and success are identified, staff can use the strategy of precorrection to promote appropriate student academic and social behavior (Colvin, Sugai, & Patching, 1993).

ISSUES RELATED TO EXPECTED OUTCOMES

In social science and education, it is generally held that recommendations to adopt a specific practice should be based on whether research has deemed the practice effective and efficient. For example, Sasso, Conroy, Peck-Stichter, and Fox (2001) have suggested that, based on the limits of the current research base, it is inappropriate to recommend the use of functional behavioral assessment (FBA) in general school-based settings. With this in mind, the degree to which schoolwide systems of behavior support, or elements of schoolwide approaches, have been found to be effective should be of concern to those who consider recommending or adopting such practices.

The following section seeks to clarify issues surrounding the outcomes that might be expected of validated schoolwide behavior support practices. Specifically, the success of such practice should focus on the system as a whole to assess how desired changes in individual student behavior predict positive outcomes in the larger system or environment. That is, intervention must not be judged simply on the basis of measures of individual behavior without also examining what effect those behaviors have on the system within which that individual operates (i.e., school, family, and community). These larger system outcomes are sometimes referred to as "lifestyle change" and involve a comparative analysis of (1) benefits for the individual and system (i.e., positive life outcomes, resource savings, social acceptance) and (2) the costs of intervention in terms of undesired outcomes (i.e., resources spent, negative side effects, negative social acceptance) (Scott, Nelson, & Zabala, 2003; Wood, 1991). Such analysis has been advocated as the key measure of "the essence of effectiveness" (Baer, Wolf, & Risley, 1987; p. 322). For the purposes of this discussion, these lifestyle issues have been organized into the categories of social order, academic achievement, and institutionalization.

Social Order Issues

In outlining desired outcomes with respect to social order that might be associated with a systemwide approach to behavior management, it is important to differentiate the issues of social order from those of school violence. The term "school violence" is nonspecific and has been shown to reflect research conducted on various issues such as crime on school campuses, victimization, and weapons possession (Furlong & Morrison, 2000). In addition, national surveys have found that school staff and students identify behaviors such as cursing, pushing, grabbing, verbal threats, and intimidation as the most pressing behavioral issues occurring on school property (Furlong et al., 1994; Petersen et al., 1998; Petersen, Beekley, Speaker, & Pietrzak, 1998). Furthermore, while the number of school incidents serious enough to warrant calling the police demonstrated a general decline from 1993 to 1997, staff and students during the same period reported feeling less safe in their school environments (U.S. Departments of Education and Justice, 1999). Finally, evidence suggests that measures aimed at deterring the most serious of school incidents have been at best ineffective and at worst counterproductive in creating safe and orderly school environments (Hyman & Perone, 1998; Mayer & Leone, 1999). All of these data suggest that, where schools are concerned, social order is a concept that includes, but goes beyond, consideration of the most violent of school incidents.

Whether social order exists in a school might be best considered as the degree to which the environment supports the ability of the school to effectively carry out its daily functions. An environment that sustains effective school activities might be expected to (1) have minimal distractions and disruptions, (2) provide maximum time involved in educational pursuits (with education defined broadly to include not only academics but also artistic achievement and social development), and (3) present a climate in which staff and students feel safe to conduct their daily activities (Northwest Regional Educational Laboratory, 2001). To warrant implementation, a systemwide approach to school discipline should serve to develop a high degree of social order in schools.

Academic Achievement Issues

Federal mandates, such as those included in the No Child Left Behind Act of 2001 (Public Law 107-110), continue to put pressure on schools to demonstrate high levels of academic achievement. As suggested above, a schoolwide approach to discipline that has an impact on social order would be expected to provide an environment that is supportive of educational pursuits, with academic achievement considered as a subset of students' educational activities.

The link between academic achievement and schoolwide systems of behavior support is often perceived as tenuous. However, Scott, Nelson, and Liaupsin (2001) have identified research that points to a strong reciprocal connection between academic achievement and problem behavior. Examples of these relationships can be found in functional assessments that investigate patterns of behavior that maintain and reinforce both social and academic failure (Dunlap, Kern, Dunlap, Clarke, & Robbins, 1991; Lewis, Sugai, & Colvin, 1998; Skiba & Peterson, 2000). On a broader scale, a meta-analysis of academic and behavior research found that (1) poor academic performance is associated with high rates of delinquent offending, (2) high academic performance is related to low rates of delinquent offending among youth, and (3) interventions that improve academic performance are associated with reductions in the prevalence of problem behavior (Maguin & Loeber, 1996). Further evidence regarding the nature of the connection between academics and achievement can be found in behavioral research that describes how academic activities can become aversive for some students (Denny, Epstein, & Rose, 1992; Gunter, Jack, DePaepe, Reed, & Harrison, 1994; Shores et al., 1994) and how student behavior (or the perception of student behavior) appears to affect the quality of instructional interactions between students and teachers (Carr et al., 1991; Johns, 2000). Finally, reactive approaches to school disciplinary problems, such as suspension and expulsion, not only reduce the amount of time students spend in academic instruction but also feed predictable patterns in which students (and teachers) are reinforced for seeking to escape or avoid difficult academic situations.

To meet the needs of schools that are under pressure to produce improvements in academic achievement, an effective schoolwide response to disciplinary issues might be expected to (1) provide proactive solutions that prevent the loss of instructional time (Brophy, 1988) and (2) show evidence of actual improvements in measures of academic achievement (Nelson et al., 2002).

Institutionalization Issues

As previously mentioned, success must be judged by how change predicts important life outcomes for the system as a whole. Institutionalization of change involves outcomes that predict (1) success for students beyond the school, (2) perceptions of success among varied stakeholder groups, and (3) sustained use of positive practices in the school. To be certain, there is great overlap between social order, academic achievement, and institutional change. Evidence strongly suggests that social order positively affects academic achievement (e.g., Colvin, Kame'enui, & Sugai, 1993; Najaka, Gottfredson, & Wilson, 2002), that academic achievement positively affects social order (e.g., Gersten, Darch, & Gleason,. 1988; Nelson, Johnson, & Marchand-Martella, 1996; Scott & Shearer-Lingo, 2002), and that both social order and academic achievement positively affect student success in the community (e.g., Snyder, 2001; Sprague et al., 2001).

But institutionalization analysis takes this assessment a step further. Institutionalization has occurred when adults in the system see their actions as contributing to these successful outcomes, which in turn leads to positive judgments of the system or institution itself. This may be measured by stakeholder satisfaction surveys, reduced student and staff absenteeism rates, increased parent participation in the school, numbers of positive referrals, or the degree of staff engagement with schoolwide decision making and goal setting. In addition, positive institutional change can be measured by the ability of a system to sustain processes and procedures that have been collaboratively developed as part of the systemic effort. Successful institutions are effectively reinforced for their behavior and therefore are more likely to continue.

Although a school may elect to simply follow disciplinary referral rates as the sole measure of the effect of schoolwide behavior support efforts, such limited focus may provide poor or inaccurate assessment of lifestyle change in the system. For example, consider a school in which the administrator strictly admonishes the staff to avoid referring students for discipline. Simple drops in referral rates in this school will not necessarily be reflective of positive overall change among either students or staff. In fact, student disruptions in the classroom may worsen the learning environment for all students and result in less time engaged in instruction—prompting teachers to abandon systematic schoolwide efforts over time. On the other hand, it is possible that simply cutting back on referrals keeps students in the classroom, which can in turn translate to higher rates of academic achievement. The true benefits of the systemic process can only be measured by considering lifestyle changes across social order, academic achievement, and institutionalization.

CURRENT FINDINGS RELATED TO POSITIVE OUTCOMES

The research literature offers information related to several positive student and school outcomes when schoolwide systems of behavior support are implemented. The following discussion will highlight some of this research specific to social order outcomes, academic achievement outcomes, and institutionalization outcomes.

Social Order Outcomes

While the research theoretically supporting the various characteristics of schoolwide systems of behavior support has been developed over the past 50 years, the combination of these lines of research into a systems model of schoolwide behavior management is relatively new. Despite this novelty, the literature demonstrating the ability of such a model to positively affect social order in schools is relatively strong and continues to grow. Rather than describing the outcomes of individual studies, this section will describe the breadth of the research literature related to positive social order outcomes in the areas of (1) research designs, (2) measures of effectiveness, and (3) implementation across organizational levels (i.e., within-school settings, schools, districts, and states).

Three research approaches have generally been used in demonstrating the effectiveness of schoolwide models of behavior support in creating positive social order outcomes. These include case studies, single-subject research, and combination designs. First, case studies that are largely descriptive have added to the data base by describing the difficulties encountered during implementation and the impact on future practice. For instance, Colvin and Fernandez (2000) describe how the schoolwide team at an elementary school encountered difficulties in maintaining a focus on sequential implementation of a plan in the face of staff pressures to have the entire plan in place. Case studies that include experimental data related to social order outcomes are also present in the literature and report findings such as reductions in office referrals (Nelson, Colvin, & Smith, 1996; Nelson, Martella, & Galand, 1998; Scott, 2001) and reductions in long and short-term suspensions (Turnbull, Edmonson, & Griggs, 2002). Single-subject research designs also have been used to document the positive outcomes of schoolwide systems of behavior support (Colvin, Sugai, Good, & Lee, 1997; Lewis, Colvin, & Sugai, 2000; Lewis, Powers, Kelk, & Newcomer, 2002; Lewis et al., 1998). This type of research is particularly well suited for the study of implementation effectiveness in specific school settings and where frequent measurement of specific behaviors is desired. For example, Lewis et al. (1998) used a multiple baseline across settings design to demonstrate the effectiveness of a schoolwide social skills training program in reducing the frequency of student problem behavior across three nonclassroom settings (cafeteria, playground, and hallway). In another study, Lewis et al. (2000) used a multiple baseline across groups design to investigate the effects of a positive behavioral support plan (reviewing behavioral expectations with students and providing increased active supervision) on the frequency of problem behavior exhibited in an elementary school playground setting.

A small number of studies exploring social order outcomes have implemented a combination of research designs (i.e., some combination of descriptive and single-subject research). Metzler, Biglan, Rusby, and Sprague (2001) evaluated the development of social order in a middle school through the use of a comprehensive design that included a case study description, a quasi-experimental single-subject design, and multiple procedural validity and stakeholder perception measures. In their review of the initial behavioral outcomes of the Peace-Builders program, Flannery et al. (2003) designed a large-scale, multiyear follow-along study that included four matched sets of schools (eight schools) with delayed implementation across one school in each of the four matched sets. Both of these studies represent major investments in research resources (i.e., time, money) that may not typically be available.

Several measures of effectiveness have been collected in an effort to document positive outcomes in the area of social order. As described above, studies using single-subject research designs to explore implementation effects in specific settings have collected data on rates of problem and appropriate behavior (e.g., Lewis et al., 2000; Lewis et al., 1998). However, studies have most often reported the use of indirect measures (e.g., surveys and teacher reports) with archival data, such as office referrals and suspensions being the most frequently reported measures of effectiveness (e.g., Sugai et al., 2000).

There are at least two reasons that office disciplinary referrals may be the most frequently used measure of social order outcomes. First, the process of schoolwide behavior support strongly suggests that schools collect and analyze office referral data; if schools are involved in implementing a schoolwide system of behavior support, these data will be available (Sprague, Sugai, Horner, & Walker, 1999; Sugai et al., 2000; Tobin, Sugai, & Colvin, 2000). Second, office referrals are generally considered representative of the frequency of problem behaviors in schools. Third, it has been suggested that the level of office referrals in a school may be indicative of the school's overall social climate (Warren et al., 2003).

It should be noted that questions have been raised regarding the valid use of office referrals as a research measure. In a study examining the referral records of students who met borderline or clinical cutoff scores on the Teacher Report Form of the Child Behavior Checklist (Achenbach, 1991), Nelson et al. (2002) found a relatively high number of false negatives, suggesting that office discipline referrals are not a viable tool for identifying students who require targeted or intensive intervention services. Further, schools are likely to alter elements of their office referral process as one aspect of implementing a schoolwide system of behavior support (Sugai et al., 2000). Such changes in process may cause office referral rates to rise or fall prior to full implementation of a schoolwide behavior management plan. Studies reporting positive social order outcomes based solely on first-year implementation data should be considered with this issue in mind.

One of the great strengths of a systematic schoolwide approach to behavior support is that it involves a "scalable" process that can be applied across the range of organizational levels involved in education, from specific with-in school environments, to whole schools, and to even larger systems encompassing multiple schools. Positive results in terms of social order have been demonstrated across a variety of specific school environments, including classrooms (Colvin et al., 1997), playgrounds (Lewis et al., 2000; Lewis et al., 2002), and common areas (Kartub et al., 2000; Lewis et al., 1998; Nelson et al., 1996). At the level of the individual school, studies reporting improvements in social order have been conducted in elementary (e.g., Netzel & Eber, 2003) and middle school settings (e.g., Warren et al., 2003). Beyond the individual school level, limited research has been conducted that demonstrates how schoolwide behavior support can be organized at the district (Lohrmann-O'Rourke et al., 2000; Mayer & Butterworth, 1981; Nersesian et al., 2000; Sadler, 2000) and state levels (Nakasato, 2000) to achieve positive social order outcomes in multiple schools.

Academic Achievement Outcomes

There have been many studies of schoolwide behavior support and its positive effect on student behavior and other social measures (e.g., office referrals, suspensions) across preschool (e.g., Fox & Little, 2001), elementary (e.g., Netzel & Eber, 2003; Scott, 2001) and middle school settings (e.g., Nakasato, 2000; Warren et al., 2003); however, few studies have been published that also measured student academic achievement. Several reasons exist as to why so few studies have been published to date. First, although positive behavior support and schoolwide plans are not new, there has been an increased focus on these approaches. Schools strive to provide students with safe and appropriate learning environments in which students' social and academic achievements can be measured, as mandated by the 1997 amendments to IDEA, the No Child Left Behind Act of 2001 (Public Law 107-110), and other federal and state legislation and policies. Second, the process of a school designing, implementing, and monitoring a schoolwide system of behavior support is a time-intensive process with school commitments of multiple years (Warren et al., 2003). Thus, it is possible that studies that have measured both academic and social student behaviors have not yet made it through the publishing maze. Third, the initial focus of the school may be to decrease the number of student problem behaviors and office referrals before looking at academic performance. Because schoolwide systems of behavior support grew from the need for schools to prevent student problem behavior, it is likely that schools have focused on more traditional forms of problematic behaviors such as noncompliance, disruption, and aggression rather than academic achievement behaviors such as reading and math performance or the relationships between social and academic performance.

However, there are a few studies that have measured academic achievement. For example, Nelson et al. (2002) studied the effects of a 2-year schoolwide behavior support plan on student's academic and social performance. They found that students whose schools implemented a schoolwide behavior support plan had (1) higher gain scores in all areas except math, as measured by the fourth-grade CTBS; (2) higher gain scores in reading and mathematics, as measured by the state criterion-referenced test, the Washington Assessment of Student Learning; and (3) improvements in broad reading dictation and calculation subtests of the Woodcock–Johnson—revised, when compared to students from nonparticipating schools. In addition, there was a significant decrease in the number of disciplinary referrals. Overall, Nelson and colleagues suggest that the positive academic achievement outcomes were a result of the relationship between fewer student disruptive behaviors and improved student behaviors and consequently more time spent in instructional activities. In addition, Nelson et al. state that future studies need to simultaneously focus on academic as well as social outcome measures.

Student academic achievement as an outcome goal also is embedded within the High Five Program (Taylor-Greene & Kartub, 2000). Taylor-Greene and Kartub describe the outcomes of a schoolwide behavior support plan implemented in a middle school in 1994. Although no specific academic variables were measured, "improving student attendance and grades" (p. 234) were a primary goal of the plan and well achieved during the 5 years of implementation. In addition, Colvin and Fernandez (2000) describe how an elementary school that has implemented a schoolwide behavior support plan for the past several years has recently added an academic achievement outcome measure to the overall plan. Colvin and Fernandez state that "the school has learned that behavior support alone is not sufficient to assist all students; some students will display inappropriate behavior because they are unable to do the required work. Over the past 2 years, data have been taken regularly on reading performance for all students" (p. 253).

Thus, although student academic achievement outcomes may not have been the impetus for implementing systematic schoolwide behavior support efforts, more schools are now embedding academic achievement measures into their plans. In addition, there is initial data to suggest a strong empirical connection between schoolwide behavior support and academic achievement.

Institutionalization Outcomes

Along with social order and academic achievement, institutionalization is a key component of schoolwide behavior support in accomplishing large-scale lifestyle change.

Initially, effective schoolwide systems of behavior management should promote positive stakeholder perceptions of the system, thereby generalizing to successful outcomes for students outside of the school environment. Such change is institutionalized when these outcomes act as the catalyst for stakeholders to develop practices that are sustained after the initial intervention agents have been withdrawn.

Stakeholder perceptions of schoolwide systems of behavior support are valuable in demonstrating the positive climate outcomes that can be achieved through schoolwide approaches to behavior management. A number of studies have provided descriptive information regarding the social validity of implementation efforts (see Clarke, Worcester, Dunlap, Murray, & Bradley-Klug, 2002; Scott & Barrett, 2004; Wood, 1991). Additional studies have provided experimental data through the use of teacher satisfaction surveys (Nelson et al., 2002) and climate surveys directed at both teachers and students (Metzler et al., 2001). However, to date, the degree to which the views of parents and support staff have been taken into consideration is unclear; studies often use the term "school staff" without differentiating among staff roles. Chapman and Hofweber (2000) included parents as part of the team that developed a schoolwide approach to discipline, but data were not taken on the specific perspectives of parents.

Schoolwide behavior support is designed to employ a systems approach to develop a host environment in which practices are sustained. In other words, it is expected that schoolwide behavior interventions that are made through changes to overall policies, routines, and physical arrangements are likely to be maintained over long periods of time (Sugai, Horner, et al., 1999), and sustained postschool by existing community organizations and supports (Chapman & Hofweber, 2000). That is, effective schoolwide systems of behavior support create success in the school, with the responsibility being transferred to effective community-based systems such as mental health, Medicare, and public assistance once students leave the school setting. Although there is certainly ample evidence that it is possible to make such systems-level change within schools (e.g., Taylor-Greene & Kartub, 2000; Nelson et al., 2002), the literature currently contains only limited evidence to suggest that the systems changes, and the outcomes associated with those systems changes, actually do maintain over time. Among the scant evidence, Metzler et al. (2001) and Flannery et al. (2003) each measured sustained implementation of practices over a 2-year period, and Taylor-Greene and Kartub (2000) demonstrated the durability of implementation over a 5-year period.

As noted above, there is strong evidence to support the idea that schools can indeed develop environments that support high levels of social order. One might hope that these improvements within the school environment would translate into successful lifestyle outcomes for students outside of the confines of the school. Some studies have included reports of positive out-of-school outcomes for individual students (e.g., Turnbull et al., 2002). However, the literature does not yet include studies that show broad evidence of positive out-of-school or postschool outcomes related to schoolwide systems of behavior support.

A review of the literature with an eye toward institutionalization of lifestyle change appears to support the notion that a process of schoolwide behavior support can be sustained over multiple years and can result in positive stakeholder perceptions of the process. However, future research should be directed at evaluating the impact of schoolwide practices across a broader range of stakeholders and attempt to determine the effects of such practices on students in out-of-school settings and in their postschooling success.

DIRECTIONS FOR FUTURE RESEARCH

The ability of schoolwide systems of behavior support to produce positive outcomes in the area of social order appears well documented. However, the effect of the implementation of schoolwide systems of behavior support on (1) the reciprocal connection between social order and achievement and (2) the institutionalization of systems changes, while understood theoretically, has yet to be well established through the analysis of outcomes data. This may be, in part, because social order is the direct target of systems of positive behavior support, while academic achievement and institutionalization are valued "secondary outcomes" that are expected in orderly school environments. Two approaches to elucidating these as yet tenuous connections should be explored by researchers.

First, studies pairing the implementation of schoolwide systems of behavior support with specific academic programs may provide insight into the connection between social order and academic achievement. For example, Kellam, Mayer, Rebok, and Hawkins (1998) conducted a well-controlled study in which they implemented both a schoolwide system of behavior support and a research-validated early reading program. They found implementation of the reading program to be successful only in schools that first developed an orderly school environment through a system of schoolwide behavior support. Second, researchers should seek to use multiple tools to measure changes in the perceptions of the broad range of stakeholders represented in educational communities in an effort to document the institutionalization of systematic changes in school environments.

As noted in the discussion of social order outcomes, few studies appear to have followed the effects of schoolwide behavior support for more than 2 years. Documenting the initial dramatic effects that can occur within schools is certainly necessary and should continue. However, schoolwide behavior support is a systems-change process intended to create "host" environments that will maintain and increase their capacity to deal with problematic issues over long periods of time (Sugai, Horner, et al., 1999). Given that this is the case, there is a need to demonstrate that the changes to a school's systems are indeed long-term and will continue to produce effective results. Despite the logistical problems of conducting such research, the literature would clearly benefit from studies that either follow schoolwide behavior support efforts for periods of 3 years or revisit schools that implemented programs in the past to determine whether changes have been institutionalized.

With respect to research designs, it should be noted that studies show positive outcomes related to schoolwide behavior support fall generally into the categories of case study and single-subject research. Metzler et al. (2001) suggest three reasons that case study and single-subject research approaches are likely to continue dominating the schoolwide behavior support literature. First, the naturalistic nature of conducting studies in schools precludes the strict controls required of more traditional group research designs. Second, case study and single-subject research are less time consuming and less costly. Third, the schoolwide model of behavior support is a process involving systems change in which no two schools are likely to develop strictly identical plans; the stringent controls required for alternative research designs, such as randomized trials, will be extremely difficult to implement.

With respect to the various educational organizational levels, examples of successful implementation in the literature appear to be plentiful at the elementary school level, less likely to be found at the middle school level, and nonexistent at the high school level. One reason for the lack of examples at the middle and high school levels may be that these environments are more organizationally complex than elementary schools. For instance, high schools are often organized into subject area departments that are insular and that operate somewhat autonomously. In spite of the difficulties of achieving consensus and taking collaborative action in such environments, schoolwide systems of behavior support hold clear promise in dealing with issues that are key in secondary environments (e.g., graduation and dropout rates, suspensions, and expulsions).

SUMMARY

Schoolwide systems of behavior support are well suited to meet the current and future challenges faced by schools in providing a successful educational experience for all students. This chapter has provided a description of the structures underlying schoolwide systems of behavior support and the literature supporting the use of such systems. The four characteristics of effective schoolwide systems of behavior support (e.g., shared vision, leadership, collaborative effort, and data-based evaluation), create the organizational environments that can support the creation and maintenance of proactive social and academic intervention strategies. The literature detailing current outcomes suggests that schoolwide behavior support can be effective in developing safe and orderly educational environments and that such environments are associated with high rates of academic achievement and perceptions of an improved school climate among students and staff. Despite the positive outcomes already established in the literature, additional research across the spectrum of issues associated with implementing schoolwide systems of behavior support is necessary to demonstrate that the promise of such approaches can positively affect not only education environments but the larger community as well.

REFERENCES

Achenbach, T. M., (1991). *Manual for the Teacher Report Form.* Burlington: University of Vermont Press.

American Psychological Association. (1993). *Violence and youth, Report of the Commission on Violence and Youth.* Washington, DC: Author.

Baer, D. M., Wolf, M. M., & Risley, T. R. (1987). Some still-current dimensions of applied behavior analysis. *Journal of Applied Behavior Analysis, 20,* 313–327.

Brophy, J. E. (1988). Research linking teacher behavior to student achievement: Potential implications for instruction of chapter 1 students. *Educational Psychologist, 23,* 235–286.

Carr, E. G., Taylor, J. C., & Robinson, S. (1991). The effects of severe behavior problems in children on the teaching behavior of adults. *Journal of Applied Behavior Analysis, 24,* 523–535.

Chapman, D., & Hofweber, C. (2000). Effective behavior support in British Columbia. *Journal of Positive Behavior Interventions, 2,* 235–237.

Clarke, S., Worcester, J., Dunlap, G., Murray, M., & Bradley-Klug, K. (2002). Using multiple measures to evaluate positive behavior support: A case example. *Journal of Positive Behavior Interventions, 4,* 131–145.

Colvin, G., & Fernandez, E. (2000). Sustaining effective behavior support systems in an elementary school. *Journal of Positive Behavior Interventions, 2,* 251–253.

Colvin, G., Kame'enui, E., & Sugai, G. (1993). Reconceptualizing behavior management and school-wide discipline in general education. *Education and Treatment of Children, 16,* 361–381.

Colvin, G., Sugai, G., Good, R. H., III, & Lee, Y. Y. (1997). Using active supervision and precorrection to improve transition behaviors in an elementary school. *School Psychology Quarterly, 12,* 344–363.

Colvin, G., Sugai, G., & Patching, B. (1993). Precorrection: An instructional approach for managing predictable problem behaviors. *Intervention in School and Clinic, 28,* 143–150.

Contenbader, V. K., & Markson, S. (1994). School suspension: A survey of current policies and practices. *NASSP Bulletin, 78,* 103–107.

Denny, R. K., Epstein, M. H., & Rose, E. (1992). Direct observation of adolescents with serious emotional disturbance and their nonhandicapped peers in mainstream vocational education classrooms. *Behavioral Disorders, 18,* 33–41.

Dunlap, G., Kern, L., Dunlap, L., Clarke, S., & Robbins, F. (1991). Functional assessment, curricular revision and severe behavior problems. *Journal of Applied Behavior Analysis, 24,* 387–397.

Eber, L., Sugai, G., Smith, C. R., & Scott, T. M. (2002). Wraparound and positive behavioral interventions and supports in the schools. *Journal of Emotional and Behavioral Disorders, 10,* 171–180.

Embry, D. D., Flannery, D. J., Vazsonyi, A. T., Powell, K. E., & Atha, H. (1996). PeaceBuilders: A theoretically driven, school-based model for early violence prevention. *American Journal of Preventive Medicine, 12,* 91–100.

Flannery, D. J., Vazsonyi, A. T., Liau, A. K., Guo, S., Powell, K. E., Athu, H., et al. (2003). Initial behavior outcomes for the PeaceBuilders Universal School-based Violence Prevention Program. *Developmental Psychology, 39,* 292–308.

Fox, L., Dunlap, G., & Cushing, L. (2002). Early intervention, positive behavior support, and transition to school. *Journal of Emotional and Behavioral Disorders, 10,* 149–157.

Fox, L., & Little, N. (2001). Starting early: Developing school-wide behavior support in a community preschool. *Journal of Positive Behavior Interventions, 3,* 251–254.

Freeman, R. L., Smith, C. L., & Tieghi-Benet, M. (2003). Promoting implementation success through the use of continuous systems-level assessment strategies. *Journal of Positive Behavior Interventions, 5,* 66–70.

Furlong, M. J., & Morrison, G. M. (2000). The school in school violence: Definitions and facts. *Journal of Emotional and Behavioral Disorders, 8,* 71–82.

Furlong, M. J., Morrison, G. M., & Dear, J. D. (1994). Addressing school violence as part of schools' educational mission. *Preventing School Failure, 38,* 10–17.

Gersten, R. M., Darch, C., & Gleason, M. (1988). Effectiveness of a direct instruction academic kindergarten for low-income students. *Elementary School Journal, 89,* 227–240.

Gunter, P. L., Jack, S. L., DePaepe, P., Reed, T. M., & Harrison, J. (1994). Effects of challenging behaviors of students with EBD on teacher instructional behavior. *Preventing School Failure, 38,* 35–39.

Horner, R. H., Sugai, G., Todd, A. W., & Lewis-Palmer, T. (in press). School-wide positive behavior support: An alternative approach to discipline in schools. In

L. Bambara & L. Kern (Eds.), *Positive behavior support*. New York: Guilford Press.

Hyman, I. A., & Perone, D. C. (1998). The other side of school violence: Educator policies and practices that may contribute to student misbehavior. *Journal of School Psychology, 36,* 7–27.

Johns, B. (2000). Reaching them through teaching them: Curriculum and instruction for students with E/BD. *Beyond Behavior, 10,* 3–6.

Kartub, D. T., Taylor-Greene, S., March, R. E., & Horner, R. H. (2000). Reducing hallway noise: A systems approach. *Journal of Positive Behavior Interventions, 2,* 179–182.

Kellam, S. G., Mayer, L. S., Rebok, G. W., & Hawkins, W. E. (1998). Effects of improving achievement on aggressive behavior and of improving aggressive behavior on achievement through two preventive interventions: An investigation of causal paths. In B. P. Dohrenwend (Ed.), *Adversity, stress, and psychopathology* (pp. 486–505). New York: Oxford University Press.

Knoff, H. M., & Batsche, G. M. (1995). Project ACHIEVE: Analyzing a school reform process for at-risk and underachieving students. *School Psychology Review, 24,* 579–603.

Lewis, T. J., Colvin, G., & Sugai, G. (2000). The effects of pre-correction and active supervision on the recess behavior of elementary students. *Education and Treatment of Children, 23,* 109–121.

Lewis, T. J., Powers, L. J., Kelk, M. J., & Newcomer, L. L. (2002). Reducing problem behaviors on the playground: An investigation of the application of school-wide positive behavior supports. *Psychology in the Schools, 39,* 181–190.

Lewis, T. J., & Sugai, G. (1999). Effective behavior support: A systems approach to proactive schoolwide management. *Focus on Exceptional Children, 31*(6), 1–24.

Lewis, T. J., Sugai, G., & Colvin, G. (1998). Reducing problem behavior through a school-wide system of effective behavioral support: Investigation of a school-wide social skills training program and contextual interventions. *School Psychology Review, 27,* 446–459.

Lohrmann-O'Rourke, S., Knoster, T., Sabatine, K., Smith, D., Horvath, B., & Llewellyn, G. (2000). School-wide application of pbs in the Bangor area school district. *Journal of Positive Behavior Interventions, 2,* 238–240.

Maguin, E., & Loeber, R. (1996). Academic performance and delinquency. In M. Tonry (Ed.), *Crime and justice: A review of research* (pp. 145–264). Chicago: University of Chicago Press.

Mayer, G. R., & Butterworth, T. W. (1981). Evaluating a preventive approach to reducing school vandalism. *Phi Delta Kappan, 62,* 498–499.

Mayer, M., & Leone, P. E. (1999). A structural analysis of school violence and disruption: Implications for creating safer schools. *Education and Treatment of Children, 22,* 333–356.

Metzler, C. W., Biglan, A., Rusby, J. C., & Sprague, J. R. (2001). Evaluation of a comprehensive behavior management program to improve school-wide positive behavior support. *Education and Treatment of Children, 24,* 448–479.

Najaka, S. S., Gottfredson, D. C., & Wilson, D. B. (2002). A meta-analytic inquiry into the relationship between selected risk factors and problem behavior. *Prevention Science, 2,* 257–271.

Nakasato, J. (2000). Data-based decision making in Hawaii's behavior support effort. *Journal of Positive Behavior Interventions, 2,* 247–251.

Nelson, J. R., Benner, G. J., Reid, R. C., Epstein, M. H., & Currin, D. (2002). The convergent validity of office discipline referrals with the cbcl-trf. *Journal of Emotional and Behavioral Disorders, 10,* 181–188.

Nelson, J. R., Colvin, G., & Smith, D. J. (1996). The effects of setting clear standards on students' social behavior in common areas of the school. *Journal of At-Risk Issues, 3*(1), 10–18.

Nelson, J. R., Johnson, A., & Marchand-Martella, N. (1996). A comparative analysis of the effects of direct instruction, cooperative learning, and independent learning practices on the disruptive behaviors of students with behavior disorders. *Journal of Emotional and Behavioral Disorders, 4,* 53–63.

Nelson, J. R., Martella, R., & Galand, B. (1998). The Effects of teaching school expectations and establishing a consistent consequence on formal office disciplinary actions. *Journal of Emotional and Behavioral Disorders, 6,* 153–161.

Nelson, J. R., Martella, R. M., & Marchand-Martella, N. (2002). Maximizing student learning: The effects of a comprehensive school-based program for preventing problem behaviors. *Journal of Emotional and Behavioral Disorders, 10,* 136–148.

Nersesian, M., Todd, A. W., Lehmann, J., & Watson, J. (2000). School-wide behavior support through district-level system change. *Journal of Positive Behavior Interventions, 2,* 244–247.

Netzel, D. M. & Eber, L. (2003). Shifting from reactive to proactive discipline in an urban school district: A change of focus through PBS implementation. *Journal of Positive Behavior Interventions, 5,* 71–79.

Northwest Regional Educational Laboratory (2001, January). *Research you can use to improve results.* Retrieved May 17, 2003, from *http://www. nwrel.org/scpd /sirs/rycu/index.html.*

Panko-Stilmock, J. (1996). Teacher gender and discipline referral rates for middle level boys and girls. Unpublished doctoral dissertation, University of Nebraska–Lincoln.

Petersen, G. J., Beekley, C. Z., Speaker, K. M., & Pietrzak, D. (1998). An examination of violence in three rural school districts. *Rural Educator, 19,* 25–32.

Petersen, G. J., Pietrzak, D., & Speaker, K. M. (1998). The enemy within: A national study on school violence and prevention. *Urban Education, 33,* 331–359.

Rylance, B. J. (1997). Predictors of high school graduation or dropping out for youths with severe emotional disturbances. *Behavioral Disorders, 23,* 5–17.

Sadler, C. (2000). Effective behavior support implementation at the district level: Tigard–Tualatin School District. *Journal of Positive Behavior Interventions, 2*, 241–243.

Sasso, G. M., Conroy, M. A., Peck-Stichter, J., & Fox, J. J. (2001). Slowing down the bandwagon: The misapplication of functional assessment for students with emotional or behavioral disorders. *Behavioral Disorders, 26*, 282–296.

Scott, T. M. (2001). A school-wide example of positive behavioral support. *Journal of Positive Behavior Interventions, 3*, 88–94.

Scott, T. M., & Barrett, S. (2004). Using cost/benefit analysis with school-wide positive behavior support: A sample evaluation of lifestyle change at the systems level. *Journal of Positive Behavior Interventions, 6*(1), 21–28.

Scott, T. M., & Hunter, J. (2001). Initiating school-wide support systems: An administrator's guide to the process. *Beyond Behavior, 11*, 13–15.

Scott, T. M., Nelson, C. M., & Liaupsin, C. J. (2001). Effective instruction: The forgotten component in preventing school violence. *Education and Treatment of Children, 24*, 309–322.

Scott, T. M., Nelson, C. M., & Zabala, J. S. (2003). Functional behavior assessment training in public schools: Facilitating systemic change. *Journal of Positive Behavior Interventions, 5*(4), 216–224.

Scott, T. M., & Shearer-Lingo, A. (2002). The effects of reading fluency instruction on the academic and behavioral success of middle school students in a self-contained EBD classroom. *Preventing School Failure, 46*, 167–173.

Shores, R. E., Jack, S. L., Gunter, P. L., Ellis, D. N., DeBriere, T. J., & Wehby, J. H. (1994). Classroom interactions of children with behavior disorders. *Journal of Emotional and Behavioral Disorders, 1*, 27–39.

Skiba, R. J., & Peterson, R. L. (2000). School discipline at a crossroads: From zero tolerance to early response. *Exceptional Children, 66*, 335–346.

Skiba, R. J., Peterson, R. L., & Williams, T. (1997). Office referrals and suspension: disciplinary intervention in middle schools. *Education and Treatment of Children, 20*, 295–315.

Snyder, H. (2001). Child delinquents. In L. Loeber & D. P. Farrington (Eds.), *Risk factors and successful interventions*. Thousand Oaks, CA: Sage.

Sprague, J. R., Sugai, G., Horner, R. H., & Walker, H. M. (1999). *Using office discipline referral data to evaluate school-wide discipline and violence prevention interventions* (022 Collected Works—Serials; 142 Reports—Evaluative). Eugene, OR: Oregon School Study Council.

Sprague, J. R., Walker, H. M., Stieber, S., Simonsen, B., Nishioka, V., & Wagner, L. (2001). Exploring the relationship between school discipline referrals and delinquency. *Psychology in the Schools, 38*, 197–206.

Stephenson, J., Linfoot, K., & Martin, A. (2000). Behaviours of concern to teachers in the early years of school. *International Journal of Disability, Development and Education, 47*, 225–235.

Sugai, G., & Horner, R. H. (2002). Introduction to the special series on positive behavior support in schools. *Journal of Emotional and Behavioral Disorders, 10*, 130–135.

Sugai, G., Horner, R. H., Dunlap, G., Hieneman, M., Lewis, T. J., Nelson, C. M., et al. (1999). *Applying Positive Behavioral Support and Functional Behavioral Assessment in Schools. Technical Assistance Guide 1, Version 1.4.3* (141 Reports—Descriptive). Washington, DC: Center on Positive Behavioral Interventions and Support, Office of Special Education Programs, U.S. Department of Education.

Sugai, G., Lewis-Palmer, T., Todd, A. W., & Horner, R. H. (1999). *School-wide evaluation tool.* Eugene: University of Oregon, Positive Behavioral Interventions and Supports Technical Assistance Center.

Sugai, G., Sprague, J. R., Horner, R., & Walker, H. M. (2000). Preventing school violence: The use of office discipline referrals to assess and monitor school-wide discipline interventions. *Journal of Emotional and Behavioral Disorders, 8*, 94–101.

Taylor-Greene, S., & Kartub, D. T. (2000). Durable implementation of school-wide positive behavior support: The high five program. *Journal of Positive Behavior Interventions, 2*, 233–235.

Tobin, T., Sugai, G., & Colvin, G. (2000). Using discipline referrals to make decisions. *NASSP Bulletin, 84*(616), 106–117.

Turnbull, A. P., Edmonson, H., & Griggs, P. (2002). A blueprint for school-wide positive behavior support: Implementation of three components. *Exceptional Children, 68*, 377–402.

U.S. Departments of Education and Justice. (1999). Indicators of School Crime and Safety, 1999. (NCES 19989-057/NCJ-178906). Washington, DC: Authors.

Van Acker, R., Grant, S. H., & Henry, D. (1996). Teacher and student behavior as a function of risk for aggression. *Education and Treatment of Children, 19*, 316–334.

Walker, H. M., Colvin, G., & Ramsey, E. (1995). *Antisocial behavior in school: Strategies and best practices*. Pacific Grove, CA: Brooks/Cole.

Warren, J. S., Edmonson, H. M., Griggs, P., Lassen, S. R., McCart, A., Turnbull, A., & Sailor, W. (2003). Urban applications of school-wide positive behavior support: Critical issues and lessons learned. *Journal of Positive Behavior Interventions, 5*, 80–91.

Wehby, J. H., Symons, F. J., & Shores, R. E. (1995). A descriptive analysis of aggressive behavior in classrooms for children with emotional and behavioral disorders. *Behavioral Disorders, 20*, 87–105.

Wood, F. H. (1991). Cost considerations in managing the behavior of students with emotional/behavioral disorders. *Preventing School Failure, 35*, 17–23.

26

Collaboration with Other Agencies

Wraparound and Systems of Care for Children and Youths with Emotional and Behavioral Disorders

LUCILLE EBER *and* SANDRA KEENAN

SYSTEM OF CARE: THEORY TO PRACTICE

Many youths with emotional and behavioral disorders (EBD) traverse through special education, mental health, juvenile justice, and child welfare with historically dismal outcomes. The need for collaborative approaches that link multiple stakeholders in efficient and effective interventions are demonstrated through the repeated failures of individual systems, such as education and mental health, to unilaterally effect positive change (Koyanagi & Gaines, 1993). It is clear that the traditionally separate systems that respond to the home, school, and community life of children with EBD must link together through collaborative structures and practices.

Over the past 20 years, advocates, researchers, and practitioners have been focusing on how to actualize a coordinated multi-agency network that makes the full range of supports and services available as needed by children with mental health problems and their families. The concept of a comprehensive system of care that is responsive to the needs and preferences of the child/family from a strength-based perspective is relatively easy to support in theory. But it is

much harder to fully implement these systems of care within and across the various agencies involved with children with EBD and their families. Can the locus and management of services truly be derived from multiagency collaboration? What activities on both the infrastructure level and service delivery level are required to make this happen? How do we know when a system of care is working? These and similar questions continue to be raised, not only by critics but also by practitioners who are deeply involved in doing the work.

This chapter describes the history and development of interagency systems of care and the wraparound approach, a widely used tool for building constructive relationships and support networks among children with EBD and their families, teachers, and other caregivers. Examples of models that recognize the importance of connecting families, schools, and human service partners to collaboratively address the comprehensive needs of students with emotional and behavioral challenges are provided. Emerging interagency school and community-based models that connect effective learning and behavior change with system-of-care principles are also discussed. Evaluation data of these initiatives are presented, as are recommendations for needed research to guide system development and practices across disciplines.

A HISTORY OF FRAGMENTATION

Special education, mental health, primary health, child welfare, and juvenile justice are the primary systems that attempt to support students with serious mental health needs and their families. Unfortunately, these separate systems have very different structures, tools, and even philosophies, and historically they have not connected very well on behalf of children and families. Differences in eligibility criteria, definitions, policies, and intervention approaches often create dissonance and confusion for children, families, teachers, and other service providers. Passing from one system to the other while symptoms worsen and problems escalate is unfortunately a common experience for many youths and families. The fragmentation among systems has even resulted in families being forced to relinquish custody to the child welfare system as a last resort to allow their child to access treatment (Freisan, Giliberti, Katz-Levy, Osher, & Pullmann, 2003). The juvenile justice system has, also by default, responsibility for three to five times more youths (30–40% of the general population) with EBD than public schools (Leone & Miesel, 1997). Each year, there are over 150 million visits to primary care pediatricians, who prescribe the majority of psychotropic drugs and often counsel families about emotional and behavioral problems. Most children with mental health needs see their primary care providers rather than a mental health specialist. This may be the only contact with a "system" for many preschool children (Kelleher, 2002).

Overall, these individual systems working in isolation of each other have repeatedly failed to address the complex needs presented by youths with EBD and their families. In fact, many children/youths with serious emotional/behavioral problems are not receiving any specialized services from schools or mental health systems (Friedman, Katz-Levy, & Sondheimer, 1996; Hoagwood & Erwin, 1997; Knitzer, Steinberg, & Flesch, 1990; Leaf et al., 1996). And those that do receive services have experienced dismal outcomes, including low academic achievement, high dropout rates, poor postschool adjustment, and high use of restrictive placements and incarcerations (Blackorby & Wagner, 1996; Carson, Sitlington, & Frank, 1995; Koyanagi & Gaines, 1993; Wagner, 1995; U.S. Department of Education, 1998).

Although the Joint Commission on Mental Health identified the need to address children's mental health in 1969, not much has happened in the ensuing years. In 1974, every federally-funded Community Mental Health Center was required to provide children's services, but funding was insufficient. Additional unfunded mandates that were never implemented included the 1978 President's Commission on Mental Health and the Mental Health System Act of 1980. The Education for All Handicapped Children Act (Public Law 94-142; U.S. Department of Education, 1997) in 1975, intended to ensure appropriate services for all students with disabilities, may have inadvertently slowed down progress for this population as state mental health agencies actually decreased their focus on children, assuming special education would serve as the children's mental health service system (Duchnowski, Kutash, & Friedman, 2002). Over time, the education sector has been observed to be a primary player in providing what few mental health services are provided to youths with EBD (Burns et al., 1997; Farmer, Stangl, Burns, Costello, & Angold, 1999; Leaf et al., 1996). Unfortunately, as previously stated, the outcomes have not been good. Over 25 years later, students with EBD continue to be the most underidentified and inadequately served of all disability groups (Forness, 2002).

SEEDS OF CHANGE: THE SYSTEM-OF-CARE CONCEPT

Jane Knitzer's seminal document *Unclaimed Children* (Knitzer, 1982) first exposed the woeful inadequacies of children's mental health, child welfare, and juvenile justice systems in America. She proposed that a seamless "system of care" was needed and is credited with setting into motion the idea that "children and adolescents with SED [serious emotional disturbances] should have access to community-based services and supports" (Hernandez & Hodges, 2003, p. 21). In 1983, The National Institute of Mental Health responded by funding the Child and Adolescent Service System program (CASSP), an initiative that provided funds and technical assistance to all 50 states, several territories, and some local jurisdictions to plan and develop systems of care for children with EBD. Recognizing the multiple systems involvement of these children, a core factor of CASSP was interagency collaboration (National Institute of Mental Health, 1983).

Stroul and Freidman wrote their landmark monograph *A System of Care for Children and Youth with Serious Emotional Disturbance* (Stroul & Friedman, 1986) that further described Knitzer's concept of a full continuum of care. They outlined a set of values and principles that emphasized access to a full continuum of culturally relevant services in community settings (see Table 26.1). The emphasis of the system-of-care rhetoric was on a community-based service delivery process and an underlying philosophical base of flexibility to meet family/child needs rather than agency needs (Hernandez & Hodges, 2003).

The system-of-care concept created a vision of a comprehensive service system for youths and families. The charge was to increase collaboration and ensure access to a full array of community-based culturally relevant services rather than limiting treatment options to residential or other restricted settings. Active coordination and collaboration across all child-serving agencies was the primary goal. Mental health, child welfare, education, special education, juvenile justice, health, and vocational rehabilitation would be organized into a coordinated network. This included more accessible, family-friendly options, and suggested integrated

TABLE 26.1. System of Care Values and Guiding Principles

Core values

1. The system of care should be child centered and family focused, with the needs of the child and family dictating the types and mix of services provided.
2. The system of care should be community based, with the locus of services as well as management and decision-making responsibility resting at the community level.
3. The system of care should be culturally competent, with agencies, programs, and services that are responsive to the cultural, racial, and ethnic differences of the populations they serve.

Guiding principles

1. Children with emotional disturbances should have access to a comprehensive array of services that address the child's physical, emotional, social, and educational needs.
2. Children with emotional disturbances should receive individualized services in accordance with the unique needs and potentials of each child and guided by an individualized service plan.
3. Children with emotional disturbances should receive services within the least restrictive, most normative environment that is clinically appropriate.
4. The families and surrogate families of children with emotional disturbances should be full participants in all aspects of the planning and delivery of services.
5. Children with emotional disturbances should receive services that are integrated, with linkages between child-serving agencies and programs and mechanisms for planning, developing, and coordinating services.
6. Children with emotional disturbances should be provided with case management or similar mechanisms to ensure that multiple services are delivered in a coordinated and therapeutic manner and that they can move through the system of services in accordance with their changing needs.
7. Early identification and intervention for children with emotional disturbances should be promoted by the system of care in order to enhance the likelihood of positive outcomes.
8. Children with emotional disturbances should be ensured smooth transitions to the adult service system as they reach maturity.
9. The rights of children with emotional disturbances should be protected, and effective advocacy efforts for children and youth with emotional disturbances should be promoted.
10. Children with emotional disturbances should receive services without regard to race, religion, national origin, sex, physical disability, or other characteristics, and services should be sensitive and responsive to cultural differences and special needs.

Note. Data from Stroul and Friedman (1986).

policies and funding structures that still remain elusive in many communities and states today (Hernandez & Hodges, 2003).

Communities and states initially responded with what Lourie (1994) described as "incremental optimism," developing whatever services consistent with system-of-care principles and values they could get resources to support. Services such as case management, respite care, day treatment, and in-home supports became more readily available. Sometimes these new services were offered through interagency networks, but in some states and communities new services were offered through single agencies and not necessarily with a coordinated approach. From 1989 to 1993, the Robert Wood Johnson Foundation's *Mental Health Services Program for Youth* (MHSPY) funded 27 state and local initiatives that introduced managed care technologies to the development of systems of care. The *Comprehensive Community Mental Health Services for Children and Their Families Program* was created in 1992 through federal legislation. Since then, this program has funded 85 state and local communities, including tribal sites and territories, to build systems of care. The core of this program is the development of a comprehensive array of community-based services and supports. Increasing access and satisfaction while decreasing use of restrictive and costly placements were system outcomes reported for these system-of-care initiatives (Hoagwood, Burns, Kiser, Ringeisen, & Schoenwald, 2001). This was a major shift in thinking and focus for the field of children's mental health services.

SYSTEMS OF CARE AND SCHOOLS

Although schools were not a major player in the early system-of-care innovations, education for students with disabilities was being redefined with the passage of Public Law 94-142 in 1975. Students could not be excluded from school because of a disability, and all students, including those identified as "seriously emotionally disturbed" (SED), were now provided access to appropriate services to ensure educational success, including related services such as counseling and classroom modifications. Consistent with the community-based philosophy of systems of care, the least restrictive environment (LRE) assurances directed schools to develop the services needed for students with disabilities, including those with SED, to be educated with their nondisabled peers.

Similar to mental health's experiences with systems of care, the concept of LRE has proven challenging for educators, especially with regard to students identified as EBD (Forness, 2002). *At the Schoolhouse Door* (Knitzer et al., 1990) documented how special education programs for these identified children (a small segment of those who actually should qualify for special services) also were far from effective and perhaps even exacerbated problems for children, given the overemphasis on behavior control at the expense of instruction. *At the Schoolhouse Door* made it clear that, due to the complex needs of these children, coordinated supports and services across home, school, and community are necessary. Providing special school programs without integrating treatment for their emotional/behavioral challenges and supports for families and without careful transitions across settings is not enough. Knitzer reiterated that no system alone can begin to address the challenges presented by this population, and a collaborative system of care must be the priority for education as well as mental health and the other systems involved with these children and their families.

In 1994, the U.S. Department of Education proposed a *National Agenda for Achieving Better Results for Children and Youth with Serious Emotional Disturbance* (U.S. Department of Education, 1994) that coincided with the system-of-care initiatives coming from the mental health field. The need for collaborative and comprehensive systems that partnered with families in organizing relevant and effective services was recognized in this agenda introduced from the field of education (Smith & Coutinho, 1997). Concurrently with the development of the *National Agenda*, the Office of Special Education Programs (OSEP) of the U.S. Department of Education funded a series of school-initiated demonstration projects based on community-based system-of-care principles (Kallas, 1992). Developing the skills and capacities of schools and communities to effectively respond to and prevent SED so that these students could succeed academically and socially was recognized. Collaboration across service sectors and with families was the crosscutting theme.

There are provisions within the 1997 reauthorization of the Individuals with Disabilities Education Act (IDEA) that support the development of community-based collaboration and systems of care. Section 300.244, Coordinated Services System, allows a school system to use federal funds to develop and implement a coordinated services system designed to improve results for children and families that includes interagency agreements. Section 300.235, Permissive Use of Funds, allows nondisabled children to benefit and have access to services or programs in which school districts use special education personnel in classwide or schoolwide behavioral and emotional support programs. Section 300.306, Nonacademic Services, requires the provision of nonacademic and extracurricular services such as counseling services, health services, and referrals to agencies. Section 300.142, Methods of Ensuring Services, requires each state to establish responsibility for services and other mechanisms for interagency coordination, which helps to define the financial responsibility of each agency for providing services. IDEA clearly states that the financial responsibility of each noneducational public agency, including the state Medicaid agency and other public insurers of children with disabilities, must precede the financial responsibility of the local education agency. This provision has allowed some states to develop a wide array of services that are Medicaid eligible and complement the school-based services (Pumariega & Winters, 2003).

New provisions under the federal *No Child Left Behind Act of 2002, Subpart 14, Section 5541*, allow funds to be used to enhance or develop collaborative efforts between school-based service systems and mental health service systems for prevention, diagnosis, referral, and treatment services for students, as well as the availability of crisis intervention services. This legislation also allows funds to be used for training school personnel and mental health professionals as well as provides technical assistance and consultation to school systems and mental health agencies and families (U.S. Department of Education, 2002).

All of these provisions can help facilitate interagency collaboration, shared or blended funding, and better outcomes for students. However, relatively few communities have taken advantage of these opportunities. This is most likely due to a lack of state funding to support planning, collaboration, and the development of services.

WRAPAROUND: A SYSTEM-OF-CARE TOOL

Neither the system-of-care principles nor the National Agenda for SED described or prescribed the actual changes in practices needed to improve child/youth functioning. What do practitioners need to do to ensure that community-based services are based on the strengths, needs, and preferences of the children and families, many of whom have experienced multiple failed attempts of various agencies to provide effective interventions? What should practitioners do differently so that children with very intensive and comprehensive emotional and behavioral needs can be successful in their homes, schools, and communities? What does it look like when the services offered, the agencies participating, and the programs generated are responsive to the cultural context and characteristics of the individual children and their families? During the 1980s and 1990s, the wraparound approach emerged as a grassroots response to the shift in thinking and practice that was needed to implement system-of-care values and principles.

Burchard and his colleagues (2002) explain how wraparound evolved as practitioners sought alternatives to more medically oriented models that "failed to recognize the importance of context and normative roles on behavioral adjustment and development" (Burchard, Bruns, & Burchard, 2002, p. 70). They refer to the "wraparound theory of change" that has emerged as consistent with existing psychosocial child development theories such as Bronfenbrenner's (1979) social-ecological theory, Bandura's (1977) social learning theory, and Munger's (1998) systems change theory. Burchard et al. (2002) describe the wraparound theory of change as follows: "Children with severe emotional and behavioral problems will develop a more normal lifestyle if their services and supports are family centered and child focused, strength-based, individualized, community-based, interagency coordinated, and culturally competent" (p. 70).

It was estimated in 1998 that over 200,000 youths and their families were engaged in the wraparound process in 88% of the U.S. territories and states (Faw, 1998). Consensus about the definition of wraparound programmatic values, elements, and practices was documented by the Center for Mental Health Services (CMHS) as part of a series of monographs documenting promising practices in children's mental health (Burns & Goldman, 1999). Burns and Goldman documented an experienced group of wraparound implementers' and evaluators' consensus that wraparound is a philosophy and approach with a defined planning process that is family-centered, strength-based, flexible, and collaborative. Through the wraparound process, a uniquely designed child/family team that includes natural support persons as key players is developed with the family. The team designs a unique and culturally relevant set of individualized community services and natural supports so that a specific child and family can achieve a unique set of outcomes (Burns & Goldman, 1999, p. 13). Table 26.2 provides the core elements of wraparound.

Consistent with system-of-care philosophy, wraparound plans are uniquely designed to fit individual needs, as opposed to attempting to make a youth and family fit into a prescribed program (Eber, Nelson, & Miles, 1997). Ownership of the plan by the youth and family and those who spend the most time with and have the most responsibility for the youth (i.e., teachers, other caregivers) are hallmark traits of the process that these stakeholders have frequently reported to be critical to successful outcomes (Eber, 2003). Stepping outside of the box of the usual categorical service options, teams create or reorganize services based on unique needs and circumstances of students with complex needs. Services are created on a "one student at a time" basis to support normalized and inclusive options. Natural supports (i.e., child care, transportation, mentors, parent-to-parent support) are combined with traditional interventions (i.e., positive behavioral interventions, teaching social skills, reading instruction, medication, therapy). Examples of supports and services in wraparound plans include respite, mentors, peer supports, parent partners, and assistance for families in need of basic supports such as housing, transportation, job assistance, child care, and health and safety supports. School components of wraparound plans include strength-based academic, behavioral, and social skills instructional strategies and reinforcement, as well as consultation and supports for teachers (Eber, 1996, 2003).

As a broadly used tool for implementing a system of care (Burns & Goldman, 1999), the wraparound process has resulted in new ways to organize supports and interventions for youths with emotional/behavioral challenges, their families, teachers, and other service providers and caregivers. Often reaching beyond the bounds of traditional categorical program structures, wraparound

---

TABLE 26.2. Elements of Wraparound

1. Community based
2. Individualized and strength based
3. Culturally competent
4. Families as full and active partners
5. Team-based process involving family, child, natural supports, agencies, and community supports
6. Flexible approach and funding
7. Balance of formal and informal community and family resources
8. Unconditional commitment
9. Development and implementation of an individualized service/support plan based on a community/neighborhood, interagency, collaborative process
10. Outcomes determined and measured through the team process

plans alter ecological variables across settings and create consensus on needs and behaviors targeted for change, thereby creating a context where effective interventions are more likely to be applied and evaluated. An important by-product of wraparound, and a critical aspect of effective interventions for these young people, is alignment of families with teachers and other service providers in productive and proactive partnerships (Eber, Sugai, Smith, & Scott, 2002).

WRAPAROUND AND SPECIAL EDUCATION

Educators' involvement with collaborative systems of care initiatives has been described as marginal and cautious (Lourie, 1994), and integration between education and other child-serving agencies has been limited (Woodruff et al., 1999). Yet, as discussed previously, the federal mandates of special education are consistent with system-of-care values and principles. For example, a similarity is that both the individualized education program (IEP) planning process and wraparound planning assure that interventions are designed and resources provided on the basis of individual need rather than predetermined program or setting resources. The least restrictive environment and family rights components of the federal special education mandate provide further consistency with the community-based, family centered aspects of system of care. However, there may be some differences between the intent of the original Public Law 94-142 and the actual practices of special education that have evolved over the past 30 years. Perhaps feeling the burden of being a mandated provider has prevented some school systems from embracing a process that doesn't necessarily separate mental health, medical, and family needs from educational needs as a plan of support is developed. However, high rates of restrictive placements in special education for students with EBD, as well as due process procedures between families and schools disputing appropriateness of interventions, suggest that more collaborative models should be considered.

The wraparound process has noted links to special education practices for children with developmental disabilities, including person-centered planning and positive behavior supports (Carr et al., 2002; Clark & Heinemann, 1999; Scott & Eber, 2003; VanDenBerg, 1998). Similarities between wraparound plans and the individual family service plans (IFSP) that guide cross-system planning in early childhood education are also evident. Key elements that connect these special education practices and wraparound include: (1) having families (including the student) define outcomes based on their quality-of-life choices, (2) identifying and arranging the supports the adults (i.e., families, teachers, other caregivers) need to effectively implement interventions for the child, (3) using a collaborative teaming process that includes natural support persons and cross-agency providers, and (4) taking steps to ensure that the values and skills of those implementing the interventions are compatible with the plan designed.

A wraparound plan addresses all life domains that affect the quality of life of the student and family at home, in school, and in the community. However, not all supports and services included in a wraparound plan must be included in the IEP. Services for other family members (parents, siblings) or basic living assistance for families are often important components of a youth's wraparound plan but are not necessarily part of the IEP. Wraparound plans often involve more frequent team meetings than typically associated with the IEP process, as interventions are monitored closely and new domains are addressed after high-priority needs are met. The cohesive and dynamic team approach ensures that the team meetings themselves are viewed as supportive and helpful to the youth, family, and teacher and that problem solving occurs as needed to ensure optimum success. Unique aspects of wraparound planning that make it different than typical school-based programming for students with EBD are further described in other publications (Eber, 2003, Eber et al., 1997, 2002).

TRAINING WITHIN A SYSTEM OF CARE: DEVELOPING SKILLS FOR COLLABORATION

Implementation of a system of care requires significant changes in not only system structures and program design but also changes in practices across disciplines. Repositioning and retraining personnel to move from deficit-based approaches to strength-based proactive interventions that draw on natural supports is a critical component of system-of-care implementation. Practitioners need a blend of values and skills to implement system-of-care principles. These include learning how to develop respectful partnerships with families as equal decision makers; building collaborations among providers, families, and natural support persons; and being aware of how to ensure that effective interventions are designed and implemented (Eber, 2003; Duchnowski et al., 2002). Although some states, communities, and universities have developed interagency training processes and programs, formalized training procedures and materials based on research-tested skill sets are lacking. If practitioners trained to facilitate wraparound teams emerge from a variety of fields (i.e., mental health, education, probation), consistent training structures that consider the nuances of these historically separate fields are needed.

Nonetheless, training curricula based on a common definition and key elements of wraparound have been developed by leaders in the field (Burns & Goldman, 1999). Training for practitioners on how to guide the development of effective wraparound teams that represents the strengths, culture, preferences, and needs of an individual child and family is typically ongoing in system-of-care communities. This is especially the case in the 85 CMHS[RR1] grant-funded communities where training and technical assistance for implementing system of care principles are required components. Accessing community resources, developing natural supports, building and using strengths, and identifying interventions that are acceptable across multiple settings with the key people who interact with the child may be skill areas that some professionals have not been exposed to through previous training or experience. Examples of specific skill sets needed for those facilitating wraparound teams (Eber, 2003) include:

• *Initial conversations* as the initial step in engaging the family by listening to their story. The facilitator is trained to learn about the families' (and teachers' and other

service providers') past experiences, needs, fears, natural supports, quality-of-life preferences, and hopes and dreams for their child and family.

• *Blending perspectives* of different team members to define specific outcomes that family members, teachers, and other professionals can agree on to problem-solve together in a nonblaming, nonjudging manner. Obtaining data (i.e., strengths, needs) from multiple perspectives is needed before a team, a plan, and interventions are developed.

• *Needs versus services* is an important distinction that wraparound team members need to understand, as many family members and service providers often state needs in terms of services. For example, they may think they are stating needs when they say "The child needs counseling" or "The family needs a residential placement for their child." Helping teams clarify needs (i.e., the child needs to learn new ways to get attention from adults; the child needs to have friends to play with; the family needs to feel that all of their children are safe) is an important skill for wraparound teams.

An example of new partnerships that are forming out of the system of care work being done across this country involves families taking on new roles as trainers and faculty. In *A Shared Agenda* (NASDSE, 2002) family members were identified as playing a potent role in teaching practitioners about how to make their systems and services more family-friendly. Having family members as faculty gives providers and professionals the invaluable opportunity to hear firsthand about what has worked from families who have designed and developed effective services for their children. Their personal experience brings to life what providers and administrators can only partially learn through textbooks. Family as faculty, and the curricula offered by family-run organizations, provides families an opportunity to develop strategies that dissolve some of the barriers that make it difficult for local systems and providers to be creative in designing services and supports for children and their families (Osher, deFur, Nava, Spencer, & Toth-Dennis, 1999). Other examples of family involvement in teacher training include parents giving guest lectures to preservice teachers on issues related to parenting, child care, raising a child with special needs, and transitioning children into the school system; parents designing teacher education programs; and working with pre-service teachers who are assigned to work closely with a single family for several weeks and keep a journal of their activities (Shartrand, Weiss, Kreider, & Lopez, 1997).

Having family members as trainers in school and agency personnel preparation models the collaboration required in a system of care. In North Carolina, family members assist training teams and faculty in the development, review, and critique of university curriculum, and effectively team-teach in university classrooms. They integrate system-of-care principles and practices into graduate and undergraduate curricula. Faculty members noted that, while student attitudes toward families were generally positive at the beginning of the class, by the end they were even less blaming and more community-oriented. Surveys taken at the end of the class all had positive comments regarding the co-teaching model and suggested that more classes be structured on the basis of a similar model (Osher et al., 1998).

IMPLEMENTING SYSTEMS OF CARE: WHAT ARE THE OUTCOMES?

Program evaluation results of system-of-care initiatives over the past 20 years have offered insights about implementation strategies, and the early results are described as encouraging (see, for example, Burns & Goldman, 1999; Burns & Hoagwood, 2002; Epstein, Kutash, & Duchnowski, 1998; Stroul, 1993). Examples of system outcomes include reductions in use of restrictive placements and greater access to a broader array of services. Consumer outcomes include increased parent and child satisfaction and functioning outcomes that include improved behavioral/emotional functioning at home, in school, and in the community. Lack of controlled studies is a recognized weakness, as most results are simply pre–post design studies done as program evaluation rather than research.

CMHS Demonstration Projects

National evaluation data, gathered from through August of 1999, focused on 31

grant communities that developed systems of care for approximately 40,029 children and their families. Over half of the children (55%) had an individualized education program (IEP), and 62% of those with IEPs had a designation of EBD. The outcomes, published in the *Evaluation of the Comprehensive Community Mental Health Services for Children and Their Families Program: Annual Report to Congress 1999* (Center for Mental Health, 1999), are divided into clinical and functional categories. One important clinical outcome was the reduction of behavior and emotional problems in 42% of the children who had received 2 years of services. Of these 42%, 70% were reduced to below clinical levels and were no longer classified as clinically impaired in their social functioning. Although boys and girls entering the system with comparable levels of functional impairment made improvements, girls showed faster and larger improvements in functioning than boys.

In addition, school attendance and performance improved. After 1 year in the program, regular school attendance improved from 85.9% to 89.4%. For students remaining in the program for up to a year, grades that were average or above-average increased by 20%. Another measure of the effectiveness of the system was the children's interaction with law enforcement, which dropped by 25% among children who participated in services for more than a year.

About 17% of the children in communities funded in 1993 and 1994 had a dual diagnosis of substance abuse and a mental disorder. Although these children were confronted with greater obstacles, they made the largest improvements in functioning after 1 year in the program. These children showed a 29-point decrease, overall, in scores on the Child Adolescent Functioning Assessment Scale (Hodges, 1994), in comparison to a 12-point reduction for children without a substance abuse diagnosis.

A review of the 85 projects funded by CMHS has shown several common factors in school-based programs that have proven effective. These include the use of clinicians and other student support providers in the schools; a profamily approach to services, with significant family involvement; community-based support and training across regular and special education, mental health, social service, and juvenile justice professionals; and diverse groups working together to achieve cultural competency. All of these school-based programs incorporated some form of the wraparound approach.

School-Based Wraparound

The experiences of the La Grange Area Department of Education's (LADSE) implementing the wraparound process have been reported as an early example of education taking a lead role in coordinating system-of-care principles through a multiple agency network (Duchnowski, Kutash, & Friedman, 2002). Funded through an Office of Special Education Programs systems change grant in 1991, a coalition of providers from multiple agencies both private and public (education, mental health, juvenile justice, child welfare) and family members was convened to support implementation. Individual wraparound teams were initially developed for children returning from hospital and residential placements with families in lead decision-making roles. After 2 years, LADSE restructured its special education programs, using wraparound as the planning process to develop individualized plans that were strength-based and involved multiple life domain strategies using natural supports as well as traditional mental health and educational strategies. Reductions in use of out-of-home settings and self-contained classrooms were reported as the primary model for students with EBD (Eber, 1996).

Lehigh Valley Council for Youth

An unusual partnership between United Way of Greater Lehigh Valley, Pennsylvania, and local school districts resulted in implementation of the wraparound process through school-based teams. Different from the LADSE project, where school social workers where retrained and repositioned to facilitate wraparound teams, the Lehigh Valley United Way hired, trained, and supervised the wraparound team facilitators who were placed in schools through collaborative agreements in which schools gradually assumed funding responsibility for the positions. Annual reports for 2000–2001 and 2001–2002 show increases in school attendance, improved social/emotional functioning based on the CAFAS, increases in academic averages, and increases in assets reported by youths (i.e., constructive use of time, adult support, family support, homework completion, conflict resolution, hopes about the future). Collaboration with juvenile probation during 2001–2002 yielded significant reductions in suspensions and absences from school among 23 youths who were on probation.

Westerly, Rhode Island

This Rhode Island school system created school- and systemwide supports for all students, providing early intervention for students who are at risk and more intensive services to address the needs of students with EBD. A continual system of care from early elementary school through high school was created and supported by "planning center" models that connect the school and community with social services agencies as well as providing many resources for individual student support needs (Woodruff et al., 1999). The results of the program included decreases in truancies, suspensions, penalization retentions, failing grades, and major aggressive episodes, whereas passing grades, school attendance, number of special-needs students who made the honor roll, student mediation, and satisfied staff and parents increased (Keenan, 1997).

LINKS FROM THE PAST, HOPES FOR THE FUTURE
School-Based Systems of Care

Even though school and mental health partnerships have been underutilized, schools are recognized as potentially powerful in effecting better outcomes for students with or at risk of EBD due to the "scope of influence" they have on the lives of children (Duchnowski et al., 2002). Effective behavioral interventions for students with EBD are available (Peacock Hill Working Group, 1992). Getting these interventions implemented in schools has been the challenge. To be successful, a system of care must have the capacity to design, implement, and evaluate interventions likely to produce positive change in the quality and life experiences of individual children and their families. Ensuring that those who spend the most time interacting with children with EBD (i.e., educators and families) are equipped with the knowledge about effective interventions is critical.

In Chapter 25 of this volume, by Liaupsin, Jolivette, and Scott, a schoolwide intervention model has been presented to guide educators in conceptualizing and applying positive behavior supports (PBS) across the whole school population. System-of-care approaches such as wraparound are an important component of schoolwide systems of PBS (see Scott & Eber, 2003) and offer promising direction for school and mental health partnerships. The emerging knowledge of how to implement schoolwide PBS across all school settings for all students, including those with EBD, together with family-centered collaborative approaches that bring community supports into active partnerships with teachers and families offer much promise for systemic change that affects schools, families, and communities. The 2000 Surgeon General's Conference on Children's Mental Health (U.S. Public Health Service, 2002) referenced the three-tiered schoolwide system of PBS among their goals and action steps, many of which related to systems of care and interagency collaboration.

Systems of care and wraparound build on a key concept of PBS introduced by Carr and his colleagues (1994) that intervention involves changing the social systems, not simply the individual. Schools involved with schoolwide positive behavior supports are learning that the goal is not just to change the individual but to alter the environment around them so that positive behaviors are more likely to occur. This knowledge can become a powerful tool for wraparound teams committed to unconditional support for youth.

Walker and his colleagues (1996) propose that interventions for students with the most complex needs will be strengthened by building consistent structures for organizing and applying effective behavior interventions throughout school environments. Data from Illinois PBS schools support this concept. In an end-of-year report, Lewis-Palmer, Horner, Sugai, and Eber (2002) indicated that PBS schools that report 80% or more of staff involved in schoolwide universal strategies also report greater effectiveness (60%) with their wraparound-based interventions

for students with significant challenges than schools with less than 80% involvement with universal strategies (40%). These findings suggest that investing in building schoolwide systems of positive behavior support around all students can increase school personnel's confidence and ability to effectively educate students with the most challenging emotional/behavioral needs. Combining the technology of effective behavior change with interagency collaborative approaches may be a useful way to structure systems of care in schools.

Communities and states involved with the CMHS system of care grants have begun expanding their collaborations with their education partners to include schoolwide systems of PBS. Some states (i.e., New York, New Hampshire, North Carolina, and Delaware) have active interagency planning and implementation of schoolwide systems of PBS with joint leadership from at least mental health and education. These education/mental health partnerships actively assist schools to establish consistent practices that promote prosocial skills of all students and reduce reliance on reactive discipline measures. The focus is on establishing school environments where strength-based interventions that rearrange environments around students with EBD to ensure their success in natural school settings can more readily occur. Several CMHS grant communities are using the schoolwide system of PBS as a key structure for implementation of system of care for students with EBD (e.g., Chicago, eastern Kentucky), while other CMHS demonstration sites are adding the schoolwide system of PBS to their local system-of-care implementation plan (i.e., Tampa, Florida; Worcester, Masssachusetts). The current task for these communities is to establish an effective role for families, mental health professionals, and other community providers in school-based systems of care that recognize that prevention and early intervention are critical parts of the system.

Systems of Care for Infants and Toddlers

Jane Knitzer (1995) challenged the field by focusing on the mental health needs of the youngest and most vulnerable children and the need for integrated early childhood systems of care. At the 2000 Surgeon's General Conference (U.S. Public Health Service, 2002), she stressed the importance of building a knowledge-based system to promote emotional wellness and resilience in infants, toddlers, and preschoolers facing a range of challenges. The lack of appropriate services persists despite clear evidence that the prevalence rates for serious disorders in young children are similar to those of older children.

A study of more than 3,800 preschool-age children reported that 21% of the sample met the criteria for a psychiatric disorder and 9.1% met the criteria for a severe emotional disorder (Lavigne, 1996). The number of children living in one-parent homes continues to grow, as does the number of children whose lives are affected in some way by substance abuse, mental illness, and HIV. In addition, one child in six has no health insurance; one in seven has a working family member but is still poor; and one in thirteen is born with low birth weight. Three of five preschoolers are in child care every day, and of all children under age 5, 41% spend 35 or more hours in child care each week (Children's Defense Fund, 2000). Recent research shows that early childhood is a critical period for supporting the mental, emotional, and behavioral development of very young children.

The main goal of an early childhood system of care is to create an environment in which young children who are at risk and those with established developmental delays or emotional disturbances can achieve optimal biological, psychological, and social development (Pumariega & Winters, 2003). High-quality early childhood programs may protect children from the effects of exposure to risk factors and may also create or enhance protective factors for children considered to be at risk of EBD (Knitzer, 1995). Systems of care serving young children and their families are guided by values and practice guidelines that are similar to those of systems of care for older children, but with the addition of knowledge and expertise related to early childhood developmental needs and the importance of nurturing environments. Program developments in early childhood mental health services have been guided by research showing that early intervention can systematically reduce later developmental challenges for children when the interventions are offered during the first 5 years of life.

GUIDING THE FUTURE: A NEED FOR RESEARCH

There is clearly a need to establish consensus about effective interventions and treatment among various care providers (i.e., family, school, mental health, primary health, juvenile justice, etc.). Researchers have proposed types of outcomes that need to be addressed in studies comparing system of care to traditional service delivery models. System outcomes include utilization of restrictive settings, cost, and reinvestment of system resources. Child/family categories such as clinical diagnosis; functioning or adaptability across home, school, and community; satisfaction or quality of life; and safety have been proposed (Duchnowski et al., 2002). But how do we clearly connect system structures and practice to child/family outcomes?

The challenges to establishing a research base for system of care and wraparound are well documented and include a lack of controlled studies as well as questions about fidelity of the intervention. How do we identify appropriate comparison groups for communitywide evaluation of system of care? How do researchers capture consistent application of interventions that are based on the unique needs, culture, and strengths of each youth and family? Further complicating the situation is that the term "wraparound" has been sometimes used to describe interventions that are not consistent with the original approach and do not meet the definitional criteria (Burchard et al., 2002). How do we differentiate studies that purport to study system of care and wraparound but just increase access and flexibility while applying more of the same clinical practices (i.e., therapy)?

Participants at the Surgeon General's Conference provided some of the answers to these questions in 2000. The report calls for investing in early childhood mental health through system-of-care approaches and refocusing research from system-level changes and performance to an examination of the effects of system change on individual outcomes. Evaluating effectiveness is especially important given managed care, calls for accountability, and decreasing state and local budgets. It will require leaders in the field to define what are appropriate child and family outcomes and what are realistic time frames for achieving these outcomes (Pumariega & Winters, 2003). The need to provide effective, comprehensive networks of supports and services to all children with or at risk of EBD and their families is a daunting task for all child-serving agencies. Expanded policy, funding, and research that prioritize collaborative systemwide prevention and early intervention as critical components of systems of care, rather than through reactive approaches of individual agencies, offers promise for better outcomes for children, families, and communities.

REFERENCES

Bandura, A. (1977). *Social learning theory.* Englewood Cliffs, NJ: Prentice Hall.

Blackorby, J., & Wagner, M. (1996[MQ7]). Longitudinal post school outcomes of youth with disabilities: Findings from the National Longitudinal Transition Study. *Exceptional Children, 62,* 399–413.

Bronfenbrenner, U. (1979). *The ecology of human development.* Cambridge, MA: Harvard University Press.

Burchard, J. D., Bruns, E. J., & Burchard, S. N. (2002). The wraparound approach. In B. Burns & K. Hoagwood (Eds.), *Community treatment for youth: Evidence-based interventions for severe emotional and behavioral disorders.* New York: Oxford University Press.

Burns, B. J., Costello, E. J., Angold, A., Tweed, D., Stangl, D., Farmer, E. M. Z., & Erkanli, A. (1997). Children's mental health service use across service sectors. *Health Affairs, 14,* 148–159.

Burns, B. J., & Goldman, S. K. (1999). *Promising practices in wraparound for children with serious emotional disturbance and their families: Vol. 4. Systems of care: Promising practices in children's mental health.* Washington DC: Center for Effective Collaboration and Practice, American Institutes for Research.

Burns, B. J., & Hoagwood, K. (Eds.). (2002). *Community treatment for youth: Evidence-based interventions for severe emotional and behavioral disorders.* New York: Oxford University Press.

Carr, E. G. Dunlap, G., Horner, R. H., Koegel, R. L., Turnbull A. P., Sailor, W., Anderson, J. L, Albin, R.W., Koegel, L. K., & Fox, L. (2002). Positive behavior support: Evolution of an applied science. *Journal of Positive Behavior Interventions, 4,* 4–16.

Carr, E. G., Levin, L., McConnachie, G., Carlson, J. I.,

Kemp, D. C., & Smith, C. E. (1994). *Communication-based intervention for problem behavior: A user's guide for producing change.* Baltimore: Brookes.

Carson, R. R., Sitlington, P. C., & Frank, A. R. (1995). Young adulthood for individuals with behavior disorders: What does it hold? *Behavioral Disorders, 20,* 127–135.

Center for Mental Health Services. (1999). *Annual report to Congress on the evaluation of the Comprehensive Community Mental Health Services for Children and Their Families Program, 1999.* Atlanta, GA: ORC Macro.

Children's Defense Fund. (2000). *The state of America's children yearbook 2000.* Available at *http://www.childrensdefense.org/keyfacts.html.*

Clark, H. B., & Heinemann, M. (1999). Comparing the Wraparound Process to positive behavior support: What can we learn? *Journal of Positive Behavior Interventions, 1,* 183–186.

Duchnowski, A. J., Kutash, K., & Friedman, R. M. (2002). Community-based interventions in a systems of care and outcomes framework. In B. Burns & K. Hoagwood (Eds.), *Community treatment for youth: Evidence-based interventions for severe emotional and behavioral disorders.* New York: Oxford University Press.

Eber, L. (1996). Restructuring schools through wraparound approach: The LADSE experience. In R. J. Illback & C. M. Nelson (Eds), *School-based services for students with emotional and behavioral disorders* (pp. 139–154). Binghamton, NY: Haworth.

Eber, L. (2003). *The art and science of wraparound: Completing the continuum of schoolwide behavioral support.* Bloomington, IN: Forum on Education at Indiana University.

Eber, L., Nelson, C. M., & Miles, P. (1997). School-based wraparound for students with emotional and behavioral challenges. *Exceptional Children, 63,* 539–555.

Eber, L., Sugai, G., Smith, C., & Scott, T. (2002). Wraparound and positive behavioral interventions and supports in the schools. *Journal of Emotional and Behavioral Disorders, 10,* 171–180.

Epstein, M. H., Kutash, K., & Duchnowski, A. (1998). *Outcomes for children and youth with emotional and behavioral disorders and their families: Programs and evaluation best practices.* Austin, TX: Pro-Ed.

Farmer, E. M. Z., Stangl, D. K., Burns, B. J., Costello, E. J., & Angold, A. (1999). Use, persistence and intensity: Patterns of care for children's mental health across one year. *Community Mental Health Journal, 35,* 31–46.

Faw, L. (1998). The state wraparound survey. *Promising practices in wraparound for children with serious emotional disturbance and their families* (Vol. 4, pp. 61–65). Washington DC: Center for Effective Collaboration and Practice, American Institute for Research.

Forness, S. R. (2002). Schools and identification of mental health needs. In U.S. Public Health Service, *Report of the Surgeon General's Conference on Children's Mental Health: A National Action Agenda* (pp. 22–23). Washington, DC: U.S. Public Health Service.

Friedman, R. M., Katz-Leavy, J. W., & Sondheimer, D. L. (1996). Prevalence of severe emotional disturbance in children and adolescents. In R. W. Manderscheid & M. A. Sonnenschein (Eds.), *Mental health, United States, 1996* (pp. 71–89). Rockville, MD: Department of Health and Human Services, Public Health Services, Substance Abuse and Mental Health Services Administration, Center for Mental Health Services.

Friesan, B. J., Giliberti, M., Katz-Levy, J., Osher, T., & Pullmann, M. D. (2003). Research in the service of policy change: The custody problem. *Journal of Emotional and Behavioral Disorders, 11*, 39–48.

Hernandez, M., & Hodges, S. (2003). Building upon the theory of change for systems for care. *Journal of Emotional and Behavioral Disorders, 11*, 19–26.

Hoagwood, K., Burns, B. J., Kiser, L., Ringeisen, H., & Schoenwald, S. K. (2001). Evidence-based practice in child and adolescent mental health services. *Psychiatric Services, 52*, 1179–1190.

Hoagwood, K., & Erwin, H. (1997). Effectiveness of school-based mental heath services for children: A 10-year research review. *Journal of Child and Family Studies, 6*, 435–451.

Hodges, K. (1994). *The Child and Adolescent Functional Assessment Scale.* Available from Kay Hodges, Psychology Department, Eastern Michigan University, Ypsilanti, MI 48197.

Kallas, A. (1992). *Research in special education: Directory of current projects, 1992 edition.* Reston, VA: Council for Exceptional Children, ERIC/OSEP Special Project.

Keenan, S. (1997). Program elements that support teachers and students with learning and behavior problems. In P. Zionts (Ed.), *Inclusion strategies for students with learning and behavioral problems* (pp. 117–138). Austin, TX: Pro-Ed.

Kelleher, K. (2002). Primary care and identification of mental health needs. In U.S. Public Health Service, *Report of the Surgeon General's Conference on Children's Mental Health: A National Action Agenda* (pp. 21–22). Washington, DC: U.S. Public Health Service.

Knitzer, J. (1982). *Unclaimed children: The failure of public responsibility to children and adolescents in need of mental health services.* Washington, DC: Children's Defense Fund.

Knitzer, J. (1995). Meeting the mental health needs of young children and families: Service needs, challenges, and opportunities. In B. Stroul (Ed.), *Systems of care of children and adolescents with serious emotional disturbances: From theory to reality.* Baltimore: Brookes.

Knitzer, J., Steinberg, Z., & Flesch, B. (1990). At the school house door: An examination of programs and policies for children with behavioral and emotional problems. New York: Bank Street College of Education.

Koyanagi, C., & Gaines, S. (1993). *All systems failure: An examination of the results of neglecting the needs of children with serious emotional disturbance.* Alexandria, VA: National Mental Health Association.

Lavigne, J. V. (1996). Prevalence rates and correlates of psychiatric disorder among preschool children. *Journal of the American Academy of Child and Adolescent Psychiatry, 35*, 204–214.

Leaf, P. J., Aelgria, M., Cohen, P., Goodman, S. H., Horwitz, S. M., Hoven, C. W., Narrow, W. E., Vaden- Kiernan, M., & Regier, D. A. (1996). Mental health service use in the community and schools: Results from the four-community MECA study. *Journal of American Academy of Child and Adolescent Psychiatry, 35*, 889–897.

Leone, P. E., & Meisel, S. (1997). Improving education services for students in detention confinement facilities. *Children's Legal Rights Journal, 71*(1), 2–12.

Lewis-Palmer, T., Horner, R. H., Sugai, G., & Eber, L. (2002). An end-of-year progress report for the Illinois PBIS Initiative. Available at *www.ebdnetwork-il.org.*

Lourie, I. S. (1994). *Principles of local system development for children, adolescents, and their families.* Chicago: Kaleidoscope.

Munger, R. L. (1998). *The ecology of troubled children.* Cambridge, MA: Brookline.

NASDSE, National Association of State Mental Health Program Directors and the Policymaker Partnership for Implementing IDEA at the National Association of State Directors of Special Education. (2002). *Mental health, schools and families working together for all children and youth: Toward a shared agenda.* Alexandria, VA: Author.

National Institute of Mental Health. (1983). *Program announcement: Child and Adolescent Service System Program.* Rockville, MD: Author.

Osher, T., deFur, E., Nava, C., Spencer, S., & Toth-Dennis, D. (1999). New roles for families in systems of care. In *Systems of care: Promising practices in children's mental health* (Vol. I). Washington, DC: Center for Effective Collaboration and Practice, American Institutes for Research.

Peacock Hill Working Group. (1992). Problems and promises in the education of students with emotional and behavioral disorders. *Behavioral Disorders, 16*, 299–313.

Pumariega, A., & Winters, N. (2003). *The handbook of child and adolescent systems of care, the new community psychiatry.* San Francisco: Jossey-Bass.

Scott, T., & Eber, L. (2003). Functional assessment and wraparound as systemic school processes: Primary, secondary, and tertiary systems examples. *Journal of Positive Behavior Supports, 5*, 131–143.

Shartrand, A. M., Weiss, H. B., Kreider, H. M., & Lopez, M. E. (1997). *New skills for new schools:*

Preparing teachers in family involvement. Cambridge, MA: Harvard Family Research Project, Harvard Graduate School of Education.

Smith, S. W., & Coutinho, M. J. (1997). Achieving the goals of the national agenda: Progress and prospects. *Journal of Emotional and Behavioral Disorders, 5,* 2–5.

Stroul, B. A. (1993). *Systems of care for children and adolescents with severe emotional disturbances: What are the results?* Washington, DC: Georgetown University Child Development Center.

Stroul, B. A., & Friedman, R. M. (1986). *A system of care for children and youth with severe emotional disturbances* (rev. ed.). Washington, DC: Georgetown University Child Development Center, CASSP Technical Assistance Center.

U.S. Department of Education. (1994). *National agenda for achieving better results for children and youth with serious emotional disturbance.* Washington, DC: Office of Special Education Programs, U.S. Department of Education.

U.S. Department of Education. (1997). *Public Law 94-142: The Individuals with Disabilities Education Act.* Washington, DC: Author.

U.S. Department of Education. (1998). *Twentieth annual report to Congress on the implementation of IDEA: The Individuals with Disabilities Education Act.* Washington, DC: U.S. Government Printing Office.

U.S. Department of Education. (2002). *Public Law 107-110: The No Child Left Behind Act of 2001.* Washington, DC: Author.

U.S. Public Health Service. (2002). *Report of the Surgeon General's Conference on Children's Mental Health: A national action agenda.* Washington, DC: Author.

VanDenBerg, J. (1998). History of the wraparound process. In B. J. Burns & S. K. Goldman (Eds.), *Promising practices in wraparound for children with serious emotional disturbance and their families: Vol 4. Systems of care: Promising practices in children's mental health* (pp. 1–8). Washington DC: Center for Effective Collaboration and Practice, American Institutes for Research.

Wagner, M. M. (1995). Outcomes for youths with serious emotional disturbance in secondary school and early adulthood. *Critical Issues for Children and Youths, 5,* 90–112.

Walker, H. M., Horner, R. H., Sugai, G., Bullis, M., Sprague, J. R., Bricker, D., & Kaufman, M. J. (1996). Integrated approaches to preventing antisocial behavioral patterns among school-age youth and children. *Journal of Emotional and Behavioral Disorders, 4,* 193–256.

Woodruff, D. W., Osher, D., Hoffman, C. C., Gruner, A., King, M. A., Snow, S. T., & McIntire, J. C. (1999). The role of education in a system of care: Effectively serving children with emotional or behavioral disorders. *Systems of care: Promising practices in children's mental health* (Vol. 1, p. 40). Washington, DC: Center for Effective Collaboration and Practice, American Institutes for Research.

PART V

RESEARCH METHODOLOGY

Introduction

Eleanor Guetzloe

My personal introduction to research in the field of emotional and behavioral disorders (EBD) took place in 1966. I was then a new graduate student at the University of South Florida (USF) pursuing a master's degree in the field of special education. My assignment was to become familiar with the literature related to one category of disability, and I chose to study students with EBD.

The very first research report I read was *Public School Classes for the Emotionally Handicapped: A Research Analysis* by William C. Morse, Richard L. Cutler, and Albert H. Fink (Morse, Cutler, & Fink, 1964). My next choice was Eli M. Bower's *The Education of Emotionally Handicapped Children* (1961). In a very short time, I was caught up in the excitement of this relatively new but quickly expanding field of study.

A FEW OF MY FAVORITE THINGS

In fact, the literature in this field and its related disciplines became the deciding factor in my choice to make the education and treatment of students with EBD my life's work. As I began to write this introduction, I gathered a few of the older texts from my bookshelves. They are like old friends: *The Aggressive Child* (Redl & Wineman, 1957), *On Becoming a Person* (Rogers, 1961), *Educating Emotionally Disturbed Children* (Haring & Phillips, 1962), *Conflict in the Classroom* (Long, Morse, & Newman, 1965),

The Emotionally Disturbed Child in the Classroom (Hewett, 1968), *Educating Emotionally Disturbed Children* (Dupont, 1969), *Educating the Emotionally Disturbed* (Harshman, 1969), *Behavior Disorders in School-Aged Children* (Clarizio & McCoy, 1970), and *Psychopathological Disorders of Childhood* (Quay & Werry, 1972), to mention a few. I have often wished that they were all still in print. To attain some sense of the history of this field, our new professionals need sets of their own.

Upon graduation, I was invited to become a member of the faculty at the University of South Florida, specializing in the area of EBD. For the next 34 years, I sought the best research, articles, and texts available, believing strongly that it was my responsibility to share the most valid and reliable information with those who would enter this field, those who would serve students with EBD.

Students in our master's program were required to complete one course in research methods and design, in addition to a prerequisite course in educational measurement. The major focus in both of these courses was on becoming an efficient consumer of research, with the knowledge and skills necessary to understand research findings and apply those findings in the classroom. All of our classes required reviews of the current literature to include the practical implications of research studies. My students would often complain that the authors of research articles did not state the practical implications of their studies and that the findings were often not relevant to their own situations.

Researchers and practitioners share responsibilities for the applicability of research findings. Research data must be (1) understandable (explained in practical terms), (2) relevant (applicable in educational settings), and (3) replicable with students with EBD. Meeting these criteria is the responsibility of the researcher/author. Teachers also must have the knowledge and skills necessary to apply research findings with fidelity, which are among the practitioners' responsibilities (as well as those of the institutions that provide teacher training).

APPROPRIATE TEACHER TRAINING

As part of their preservice education, teachers need specific knowledge and skills in the interpretation and use of research findings. Courses in educational methods and materials should stress research-based instructional strategies that have been determined to be effective (e.g., the steps of direct instruction, the techniques of precision teaching, or the principles of universal design for learning).

Today, more than ever, there is a tremendous need for teachers and other education professionals to be able to understand and apply research-based instructional procedures. Prompted recently by the provisions of the No Child Left Behind Act (NCLB), the U.S. Department of Education (DOE) has called for the use of "scientifically based" instructional procedures in all classrooms, including those for students with EBD as well as other students with disabilities. The DOE has also proclaimed that only "scientifically based" research will receive funding.

The provisions of this legislation have not been accepted without controversy. Education authorities have questioned a number of the NCLB mandates; of particular concern are the requirements that statewide standardized tests be used to measure the adequate yearly progress of all students (Neill, 2003; Marshak, 2003). The mandate that is probably of greatest concern to researchers is that only "scientifically based"

research will be funded by the DOE. What is meant by the term "scientifically based?"

According to the DOE guidelines (U.S. Department of Education, 2003), research studies must meet the following criteria in order to receive federal funding:

1. Use of rigorous, systematic, and empirical methods.
2. Adequacy of data to justify the general conclusion drawn.
3. Reliance on methods that provide valid data across multiple measurements and observations.
4. Use of control groups.
5. Assurance that details allow for replication.
6. Acceptance by a peer-reviewed journal or approval by a panel of independent experts.

Odom (2003) noted that, in policies currently followed in funding competitions, the DOE seems to find acceptable only research evidence derived from randomized experimental group designs (REGD). While agreeing that REGD provides a rigorous way of proving positive outcomes of interventions, Odom expressed concern about limiting all research to this methodology, pointing out that different research questions require different research designs. Some of those different methodologies are the topics of the remaining several chapters in this text.

WHAT'S IN THIS SECTION?

In Part V of this *Handbook*, the various authors address (1) applied behavior analysis, (2) experimental research design, (3) qualitative research, and (4) data collection in research and application. Each chapter includes a review of the research literature, definitions and descriptions of the principles of the specific methodology, and recommendations for improvement in the use of that research design in the study of students with EBD.

In Chapter 27, Timothy J. Lewis, Teri Lewis-Palmer, Lori Newcomer, and Janine Stichter discuss the principles and practices of applied behavior analysis (ABA) and the application of ABA to the study of individual students, classrooms, and entire schools.

These authors note the wide acceptance and classroom use of strategies based on behavioral principles. They also review ABA-based strategies commonly used with students with EBD (e.g., functional behavior assessment, positive reinforcement, response cost, and extinction).

In discussing experimental research design and its application to the study of children and youth with EBD, Richard Van Acker, Mitchell L. Yell, Renée Bradley, and Erik Drasgow in Chapter 28 provide overviews of two research designs (true experiments and quasi-experimental designs) and their application to the scientific study of students with EBD. Based upon their review of the literature, they make a number of specific recommendations for strengthening experimental designs in research related to students with EBD.

In Chapter 29, Edward J. Sabornie addresses the contributions of qualitative research to our knowledge of students with EBD. He calls for the acceptance of both qualitative and quantitative research methods in the field of special education. He presents an overview of the five most commonly used qualitative research designs, together with examples of how each technique can be used to address various problems in the field of EBD. He also provides a review of the limited number of published qualitative research studies that have dealt with issues in the field of EBD.

Philip L. Gunter and R. Kenton Denny, in the final chapter, discuss data collection in research and the application of data in the instruction of students with EBD. They present a strong case for formative evaluation of student progress (i.e., frequent and repeated measurement) rather than summative evaluation only (e.g., published norm-referenced test results). They cite the need, as described by the National Council for Accreditation of Teacher Education (NCATE, 2000), for teachers-in-training to (1) collect and analyze data and (2) use those data to support and improve student learning. They stress the importance of teacher training in the use of behavioral techniques and address the application of technology in data collection research procedures. They discuss specific technologies that are being applied to data collection, including descriptions of the various computer software systems.

SUMMARY

In legislation, rules, and regulations, the United States government has called for the use of scientifically based practices in all of our nation's schools. The authors of this section have addressed research methods that are useful in providing valid and reliable information related to the characteristics and needs of students with EBD, as well as their progress in school and classroom programs.

REFERENCES

Bower, E. M. (1961). *The education of emotionally handicapped children.* Sacramento: California State Department of Education.

Clarizio, H. F., & McCoy, G. F. (1970). *Behavior disorders in school-aged children.* Scranton, PA: Chandler.

Dupont, H. (1969). *Educating emotionally disturbed children.* New York: Holt.

Haring, N. G., & Phillips, E. L. (1962). *Educating emotionally disturbed children.* New York: McGraw-Hill.

Harshman, H. W. (1969). *Educating the emotionally disturbed.* New York: Crowell.

Hewett, F. M. (1968). *The emotionally disturbed child in the classroom.* Boston: Allyn & Bacon.

Long, N. J., Morse, W. C., & Newman, R. G. (1965). *Conflict in the classroom.* Belmont, CA: Wadsworth.

Marshak, D. (2003, November). No Child Left Behind: A foolish race into the past. *Phi Delta Kappan, 85,* 229–231.

Morse, W. C., Cutler, R. L., & Fink, A. H. (1964). *Public school classes for the emotionally handicapped: A research analysis.* Washington, DC: Council for Exceptional Children.

National Council for Accreditation of Teacher Education. (2003). *Professional standards for the accreditation of schools, colleges, and departments of education.* Washington, DC: Author.

Neill, M. (2003, November). Leaving children behind: How No Child Left Behind will fail our children. *Phi Delta Kappan, 85,* 225–228.

Odom, S. (2003, July). Education, science, and the teeth of Aristotle's wives. *Focus on Research, 16*(4), 1–2, 4.

Quay, H. C., & Werry, J. S. (1972). *Psychopathological disorders of childhood.* New York: Wiley.

Redl, F., & Wineman, D. (1957). *The aggressive child.* Glencoe, IL: Free Press.

Rogers, C. R. (1961). *On becoming a person.* Cambridge, MA: Riverside Press.

U.S. Department of Education (2003). *No Child Left Behind: A toolkit for teachers.* Washington, DC: U.S. Department of Education.

27

Applied Behavior Analysis and the Education and Treatment of Students with Emotional and Behavioral Disorders

TIMOTHY J. LEWIS, TERI LEWIS-PALMER,
LORI NEWCOMER, *and* JANINE STICHTER

Students with emotional and behavioral disorders (EBD) represent a very heterogeneous group of students who may share a common educational label but little else. As the field of behavior disorders within special education began to establish itself as a distinct discipline—separate from mental health, medicine, and general education—in the early 1950s and 1960s, the field was in need of a science that lent itself to the idiosyncratic nature of each student's disability and "fit" within an instructional context. Initially, most classrooms for children and youths with EBD modeled practices based on mental health and therapeutic approaches such as the League School founded by Carl Fenichel or Nicholas Long's Michigan Fresh Air Camps. However, in the early 1960s the field began applying behavioral psychological principles based on the work of Watson, Thorndike, and Skinner with children with disabilities who displayed high rates of problem behavior. The outcome of this work brought us Bijou's writings on the effect of instruction and reinforcement, Lovaas's work using the principles of positive reinforcement and punishment on shaping severely disabled children's self-injurious

behavior, and Hewitt's application of behavioral psychology to form the "engineered classroom." In 1968 the *Journal of Applied Behavior Analysis* was established and began publishing research reports focusing on the outcomes of investigations using principles and practices of applied behavior analysis (ABA) primarily with subjects with severe disabilities. In the first issue of the journal, a seminal article outlining the essential features of ABA by Baer, Wolf, and Risley (1968) was published. Since then, a significant body of work has been done with ABA focusing on individuals with disabilities who display problem behavior.

ABA is a set of principles and practices that are used to understand current patterns of problem behavior and alter present patterns to lead to higher rates of appropriate behavior. Based on the work of Baer, Wolf, and Risley and others, Cooper, Heron, and Heward (1987) defined ABA as follows:

> Applied behavior analysis is the science in which procedures derived from the principles of behavior are systematically applied to improve socially significant behavior to a meaningful degree and to demonstrate experimen-

tally that the procedures employed were responsible for the improvement in behavior. (p. 14)

The first important principle is the notion that ABA is an "applied" science, meaning the behavior(s) under study must be meaningful to the person within the problem context (e.g., classroom, home, community). Within schools, the emphasis is on those behaviors that will allow children and youths to be more academically and socially successful. As mentioned earlier, ABA has its roots in "behavioral" psychology, specifically operant behaviors as defined by the work of B. F. Skinner. Finally, ABA is "analytic" in that all research in this discipline must demonstrate clear functional relationships between the variable under study and the student's behavior as measured through direct observation.

The majority of research in ABA to date has been conducted with individuals with developmental disabilities. However, in the past three decades more work using ABA principles across a range of individuals with mild disabilities, including EBD, have emerged. Within the past two decades professional periodicals such as the *Journal of Behavioral Education, Behavioral Disorders*, the *Journal of Emotional and Behavioral Disorders, Education and Treatment of Children*, and, most recently, the *Journal of Positive Behavioral Interventions* have published numerous research reports using ABA principles and research designs. The purpose of this chapter is to discuss the important contribution ABA has made in the field of EBD and the larger field of addressing problem behavior within educational settings. Following the three essential features of ABA as outlined above, basic principles of behavior are first presented, followed by an overview of basic ABA research designs. The remainder of the chapter then focuses on the application of ABA principles and research at the individual student, classroom, and schoolwide level. Implications for current and future research and practice are then discussed.

BASIC PRINCIPLES OF ABA

A fundamental assumption of behavioral theory is that all behavioral sequences consist of antecedents, behavior, and consequences (A–B–C). Operant behavior is defined by this three-term contingency that specifies the temporal and functional relationships between antecedent stimuli, behavior, and consequences. Behavioral response is dependent on the antecedent stimuli and an individual's previous learning history in the presence of similar stimuli. When an event occurs with specified probability with another event (e.g., an infant cries and is then picked up by an adult) the covariation between the two events can be used to predict that one will occur based on the presence of the other. Applied behavior analysis is used to determine those variables that occasion (discriminative stimulus) and maintain (positive/negative reinforcement) behavior. This basic model of behavior analysis enables us to predict and control behavior by altering the probability that a specific behavior will occur. Behavior change procedures operationalize principles of behavior to teach replacement behavior, to alter the environment, and to reduce problem behavior.

A functional relationship exists when one event can be made to reliably occur by the manipulation of the other event. Applied behavior analysis principles and procedures can define the functional relationship between behavior and environmental events through the examination of observed behaviors and environmental factors. The identification of functional relationships is critical to the development of effective positive behavior support plans for students with EBD.

Antecedent stimuli are those stimuli that come before the response or behavior, such as prompts or directions a teacher may make in the classroom. The stimulus that signals the performance of a desired response is called a discriminative stimulus (S^D). *Stimulus control* exists when a specific response will appear predictably in the presence of a given stimulus but not in the presence of other stimuli. Take the example of the teacher who uses an attention signal in her classroom. She raises her hand and says, "Eyes up front, please." When she has everyone's attention, the teacher says "Thank you for your cooperation." Her prompt is the S^D that signals the class to direct their attention to the teacher. The consequences that follow a behavior in the presence of specific antecedent stimuli influence the likelihood that the behavior will occur again. In our example, the teacher provided verbal praise (i.e., positive reinforcement) to the students when they demonstrated the desired behavior. Stimulus control is achieved by the (1) effective use of discriminative stimuli, (2) systematic and contingent presentation of a reinforcing stimuli following a behavior, and (3) withholding reinforcing stimuli when the desired behavior does not occur.

Reinforcement and punishment are pervasive in behavior change procedures. The rate of operant behavior is either increased or decreased through the manipulation of consequent stimuli based on these principles. *Reinforcement* describes the functional relationship between an increase in the frequency of a behavior paired with the subsequent presentation or removal of a stimulus following the behavior. *Positive reinforcement* occurs when the consequence or stimulus that follows a behavior is associated with an increase in the behavior. *Negative reinforcement* occurs when the removal of an aversive stimulus is associated with an increase in the student's behavior. *Punishment* is defined as a functional relationship between a consequent stimulus and a decrease in the probability of a subsequent occurrence of the behavior it follows. There are two types of punishment procedures, Type I and Type II. *Type I punishment* is the contingent presentation of an aversive stimulus that results in a decrease in the occurrence of a behavior. *Type II punishment* is the contingent withdrawal of a reinforcing stimuli that results in a decrease in the occurrence of behavior.

Setting events refer to controlling variables that are often far more complex than simple antecedent stimuli. Bijou and Baer (1961) defined a setting event as a stimulus-response interaction that simply because it has occurred, will affect other stimulus-response relationships that follow it. Setting events are those events in the surrounding context of the behavior that influence the relation among the three-term contingency of antecedent, behavior, and consequence. By operating on one or more components of the three-term contingency, setting events can either increase or decrease the probability of

the occurrence of a specific behavior. Consider the teenage student who did not get enough sleep. His lack of sleep and feeling tired can be a setting event that influences his response to various antecedents in the environment, such as a teacher reprimand or attention as well as altering the "value" of reinforcing stimuli.

The behavior patterns of a student are the result of previous experiences with various contingencies of reinforcement and punishment the student has encountered. These response patterns make up a behavior repertoire for the student that functions to access reinforcing stimuli or to escape/avoid aversive stimuli. To support students with EBD, it is important to observe, measure, and analyze how the problem behavior "works" as a function of environmental variables and to consider the learning history of the student. The scientific method is the best way to discover the functional relationships between behavior and the environment. Applied behavior analysis provides a technology made up of highly efficient procedures to assess the functional relationships between behaviors and the environment and the techniques to arrange consequences that increase and decrease behavior in a precise, measurable, and accountable manner.

The sections that follow will provide an overview of basic research designs used within the field of ABA, the use of ABA principles to assess and understand problem behavior, and applications of ABA research at the individual student, classroom, and schoolwide levels.

ABA-BASED RESEARCH DESIGNS

Despite the prevalent use of labels in education and mental health, it is well understood that *individuals* with EBD are by no means a homogenous group. Additionally, despite the specific terminology in the label, the needs of students with EBD do not reside in a "behavior vacuum." Instead, the issues of concern occur within a context and span from social to academic needs. To further understand the impact of this disorder and the related support necessitated, a significant amount of study related to students with EBD has been done utilizing large-scale, indirect research methodology (i.e., surveys, rating scales, interviews) that provide correlational data on specific factors of interest. This methodology is very helpful in providing data on the effectiveness of large-scale interventions as well as risk factors and other general precursors to academic and social behaviors. However, as with all research methodology, these assessments have limitations, primarily due to difficulties in accounting for and controlling variables that may affect the results, as well as limitations in accounting for attributes specific to intra-subject and specific context factors. Therefore, at the individual level, this type of inquiry provides little more than a "conditional probability" regarding the likelihood of a specific behavior or the effectiveness of a specific intervention. Applied behavior analysis has long demonstrated that identifying the interactions between an individual and the context within which they are functioning is essential to predict and affect the behavior of the individual (Cooper et al., 1987). Furthermore, when such analysis is done correctly, the repeated results of such experimentation can provide generalized information that can lead to effective practices designed to increase the likelihood of teaching and promoting desired behavior. By design, such research inherently requires a considerable amount of control and, often, repeated measures of the dependent variable. This is done to ensure that ensuing results are not due to the effect of participating in a novel experimental situation (i.e., to make sure that it is not the presence of additional persons or materials that is causing the change, instead of the designed intervention).

To demonstrate the level of control, single-subject experiments require a great deal of detail in their description to document internal validity (e.g., to assure that the procedures designed are implemented as described) and provide sufficient information for generalization and replication. These studies are typically done with small numbers of participants—as few as one subject at a time—and are most commonly referred to as single-subject designs (SSD) (Tawney & Gast, 1984). ABA research designs typically employ a small number of subjects for two main reasons: (1) the degree of control necessary often prevents the use of large groups of participants in natural settings, and (2) because

ABA designs can be tailored to specific contexts and independent variables, they are often employed to address a specific problem and hence randomization is not employed or desirable (as it is in group design).

Single-subject research demonstrates functional relationships through the use of two critical components. The first is the use of baseline measurement; the second is repeated introduction of the independent variable(s) (Johnston & Pennypacker, 1980). Under baseline conditions a behavior(s) is operationally defined such that it can be accurately and reliably observed. Following baseline, an intervention (independent variable) phase is then introduced. Direct observation data points collected over time and conditions are plotted and visually analyzed for clear within- and across-phase patterns related to (1) level (i.e., the overall amount of behavior within a condition), (2) trend (i.e., patterns of behavior over time—increasing, decreasing, or the same), and (3) variability (i.e., less variability in data lending to firmer conclusions). Data within each phase of a single-subject study should indicate a steady predictive pattern prior to introduction of subsequent phases. At present there are no standards for determining a sufficient number of baseline data points prior to intervention. However, the failure to establish a clear pattern during baseline severely limits the conclusions that can be drawn regarding the impact of the independent variable.

> Establishing stable responding is thus an index of the rigor of experimental control. If sufficiently stable responding cannot be obtained, the experimenter is in no position to add an independent variable of suspected but unknown influence. To do so would be to compound confusion and lead to further ignorance. (Johnston & Pennypacker, 1980, p. 229)

Although the contributions of ABA research designs have long been acknowledged, there continue to be concerns regarding the plausibility of conducting ABA single-subject research with students identified as EBD. This hesitation is verified by the paucity of EBD (as compared to developmental disabilities) single-subject research over the past 20 years (Clarke, Dunlap, & Stichter, 2002). Yet, despite concerns regarding the realistic application of directly measuring and manipulating the behavioral context of higher-functioning students in natural settings, close inspection of the EBD literature provides successful examples of various single-subject designs employed with individuals identified with EBD. The most commonly employed ABA research designs are withdrawal, multiple-baseline, and alternating-treatment designs. The next section will provide definitions of each design, recent published examples across social and academic behaviors, and limitations of each design, specifically related to students with EBD. Each of the designs allows the relationship between the intervention and student behavior to be experimentally documented by demonstrating change a minimum of three times. Additionally, the three demonstrations of change need to occur at three different points in time to help control for possible confounding events (e.g., student illness, change in teachers).

Withdrawal Designs

The withdrawal design serves as the "foundation" of all single-subject designs in that it meets the basic assumptions of single-subject research, allowing the researcher to draw conclusions about functional relationships between the intervention and student behavior. By definition a withdrawal design (A–B–A) presents an intervention and then withdraws it to assess impact (see Figure 27.1 for a sample design). This is typically done with a baseline condition, then an intervention phase, and then a repetition of baseline and intervention phases. Since the baseline phases are repeated, the internal validity is enhanced sufficiently to potentially interpret a functional relationship between the independent and dependent variables. Within applied research this design is typically done to verify the effects of certain variables or conditions, often on problematic behavior. For example, if it were hypothesized that the student with EBD became increasingly agitated or verbally abusive when presented with difficult math work, an A–B–A design might be used to measure behavior during typical math work (A), then when asked to do more challenging work (B), and then again when presented with typical work (A). For ethical and practical reasons, the withdrawal design is typically not constructed in

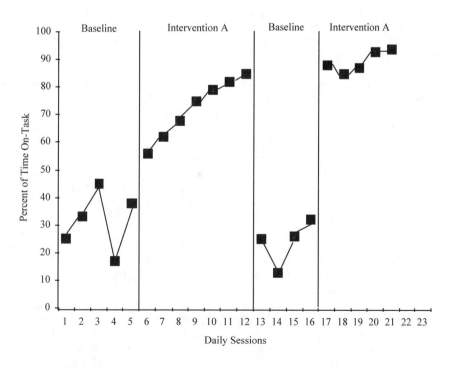

FIGURE 27.1. Sample data from an A–B–A–B, or withdrawal, design.

applied research in a way that intervention assumed to have a positive effect is withdrawn. Instead, one of two options is more typically employed.

Jolivette, Wehby, Canale, and Massey (2001) demonstrated one of these options in their withdrawal design to assess the effects of choice and no choice on student engagement and disruption during math work. Jolivette and her colleagues began with choice, withdrew choice, and then returned to choice, as it was hypothesized that choice would have a positive impact on the dependent variables assessed for the students with EBD. By providing the intervention first and then removing it, the researchers addressed potential ethical and practical issues for the teacher. However, given that they began with intervention, they ran the risk of a compromised "baseline condition." To increase the internal validity of their study, Jolivette et al. embedded their withdrawal design within a multiple baseline design across three students identified with EBD. The second manner in which to address the potential limitations identified above for the withdrawal design is to employ what is more typically referred to as the reversal design (A–B–A–B). This design supports the traditional baseline to intervention to withdrawal/ return to baseline but then reintroduces the intervention in the final phase. It should be noted that, although the prior explanations of reversal design depict those most commonly found in education research, they do not reflect the original intent of the reversal design. For a complete discussion of reversal designs, see Tawney and Gast (1984).

The A–B–A–B design affords increased internal validity and provides the students with additional exposure to the intervention. Kern, Bambara, and Fogt (2002) utilized the reversal design to assess the effects of classwide curricular modifications on the prosocial and challenging behavior of six students identified with severe emotional disturbance. Despite the simplicity and increased internal validity of this design when used to assess an intervention designed to increase desired behavior, even short periods of withdrawal can create increased concerns for practitioners within applied research settings. Additionally, certain behaviors such as those that are dangerous and certain independent variables that cannot be "un-

learned" are not appropriate for withdrawal designs.

Multiple-Baseline Designs

Multiple-baseline designs were introduced to support research question(s) that seek the analysis of more than one dependent variable (Kazdin, 1982). Typically, multiple baselines are conducted across individuals, stimulus conditions (i.e., settings), or specific behaviors. Figure 27.2 provides an illustration of a multiple-baseline design. For example, one might want to assess the impact of an intervention strategy on more than one academic behavior or more than one student. Cade and Gunter (2002) employed such a design when researching the effects of instruction in the use of a mnemonic strategy on the percentage of division facts calculated correctly. These researchers assessed the percentage of correct division facts across three students identified as seriously emotionally disturbed (SED) with staggered baselines of 3, 8, and 18 days. This design is considered particularly effective for such dependent variables as academic strategies that are learned and other interventions that can or should not be withdrawn (Alberto & Troutman, 2003). This is particularly relevant for students with EBD who are considered "high-functioning" and for whom "withdrawing" the independent variable may not produce reductions in the target behavior (e.g., where one will not "unlearn" a social skill). In addition, by staggering the baseline time, one can better argue the effects of the independent variable across individuals, settings, and/or behaviors through decreasing the likelihood that timing or other temporally specific variables affected the change in the dependent variable. Myaard, Crawford, Jackson, and Alessi (2000) employed a multiple-baseline design to assess the effects of a wraparound process on four adjudicated youths. This particular study highlights that multiple-baseline designs, when well developed through clear operational definitions of independent and dependent variables, can measure multiple dependent measures across subjects or potential settings. In this case the authors employed the multiple-baseline design across subjects. However, within this design, they also measured the effects of the wraparound

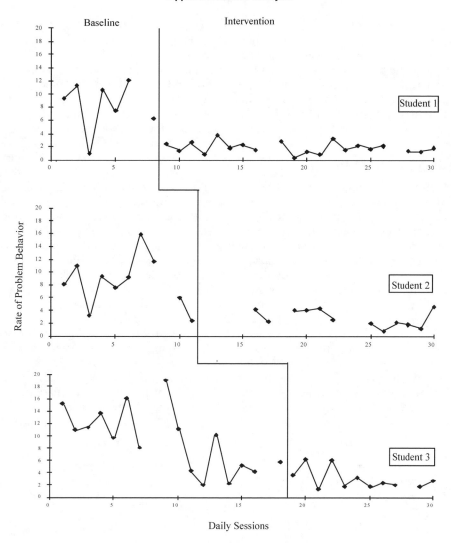

FIGURE 27.2. Sample multiple-baseline across-student design.

process for each youth across five dependent measures (i.e., compliance, appropriate peer interactions, physical aggression, alcohol/ drug use, and verbal abuse).

This latter study was extensive in regard to time, spanning across 52 weeks, with one student tracked across 22 weeks of baseline. This highlights one of the potential limitations of a multiple-baseline design for students with EBD. To adequately control for and potentially determine a functional relationship, an extended amount of baseline data collection time may be necessary. Under certain circumstances it may be deemed dangerous or unethical to simply observe and

collect data on certain behaviors for extended periods of time. Additionally, when a student cannot perform a desired behavior to any significant degree it may be rather unwarranted to extend observation of low levels of proficiency with no intervention for the sake of a multiple baseline (e.g., computing multiplication facts). However, because multiple baselines require no withdrawal of intervention (as with some other ABA designs), and because it can be designed to assess behavior in multiple settings or across a number of individuals, it is often considered a well-suited design for natural settings such as schools and classrooms. Furthermore, because students with EBD are more likely than students with developmental disabilities to exhibit a larger repertoire of behaviors (i.e., multiple topographies) for the same behavioral function, utilizing the multiple-baseline design to assess the impact of an intervention across settings/contexts can be particularly beneficial.

Alternating-Treatment Designs

Whereas multiple-baseline designs assist the investigator in assessing the impact of one intervention on various dependent variables; alternating-treatment designs support the assessment of the impact of multiple interventions on one dependent variable (Kazdin, 1982). This design is particularly popular in applied settings when practitioners are challenged to find which intervention will be the most effective. This design can be employed in a variety of ways as long as each treatment condition is presented an equal amount of times or the rotation is repeated (Tawney & Gast, 1984). This may look like an A–B–A–B configuration where A and B are each different interventions, or can look

like A–B–C–A–B–C. These designs typically include a baseline prior to the introduction of the variables under study (see Figure 27.3 for a sample alternating-treatment design). Miller, Gunter, Venn, Hummell, and Wiley (2003) employed this design to assess the effects of curriculum modifications on the engagement and academic responding of three students identified as having EBD. The researchers were interested in assessing the effects of four different academic conditions and utilized an A–B–A–C–D–C–D design across approximately 49 days to determine differences across the four conditions. Kern, Delaney, Clarke, Dunlap, and Childs (2001) developed two different alternating-treatment designs (A–B–A and A–B–A–C–D–C) to assess the rate of on-task and problematic behavior for two boys identified as having EBD. Functional assessment was used to identify curricular variables that affected the rates of problematic behaviors for both students. These variables were then modified and assessed in the appropriate alternating-treatment design as developed, based on the number of modified curricular variables. In applied research, an alternating-treatment

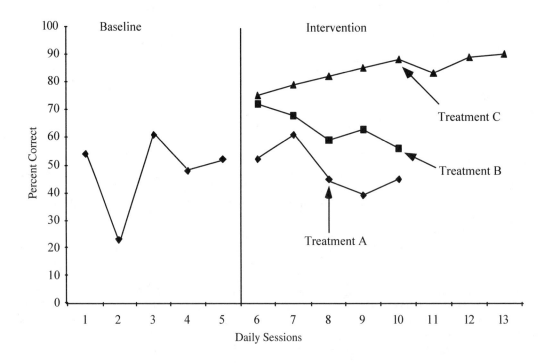

FIGURE 27.3. Sample alternating-treatment design.

design is very practical, as it mirrors, in an organized and controlled manner, practices that occur in schools and other applied settings, trying different approaches to assess which one is most effective. However, as with all research designs, it is important to match the usefulness of this design with the specific dependent variable and students. If the specific student with EBD does not tolerate change or exhibits a dangerous or highly disruptive behavior, it may be best to fine-tune assessments to develop one well-constructed intervention and more formally assess its effectiveness through a multiple-baseline design.

This description of common ABA research designs is not meant to reflect an exhaustive list of potential means for assessing and concluding functional relationships between independent and dependent variables; nor are the examples meant to signify exemplar status—such a review is not our intention in this section. Nevertheless, as demonstrated by the examples, the use of ABA research designs can and has afforded researchers and practitioners with a wealth of information on evidence-based practices for students with EBD. Furthermore, these designs provide a substantial continuum from which to investigate, with substantial rigor, the effects of procedures and interventions on a small and large scale. The widespread transfer of applied behavior analysis in the area of disability research from its more clinical, developmental disabilities roots to educational settings with students identified as having EBD is relatively recent. Given this reality, it is important to keep in mind that educational research in ABA for students with EBD continues to evolve. The application of functional assessment within the EBD research literature is currently serving as a poignant case example of this process.

APPLICATION OF ABA PRACTICES IN THE FIELD AT THE INDIVIDUAL STUDENT LEVEL

Research in the field of EBD using the principles of ABA has brought a wealth of empirically validated behavior change strategies. The overwhelming majority of behavior management textbooks on the market today all outline and advocate strategies that are firmly rooted in behavioral principles. Across North America, classrooms serving children and youths with EBD typically employ many strategies grounded in ABA research. The following section provides a brief review of some of the more common strategies and examples of research using single-subject designs.

Positive Reinforcement

A central principle of behavioral theory is that behavior is influenced by the resulting consequences. Events, or consequences, that follow the occurrence of a behavior can function in one of three ways. The event can (1) strengthen and increase the behavior, (2) weaken or decrease the behavior, or (3) maintain the behavior at current levels. Reinforcement is a term that describes the relationship between the behavior (response) and the event (consequence) that follows. The principles of reinforcement are central to all ABA-based behavior change procedures. Reinforcement is said to occur only if the behavior increases or maintains its rate as a result of the consequence. Positive reinforcement occurs if the contingent presentation of a consequence increases behavior. Negative reinforcement occurs when the removal of an aversive stimulus or event also results in an increase in behavior. Skinner (1953, 1969, 1971) argued that the behavior of an individual is dependent on his or her history of reinforcement. Both "problem" behaviors and "desirable" behaviors are learned and maintained through the same environment–behavior interactions. The use of reinforcement contingent upon behavior, in conjunction with assessment and systematic teaching of replacement behaviors, is the foundation of many strategies to influence and change behavior. The acquisition of academic and social behaviors can be facilitated by careful selection of appropriate reinforcers, providing sufficient amounts of reinforcement, and using continuous and intermittent schedules of reinforcement.

Many of the strategies used to develop desired replacement behaviors are often supported by appropriate use of reductive techniques. Reductive techniques are those that will temporarily stop or repress behavior excesses, allowing the teacher to build appropriate replacement skills using positive reinforcement procedures. There are three classes of reductive procedures using reinforcers: (1) differential reinforcement of low rates of behavior (DRL), (2) differential reinforcement of other behavior (DRO), and (3) differential reinforcement of incompatible or alternative behavior (DRI/DRA). DRO and DRL often involve contingent removal or delay of a reinforcer, while DRI and DRA target desirable behaviors to reinforce.

DRL studies in the past have involved the provision of a reinforcer following fewer episodes of an appropriate target behavior displayed at too high of a rate during a specified interval. In addition to the classic model, full-interval DRL and interval DRL have proven effective in reducing undesirable behavior. Full-interval DRL sets the upper limit for response and provides a reward if the criterion is not exceeded (Dietz & Repp, 1973, 1974; Trice & Parker, 1983). Interval DRL sets the criterion at greater than one response per interval, but resets the interval as soon as the criterion is exceeded (Deitz & Repp, 1973; Deitz et al., 1978).

DRO provides reinforcement contingent on no displays of the problem behavior for a specified period, with a contingent resetting of a timer. The procedure provides for a delay of reinforcement contingent on a response before the interval ends (Chiang, Iwata, & Dorsey, 1979; Homer & Peterson, 1980; Poling & Ryan, 1982; Repp, Barton, & Brulle, 1983).

DRI focuses on reinforcing the occurrence of desirable behaviors, thereby reducing targeted problem behaviors. Techniques include differential attention in the classroom (Becker, Madsen, Arnold, & Thomas, 1967; Broden, Bruce, Mitchell, Carter, & Hall, 1970; Kazdin, 1973, 1977; Madsen, Becker, & Thomas, 1968; Witt & Adams, 1980), differential peer attention (Solomon & Wahler, 1973), and home-based contingencies (Budd, Leibowitz, Riner, Mindell, & Goldfarb, 1981; Lahey et al., 1977; Todd, Scott, Bostow, & Alexander, 1976; Trice, Parker, Furrow, & Iwata, 1983). DRA has been effective at reducing disruptive behavior as well as increasing academic performance by rewarding time on task (Ferritor, Buckholdt, Hamblin, & Smith, 1972; Marholin & Steinman, 1977; Allyon & Roberts, 1974).

Point Systems

For many problem behaviors, basic contingent reinforcement procedures are employed. Point systems or "token economies" are widely used for students with behavior disorders (e.g., Allyon & Azrin, 1968; Wood & Flynn, 1978). In point systems, points are awarded as a secondary reinforcer if and when appropriate target behaviors occur, allowing an association to be established between the reinforcer (point) and the behavior. Points thus awarded additionally serve as generalized reinforcers in that specified amounts can be accumulated and exchanged for other items that have proven to have reinforcing value to the student. Point systems have several advantages. As a generalized reinforcer, points allow contingent and immediate reinforcement of target behaviors. The points can also be used to maintain performance over extended periods of time (Kazdin, 1977; Kazdin & Bootzin, 1972).

Level Systems

A level system lists and organizes behavioral targets and their consequences in a hierarchy of levels, with increasing expectations for behavioral improvement and decreasing behavioral structure (Scheuermann, Webber, Partin, & Knies, 1994). Many of the more restrictive educational programs for students with behavior disorders are organized around a level system that functions as an adaptation of a token economy (Smith & Farrell, 1993). The levels provide a framework for shaping the academic and social skills of students to help them progress through a sequence of levels. Each level is associated with higher academic and social behavior expectations, greater autonomy, and more access to natural reinforcers. Students on the lowest level have only basic privileges, little freedom or choice in activities, and access to a limited range of reinforcers. Students are periodically assessed and move through the levels as they meet the various performance criteria of each level. The highest level is considered a transition stage for movement to a more inclusive setting (Barbetta, 1990); however, the efficacy of level systems in promoting successful transitions to less restrictive environments has not been demonstrated (Scheuermann et al., 1994; Smith & Farrell, 1993).

Level systems should be individualized for a given student, based on individual assessment of academic, social, and behavior deficits, with each student having a set of individualized criteria and behavior requirements. Level systems that restrict access to the least restrictive environment as a privilege and do not take into consideration whether or not the student could benefit from participation in that environment may violate legal requirements associated with due process and the least restrictive environment regulations of IDEA (Scheuermann et al., 1994).

Response Cost

A response cost procedure removes points, tokens, privileges, activities, or other reinforcers previously earned by the student following the occurrence of a specific behavior (Rutherford, 1983). Response cost procedures are frequently used in conjunction with a point system or token economy to decrease or eliminate problem behaviors that compete with the desirable replacement behaviors. Variables that influence the success of response cost include the ratio of fines to reinforcers and the amount of cost imposed (Polsgrove & Reith, 1983). Response cost procedures have been found to compare favorably with positive reinforcement as a behavior management strategy (Hundert, 1976; Iwata & Bailey, 1974) and have been used to modify social behaviors such as rule violation and off-task behavior (DuPaul, Guevremont, & Barkley, 1992; Rapport, Murphy, & Bailey, 1982; Salend, 1988), aggressive behavior (Reynolds & Kelley, 1997), and classroom disruption (Kelley & McCain, 1995; Proctor & Morgan, 1991). Response cost procedures have proven effective in quickly reducing problem behavior, particularly when part of a powerful point or token system (Alexander, Corbett, & Smigel, 1976).

Extinction

Extinction involves withholding reinforcement that is currently maintaining problem behavior. In the classroom, extinction is most often used to decrease behaviors that are maintained by teacher or peer attention. The procedure has been successful in reduc-

ing mild disruptive behavior in the classroom (Andorfer, Miltenberger, Woster, Rortvedt, & Gaffaney, 1994; Zimmerman & Zimmerman, 1962), obscene language (Salend & Meddaugh, 1985), off-task behavior (Hall, Lund, & Jackson, 1968), and noncompliant, self-injurious behavior (Zarcone, Iwata, Mazaleski, & Smith, 1994). Extinction is almost always combined with reinforcement of other appropriate behaviors to increase the likelihood of meaningful behavior change.

Time Out

Time out from positive reinforcement is an effective response-weakening consequence when used properly (Brantner & Doherty, 1983; Polsgrove & Reith, 1983). Like extinction, time out is a procedure that denies access to reinforcers. Time out can be either exclusionary or nonexclusionary. Exclusionary time out removes the student from the instructional setting by taking the student outside the classroom or activity. Seclusionary time out removes the student to a separate area of the school, typically outside of the instructional area. Exclusionary forms of time out are highly intrusive and restrictive and should be used only when less intrusive means fail.

Inclusionary time-out procedures that can be used in the instructional setting include "planned ignoring," reduction of response maintenance stimuli, and contingent observation. Planned ignoring involves withholding attention for inappropriate behavior and is useful when behavior is not harmful or dangerous to others in the environment or is not self-destructive. Planned ignoring is appropriately applied if teacher attention during time-in is associated with positive reinforcement. Risley and Wolf (1967) eliminated out-of-seat, disruptive, and off-task behavior of children during language training sessions by looking away from the child when disruptive behavior occurred. Foxx and Shapiro (1978) used reduction of response maintenance stimuli by systematically enriching the time-in setting, using differential reinforcement for behaviors incompatible with the target behavior. Students were given "time-out ribbons" to wear. While wearing the ribbons, the students received high rates of reinforcement. If the student misbehaved, the ribbon was removed and reinforcement was withheld for 3 minutes. Porterfield, Herbert-Jackson, and Risley (1976) implemented contingent observation by removing children to the side of the play area where they could observe the group without participating or receiving reinforcement for a brief period of time. However, a critical component of all time-out strategies is for the "time-in" setting to be reinforcing to the student.

Functional Behavioral Assessment

One of the most powerful tools ABA has given the field is functional behavioral assessment (FBA). Functional behavioral assessment has been defined as a set of procedures to identify contextual variables that promote and maintain challenging behavior (Lennox & Miltenberger, 1989). In the process, hypotheses are developed that describe the relationship between the predictor events, the problem behavior, and the maintaining consequences (O'Neill et al., 1997). Although there are variations in techniques used, all assessments are based on three basic assumptions: (1) environmental factors are directly related to problem behaviors, (2) variables can be identified through assessment, and (3) systematic manipulation of variables either reduces problem behavior or supports the development of appropriate functionally equivalent skills (Sasso, Conroy, Stichter, & Fox, 2001). The procedure generally involves three phases: (1) hypothesis development, in which data from interviews and direct observation are combined without any manipulations performed to develop an hypothesis; (2) hypothesis confirmation, in which formal baseline data are collected and variables are manipulated to confirm or deny the hypotheses; and (3) hypothesis testing, in which an intervention based on the hypothesis is tested, thereby affirming or denying the predictive validity of the first two phases. The methodology has been applied in both analogue and natural settings to investigate interventions based on antecedent and consequent events.

Researchers in the area of applied behavior analysis first emphasized the importance of functional analysis to identify environmental variables associated with the occurrences of students' challenging behavior in the mid-1960s (Bijou, Peterson, & Ault,

1968; Wolf, Risley, & Mees, 1966). Carr (1977) identified functional relationships between dependent and independent variables in the literature on self-injurious behavior (SIB). He proposed three hypotheses—positive reinforcement, negative reinforcement, and self-stimulation—as controlling conditions of SIB. Iwata and his colleagues extended the work of Carr and set the paradigm for a standardized approach to analogue functional assessment (Bijou et al., 1968; Iwata, Dorsey, Slifer, Bauman, & Richman, 1982; Iwata, Pace, Kalsher, Cowdery, & Cataldo, 1990; Wolf et al., 1966).

The function of challenging behavior has been categorized into broad categories of escape behavior, attention-seeking behavior and sensory regulation (Carr & Durand, 1985; O'Neill et al., 1997). Means of escape/avoidance (negative reinforcement) occur when a demand or task is presented that the student finds to be aversive and when the termination of the demand or task has reinforced the student's challenging behavior (Carr & Durand, 1985). In the classroom setting, instructional demands frequently function as aversive stimuli. Problem behaviors such as aggression, tantrums, and self-injury may serve as escape behaviors that effectively provide a means for avoidance of participation in instructional tasks (Carr & Durand, 1985; Durand & Carr, 1991; O'Neill et al., 1997). Social reactions to problem behavior are generically referred to as attention. Attention contingent on problem behavior (positive reinforcement) reinforces the challenging behavior of students (Carr & Durand, 1985; Durand & Carr, 1991; O'Neill et al., 1997; Taylor & Romanczyk, 1994). DuPaul and Ervin (1996) included two other possible functions for challenging behaviors exhibited by students in the classroom setting: (1) gaining access to an object or activity (positive reinforcement) (e.g., food, toys, television) and (2) attaining sensory regulation (homeostasis).

The research base on FBA primarily reflects work with students with developmental disabilities (Blakeslee, Sugai, & Gruba, 1994; Nelson, Roberts, Mathur, & Rutherford, 1999). Recently, research has extended the literature, to a limited extent, to include school-based problem behaviors with higher-incidence populations, including students with or at risk for emotional behavioral disorders who have mild or no cognitive disabilities (Blair, Umbreit, & Bos, 1999; Clarke et al., 1995; Dunlap, Kern-Dunlap, Clarke, & Robbins, 1991; Ervin, DuPaul, Kern, & Friman, 1998; Kamps et al., 1995; Kern, Dunlap, Clarke, & Childs, 1994; Lee, Sugai, & Horner, 1996; Lewis & Sugai, 1996b; Meyer, 1999; Northrup et al., 1995; Umbreit, 1995).

Several methodologies have emerged to conduct FBA in analogue and applied settings. While there is no consensus across research studies regarding the specific technology and measures used to generate hypotheses, all employ multiple data sources. Most studies use a combination of indirect or descriptive analyses and structured observation that include structured interviews or teacher rating scales, direct observation of antecedents, target behaviors and consequences, and hypothesis development and validation. Hypotheses are then validated by systematically manipulating variables associated with occurrences of problem behavior and observing the effects on the behavior.

Descriptive data are collected through structured student, parent, and teacher interviews (Dunlap et al., 1991; Kern, Childs, Dunlap, Clarke, & Faulk, 1994; O'Neill et al., 1997; Reed, Thomas, Sprague, & Horner, 1997), behavior checklists, or teacher rating scales (Durand & Crimmins, 1988; Lewis, Scott, & Sugai, 1994; O'Neill et al., 1997). Direct methods of data collection include scatter plots, antecedent–response–consequence records, and direct observation (Bijou et al., 1968; Lewis & Sugai, 1996a; Repp, Felce, & Barton, 1988; Symons, McDonald, & Wehby, 1998; Touchette, MacDonald, & Langer, 1985). Experimental data are collected through direct manipulation of variables that affect behavior (Ervin et al., 1998; Iwata et al., 1982; Northrup et al., 1995; Umbreit, 1995). The assumption is that compiling information from a variety of sources creates a more accurate hypothesis.

Functional Interventions

The value of FBA has rested on the assumption that treatment effectiveness increases if the treatment matches the function of the target behavior. Thus, conducting an FBA results in behavior interventions that are effective, individualized. and appropriate (Karsh, Repp, Dahlquist, & Munk, 1995). Kern and Dunlap (1999) maintain that assessment-based interventions can be grouped into two categories: (1) teaching functionally equivalent behaviors as alternatives to problem behaviors when data indicate specific behaviors are maintaining the problem, and (2) changing environmental stimuli when assessment data indicate that particular setting events or antecedents are exerting stimulus control over problem behavior. Researchers have designed interventions based on FBA to address challenging behavior by eliminating the identified reinforcement, changing antecedent and setting events, or teaching alternative behaviors. By identifying these variables through FBA, researchers have modified curricular features to reduce or eliminate challenging behavior.

Studies focusing on antecedent events report reductions in problem behaviors through systematic curricular accommodations (Colvin, Sugai, & Patching, 1993; Dunlap, White, Vera, Wilson, & Panacek, 1996; Umbreit, 1995). Dunlap and colleagues (1991) identified curricular variables that occasion disruptive behavior when investigating the relationship between problem behaviors and two conditions, student choice of task, or teacher assignment of task. Disruptive behavior occurred 39–75% of the time during no-choice conditions. Allowing students to choose the task resulted in no disruptive behavior and an increase in on-task behavior. Dunlap, Foster-Johnson, Clarke, Kern, and Childs (1995) found that some children were especially disruptive during particular academic activities but that their disruptions were reduced when the assignments were modified to incorporate the students' idiosyncratic interests. Winterling, Dunlap, and O'Neill (1987) reported a reduction in challenging behavior when students were presented a variety of tasks in a distributed fashion, as opposed to presenting one task repeatedly. Meyer (1999) investigated the effect of task difficulty and level of adult attention as antecedents to problem behavior. Results revealed higher rates of off-task behavior during difficult tasks and improved behavior when students were taught an alternative behavior that matched assessment results. Weeks and Gaylord-Ross (1981) also established a relationship between task difficulty and problem behavior through their investigation in which the rate of problem behaviors decreased when the level of task difficulty was reduced. Carr and Durand (1985) provide additional evidence that difficult tasks that result in failure can serve as discriminative stimuli for problem behavior. They successfully reduced problem behaviors during their investigation by teaching students to ask for assistance when presented with a difficult task. Similarly, lower rates of challenging behavior occurred when task length was reduced (Dunlap et al., 1991; Kern, Childs, et al., 1994). Horner, Day, Sprague, O'Brien, and Heathfield (1991) found that interspersing low-probability requests with high-probability requests reduced high rates of SIB and aggression. Results of their investigation indicate that rates of problem behaviors were significantly reduced during difficult tasks when commands to do hard tasks were interspersed with commands to do easy tasks. Several studies have also included data to support the long-term effectiveness of these interventions (Dunlap et al., 1991; Horner et al., 1991; Kern, Childs, et al., 1994).

Results from other studies have established the benefit of developing interventions based on the maintaining functions of the behavior. Kamps et al. (1995) and Schill, Kratochwill, and Elliott (1998) investigated interventions that manipulated the environmental variables of receiving immediate tangible rewards and adult attention to successfully improve compliance and decrease misbehavior. Northrup and his colleagues (Broussard & Northrup, 1997; Northrup et al., 1991) measured teacher and peer attention as a maintaining function of disruptive classroom behavior. Lewis and Sugai (1996a, 1996b) also investigated the functional relationship of peer attention to social behavior in the classroom. Other studies have established avoidance and escape from adults and peers as a maintaining consequence (Shores, Gunter, Denny, & Jack, 1993) as well as avoidance of tasks or responsibilities (Dunlap et al., 1993; Hendrickson, Gable, Novak, & Peck, 1996; Kern, Childs, et al., 1994; Umbreit, 1995).

Recent research in FBA and assessment-based interventions has demonstrated that developing specific hypotheses about controlling environmental variables and making programmatic changes specific to those variables can be an effective approach to intervention development. It is arguable that FBA is a more effective approach for supporting children at risk and with emotional/behavioral disorders than a "cookbook" approach where reductive procedures (e.g., time out, DRO) are selected from an array of known interventions based on the topography of the behavior (Kern & Dunlap, 1999). However, in a recent meta-analysis, Stage and Quiroz (1997) concluded that interventions based on group contingencies, self-management, and differential reinforcement tended to be more effective than interventions based on FBA.

Limitations in Current FBA Research Base

Recent reviews in the literature regarding FBA for students with or at risk for EBD in general education settings and who have mild or no cognitive disabilities suggest that our knowledge regarding FBA for this population is limited (Fox, Conroy, & Heckaman, 1998; Heckaman, Conroy, Fox, & Chait, 2000; Nelson et al., 1999; Sasso, Conroy, Stichter, & Fox, 2001). Within the body of research that does exist, questions of external validity focus on the limitations of the findings and the degree to which outcomes based on FBA can be generalized to settings, practitioners, and behaviors across time. One threat to the external validity of existing research centers on the representativeness of participants identified through recent reviews of the literature. Sasso et al. (2001) reveal that existing research has been conducted on a relatively small and narrow sample of participants. When focusing on empirical studies in which FBA was used to develop hypotheses for students identified with or at risk for EBD, their review of the existing research base produced only 40 students, ranging in age from 4 to 14 years. No studies have included students above the age of 14. In those studies, externalizing behaviors were identified exclusively as the target behaviors. Based on the limited number of participants in the existing research, generalizability across ages, types of behavior, and disability category has not been established.

Another criticism of the external validity

of existing research is the degree to which outcomes based on functional assessment can be generalized to settings and behaviors, since the existing data base does not reflect the use of a single functional assessment instrument or technique consistently across studies. Sasso et al. (2001) caution "to empirically investigate and scientifically analyze a phenomenon, we must clearly define that phenomenon" (p. 289). Instead, current practice appears to be based on a variety of procedures specific to various researchers and situations. The research literature has not established an operational definition of the procedures and instruments or how data collected are analyzed separately and together to determine the function of the behavior. There is also a limited amount of research comparing the results of different approaches such as interviews and questionnaires, descriptive observation, and experimental analyses (Cunningham & O'Neill, 2000; Kratochwill & McGivern, 1996; Sturmey, 1995; Vollmer & Smith, 1996), or even the usefulness of a single method versus a multivariate assessment (Conroy & Fox, 1994).

FBA-based support plans are most likely to succeed within a framework in which school personnel routinely reinforce positive behavior and dedicate as much time and effort to teaching social skills as academic skills (Sugai et al., 2000). A systems perspective provides support for the adoption and sustained use of effective practices (Sugai, Horner, & Sprague, 1999). As schools cultivate the systems and skills to promote a range of positive and academic supports and disciplinary practices, such efforts must include the team problem-solving process of FBA.

APPLICATION OF ABA PRINCIPLES TO CLASSROOMS AND SCHOOLWIDE SYSTEMS

Classrooms

Similar to research on students with EBD and their families, ongoing investigations have provided the field with compelling data to indicate that all too frequently coercive relationships are perpetuated between teachers and students exhibiting problem behavior (Wehby, Symons, & Canale, 1998).

These coercive relationships also extend to the student and instructional contexts, reinforcing the ineffective use of aversive management practices by the teacher and increased antisocial and aggressive behavior by the student (Kauffman, 2000). Additional experimental analysis has further investigated the relationship between contextual factors such as environmental characteristics and instructional cues and specific students (for a review see Conroy & Stichter, 2003; Stichter, Clarke, & Dunlap, in press). In addition, as the rate of students considered at risk when entering school has increased, a clearer understanding of the precursors within home and community settings has emerged. This body of work has established the existence of a relationship between temporally distant (e.g., what happens at home before school) and environmentally specific factors (e.g., classroom demands or lack of structured tasks) to either promote prosocial behavior or reinforce antisocial behavior.

Applied behavior analysis has made a major contribution to this research base and, as with FBA, has provided a framework for assessing and developing effective classroom management. More specifically, operant conditioning describes the relationship between behavior and environmental events. To effectively identify this relationship one must assess the antecedents (what happens prior to the behavior), the specific behavior, and the consequences (what happens after the behavior). Historically schools and classrooms have focused on the consequence aspect of the A–B–C model. In other words, what will happen if a student violates rules? This form of consequence, commonly referred to as punishment, is by definition a consequence that decreases the likelihood a behavior will occur. However, as many teachers will attest, there are some students, frequently those identified as antisocial or at risk, for whom punishment must be used frequently. Again, by definition, punishment must not be working in these cases, as it is not consistently decreasing the target behavior. Another form of consequence is reinforcement. By its definition it is designed to increase the likelihood of a behavior either through access to something desirable (e.g., extra recess) or through the removal of something undesirable (e.g., no homework that day) when the behavior occurs. ABA tells us that if a behavior maintains or increases it is somehow being reinforced. A significant contribution of functional assessment is an empirically based understanding that what is reinforcing to one student with EBD may not be to another, or those things considered reinforcing under some conditions are not under others. Additionally, reinforcement or even punishment is not effective when inconsistently applied. Inconsistent behavior management is one of the most frequently identified contributors to students' behavior problems within schools (Kauffman, 2000; Mayer, 1995, 2002). Finally, a classroom management system with an emphasis on inflexible rules and consequences, and or with a heavy emphasis on artificial reinforcement (e.g., stickers), typically does not maintain and generalize effectively to other settings.

As the operant model demonstrates, the conditions under which behaviors occur help predict the resulting behavior and therefore the impact of the paired consequences. For this reason, as discussed above, an increased emphasis has been placed on research and practice designed to assess the classroom environment. Instead of an emphasis on the consequence of undesired behavior, the focus is on prevention. The literature is replete with documentation regarding the positive impact of prevention (early intervention) in partnership with ongoing remediation of antisocial behavior patterns (Sugai et al., 2000). By employing effective instruction as a management tool, the emphasis shifts to increasing the likelihood of students' success. This is accomplished by examining classroom situations that appear to elicit increased problematic behavior and assessing ways in which students can be best taught, modeled, and reinforced for desired behavior. By altering unsuccessful contexts through increased predictability and structure, a teacher exerts stimulus control. This also provides the student with increased ability to accurately predict the success of a response within a given situation. By preplanning and assessing potential situations, the teacher can provide appropriate precorrects (Colvin, Sugai, et al., 1993) as well as effective prompts and cues to increase student success. The stage is then set to offer reinforcement for the desired behavior and reduce the potential for a coercive behavior cycle between the student and teacher. Just as with family and community, students with EBD benefit the most from healthy classrooms with an emphasis on prevention as means to develop effective classroom climates.

Schoolwide Systems

Fighting, violence, gangs, lack of discipline, lack of funding, and use of drugs are consistently rated as the greatest problems facing local schools (Rose & Gallup, 1998). Additionally, two-thirds of parents do not feel that their children are safe while at school or in surrounding neighborhoods (Rose & Gallup, 1998). However, discipline patterns indicate that a relatively small number of students in a school building engage in the most serious and/or chronic problem behaviors (e.g., Taylor-Greene et al., 1997). The disruptive behavior of individual students in schools, however, is detrimental to students, schools, and communities.

This chapter has focused on supporting students with EBD individually and through increased classroom instruction and management. To establish a full-continuum of support within a school, it is necessary to build a schoolwide foundation designed to increase the ability of schools to educate all students, especially students with challenging social behaviors, by establishing an efficient and effective model of (1) systems that support staff, (2) practices that support students, and (3) data that guide decision making (Lewis & Sugai, 1999; Sugai et al., 2000; Sugai & Horner, 1994, 1999).

There are several challenges impeding a school's ability to support students with EBD. First, problem behaviors are high intensity and/or frequency. Second, students in need of support are difficult to identify, and once identified their problem behaviors are difficult to understand (i.e., determine when and why they occur). Third, while a small number of students account for the majority of behavior problems, there are still too many students displaying significant problem behavior at any one time. Fourth, these problem behaviors are disrupting learning and teaching environments for all students. Finally, educating individual students with EBD requires highly individualized, specialized, and intensive behavioral supports.

Increasing disciplinary challenges coupled by decreasing resources has made it even more difficult to provide individual students with the level of support required. One response is for schools to adopt a systems approach to addressing discipline. Establishing proactive schoolwide disciplinary systems within a school is unlikely to have an immediate and direct impact on students with EBD. However, building schoolwide systems increases the likelihood of success through a series of capacity-building steps. First, schools need to build a foundation that prevents students from becoming at risk for school failure. Next, schools need to build systems that organize the many initiatives, programs, and policies to work efficiently. Third, schools need to build the capacity to identify students with intense needs and provide them with the individualized and specialized support necessary for their success.

Gottfredson, Gottfredson, and Hybl (1993) implemented a systems approach to discipline within eight middle schools. Level of implementation varied across the eight schools, resulting in three being rated as high implementation, three as medium implementation, and two as low implementation. The mixed success for fidelity of implementation is indicative of the difficulty schools face in implementing schoolwide initiatives. Pre–post findings resulted in positive changes for high implementation schools only. Knoff and Batsche (1995) tracked and compared a school implementing a systems approach to discipline with a control school for 3 years. After 3 years of implementation the target school had reductions in referrals and placement of at-risk students into special education, office-discipline referrals, grade retention, and out-of-school suspension. Furthermore, the target school observed increases in academic performance.

Taylor-Greene et al. (1997) implemented a comprehensive schoolwide disciplinary system in response to high rates of office-discipline referrals. Prior to implementation the 530 middle schools students accounted for 2,628 or 15 office-discipline referrals (ODR) per day. After implementation the ODRs decreased by about 50%, or to 8.7 ODRs per day. Prior to implementation, 6% of the students had 20 or more ODRs and accounted for 52% of all ODRs. These 34 students re-mained the most frequently referred after implementation; however, there was a 65% reduction in their overall number of ODRs. Similar results have been reported at the school level (e.g., Colvin, Kameenui, & Sugai, 1993) and when applied to specific settings within a school, such as the cafeteria, playground, hallways, etc. (Colvin, Sugai, Good, & Lee, 1997; Lewis, Sugai, & Colvin, 1998).

There is a growing literature base indicating the ability of schools to implement schoolwide disciplinary systems that result in the reduction of overall rates of problem behavior. While results need to be replicated in elementary and middle schools and expanded to high schools, the results are promising. Further research is required to identify the variables within a school that support fidelity and sustainability of implementation. Finally, while schoolwide systems are viewed as a foundation for providing more specialized attention to students with EBD, research is needed to verify this premise. Research examining the impact of schoolwide disciplinary systems on students with EBD should focus on both academic and behavioral outcomes. For example, the effects of early identification, modeling of appropriate behavior, and establishing routines and environments that are discriminative stimuli for appropriate behavior must be determined.

CONCLUSION

The purpose of this chapter was to provide an overview of applied behavior analysis's impact on the education and treatment of individuals with EBD. Applied behavior analysis began influencing the field of EBD in the 1960s through the application of behavioral principles and practices. Specifically, the field incorporates the principles associated with the three-term contingency. Instructional practices, stimulus control, and shaping procedures enhance the acquisition of academic and social skills, while punishment and reinforcement support the reduction of problem behavior and maintenance and generalization of more appropriate behaviors. The seminal 1968 article by Baer, Wolf, and Risley further influenced the field by providing guidelines for applying and adapting strategies to fit varying contexts and addressing important issues. Furthermore, the field of applied behavior analysis has provided a series of research designs (i.e., withdrawal, multiple-baseline, and alternating-treatments) to test the efficacy of strategies across settings, individuals, and behaviors. The adoption of single-subject methodology is critical for the education and treatment of individuals with EBD for several reasons. First, a primary focus is on the impact on individuals and not on groups. Single-subject research designs are uniquely designed to use the individual as their own comparison to determine outcomes specific to the individual. Second, the in-depth focus on individuals provides the opportunity to complete a fine-grained analysis of the independent variable. Finally, the emphasis of applied behavior analysis is on functional relationships that single-subject methodology is able to assess.

Recently, the guidelines set forth by Baer, Wolf, and Risley are being applied to classrooms and schools. Not only has the expansion helped to establish a continuum of support, but also it has increased the focus on prevention over remediation. At the individual student level, this is most noticeable in the use of functional behavioral assessment and the application of functional interventions to support the behavioral needs of students with EBD. At the classroom level, applied behavior analysis has provided the framework for understanding the coercive pattern of interaction frequently observed between teachers and students with EBD. Instructional and behavior management strategies are combined to establish classroom environments that foster academic and behavioral success for students. Finally, at the school level, the field of applied behavior analysis has provided a foundation to support the adoption, implementation, and sustainability of practices at both the individual and classroom levels. Schoolwide interventions decrease the number of students requiring intensive support and increase the availability of resources and support staff in their implementation of strategies.

Although the field of applied behavior analysis has had a positive impact on the field of EBD, additional research is needed. While not specifically addressed in this chapter, research on comprehensive systems that incorporate all students, all settings, and adapted to all levels of support—individual, classroom, school—are needed to increase the sustainability of effective practices.

Future research focused on changing individual student behavior, in particular functional behavior assessment and functional intervention studies, should continue to expand generalization through direct and systematic replication across settings, practitioners, and behavior. Particular attention should be focused on the representativeness of participants. Only very limited research is available on students older than 15 years and on students with less overt or internalizing problem behaviors. Finally, research needs to continue to define and refine the FBA process, including methods, measures, and steps.

Research on effective teaching practices have defined critical variables and levels necessary to foster student success. However, maintaining teachers' use of these strategies continues to be an issue. Future research should focus on sustaining teacher/practitioner behaviors that increase fidelity and maintenance of implementation. Finally, at the schoolwide level, results remain preliminary and direct, and systematic replication is required to evaluate the immediate and long-term impact on student behavior. Similar to issues at the classroom level, the fidelity and sustainability of practices remain challenges and need further research. To date schoolwide research has focused on general changes within the school and has implied benefits to students with EBD. Further efforts should focus on confirming the necessity of a schoolwide foundation to support more intensive strategies and practices. It will be important to understand what features of schoolwide disciplinary systems benefit students with EBD and how.

The education and treatment of individuals with EBD has been improved by the application of the theories, methodologies, and practices of applied behavior analysis. Both academic and behavioral gains are based on applied behavior analysis and impact individual students, classrooms, and schools. The continued reliance on applied behavior analysis will allow the field to validate, expand, and extend the current state of support for students with EBD.

REFERENCES

Alberto, P., & Troutman, A. (2003). *Applied behavior analysis for teachers*. Columbus, OH: Merrill/Prentice Hall.

Alexander, R. N., Corbett, T. F., & Smigel, J. (1976). The effects of individual and group consequences on school attendance and curfew violations with predelinquent adolescents. *Journal of Applied Behavior Analysis, 9*, 221– 226.

Allyon, T., & Azrin, N. (1968). *The token economy: A motivational system for therapy and rehabilitation*. New York: Appleton-Century-Crofts.

Allyon, T., & Roberts, M., (1974). Eliminating discipline problems by strengthening academic performance. *Journal of Applied Behavior Analysis, 7*, 72–76.

Andorfer, R., Miltenberger, R., Woster, S., Rortvedt, A., & Gaffaney, T. (1994). Home-based descriptive and experimental analysis of problem behaviors in children. *Topics in Early Childhood Special Education, 14*, 64–87.

Baer, D. M., Wolf, M. M., & Risley, T. R. (1968). Some current dimensions of applied behavior analysis. *Journal of Applied Behavior Analysis, 1*, 91–97.

Barbetta, P. (1990). GOALS: A group oriented adapted levels system for children with behavior disorders. *Academic Therapy, 25*, 645–656.

Becker, W., Madsen, C., Arnold, C. & Thomas, D. (1967). The contingent use of teacher attention and praise in reducing classroom behavior problems. *Journal of Special Education, 1*, 287–308.

Bijou, S. W., & Baer, D. M. (1961). *Child development: Vol. 1. A systematic and empirical theory*. New York: Appleton-Century-Crofts.

Bijou, S. W., Peterson, R. F., & Ault, M. H. (1968). A method to integrate descriptive and experimental field studies at the level of data and empirical concepts. *Journal of Applied Behavior Analysis, 1*, 175–191.

Blair, K., Umbreit, J., & Bos, C. (1999). Using functional assessment and children's preferences to improve the behavior of young children with behavioral disorders. *Behavioral Disorders, 24*, 151–166.

Blakeslee, T., Sugai, G. M, & Gruba, J. (1994). A review of functional assessment use in data-based intervention studies. *Journal of Behavioral Education, 4*, 397–413.

Brantner, J. R., & Doherty, M. A. (1983). A review of timeout: A conceptual and methodological analysis. In S. Axelrod & J. Apsche (eds.), *The effects of punishment on human behavior*. New York: Academic Press.

Broden, M., Bruce, C. Mitchell, M., Carter, V., & Hall, R. (1970). Effects of teacher attention in attending behavior of two boys at adjacent desks. *Journal of Applied Behavior Analysis, 3*, 199–203.

Broussard, C., & Northrup, J. (1997). The use of functional analysis to develop peer interventions of disruptive classroom behavior. *School Psychology Quarterly, 12*, 65–76.

Budd, K., Leibowitz, J., Riner, L., Mindell, C., & Goldfarb, A. (1981). Home based treatment of severe disruptive behaviors: A reinforcement package for preschool and kindergarten children. *Journal of Behavior Modification, 5*, 273–298.

Cade, T., & Gunter, P. H. (2002). Teaching students with severe emotional or behavioral disorders to use a musical mnemonic technique to solve basic division calculations. *Behavioral Disorders, 27*, 208–214.

Carr, E. G. (1977). The motivation of self-injurious behavior: A review of some hypotheses. *Psychological Bulletin, 84*, 800–816.

Carr, E. G., & Durand, V. M. (1985). Reducing behavior problems through functional communication training. *Journal of Applied Behavior Analysis, 18*, 111–126.

Chiang, S., Iwata, B., & Dorsey, M. (1979). Elimination of disruptive bus riding behavior via token reinforcement on a "distance-based" schedule. *Education and Treatment of Children, 2*, 101–109.

Clarke, S., Dunlap, G., Foster, J. L., Childs, K., Wilson, D., White, R., & Vera, A. (1995). Improving the conduct of students with behavioral disorders by incorporating student interests into curricular areas. *Behavioral Disorders, 20*, 221–231.

Clarke, S., Dunlap, G. & Stichter, J. P. (2002). Twenty years of intervention research in emotional and behavioral disorders: A descriptive analysis and a comparison with research in developmental disabilities. *Behavior Modification, 25*, 659–683.

Colvin, G. C., Kameenui, E. J., & Sugai, G. M. (1993). Reconceptualizing behavior management and school-wide discipline in general education. *Education and Treatment of Children, 16*, 361–381.

Colvin, G., Sugai, G. M.., Good, R. H., & Lee, Y. (1997). Using active supervision and precorrection to improve transition behaviors in an elementary school. *School Psychology Quarterly, 12*, 344–363.

Colvin, G., Sugai, G. M., & Patching, B. (1993). Precorrection: An instructional approach for managing predictable problem behaviors. *Intervention in School and Clinic, 28*, 143–150.

Conroy, M. A., & Fox, J. J. (1994). Setting events and challenging behavior in the classroom: Incorporating contextual factors into effective intervention plans. *Preventing School Failure, 38*, 29–34.

Conroy, M. A., & Stichter, J. P. (2003). A review of the last twenty years of setting events research for students with EBD. *Journal of Special Education, 37*, 15–25.

Cooper, J. O., Heron, T. E., & Heward, W. L. (1987). *Applied behavior analysis*. Columbus, OH: Merrill.

Cunningham, E., & O'Neill, R. (2000). Comparisons of results of functional assessment and analysis methods with young children with autism. *Education and Training in Mental Retardation and Developmental Disabilities, 35*, 406–414.

Dietz, S., & Repp, A., (1973). Decreasing classroom misbehavior through the use of DRL schedules of reinforcement. *Journal of Applied Behavior Analysis*, *6*, 457–463.

Dietz, S., & Repp, A., (1974). Differentially reinforcing low rates of misbehavior with normal elementary school children. *Journal of Applied Behavior Analysis*, *7*, 622.

Dietz, S., Slack, D., Schwarzmueller, E., Wilander, A., Weatherly, L., & Hilliard, G. (1978). Reducing inappropriate behavior in special classrooms by reinforcing average interresponse times: Interval DRL. *Behavior Therapy*, *1*, 37–46.

Dunlap, G., Foster-Johnson, L., Clarke, S., Kern, L., & Childs, K. (1995). Modifying activities to produce functional outcomes: Effects on the disruptive behaviors of students with disabilities. *Journal of the Association for Persons with Severe Handicaps*, *20*, 248–258.

Dunlap, G., Kern, L., dePerczel, M., Clarke, S., Wilson, D., Childs, K. E., White, R., & Falk, G. (1993). Functional analysis of classroom variables for students with emotional and behavioral disorders. *Behavioral Disorders*, *18*, 275–291.

Dunlap, G., Kern-Dunlap, L., Clarke, S., & Robbins, F. R. (1991). Functional assessment, curricular revision, and severe behavior problems. *Journal of Applied Behavior Analysis*, *24*, 387–397.

Dunlap, G., White, R., Vera, A., Wilson, D., & Panacek, L. (1996). The effects of multi-component, assessment-based curricular modifications on the classroom behavior of children with emotional and behavioral disorders. *Journal of Behavioral Education*, *6*, 481–500.

DuPaul, G., & Ervin, R. (1996). Functional assessment of behaviors related to attention-deficit/hyperactivity disorder: Linking assessment to intervention design. *Behavior Therapy*, *27*, 601–622.

DuPaul, G., Guevremont, D., & Barkley, R. A. (1992). Behavioral treatment of attention-deficit hyperactivity disorder in the classroom. *Behavior Modification*, *16*, 204–225.

Durand, V. M., & Carr, E. G. (1991). Functional communication training to reduce challenging behavior: Maintenance and application in new settings. *Journal of Applied Behavior Analysis*, *24*, 251–264.

Durand, V. M., & Crimmins, D. (1988). Identifying the variables maintaining self-injurious behavior. *Journal of Autism and Developmental Disorders*, *18*, 99–117.

Ervin, R. A., DuPaul, G. J., Kern, L., & Friman, P. (1998). Classroom-based functional and adjunctive assessments: Proactive approaches to intervention selection for adolescents with attention deficit hyperactivity disorder. *Journal of Applied Behavior Analysis*, *31*, 65–78.

Ferritor, D., Buckholdt, D., Hamblin, R.L., & Smith, L. (1972). The noneffects of contingent reinforcement for attending behavior on work accomplished. *Journal of Applied Behavior Analysis*, *5*, 7–17.

Fox, J. J., Conroy, M. A., & Heckaman, K. (1998). Research issues in functional assessment of the chal-

lenging behaviors of students with emotional and behavioral disorders. *Behavioral Disorders*, *24*, 26–33.

Foxx, R. M., & Shapiro, S. T. (1978). The timeout ribbon: A nonexlusionary timeout procedure. *Journal of Applied Behavior Analysis*, *11*, 125–136.

Gottfredson, D. C., Gottfredson, G. D., & Hybl, L. (1993). Managing adolescent behavior: A multiyear, multi-school study. *American Educational Research Journal*, *30*, 179–215.

Hall, R. V., Lund, D., & Jackson, D. (1968). Effects of teacher attention on study behavior. *Journal of Applied Behavior Analysis*, *1*, 1–12.

Heckaman, K., Conroy, M. A., Fox, J. J., & Chait, A. (2000). Functional-assessment based intervention research on students with or at risk for emotional and behavioral disorders in school setting. *Behavioral Disorders*, *25*, 196–210.

Hendrickson, J. M., Gable, R. A., Novak, C., & Peck, S. (1996). Functional assessment as strategy assessment for teaching academics. *Education and Treatment of Children*, *19*, 257–271.

Homer, A., & Peterson, L. (1980). Differential reinforcement of other behavior: A preferred response elimination procedure. *Behavior Therapy*, *11*, 449–471.

Horner, R., Day, H. M., Sprague, J., O'Brien, M., & Heathfield, L. T. (1991). Interspersed requests: A nonaversive procedure for reducing aggression and self-injury during instruction. *Journal of Applied Behavior Analysis*, *24*, 265–278.

Hundert, J. (1976). The effectiveness of reinforcement, response cost, and mixed programs on classroom behaviors. *Journal of Applied Behavior Analysis*, *9*, 107–117.

Iwata, B. A., & Bailey, J. S. (1974). Reward versus cost token systems: An analysis of the effects on students and teacher. *Journal of Applied Behavior Analysis*, *7*, 567–576.

Iwata, B. A., Dorsey, M. F., Slifer, K. J., Bauman, K. E., & Richman, G. S. (1982). Toward a functional analysis of self injury. *Analysis and Intervention in Developmental Disabilities*, *2*, 3–20. Reprinted in *Journal of Applied Behavior Analysis*, *27*, 197–209.

Iwata, B. A., Pace, G., Kalsher, M., Cowdery, G., & Cataldo, M. (1990). Experimental analysis and extinction of self-injurious escape behavior. *Journal of Applied Behavior Analysis*, *23*, 11–27.

Johnston, J. M., & Pennypacker, H. S. (1980). *Strategies and tactics of human behavioral research*. Hillsdale, NJ: Erlbaum.

Jolivette, K., Wehby, J. H., Canale, J., & Massey, G. (2001). Effects of choice making opportunities on the behavior of students with emotional and behavioral disorders. *Behavioral Disorders*, *26*, 131–145.

Kamps, D., Ellis, C., Mancina, C., Wyble, J., Greene, L., & Harvey, D. (1995). Case studies using functional analysis for young children with behavior risks. *Education and Treatment of Children*, *18*, 243–260.

Karsh, K. G., Repp, A., Dahlquist, C. M., & Munk, D. (1995). In vivo functional assessment and multi-element interventions for problem behaviors of students with disabilities in classroom settings. *Journal of Behavioral Education, 5*, 189–210.

Kauffman, J. M. (2000). *Characteristics of emotional and behavioral disorders of children and youth* (7th ed.). Upper Saddle River, NJ: Merrill/Prentice Hall.

Kazdin, A. (1973). The effect of vicarious reinforcement on attentive behavior in the classroom. *Journal of Applied Behavior Analysis, 6*, 71–78.

Kazdin, A. E. (1977). *The token economy: A review and evaluation.* New York: Plenum.

Kazdin, A. E. (1982). *Single-case research designs.* New York: Oxford University Press.

Kazdin, A. E., & Bootzin, R. R. (1972). The token economy: An evaluative review. *Journal of Applied Behavior Analysis, 5*, 343–372.

Kelley, M. L., & McCain, A. (1995). Promoting academic performance in inattentive children. *Behavior Modification, 19*, 357–375.

Kern, L., Bambara, L., & Fogt, J. (2002). Class-wide curricular modifications to improve the behavior of students with emotional or behavioral disorders. *Behavioral Disorders, 27*, 317–326.

Kern, L., Childs, K. E., Dunlap, G., Clarke, S., & Falk, G. D. (1994). Using assessment based curricular intervention to improve the classroom behavior of a student with emotional and behavioral challenges. *Journal of Applied Behavior Analysis, 27*, 7–19.

Kern, L., Delaney, B., Clarke, S., Dunlap, G., & Childs, K. (2001). Improving the classroom behavior of students with emotional and behavioral disorders using individualized curricular modifications. *Journal of Emotional and Behavioral Disorders, 9*, 239–247.

Kern, L., & Dunlap, G. (1999). Assessment-based interventions for children with emotional and behavioral disorders. In A. Repp & R. H. Horner (Eds.), *Functional analysis of problem behavior: From effective assessment to effective support* (pp. 197–218). Belmont, CA: Wadsworth.

Kern, L., Dunlap, G., Clarke, S., & Childs, K.E. (1994). Student-assisted functional assessment interview. *Diagnostique, 19*(2–3), 29–39.

Knoff, H. M., & Batsche, G. M. (1995). Project ACHIEVE: Analyzing a school reform process for at-risk and underachieving students. *School Psychology Review, 24*, 579–603.

Kratochwill, T. R., & McGivern, J. E. (1996). Clinical diagnosis, behavioral assessment, and functional analysis: Examining the connection between assessment and intervention. *School Psychology Review, 25*, 342–355.

Lahey, B., Gendrich, J., Gendrich, S., Schnelle, J., Gant, G., & McNees, P. (1977). An evaluation of daily report cards with minimal teacher and parent contacts as an efficient method of classroom intervention. *Behavior Modification, 1*, 381–394.

Lee, Y., Sugai, G., & Horner, R. H. (1996). Using an instructional intervention to reduce problem and off-task behaviors. *Journal of Positive Behavior Interventions, 1*, 195–204.

Lennox, D. B., & Miltenberger, R. (1989). Conducting a functional assessment of problem behavior in applied settings. *Journal of the Association for Persons with Severe Handicaps, 14*, 304–311.

Lewis, T. J., Scott, T., & Sugai, G. (1994). The problem behavior questionnaire: A teacher based instrument to develop functional hypotheses of problem behavior in general education classrooms. *Diagnostique, 19*, 103–115.

Lewis, T. J., & Sugai, G. (1996a). Functional Assessment of Problem Behavior: A pilot investigation of the comparative and interactive effects of teacher and peer social attention on students in general education settings. *School Psychology Quarterly, 11*, 1–19.

Lewis, T. J., & Sugai, G. (1996b). Descriptive and experimental analysis of teacher and peer Attention and the use of assessment based intervention to improve the pro-social behavior of a student in a general education setting. *Journal of Behavioral Education, 6*, 7–24.

Lewis, T. J., & Sugai, G. (1999). Effective behavior support: A systems approach to proactive school-wide management. *Focus on Exceptional Children, 31*(6), 1–24.

Lewis, T. J., Sugai, G. M., & Colvin, G. (1998). Reducing problem behavior through a school-wide system of effective behavioral support: Investigation of a school-wide social skills training program and contextual interventions. *School Psychology Review, 27*, 446–459.

Madsen, C., Becker, W., & Thomas, D. (1968). Rules, praise, and ignoring: elements of elementary classroom control. *Journal of Applied Behavior Analysis, 1*, 139–150.

Marholin, D., & Steinman, W. (1977). Stimulus control in the classroom as a function of the behavior reinforced. *Journal of Applied Behavior Analysis, 5*, 465–478.

Mayer, G. R. (1995). Preventing antisocial behavior in the schools. *Journal of Applied Behavior Analysis, 28*, 467–478.

Mayer, G. R. (2002). Behavioral strategies to reduce school violence. *Child and Family Behavior Therapy, 24*, 83–100.

Meyer, K. (1999). Functional analysis and treatment of problem behavior exhibited by elementary school children. *Journal of Applied Behavior Analysis, 32*, 229–232.

Miller, K., Gunter, P. H., Venn, M., Hummel, J., & Wiley, L. (2003). Effects of curricular and materials modification on academic performance and task engagement of three students with emotional disorders. *Behavioral Disorders, 28*, 130–149.

Myaard, M., Crawford, C., Jackson, M., & Alessi, G. (2000). Applying behavior analysis within the wraparound process: A multiple baseline study. *Journal of Emotional and Behavioral Disorders, 8*, 216–229.

Nelson, J. R., Roberts, M. L., Mathur, S. R., & Rutherford, R. B. (1999). Has public policy exceeded our knowledge base: A review of the functional behavioral assessment literature. *Behavioral Disorders, 24,* 169–179.

Northrup, J., Broussard, C., Jones, K., George, T., Vollmer, T., & Herring, M. (1995). The differential effects of teacher and peer attention on the disruptive classroom behavior of three children with a diagnosis of attention deficit hyperactivity disorder. *Journal of Applied Behavior Analysis, 28,* 227–228.

Northrup, J., Wacker, D., Sasso, G., Steege, M., Cigrand, K., Cook, J., & DeRaad, A. (1991). A brief functional analysis of aggressive and alternative behavior in an outclinic setting. *Journal of Applied Behavior Analysis, 24,* 509–522.

O'Neill, R. E., Horner, R. H., Albin, R. W., Sprague, J. R., Storey, K., & Newton, J. S. (1997). *Functional assessment and program development for problem behavior: A practical handbook.* Pacific Grove, CA: Brooks/Cole.

Poling, A., & Ryan, C. (1982). Differential reinforcement of other behavior schedules. *Behavior Modification, 6,* 3–21.

Polsgrove, L., & Reith, H. J. (1983). Procedures for reducing children's inappropriate behavior in special education settings. *Exceptional Education Quarterly, 3,* 20–33.

Porterfield, J. K., Herbert-Jackson, E., & Risley, T. R. (1976). Contingent observation: An effective and acceptable procedure for reducing disruptive behavior of young children in a group setting. *Journal of Applied Behavior Analysis, 9,* 55–64.

Proctor, M., & Morgan, D. (1991). Effectiveness of a response cost raffle procedure on the disruptive classroom behavior of adolescents with behavior problems. *School Psychology Review, 20,* 97–109.

Rapport, M., Murphy, A., & Bailey, J. (1982). Ritalin vs. response cost in the control of hyperactive children: A within-subject comparison. *Journal of Applied Behavior Analysis, 15,* 205–216.

Reed, H., Thomas, E., Sprague, J. R., & Horner, R. H. (1997). The student guided functional assessment interview: An analysis of student and teacher agreement. *Journal of Behavioral Education, 7*(1), 33–49.

Repp, A. C., Barton, L. E., & Brulle, A. R. (1983). A comparison of two procedures for programming the differential reinforcement of other behavior. *Journal of Applied Behavior Analysis, 16,* 435–445.

Repp, A. C., Felce, D., & Barton, L. E. (1988). Basing the treatment of stereotypic and self-injurious behavior on hypotheses of their causes. *Journal of Applied Behavior Analysis, 21,* 281–289.

Reynolds, L., & Kelley, M. L. (1997). The efficacy of a response cost-based treatment package for preschoolers. *Behavior Modification, 21,* 216–230.

Risely, T. R., & Wolf, M. M. (1967). Establishing functional speech in echolalia children. *Behavior Research and Therapy, 5,* 73–88.

Rose, L. C., & Gallup, A. M. (1998). The 30th annual Phi Delta Kappan/Gallup poll of the public's attitude toward the public schools. *Kappan, 79,* 41–56.

Rutherford, R. B. (1983). Theory and research on the use of aversive procedures in the education of moderately behaviorally disordered and emotionally disturbed children and youth. In F. H. Wood & K. C. Lakin (Eds.), *Punishment and aversive stimulation in special education* (pp. 41–64). Reston, VA: Council for Exceptional Children.

Salend, S. (1988). Effects of a student-managed response cost system on the behavior of two mainstreamed students. *Elementary School Journal, 89,* 89–97.

Salend, S., & Meddaugh, D. (1985). Using a peer-mediated extinction procedure to decrease obscene language. *The Pointer, 30,* 8–11.

Sasso, G. M., Conroy, M. A., Stichter, J. P., & Fox, J. J. (2001). Slowing down the bandwagon: The pseudovalidation and misapplication of functional assessment for students with EBD. *Behavioral Disorders, 26,* 282–296.

Scheuermann, B., Webber, J., Partin, M., & Knies, W. C. (1994). Level systems and the law: Are they compatible? *Behavioral Disorders, 19,* 205–220.

Schill, M., Kratochwill, T. R., & Elliott, S. N. (1998). Functional assessment in behavioral consultation: A treatment utility study. *School Psychology Quarterly, 13,* 116–140.

Shores, R. E., Gunter, P., Denny, R. K., & Jack, S. L. (1993). Classroom influences on aggressive and disruptive behaviors of students with emotional and behavioral disorders. *Focus on Exceptional Children, 26*(2), 1–10.

Skinner, B. F. (1953). *Science and human behavior.* New York: MacMillan.

Skinner, B. F. (1969). *Contingencies of reinforcement: A theoretical analysis.* New York: Appleton-Century-Crofts.

Skinner, B. F. (1971). *Beyond freedom and dignity.* New York: Knopf.

Smith, S., & Farrell, D. (1993). Level system use in special education: Classroom intervention with prima facie appeal. *Behavioral Disorders, 18,* 251–264.

Solomon, R. & Wahler, R. (1973). Peer reinforcement control of classroom problem behavior. *Journal of Applied Behavior Analysis, 6,* 49–56.

Stage, S. A., & Quiroz, D. R. (1997). A meta-analysis of interventions to decrease disruptive classroom behvior in public education settings. *School Psychology Review, 26,* 333–368.

Stichter, J. P., Clarke, S., & Dunlap, G. (in press). Twenty-two years of assessment-based and antecedent-based interventions across behavioral and developmental disabilities. *Education and Treatment of Children.*

Sturmey, P. (1995). Analog baselines: A critical review of the methodology. *Research in Developmental Disabilities, 16,* 269–284.

Sugai, G., & Horner, R. H. (1994). Including students with severe behavior problems in general education settings: Assumptions, challenges, and solutions. In J. Marr, G. Sugai, & G. Tindal (Eds.), *The Oregon Conference Monograph* (pp. 109–120). Eugene, OR: College of Education, University of Oregon.

Sugai, G., & Horner, R. (1999). Discipline and behavioral support: Practices, pitfalls, and promises. *Effective School Practices, 17,* 10–22.

Sugai, G., Horner, R. H., Dunlap, G., Hieneman, M., Lewis, T. J., Nelson, C. M., Scott, T., Liaupsin, C. , Sailor, W. , Turnbull, A., Trunbull, H. R., Wickham, D., Wicox, B., & Ruef, M. (2000). Applying positive behavior support and functional behavioral assessment in schools. *Journal of Positive Behavior Interventions, 2,* 131–143.

Sugai, G., Horner, R., & Sprague, J. (1999). Functional-assessment-based behavior support planning: Research to practice to research. *Behavioral Disorders, 3,* 253–257.

Symons, F. J., McDonald, L. M., & Wehby, J. H. (1998). Functional assessment and teacher data collection. *Education and Treatment of Children, 21,* 135–139.

Tawney, J. W., & Gast, D. (1984). *Single subject research in special education.* Columbus, OH: Merrill.

Taylor, J. C., & Romanczyk, R. G. (1994). Generating hypotheses about the function of student problem behavior by observing teacher behavior. *Journal of Applied Behavior Analysis, 27,* 251–265.

Taylor-Greene, S., Brown, D., Nelson, L., Longton, J., Gassman, T., Cohen, J., Swartz, J., Horner, R. H., Sugai, G., & Hall, S. (1997). School-wide behavioral support: Starting the year off right. *Journal of Behavioral Education, 7,* 99–112.

Todd, D., Scott, R., Bostow, D., & Alexander, S. (1976). Modification of the excessive inappropriate classroom behavior of two elementary school students using home based consequences and daily report card procedures. *Journal of Applied Behavior Analysis, 9,* 465–478.

Touchette, P. E., MacDonald, R. F., & Langer, S. N. (1985). A scatter plot for identifying stimulus control of problem behavior. *Journal of Applied Behavior Analysis, 18,* 343–351.

Trice, A., & Parker, F. (1983). Decreasing adolescent swearing in an instructional setting. *Education and Treatment of Children, 6,* 19–35.

Trice, A., Parker, F., Furrow, F., & Iwata, M., (1983). An analysis of home contingencies to improve behavior with disruptive adolescents. *Education and Treatment of Children, 6,* 389–399.

Umbreit, J. (1995). Functional assessment and intervention in a regular classroom setting for the disruptive behavior of a student with attention deficit hyperactivity disorder. *Behavioral Disorders, 20,* 267–278.

Vollmer, T., & Smith, R. G. (1996). Some current themes in functional analysis research. *Research in Developmental Disabilities, 17,* 229–249.

Weeks, M., & Gaylord-Ross, R. (1981). Task difficulty and aberrant behavior in severely handicapped students. *Journal of Applied Behavior Analysis, 14,* 449–463.

Wehby, J. H., Symons, F. J., & Canale, J. A. (1998).Teaching practices in classrooms for students with emotional and behavioral disorders: Discrepancies between recommendations and observations. *Behavioral Disorders, 24,* 51–56.

Winterling, V., Dunlap, G., & O'Neill, R. E. (1987). The influence of task variation on the aberrant behaviors of autistic students. *Education and Treatment of Children, 10,* 105–119.

Witt, J. C., & Adams, R. M. (1980). Direct and observed reinforcement in the classroom: The interaction between information and reinforcement for socially approved and disapproved behaviors. *Behavior Modification, 4,* 321–336.

Wolf, M., Risley, T., & Mees, H. (1966). Application of operant conditioning procedures to the behavior problems of an autistic child. In R. Ulrich & T. Stachnik & J. Mabry (Eds.), *Control of human behavior: Expanding the behavioral laboratory.* Glenview, IL: Scott, Foresman.

Wood, R., & Flynn, J. M. (1978). A self-evaluation token system versus and external evaluation token system alone in a residential setting with predelinquent youth. *Journal of Applied Behavior Analysis, 11,* 503–512.

Zarcone, J., Iwata, B., Mazaleski, J., & Smith, R. (1994). Momentum and extinction effects on self-injurious behavior and noncompliance. *Journal of Applied Behavior Analysis, 27,* 649–658.

Zimmerman, E. H., & Zimmerman, J. (1962). The alteration of behavior in a special classroom situation. *Journal of the Experimental Analysis of Behavior, 5,* 59–60.

28

Experimental Research Designs in the Study of Children and Youth with Emotional and Behavioral Disorders

RICHARD VAN ACKER, MITCHELL L. YELL,
RENÉE BRADLEY, *and* ERIK DRASGOW

Over the past few years, there have been increased efforts to ensure that teachers across the nation use instructional procedures that have been validated as effective by scientific research. For example, the National Research Council (2002) and the Coalition for Evidence-Based Policy (2002) issued reports stating that education will only see progress if we build a knowledge base of educational practices that have proven effective by rigorous experimental research. These clarion calls led to a central principle in the recently enacted No Child Left Behind Act of 2001 (NCLB) that requires that federal funds be expended only to support educational activities that are backed by scientifically based research.

What constitutes sound scientific research? The National Research Council (2002) reports that for a research design to be scientific it must allow for direct experimental investigation of important educational questions. In this chapter, we will provide an overview of experimental research designs and review how such designs have been applied to the scientific study of children and programs for children with emotional and behavioral disorders (EBD). To

do this, we first review basic concepts in experimental research. Second, we examine factors that often affect experimental design in educational research. Finally, we offer recommendations for conducting rigorous experimental research in the field of EBD.

EXPERIMENTAL RESEARCH

Educational research refers to the systematic collection and analysis of data in order to develop valid and generalizable descriptions, interventions, and explanations related to various aspects of education (Gall, Borg, & Gall, 2003). In experimental research, the participants in the experiment are typically placed into one or more groups, and a researcher manipulates certain attributes, treatments, stimuli, or conditions of interest. The researcher then observes the effect that the manipulations have on the condition or behavior of the participants in the study.

Experimental research is the only type of research in which the researcher can test a hypothesis to establish cause-and-effect relationships (Gay & Airasian, 2003). In experimental research, the researcher (1) manipulates an independent variable, (2) controls extraneous variables, and (3) observes the effect of the manipulation of the independent variable on the dependent variable. If a research experiment is planned and conducted properly, and the data analyzed appropriately, the researcher can conclude that the manipulated variable caused, or did not cause, a change in the variable being observed.

There are three types of research that are generally considered to be experimental research: (1) true experiments, (2) quasi-experiments, and (3) single-subject research (Gall et al., 2003; Gay & Airasian, 2003; Martella, Nelson, & Marchand-Martella, 1999). In this chapter, we will examine true experiments and quasi-experiments and their application to the study of children and youth with EBD. Lewis, Lewis-Palmer, Newcomer, and Stichter (Chapter 27, this volume) examine single-subject research; therefore, we will not cover these designs. To begin our exploration of experimental research designs, we first briefly describe the experimental process and then review some basic concepts in experimental research. In experimental research the researcher begins with a hypothesis that predicts a causal or functional relationship between two variables. The purpose of the experiment is to support or refute this hypothesis.

The Experimental Process

The experimental process usually consists of four steps. First, the researcher selects the participants in the study. In this step, the researcher controls the selection of the participants. This means that the participants are selected from a well-defined population. Second, the researcher assigns the participants to either a treatment or control group. In this step, the researcher attempts to ensure that the two groups are as similar as possible, often by randomly assigning participants to the groups. Third, the experimental group is exposed to the treatment or intervention, also called the independent variable, whereas the control group is exposed to either (1) no treatment, (2) a different level of the same treatment, or (3) an alternative treatment. The direct manipulation of at least one independent variable is a distinguishing characteristic of experimental research (Gay & Airasian, 2003). In this step, the researcher attempts to remove the influence of any variable, other than the independent variable, that might affect the performance of the groups. Fourth, the researcher compares the experimental and control groups' performance on some measure of interest that is related to the treatment. This measure is called the dependent variable, because it is presumed to be dependent on the treatment introduced by the researcher (Gall et al., 2003). The researcher uses statistical analysis to determine whether the treatment resulted in a significant difference between the two groups.

Basic Concepts in Experimental Research

Subject Selection and Assignment to Treatment Condition

One of the most important decisions the researcher makes in the development of his or her study is the selection and assignment of subjects to treatment levels. As we shall discuss throughout this chapter, the validity of the inferences drawn from any study will be greatly influenced by the care the researcher takes to ensure the equivalence of the groups assigned to the various treatment levels. One of the most effective ways to control for group equivalence and the impact of extraneous variables, as well as to protect against many of the threats to internal validity, involves the random selection and the random assignment of subjects to treatment levels.

Random assignment differs from random selection of subjects. In random selection the researcher attempts to select subjects from the population of possible subjects in such a way that each member of the population has an equal chance of being selected. Once the sample is selected, random assignment refers to the placement of subjects within the various treatment groups in such a way that each subject has an equal chance of being placed into each condition. Random assignment enhances the equivalence of groups prior to exposure to the independent variable by distributing all extraneous variables into the groups by chance alone.

Another common strategy for the selection of subjects involves comparing identified or treated students with matched students in the general population. Students with an educational disability of emotional disturbance or some other mental health disability (e.g., conduct disorder [CD], oppositional defiant disorder [ODD]) are compared with a group of children drawn from the general population. The subjects in the comparison group are typically matched to the "clinical" subjects on the basis of specified demographic variables (e.g., age, gender, socioeconomic status). The comparison group children differ in that they are typically excluded from involvement if they have a mental health diagnosis similar to that of the clinical sample. Studies employ a variety of procedures to identify the comparison group subjects. For example, Gibb, Allred, Ingram, Young, and Egan (1999), in their study to examine the effects of inclusion within the general education classroom on students with EBD, targeted 14 students with EBD who were recently included within the general education program of a suburban junior high school. Prior to the start of the study, these students had been taught in self-contained classrooms. Twenty general education students constituted the comparison group. These students were randomly selected from the population of junior high school students who had been assigned to at least one of the same general education classes as the target students with EBD. Each student in this population was assigned a number, and a table of random numbers was then employed to select the 20 comparison subjects.

Some researchers seek comparison subjects through various means of securing volunteers. Melnick and Hinshaw (1996), in a study exploring the social goal attainment behavior of boys with attention-deficit/hyperactivity disorder (ADHD) and non-diagnosed boys during small-group play, employed 27 subjects with ADHD who were recruited from local pediatricians, mental health clinics, and parent support groups. The 18 comparison subjects were recruited from advertisements in local newspapers. Inclusion and exclusion criteria for the comparison group subjects were the same as the ADHD group, with the exception that comparison group subjects could not have a clinical diagnosis of ADHD, oppositional defiant disorder (ODD), or conduct disorder (CD). Examination of the known demo-

graphic variables of the subjects in the two groups found they did not differ significantly on any sociodemographic or cognitive variable except verbal intelligence scores on the Wechsler Intelligence Scale for Children—Revised (WISC-R) (comparison boys scored higher). Obviously, subjects who volunteer for participation in a study may differ dramatically from subjects referred to a clinical setting or assigned to a given diagnostic category on the basis of their disability. These differences may detract greatly from group equivalency and may introduce extraneous variables. For example, in the Melnick and Hinshaw (1996) study, one might anticipate that increased verbal intelligence might significantly impact social goal setting and goal attainment above and beyond the variance that could be attributed to the diagnostic criteria of ADHD. As researchers move away from random selection and random assignment of subjects to treatment level, error variation may be introduced that, as we shall see later, may detract from the validity of the study. Once the subjects are selected and assigned to their respective treatment conditions, the researcher must implement a series of procedures to systematically manipulate the presentation of the independent variable and observe the outcome on the dependent measures. Next we will review independent and dependent variables.

Independent Variables

An independent variable, sometimes called the experimental or treatment variable, is an activity or characteristic that a researcher believes will make a difference with respect to some behavior (Gay & Airasian, 2003). In an experiment, the researcher manipulates the independent variable to see if it results in change in the behavior. In the previous example, the researchers decided that the choice-making interventions would be the independent variable. Thus, a researcher has direct control over what the independent variable will be, when participants receive the independent variable, and how much each participant will receive (McMillan, 2004). Table 28.1 lists a sample of experimental studies involving students with EBD and the independent variables used in the research.

TABLE 28.1. Experimental Research

Study	Purpose	Independent variable(s)	Dependent variable(s)	Results
Babyak, Koorland, & Mathes (2000)	• To examine the effects of story mapping instruction on the reading comprehension of students with EBD.	• Story mapping intervention taught by direct instruction, guided practice, and independent practice.	• Story retells. • Comprehension questions. • Main idea probes.	• The story mapping instruction improved the reading comprehension of all participants.
Dawson, Venn, & Gunter (2000)	• To examine the effects of modeling on the reading performance of students with EBD. • To compare the effectiveness of models provided by a teacher versus models provided by a computer.	• Using a computer with a synthesized voice as a model. • Using the teacher as the model.	• The number of correct words read per minute. • The mean percentage of words read correctly.	• Students read more words correctly when the teacher modeled the reading passage than when no model was provided. • Students read more words correctly when the computer modeled the reading passage than when no model was provided. • Students read more words correctly when the teacher, rather than the computer, modeled the reading passage.
Jolivette, Wehby, Canale, & Massey (2001)	• To examine the effects of choice making on academic and social behaviors of elementary students with EBD.	• Providing students with choice of academic assignment.	• Direct observation of task engagement. • Direct observation of disruption. • Direct observation of off-task behavior • Attempted task problems. • Problems correct.	• Two of the three students demonstrated moderate positive effects on task engagement, disruption, off-task behavior, and academic productivity when given a choice of activities.
Kern, Bambara, & Fogt (2002)	• To examine the effects of classwide curricular modifications on the engagement and challenging behaviors of students with EBD.	• Providing opportunities for individual and group choice making. • Incorporating high-interest activities into a lesson.	• Direct observation of student engagement. • Direct observation of destructive behavior.	• When the choice making and high-interest activities were introduced classwide, student engagement increased and destructive behavior decreased.
Lane, O'Shaughnessy, Lambros, Gresham, & Beebe-Frankenberger (2001)	• To examine the effectiveness of a reading intervention program for first-grade students at risk of developing conduct and attention problems.	• Phonological awareness training for reading.	• A measure of nonsense word fluency. • A curriculum-based measure of oral reading fluency. • Direct observation of disruptive behaviors and negative social interactions.	• All students who participated in the phonological awareness training experienced substantial growth in word attack and oral reading fluency. • There was evidence of a reciprocal relationship between improvements in phonemic awareness skills and decreases in maladaptive behaviors.
Lane et al. (2003)	• To examine the effectiveness of social skills instruction for students at risk for antisocial behavior who were unresponsive to a schoolwide primary intervention program.	• Explicit instruction in social skills during small-group sessions.	• Direct observation of total disruptive behaviors. • Direct observation of academic engaged time. • Direct observation of negative social interactions on the playground. • Measure of oral reading fluency.	• The social skills instruction program was effective in decreasing disruptive behaviors in the classroom and improving social interactions on the playground. • The social skills instruction program was associated with improved academic engaged time.

(continued)

TABLE 28.1. (*continued*)

Study	Purpose	Independent variable(s)	Dependent variable(s)	Results
Levendoski & Cartledge (2000)	• To examine the effects of a self-monitoring procedure on the on-task behavior and academic productivity of students with EBD.	• Self-monitoring training using cards and a self-monitoring procedure once every 10 minutes.	• Direct observation of time on-task. • Number of math problems completed correctly.	• When self-monitoring was in place, students demonstrated increases in on-task time and academic productivity while performing newly taught math problems.
Sutherland, Wehby, & Copeland (2000)	• To examine the effect of an observation-feedback intervention on the rates of a teacher's behavior-specific praise of students with EBD. • To examine the effect of observation on the rate of teacher behavior-specific praise for the on-task behavior of students with EBD.	• Observing and providing feedback on a teacher's use of behavior-specific praise.	• The teacher's non-behavior-specific praise rates. • The teacher's behavior-specific praise rates. • Direct observation of on-task behavior.	• The teacher's baseline rates of behavior-specific praise rates were high during baseline; they were not maintained during the withdrawal phase. • The percentage of on-task intervals increased for students and increased when the rates of behavior-specific praise was increased. • The percentage of on-task intervals decreased for students and increased when the rates of behavior-specific praise was decreased.
Trout, Epstein, Mickelson, Nelson, & Lewis (2003)	• To examine the outcomes of a supplemental daily direction instruction reading curriculum and a fluency building program on the reading skills of students at risk for emotional disturbance and reading deficits.	• A daily half-hour one-on-one tutoring session over a 7-month period using two direct instruction reading programs.	• A 1-minute curriculum-based measure of letter sounds. • A 1-minute curriculum-based measure of blends. • A 1-minute curriculum-based measure of high-frequency sight words.	• The supplemental daily direction/instruction reading curriculum and fluency-building program were effective methods for increasing students' phonemic awareness and basic reading skills in letter sounds, blends, and high-frequency sight words.

Dependent Variables

A dependent variable, sometimes called the criterion or outcome variable, refers to the change or difference in behavior that occurs as a result of the independent variable (Gay & Airasian, 2003; McMillan, 2004). It is the variable that is measured to see if an intervention has resulted in the expected change. The effect on the dependent variable is "dependent" on what happens when the independent variable is manipulated.

When researchers choose the dependent variable, they look for variables that are sensitive to changes in behavior and are easy to use. Additionally, researchers want dependent variables that are reliable and valid. Table 28.1 lists selected experimental studies involving students with EBD and the dependent variables used in the research.

Extraneous Variables

The goal of experimental research is the unequivocal demonstration that changes in the dependent variable are related to systematic manipulations of the independent variable (Gresham, MacMillan, Beebe-Frankenberger, & Bocian, 2000). If extraneous variables are allowed to intrude during an experiment, the researcher will not be able to determine whether changes in the dependent variable are properly attributable to manipulations of the independent variable or rather to the presence of the extraneous variables (Gall et al., 2003). According to Gay and Airasian (2003), extraneous variables may be participant variables (i.e., variables on which the participants in an experiment differ) or environmental variables (i.e., differences in the environment that might cause unwanted differences between groups in a study). In experimental studies, researchers attempt to control or eliminate all extraneous variables so that any changes in the dependent variable may be properly attributed solely to manipulation of the independent variable. When a researcher can demonstrate that the independent variable produced changes in the dependent variable, while decreasing the possibility that extraneous factors produced the results, he or she is said to have demonstrated experimental control (Martella et al., 1999). These extraneous or confounding variables represent threats to experimental validity that researchers must take steps to minimize. Two major categories of confounding variables that threaten experimental validity are threats to (1) internal validity and (2) external validity (Campbell & Stanley, 1971). We next discuss these threats.

Threats to Internal Validity. When a study has internal validity, we can say with confidence that changes in the dependent variable were due to the manipulation of the independent variable. Threats to internal validity are confounding variables that could have accounted for changes in the dependent variable. Thus, internal validity threats can be rival explanations for changes in the participants. Campbell and Stanley (1971) and Cook and Campbell (1979) identified a number of major threats to internal validity. Table 28.2 lists and provides a description of each threat to internal validity. Although it is very difficult to eliminate threats to internal validity totally, the use of appropriate research designs can largely eliminate or lessen the effects of extraneous variables and, thus, overcome these threats.

Threats to External Validity. Research has external validity if the results can be generalized to other persons, settings, and times. This is a crucial question for educators and researchers attempting to translate research to practice. According to Bracht and Glass (1968), researchers should consider two general classes of external validity: population validity and ecological validity. *Population validity* refers to the degree to which the results of a research study can be generalized from the specific sample that was studied to a larger population. The more evidence that researchers provide regarding the similarities between the sample population and the target population, the more confidence we can have in the external validity of the study. *Ecological validity* is concerned with the generalization of the study to other ecological settings. If a study has ecological validity it means that the situational and setting conditions that were present during the study are similar to the ecological conditions in the setting where the results will be applied. The more similar the experimental environment is to the target environment, the greater the ecological, and thus the external, validity of

TABLE 28.2. Threats to Internal Validity

Threat	Description
History	Events occur between the pretest and posttest that may affect the participants' performance.
Maturation	Developmental changes occur as participants grow older during the study.
Testing	Participants may show improvement on a posttest as a result of taking the pretest.
Instrumentation	Changes in the measuring instrument are made, or reliability of the measuring instrument comes into question.
Statistical regression	High scorers or low scorers tend to regress toward the mean on a posttest.
Differential selection	Participants in the experimental and control groups have different characteristics.
Selection–maturation interaction	Participants in the study mature at different rates.
Attrition	Participants drop out of the study in different numbers, which alters the composition of the groups.

the study. Table 28.3 lists and describes the threats to external validity.

These extraneous sources of variance introduce error into the study, and a researcher should attempt to control these variables whenever possible. There are a number of ways a researcher can exert such control. The first method involves holding the extraneous variable constant for all subjects. For example, Charlebois, Normandeau, Vitaro, and Berneche (1999), in their study of social skills training versus self-regulation skills training on the behavior of youths with inattentive, overactive, and aggressive behaviors, held a number of extraneous variables constant (e.g., gender, age, ethnicity, and to lesser degree culture) when they decided to limit their sample to "a homogeneous group of French-speaking Caucasian [kindergarten] boys" (p. 138). By holding these variables constant between both the treatment and the experimental group, the researcher ensures that these variables are not having a differential effect on the outcome of the study. That is, the variables that are held constant impact all conditions equally. While this is a very common practice in educational research, holding variables constant has some distinct disadvantages. Perhaps the most significant disadvantage is that it limits the generalizability of the results—reducing external validity. Charlebois and his colleagues can only generalize their findings to other French-speaking Caucasian kindergarten boys. Other disadvantages include limiting the pool of possible subjects and reducing the amount of data available—impacting statistical power. Again, Charlebois et al. began their subject selection with 550 kindergarten males. In an effort to control various extraneous variables, they employed a multiple-gate screening procedure that ultimately limited their sample to 30 boys.

Random assignment to treatment condition is another method a researcher may use to control for extraneous variables. Through random assignment, the distribution of all extraneous variables associated with the subjects is based on chance. Systematic error based on sampling bias is eliminated. For example, Pelham et al. (2000) randomly assigned the participants of the Summer Treatment Program of the larger Multimodal Treatment Study of Children with ADHD to either the behavior-intervention-only or the combined treatment (behavior intervention plus medication) condition, the two groups did not differ significantly on a variety of known demographic variables.

Matching subjects prior to assignment to the treatment condition is one of the most frequently used methods to control extraneous variables in educational research. Matched sets of individuals meeting the specified matching criteria for the extraneous variable(s) are identified. The number of individuals in each set equals the number of treatment conditions. Then, each member of the matched set is randomly assigned to one of the levels of the treatment condition (matched randomization). In a study explor-

TABLE 28.3. Threats to External Validity

Threat	Description
Pretest–treatment interactions	The pretest sensitizes participants to aspects of the treatment.
Selection–treatment interactions	The nonrandom selection of participants limits the generalizability of the study.
Multiple treatment interference	When participants receive more than one treatment, the effect of the prior treatment can affect the later treatment.
Specificity of variables	Poorly defined variables make it difficult to identify the settings and procedures to which the study can be generalized.
Treatment diffusion	Treatment groups communicate and adopt parts of each other's treatment.
Experimenter effects	Actions by the researcher affect the participants' performance and responses.
Reactive effects	The fact that they are in a study affects the participants and alters their behavior.

ing the affect regulation of adolescents with depression, Sheeber, Allen, Davis, and Sorensen (2000) identified 25 adolescent subjects with depression (either major depressive disorder or dysthymia). They were matched on race, gender, age, and neighborhood of residence with adolescents who did not meet the diagnostic criteria for any current psychiatric disorder and who had no history of mental health treatment. Most of the comparison group students ($N = 21$) were recruited via a canvassing technique in which research staff went door to door in the neighborhoods of the depressed participants. The remaining four matched subjects were recruited from referrals of the parents of the depressed participants. Posttreatment examination of the two groups indicated that there were no significant group differences on a number of important variables (besides those upon which subjects were matched), such as parent's level of education. There were, however, differences on variables such as number of households headed by a single parent and median family income—with the depressed group displaying lower income and more single-parent households. One might anticipate that these and other uncontrolled extraneous variables might impact the findings. Researchers attempt to match subjects across groups on those variables previously identified to show some significant relationship to the dependent measure.

Another possible method to control extraneous variables involves including the variable as one of the factors in the experimental design. The randomized block design isolates the effects of the extraneous variable through blocking. That is, subjects who are identified as being relatively similar (e.g., greater variance between groups than within groups) with respect to a specific extraneous variable are assigned to the same block. Once the blocks have been formed, treatments are randomly assigned to the experimental units within each block. Ideally, the net result will be treatment groups with an equal number of members from each block.

Huesmann et al. (1998) employed a randomized block design when they investigated the relative efficacy of a multicomponent preventative trial to address the development of antisocial behavior in urban children. Sixteen schools were recruited to participate in the study. The schools were blocked on the basis of pretest aggression, ethnic composition, socioeconomic status, and normative beliefs about aggression. Then schools from each block were randomly assigned to one of four conditions: (1) no treatment control, (2) classroom enhancement (teacher seminars on positive classroom management plus a social problem-solving curriculum for the students), (3) classroom enhancement plus a small-group peer-based social skills program, or (4) classroom enhancement, small-group peer social skills, plus a family intervention program.

If a researcher wishes to isolate the effects of two extraneous variables, a Latin square design can be employed. In this design, experimental units are blocked on both variables prior to random assignment to treatment. Typically a matrix is developed with the number of rows and columns equal to the number of treatments. The levels of the first extraneous variable are assigned to the rows of the matrix; the levels of the second extraneous variable are assigned to the columns. The levels of the treatment are then assigned to the cells such that each level of the treatment is assigned to each type of cell in the matrix. For example, Taylor, Gunter, and Slate (2001) employed a Latin square design when they explored teacher perceptions of inappropriate behavior as a function of the teacher's and the student's gender and ethnic background. Teachers (preservice and in-service) were initially blocked for gender and ethnicity and then randomly assigned to one of four groups. Each group was then asked to view four videos in different order (see Figure 28.1). Prior to analyses for ethnic and gender differences, an analysis was completed to determine if the order of presentation of video tapes had an effect on respondents' ratings. No significant differences were reported based on order; therefore, the data could be combined across the four groups to explore gender and ethnicity differences.

Bryan (1997) employed a variation of the Latin square design in a study exploring the sexual behavior of high-risk youths. As part of the study, Bryan presented incarcerated adolescents (who tend to be younger at first intercourse, have a greater number of sex partners, and lower rates of condom use than adolescents in general) with a series of scenarios depicting various levels of trust in the relationship, length of relationship, and

	Group 1	Group 2	Group 3	Group 4
1st tape viewed	Tape A	Tape B	Tape C	Tape D
2nd tape viewed	Tape B	Tape C	Tape D	Tape A
3rd tape viewed	Tape C	Tape D	Tape A	Tape B
4th tape viewed	Tape D	Tape A	Tape B	Tape C

FIGURE 28.1. Latin square design as employed by Taylor, Gunter, and Slate (2001) to counterbalance the extraneous variables of order of tape presentation on rating of video sequences of student behavior. Teacher groups were blocked and randomly assigned to presentation order on the basis of gender and ethnicity of teacher.

frequency of intercourse in a $2 \times 2 \times 2$ within-subjects Greco-Latin square design (formed by superimposing Latin square designs upon one another). There were significant effects for both trust and frequency of intercourse on the participant's judgment of whether or not condoms would be used.

The final method a researcher may use to control extraneous variables involves statistical control. Subjects are provided pretest measures on one or more concomitant variables (also called covariates) in addition to the dependent variable. These concomitant variables are extraneous variables thought to affect the dependent variable that has not been controlled for in the experiment. Through the use of a statistical procedure called the analysis of covariance, the dependent variable can be adjusted statistically to remove the effects of the uncontrolled source(s) of variation represented by the covariates. This procedure parcels the variance across the variables under consideration. Each variable is allotted the amount of variance that it contributes to the overall variance in the outcome. Thus, the researcher can identify the specific amount of the change any given variable contributes independent of the other variables involved (see, for example, Kirk, 1995).

Lack of Treatment Integrity

The goal of experimental research is to demonstrate that changes in the dependent variable were due to manipulations of the independent variable and not due to the influence of extraneous variables. Researchers design their experiments and then collect and analyze the data. In many situations, however, the researcher depends on others to actually administer the experimental treatments. For example, in educational research a classroom teacher may be given the responsibility of ensuring that the experimental protocol is followed. Unfortunately, the most carefully designed experiment can go awry if the person implementing the treatments fails to follow the exact procedures specified by the researcher. When this happens, the experiment is said to lack treatment integrity (Gresham et al., 2000).

Treatment integrity, also termed "treatment fidelity," refers to the degree to which a treatment is implemented as planned (Gresham et al., 2000). According to Gresham (1989), establishing the integrity of the treatment is one of the most important aspects of scientific research. Lack of treatment integrity is a critical problem in conducting and interpreting experiments because the experiment will be compromised if the intervention actually implemented is different from that planned intervention.

Researchers should work to ensure that treatments are implemented as planned to maximize treatment integrity. Unfortunately this often does not happen in educational research (Gall et al., 2003; Gresham, 1989; Gresham, 1997; Gresham, Gansle, & Noell, 1993; Gresham, Gansle, Noell, Cohen, & Rosenblum, 1993). For example, Gresham et al. (2000) found that only 18.5% of 65 intervention studies reported in three major learning disabilities journals over the past 5 years reported measures of treatment integrity.

Researchers can help to ensure that their experiments have good treatment integrity by (1) developing a protocol specifying the treatment components, (2) training the individuals who will implement the treatments, (3) collecting data on the implementation of the treatments, and (4) providing booster training sessions on treatment implementation if needed. Moreover, researchers should report data on treatment integrity when publishing their findings.

Educational research conducted by Lane et al. (2003) provides an excellent example of a study that maximized treatment integrity through careful training and assessment. In their experiment, the researchers sought to investigate the effectiveness of group social skills instruction for students at risk for antisocial behavior. To ensure treatment integrity in delivery of the intervention, the researchers (1) provided a 2-hour training session for teachers prior to the study, (2) conducted weekly supervision and training during the instruction phase of the study, (3) supplied teachers with behavioral scripts, and (4) collected treatment integrity data in 25% of the intervention sessions. Furthermore, Lane et al. reported the treatment information in their study.

EXPERIMENTAL DESIGNS

The selection of an appropriate experimental design can be rather daunting. The design must be structurally congruent with the research question and compatible with available resources (e.g., sufficient subject availability and time). Over the years, researchers have generated a number of excellent blueprints for the procedures one can employ when attempting to test a hypothesis. A complete discussion of experimental design would be far too ambitious an undertaking for this chapter. Therefore, only a few of the more common and promising approaches will be examined. For a more complete treatment of the subject of experimental design, the interested reader is referred to Brown and Melamed (1990), Campbell and Stanley (1971), Cook and Campbell (1979), Kirk (1995), Shadish, Cook, and Campbell (2002), and Timm (1975).

A *"true" experimental design* requires random assignment of subjects to the treatment levels and the provision for a valid comparison between treatment levels. In the presentation of some of the more common experimental designs below, we will assume the researcher has randomly assigned subjects to treatment levels. If the assignment of subjects to treatment levels is other than random, a study is said to employ a *quasi-experimental design*. In this section, each design is equally applicable for use with or without randomization. If randomization is not feasible, however, group equivalency and the added introduction of error must be taken into consideration.

Experimental design identifies the assignment of subjects to groups, the measurement of dependent variables, and implementation of the independent variable. All experimental designs require a posttest measurement of the dependent variable(s) to determine the effects of the experimental treatment. Some designs also call for a measure or test to be administered to the subjects prior to exposure to the independent variable. To aid understanding, each design will be diagrammed using a symbol system modified from that developed by Campbell and Stanley (1971):

X = exposure of a group to an experimental (treatment) variable

C = exposure of a group to the control or placebo condition

O = observation or test to measure dependent variable (subscript "pre" = pretest and subscript "post" = posttest)

Posttest-Only Control-Group Design

One of the most efficient experimental designs is the posttest-only control-group design. Subjects are randomly assigned to either the treatment condition or to the control condition. If assignment to condition is not random, the design is termed a static-group comparison design. Following exposure of the treatment group to the independent variable(s) both groups are assessed on the dependent measure to see if they demonstrate statistically significant differences. The diagram for this design is provided below.

$$X \quad O_{post}$$
$$C \quad O_{post}$$

The posttest-only control-group design/static-group comparison design can be extended to involve more than a single treatment condition. The subjects would be assigned to the multiple groups, and the effects of the various experimental conditions could be investigated through a variety of statistical tests. The expanded design can be diagrammed as:

$$X_1 \ O_{post}$$
$$X_2 \ O_{post}$$
$$C \ \ O_{post}$$

Pretest–Posttest Control-Group Design

By adding a pretest assessment of the dependent measure prior to the administration of the independent variable to the previous design, the researcher employs the pretest–posttest control-group design. When applied to groups that were not randomly assigned to their condition, the design is termed a nonequivalent control-group design. The addition of the pretest allows the researcher to compare the gain scores of the groups. If a researcher feels that the groups may lack equivalency of critical variables, pretest measures of these variables can be used in an analysis of covariance to statistically control for differences between the groups on these variables. The diagram for the simplest type of pretest–posttest control-group design would appear as:

$$O_{pre} \ X \ \ O_{post} \ \ O_{post} - O_{pre} = X \text{ gain score}$$
$$O_{pre} \ C \ \ O_{post} \ \ O_{post} - O_{pre} = C \text{ gain score}$$

The pretest–posttest control-group design also can be extended to have as many treatment levels as desired plus a control group. This is a strong design; however, the possibility of influencing the outcome through the introduction of the pretest may be a possibility.

Serna, Lamros, Nielsen, and Forness (2002) employed this design in their investigation of a primary prevention program to address the needs of students at risk for the development of EBD. Although random assignment was not possible, children were assigned to either classrooms that delivered the *Learning with Purpose: A Life-Long Learning Approach to Self-Determination*

program or a "no-treatment" control classroom. The study relied upon teachers volunteering to allow the delivery of the intervention in their classrooms. As it turns out, eight of the high-risk subjects were assigned to classrooms that elected to engage in the experimental condition, and only one high-risk student was assigned to the control classroom. This type of problem often arises when subjects or experimental units (e.g., classrooms) are allowed to select their assignment to condition (see interaction of selection and treatment effects).

Solomon Four-Group Design

By combining the pretest-only control-group design and the pretest–posttest control-group design, a researcher employs what has been termed the Solomon four-group design. This design calls for a minimum of two groups assigned to the control condition and two groups assigned to each level of the treatment. In its four-group form, only one of the control groups and one of the treatment groups are pretested; however, all four groups are posttested at the close of the experiment. The Solomon four-group design can be diagrammed as:

$$O_{pre} \ \ \ X \ \ \ O_{post}$$
$$O_{pre} \ \ \ C \ \ \ O_{post}$$
$$\quad\quad\ \ X \ \ \ O_{post}$$
$$\quad\quad\ \ C \ \ \ O_{post}$$

The advantage of the Solomon four-group design is that it allows the researcher to check on the possible effects of pretesting and the interaction of pretesting with the experimental treatment. The downside of using this design is the need for more groups, thus more subjects. The design can be extended to include multiple treatment levels plus a control group condition, but for each level of treatment two additional groups are required.

Ullman, Stein, and Dukes (2000), as part of an evaluation of the Drug Abuse Resistance Education Program (DARE) employed a Solomon four-group design to examine the effects of the program on the subjects' self-esteem, resistance to peer pressure, institutional bonds (with family and school), and acceptance of risky behavior. Interestingly, these researchers report that pretest sensitivity significantly impacted the outcome for two of the DARE core constructs, namely, acceptance of risky behavior and institutional bonds.

Factorial Designs

When a researcher is interested in evaluating two or more independent variables simultaneously. This allows the researcher to explore the effect of each variable independently as well as examine the interaction of the variables upon the outcome. *Interaction* occurs when the effect on the dependent variable for one independent variable fails to remain constant over the levels of the other. For example, Tashman, Weist, Nabors, and Shafer (1998), in a study of the impact of involvement in meaningful activities and the self-reported aggression and delinquency among inner-city adolescents, found gender versus activity level interaction effects. Males with higher levels of meaningful activity had significantly lower scores on aggression and delinquency behavioral subscales than males with lower levels of meaningful activity. This relationship, however, was not found in females; level of involvement in meaningful activities had no impact on the aggression and delinquency scores of females.

In its simplest form the factorial design would have two independent variables, with two levels of each variable. This would be known as a 2 × 2 factorial design. Theoretically, there could be any number of independent variables with any number of levels for each. The numerical designation of the factorial design indicates the number of independent variables and the number of levels for each. For example a 2 × 3 × 6 factorial design would have three independent variables (represented by the use of three separate integers) and 2, 3, and 6 levels for each of the three independent variables, respectively. The number of treatment combinations will equal the product of the number of levels of each of the treatments. Thus, our 2 × 2 factorial design would require 4 groups, while the 2 × 3 × 6 factorial design would require 36 groups. Each possible combination of the independent variables is tested, so each requires an independent group of subjects.

In a completely randomized factorial design, subjects are randomly assigned to each group or cell in the design. A partially randomized design exists if random assignment is not feasible for one or more of the independent variables, but possible for others.

This design allows the researcher greater ability to manipulate or control variables by assigning more than one independent variable. The addition of more independent variables, however, requires increased numbers of groups/subjects. The inclusion of additional independent variables also can add to problems in the interpretation of the results. Three- and four-way interactions can become almost impossible to interpret.

Lovaas and his colleagues (Lovaas, 1996; McEachin, Smith, & Lovaas, 1993) employed a 3 × 3 split-plot factorial design to evaluate the treatment outcomes in the Early Intervention Project (EIP), a study exploring the effects of a discrete-trial treatment program for students with autism. There were three levels of the between-subject variable (Experimental, Control Group 1, and Control Group 2) and three levels of the within-subject variable (in-take, follow-up, and long-term follow-up). Figure 28.2 displays a diagram to depict this 3 × 3 factorial design.

Repeated-Measures Designs

When a researcher wants to measure outcomes on the dependent variable(s) on some sort of ongoing or repeated basis beyond just a single pre- and posttest. Longitudinal research and many of the current epidemiological and prevention research studies often involve an intervention delivered over several years with repeated measurement on various dependent variables across the duration of the study. There will be times when the researcher is concerned about the maintenance of treatment effects or the long-term outcomes from exposure to a given treatment. These studies will employ a repeated-measures design.

One example of a repeated-measures design simply extends one of the earlier designs by continuing the measurement of the dependent measure in time. This approach is illustrated below as an extension of the pretest–posttest control-group design. The subscript numerals indicate the repeated administrations of the posttest over time.

Treatment

	Experimental Group Consisted of 19 students and received more than 40 hours per week of discrete trial one-to-one treatment.	Control Group 1 Consisted of 19 students who received 10 hours or less per week of discrete trial one-to-one treatment.	Control Group 2 Consisted of 21 students who did not receive treatment as part of the individualized education program.
Intake Assessment Assessment of subjects immediately prior to treatment.			
Follow-Up Assessment Assessment as the subjects entered elementary school following the 3-year project period.			
Long-Term Follow-Up Assessment in early adolescence.			

FIGURE 28.2. Diagram of the 3 × 3 factorial design (group × time) employed in the Early Intervention Project (Lovaas, 1996; McEachin, Smith, & Lovaas, 1993).

O_{pre} X O_{post-1} O_{post-2} O_{post-3} O_{post-4}

O_{pre} C O_{post-5} O_{post-6} O_{post-7} O_{post-8}

Kellum, Rebok, Ialongo, and Mayer (1994) employed a repeated measures design that explored the development and malleability of aggressive behavior in children as they matured following the delivery of a developmental epidemiologically based prevention trial. They implemented their intervention across a number of years while the students were in elementary school and followed the impact of the intervention through adolescence and early adulthood. Lane et al. (2003) also employed this type of repeated measures design (assessing students on five separate occasions following intervention) in their study exploring the lasting effects of a social skills instructional program for students identified by their teachers as at risk for the development of antisocial behavior.

In longitudinal intervention studies, epidemiological studies, and prevention trials, researchers often monitor the impact of the intervention simultaneously with the ongoing delivery of the intervention. This type of repeated-measures approach can be applied to any of the previously discussed designs. Below it is diagramed as applied to a Solomon four-group design. Again, the subscript numerals indicate the sequential nature of the intervention delivery and posttest measurement.

O_{pre} X_1 O_{post-1} X_2 O_{post-2} X_3 O_{post-3}

O_{pre} C O_{post-4} C O_{post-5} C O_{post-6}

     X_7 O_{post-7} X_8 O_{post-8} X_9 O_{post-9}

     C O_{post10} C $O_{post-11}$ C $O_{post-12}$

The Fast Track Project (Conduct Problems Prevention Research Group, 2002) employed a series of assessments at the start and close of each academic year across three separate cohorts of students over the course of the 10-year intervention program. Subjects were provided preintervention assessment on a variety of variables including academic and social performance; these assessments were readministered periodically during the multiyear intervention phase as well as following intervention in a follow-up or maintenance phase of the investigation. This allowed the investigators to identify the impact of the intervention on subjects during the process of the study (increasing the probability of identifying mediating and moderating variables) as well as the long-term impact of the intervention on the subjects' academic and social behavior. This design enabled the researchers to examine change across multiple points in time and across cohorts.

The experimental designs discussed above form the basic building blocks for most of the current research designs implemented in experimental group research. Coupled with the procedures discussed for controlling extraneous and confounding variables (e.g., randomized block designs, Latin square/counter-balanced designs), these designs should allow most researchers to design a study that will allow them to draw valid conclusions about the existence and nature of the experimental effect.

CHALLENGES IN EXPERIMENTAL RESEARCH

There is no doubt that the field of behavioral disorders has benefited and will continue to benefit from quality experimental research. The nature of educational and behavioral research, however, presents the researcher with a number of interesting challenges. In this section we will explore four of these challenges—the random selection and assignment of subjects to experimental conditions, the identification of mediating and moderating variables, the nesting of variables, and dealing with missing data. While these issues are not unique to educational research, they are common and are all too often overlooked.

The Challenge of Employing Random Selection and/or Random Assignment

The ability to employ randomization in educational research is often hindered by the fact that the researcher cannot typically ensure random assignment to treatment due to factors such as educational placement or the natural distribution of specified attributes (e.g., disability). Preexisting groups of subjects (e.g., classroom groups) will naturally include individuals whose attributes, attitudes, and experiences differ markedly.

An examination of several journals known to publish research in the area of emotional and behavioral disorders found very few studies that employed random selection or even random assignment of subjects to treatment levels. There were some studies, however, that, despite the obstacles of doing so, managed to employ true random assignment. As mentioned in our earlier discussion of random assignment, Pelham et al. (2000) in their study of behavioral treatment with and without medication is an excellent example of the use of random assignment of subjects to condition.

A common practice in educational research involves the random assignment of condition to an experimental unit such as a school or a classroom rather than individual subjects. For example, Kamps, Tankersley, and Ellis (2000), in a study designed to explore the impact of a follow-up prevention program for Head Start kindergarten and first-grade students with EBD, randomly assigned classrooms, rather than individual students, to either the treatment or the no-treatment control condition since the treatment interventions were delivered to classroom groups. Random assignment of the class or school is often a necessity. It is unreasonable to think a researcher could randomly assign subjects to a particular school or classroom. Obviously, this procedure provides far less assurance of group equivalency than does random assignment of subjects. Schools and classrooms represent physical and social contexts that may exert any number of forces upon the students assigned to the school or classroom. Each of these extraneous variables serves as a means to increase the estimate of error variance in the study and can add to problems in the valid inference of outcomes (see our discussion of nesting, below). Other approaches to isolate or partial out some of the individualized effects that can contribute to error due to an inability to randomly assign subjects include the use of matching, the use of a randomized block design, the use of a Latin square design, or through statistical control.

Mediating and Moderating Variables

Extraneous variables can sometimes have a bearing on the relationship of the independent and dependent variables. Over the past decade, researchers have become increasingly aware how one variable can influence the direction, strength, or even the display of any impact at all of the independent variable. For example, in a study exploring the effects of social skills training versus self-regulation skills training on trainers' management strategies and the behaviors exhibited by boys identified as inattentive, overactive, and aggressive (IOA), Charlebois et al. (1999) found that significant improvement in the learning of social skills was influenced by the subject's capacity to concentrate on the task. Thus, the social skills intervention was more effective if it first strengthened the student's capacity to attend to the learning task. Interestingly, this was not true for the self-regulation skills training condition. Variables that influence the strength or direction of a relationship between an independent variable and the dependent variable are termed *moderating variables*. In this study, the capacity of the student to attend to the learning task modulated (determined the strength of) the impact of the social skills training intervention on the learning of social skills.

When one variable (not the independent variable under consideration) accounts for the relationship between the independent variable and the dependent variable, it is called a *mediating variable*. For example, if teachers participate in an in-service education program designed to reduce ethnic bias on referral rates for EBD evaluations, the impact of the in-service education on teacher beliefs about behavior and ethnicity may serve as a mediating variable. Without the mediating variable (change in teacher beliefs), there is no effect of the treatment (in-service education program) on the dependent variable (ethnic bias in the referral rates for EBD) except through the treatment's impact on the mediating variable, and the mediating variable, in turn, impacts the dependent variable. The Conduct Problems Prevention Research Group (1997) demonstrated that the effects of an intensive psychosocial, parent–school preventative intervention for conduct problems on the outcome of school-based special services was partially mediated by the effects of the treatment on several family-level variables (e.g., parental discipline, warmth, and attitude toward the child). That is, when the effects of treatment on these parental mediators were taken into account, intervention effects on

reducing special education placement were attenuated. Likewise, Vitaro, Brendgen, Pagani, Tremblay, and McDuff (1999) demonstrated in a randomized clinical preventative intervention that reduction of risk for conduct disturbance was at least partially mediated by enhancing the quality of peer relationships.

The identification of possible mediating and/or moderating variables should be undertaken when exploring the outcome of educational research. The complexity of the social context of the school makes the existence of these variables a critical consideration when interpreting the results of any study.

Nesting of Variables and Hierarchical Experiments

As mentioned above, it is not unusual for educational research to employ experimental units that include numerous observational units or subjects. For example, many studies assign condition to classrooms or even to entire schools. In cases such as these, the individual subjects are nested within these larger experimental units. For example, in the Metropolitan Area Child Study, Huesmann et al. (1998) blocked the participating schools on the variables of pretest levels of aggression, normative beliefs about aggression, ethnic makeup of the schools, and socioeconomic status of the school's catchment area. Schools in each block were then randomly assigned to condition. Thus, each target grade classroom (grades 2, 3, 5, and 6) in the entire school was assigned to the same specified treatment condition or a no-treatment control condition. Consequently, each student within each classroom was assigned to the specified condition. Students and teachers (the observational units) were nested within classrooms, and classrooms were nested within schools (the experimental unit). Each classroom would be impacted by school-based variables (e.g., governance style, environmental factors, school climate), and each student and teacher would be additionally impacted by classroom-based variables (e.g., classroom climate, teaching style, physical setting). The potential impact of these extraneous variables experienced by groups of subjects assigned to different conditions cannot be overlooked. Nesting also can impact the independence of the individual subject scores on specific dependent variables. For example, if opportunities to respond to an oral question were the dependent variable, the fact that student A in the classroom is provided the opportunity to respond impacts the ability of Student B to respond to that question. Huesmann and his colleagues (1998) were required to employ a model with four hierarchical levels—individual student, class group, teacher, and school—in their assessment of a program to prevent the development of aggression in urban children. Failure to consider the multiple levels of the data can result in an overestimation of the variance belonging to the variables that are included in the model (Opdenakker & Van Damme, 1998).

A common error in the analysis of this type of research is to ignore the extraneous variable resulting from nesting and to treat the study as if subjects, not classrooms, were assigned to treatment levels. Failure to consider the impact of nesting could introduce error variance in the assessment of the treatment holding the nested variable. Hierarchical designs constructed from completely randomized designs and multilevel analyses are appropriate when nested variables exist. A correct analysis takes into account the effects of the nested variable and makes the analysis congruent with the way the experiment was actually carried out. Two commonly used multilevel models for analyses of nested data include the multilevel regression model and the model for multilevel covariance structure analysis (Hox, 2002). A complete discussion of hierarchical designs and analyses is beyond the scope of this chapter. The interested reader is directed to consult an advanced experimental research text (see, e.g., Hox, 2002; Kirk, 1995).

Missing Data

Missing data are common in most studies, especially when subjects are followed over time (e.g., repeated measures and longitudinal research). These missing data can jeopardize the validity of the study due to the reduced power to detect differences. Moreover, the subjects who are lost to follow-up may differ considerably from those who

remain available for multiple posttests. Missing data can be either randomly missing data that results from the random loss of subjects or due to various individual subjects being unavailable for one or more of the assessments. Missing data also can be nonrandom missing data. These result from a systematic loss of subjects from one or more conditions (e.g., the condition places extensive demands on subjects, resulting in a highly uneven attrition across conditions) or the loss of a group of subjects on a particular measure (e.g., a classroom fails to complete an assessment). In a study exploring the development of aggressive behavior in children with and without comorbid anxious symptoms, Ialongo, Edelsohn, Werthamer-Larsson, Crockett, and Kellam (1996) were missing data from approximately 27% of the subjects on at least one measure. Of the 570 children initially assessed during the fall of first grade, only 531 were still available in the spring (e.g., students left the school). An additional 116 students failed to complete at least one assessment. In 34 cases, the parents rescinded consent for participation, and in the remaining cases the subjects were either absent from school or otherwise unable to complete at least one measure. Such a significant loss of data clearly threatens the validity of a study.

There are several approaches to handling missing data. For random missing data, some of the most common include (1) listwise deletion, (2) pairwise deletion, (3) mean imputation, (4) regression imputation, and (5) multiple imputation. In listwise deletion (a common default method of addressing missing data in many statistical packages) researchers eliminate all scores for any subject missing data on any predictor or criterion variable. This can result in the loss of considerable data. Pairwise deletion uses those observations that have no missing values to compute the correlations for a given variable. Thus, it preserves information that would be lost when using listwise deletion. However, since different sample sizes are used to compute the various correlations, the resulting correlation matrix may not be positive (a requirement for some statistical analyses). Mean imputation involves substituting the mean for a particular variable from those cases with data for the missing value. Replacement with the group mean, however, leads to an underestimate of the standard deviation and inflation of the Type I error rate (Steiner, 2003). The regression-based procedure takes into account the relationship among variables in the estimation of the various missing data points. This process reduces, but does not eliminate, the concerns raised with mean imputation. Multiple imputation as a "process replaces each missing data point with a set of $m > 1$ plausible values to generate m complete data sets. These complete data sets are then analyzed by standard statistical software, and the results are combined to give parameter estimates and standard errors that take into account the uncertainty due to the missing data values (Sinharay, Stern, & Russell, 2001, p. 317). Thus, this method represents the most statistically efficient approach. When addressing *nonrandom* missing data, two methods of estimating scores have been suggested: the joint maximum likelihood estimation (JMLE) and the marginal maximum likelihood estimation (MML) (DeMars, 2002). Researchers will want to take care in the selection of an appropriate means to address missing data in an effort to maintain statistical power without compromising the validity of the study.

RECOMMENDATIONS AND FUTURE DIRECTIONS

In their review of research in EBD, Dunlap and Childs (1996) indicated that single-subject designs were the most frequently used approach. On the basis of our review of the current literature, this remains true today, especially in the educational literature. Whereas there has been a modest increase in the number of group research design studies, the majority of these studies are reported in the psychological literature.

There is a significant need for increased research efforts in the field of EBD. The existing outcome data for this population of students does not suggest that we currently possess the information needed to ensure their success (Wagner, Valdes, & Associates, 1993). There is far too little research guiding many of the common practices being implemented in the name of "best practices" for students with EBD (Simpson, 1999). The President's Commis-

sion on Excellence in Special Education noted eight findings in their report, *A New Era: Revitalizing Special Education for Children and Their Families* (U.S. Department of Education, 2002). One addressed research, stating: "Research on special education needs enhanced rigor and the long-term coordination necessary to support the needs of children, educators and parents. In addition, the current system does not always embrace or implement evidence-based practices once established" (p. 8).

With the passage of Public Law 107-110, the NCLB, and the Education Sciences Reform Act of 2002, the federal government is demanding that educators use "scientifically based research practices" in the identification of effective and efficient educational interventions. In the federal guidelines related to NCLB, the U.S. Department of Education (USDOE) stresses the need for randomized control experiments as a means of improving the quality and impact of educational research.

> *No Child Left Behind* sets forth rigorous requirements to ensure that research is scientifically based. It moves the testing of educational practices toward the medical model used by scientists to assess the effectiveness of medications, therapies and the like. Studies that test random samples of the population and that involve a control group are scientifically controlled. To gain scientifically based research about a particular educational program or practice, it must be the subject of such a study. (U.S. Department of Education website, *www.ed.gov/nclb/methods/whatworks/edpicks.jhtml*)

The preference for this type of research is evident in the U.S. Department of Education's Strategic Plan that is citing the "use of randomized experimental designs" as a performance measure for improving the "Quality and Rigor of Department-funded Research" (USDOE, 2002). In addition, several research funding opportunities in the Office of Special Education Programs gave competitive preference points for randomized experimental designs.

Although this type of research is not particularly common in educational research over the past decade, there have been a number of large preventative trials funded that employed randomized controls to test interventions designed to impact aggression and antisocial behavior (e.g., Huesmann et al., 1998; Conduct Problems Prevention Research Group, 1997), ADHD (Pelham et al., 2000), and autism (McEachin, Smith, & Lovaas, 1993). These research efforts often use large samples of students and intervene across multiple contexts for an extended period of time. Considerable effort and fiscal support is necessary to conduct this type of research. Nevertheless, the potential benefits cannot be underestimated.

Obviously, researchers should strive to increase the scientific rigor of their studies. However, there are "real-world" considerations that may make the use of randomized control experiments less than desirable. Indeed, the National Research Council report *Scientific Research in Education* (2002) recognizes the value of randomized controls in addressing causal questions but also encourages the use of multiple methods to both supplement the randomized trials and to address some other important questions that are not appropriately addressed by a randomized design. Moreover, there are a number of ethical and practical implications for efforts to employ "true random assignment" within educational research. Some research questions do not lend themselves to random assignment of subjects. In some cases, random assignment of subjects to condition might increase the internal validity of the study but detract from the external validity—the ability to generalize the findings to the real school and classroom.

Based upon the literature in EBD reviewed to prepare this chapter, there are a number of recommendations we can make (in addition to a greater use of randomized controls in experimental research) that might benefit the design of the research and the reporting of outcomes. These include:

- Researchers need to identify how subjects were selected from the population and assigned to treatment conditions. In far too many studies, the information was missing altogether or provided in a manner that would not permit the reader to draw adequate information that might help in determining the potential generalizability of the findings.
- Care should be taken to collect and report on the integrity of the delivery of the intervention or treatment.
- When treatment condition is assigned to experimental units such as the classroom or the school, rather than to individual subjects, statistical analyses should control for the nesting of subjects (e.g., students nested within classrooms, nested within schools). Often the lack of independence of data points was ignored during analysis. This introduces a new source for error.
- Studies should report information on attrition and missing data and indicate the steps taken to address these issues when analyzing the outcome data.
- Researchers should take care to anticipate the potential of moderating or mediating variables and design their studies in such a way as to capture the impact of these important variables.
- When possible, researchers should attempt to expand the settings from which subjects are drawn for research in emotional and behavioral disorders. Dunlap and Childs (1996) criticized the field for its rather restrictive use of settings (e.g., clinical settings and self-contained classrooms) in the research published between 1980 and 1993. There remains a tendency in the field to use these populations despite the fact that the majority of students with EBD are educated within the general education classroom for the majority of their day.

The education and treatment of children and youths with EBD requires increased guidance from empirical research. As indicated above, federal legislation requires that educational practices be "scientifically based." Unfortunately, there is sometimes little science supporting the actions of educators serving the needs of students with EBD. Some of the areas identified in the literature in need of increased research include:

- The further identification of "best practices." In some cases this might include the application of group research design to practices identified as promising through single-subject research. Research should explore both the efficacy and efficiency of practices.

- Prevention and early intervention research that targets multiple contexts impacting the development of challenging behaviors, with longitudinal outcome analysis.
- The identification of ways to improve the adoption of best practices by parents (Gunter & Denny, 1996; Hester & Kaiser, 1998), special education practitioners, and regular educators (Walker, Zeller, Close, Webber, & Gresham, 1999).
- The examination of teacher education practices to promote the development of teachers (both special and general education teachers) properly equipped to meet the needs of this challenging population of students (Landrum & Tankersley, 1999). The impact of recent trends in many states to promote the certification of "multi-category" specialists needs to be examined. Additionally, many states are adopting a wide array of alternative certification programs. Are these approaches to teacher certification resulting in the development of teachers capable of meeting the demands of the EBD population?
- Exploring effective and efficient models of inter- and multiagency collaboration in efforts to provide integrated services to students with EBD and their families (Walker et al., 1999).
- The relative efficacy of behavioral, pharmacological, and combined intervention procedures with students displaying various types of challenging behaviors and/or behavioral syndromes (Forness, Kavale, Sweeney, & Crenshaw, 1999).
- Conducting longitudinal research to explore the lasting impact of intervention studies.

CONCLUSION

There are significant needs to identify effective and efficient ways to intervene with students with EBD. We have attempted to identify how experimental research methods have been used to answer important research questions in the field. Great strides have been made to guide practice empirically. Nevertheless, group research methods provide a means to explore questions that could supply even greater opportunities for educators and other professionals to help these children and youths to succeed.

There are federal mandates that support the increased use of experimental research to identify effective educational practices. Perhaps, if federal and private funding sources can be identified, the time is right for a giant leap in our understanding of EBD. Researchers should embrace these new opportunities and be prepared to undertake the most rigorous, yet contextually valid, studies designed to answer the important questions that continue to present themselves in this field. Experimental research methods such as those discussed here will play an important, though not exclusive, role in this effort.

REFERENCES

Babyak, A. E., Koorland, M., & Mathes, P. G. (2000). The effects of story mapping instruction on the reading comprehension of students with behavioral disorders. *Behavioral Disorders, 25,* 239–258.

Bracht, G. H., & Glass, G. V. (1968). The external validity of experiments. *American Education Research Journal, 5,* 437–474.

Brown, S. R., & Melamed, L. E. (1990). *Experimental design and analysis: Quantitative applications in the social sciences.* Newbury Park, CA: Sage.

Bryan, A. D. (1997). *Psychosocial and contextual determinants of condom use among incarcerated adolescents.* Unpublished doctoral dissertation, Arizona State University, Tempe, AZ.

Campbell, D. T., & Stanley, J. C. (1971). *Experimental and quasi-experimental designs for research.* Chicago: Rand McNally.

Charlebois, P., Normandeau, S., Vitaro, F., & Berneche, F. (1999). Skills training for inattentive, overactive, aggressive boys: Differential effects of content and delivery method. *Behavioral Disorders, 24,* 137–150.

Coalition for Evidence-Based Policy. (2002). *Bringing evidence-driven progress to education.* Available at http://www.excelgov.org/displaycontent.asp?keyword=prppcEvidence.

Conduct Problems Prevention Research Group. (1997, April). *Testing developmental theory through prevention trials.* Paper presented at the biennial meeting of the Society for Research in Child Development, Washington, DC.

Conduct Problems Prevention Research Group. (2002). The implementation of the Fast Track Program: An example of a large scale prevention science efficacy trial. *Journal of Abnormal Child Psychology, 30,* 1–17.

Cook, T. D., & Campbell, D. T. (1979). *Quasi-experimentation, design and analysis issues for field settings.* Chicago: Rand McNally.

Dawson, L., Venn, M. L., & Gunter, P. L. (2000). The effects of teacher versus computer reading models. *Behavioral Disorders, 25*, 105–113.

DeMars, C. (2002). Incomplete data and item parameter estimates under JMLE and MML estimates. *Applied Measurement in Education, 15*(1), 15–31.

Dunlap, G., & Childs, K. E. (1996). Intervention research in emotional and behavioral disorders: An analysis of studies from 1980–1993. *Behavioral Disorders, 21*, 125–136.

Forness, S. R., Kavale, K. A., Sweeney, D. P., & Crenshaw, T. M. (1999). The future of research and practice in behavioral disorders: Psychopharmacology and its school implications. *Behavioral Disorders, 24*, 305–318.

Gall, M. D., Borg, W. R., & Gall, J. P. (2003). *Educational research: An introduction* (7th ed.). Boston: Allyn & Bacon.

Gay, L. R., & Airasian, P. (2003). *Educational research: Competencies for analysis and application* (7th ed.). Upper Saddle River, NJ: Merrill/Prentice Hall.

Gibb, S. A., Allred, K., Ingram, C. F., Young, J. R., & Egan, W. M. (1999). Lessons learned from the inclusion of students with emotional and behavioral disorders in one junior high school. *Behavioral Disorders, 24*(2), 122–136.

Gresham, F. M. (1989). Assessment of treatment integrity in school consultation and prereferral intervention, *School Psychology Review, 18*, 37–50.

Gresham, F. M. (1997). Treatment integrity in single-subject research. In R. Franklin, D. Allison, & B. Gorman (Eds.), *Design and analysis of single-subject research* (pp. 93–117). Mahwah, NJ: Erlbaum.

Gresham, F. M., Gansle, K., & Noell, G. (1993). Treatment integrity in applied behavior analysis with children. *Journal of Applied Behavior Analysis, 6*, 257–263.

Gresham, F. M., Gansle, K., Noell, G., Cohen, S., & Rosenblum, S. (1993). Treatment integrity in school-based intervention studies: 1980–1990. *School Psychology Review, 22*, 254–272.

Gresham, F. M., MacMillan, D. L., Beebe-Frankenberger, M. E., & Bocian, K. M. (2000). Treatment integrity in learning disabilities intervention research: Do we really know how treatments are implemented? *Learning Disabilities Research and Practice, 15*, 198–206.

Gunter, P. L. & Denny, R. K. (1996). Research issues and needs regarding teacher use of classroom management strategies. *Behavioral Disorders, 22*, 15–20.

Hester, P. P., & Kaiser, A. P. (1998). Early intervention for the prevention of conduct disorder: Research issues in early identification, implementation, and interpretation of treatment outcome. *Behavioral Disorders, 24*, 57–65.

Hox, J. J. (2002). *Applied multilevel analysis: Techniques and applications.* Mahwah, NJ: Erlbaum.

Huesmann, L. R., Maxwell, C. D., Eron, L., Dahlberg, L. L., Guerra, N. G., Tolan, P. H., Van Acker, R., & Henry, D. (1998). Evaluating a cognitive/ecological program for the prevention of aggression among urban children. *American Journal of Preventative Medicine, 12*(5, Suppl.), 120–128.

Ialongo, N., Edelsohn, G., Werthamer-Larsson, L., Crockett, L., & Kellam, S. (1996). The course of aggression in first-grade children with and without comorbid anxious symptoms. *Journal of Abnormal Child Psychology, 24*, 445–456.

Jolivette, K., Wehby, J. H., Canale, J., & Massey, N. G. (2001). Effects of choice-making opportunities on the behavior of students with emotional and behavioral disorders. *Behavioral Disorders, 26*, 131–145.

Kamps, D. M., Tankersley, M., & Ellis, C. (2000). Social skills interventions for young at-risk students: A 2-year follow-up study. *Behavioral Disorders, 25*, 310–324.

Kellum, S. G., Rebok, G. W., Ialongo, N., & Mayer, L. S. (1994). The course and malleability of aggressive behavior from early first grade into middle school: Results of a developmental epidemiologically-based preventative trial. *Journal of Child Psychology and Psychiatry and Allied Disciplines, 35*, 259–281.

Kern, L., Bambara, L., & Fogt, J. (2002). Class-wide curricular modification to improve the behavior of students with emotional or behavioral disorders. *Behavioral Disorders, 27*, 317–326.

Kirk, R. E. (1995). *Experimental design: Procedures for the behavioral sciences.* Pacific Grove, CA: Brooks/Cole.

Landrum, T. L., & Tankersley, M. (1999). Emotional and behavioral disorders in the new millennium: The future is now. *Behavioral Disorders, 24*, 319–330.

Lane, K. L, O'Shaughnessy, T. E., Lambros, K. M., Gresham, F. M., & Beebe-Frankenberger, M. E. (2001). The efficacy of phonological awareness training with first-grade students who have behavior problems and reading difficulties. *Journal of Emotional and Behavior Disorders, 9*, 219–231.

Lane, K. L., Wehby, J. H., Menzies, H. M., Doukas, G. L., Munton, S. M., & Gregg, R. M. (2003). Social skills instruction for students at risk for antisocial behavior: The effects of small group instruction. *Behavioral Disorders, 28*, 229–248.

Levendoski, L .S., & Cartledge, G. (2000). Self-monitoring for elementary school children with serious emotional disturbances: Classroom applications for increased academic responding. *Behavioral Disorders, 25*, 211–224.

Lovaas, O. I. (1996). The UCLA young autism model of service delivery. In C. Maurice, G. Green, & S. Luce (Eds.), *Behavioral intervention for young children with autism: A manual for parents and professionals* (pp. 241–248). Southborough, MA: New England Center for Autism.

Martella, R. C., Nelson, J. R., & Marchand-Martella, N. (1999). *Research methods: Learning to become a critical research consumer.* Boston: Allyn & Bacon.

McEachin, J. J., Smith, T., & Lovaas, O. I. (1993). Long-term outcomes for children with autism who received intensive behavioral treatment. *American Journal of Mental Retardation, 97,* 359–372.

McMillan, J. H. (2004). *Educational research: Fundamentals for the consumer* (4th ed.). Boston: Allyn & Bacon.

Melnick, S. M., & Hinshaw, S. P. (1996). What they want and what they get: The social goals of boys with ADHD and comparison boys. *Journal of Abnormal Child Psychology, 24,* 169–185.

National Research Council. (2002). Scientific research in education. Committtee on Scientific Principles for Education Research. R. J. Shavelson & L. Towne (Eds.), *Center for Education: Division of Behavioral and Social Sciences and Education.* Washington DC: National Academy Press.

No Child Left Behind Act of 2001. 20 U.S.C. § 6301 et seq.

Opdenakker, M. C., & Van Damme, J. (1998, April). *The importance of identifying levels in multilevel analysis: An illustration of the effects of ignoring the top or intermediate levels in school effectiveness research.* Paper presented at the annual meeting of the American Educational Research Association, San Diego, CA.

Pelham, W. E., Gnagy, E. M., Greiner, A. R., Hoza, B., Hinshaw, S. P., Swanson, J. M., Simpson, S., Shapiro, C., Bukstein, O., Baron-Myak, C., & McBurnett, K. (2000). Behavioral versus behavioral and pharmacological treatment in ADHD children attending a summer treatment program. *Journal of Abnormal Child Psychology, 28,* 507–525.

Serna, L. A., Lamros, K., Nielsen, E., & Forness, S. R. (2002). Head Start children at risk for emotional or behavioral disorders: Behavior profiles and clinical implications of a primary prevention program. *Behavioral Disorders, 27,* 137–141.

Shadish, W., Cook, T., & Campbell, D., (2002). *Experimental and quasi-experimental designs for generalized causal inference.* New York: Houghton-Mifflin.

Sheeber, L., Allen, N., Davis, B., & Sorensen, E. (2000). Regulation of negative affect during mother–child problem-solving interactions: Adolescent depressive status and family processes. *Journal of Abnormal Child Psychology, 28*(5), 467–479.

Simpson, R. L. (1999) Children and youth with emotional and behavioral disorders: A concerned look at the present and a hopeful eye to the future. *Behavioral Disorders, 24,* 284–292.

Sinharay, S., Stern, H. S., & Russell, D. (2001). The use of multiple imputations for the analysis of missing data. *Psychological Methods, 6,* 317–329.

Steiner, D. L. (2003). The case of the missing data: Methods of dealing with dropouts and other research vagaries. *Canadian Journal of Psychiatry, 47,* 70–77.

Sutherland, K. S., Wehby, J. H., & Copeland, S. R. (2000). Effect of varying rates of behavior specific praise on the on-task behavior of students with EBD. *Journal of Emotional and Behavior Disorders, 8,* 2–8.

Tashman, N. A., Weist, M. D., Nabors, L. A., & Shafer, M. E. (1998). Involvement in meaningful activities and self-reported aggression and delinquency among inner-city teenagers. *Journal of Clinical Psychology in Medical Settings, 5,* 239–248.

Taylor, P. B., Gunter, P. L., & Slate, J. R. (2001). Teacher's perceptions of inappropriate student behavior as a function of teachers' and students' gender and ethnic background. *Behavioral Disorders, 26,* 147–151.

Timm, N. H. (1975). *Multivariate analysis with applications in education and psychology.* Monterey, CA: Brooks/Cole.

Trout, A. L., Epstein, M. H., Mickelson, W. T., Nelson, J. R., & Lewis, L. M. (2003). Effects of a reading intervention for kindergarten students at risk for emotional disturbance and reading deficits. *Behavioral Disorders, 28,* 313–426.

Ullman, J. B., Stein, J. A., & Dukes, R. L. (2000). Evaluation of D.A.R.E. (Drug Abuse Resistance Education) with latent variables in context of a Solomon Four Group Design. In J. S. Rose, L. Chassin, C. C. Presson, and S. J. Sherman (Eds.), *Multivariate applications in substance use research: New methods for new questions* (pp. 203–231). Mahwah, NJ: Erlbaum.

U.S. Department of Education, Office of Special Education and Rehabilitative Services. (2002). *A new era: Revitalizing special education for children and their families.* Washington, DC: U.S. Printing Office.

Vitaro, F., Brendgen, M., Pagani, L., Tremblay, R., & McDuff, P. (1999). Disruptive behavior, peer associations, and conduct disorder: Testing the developmental links through early intervention. *Development and Psychopathology, 11,* 287–304.

Wagner, M., Valdes, K., & Associates. (1993). *National longitudinal study of special education students.* Stanford, CA: Stanford Research Institute.

Walker, H. M., Zeller, R. W., Close, D. W., Webber, J., & Gresham, F. M. (1999). The present unwrapped: Change and challenge in the field of behavior disorders. *Behavioral Disorders, 24,* 293–304.

29

Qualitative Research and Its Contributions to the Knowledge of Emotional and Behavioral Disorders

EDWARD J. SABORNIE

The contributions of qualitative research to the study of emotional and behavioral disorders (EBD) are far from abundant and relatively recent. This chapter discusses qualitative, or "naturalistic," research by (1) contrasting it with quantitative empiricism, (2) examining several methods typical of qualitative inquiry, (3) reviewing the qualitative research literature pertaining to EBD, and (4) providing implications for EBD drawn from the available research. As a starting point for this chapter, perhaps it is wise to explain why qualitative research has been relatively ignored in investigations involving children and youths with EBD. First, qualitative research has taken a back seat to quantitative experimentation in EBD because most of the leading experts in EBD of the late 1900s and the present were trained solely in the latter, that is, group-design and single-subject research. Lacking knowledge of qualitative research, much less using it in actual studies, the experts and pioneers in EBD did not pass this legacy to their protégés. Moreover, qualitative investigation in *special education* did not really gain appreciation until two decades ago when Stainback and Stainback (1984) concluded that qualitative research can broaden perspective and add much to our understanding

of children and youths identified as exceptional. The Stainbacks' conclusions at that time, however, were not unanimously accepted as the proper route for special education research (see Simpson & Eaves, 1985). Prior to the Stainbacks' seminal article, it is safe to say the only qualitative research familiar to most special educators consisted of Itard's examination of Victor, the *Wild Boy of Aveyron* (Itard, 1962), and Freud's case studies (see Freud, 1952).

Over time, quantitative research in EBD has continuously examined difficult behaviors in individuals and ways in which to change or eliminate them. While naturalistic research can focus on challenging behaviors and emotions (e.g., Freud, 1952; Wolcott, 1983), much, if not most, of its concern in EBD has been on rich descriptions of individuals and interpreting their dialogue, and meticulous examinations of the social contexts in which problem behaviors exist. Group-design and applied behavior analysis research in EBD have *tested* hypotheses concerned with objective descriptions of problem behaviors and ways to treat them. Qualitative research, because of its open-ended nature, *generated* hypotheses related to individuals and their inappropriate behavior and feelings. Quantitative research is typically concerned with the overt manifestation of behavior in an environment along with its frequency and intensity. Qualitative research, however, is more interested in an examination of a person's feelings for *why* he or she acted in a certain way, determined via in-depth interviewing over time. Quantitative research is concerned with the ability to generalize findings to other, similarly affected children and youths, but qualitative research has a *local* focus that is "grounded" in the actual phenomena under investigation (Peck & Furman, 1992).

Contrary to some of the leading experts in qualitative inquiry (e.g., Lincoln & Guba, 1985), I believe that quantitative and naturalistic research can coexist in the field of EBD. However, I do not favor the use of qualitative inquiry in EBD over its counterpart, quantitative research. Including qualitative research in the examination of human behavior simply leads to a more comprehensive picture of EBD, even though qualitative research may not be considered by some as scientific because of its interpretative view of the nature of knowledge (Kavale & Forness, 1998; Simpson & Eaves, 1985).

What is often ignored is that the two paradigms of empirical study share similarities. For example, both depend on varying amounts of direct observation of behavior and context. Without extensive observation, both quantitative and qualitative research would contribute little to science—regardless of how science is defined or practiced. A second area of similarity between quantitative and qualitative research concerns the dependence on repeated measurements. The hallmark of applied behavior analysis research is repeated measurement of behavior under baseline and various treatment conditions, and group research is also known for its repeated-measures analysis of variance designs. Continuous observation of behavior and its context is also the mainstay of different types of qualitative research. Some approaches to naturalistic inquiry require the researcher (or "inquirer") to immerse him- or herself into an environment as a "participant observer" so that nuances of the phenomenon under study are experienced by the researcher and interpreted and exposed in text. Both types of investigation also share an interest in how reliability of measurement is involved with research design. Group-

design research is concerned with stability of measurement as a function of any investigation. Applied behavior analysis research involves interobserver agreement coefficients and checks for fidelity of treatment in its designs and concern for reliability. Some qualitative research incorporates a sense of reliability through *triangulation*, which involves using (1) several data sources, (2) different data collectors, and (3) multiple interpreters of data (Denzin & Lincoln, 2003). Social validity has grown in importance in behavioral research over the years (see Kazdin, 1977; Wolf, 1978), while it has always been the sine qua non of qualitative inquiry. Last, quantitative researchers use SAS and SPSS software to analyze data, while qualitative inquiry often requires NUD*IST and The Ethnograph software for text analyses. In other words, quantitative and naturalistic research share more traits than most devotees of either approach care to admit.

Because qualitative research in EBD is a contemporary trend and its specific methods may not be well known, the discussion now turns to an exploration of the most frequently used "traditions" (Creswell, 1998) of qualitative research: (1) biographical, (2) phenomenological, (3) grounded theory, (4) ethnography, and (5) case study. An example of how the naturalistic inquiry could be applied with students or individuals with EBD is also included with each type of research.

A QUALITATIVE INQUIRY PRIMER

Biographical Research

A biographical qualitative study is one in which a single person's experiences, labors, and life's journeys are told to a researcher and then brought to text. What is unique in a biographical research report is the description of a special incident in a person's life, interpreted by another person (i.e., the researcher), that served as a turning point. Biographical inquiry can include autobiographies, oral histories, life histories, and the most common, individual biographies (Creswell, 1998).

In the general type of interpretive biography, the researcher would begin by searching written documents and records, including data of a quantitative type, that describe a person and begin to set the stage of an individual's life. The archival search and interpretation of such records forms the introductory narrative of the article, chapter, or book about the person of interest. The researcher also describes the relationship that he or she has developed with the person under study in any biographical research report. The bulk of the data involved in a biographical inquiry, however, originate with numerous interviews and conversations the researcher has with the person of interest. In these conversations, the individual typically tells the inquirer of some unusual occurrence that led to a significant change in the person's life. Next, the researcher would visit the place where the noteworthy event occurred in the person's life, attempt to understand the nuances and context of the environment, and describe it with verisimilitude so that the consumer of the research feels alive in the environment. The investigator attempts to interpret the meaning of the life-changing event for the reader and reflects on his or her own impressions of the event and context. Last, the researcher attempts to connect the person's special event to the larger world and extant literature, and closes the study with "lessons learned" (Lincoln & Guba, 1985).

Biographical Research Example

A 12-year-old student with EBD, Ralph, informs a naturalistic researcher of his life history in school through the sixth grade. The researcher examines Ralph's school cumulative folder to find information concerning his grades, number of disciplinary referrals, days absent, when he was first identified by the school district as having EBD, and so on related to school functioning. Ralph then has a series of 20 lengthy conversations with the researcher in which he describes experiences in and out of school. The researcher audiotapes all of the talks with Ralph. During the interviews Ralph repeatedly mentions his sixth-grade English teacher as the person responsible for changing his view of school. The teacher, Ms. Jones, was extremely helpful, in Ralph's opinion. She went out of her way to teach him one-on-one, made sure that he had a peer to help him every day in class if necessary, and constantly reinforced him for work completed and appropriate behavior rather

than punishing him for his misbehavior, as did so many of his other teachers. Ms. Jones made it possible for Ralph to enjoy school, hence, Ralph did not misbehave in Ms. Jones's English class and received a final grade of A. Ms. Jones's class was *the* significant educational event for Ralph. In all of Ralph's other classes he was frequently absent and exhibited inappropriate behavior. The researcher then spends an entire month in Ms. Jones's class writing field notes on events that occur. The investigator attempts to "get a feel" for what it is like to be a student in the class, and discusses teaching philosophy with Ms. Jones. The experimenter also spends extended periods of time in Ralph's other classes in an attempt to capture the essence of why he had problems in those environments. Finally, the researcher interprets all the events in a manuscript that attempts to determine the context related to Ralph's appropriate and inappropriate behavior in and out of Ms. Jones's class.

Phenomenological Research

The phenomenological approach is perhaps the most controversial form of naturalistic inquiry (from the viewpoint of the non-qualitative researcher) because of its heavy reliance on interpretative techniques and postmodern perspectives. "Phenomenologists reject scientific *realism* [emphasis in original] and the accompanying view that the empirical sciences have a privileged position in identifying and explaining features of a mind independent world" (Schwandt, 2001, p. 191). The specific meaning of a "mind independent world" is not exactly clear, but a distinguishing characteristic of phenomenology is the researcher's attempt to describe the subjective impressions of research participants, and to structure and derive meaning from such statements. Unlike the positivistic experimenter describing data, facts, and findings in an objective manner, the phenomenological researcher describes subjective feelings and reactions of research participants to some phenomenon all have experienced. The participants' individual emotional reactions to a phenomenon are the data source, and the researcher attempts to find some underlying structure to all of the participants' feelings toward and interactions with the phenomenon.

A phenomenological study begins with the researcher and his or her philosophical ideas concerning the phenomenon (e.g., a very positive, helping, and conscientious teacher; see following example) under study. This leads to the researcher attempting to see the phenomenon through the eyes of the participants, relating to the phenomenon as they do, and attempting to derive meaning from contact with the phenomenon primarily from the view of the research participant. The researcher "lives" how all the participants live when the phenomenon is present. Throughout the researcher's experience with the phenomenon he or she also conducts extensive interviews (usually audiotaped or preserved digitally as a permanent product) with participants. Next, the researcher annotates important participant statements and feelings when describing the phenomenon; these verbalizations are then categorized into themes to derive some uniform meaning. Last, the phenomenologist describes the themes in a narrative to give structure to the way participants' form opinions about the phenomenon under examination. The underlying notion of phenomenological inquiry is that there is a specific configuration to participants' subjective impressions of the phenomenon of interest.

Phenomenological Research Example

A phenomenological investigator wants to determine why all students with EBD at Anywhere Middle School consider Ms. Jones such a positive, reinforcing, and inspiring teacher, and the best instructor they ever had. In other words, the "phenomenon" under study is Ms. Jones's affirmative, respectful, highly acclaimed teaching style.

The researcher first begins to think philosophically, and speculates why all sixth-grade students with EBD love Ms. Jones so much. Such beliefs would be presented in the introduction of a manuscript of the study. The researcher then spends every day for 1 month observing the teaching style of Ms. Jones in an attempt to understand exactly what takes place in the classroom, how the instruction is provided, how she interacts with the students, and so on. The researcher is present in the classroom just as any student would be, engages in the same activities, and enjoys all the privileges of any of

Ms. Jones's pupils. While observing for the 1-month period, the investigator also selects and interviews (several times) five different students with EBD who have Ms. Jones for English at least one period per day. The researcher asks the students various prepared questions about Ms. Jones and her teaching style, allows students to describe her teaching extemporaneously, and transcribes and audiotapes the students' responses. Next, the phenomenologist reads and listens to all the responses of the students, and reduces the verbal responses to important statements concerning the teaching style of Ms. Jones. These statements are next searched for meanings and then divided into themes (e.g., level of respect for students, patience with all responses, wanting to make students feel successful, etc.). For comparison purposes, the same five students with EBD are asked identical questions about the teaching style of Mr. Greene, who is not the most respected or well-liked teacher and presents the phenomenon of "ineffective teaching." The pupils' statements about Mr. Greene are then treated in the same way as those for Ms. Jones, and the researcher compares and contrasts the two very different teaching styles from the students' impressions. The researcher then interprets the narrative findings, clusters the data pointing to what is effective or ineffective teaching from the subjective statements of the participants, and derives meaning for teaching students with EBD at the middle school level. In essence, the phenomenologist simply categorizes and organizes the subjective expressions and searches for order in the participants' responses.

Grounded Theory Research

Perhaps one of the more difficult and certainly less interpretative types of qualitative research is the production of grounded theory. A theory is a relationship among concepts and sets of concepts (Strauss & Corbin, 1994). In this style of naturalistic inquiry the researcher has some questions about a topic or item of interest (i.e., the phenomenon), spends some time in the field collecting data related to the phenomenon, then spends a moment analyzing and reconstructing the data, and then back to data collection—ad nauseam—until he or she is satisfied that it is time to end the research activity with a tentative theory. The intent of the back-and-forth iterative process of data collection and analysis is to formulate, verify, redesign, and ascertain a theory that is closely related and accurate of a phenomenon. Grounded theory qualitative research was originally developed in the 1960s by sociologists Glaser and Strauss (1967).

To begin this type of inquiry, the experimenter travels to a research site to conduct numerous interviews with research participants who are involved with a phenomenon. The interview data are used to uncover information about the phenomenon from participants' perspectives and to construct *categories*, which are units filled with descriptions of the phenomenon. The researcher may also observe the participants engaged in interactions with the phenomenon, but this step in data collection is rare in grounded theory investigations. At the same time that interview data are being collected and recorded the researcher is beginning preliminary analyses to form theoretical constructs. The researcher continues the interview data gathering and analysis back and forth until the categories are *saturated* and the phenomenon is exposed in its entirety. Creswell (1998) refers to the data collection and formation of the changing categories as "constant comparative" data analysis.

Grounded theory data analysis follows a standard format. The researcher begins with *open coding*, which is the formation of initial categories. Subcategories are also created with associated dimensions to describe the phenomenon. Subsequent to open coding is *axial coding,* where new categories are formed and a central category of the phenomenon established. The context of the phenomenon and specific consequences of its presence and actions are also noted in axial coding. Axial coding is followed by *selective coding*, in which the researcher creates a narrative where the categories and subcategories are merged and tentative hypotheses are created. At the end of all the rounds of data collection and analysis the researcher finally presents the theory in a narrative (research article) explaining the phenomenon under examination. Unlike other types of qualitative investigation, grounded theory requires the researcher to suppress his or her preconceived notions so that a pure view of the phenomenon and a theory concerning it emerges from a systematic process.

Grounded Theory Research Example

A researcher is interested in the use of time out (the phenomenon) in a self-contained classroom serving nine elementary-level students with EBD. The teacher in the classroom, Mr. Greene, admits to being a devotee of the treatment for inappropriate student behavior and uses it often with all of his students. Problem behaviors of varying frequency and intensity are followed with periods spent in a small room in the corner of Mr. Greene's classroom that is meant for time out and nothing else.

The researcher first begins by spending a great deal of time collecting impressions of time out via lengthy interviews with each of the nine students, the paraprofessional in the classroom, and Mr. Greene. After this period of data collection the grounded theorist engages in open coding, where categories are formed with related descriptions of time out from all the available student and teacher perspectives. One category, for example, is called "fright" (filled with students' reactions), another is called "threat" (the teacher's viewpoint), and another is "time management" (filled with the paraprofessional's perspective). The researcher travels back to the classroom for additional interviews with the students to determine how they feel while in the time-out room for punishment. The experimenter learns that a subcategory of student fright is shame and worry while the pupil is confined during the time-out period. While students are placed in the time-out area the researcher learns that Mr. Greene feels a sense of power and confusion regarding whether he is using the right intervention. Mr. Greene also feels a sense of relief that the misbehaving student is no longer bothering him or the class. Through axial coding the researcher learns that a feeling of trepidation pervades the feelings of all (i.e., students, teacher, and paraprofessional) toward the concept and physical presence of the time-out room and treatment.

Data collection continues in an effort to determine the consequences of the use of time out from the perspective of all in the classroom. The researcher merges this information with what has already been gathered to form a tentative proposition: time out appears to be an ineffective treatment as used in a manner similar to Mr. Greene's. The researcher then creates the narrative with hard examples of why it appears ineffective from interviews of all the participants in the classroom. The researcher provides the grounded theory that Mr. Greene's use of time out is improper because he (1) rarely, if ever, uses positive reinforcement when his students are behaving appropriately in the classroom, (2) uses it capriciously with no regard to fairness for offense and time spent in the room, and (3) fails to see that the use of time out has no relationship with decreased levels of student misconduct.

Ethnographic Research

The ethnographic approach to qualitative inquiry is probably the best known of all methods because of its use in anthropology. Margaret Mead (1963) was one of a few 20th-century anthropologists who popularized the techniques found in ethnography when she lived with and comprehensively studied primitive societies, among other groups. Ethnographic research is the origin of the participant observer found in other types of naturalistic inquiry. Recently, however, there has been no strict format of ethnography, for it has morphed into different shapes and has been embraced by the scholarship and philosophies of Marxism, feminism, women's studies, and postmodernism, among other epistemologies (Creswell, 1998; Tedlock, 2003).

To conduct a traditional ethnographic study the researcher must be immersed in a particular coterie. This type of inquiry is a description and interpretation of a system within a group, or *culture*. The investigator observes people doing ordinary things in typical environments and examines the data in such a way as to expose the culture and life cycles of the group. The researcher records what people do and say as well as the products they create and stories they tell. Any artifacts, myths, and patterns to daily life can be deconstructed to give additional meaning to the peculiarities and functions of the culture.

In order to obtain a comprehensive picture of a culture the ethnographer must stay in the field for extensive periods of time and collect data through any means possible—typically interviews and observations, using field notes. The researcher interviews and observes influential members of the group or culture so that the perspectives of the leaders can be captured and compared to ordinary members of the "culture-sharing group." In an ethnography the culture and its members are described in great detail, their actions and contributions to the greater good of the culture are scrutinized, and the researcher interprets meaning from the culture. What emerges in the final ethnographic report is a literary, holistic portrait of the culture and group under examination—with all the warts and complexities.

Ethnographic Research Example

Ms. Jones is a special education teacher of students with EBD in a high school. To add spice to her teaching experience she wants to examine what the school-related "culture" of students with EBD is all about, so she conducts an ethnographic investigation. She takes time every day to interview her students concerning their perspective on receiving special education for students with EBD, observes what they do and say in all special and general education classrooms, and follows them around the high school campus to observe them outside of class. Ethnographer Jones examines the students' cumulative and special education confidential folders looking for artifacts that the students may have contributed over the course of their school careers. Ms. Jones compiles extensive field notes and interview data on all her high school students, and does the same with other groups identified as having EBD at the middle school and elementary school levels. She interviews and observes a total of 150 students with EBD across all school levels in the district. For every minute Ms. Jones spends interviewing students with EBD she also spends an equal amount of time observing their actions in various environments. She begins the difficult task of interpretation of her field notes and observations after one very long year of immersing herself into the school lives of pupils identified with EBD. What emerges from Ms. Jones's 1-year project, spiced with numerous direct quotes from the interviews with the students, is a story providing holistic meaning to the local school-related lives of pupils with EBD.

Case Study Research

The last type of commonly used qualitative research considered here is the case study. A "case" need not pertain solely to individuals; it can include an event, activity, or program as long as it is bordered by time and place (Creswell, 1998; Stake, 1994, 1995). A case study can examine (1) multiple examples of the same phenomenon (e.g., self-contained special education classes serving students with EBD—a multisite or collective case investigation including cross-case analysis), (2) one program or type of treatment (e.g., a special school serving only students with EBD—a within-site study), or (3) one bounded system to illustrate the entire population of similar cases (e.g., an itinerant teacher of students with EBD—an instrumental case study).

The data collection in case studies can be burdensome, for it includes traditional and participant observations, in-depth interviews of the players involved in the case, and artifact, document, and archival record perusal. The data collection time frame is open ended, and the researcher may choose to engage in *purposeful sampling*, or selecting a variety of cases that show different perspectives on the same phenomenon. The investigator may choose to analyze the case(s) in holistic fashion, where the entire phenomenon is exposed (e.g., the trials and tribulations of general educators), or through *embedded analysis*, where a specific quality of the case is examined (e.g., general educators serving only students with EBD in regular classrooms). Case study implementation requires the researcher to create extensive field notes, or anecdotal written records, that describe the case in totality, document the researcher's relationship to the phenomenon, and paint a picture of the context in which the case exists. Chronologies of events that interact with the case are part of the typical modus operandi and are noted by the case study investigator. Subsequent to data collection, the investigator is busy interpreting his or her findings while attempting to find meaning and lessons learned from the case.

Data analysis involves a search for themes in the field notes and observations while keeping in mind the social context in which the case exists.

Case Study Research Example

A researcher wants to conduct a multisite examination of special education in a cross-categorical resource room (CCRR) placement serving students with EBD. The "case" in this scenario is the public school CCRR option in which students identified with EBD, learning disabilities, mild intellectual disabilities, and attention-deficit/hyperactivity disorders (ADHD) are educated. The researcher engages in purposeful sampling in that three different CCRRs are selected for examination and data collection: one at the elementary level, one at the middle school level, and one at the high school level in three different school districts. By selecting three different CCRRs at three different levels across different districts the experimenter is attempting to depict the case in an array of contexts with a variety of missions.

The researcher first visits the historical records of each school district to determine the sequence of events that led to the creation of CCRRs. In this data search, the investigator finds school histories, district-level memoranda, minutes from meetings involving special educators, administrators, and parents, regulations concerning class size, and even state-level documents with procedures for implementation of CCRRs. These documents describe the nascence and nuances of the CCRR program for students with EBD in each district. Later, the historical artifacts will also be used to describe part of the social context in a manuscript about the study.

Next, the case study researcher immerses him- or herself into the daily workings of each of the three CCRRs by playing the part of participant observer, or paraprofessional, in each classroom for 2 months. At the direction of the teachers, the researcher engages in individual and small-group instruction, classroom management, disciplinary techniques, scheduling, and collaboration with general educators, among other tasks. While a participant observer, the researcher keeps a daily journal of important events that occur in the classroom. After this experience the investigator begins traditional observation for 2 months in each CCRR while compiling copious field notes and anecdotal recordings of the day-to-day rhythm found in each setting. During the traditional observation period, the researcher also audiotapes interviews with all the players (i.e., students, teachers, paraprofessionals, regular educators collaborating with the CCRR teachers, school principals, parents, etc.) found in contact with the CCRRs. Permanent products of the behavior demonstrated at the research sites are also collected and used later for analyzing and understanding social context.

After the researcher is satisfied with the amount and quality of the data collected, he or she begins the task of analyzing the data for themes and meaning, and thoroughly describing the CCRRs in a research narrative. Similarities and differences across the CCRRs, teachers, students, and specific traits of each program are illustrated in the research report. The case is described in a chronology from its beginnings in theory to its present-day position and health. The research manuscript ends with a discussion of the social context and meaning of CCRRs for students with EBD, and any lessons learned by the researcher in the quest for knowledge about cross-categorical resource rooms.

QUALITATIVE RESEARCH STUDIES IN EBD

As stated above, the quantity of *published* qualitative research studies with persons having EBD is not voluminous. The few studies that do exist originated in the 1990s and early 2000s, and the scope of these experiments is broad. What follows in the next section is a review of the published studies dealing with many different issues in EBD. There is no pattern to these studies, and with some investigations specific findings or implications related solely to persons or students with EBD are not available. Some studies are on the periphery of important issues related to EBD (e.g., Adams, Bosley, & Cooper, 1995), but collectively they show the type of knowledge naturalistic inquiry can add to the field of EBD. In keeping with the tradition of naturalistic inquiry, the research below is explained by using authentic narrative from the participants found in the reports. Studies are reviewed without judging quality or magnitude of contribution; it is left to the reader to decide these important parameters concerning this corpus of research.

A Phenomenological Study of Aggression

In a very informal phenomenological study concerning the effects on the family of a child who is aggressive and violent, Adams et al. (1995) interviewed family members and other caregivers regarding how they manage day to day with an aggressive child. Twenty-three different family members of an aggressive child (age unspecified) were polled using prepared open-ended questions concerning (1) defining aggression, (2) planning for violent episodes, (3) the aftermath of a violent exchange, (4) managing during a violent outburst, (5) supports that have helped the family cope with the aggressive child, and (6) advice family members would give others concerning management of childhood aggression. The exact number of interviews conducted by the researchers was not specified, nor was the place or total time length of the interview data collection. There was no mention of the researchers living with the interview participants to obtain a participant observer view of the aggressive child, nor was triangulation of data interpretation mentioned in the article. Many important statements provided by the participants concerning the violent child were noted and included in the narrative, including:

> You can't be a normal family when you are waiting for a bomb to explode. (p. 10)
>
> My brother lies about our parents. He says they are evil. He is mean. He was never sorry. (p. 10)
>
> My husband doesn't care, so I just tried to love her double. (p. 10)
>
> Nobody knows how to help us. (p. 9)
>
> It is a war to have a child like this; you walk on eggs. (p. 8)

The report is full of direct quotes of important interview statements and feelings, and ends with participant comments concerning advice to other families with a child who is violent. Unlike other phenomenological inquiry, however, the researchers did not attempt to form structure with the interview responses other than organizing the narrative into answers to the open-ended questions. Based on the data presented from the interviews, it is safe to say that the family participants struggle to deal any way they can—mostly unsuccessfully—with violence in the family.

Grounded Theory of Parental Perspectives

Kolb and Hanley-Maxwell (2003), using grounded theory research, explored the critical social skills perspectives of 11 parents of adolescents with high-incidence disabilities. Two of the 11 parents had offspring with EBD, and the others were parents of children with high-incidence disability (i.e., learning disabilities, mild intellectual disability). Responses were not separated by category of disability of the respondent but were grouped simply into those of parents of early adolescents with high incidence disability. The 11 children of the parent respondents ranged in age from 12 to 15, and all originated from the same middle school in a small midwestern town. The phenomenon for grounded theory creation in this study was social skills: what parents think about the meaning of social skills and what parents think their offspring should learn about them in school.

Data from in-depth semistructured interviews of parents, phone conversations, informal talks, and field notes were collected and used in the analysis. Connie, a parent of an adolescent girl with EBD, had this to say about her daughter in an interview: "I think she's been rejected and not part of [peer social activities], and it hasn't been until this school year that anyone has ever called her on the phone or that she has been invited over to a friend's house" (Kolb & Hanley-Maxwell, 2003, p. 169).

Total contact with each parent participant lasted between 3 and 4 hours, and the researchers collected study-related data for over 1 year. All interview comments by each parent respondent were audiotaped and transcribed verbatim. After each parent interview the primary investigator wrote field notes to summarize the interview and its noteworthy exchanges.

The researchers were comprehensive in their data coding in that they used open, axial, and selective coding until saturation of categories, and also asked participants to review the final version of coding findings (i.e., "member checks"). Triangulation was performed by using "multiple sources of data" (Whitt & Kuh, 1993, p. 261) in examining the parents' perspectives on social skills. The grounded theory that emerged from the data analysis indicated that parents want their adolescent offspring with high-incidence disabilities to be successful in the social domain by acquiring intuition, empathy, and discernment. Parents also want teaching of social skills to be woven into academic instruction and "teachable moments." The authors closed by discussing the age-old problem surrounding the instructional time spent teaching social skills and the time spent emphasizing academic skills. The Kolb and Hanley-Maxwell study is perhaps one of the better designed special education grounded theory investigations, but foci endemic only to persons with EBD were not included.

Behavior Disorders in Ethnographic Studies

Crowley (1993) used ethnographic research procedures to examine the perceptions of six adolescents with EBD about helpful general education teacher behaviors. The 2 female and 4 male participants (1 African American, 5 whites) were between the ages of 13 to 18. The adolescents were selected because they had a history of aggression in school, which led to their identification as having EBD, and they spent at least one school period a day in general education classes. The participants attended a suburban high school that enrolled between 1,600 and 1,800 students.

The ethnographic research procedures consisted of between four and eight 50-minute structured interviews with each participant over 6 months. The interview questions were selected a priori and consisted of such questions as "What kinds of things do teachers do that you find helpful in your general education classes?" The interviews were audiotaped and later transcribed using computer software. Following the suggestions of Patton (1980), Crowley also used direct observations of the six participants in their general education placements. Using a prepared observation guide, she observed a total of thirty-six, 50-minute content area class periods involving the participants. Through an iterative process at the conclusion of data analysis Crowley constructed themes and subthemes to give meaning to the interviews and field observations. In an unusual break from methods typically found in qualitative research, Crowley also performed an interrater reliability check (see Alberto & Troutman, 2003) and an internal validity check on the assignment of data to themes and subthemes.

The results of Crowley's extensive treatment of the data allowed for six themes to emerge; three themes were related to helpful teacher behavior, two themes were found to be associated with unhelpful teacher interactions with students, and one overarching theme was linked with student anger. Teacher–student communication, flexible academic programming, and flexible behavioral programming were associated with helpful teacher behavior. Teacher rigidity and teachers' use of punitive discipline were joined with unhelpful instructor behavior. The general student anger theme had four subthemes: (1) general pervasive anger (e.g., "It [school] sucks. The administration sucks, some of the teachers suck, the rules suck, curriculum sucks, the way they have it set up sucks" [p. 142]); (2) anger toward peers; (3) anger toward teachers (e.g., "They're [the teachers] just goofballs in the travesty of the game called school, and it's all ridiculous. And they're all stupid and they're all very easy to manipulate. It's stupid and it's so dumb" [p. 143]); and (4) anger toward the administration. Crowley concluded that students with EBD can be a valuable source for important opinions about treatments meant to assist them. This study also shows, surprisingly, that a combination of quantitative and qualitative research methods can be used effectively to increase knowledge of students with EBD.

Todis, Bullis, Waintrup, Schultz, and D'Ambrosio (2001) used ethnographic life histories to examine resilience among 15 formerly incarcerated adolescents (8 males and 7 females). One truly remarkable feature of this study is that it examined participants' lives and resilience over a period of 5 years. Initially, the researchers used 1- to 1½-hour audiotaped interviews of the par-

ticipants and 44 "knowledgeable others" (e.g., family members, teachers, friends) to gain insight into the lives of the formerly incarcerated youth. During year 1, every other week the researchers used participant observation in homes, places of work, and other environments that were frequented by the youths. These observations lasted about 3 hours during the first year of the study, and field notes were also taken related to the observations. After the first year of the investigation the observations and interviews were reduced to one per month. Data analysis coincided with data collection, and computer software was used to manage the interview and observation field notes. The data analysis involved the formation of categories and subcategories as the data were reduced, and diagrams and matrices were also used to depict respondent relationships and represent tentative theories.

Results were framed with extensive descriptions of the participants' life histories beginning with the predelinquent years, involvement with the legal and corrections system, and up to current life status. The researchers categorized the life histories of the 15 youths into three categories: succeeders ($n = 6$), drifters ($n = 7$), and strugglers ($n = 2$). Interview comments from Gary, a succeeder, included: "I'm always looking for the next thing, the next step I can take forward. I just want to see how far I can get in the world" (p. 135). Sally, a drifter, stated: "I have to change a whole lot of things before [the baby is born in] December, you know? Sometimes it makes me really sad how I'm gonna have to be grown-up, but man, I haven't been doing good as a teenager anyway. It's not like I've been making real good choices anyway" (p. 136). In order for formerly incarcerated youth to become "succeeders," Todis et al. concluded that transition supports need to be improved, parent and adult support needs to increase, and schools need to take more of a positive and active role in participants' lives. That Todis et al. spent 5 years involved in this one study is remarkable and shows that some qualitative research is far from ephemeral.

Case Study Research in EBD

Epstein and Quinn (1996) provided a case study of a 15-year-old with EBD, Fred, and his experiences with a system of care. The participant had a history of attention deficit disorder, trouble completing assignments at school, aggressive behavior, theft, and arson. He was identified as having EBD when he was in elementary school. The case study narrative included data from archival records, and parent and participant interviews. Total number and length of the interviews were not provided. Two different data collectors checked the interview summaries to ensure that accuracy and important information from each interview were highlighted and preserved. Member checks were also performed on the data in that interviewees were given a written summary of their interview and asked to check it for accuracy. Multiaxial timelines were constructed that depicted a chronology of the participant's problems, life events, and involvement with local or state care agencies, as well as the cost of services. The timelines provided a multidimensional portrait of Fred's history through various systems of care. From the age of 9 the participant's care consisted of a full year at a state mental hospital, 2 years at an out-of-state residential facility, weekly counseling, placement in a special education alternative school while returning to live at home, and back to a local residential care facility.

The intent of the Epstein and Quinn study was to document the relationship between a family, a child in need of robust behavioral and emotional assistance, and the services provided by a system of care. Results showed that the system of care provided to Fred, in its entirety, was not very successful in improving his externalizing behaviors. The participant did not regularly participate in planning meetings meant to coordinate care for him. The cost of Fred's out-of-community care was over $290,000, with little if any improvement in his externalizing EBD. This qualitative case study depicted a continuum of available treatment options and how a system of care responds to an individual and family in crisis. Though the system was not successful, the study shed light on a situation that would not have had a chance to be exposed in such detail in a quantitative investigation.

Focus Group Research in EBD

Another qualitative research methodology not discussed above is use of *focus groups*. This type of research is a tool for group interviewing a select number of well-informed persons who have expert information or experience on a topic or phenomenon. Blumer (1969) stated that a small group of experts gathered for discussion on a topic within their expertise is often more informative than a randomly selected or representative sample. The group interviewer interacts with the focus group interviewees in a structured or unstructured manner, depending on the purpose of the research, and responses are coded similarly to other naturalistic inquiry while searching for themes, structure, meaning, and context.

Morningstar, Turnbull, and Turnbull (1995) used focus groups, or purposive sampling, to examine student perspectives on the importance of family involvement in the transition process from school to adult life. Thirteen adolescents with EBD, ages 13–19, were selected as members of three out of four focus groups; youths with learning disabilities ($n = 18$) and mild intellectual disabilities ($n = 9$) also made up the membership in the four focus groups. The responses specific to students with EBD were not partialed out of the total data set of focus group responses.

Each focus group was interviewed for approximately 2 hours, and participants were reinforced with edibles prior to or immediately following the focus group session. A moderator guided students' discussion and answers to open-ended queries, and all focus group responses were audiotaped. An observer operated the audiotaping system and wrote field notes during the focus group sessions. Data were analyzed by summarizing participants' responses and checking field notes, and by sorting responses into categories. Raw data and categories were analyzed from a within and across the four focus groups perspective, and final conclusions from respondent comments and categories were checked for verifiability by two different researchers.

Results allowed for collapsing the responses across all the focus groups into the categories of (1) creation of a vision for the future, (2) family and student involvement in the transition process, and (3) family involvement in facilitating self-determination. It was apparent that the family had a strong guiding effect on the youths in the transition process, and many students were considering careers related to what a family member had chosen (e.g., nurse, diesel mechanic, cosmetologist). Following is an example of this rhetoric.

> Student: "I plan to move to Nevada and become a cosmetologist."
>
> Moderator: "Why do you want to move to Nevada?"
>
> Student: "Because my aunt lives there and she's a cosmetologist." (Morningstar et al., 1995, p. 252)

Unfortunately, the focus group participants were not actively involved in any systematic transition planning, and many had not begun planning for their future. Many students were invited to their transition-oriented individualized education program (IEP) meetings but decided not to attend. Participants found the IEP meetings meaningless. The focus group responses were mixed concerning self-determination. Some students were allowed some autonomy in making personal decisions, while decisions for others were mostly controlled by family members. The most important methodological contribution of the Morningstar et al. study is that focus groups can be used as another vehicle to give voice to important student perspectives.

Lehman and Fredericks (1997), in a 1-year study, used focus group and interview methods to produce grounded theory and determine the characteristics of effective service coordination for families of children with EBD. Purposive sampling methods were used to ensure that respondents were experienced in issues concerning service coordination. Respondent selection led to eight parents who agreed to participate in the study and six professionals thought to be helpful in the process of service coordination. Data collection consisted of a 1½- to 2-hour focus group meeting with the 14 participants and in-depth interviews of the same length of time. Both types of interactions with the participants were audiotaped and transcribed verbatim. The focus group data were analyzed prior to the interviews to ensure that all the important aspects of service coordination would be covered in at least one type of data collection. Member checks were performed by sending all participants

transcripts of interviews to be checked for authenticity. Triangulation of data occurred in that two different sources of respondents were providing perspectives on the same phenomenon (i.e., service coordination for students with EBD).

Initial coding of the focus group and in-depth interviews led to clustering of text phrases and subsequent creation of categories and themes. Results indicated that three primary themes emerged when experts provided their perspective on effective service coordination for students with EBD: (1) personal characteristics of the professionals working with the family, (2) characteristics of the organization in which the professional is employed, and (3) characteristics of the larger community system. Personal characteristics of professionals that were deemed helpful in service coordination included genuine care for the child and family, and availability when needed, among other traits. One parent described a particularly helpful professional:

> She understood the problem and she worked with it. She knew and was real clear what all the troubled pieces were and she was very caring. And also, she was very good at being where the buck stops. . . . She was available 24 hours a day. If I needed her I could call her. (Lehman & Fredericks, 1997, p. 14)

Barriers that inhibited effective service provision included blaming and judging the parent(s) of the child with EBD and not being familiar with current best practices. The grounded theories that surfaced in the study included the characteristics of professionals that identify them as effective service coordinators and the perceived system limitations that militate against child-centered and family-focused coordinated support.

The qualitative research findings of Lehman and Fredericks are slightly related to those of Epstein and Quinn (1996), at least at the local level, where both studies were conducted. Epstein and Quinn found that one youth with EBD required quite an extensive system of support and that an expensive system did not necessarily guarantee success. Lehman and Fredericks showed that individuals providing the support and coordination of services in the system can make a difference in the eyes of the recipients of assistance.

CONCLUSIONS

The contributions of qualitative research to the development of knowledge in special education have been defended previously (e.g., Crowley, 1994–1995; MacArthur, 2003; Peck & Furman, 1992; Scruggs & Mastropieri, 1995). There appears to be a place for qualitative research in the field, but it is clear that interpretative inquiry in EBD has much more to accomplish before its true value is appreciated. The naturalistic studies that have been published up to this point in time, collectively, are scattered in foci and may not be universally viewed as important to the field. Qualitative research exists to add subjective understanding to the social context and nuances of EBD and related phenomena; perhaps over time such contributions will be better appreciated. Of particular need and interest to the field would be biographies and case studies dealing with what it is like to be identified as having EBD and what it is like to teach such students, from a phenomenological or ethnographic perspective. Such studies cannot lead to conclusions about how to prevent EBD, or the causes of EBD, or even whether certain interventions are effective in improving behavior and emotions. Green and Shane (1994) warned earlier of the folly in depending on qualitative research for answers to etiology and treatment. The types of qualitative studies suggested above, however, could assist others in knowing what it is like to have the condition and what to expect when trying to help such youths in school. Preservice teachers would be particularly interested in the latter because of their curiosity about what it takes to be effective in the classroom.

A limitation of qualitative research that cannot be ignored is the trade-off between having local knowledge of a phenomenon in naturalistic inquiry and the generalizability of findings that are offered in quantitative research. The term "generalizability" holds no meaning to most qualitative researchers (Glesne & Peshkin, 1992). Local knowledge is indeed vital for individuals interacting directly with a phenomenon but insufficient to a larger population who are facing the same experience. One wonders how many objective scientists reject interpretive research for this reason alone.

Another limitation of naturalistic inquiry concerns the notion of the researcher as the "instrument" (Lincoln & Guba, 1985). Humans can make mistakes and, just like any other instrument such as a scale, pitch pipe, or stopwatch, their subjective viewpoints need to be frequently "calibrated" in order to present a clear picture of any context—for safety reasons if for no other. While a qualitative researcher is attempting to extract meaning from observations, field notes, and interviews, ultimately he or she could be wrong. Granted, from the postmodern perspective that is closely associated with naturalistic inquiry, no personal impressions are believed to be totally erroneous. But what if the violent behavior of a person with EBD were present in an environment and the local threat were misdiagnosed because of inaccurate intuition by the research instrument (data collector)? The resultant danger for all in the setting could be exacerbated, and physical well-being could suffer. In other words, qualitative research, because of its enthusiastic dependence on human judgment, is not immune to making missteps.

Other limitations of qualitative research are related to specific types of interpretive inquiry. What if there is no structure to participants' reaction to some occurrence in phenomenological investigations? Is it proper for the researcher to then force structure because, after all, it is the interpretation of the investigator that forms the structure? In grounded theory research, what if the data categories are not sufficiently saturated, and the researcher decides to end data collection thinking that they are? It could be that continuing data collection may lead to additional categories that lend considerably more, and different, meaning. It helps to keep in mind that there is no such thing as a "perfect study," and qualitative inquiry is just as prone to problems in design, execution, and findings as any other type of research exploration.

The last limitation of qualitative research that is necessary to remember is related to the concept of significance. Quantitative investigations search for statistical significance in comparisons across groups, treatments, and so on. A quantitative study would have difficulty in the peer review process of journal publication if the entire research report included only nonsignificant findings. The next step would be to determine if the nonsignificant findings held any *practical* significance. Some positivistic studies do indeed withstand the rigors of the review process—because of practical significance—even though the major findings of the study showed no difference statistically (e.g., Sabornie & Kauffman, 1986). Not so with qualitative research, unfortunately, for there is no real way to judge the findings in terms of practical significance. Is practical significance related to the number of individuals involved in a focus group? The length of time involved in data collection of a biographical portrait? The number of themes structured in a phenomenological investigation? What about the number of theories that surfaced in a grounded study experiment? Some quantitative researchers continue to reject naturalistic inquiry because it has a history that lacks a strong response to the "So what?" question, and the practical significance of its findings. If qualitative researchers could consistently provide a beefy response to the need for understanding the practical significance of local—and only local—knowledge of a phenomenon, perhaps it would not be considered nonsense by so many positivistic researchers.

It appears that qualitative research has yet to find a sturdy home in the study of EBD. Perhaps critical masses of naturalistic researchers devoted solely to EBD do not yet exist in the field. An interpretative researcher recently said that "Positivism is dead" (actual comment by a colleague of the author), while another highly respected quantitative investigator countered with "Qualitative inquiry may be research, but it sure isn't science" (actual comment by another colleague of the author). Until we understand and accept the premises on both sides of the research aisle, lack of understanding and criticism of both types of inquiry will continue to thrive, and progress in expanding the knowledge base in EBD will be delayed. If the field of EBD is to advance, we must find ways to foster consequential knowledge rather than inhibit it, and qualitative research can broaden local knowledge

so that some fortunate persons with EBD can benefit.

REFERENCES

Adams, J., Bosley, P., & Cooper, R. (1995). Families who love violent children. *Reclaiming Children and Youth*, 4(1), 6–10.

Alberto, P. A., & Troutman, A. C. (2003). *Applied behavior analysis for teachers* (6th ed.). Upper Saddle River, NJ: Prentice Hall.

Blumer, H. (1969). *Symbolic interactionism: Perspective and method*. Englewood Cliffs, NJ: Prentice Hall.

Creswell, J. W. (1998). *Qualitative inquiry and research design: Choosing among five traditions*. Thousand Oaks, CA: Sage.

Crowley, E. P. (1993). A qualitative analysis of mainstreamed behaviorally disordered aggressive adolescents' perceptions of helpful and unhelpful teacher attitudes and behaviors. *Exceptionality*, 4, 131–151.

Crowley, E. P. (1994–1995). Using qualitative methods in special education research. *Exceptionality*, 5, 55–69.

Denzin, N. K., & Lincoln, Y. S. (Eds.). (2003). *Strategies of qualitative inquiry* (2nd ed.). Thousand Oaks, CA: Sage.

Epstein, M. H., & Quinn, K. P. (1996). A case study approach to analyzing the relationship between children and services in a system of care. *Journal of Emotional and Behavioral Disorders*, 4, 21–29.

Freud, S. (1952). *The case of Dora, and other papers: Translations of Joan Riviere and others*. New York: Norton.

Glaser, B., & Strauss, A. (1967). *The discovery of grounded theory*. Chicago: Aldine.

Glesne, C., & Peshkin, A. (1992). *Becoming qualitative researchers: An introduction*. White Plains, NY: Longman.

Green, G., & Shane, H. C. (1994, April 13). Questioning the validity of research on autism. *The Chronicle of Higher Education*, 40(32), B2.

Itard, J. M. G. (1962). *The wild boy of Aveyron* (G. Humphrey & M. Humphrey, Trans.). New York: Prentice Hall.

Kavale, K. A., & Forness, S. R. (1998). The politics of learning disabilities. *Learning Disability Quarterly*, 21, 245–273.

Kazdin, A. E. (1977). Assessing the clinical or applied importance of behavior change through social validation. *Behavior Modification*, 1, 427–449.

Kolb, S. M., & Hanley-Maxwell, C. (2003). Critical social skills for adolescents with high incidence disabilities. *Exceptional Children*, 69, 163–179.

Lehman, C. M., & Fredericks, H. D. (1997). *Qualitative investigation of effective service coordination for children and youth with emotional and behavioral disorders* (Report No. EC 305831, ERIC Document Reproduction Service No. ED411640). Monmouth, OR: Western Oregon State College.

Lincoln, Y., & Guba, E. (1985). *Naturalistic inquiry.* Beverly Hills, CA: Sage.

MacArthur, C. (2003). What have we learned about learning disabilities from qualitative research?: A review of studies. In H. L. Swanson, K. R. Harris, & S. Graham (Eds.), *Handbook of learning disabilities* (pp. 532–549). New York: Guilford Press.

Mead, M. (1963). *Sex and temperament in three primitive societies.* New York: Morrow.

Morningstar, M. E., Turnbull, A. P., & Turnbull, H. R. (1995). What do students with disabilities tell us about the importance of family involvement in the transition from school to adult life? *Exceptional Children, 62,* 249–260.

Patton, M. Q. (1980). *Qualitative evaluation methods.* Beverly Hills, CA: Sage.

Peck, C., & Furman, G. C. (1992). Qualitative research in special education: An evaluative review. In R. Gaylord-Ross (Ed.), *Issues and research in special education* (Vol. 2, pp. 1–42). New York: Teachers College Press.

Sabornie, E. J., & Kauffman, J. M. (1986). Social acceptance of learning disabled adolescents. *Learning Disability Quarterly, 9,* 55–60.

Schwandt, T. A. (2001). *Dictionary of qualitative inquiry* (2nd ed.). Thousand Oaks, CA: Sage.

Scruggs, T. E., & Mastropieri, M. A. (1995). Qualitative research methodology in the study of learning and behavioral disorders: An analysis of recent research. In T. E. Scruggs & M. A. Mastropieri (Eds.), *Advances in learning and behavioral disabilities* (Vol. 9, pp. 249–272). Greenwich, CT: JAI Press.

Simpson, R. G., & Eaves, R. C. (1985). Do we need more qualitative research or more good research? A reaction to Stainback and Stainback. *Exceptional Children, 51,* 325–329.

Stainback, S., & Stainback, W. (1984). Broadening the research perspective in special education. *Exceptional Children, 50,* 400–408.

Stake, R. E. (1994). Case studies. In N. Denzin & Y. Lincoln (Eds.), *Handbook of qualitative research* (pp. 236–247). Thousand Oaks, CA: Sage.

Stake, R. E. (1995). *The art of case study research.* Thousand Oaks, CA: Sage.

Strauss, A., & Corbin, J. (1994). Grounded theory methodology: An overview. In N. Denzin & Y. Lincoln (Eds.), *Handbook of qualitative research* (pp. 273–285). Thousand Oaks, CA: Sage.

Tedlock, B. (2003). Ethnography and ethnographic representation. In N. Denzin & Y. Lincoln (Eds.), *Handbook of qualitative research* (2nd ed., pp. 165–213). Thousand Oaks, CA: Sage.

Todis, B., Bullis, M., Waintrup, M., Schultz, R., & D'Ambrosio, R. (2001). Overcoming the odds: Qualitative examination of resilience among formerly incarcerated adolescents. *Exceptional Children, 68,* 119–139.

Whitt, E. J., & Kuh, G. D. (1993). Qualitative methods in a team approach to multiple-institution studies. In D. G. Smith (Series Ed.) & C. Conrad, A. Neumann, J. G. Haworth, & P. Scott (Vol. Eds.), *Qualitative research in higher education: Experiencing alternative perspectives and approaches* (pp. 253–266). Needham Heights, MA: Ginn Press.

Wolcott, H. F. (1983). Adequate schools and inadequate education: The life history of a sneaky kid. *Anthropology and Education Quarterly, 14*(1), 3–32.

Wolf, M. M. (1978). Social validity: The case for subjective measurement of how applied behavior analysis is finding its heart. *Journal of Applied Behavior Analysis, 11,* 203–214.

30

Data Collection in Research and Applications Involving Students with Emotional and Behavioral Disorders

PHILIP L. GUNTER *and* R. KENTON DENNY

"If you don't know where you are, you're lost, and it doesn't matter that you know where you want to go" (Bushell & Baer, 1994, p. 4). Perhaps these words are representative of the logic of law and policymakers in this country of late regarding the need for public schools to collect and analyze student academic achievement data. We have entered an era in which accountability for positive outcomes for public school students has been highlighted and mandated (Cochran-Smith, 2003). Cochran-Smith (2003) indicates that whether or not teacher trainers are in agreement, such legislative actions as the reauthorization of the Elementary and Secondary Education Act in 2001, better known as No Child Left Behind (NCLB), have moved student performance on standardized academic achievement evaluations to the forefront. Additionally, it appears that professional judgment, or even clinical judgment, as a measure of student outcomes will no longer be sufficient. "Professional judgment is valuable, but it is different from measurement. Professional judgment is often correct, but its reliability at any given moment is unknown" (Bushell & Baer, 1994, pp. 4–5).

The National Association of State Direc-

tors of Special Education (2002) reports that NCLB mandates student improvement to ensure that within 12 years all students will meet or exceed proficiency on each state's standardized academic achievement assessment. Additionally, current proposals for the reauthorization of the Individuals with Disabilities Education Act (IDEA) require the participation of all students with disabilities within each state's accountability system (Council for Exceptional Children, 2003). It is clear that public schools will be held accountable for the adequate yearly progress (AYP) of all students.

This emphasis on measurement also has been recognized via the recently revised standards of the National Council for Accreditation of Teacher Education (NCATE, 2000); all teachers-in-training are expected to exhibit the skills to "accurately assess and analyze student learning, make appropriate adjustments to instruction, monitor student learning, and have a positive effect on learning for all students" (p. 16). School personnel are to "collect and analyze data . . . and use research . . . to support and improve student learning" (p. 16). It appears from reviews and critiques of NCLB that end-of-year assessments will be used to measure

AYP (Cochran-Smith, 2003). Such measures may be aptly described as summative evaluations.

Summative evaluation procedures, especially related to children with disabilities, have been criticized. Summative evaluation is a static evaluation process to monitor "progress by measuring and comparing student performance at two points in time. It evaluates teaching and learning post hoc" (Tawney & Gast, 1984, p. 80). Such measures have been presented as insufficient in relationship to the academic and social needs of students with disabilities (Fuchs & Fuchs, 1986). Shinn and Hubbard (1994) proposed that most summative measurement tools (e.g., published norm-referenced tests) lack sufficient content validity, lack sufficient items to detect patterns of response, and in general serve only to reaffirm the severity of an academic problem in relation to a normed sample.

Tawney and Gast (1984) indicate that formative evaluation measures are needed to guide instruction of students with disabilities, defining formative evaluation as a dynamic process that "emphasizes the frequent and repeated measurement of student performance . . . over time" (p. 81). Data support not only the evaluative function of such measures but indicate the educative relationship between formative assessment measures and improved academic achievement (Fuchs & Fuchs, 1986).

Alberto and Troutman (2003) suggest three reasons to collect classroom data in the formative evaluation fashion prescribed by applied behavior analysts. First, they suggest that formative evaluation data collection allows teachers to assess the effectiveness of their instruction. Second, formative data collection procedures allow modifications in instructional programming while the instruction is in progress rather than waiting until instruction is completed. Finally, they suggest that "collecting and reporting effect-based data is the ultimate tool of accountability" (p. 90).

In this chapter, literature will be reviewed regarding data collection procedures used in empirical investigations and classroom applications involving children and youth with emotional and behavioral disorders (EBD). The historical development and adoption of applied behavior analysis procedures for evaluation of intervention effectiveness will form the foundation for the content. Applications of a variety of simple and exhaustive data collection systems for research will be reviewed. The pragmatics of the utilization of data collection procedures in daily therapeutic and naturalistic settings will be reviewed with a focus on how to potentially impact more widespread application of the tools. The need to evaluate the efficacy and efficiency of data collection procedures for generalized applications will be discussed. Links relating research and application of procedures of data collection will be explored. Finally, recommendations will be presented for future research needs regarding development and implementation of formative evaluation data collection procedures.

DEVELOPMENT OF SYSTEMATIC FORMATIVE MEASUREMENT SYSTEMS

Data collection procedures used in research and instruction involving students with EBD have been strongly influenced in the past through the ongoing application of techniques developed by applied behavior analysts. For over 30 years, the principles and procedures used by applied behavior analysts, including measurement procedures, have been applied to successfully address social and academic needs of a wide range of students with disabilities. The basic principles of measurement associated with this approach are simply to measure behavior and to measure it directly and frequently.

One of the most recognized contributors to measurement systems in school settings is Ogden Lindsley. Lindsley (1971a) developed the system of measurement and interpretation widely known as "precision teaching." Lindsley (1971b) indicated that precision teaching is an instructional approach based on seven principles:

1. Teachers learn best by studying the behavior of their students.
2. Rate of response is the universal measure of behavior.
3. Student performances are measured on a standard "celeration" chart.
4. Direct and continuous monitoring is emphasized.

5. Behaviors and processes are described and functionally defined.
6. Building behavior is emphasized.
7. Impact of environmental influences on behavior is analyzed.

Research regarding the implementation of the principles of precision teaching in classroom settings indicates that teachers and students collect academic performance data, they graph their performances, and teachers use the data to support more appropriate decision making (Haring, Liberty, & White, 1980; Howell & Lorson-Howell, 1990; West, Young, & Spooner, 1990).

Deno and his colleagues extended the basic procedures of precision teaching by linking the instructional and data collection/analysis procedures with school curriculum (Deno, 1985; Deno, 1986; Deno & Mirkin, 1977). In their early work, they implemented data collection and analysis by specially trained special education resource teachers (SERTs). These individuals were taught to identify skills, collect rate data on student performance, index these performances to classmate performances, and systematically intervene based on analysis of the data (Deno & Mirkin, 1977). The emphasis on formative assessment evolved into a model known as curriculum-based measurement (Deno, 1985). In this model, teachers administer "academic probes" to collect performance data on students' academic skills on a daily or weekly basis. The students' data are graphed and analyzed to provide instructional suggestions for program changes (Fuchs, Fuchs, & Hamlett, 1989).

The educative impact of data collection and analysis procedures such as those described above seems to be beyond question (Gunter, 2001). For example, Fuchs and Fuchs (1986) indicate that "one can expect handicapped students whose individualized educational programs are monitored systematically and developed formatively over time to achieve, on average, .7 standard deviation units higher than students whose programs are not systematically monitored and developed formatively" (p. 205). Data from the Fuchs and Fuchs meta-analysis were reported from studies involving students with disabilities ranging from mild to moderate levels and in grades from preschool through high school. The frequency of measurement (formative evaluation) ranged from twice per week to daily. The impact of formative evaluation procedures was equally effective regardless of disability level, age, or frequency of measurement.

Nelson and Polsgrove (1984) wrote that

> behavioral teachers (those using principles of applied behavior analysis) select and pace instructional procedures according to student progress data rather than according to curriculum guides, teacher's manuals, or programmed instructional sequences. The data, not publisher's manuals, are their authority. (p. 10)

One of the earliest and most comprehensive applications of behavioral principles to the education of students with EBD was Hewett's (1968) "engineered classroom." It was within this clinical setting that many of the then tentative principles of the experimental analysis of behavior, including direct and frequent measurement, were systematically applied in classrooms for students with emotional disturbance. In these early applications of behavior analytic procedures, the foundations for instructional applications of data collection were developed for work with students with EBD. Since that time development of data collection tools and procedures, particularly for research, involving students with EBD has progressed in complexity. One of the main influences in the progression has been the application of computer-assisted technologies.

APPLICATION OF TECHNOLOGY TO DATA COLLECTION PROCEDURES FOR RESEARCH

"It is possible that the greatest potential for the application of technology to education may lie in the area of instructional measurement" (Hawkins, Sharpe, & Ray, 1994, p. 243). Hawkins et al. (1994) indicate that application of computer-driven data collection systems may hold promise for the analysis of the interaction of complex and rapid teacher/student exchanges that occur in classroom settings in which the context, or setting factors, are constantly changing. Certainly, the application of these systems in settings in which students with EBD are taught has begun to support the importance of a better understanding of these complex behavioral exchanges.

Recently, Thompson, Felce, and Symons (2000) collected descriptions of computer-assisted observation devices and programs from researchers engaged in behavioral observation research. The range of devices included laptop computers (Wehby, Symons, & Shores, 1995), palm-held computers (Emerson, Reeves, & Felce, 2000), bar-code readers (Tapp & Wehby, 2000), and units that allow data collection from videotapes utilizing a computer-playback interface (Tapp & Walden, 2000).

Technologies applied to data collection appear to fall into four categories: dedicated data collection devices and software, software systems with open designs, software systems with closed designs, and hybrid systems. *Dedicated data collection devices* have software built in and allow for limited modification of the application. An example of such a system is the Datamyte and its modern-day equivalents. Systems utilizing adapted barcode readers (e.g., Timewand I or Duratrax) would be considered dedicated data collection devices. In such systems coding and entry of data may be represented numerically and can be adapted to a wide range of situations. Data may be collected in real time (i.e., continuous) or using an interval system.

Software systems with open designs driven by laptop or palm-held computers allow specific behaviors, context, or events to be defined by the user. They generally allow data to be recorded as frequency, duration, interval (including time sample), and anecdotal. An example of such a system is the MOOSES (Multiple Option Observation System for Experimental Studies) developed by John Tapp (Tapp & Wehby, 2000), which will be described in detail in a later section regarding its application to research involving students with EBD.

Software systems with closed designs are supported systems that incorporate the "what" as well as the procedure. An example is the EBASS (Ecobehavioral Assessment Systems Software) developed by Greenwood, Carta, Kamps, and Delquadri (1997). In this system, the context, participants, and target behaviors are specified within a standard observation protocol (e.g., interval re-

cording). The EBASS systems have been used most extensively in specifically addressing classroom ecologies. Their interval-driven recording system, in combination with an extensive taxonomy of context, teacher, and student behaviors, has provided much support for understanding the relevant interactions of contextual and teacher variables. The 101-item code system, while somewhat cumbersome for day-to-day use, does provide an excellent menu for selection of potentially relevant instructional variables.

Hybrid systems are generally formative assessment data collection systems or computerized assessment systems (CAS). They integrate the presentation of an instructional stimulus (question, problem, or passage) and allow the response made by the individual to be recorded. The most notable example to date is the Monitoring Basic Skills Progress program (Fuchs, Hamlett, & Fuchs, 1997). This program allows easy collection of rate data and supports graphing and analysis of collected data. It provides perhaps the most useful model for automatic data collection of student academic performance on a routine basis. The student is presented with instructional stimuli in math, reading, or spelling by the computer. The child then responds to a series of instructional prompts/probes and saves his or her completed lesson. The teacher is able to retrieve the raw data as correct and error responses and graph the data. The program provides a rudimentary decision prompt to the teacher when the data indicate a trend based on correct and error rates.

TECHNOLOGY SPECIFICALLY APPLIED TO RESEARCH INVOLVING STUDENTS WITH EBD

The application of computer-assisted and -driven technology has certainly impacted the empirical literature regarding students with EBD. In an early study, Gunter, Fox, Brady, Shores, and Cavanaugh (1988) analyzed the social interaction exchanges of social bids, responses to social bids, and ongoing exchanges between students with autism and chronologically similar-age peers without disabilities. Audiotape recordings of verbal codes for behaviors were made in the research classrooms. These recordings were played back and hand-entered into a TRS-80 Model III desktop computer for analysis using the Computer Assisted Research in Teacher Outcomes, or CARTLO, software for query analysis (Semmel & Frick, 1980). Since that time, a variety of computerized data collection systems have evolved, ranging from the Behavioral Evaluation Strategy and Taxonomy (BEST) system (Hawkins et al., 1994) to the MOOSES system previously mentioned and that has been widely used in classroom research involving students with EBD (e.g., Sutherland & Wehby, 2001; Sutherland, Wehby, & Yoder, 2001; Wehby, Dodge, Valente, & Conduct Problems Research Group, 1993; Wehby & Hollahan, 2000; Wehby, Symons, Canale, & Go, 1998; Wehby et al., 1995).

The systems have provided opportunities to enhance the exhaustive nature of observational codes and analysis of social and educational interactions represented by those codes within predetermined classroom conditions referred to as settings. Shores and his colleagues have used the MOOSES system to analyze the relationship of behaviors in classrooms for students with EBD in terms of proportional relationships using lag-sequential analysis procedures (e.g., Gunter, Jack, Shores, Carrell, & Flowers, 1993; Gunter, Shores, Jack, Denny, & DePaepe, 1994; Jack et al., 1996; Shores et al., 1993). That is, they have described teacher, student, and peer interactions in terms of the likelihood of a specific behavior occurring in response to any other given behavior on which data were gathered.

ISSUES IN TRANSFERRING DATA COLLECTION SYSTEMS FROM RESEARCH APPLICATIONS TO APPLIED APPLICATIONS

One issue that must be addressed is the complexity of the coding systems and analyses involved when implementing computerized data collection systems. While each of these systems may represent marked improvements in some aspects over paper and pencil recording systems of the past, they have not been designed for the practicing teacher or even most instructional support specialists to employ on a regular basis. For example,

Gunter et al. (1993) suggested that the use of computerized data collection systems such as MOOSES, while extremely beneficial for insight into interactive social exchanges from a research perspective, were likely not practical for use in classroom settings for students with EBD due to the complexity involved in data entry and analysis.

It also must be noted that while the use of real-time and simultaneous recording of contextual, event, and behavioral data for multiple individuals opens many doors for better understanding complex classroom interactions, they are obviously not tools for the teacher to use in their current forms to make day-to-day instructional decisions in the classroom. To be fair, most developers of observational and analysis software indicate that the primary purpose of their systems is research as opposed to direct clinical application. However, it is possible that several of the programs could be readily adapted to be more usable by a classroom teacher, given additional work toward those applications.

TEACHERS' USE OF FORMATIVE ASSESSMENT PROCEDURES

Alberto and Troutman (2003) report that teacher reactions to suggestions that they collect data in their classrooms are summarized in such statements as: "I don't have time to write down everything anyone does." "I just don't think I can manage shuffling all those sheets of paper, handling stopwatches, wrist counters, giving proper cues." "When am I supposed to concentrate on teaching?" (p. 89). Alberto and Troutman (2003) suggest that some of the applied behavior analysis data collection systems advocated in teacher training texts are, in fact, not practical for everyday use in classrooms; however, they indicate that understanding the procedures may be necessary for teachers to interpret educational research that could be very applicable to their classrooms. Therefore, it seems professionally appropriate to include in teacher training programs outcomes to enhance teachers' abilities to construct a framework for the pragmatics of data management, including how to collect, organize, analyze, interpret, and disseminate classroom data.

Gunter, Callicott, Denny, and Gerber

(2003) indicated that ease of use, comfort level, and minimal time commitment are critical variables predictive of whether or not teachers will use various treatment and data collection procedures. It appears that the data collection procedures should be concise to allow teachers to use them in a prescribed fashion. For example, Allinder and Oats's (1997) summary of the effectiveness of implementation of curriculum-based measurement procedures indicates that students with disabilities made similar gains in math and reading achievement in classrooms in which the teacher did not employ curriculum-based measurement procedures as in those classes in which the procedures were implemented with less than high levels of fidelity.

McLaughlin (1993) reviewed the types of data collection procedures used by teachers in training to complete field-based projects. He found that a slight majority of the teachers (N = 69) used direct observation procedures. However, 47.2% of the projects used permanent product data collection. The primary and secondary types of observational data collection used were random time sampling and frequency recording, respectively, accounting for 10.1% of the observational procedures used. McLaughlin recommended that the focus on observational data collection in teacher training programs should be on time sampling procedures, with about an equal amount of time spent on permanent product data collection. However, it appears that no direct observation measures of formative evaluation procedures used by teachers in classrooms for students with EBD are readily available.

MAKING DATA COLLECTION FOR INSTRUCTION MANAGEABLE

Even though we appear to lack a clear understanding of the data collection practices of teachers of students with EBD, it appears that teachers' perceptions of the manageability of the data collection process may be accurate. As mentioned previously, teachers often report that data collection procedures advocated in many teacher training programs are overly cumbersome and unrelated to the teaching process (Alberto & Troutman, 2003; Cooper, Heron, & Heward, 1987).

Perhaps one of the most important issues to be addressed regarding data collection procedures has to do with identifying the target behaviors, or perhaps topographies of target behaviors. Gunter and Denny (1996, 1998) have reflected a common realization in observing that problem behavior and instructional behaviors of students with EBD and their teachers are intertwined. In fact, they have suggested that research may support the conclusion that correct student responding may be one of the most pivotal target behaviors to be addressed in classrooms for students with EBD. One of the major contributions of current research to data collection procedures for instruction should be the identification and validation of the most important behaviors (i.e., those that lead to reinforcement and achievement in classrooms) for teachers to measure.

In addition to improving our decisions on what to measure, we should also examine our metric for measuring. Gunter and Denny (1998) indicate that the most appropriate metric to measure academic performance of students with mild disabilities is rate of correct performance, that is, the frequency of accurately performed tasks divided by time. Lindsley (1990) argued that measures of accuracy, in isolation, ignore the measures of speed and fluency, producing students who are painfully slow and fearful of making errors. Gunter and Denny's (1998) recommendation seems to be supported by the work of Binder, Haughton, and Van Eyk (1990). Binder et al. present the importance of building fluency of performance of academic tasks. They suggest that measurement of fluency is important to ensure automaticity in performance of tasks. Further research is needed to extend these findings to students with EBD.

Gunter and Denny's (1998) contention is in contrast to data reported in many research studies with students with EBD where time on task is often the metric used to measure academic performance even though collectively research indicates that time on task is not as good an indicator of academic performance as is rate of correct active responding (Good & Brophy, 2000). One positive aspect of these findings is the relative ease of collecting correct response data as compared to collection of on-task data. Frequency of response data may be gathered by simply scoring independent seatwork and dividing the number of correctly completed problems by the time required to complete the problems. However, to gather time-on-task data, at the least, some type of interval data will be required which will necessitate that the teacher (or other data collector) make rather frequent observations of student behavior.

Certainly, if procedures are in place to simplify data collection and analysis procedures, it is logical that those procedures might be more widely used (Gunter, 2001; Taylor & Romanczyk, 1994). Such efforts have already begun. For example, Deno and Espin (1991) indicate that "in reading, the most common method of data collection is to count the number of words the student reads in 1 minute" (p. 87); this conceptualization of the simplicity and limited time constraints of formative evaluation are highlighted by Witt and Beck (1999) in their text, *One-Minute Academic Functional Assessment and Interventions: "Can't" Do It . . . or "Won't" Do It?*

Recently, several procedures to further enhance the likelihood that formative evaluation measures will be implemented in classrooms for students with EBD have been proposed and evaluated (Gunter, Hummel, & Venn, 1998; Gunter, Miller, Venn, Thomas, & House, 2002; Gunter & King, 2003; Gunter, Venn, Patrick, Miller, & Kelly, 2003; Sugai, Sprague, Horner, & Walker, 2000). Descriptions of four of those efforts: to reduce the number of variables on which to gather data, to reduce the amount of time required for data collection, to involve students in the analysis and graphic display of their formative evaluation data, and to combine data collection activities across larger units (e.g., from individuals to class levels or school levels) follow.

Limiting Targeted Behaviors for Data Collection

Taylor and Romanczyk (1994) wrote that "by increasing the efficiency of direct observation and reducing the labor, resources, and expertise required to use it, we may increase its utility" (p. 252). In their evaluation, to demonstrate the efficacy of reducing the variables for direct observation with which to develop hypotheses for functional

analyses, they simply observed one variable, teacher attention to students. Based on their observations, the hypotheses they developed were supported for 14 of the 15 students involved.

Based on this notion of limiting the number of variables targeted for data collection, Gunter et al. (1998) identified correct student academic responses as a pivotal classroom behavior that would be predictive of effective interactions between teachers and their students with EBD. The protocol they developed and used to provide descriptive analyses of general education classrooms utilized only 5-minute observations of the frequency of correct responses made by students (Gunter, Reffel, Barnett, Lee, & Patrick, in press). In a second study, Gunter, Adams, et al. (2002) found that teachers using the protocol to self-evaluate their own instruction—again based on only 5-minute observations of the frequency of correct responses of student's with disabilities—were able to modify their instruction to increase the rate of students' correct responding. These increases were occasioned by increased rates of teacher praise statements and decreased rates of undesirable student behaviors. Based on the findings, they highlight the importance of this one behavior, the correct academic response, as a critical variable to target for observation and data collection.

Student Self-Evaluation and Analysis of Performance

Gunter, Miller, et al. (2002) presented information regarding procedures to implement data collection for correct academic responding, which allowed students with disabilities to develop graphic representations of their daily data using readily available spreadsheet software. Based on the findings of Fuchs and Fuchs (1986) indicating that "when data were graphed, effect sizes were higher (.8 std dev units over control group) than when data simply were recorded" (p. 205), Gunter, Miller, et al. (2002) provided a case description of teaching a student with EBD to graph her own oral reading data. The student was taught to use Microsoft Excel software to record her rate of words read correctly per minute. This study employed an adaptation of procedures for graphing data presented by Carr and Burkholder (1998). Displays of data collected using such software produces an equal-interval graphic rather than a semilogarithmic graph recommended in precision teaching procedures (cf. Deno & Espin, 1991). Deno and Espin evaluated the research comparing student achievement when the two different graphing systems were used and found little difference; however, they also reviewed research indicating that equal-interval graphic displays may be easier for teachers to use and understand. Based on their findings, they suggested that the logistical considerations regarding teacher preference for the equal-interval system should be weighted heavily, considering the little difference in impact on student achievement between the two.

Moxley (1998) reviewed literature regarding the impact of students' self-recording (graphing) their performance and indicated that "research in a wide variety of areas indicates that self-recording in itself tends to have a favorable effect on improving the performances that are recorded" (p. 44). Moxley (1998) acknowledges that some teachers will express concern that the time necessary to teach students to self-record may take time away from academic instruction; however, he suggests that this is needless worry. "If it takes more time to introduce young children to self-recording, this means those children will learn more academic skills through the very activity of self-recording" (p. 57).

Gunter and King (2003) completed a series of studies to extend the reported finding of Gunter, Miller, et al. (2002) by evaluation of the impact of various aspects of self-graphing and self-evaluation of reading fluency of students with EBD. In all of the studies reported, students recorded their own oral reading using the digital audio recording function of a desktop computer. In one study, students were taught to play back the audio recording and self-evaluate the correctness of the words read. Because the default recording time was 1-minute, the students only had to count the number of words correct on the recording to complete the self-evaluation of words read correctly per minute. This self-evaluation phase was compared to a self-evaluation and self-graphing phase. Unlike the results previously reported by Gunter, Miller, et al.

(2002), the self-graphing alone did not result in sustained, steady improvement of reading fluency. However, when the students read the passage twice and continued self-evaluation and self-graphing, sustained and steady increases in words read correctly per minute were reported.

Dunlap, Dunlap, Koegel, and Koegel (1991) present self-monitoring as a way to increase student independence and decrease the need for adult time required to gather data on students' classroom activities. O'Leary and Dubey (1979) report that, even when students are not entirely accurate with their self-monitoring activities, improvements are still evident. Improvements in students' social and academic skills have been equally responsive to self-monitoring interventions (Dunlap et al., 1991).

Carr and Punzo (1993) reported that extremely nonintrusive self-monitoring data collection systems can have positive effects on academic and social behaviors of students with EBD. In their study, they evaluated the impact of having three students daily self-monitor their accuracy and productivity on reading, math, and spelling assignments. The students simply recorded their academic performance based on the teacher's evaluation of response correctness to items on worksheets scored at the end of each class period. Students' academic performance accuracy and productivity increased, as well as their on-task behavior.

It appears that having students involved in the formative evaluation of their own performance holds much promise. The advantages of students' self-evaluation appear twofold. First, teachers may be freed from data collection they indicate reduces their instructional time. Second, students may experience an instructional benefit, as well as a motivational effect, from the self-evaluation process.

Momentary Time Sampling

While Gunter and Denny (1998) cautioned the applicability of measures of time on task, they also noted the continued and widespread use of such measures as percent of time on task to report achievement and social behavior of students with EBD. One of the cautions presented by Gunter and Denny (1998) when using such measures is the teacher time required for observations. To address this issue, Gunter, Venn, et al. (2003) evaluated the efficacy of using various interval lengths for recording time-on-task data using momentary time sampling (MTS) procedures. They evaluated interval lengths of 2, 4, and 6 minutes to determine if differences were evident in data trends resulting from the various interval lengths. Their data indicated that the 2- and 4-minute interval lengths correlated highly with a continuous measure of academic engagement of three boys identified with EBD. They suggest that rather than completing a continuous 20-minute observation to determine the percent of time a student is on-task behavior, a teacher could use a 4-minute MTS interval and only have to observe and record the student's behavior at 5 brief instances in 20 minutes. The 4-minute MTS procedure would take approximately 15 seconds to complete and may produce a sample similar to the 20-minute continuous record. Certainly, this system would help address teachers' concerns regarding the time constraints necessary for data collection procedures.

Schoolwide Data Systems

Recently, great efforts have been dedicated to broadening data collection procedures for addressing entire classrooms, and particularly entire schools (e.g., Sugai et al., 2000; Tobin & Sugai, 1999). Horner, Sugai, and Todd (2002) offer the School-wide Information System (SWIS™) as a software system to allow data from office discipline referrals to be collected and analyzed for decisions regarding intervention effectiveness at the school level. Sugai et al. (2000) present office discipline referrals as one of the most common data sources across schools, providing a readily available source of information concerning behavior problems. They contend that office discipline referral data can be a simple, available, and useful data source to assist with understanding the social nature of disciplinary problems. However, at the same time, they offer the perspective that office discipline referral data should be used with caution due to the idiosyncratic manner in which different schools and personnel within schools define undesirable behavior and apply referrals to the infractions (problems of reliability of the measures). The SWIS program allows office discipline referral data to be easily placed in a graphic form for analysis because infractions reported on office discipline referrals are entered into a web-based software program.

In reviewing the continual evolvement of data collection procedures for use in classrooms for students with EBD, at least a few generalities may be drawn. We appear as a field to have accepted rate as a superior measure of behavior to most alternatives. While accuracy and percentages have utility, rate as a measure of performance has superior qualities in sensitivity to small changes in behavior and provides a cross-study measure in that rates may be compared across students, materials, and interventions. Second, most research supports that teachers (and students) can be trained to collect direct performance data and with assistance apply those data for the improvement of instruction. Third, efforts to broaden the application of formative assessment to larger populations of students are growing in acceptance. These efforts focus on standardized data collection of individual child performance reported at a school level and, based on the research reviewed, will likely result in improved academic and social skill performance of students with EBD that can be traced to effective teacher behavior.

FUTURE RESEARCH NEEDS

Obviously, the application of procedures derived from the applied behavior analysis tradition for formative evaluation purposes holds a great deal of promise. However, we strongly believe that there is a continuing need to empirically concretize the relationship of formative evaluation procedures and summative outcome measures of academic and social achievement. The potential reinforcement (both positive and negative) and potential for punishment for schools' demonstrated effectiveness, or lack of effectiveness, are based on outcomes of summative evaluations. It may be more likely that administrative and teaching personnel in those schools will seek and implement procedures likely to lead to reinforcement contingencies (e.g., being identified as "high-performing" schools). Therefore, there is potential that schools could become environments supporting the use of systematic formative assessment measures.

As discussed earlier, teachers often believe that formative data collection procedures are not necessarily related to teaching procedures, and ultimately not related to academic or social behavior of students with disabilities. Perhaps such opinions are related to the reinforcing value or the response cost of using formative evaluation procedures. Teachers, as well as students, may select their behavior based on the efficiency of that behavior in gaining reinforcement within the school environment. That is, if teachers find that the social benefits of using formative evaluation procedures are limited in comparison to the benefits of not using the procedures (e.g., extra time to tutor students in reading), they will likely choose the behavior with the lower response cost. The questions of which behaviors are positively reinforced for teachers in the natural environment remain largely unanswered in observational research. Social reinforcement in the form of positive or negative attention from peers or supervisors may indeed be one of the most powerful reinforcers available within an instructional environment.

Mager and Pipe (1970) proposed a framework for the systematic evaluation of performance problems such as the one described in teachers' decisions whether or not to use formative measure procedures. They suggest performance problems fall into two, now well accepted, categories: a skill deficit or a motivational deficit. If we eliminate the possibility of skill deficits through adequate teacher training, then we are confronted with the challenge of identifying the function of teacher behavior. Currently the literature describing formative evaluation procedures used by teachers of students with EBD is extremely limited. Additionally, while the limited literature regarding the impact of formative evaluation procedures, when used with students with EBD, is promising, however, much more evidence of how to best implement those procedures is needed.

We suggest that research needs to examine teacher behavior from a perspective of and analysis of competing behaviors. For example, we need to identify the contingencies within the instructional environment that support or hinder teachers' formative assessment behaviors (i.e., systematic data collec-

tion behaviors). Some have suggested (e.g., Shores, Stowitschek, Kerr, & Salzberg, 1979) that student learning may be insufficient reinforcement for teachers' consistent use of formative data collection behaviors. Others have indicated that use of those behaviors might be maintained only under a negative reinforcement paradigm (e.g., Gunter & Coutinho, 1997). For example, a teacher may be more like to collect systematic performance data to support a recommendation for a change in placement of a student exhibiting learning and behavioral problems. Yet, if the procedures for the documentation of placement change require too great of a response cost, it may be likely that the formative measure procedures will not be implemented correctly (surface compliance) or not implemented at all.

Nowhere in special education is the issue of data collection more prominent than as it relates to functional behavioral assessment and analysis (see also Fox and Gable, Chapter 8, this volume). "Functional assessment is viewed most accurately as a systematic process used to identify the conditions that motivated the child to engage in problem behavior, the events that trigger the occurrence of the behavior, and the events that result from occurrences of the behavior that reinforce it" (Sasso, Conroy, Stichter, & Fox, 2001, p. 283). One of the primary tenants of functional behavioral assessment is the foundation of applied behavior analysis, that stimuli are observable and measurable. However, in their national survey of leaders in program development for students with EBD, Scott, Meers, and Nelson (2000) reported that "when asked whether hypotheses should include observable actions or events . . . a surprising 25% responded with sometimes or never" (p. 284). Overall, they reported little consistency regarding the components of a functional behavioral assessment for students with EBD. Sharing the concerns of Scott et al. (2000), Sasso et al. (2001) indicated that the technology for completion of functional behavioral assessments and analyses lacks sufficient evaluation for widespread implementation to address behavioral difficulties of many students with EBD.

Kauffman (2001) concludes that preparing teachers to use functional assessment is time-consuming and difficult. Miller, Gunter, Venn, Hummel, and Wiley (2003) also addressed this concern when reviewing literature regarding completed implementation of functional behavioral assessment procedures with students with EBD. For example, they expressed concern regarding some reports of up to 5 weeks to complete functional assessment procedures with some students with EBD in public school classroom settings (cf. Dunlap, Kern-Dunlap, Clarke, & Robbins, 1991). This provides an example in which a "no response" from the teacher may be selected due to an exceptionally high response cost, as opposed to a response to implement functional behavioral assessment procedures that are obviously complex and time-consuming. If the available reinforcement is the same for either response, it may be likely that the response with the greater response cost (e.g., amount of work required) will not be chosen. To date, it may be that little, if any, reinforcement difference has been available for the teacher choosing to implement interventions with evidence-based fidelity. However, with the implementation of NCLB referred to earlier and the required evaluation of "adequate yearly progress" for all students, it may be that reinforcement contingencies, both positive and negative, will be viewed differently by teachers. That is, in this era of accountability, teachers may be contingently reinforced for implementing procedures that result in improved student performance.

Obviously, an additional area of needed research relates to the manageability of data collection (i.e., lowering the response costs). Efforts will likely be necessary to evaluate systems that may enhance their use by teachers or other school personnel. For example, the SWIS data system removes many of the decisions required to implement the collection of behavioral data through standardized definitions, analysis, and reporting procedures. This recognizes that instructional personnel may be more likely to review and act upon data if the data are presented in an understandable and consistent format (i.e., a graphic display).

The SWIS program is a technological web-driven program. With increases in computer storage capacity, higher transmission speeds, and widespread access to the Internet, more and more data collection programs are migrating to the World Wide Web (e.g. SWIS; DIBELS). Although no web-based behavioral data sites were found, the potential for migrating systems from laptops or palm-held computers to an Internet base appears possible.

SUMMARY AND COMMENTS

We believe the foregoing information presents a compelling argument for the continued use of formative evaluation research. Given the current social and political context of accountability, researchers evaluating practices for use with students with EBD have a unique opportunity to contribute methodologies refined over the past 30 years, not only for the benefit of those students but also for the benefit of an even larger audience of teachers and students. While technology has provided a means for addressing increasingly complex instructional interactions, we must not ignore the need to support the adoption and maintenance of adequate measurement procedures by practicing teachers and clinicians. By increasing the use of formative assessment procedures by all teachers, we have the potential to create a context where performance data are valued and supported. However, until we are sure that formative procedures have been made as manageable as possible, while still maintaining validity of the process, widespread implementation may be limited. Related to this issue is the need to ensure that formative measurement procedures are taught as an integral part of teacher training programs and that the teachers leave those programs fluent in their use. Finally, after ensuring that formative evaluation procedures contribute to desired outcomes of improved student academic achievement and that teachers can implement the procedures with high fidelity, we must determine the level of implementation that can be maintained by contingencies available in school settings. Unless each of these issues is addressed, explained, and understood, we may continue to know where we want to go in bringing all students to high levels of achievement; however, we may also continue to not know where we are in that process.

REFERENCES

Alberto, P. A., & Troutman, A. C. (2003). *Applied behavior analysis for teachers* (6th ed.). Upper Saddle River, NJ: Prentice-Hall.

Allinder, R. M., & Oats, R.G. (1997). Effects of acceptability on teachers' implementation of curriculum-based measurement and student achievement in mathematics computation. *Remedial and Special Education, 97,* 113–121.

Binder, C., Haughton, E., & Van Eyk, D. (1990). Increasing endurance by building fluency: Precision teaching attention span. *Teaching Exceptional Children, 22,* 24–27.

Bushell, D., & Baer, D. M. (1994). Measurably superior instruction means close, continual contact with the relevant outcome data. Revolutionary! In R. Gardner, D. M. Sainato, J. O. Cooper, T. E. Heron, W. L. Heward, J. Eshleman, & T.Grossi (Eds.), *Behavior analysis in education: Focus on measurably superior instruction* (pp. 3–10). Pacific Grove, CA: Brooks/Cole.

Carr, J. E., & Burkholder, E. O. (1998). Creating single-subject design graphs with Microsoft Excel. *Journal of Applied Behavior Analysis, 31,* 245–251.

Carr, S. C., & Punzo, R. P. (1993). The effects of self-monitoring of academic accuracy and productivity on the performance of students with behavioral disorders. *Behavioral Disorders, 18,* 241–250.

Cochran-Smith, M. (2003). The unforgiving complexity of teaching: Avoiding simplicity in the age of accountability. *Journal of Teacher Education, 54,* 3–5.

Cooper, J. O., Heron, T. E., & Heward, W. L. (1987). *Applied behavior analysis.* Upper Saddle River, NJ: Merrill/Prentice Hall.

Council for Exceptional Children. (2003, May 27). *House approves IDEA Bill by a vote of 251 to 171.* Retrieved May 27, 2003, from *http://www.cec.sped. org/.*

Deno, S. L. (1985). Curriculum based measurement: The emerging alternative. *Exceptional Children, 52,* 219–232.

Deno, S. L. (1986). Formative evaluation of individual student programs: A new role for school psychologists. *School Psychology Review, 15,* 358–374.

Deno, S. L., & Espin, C. A. (1991). Evaluating strategies for preventing and remediating basic skills deficits. In G. Stoner, M. R. Shinn, & H. M. Walker (Eds.), *Interventions for achievement and behavior problems* (pp. 79–97). Silver Spring, MD: National Association of School Psychologists.

Deno, S. L., & Mirkin, P. (1977). *Data based program modification.* Reston, VA: Council for Exceptional Children.

Dunlap, G., Kern-Dunlap, L., Clarke, S., & Robbins, F. (1991). Functional assessment, curricular revision, and severe behavior problems. *Journal of Applied Behavior Analysis, 24,* 387–397.

Dunlap, L. K., Dunlap, G., Koegel, L. K., & Koegel, R. L. (1991). Using self-monitoring to increase independence. *Teaching Exceptional Children, 23*(3), 17–22.

Emerson, E., Reeves, D. J., & Felce, D. (2000). Palmtop computer technologies for behavioral observation research. In T. Thompson, D. Felce, & F. J. Symons (Eds.), *Behavioral observation: Technology and applications in developmental disabilities* (pp. 47–60). Baltimore: Brookes.

Fuchs, L. S., & Fuchs, D. (1986). Effects of systematic formative evaluation: A meta-analysis. *Exceptional Children, 53,* 199–208.

Fuchs, L. S., Fuchs, D., & Hamlett, C. L. (1989). Effects of instrumental use of curriculum-based measurement to enhance instructional programs. *Remedial and Special Education, 10,* 43–52.

Fuchs, L. S., Hamlett, C. L., & Fuchs, D. (1997). *Monitoring basic skills progress* (2nd ed.). Austin, TX: Pro-Ed.

Good, T. L., & Brophy, J. E. (2000). *Looking in classrooms* (8th ed.). New York: Longman.

Greenwood, C. R., Carta, J. J., Kamps, D., & Delquadri, J. (1997). *Echobehavioral Assessment Systems Software (EBASS Version 3.0): Practitioners manual.* Kansas City, KS: University of Kansas, Juniper Gardens Children's Project.

Gunter, P. L. (2001). Data-based decision-making to ensure positive outcomes for children/youth with challenging behaviors. In L. M. Bullock & R. A. Gable (Eds), *Addressing social, academic, and behavioral needs within inclusive and alternative settings* (pp. 49–52). Reston, VA: Council for Exceptional Children.

Gunter, P. L., Adams, K., Campbell, C., Isler, P., Sellers, J., Thomas, T., Venn, M. L., & Reffel, J. (2002). *Effects of teacher's data-based reflection on students' correct academic responses.* Paper presented at the Teacher Education Division (TED) of the Council for Exceptional Children 25th Annual Conference, Savannah, GA.

Gunter, P. L., Callicott, K., Denny, R. K., & Gerber, B. L. (2003). Finding a place for data collection in classrooms for students with emotional/behavioral disorders. *Preventing School Failure, 48*(1), 4–8.

Gunter, P. L., & Coutinho, M. J. (1997). The growing need to understand negative reinforcement in teacher training programs. *Teacher Education and Special Education, 20,* 249–264.

Gunter, P. L., & Denny, R. K. (1996). Research issues and needs regarding teacher use of classroom management strategies. *Behavioral Disorders, 22,* 15–20.

Gunter, P. L., & Denny, R. K. (1998). Trends, issues, and research needs regarding academic instruction of students with emotional and behavioral disorders. *Behavioral Disorders, 24,* 44–50.

Gunter, P. L., Fox, J. J., Brady, M. P., Shores, R. E., & Cavanaugh, K. (1988). Nonhandicapped peers as multiple exemplars: A generalization tactic for promoting autistic students' social skills. *Behavioral Disorders, 3,* 116–126.

Gunter, P. L., Hummell, J. H., & Venn, M. L. (1998). Are effective academic instructional practices used to teach students with behavior disorders? *Beyond Behavior, 9*(3), 5–11.

Gunter, P. L., Jack, S. L., Shores, R. E., Carrell, D., & Flowers, J. (1993). Lag sequential analysis as a tool for functional analysis of student disruptive behavior in classrooms. *Journal of Emotional and Behavioral Disorders, 1,* 138–148.

Gunter, P. L., & King, G. (2003). *Self-evaluation and analysis of oral reading performance by students with behavior disorders.* Paper presented at the 29th annual convention for the Association for Behavior Analysis, San Francisco.

Gunter, P. L., Miller, K., Venn, M. L., Thomas, K., & House, S. (2002). Have students graph their own data with the desktop computer. *Teaching Exceptional Children, 35,* 30–34.

Gunter, P. L., Reffel, J. M., Barnett, C. A., Lee, J. M., & Patrick, J. (in press). Academic response rates in elementary school classrooms. *Education and Treatment of Children.*

Gunter, P. L., Shores, R. E., Jack, S. L., Denny, R. K., & DePaepe, P. A. (1994). A case study of the effects of altering instructional interactions on the disruptive behavior of a child identified with severe behavior disorders. *Education and Treatment of Children, 17,* 435–444.

Gunter, P. L., Venn, M. L., Patrick, J., Miller, K.A., & Kelly, L. (2003). Efficacy of using to momentary time samples to determine on-task behavior of students with emotional and behavioral disorders. *Education and Treatment of Children, 26,* 400–412.

Haring, N. G., Liberty, K. A., & White, O. R. (1980). Rules for data-based strategy decisions in instructional programs: Current research and instructional implications. In W. Sailor, B. Wilcox, & L. Brown (Eds.), *Methods of instruction for severely handicapped students* (pp. 159–192). Baltimore: Brookes.

Hawkins, A., Sharpe, T., & Ray, R. (1994). Toward instructional process measureability: An interbehavioral field systems perspective. In R. Gardner, D. M. Sainato, J. O. Cooper, T. E. Heron, W. L. Heward, J. Eshleman, & T. A. Grossi (Eds.), *Behavior analysis in education: Focus on measurably superior instruction* (pp. 241–255). Pacific Grove, CA: Brooks/Cole.

Hewett, F. M. (1968). *The emotionally disturbed child in the classroom.* Boston: Allyn & Bacon.

Horner, R. H., Sugai, G., & Todd, A. W. (2002). *"Data" need not be a four-letter word: Using data to improve school-wide discipline.* Unpublished manuscript, University of Oregon.

Howell, K. W., & Lorson-Howell, K. A. (1990). Fluency in the classroom. *Teaching Exceptional Children, 22*(3), 20–23.

Individuals with Disabilities Education Act Amendments of 1997. Public Law No. 105-17, Section 20, 111 Stat. 37 (1997). Washington, DC: U.S. Government Printing Office.

Jack, S. L., Shores, R. E., Denny, R. K., Gunter, P. L., DeBriere, T., & DePaepe, P. (1996). An analysis of the relationship of teachers' reported use of classroom management strategies on types of interactions. *Journal of Behavioral Education, 6,* 67–87.

Lindsley, O. (1971a). Precision teaching in perspective: An interview. *Teaching Exceptional Children, 3,* 114–119.

Lindsley, O. (1971b). From Skinner to precision teaching: The child knows best. In J. Jordan, & L. Robbins (Eds.), *Let's try doing something else kinda thing* (pp. 1–11). Arlington, VA: Council for Exceptional Children.

Lindsley, O. (1990). Precision teaching: By teachers for children. *Teaching Exceptional Children, 22,* 10–15.

McLaughlin, T. F. (1993). An analysis and evaluation of educator selected data collection procedures in actual school settings: A brief report. *Child and Family Behavior Therapy, 15,* 61–64.

Miller, K. A., Gunter, P. L., Venn, M. L., Hummel, J., & Wiley, L. P. (2003). Effects of curricular/materials modifications on the academic performance and task engagement of three students with emotional/behavioral disorders. *Behavioral Disorders, 28,* 130–149.

Moxley, R. A. (1998). Treatment-only designs and student self-recording as strategies for public school teachers. *Education and Treatment of Children, 21,* 37–61.

National Association of State Directors of Special Education. (2002). *Implementing the No Child Left Behind Act: What it means for IDEA.* Alexandria, VA: Author.

National Council for Accreditation of Teacher Education. (2000). *Professional standards for the accreditation of schools, colleges, and departments of education,* Washington, DC: Author.

Nelson, C. M., & Polsgrove, L. (1984). Behavior analysis in special education: White rabbit or white elephant? *Remedial and Special Education, 5,* 6–17.

O'Leary, S. G., & Dubey, D. R. (1979). Applications of self-control procedures by children: A review. *Journal of Applied Behavior Analysis, 12,* 449–465.

Sasso, G. M., Conroy, M. A., Stichter, J. P., & Fox, J. J. (2001). Slowing down the bandwagon: The misapplication of functional assessment for students with emotional or behavioral disorders. *Behavioral Disorders, 26,* 282–296.

Scott, T. M., Meers, D. T., & Nelson, C. M. (2000). Toward a consensus of functional behavioral assessment for students with mild disabilities in public school contests: A national survey. *Education and Treatment of Children, 23,* 265–285.

Semmel, M., & Frick, T. (1980). *Micro-CARTLO, module 9: Tools for teacher inquiry: Using computers to analyze observational data.* Bloomington, IN: Indiana University, School of Education, Center for Innovation in Teaching the Handicapped.

Shinn, M. R., & Hubbard, D. D. (1994). Curriculum-based measurement and problem-solving assessment: Basic procedures and outcomes. In E. Meyen, G. Fergason, & R. Whelan (Eds.). *Strategies for teaching exceptional children in inclusive settings* (pp. 243–274). Denver, CO: Love.

Shores, R. E., Jack, S. L., Gunter, P. L., Ellis, D. N., DeBriere, T., & Wehby, J. H. (1993). Classroom interactions of children with severe behavior disorders. *Journal of Emotional and Behavioral Disorders, 1,* 27–39.

Shores, R. E., Stowitschek, J. J., Kerr, M. M., & Salzberg, C. L. (1979). Evaluation of competency-based special education teacher training programs: Focus on pupil performances. *Teacher Education and Special Education, 2*(3), 68–71.

Sugai, G., Sprague, J. R., Horner, R. H., & Walker, H. M. (2000). Preventing school violence: The use of office discipline referrals to assess and monitor schoolwide discipline interventions. *Journal of Emotional and Behavioral Disorders, 8,* 94–101.

Sutherland, K. S., & Wehby, J. H. (2001). The effects of self-evaluation on teaching behaviors in classrooms for students with emotional and behavioral disorders. *Journal of Special Education, 35,* 161–171.

Sutherland, K. S., Wehby, J. H., & Yoder, P.J. (2001). An examination of the relation between teacher praise and students' with emotional/behavioral disorders opportunities to respond to academic requests. *Journal of Emotional and Behavioral Disorders, 10,* 5–14.

Tapp, J., & Walden, T. A. (2000). PROCODER: A system for collection and analysis of observational data from videotapes. In T. Thompson, D. Felce, & F. J. Symons (Eds.), *Behavioral observation: Technology and applications in developmental disabilities* (pp. 61–70). Baltimore: Brookes.

Tapp, J., & Wehby, J. H. (2000). Observational software for laptop computers and optical barcode readers. In T. Thompson, D. Felce, & F. J. Symons (Eds), *Behavioral observation: Technology and applications in developmental disabilities* (pp. 71–81). Baltimore: Brookes.

Tawney, J. W., & Gast, D. L. (1984). *Single subject research in special education.* Columbus, OH: Merrill.

Taylor, J., & Romanczyk, R. (1994). Generating hypotheses about the function of student problem behavior by observing teacher behavior. *Journal of Applied Behavior Analysis, 27,* 251–265.

Thompson, T., Felce, D., & Symons, F. J. (Eds.). (2000). *Behavioral observation: Technology and applications in developmental disabilities.* Baltimore: Brookes.

Tobin, T., & Sugai, G. (1999). Using sixth-grade school records to predict school violence, chronic discipline problems, and high school outcomes. *Journal of Emotional and Behavioral Disorders, 7,* 40–53.

Wehby, J. H., Dodge, K. A., Valente, E., & Conduct Problems Research Group. (1993). School behavior of first grade children identified as at risk for development of conduct problems. *Behavioral Disorders, 19,* 67–78.

Wehby, J. H., & Hollahan, S. M. (2000). Effects of high probability requests on the latency in initiating academic tasks. *Journal of Applied Behavior Analysis, 33,* 259–263.

Wehby, J. H., Symons, F. M., Canale, J., & Go, F. (1998). Teaching practices in classrooms for students with emotional and behavioral disorders: Discrepancies between recommendations and observations. *Behavioral Disorders, 24,* 52–57.

Wehby, J. H., Symons, F. M., & Shores, R. E. (1995). A descriptive analysis of aggressive behavior in classrooms for students with emotional and behavioral disorders. *Behavioral Disorders, 20,* 87–105.

West, R. P., Young, K. R., & Spooner, F. (1990). Precision teaching: An introduction. *Teaching Exceptional Children, 22*(3), 4–9.

Author Index

Subject Index

"f" following a page number indicates a figure; "t" following a page number indicates a table